Sports and Exercise Nutrition

Fourth Edition

WILLIAM D. McARDLE
Professor Emeritus
Department of Family, Nutrition, and Exercise Science
Queens College of the City University of New York
Flushing, New York

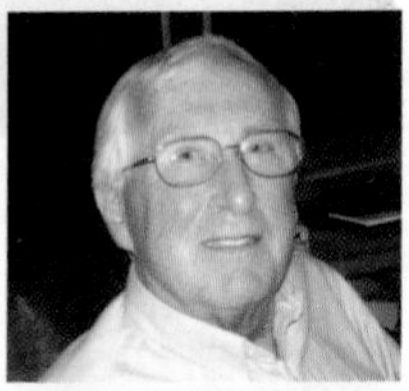

FRANK I. KATCH
Former Professor, Chair, and
Graduate Program Director of the Exercise Science Department
University of Massachusetts, Amherst
Amherst, Massachusetts

Instructor and Board Member
Certificate Program in Fitness Instruction
University of California at Los Angeles (UCLA) Extension
Los Angeles, California

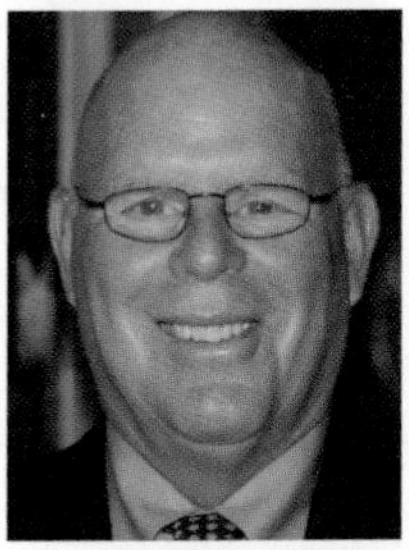

VICTOR L. KATCH
Professor, Department of Movement Science
School of Kinesiology
Associate Professor, Pediatrics
School of Medicine
University of Michigan
Ann Arbor, Michigan

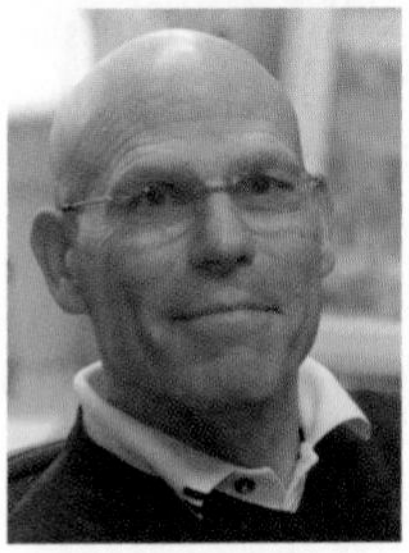

Wolters Kluwer | Lippincott Williams & Wilkins
Health
Philadelphia • Baltimore • New York • London
Buenos Aires • Hong Kong • Sydney • Tokyo

Acquisitions Editor: Emily Lupash
Product Manager: Andrea M. Klingler
Marketing Manager: Christen Murphy
Designer: Stephen Druding
Art by: Dragonfly Media Group
Compositor: s4 Carlisle

Fourth Edition

351 West Camden Street
Baltimore, MD 21201

Two Commerce Square, 2001 Market Street
Philadelphia, PA 19103

Printed in China

Library of Congress Cataloging-in-Publication Data

Katch, Frank I.
Sports and exercise nutrition / Frank I. Katch. — 4th ed.
p. ; cm.
Rev. ed. of: Sports and exercise nutrition / William D. McArdle, Frank I. Katch, Victor L. Katch. 3rd ed. c2009.
Includes bibliographical references and index.
ISBN 978-1-4511-7573-8 (alk. paper)
I. McArdle, William D. Sports and exercise nutrition. II. Title.
[DNLM: 1. Sports. 2. Energy Metabolism—physiology. 3. Exercise—physiology. 4. Nutritional Physiological Phenomena. QT 260]
613.202'4796—dc23
2011048863

To purchase additional copies of this book, call our customer service department at **(800) 638-3030** or fax orders to **(301) 223-2320**. International customers should call **(301) 223-2300**.

Visit Lippincott Williams & Wilkins on the Internet: http://www.lww.com. Lippincott Williams & Wilkins customer service representatives are available from 8:30 am to 6:00 pm, EST.

CCS0412

Dedication

To all my grandchildren, whose lives give meaning to my own:
Liam, Aiden, Quinn, Kelly, Kathleen (Kate), Dylan, Owen, Henry, Elizabeth, Grace, Claire, Elise,
Charlotte, and Sophia. May each of you become the best you can become.

—William D. McArdle (aka Grandpa)

To my wife Kerry and our three children,
David, Kevin (and his wife Kelly), and Ellen (and her husband Sean).
You truly have achieved the honorable in all of your many accomplishments.

—Frank I. Katch

To my family: Heather and Jesse; Erika and Chris (Ryan, Cameron); Leslie and Eric
To my mentors: A. D. Fleming, A. R. Behnke, and F.M. Henry
To my students: A. Weltman; P. Freedson; J. Spring; S. Sady; C. Marks;
B. Moffat; D. Ballor; D. Becque; N. Wessinger; B. Campaigne; and K. Nau

—Victor L. Katch

Dedication

Preface

In the first three editions of *Sports and Exercise Nutrition*, we were hopeful that the emergence of "sports nutrition" courses of study would meld with the established field that incorporates the exercise sciences to create a new field that we originally titled Sports and Exercise Nutrition. We are pleased this has evolved as undergraduate and graduate programs worldwide embrace coursework that now has a mainstream component that includes the science of human exercise nutrition. At full maturity, exercise nutrition (or some variant of this title) will take its deserved place as a respectable academic field of study. The evolution is far from complete, but exercise physiology and mainstream nutrition continue to become more integrated because of an ever-expanding knowledge base. Interwoven within this fabric are the clear relationships that emerge from considerable interdiscipliary research, particularly regarding sound nutritional practices, regular, moderate-intensity physical activity, and optimal health for individuals of all ages and fitness status. Students of exercise science and nutrition science now demand coursework related to the specifics of exercise nutrition, and we hope this new fourth edition of *Sports and Exercise Nutrition* contributes to this goal. The aim of this book is to provide introductory material for a one semester course in the nutritional and exercise sciences. The major focus concerns the integration of nutrition and exercise and its impact on optimal exercise performance and training responsiveness.

ORGANIZATION

As with the previous three editions, we have designed the text for a one-semester course with what we believe provides logical sequencing of material. For example, one cannot reasonably understand carbohydrate's use during exercise without first reviewing the rudiments of human digestion and then the composition and effect of carbohydrate on the body. Similarly, ergogenic aids, fluid replacement, and achieving an "optimal weight" for overall good health and sports performance (all critical topics to sports and exercise nutrition) can be evaluated best by understanding basic bioenergetics, nutrient and exercise metabolism, energy balance, and temperature regulation.

In *Sports and Exercise Nutrition, Fourth Edition*, Section I integrates information about digestion, absorption, and nutrient assimilation. Section II explains how the body extracts energy from ingested nutrients. We stress nutrition's role in energy metabolism: how nutrients metabolize, and how exercise training affects nutrient metabolism. This section ends with the measurement and quantification of the energy content of foods, and the energy requirements of diverse physical activities. Section III focuses on aspects of nutrition to optimize exercise performance and training responsiveness. We also discuss how to make prudent decisions in the nutrition–fitness marketplace. Section IV describes fundamental mechanisms and adaptations for thermal regulation during heat stress, including strategies for optimizing fluid replacement. Section V consists of two chapters on pharmacologic, chemical, and nutritional ergogenic aids. We integrate the latest published research findings related to their effectiveness and implications for health and safety. The three chapters in Section VI explain laboratory and field methods for body composition assessment, sport-specific guidelines about body composition and its assessment, energy balance, and weight control (losing and gaining weight), and the increasing prevalence of eating disorders among diverse groups of athletes and other physically active people.

NEW TO THE FOURTH EDITION

Components of the entire text have been upgraded to reflect current demographics concerning dietary- and exercise-related health issues and research findings, including updated recommendations and guidelines from federal agencies and professional nurition, medical, and sports medicine organizations regarding nutrition, physical activity, and achieving a body composition for good health and optimal exercise and sports performance.

Significant Additions and Modifications

- Inclusion of the latest dietary reference intakes, including MyPlate (strengths and limitations), incorporating new and more comprehensive approaches to nutritional recommendations for planning and assessing diets for healthy people.
- Expanded discussion about sugar intake and the blood lipid profile and associated health risks. Also included are recommended lifestyle changes to reduce type 2 diabetes risk.
- Provide the current version of the recommendations of the *Dietary Guidelines for Americans.*
- Discussion of whey protein as a dietary supplement to facilitate muscular development in response to resistance training.
- Updated discussion of potential ergogenic effects of common pharmacologic and chemical agents purported to enhance exercise performance, increase the quality and quantity of training, and augment the body's adaptation to regular exercise and training.
- Discussion of the increased prevalence and potential risks of consuming "energy drinks" that combine caffeine and malt alcohol in a beverage that commonly contains between 6 to 12% alcohol by volume.

- Expanded section about the effects of exercise (intensity, mode, duration) on gastrointestinal functions, including clinically relevant manifestitations of gastrointestinal disorders.
- Introduction of new guidelines from the American Academy of Pediatrics concerning heat stress and exercise in children and adolescents.
- Discussion of the potential role of the brain's glycogen content in resisting central fatigue in prolonged exercise coincident with dimmihshed glucose supply from the blood.
- Provide a means to evaluate the variety and balance of an individual's food choices related to current recommendations.
- Expanded discussion of portion size and portion size distortion of popular food chains (including ethnic-related food chains) and their effect on the caloric intake of the US population.
- Preoperative carbohydrate loading as a strategy to reduce postoperative stress and speed the recovery process: shorter postoperative hospital stays, faster return to normal functions, and reduced occurrence of surgical complications.
- Highlight health risks and current estimates of the financial impact of overweight and obesity. Also, an expanded discussion of the health risks of excess central fat deposition and the role of physical fitness, age, and gender on waist circumference and components of excess abdominal adipose tissue deposition.
- Inclusion of current standards for overweight and obesity in the United States and worldwide, including the most recent research evidence about statewide adult and childhood obesity rates.
- Provide the most up-to-date information on the body composition characteristics of elite male and female athletes grouped by sport category.
- Introduction of information regarding the role of brain chemicals in the genesis of disordered eating.
- Discussion of an emerging pattern of eating where individuals become so overly obsessed with healthful foods that they exhibit a form of obsessive-compulsive disorder termed *orthorexia nervosa*. As with anorexia nervosa or bulimia nervosa, this obsessive fixation on food places it in the disordered eating category.
- Discussion of the role of sleep duration and sleep quality on body weight control.
- Discussion of the overall value of progressive resistance exercise among healthy aging adults to develop additional muscle mass and increased strength to function better in daily life.
- Expansion of the concept of organic food, its meaning, classificantion, and standards, and the effect on patterns of food intake in the United States.
- Expanded information about the effects of exercise on digestive processes and functions.
- Discussion of the anhropological, experiential, economical, and psychological factors related to food choice selection.
- Provide the latest information on the topics related to nutrient timing to optimize the training response.
- Introduction of a measure to quantify the antioxidant potential of common foods consumed in the diet.
- Summary of the nutritional labeling rules for dietary supplements ("Supplement Facts" panel).
- Expanded coverage of energy beverages, sports drinks, and nutrition powders, bars, and drinks.
- Discussion of the role of ingested protein during endurance exercise on delaying processes related to fatigue.
- Provide current information about fast foods and modifications in food labeling and dietary supplement labeling.
- Updated information about the nutrient composition of different beverages with particular emphasis on sugar-sweetened beverages and disease risk.
- Introduction of the new areas of ethnic sources for poor nutriton, the hunger-obesity paradon and poverty and obesity connection to hunger and food insecurity.
- Updated information about the nutritional composition of foods from the most popular fast food restaurants.

PEDAGOGIC FEATURES

Each chapter contains numerous pedagogic features to engage the student and promote comprehension.

We have included relavant Internet links to governmental and nongovernmental websites related to nutrition, weight control, exercise and exercise training, and overall health.

Test Your Knowledge. Each chapter begins with 10 True–False statements about chapter material. Tackling these questions before reading the chapter allows students to assess changes in their comprehension after completing the chapter. This approach also provides students the opportunity to evaluate the completeness of their answers with the answer key and rationale for each answer provided at the end of each chapter.

Personal Health and Exercise Nutrition. Each chapter presents at least one case study or topic related to personal health and exercise nutrition. This unique aspect more actively engages the student in specific areas of nutritional assessment and health appraisal, application of dietary guidelines, weight control, body composition assessment, overuse syndrome, and physical activity recommendations.

Connections to the Past. Numerous individuals over the past two centuries have had a huge impact on the emerging fields of exercise, nutrition, and metabolism. A tribute to their many salient scientific contributions provides a glimpse into the exciting history of nutrition and exercise science research. Each of these individuals, in their own and unique way, has contibuted new understandings about important aspects of the emerging discipline of exercise nutrition. The impressive list includes Nobel Prize winners and research scientists and physicians on the forefronts of research and eperimentation during their era. They literally were the giants in their respective areas of inquiry upon whose shoulders future fundamental research has progressed in many interdisciplinary fields of study. All of those curently engaged in the research enterprise related to the field of exercise nutrition owe a huge debt of gratitude for their many insightful contirution.

Additional Insights. This box contains relevant inforamtion regarding aresa of controversy, confusion, and current interest related to text material. Examles of topics include: A Little Excess Weight May Not Be So Bad Above Age 70; Can Extra Vitamins Boost Ability to Generate Energy?; Waist Girth and Health Risk With Normal BMI; Probiotics: Empty Promises or the Real Deal?; Can Exercise Reallly Benefit a Weight-Loss Program?; Is Excess Sallt Really That Harmful?; and Can Exercise and Diet Preserve Muscle Mass as We Age?

Equations and Data. Important equations and data are highlighted throughout the text for easy reference.

Key Terms. Key terms are bolded within the chapter.

References. A current list of the top 25 diverse references are included at the end of every chapter, with the full reference list included on the book's website at thePoint.lww.com/MKKSEN4e.

Art Program

The full-color art program continues to be a stellar feature of the textbook. The entire art program has been updated to provide uniformity and consistency and to improve visual clarity for the reader and for clear projection during class presentations and academic seminars. More than 250 figures are included to illustrate important concepts in the text. Fourty new figures have been added, and the rest have been redrawn, expanded, or enhanced to complement the new and updated content.

ANCILLARIES

Sports and Exercise Nutrition, Fourth Edition, includes additional resources for both instructors and students, which are available on the book's companion website at thePoint.lww.com/MKKSEN4e.

Instructors and students will have access to the searchable Full Text Online.

Instructors

Approved adopting instructors will be given access to the following additional resources:

- Brownstone test generator
- PowerPoint presentations
- Image bank
- WebCT, Blackboard, and Angel cartridge

Students

Students who have purchased *Sports and Exercise Nutrition, Fourth Edition,* have access to the following additional resources via the personal code on the inside front cover:

- Animations
- Searchable Full Text Online
- Quiz bank
- Full chapter reference lists
- Appendices
- Answers to questions and scenarios in the Personal Health and Exercise Nutrition activities
- Connection to the Past boxes, with additional information to build and expand on that provided in the text boxes

How to Use This Book

This User's Guide explains all of the key features found in the third edition of *Sports and Exercise Nutrition.* Become familiar with them so you can get the most out of each chapter and gain a strong foundation in the science of exercise nutrition and bioenergetics and gain insight to how the principles work in the real world of human physical activity and sports medicine.

Introductory Section

Outlines the historical precedent for exercise nutrition, helping you strengthen and ground your knowledge of the field. The **Timeline** highlights the outstanding contributions of the early pioneeer physcians and researchers who discovered fundamental new knowledge that has greatly impacted the modern, emerging discipline of sports and exercise nutrition.

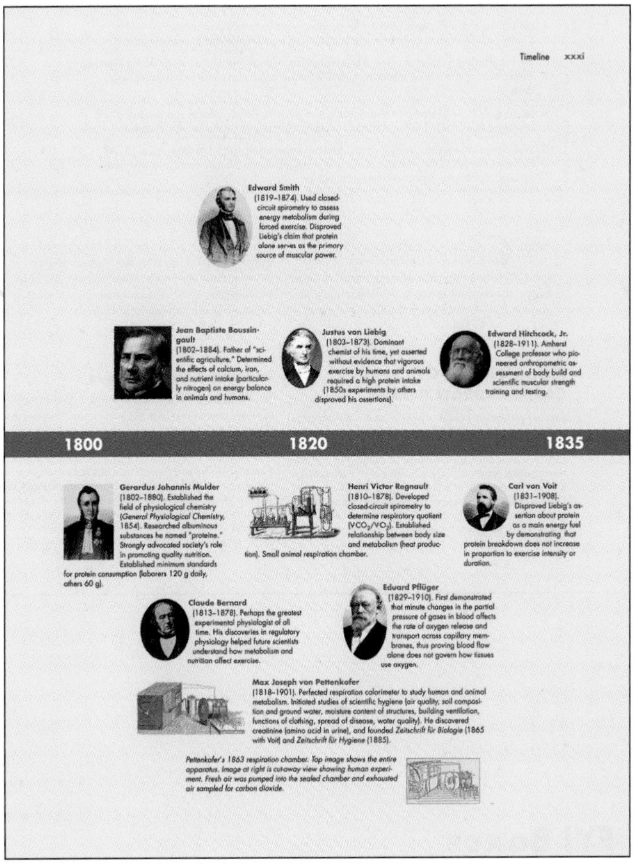
Timeline xxxi

Edward Smith (1819–1874). Used closed-circuit spirometry to assess energy metabolism during forced exercise. Disproved Liebig's claim that protein alone serves as the primary source of muscular power.

Jean Baptiste Boussingault (1802–1884). Father of "scientific agriculture." Determined the effects of calcium, iron, and nutrient intake (particularly nitrogen) on energy balance in animals and humans.

Justus von Liebig (1803–1873). Dominant chemist of his time, yet asserted without evidence that vigorous exercise by humans and animals required a high protein intake (1850s experiments by others disproved his assertions).

Edward Hitchcock, Jr. (1828–1911). Amherst College professor who pioneered anthropometric assessment of body build and scientific muscular strength training and testing.

1800 1820 1835

Gerardus Johannis Mulder (1802–1880). Established the field of physiological chemistry (*General Physiological Chemistry,* 1854). Researched albuminous substances he named "proteine." Strongly advocated society's role in promoting quality nutrition. Established minimum standards for protein consumption (laborers 120 g daily, others 60 g).

Henri Victor Regnault (1810–1878). Developed closed-circuit spirometry to determine respiratory quotient ($\dot{V}CO_2/\dot{V}O_2$). Established relationship between body size and metabolism (heat production). Small animal respiration chamber.

Carl von Voit (1831–1908). Disproved Liebig's assertion about protein as a main energy fuel by demonstrating that protein breakdown does not increase in proportion to exercise intensity or duration.

Claude Bernard (1813–1878). Perhaps the greatest experimental physiologist of all time. His discoveries in regulatory physiology helped future scientists understand how metabolism and nutrition affect exercise.

Eduard Pflüger (1829–1910). First demonstrated that minute changes in the partial pressure of gases in blood affects the rate of oxygen release and transport across capillary membranes, thus proving blood flow alone does not govern how tissues use oxygen.

Max Joseph von Pettenkofer (1818–1901). Perfected respiration calorimeter to study human and animal metabolism. Initiated studies of scientific hygiene (air quality, soil composition and ground water, moisture content of structures, building ventilation, functions of clothing, spread of disease, water quality). He discovered creatinine (amino acid in urine), and founded *Zeitschrift für Biologie* (1865 with Voit) and *Zeitschrift für Hygiene* (1885).

Pettenkofer's 1863 respiration chamber. Top image shows the entire apparatus. Image at right is cut-away view showing human experiment. Fresh air was pumped into the sealed chamber and exhausted air sampled for carbon dioxide.

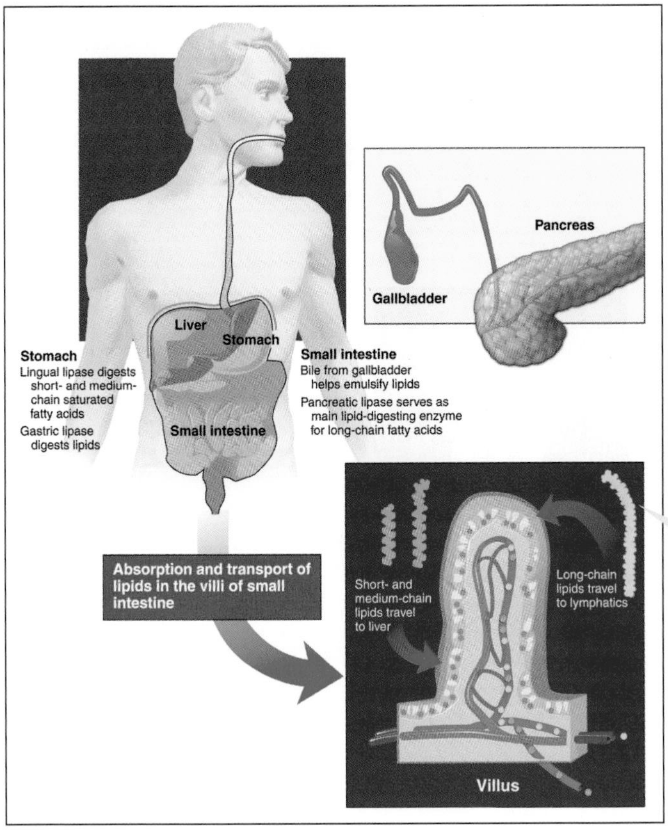

Vivid Full-Color Illustrations and Photographs

Enhance learning of important topics and add visual impact.

TEST YOUR KNOWLEDGE

Select true or false for the 10 statements below, then check out the answers at the end of the chapter. Retake the test after you've read the chapter; you should achieve 100%	True	False
1. Reduced levels of muscle glycogen induce fatigue in intense aerobic exercise.	O	O
2. It is possible to modify nutrition to "superpack" muscle with glycogen and thereby delay the onset of fatigue in prolonged intense marathon running.	O	O
3. Amino acid supplements augment muscular strength and size with resistance training.	O	O
4. L-Carnitine supplementation aids endurance athletes by enhancing fat burning and sparing liver and muscle glycogen; it also promotes fat loss in body builders.	O	O
5. Chromium, the second largest selling mineral supplement in the United States, is a well-documented "fat burner" and "muscle builder."	O	O
6. Creatine supplementation improves performance in short-duration, intense exercise.	O	O
7. Limited research indicates a potential for exogenous pyruvate as a partial replacement for dietary carbohydrate to augment endurance exercise performance and to promote fat loss.	O	O
8. The hyperhydration effect of glycerol supplementation reduces overall heat stress during exercise, lowers heart rate and core temperature, and enhances endurance performance under heat stress.	O	O
9. Because of its role in electron transport–oxidative phosphorylation, athletes supplementing with coenzyme Q_{10} (CoQ_{10}) improve aerobic capacity and exercise cardiovascular dynamics.	O	O
10. Well-designed research clearly indicates that supplementation with (−)-hydroxycitrate (HCA) facilitates the rate of fat oxidation at rest and during moderate-intensity exercise to effectively act as an antiobesity agent and ergogenic aid.	O	O

Chapter 11 highlighted that physically active individuals often resort to using banned pharmacologic and chemical agents to augment training and gain a competitive edge; they also focus on gaining a performance-enhancing advantage by consuming specific foods and food components in their daily diet. This chapter focuses on popular nutritional ergogenic aids and their impact on exercise performance and training.

MODIFICATION OF CARBOHYDRATE INTAKE

Exercise performance benefits from increased carbohydrate intake before, during, and following intense aerobic exercise and arduous training. Vigilance and mood also improve with a carbohydrate beverage administered during a day of sustained aerobic activity interspersed with rest.[114] Carbohydrate loading represents one of the more popular nutritional modifications to increase glycogen reserves. Judicious adherence to this dietary technique improves specific exercise performance, yet some aspects of carbohydrate loading could prove detrimental.

Nutrient-Related Fatigue in Prolonged Exercise

Glycogen stored in the liver and active muscle supplies most of the energy for intense aerobic exercise. Prolonging such exercise reduces glycogen reserves and causes lipid catabolism to supply a progressively greater percentage of energy from liver and adipose tissue fatty acid mobilization. Exercise that severely lowers muscle glycogen precipitates fatigue. This occurs even though active muscles have sufficient oxygen and unlimited potential energy from stored fat. Ingesting a glucose and water solution near the point of fatigue allows exercise to continue, but for all practical purposes, the muscles' "fuel

Test Your Knowledge Boxes

Offer true-false statements at the beginning of each chapter to quiz and challenge your current knowledge, allowing you to assess your comprehension after completing the chapter.

ETHNIC GROUP INFLUENCES DIABETES RISK

The high-fat and refined carbohydrate content of the Puerto Rican diet plus their sedentary lifestyle has turned Puerto Ricans into the second highest ethnic group (Native American Pima tribe is the first) in US jurisdictions afflicted with type 2 diabetes. Twenty-five percent of Puerto Ricans between ages 45 and 74 are diabetics. Fifty percent of Hispanic women and 40% of Hispanic men will develop diabetes at some point in their life. Economic, social, and nutritional changes (overnutrition and improper nutrition) over the past 20 to 30 years combined with a decline in regular physical activity link closely to the creeping epidemic of obesity, which increases diabetes risk approximately 10-fold. The figure here illustrates that not all fat is created equal, and that different forms of excess storage fat (subcutaneous, visceral, and retroperitoneal) in the abdominal region significantly contributes to diabetes risk in addition to other negative alterations in the metabolic profile.

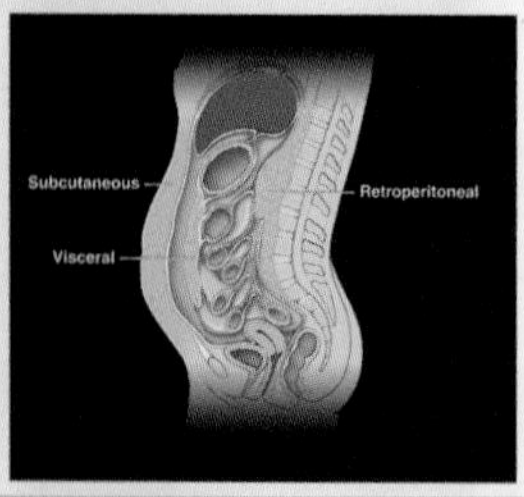

Over a broad range of BMI values, men and women with high waist circumference values possess greater relative risk for cardiovascular disease, type 2 diabetes, gallstones, cancer, cataracts (the leading cause of blindness worldwide), and all-cause mortality than individuals with small waist circumference or with peripheral obesity.

For men, the percentage of visceral fat increases progressively with age, whereas this fat deposition in women begins to increase at the onset of menopause. The waist-to-hip ratio poorly captures the specific effects of each girth measure. Waist and hip circumferences reflect different aspects of body composition and fat distribution. Each has an independent and often opposite effect on cardiovascular disease risk. Waist girth reflects central fat deposition and provides a reasonable indication of the accumulation of intra-abdominal (visceral) adipose tissue. This currently makes waist girth the trunk measure of clinical choice to evaluate health risks when more precise assessments are impractical.[65,97,120]

VARIATIONS IN VISCERAL ADIPOSE TISSUE AND WAIST CIRCUMFERENCE

Physical fitness, age, and gender alter the relation between waist circumference and abdominal adipose tissue, with men having more visceral adipose tissue than women at any waist circumference. For a given waist circumference, visceral adipose tissue also increases with age, whereas it decreases with improved physical fitness.[82,103]

TABLE 13.6 presents classification guidelines and associated disease risk for overweight and obesity based on BMI or waist girth. Men with a waist girth of 102 cm (40.2 in) or larger and women with a waist girth larger than 88 cm (36.6 in) maintain a high risk for various diseases. Waist girths of 90 cm (35.4 in) for men and 83 cm (32.7 in) for women correspond to a BMI threshold of overweight (BMI ≥ 25), whereas waist girths of 100 cm (39.4 in) for men and 93 cm (36.6 in) for women reflect the obesity cutoff (BMI ≥ 30).[96]

Documentation of a strong effect of regular exercise on reducing waist girth selectively in men may partially explain why physical activity reduces disease risk more effectively in men than in women. Both physical activity and energy intake selectively predict waist-to-hip ratio in men but not in women.

A RISKY PLACE TO STORE EXCESS BODY FAT

Central excess fat deposition, independent of excess fat storage in other anatomic areas, reflects an altered metabolic profile that increases risk of the following eight conditions:

1. Hyperinsulinemia (insulin resistance)
2. Glucose intolerance
3. Type 2 diabetes
4. Endometrial cancer
5. Hypertriglyceridemia
6. Hypercholesterolemia and negatively altered lipoprotein profile
7. Hypertension
8. Atherosclerosis

In addition to the impact of excess abdominal fat and alterations in the metabolic profile, recent research has focused on neuropeptide-adipose tissue communication and how such interactions affect intra-abdominal fat tissue physiology and disease state in that anatomic region (e.g., Crohn's disease).

Karagiannides I, et al. Neuropeptide - adipose tissue communication and intestinal pathophysiology. *Curr Pharm Des* 2011;17:1576.

Karagiannides I, Pothoulakis C. Neuropeptides, mesenteric fat, and intestinal inflammation. *Ann N Y Acad Sci* 2008;1144:127.

FYI Boxes

Highlight key concepts and facts you need to remember.

264 **Part 3** Optimal Nutrition for the Physically Active Person! Making Informed and Healthful Choices

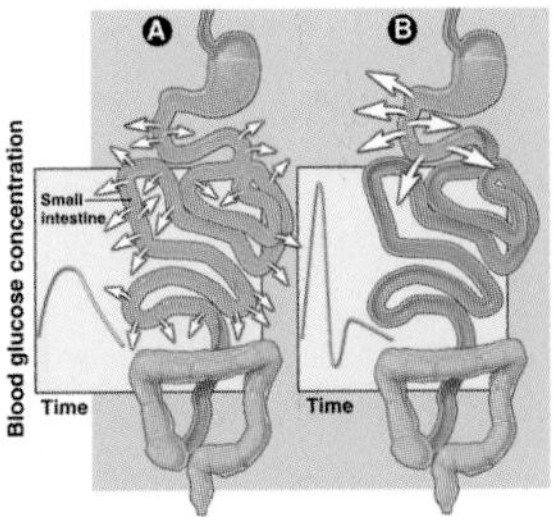

FIGURE 8.3. General response of intestinal glucose absorption following feeding of foods with either **(A)** low glycemic index or **(B)** high glycemic index such as glucose. The low-glycemic food absorbs at a slower rate throughout the full length of the small intestine to produce a more gradual rise in blood glucose.

NOT SIMPLY THE CARBOHYDRATE FORM

The glycemic index is a function of glucose appearance in the systemic circulation and its uptake by peripheral tissues, which is influenced by the properties of the carbohydrate-containing food. For example, a food's high amylose-to-amylopectin ratio or high fiber and fat content slow intestinal glucose absorption, whereas the protein content of the food may augment insulin release to facilitate glucose uptake by the cells.[90]

a ripe banana has a higher GI than a "greener" banana. Once foods are combined (i.e., a ripe banana eaten with three flavors of ice cream topped with nuts and chocolate fudge), the meal's GI for that combination of foods differs from the GI for the separate items.

The revised GI listing also includes the **glycemic load** associated with the specified serving sizes of different foods. Whereas the GI compares equal quantities of a carbohydrate-containing food, the glycemic load quantifies the overall glycemic effect of a typical food *portion*. This represents the

Connections to the Past boxes

Provide a tribute to scientists and researchers from the past two centuries who contributed new understanding about important aspects of the emerging discipline of exercise nutrition.

Connections to the Past

August Krogh (1874–1949)

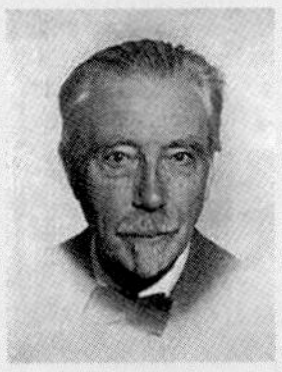

August Krogh began his career in the laboratory of the noted Danish physician-physiologist Christian Harald Bohr (1855–1911; father of physicist and 1922 Physics Nobel laureate Niels Henrik Bohr (1885-1962) and mathematician Harald Bohr; (1887–1951), who himself had been trained by physiologist Carl Ludwig (1816–1895) in Leipzig. Bohr had already clarified the dynamics of muscle contraction and solubility of oxygen in different fluids including blood. His studies of oxygen influenced Krogh's early experiments of tissue respiration in animals. Krogh devised equipment to measure respiratory gas exchange in snails, frogs, and fishes. Krogh's *An Account of the Structure and Function of the Lungs and Air Sacks of Birds*, the equivalent of a Master's thesis (1899), proved oxygen diffused rapidly through the thin pulmonary membranes, while the skin eliminated carbon dioxide. Subsequent experiments in gas transport corrected the prevailing view that lungs were gland-type structure that *secreted* oxygen and carbon dioxide. Krogh's highly accurate equipment analyzed respiratory gases, and established that pulmonary gas was exchanged by the mechanism of diffusion, not secretion. The problem solved by Krogh was whether nitrogen or nitrogenous gases were released from the body as a normal by-product of metabolism. In 1906, he proved that gaseous nitrogen remained constant, solving a vexing question in physiology. Krogh's fresh approach to this and other problems using respiratory methods to quantify nitrogen dynamics also won fame. The methods succeeded without using the traditional German method that measured nitrogen in ingested food and fluid and excreted nitrogen in feces and urine. Krogh published nearly 300 research papers, many of which are considered "classics" in exercise physiology. He also devised a bicycle ergometer with magnets and weights to quantify power output and exercise intensity. He was awarded the 1920 Nobel Prize in Physiology or Medicine for the discovery of the mechanism of regulation of the capillaries in skeletal muscle.

thePoint *Visit* thePoint.lww.com/MKKSEN4e *for more details about how Nobel Prize winner August Krogh's insightful experiments influenced basic and applied research in the biological sciences, including the emerging field of exercise physiology.*

118 **Part 1** Food Nutrients: Structure, Function, and Digestion, Absorption, and Assimilation

Additional Insights
Multivitamins and Heart Attack Protection

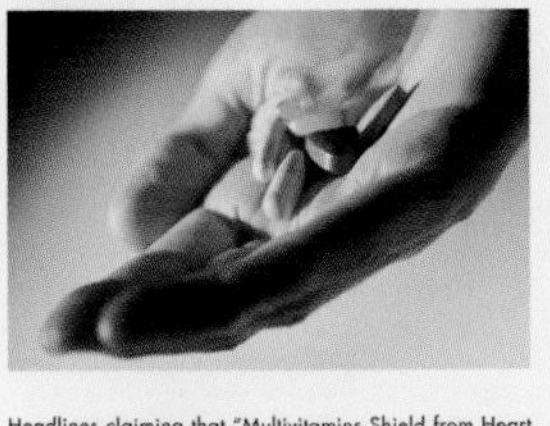

Headlines claiming that "Multivitamins Shield from Heart Attack" and "Multivitamin Use Lowers Heart Attack Risk" often tempt one to join the ranks of the more than 75 million Americans who routinely consume daily multivitamin supplements in pill and powder form at a cost that can reach $75 monthly. Much of the recent media hype comes from a 10-year follow-up study of 31,671 healthy women and 2262 women with documented cardiovascular disease (that included metabolic syndrome, hypertension, and stroke risk factors) who consumed multivitamins on a daily basis. The multivitamins were estimated to contain nutrients close to recommended daily allowances for vitamin A (0.9 mg), vitamin C (60 mg), vitamin D (5 μg), vitamin E (9 mg), thiamine (1.2 mg), riboflavin (1.4 mg), vitamin B_6 (1.8 mg), vitamin B_{12} (3 μg), and folic acid (400 μg). For the healthy women, taking multivitamins for 10 or more years coincided with a 42% lower likelihood of heart attack. Less positive results emerged for the women with heart disease, as no significant difference in heart attack incidence was associated with multivitamin and supplement use. It is important to note that this study did not *prove* that multivitamin and supplement use protects against heart attacks because this retrospective, observational study was not a randomized experiment designed to tease out cause and effect. To do so, an equal number of women with and without heart disease would be randomly assigned to a control or experimental group. The experimental group would receive supplements while the control group would not take supplements. At the end of the treatment period (e.g., 10 years), the number of deaths between the two groups would be compared. If the supplements "worked," then significantly fewer deaths would occur in the supplemented group compared to the nonsupplemented counterparts.

A plausible explanation in critique of the current observational study maintains that individuals who regularly use vitamin supplements usually live healthier overall lifestyles than nonsupplement users—they smoke less, pay more attention to their weight, remain more physically active, and generally eat a more healthful diet. The plausible reality is that multivitamin supplement use may actually be a surrogate measure of a healthy lifestyle, which in itself provides considerable heart disease protection. The bottom line is that well-controlled experiments find little or no long-lasting benefit from taking a daily multivitamin/mineral supplement on longevity; breast, ovarian, colorectal, or other cancers; coronary heart disease or stroke; viral infections; or performance on memory and cognitive tests. The best advice is to maintain a healthy lifestyle and obtain daily nutrients in a well-balanced dietary regimen and not from store-bought supplements.

Source: Rautiainen S, et al. Multivitamin use and the risk of myocardial infarction: a population-based cohort of Swedish women. *Am J Clin Nutr* 2011;93:674.

Related References

Chlebowski RT, et al Calcium plus vitamin D supplementation and the risk of breast cancer. *J Natl Cancer Inst* 2008;100:1581.

deVogel S, et al. Dietary folate, methionine, riboflavin, and vitamin B-6 and risk of sporadic colorectal cancer. *J Nutr* 2008;138:2372.

Park SY, et al. Multivitamin use and the risk of mortality and cancer: the multiethnic cohort study. *Am J Epidemiol* 2011;173:906.

Sesso HD, et al. Vitamins E and C in the prevention of cardiovascular disease in men. The Physicians' Health Study II Randomized Controlled Trial. *JAMA* 2008;300:2123.

LET NATURE DO IT

The normal process for protein digestion and absorption that provides amino acids in readily available form argues against the widespread practice advocated in body building and strength training magazines of ingesting a "predigested," hydrolyzed simple amino acid supplement to facilitate amino acid availability. The advertising hype does not justify the purchase of these products.

form. This coenzyme breakdown occurs first in the stomach and then along sections of small intestine where absorption proceeds. Effective vitamin nutrition for healthy men and women depends mainly on *consuming* a variety of vitamin-laden nutrients, not on limitations in their *absorption*.

Mineral Absorption

Both extrinsic (dietary) and intrinsic (cellular) factors control the eventual fate of ingested minerals. Overall, the body does not absorb minerals very well. Intestinal absorption

Additional Insights boxes

Contain relevant information regarding areas of controversy, confusion, and current interest related to material in the text.

314 **Part 3** Optimal Nutrition for the Physically Active Person

marketing advantage in today's consumer market but does not guarantee the product is legitimately organic. The purpose of organic certification is to protect consumers from misuse of the term and to make buying organics easier.

In the United States, federal organic legislation defines three levels of organics. Products made entirely with certified organic ingredients and methods can be labeled "100% organic." Products with at least 95% organic ingredients can use the word "organic." Both of these categories also may display the USDA organic seal. A third category, containing a minimum of 70% organic ingredients, can be labeled "made with organic ingredients."

Organic foods are supposed to be free of most chemical pesticides, fertilizers, antibiotics, hormones, and genetic engineering. Organic farmers and ranchers must enrich the soil and demonstrate humane animal treatment.

SUMMARY

1. Many factors affect food choices including traditions, early food experiences, emotions, food fears, food availability, and nutritional quality.
2. Pleasure associated with taste, texture, and aroma of food is learned within a perceptual and cultural context.
3. Many manufactures capitalize on the link between smell and taste and food pleasure by adding chemicals that mimic certain smells and tastes so one can purchase almost any "food" chemically altered to taste like something else.
4. Determining a food's nutrient density or "healthfulness" provides useful information about its nutritional quality referred to as the Index of Nutritional Quality (INQ).
5. Appetite and hunger refer to different entities. Appetite represents the desire to eat and is affected by external and psychological factors. Hunger represents an internal drive to eat largely based on central and peripheral physiologic systems.
6. New regulations from the Food and Drug Administration (FDA), under the aegis of the US Department of Agriculture's (USDA) Food Safety and Inspection Service, require manufacturers to adhere to guidelines when linking a nutrient(s) to medical or health benefits.
7. Four governmental agencies (FTC, FDA, USDA, and ATF) create the rules, regulations, and legal requirements concerning advertising, packaging, and labeling of foods and alcoholic beverages.
8. The Nutrition Labeling and Education Act of 1990 (NLEA) requires food manufacturers to strictly comply to regulations about what can and cannot be printed on food labels.
9. The format for the nutrition panel on foods must declare the nutrient content per serving as percentages of the Daily Values (the new label reference values).
10. The new "% Daily Value" comprises two sets of dietary standards: Daily Reference Values (DRVs) and Reference Daily Intakes (RDIs).
11. DRVs established for macronutrients include sources of energy (lipid, carbohydrate [including fiber], and protein) and noncalorie contributors (cholesterol, sodium, and potassium).
12. The RDI replaces the term "US RDA." The new RDIs remain the same as the old US RDAs.
13. Food labels must indicate the amount of a particular nutrient, but no requirement exists to list its relative percentage in a food.
14. As of January 1, 2012, the familiar nutrition label required on all packaged food items must appear on 40 of the most commonly purchased cuts of beef, poultry, pork, and lamb.
15. The Nutrition Facts panels must include the number of calories, the grams of total fat, and saturated fat content.
16. A manufacturer wishing to include an additive in a food must follow specific FDA guidelines to ensure the additive's effectiveness (i.e., meet its claims).
17. A list of additives that are generally recognized as safe (GRAS) currently includes about 2000 flavoring agents and 200 coloring agents.
18. The healthcare reform legislation law of 2010 (enacted in 2012) requires restaurants and similar retail food establishments with 20 or more locations to list calorie content information for standard menu items on restaurant menus and menu boards.
19. Level of income and education, racial and ethnic background, and geographic locale and personal interests influence the amount, type, and quality of food consumed by a particular group or individual in the group.
20. People who often eat at fast-food restaurants usually double their caloric intake compared with eating at home.
21. The nongovernmental watchdog organization Center for Science in the Public Interest raises public awareness about the nutritional content of favorite foods and meals, often with alarming results about high fat content (particularly saturated fat) and excessive calorie content.
22. Hunger and obesity coexist within the same person and within the same household and link closely to "malnutrition."
23. Malnutrition from undernutrition and overnutrition emerges from living in poverty with an inadequate access to nutrient dense foods.

Section Summaries

Help reinforce and review key concepts and material.

Chapter 1 The Macronutrients 35

PERSONAL HEALTH AND EXERCISE NUTRITION 1.2

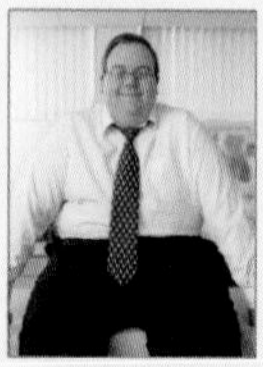

Adult Hyperlipidemia

The following data were obtained on a 58-year-old executive who has not had an annual physical examination in 5 years. He has gained weight and is now concerned about his health status.

Medical History

The patient has no history of chronic diseases or major hospitalization. He does not take medications or dietary supplements and has no known food allergies.

Family History

The patient's father died from a heart attack at age 61; his younger brother has had triple bypass surgery, and his uncle has type 2 diabetes. His mother, physically inactive for most of her adult life, classifies as obese with high serum cholesterol and triacylglycerol levels.

Social History

The patient has been overweight since high school. He has gained 15 lb during the last year, which he attributes to his job and changes in eating habits (eats out more frequently). The patient, J.M., wants to improve his diet but does not know what to do. He typically eats only two meals daily, with at least one meal consumed at a restaurant and several snacks interspersed. He drinks three to five cups of coffee throughout the day and two to three alcoholic drinks every evening. He also smokes one pack of cigarettes daily and reports high stress in his job and at home (two teenage children). Patient states he has little opportunity for exercise or leisure time activities given his present schedule.

Physical Examination/Anthropometric/Laboratory Data

- Blood pressure: 135/90 mm Hg
- Height: 6 feet (182.9 cm)
- Body weight: 215 lb (97.1 kg)
- Body mass index (BMI): 29.0
- Abdominal girth: 40.9 inches (104 cm)
- Laboratory data
  - Nonfasting total cholesterol: 267 mg·dL^{-1}
  - HDL-C: 34 mg·dL^{-1}
  - LDL-C: 141 mg·dL^{-1}
  - Blood glucose: 124 mg·dL^{-1}
- Dietary intake from 24-hour food recall
  - Calories: 3001 kcal
  - Protein: 110 g (14.7% of total kcal)
  - Lipid: 121 g (36.3% of total kcal)
  - Carbohydrate: 368 g (49% of total kcal)
  - Saturated fatty acids: 18% of total kcal
  - Monounsaturated fatty acids (MUFA): 7% of total kcal
  - Cholesterol: 390 mg·dL^{-1}
  - Fiber: 10 g
  - Folic acid: 200 μg
- General impressions: overly fat male with possible metabolic syndrome

Case Questions

1. Provide an overall assessment of patient's health status.
2. What other laboratory tests could be performed?
3. Interpret the blood lipid profile based on his history, physical examination, and laboratory data.
4. Give recommendations for improving the adequacy of patient's diet.
5. Create the best dietary approach for the patient.
6. What course of action should the patient consider to improve his blood lipid profile?

thePoint *Visit thePoint.lww.com/MKKSEN4e to review the answers to these case questions.*

Personal Health and Exercise Nutrition Activities

Engage readers in specific areas of nutritional assessment and health appraisal, application of dietary guidelines, weight control, body composition, overuse syndrome, and physical activity ecommendations.

Relevant Web Sites

Highlighted within the text, these links direct you to reliable online exercise nutrition resources.

Designer Drug Unmasked

The Department of Molecular and Medical Pharmacology at the University of California at Los Angeles (UCLA) supports the world's largest WADA-accredited sports drug-testing facility involved with athletic doping. Founded in 1982 by a grant from the Los Angeles Olympic Organizing Committee, the UCLA facility was the first US laboratory accredited by the IOC (**www.pathnet.medsch.ucla.edu/OlympicLab/index.html**). Among its many accomplishments, the laboratory unmasked a potentially illegal "designer" compound that mimics the chemical structure similar to the prohibited steroids gestrinome and trenbolone. The researchers called the discovery a new stand-alone steroid chemical entity, not a "pro-steroid" or "precursor steroid" like many performance-boosting substances on the market—a drug with no prior record of manufacture or existence. The US Anti-Doping Agency (USADA; **www.usantidoping.org**) oversees drug testing for all sports federations under the US Olympic umbrella. The USADA said an anonymous tipster provided a syringe sample of a steroid identified as tetrahydrogestrinone (THG). Athletes who test positive face 2-year suspensions that prohibit participation in international meets.

As of October 17, 2003, the National Football League (NFL) began testing players for THG to avoid the scandal that has embarrassed track and field. For at least the past

Key References

At the end of each chapter are listed the top 25 classic and up-to-date references from the chapter. The full reference lists for each chapter are available online at thePoint.lww.com/MKKSEN4e.

Key References

Angell M, Kassirer JP. Alternative medicine: the risks of untested and unregulated remedies. *N Engl J Med* 1998;339:831.

Dietz WH. Does hunger cause obesity? *Pediatrics* 1995;95:766.

Dinour LM, et al. The food insecurity–obesity paradox: a review of the literature and the role food stamps may play. *J Am Diet Assoc* 2007;107:1952.

Drewnowski A. Concept of a nutritious food: toward a nutrient density score. *Am J Clin Nutr* 2005;82:721.

Drewnowski A, Specter SE. Poverty and obesity: the role of energy density and energy costs, *Am J Clin Nutr* 2004;79:6.

Fisher JO, et al. Children's bite size and intake of an entrée are greater with large portions than with age-appropriate or self-selected portions. *Am J Clin Nutr* 2003;77:1164.

Jones SJ, et al. Lower risk of overweight in school-aged food insecure girls who participate in food assistance. *Arch Pediatr Adolesc Med* 2003;157:780.

Life Sciences Research Office, Federation of American Societies of Experimental Biology. Core indicators of nutritional state for difficult-to-sample populations. *J Nutr* 1990;120(Suppl 11):S1559.

Nestle M. *Food Politics: How the Food Industry Influences Nutrition and Health.* Berkeley, CA: University of California Press, 2002.

Nielsen SJ, Popkin BM. Patterns and trends in food portion sizes, 1977-1998. *JAMA* 2003;289:450.

Nielsen SJ, Popkin BM. Changes in beverage intake between 1977 and 2001. *Am J Prev Med* 2004;27:205.

Olson CM. Nutrition and health outcomes associated with food insecurity and hunger. *J Nutr* 1999;129(Suppl 2):S521.

Sarubin A. Government regulation of dietary supplements. In: *The Health Professional's Guide to Dietary Supplements.* Chicago: The American Dietetic Association, 1999.

Scheier LM. What is the hunger-obesity paradox? *J Am Diet Assoc* 2005;105:883.

Sitzman K. Expanding food portions contribute to overweight and obesity. *AAOHN J* 2004;52:356.

Townsend MS, et al. Food insecurity is positively related to overweight in women. *J Nutr* 2001;131:1738.

Young LR, Nestle M. The contribution of expanding portion sizes to the U.S. obesity epidemic. *Am J Public Health* 2002;92:246.

thePoint *Visit* **thePoint.lww.com/MKKSEN4e** *for a complete and thorough list of the references cited in this chapter, as well as additional references.*

Student Resources

Inside the front cover of your textbook you will find your personal access code. Use it to log on the thePoint.lww.com/MKKSEN4e, the companion website for this textbook. On the website you can access various supplemental materials available to help enhance and further your learning. These assets include the fully searchable online text, a quiz bank, animations, full chapter reference lists, expanded Conectins to the Past boxes, answers to the Personal Health and Nutrition Activities, and the Appendices from the book.

thePoint

Acknowledgments

We gratefully acknowledge the following individuals at Lippincott Williams & Wilkins for their dedication and expertise with this project: Emily Lupash, Senior Acquisitions Editor; Christen D. Murphy, Marketing Manager, for creatively promoting our text and interpreting its unique aspects to the appropriate markets; and a very special thanks to Andrea Klingler, Product Manager, for tolerating our unique idiosyncrasies, for gently keeping us focused and "on track," and for making what often becomes a difficult task a relatively enjoyable experience. We are also grateful to the numerous undergraduate and graduate students at our respective universities for keeping our "motors" going during our work on various projects related to this text.

Since the first time we conceived of formulating the material that led to the publication of the first and subsequent editions of our text, the field has lost many outstanding researchers and educators who we were priviieged to know throughout our academic careers. We hereby acknowledge these friends and respected colleagues who allowed us to benefit from their close association, continual mentoring and encouragement, and research collaborations: Captain Albert Behnke, Jr., MD; Dr. Carl Blomquist; Dr. James Bosco; Dr. Roger Burke; Dr. Elsworth Buskirk; Dr. John Cooper; Dr. Albert Craig, Jr.; Dr. Thomas K. Cureton; Dr. Chris Dawson; Dr. Marvin Eyler; Dr. Guido Foglia; Dr. Carl Gisolfi; Dr. George Grey; Dr. Donald Hagan; Dr. Franklin Henry; Dr. Steven Horvath; Dr. James Humphrey; Dr. Paul Hunsicker; Dr.Frederick Kasch; Dr. Walter Kroll; Dr. Lynn McCraw; Dr. Ernest Michael, Jr.; Dr. Michael Pollock; Dr. Larry Rarick; Dr. George Q. Rich III; Dr. Benjamin Ricci; Dr. Paola Timiras; and Dr. Brain Whipp.

Contents

Introduction

Food provides the source of essential elements and building blocks to synthesize new tissue, preserve lean body mass, optimize skeletal structure, repair existing cells, maximize oxygen transport and use, maintain favorable fluid and electrolyte balance, and regulate all metabolic processes. **"Optimal" nutrition** encompasses more than preventing nutrient deficiencies related to disease, including overt endemic diseases ranging from beriberi (vitamin deficiency disease from inadequate thiamine [vitamin B_1]; damages heart and nervous system) to xerophthalmia (caused by vitamin A deficiency and general malnutrition leading to night blindness, corneal ulceration, and blindness). It also encompasses the recognition of individual differences in the need for and tolerance of specific nutrients and the role of genetic heritage in such factors. Borderline nutrient deficiencies (i.e., less than required to cause clinical manifestations of disease) can negatively impact bodily structure and function and thus the capacity for physical activity.

Optimal nutrition also forms the foundation for physical performance; it provides the fuel for biologic work and the nutrients for extracting and transfering food's potential energy to the kinetic energy of movement. Not surprisingly, then, from the time of the ancient Olympics to the present, almost every conceivable dietary practice has been used to enhance exercise performance. Writings from the first Olympic games in 776 BC to today's computerized era provide a glimpse of what athletes consume. Poets, philosophers, writers, and the physicians of ancient Greece and Rome tell of diverse strategies athletes undertook to prepare for competitions. They consumed various animal meats (oxen, goat, bull, deer); moist cheeses and wheat; dried figs; and special "concoctions" and liquors. For the next 2000 years, however, little reliable information existed about the food preferences of top athletes (except for rowers and pedestrian walkers during the 19th century). The 1936 Berlin Olympics offered a preliminary assessment of the food consumed by world-class athletes. From the article by Schenk,[1]

> . . . the Olympic athletes competing at Berlin frequently focused upon meat, that athletes regularly dined on two steaks per meal, sometimes poultry, and averaged nearly half a kilogram of meat daily . . . pre-event meals regularly consisted of one to three steaks and eggs, supplemented with "meat-juice" extract. . . . Other athletes stressed the importance of carbohydrate. . . . Olympic athletes from England, Finland, and Holland regularly consumed porridge, the Americans ate shredded wheat or corn flakes in milk, and the Chileans and Italians feasted on pasta . . . members of the Japanese team consumed a pound of rice daily.

During the 2004 Olympic Games in Athens, about 12,000 athletes from 197 countries consumed an inordinate amount of food. During this Olympiad, some countries applied specific dietary regimens, whereas athletes from less industrialized countries had free choice of what they ate, often combining ritual with novelty foods. The majority of athletes probably consumed dietary supplements including vitamins and minerals; a smaller percentage most likely ingested stimulants, narcotics, anabolic agents, diuretics, peptides, glycoprotein hormones and analogs, alcohol, marijuana, local anesthetics, corticosteroids, β-blockers, β_2-agonists, and used blood doping, all of which the International Olympic Committee prohibits. In the war against illegal drug use, the Beijing 2008 Olympic Games performed approximately 4500 drug tests. This was a major increase compared with the 2800 tests carried out at the 2000 Sydney Games and the 3700 tests at the 2004 Athens Games. For the 2012 London Games, the London Organizing Committee will administer approximately 5000 tests under the authority of the International Olympic Committee (10% more than those conducted in Beijing in 2008, where 20 of the samples returned positive). A further 1200 tests will be carried out on a subsample of all athletes at the London 2012 Paralympics, with UK Anti-Doping also playing a role in the testing process. Experts estimate that the *percentage* of people caught

FOOD SERVICES AT THE 2012 LONDON OLYMPIC GAMES

Feeding Olympic athletes, staff, and spectators represents an enormous undertaking. For the 2012 London Games, preparations are being made over a 2-year planning period to accomplish the following at 31 competition venues over 955 competition sessions: Attend to a total workforce of 160,000 people; supply 14 million meals for 23,900 athletes and team officials and 20,600 broadcasters and press; and cater to 4800 Olympic and Paralympic family members. In the Olympic Village, plans include the following in terms of food quantities:

1. 25,000 loaves of bread
2. 232 tons of potatoes
3. 82 tons of seafood
4. 31 tons of poultry items
5. In excess of 100 tons of meat
6. 75,000 liters of milk
7. 19 tons of eggs (free range)
8. 21 tons of cheese
9. In excess of 330 tons of fruit and vegetables

Source: Data available at http://www.london2012.com/documents/locog-publications/food-vision.pdf/.

doping is between 1% and 2% (number of positive tests against the total number of tests). The World Anti-Doping Authority estimates that the *number* of people doping is in the double digits, with recent cases showing cheaters are becoming more sophisticated by turning to masking agents such as furosemide, a "water pill" (diuretic) used to reduce swelling and fluid retention by causing the kidneys to excrete water and salt into the urine.

Even today's technologically savvy world is inundated with trendy theories, misinformation, and outright quackery that links nutrition and physical performance. Accomplishments during the last 100 years of Olympic competition undeniably have improved, but no one has yet established universal ties between food and physical achievement. Athletes have every reason to desire any substance that might confer a competitive advantage because winning ensures glory and multimillion dollar endorsement contracts. Their eagerness to shave milliseconds from a run or add centimeters to a jump convinces them to experiment with nutrition and polypharmacy supplementation, including illegal drugs.

The search for the "holy grail" to enhance physical performance has not been limited to the last few decades. Athletes and trainers in ancient civilizations also sought to improve athletic prowess. Although lacking objective proof, these early athletes routinely experimented with nutritional substances and rituals, trusting that the natural and supernatural would provide an advantage. Over the past 25 centuries, the scientific method has gradually replaced dogma and ritual as the most effective approach to healthful living and optimal physical performance. The emerging field of exercise nutrition uses the ideas of pioneers in medicine, anatomy, physics, chemistry, hygiene, nutrition, and physical culture to establish a robust body of knowledge.

A sound understanding of exercise nutrition enables one to appreciate the importance of adequate nutrition and to critically evaluate the validity of claims concerning nutrient supplements and special dietary modifications to enhance physique, physical performance, and exercise training responses. Knowledge of the nutrition–metabolism interaction forms the basis for the preparation, performance, and recuperation phases of intense exercise and/or training. Not surprisingly, many physically active individuals, including some of the world's best athletes, obtain nutritional information in the locker room and from magazine and newspaper articles, advertisements, video "infomercials," training partners, health-food shops, and testimonials from successful athletes, rather than from well-informed and well-educated coaches, trainers, physicians, and physical fitness and exercise nutrition professionals. Far too many devote considerable time and energy striving for optimum performance and training, only to fall short because of inadequate, counterproductive, and sometimes harmful nutritional practices.

We hope the fourth edition of *Sports and Exercise Nutrition* continues to provide "cutting edge" scientific information for all people involved in regular physical activity and exercise training, not just the competitive athlete.

EXERCISE NUTRITION FOR THE FUTURE: A FRESH LOOK

"And if we are ignorant of our past, if we are indifferent to our story and those people who did so much for us, we're not just being stupid, we're being rude." (From 146th Beloit College Commencement. May 12, 1996. Pulitzer Prize-winner David McCollough)

The accompanying timeline presents an historical overview of selected individuals, from the Renaissance to the 21st century, whose work and scientific experiments demonstrate the intimate interconnections among medicine, physiology, exercise, and nutrition. In the *Connections to the Past* boxes in each chapter, we chronicle a select group of these pioneers. Their important accomplishments provide a powerful rationale for developing an integrated subject field of study that we call **exercise nutrition**.

Some consider an exercise nutrition curriculum (at a college or university) as a subset of nutrition, but we believe this designation requires updating. First, we recommend a change in name from "sports nutrition" to "exercise nutrition" (or physical activity nutrition). The term *exercise* encompasses more than the word *sports*, and it more fully reflects the many physically active men and women who are not necessarily athletes. An academic program would have as its core academic content applicable to the ever-increasing number of physically active individuals. Such a curriculum would be housed in neither a Department of Nutrition nor a Department of Exercise Science or Kinesiology. Rather, the curriculum deserves a unique identity. **TABLE I.1** presents six core areas for research and study that constitute exercise nutrition, with specific topics listed within each area.

The focus of exercise nutrition is cross-disciplinary by necessity. It synthesizes knowledge from the separate but related fields of nutrition and kinesiology. A number of existing fields take a cross-disciplinary approach. Biochemists do not receive in-depth training as chemists or biologists. Instead, their training as biochemists makes them more competent biochemists than more narrowly focused chemists or biologists. The same inclusivity characterizes a biophysicist, a radio astronomer, a molecular biologist, and a geophysicist.

Historic precedents exist for linking two fields: those involving nutrition and those involving exercise. The chemist Lavoisier, for example, employed exercise to study respiration, probably not thinking that his discoveries would impact fields other than chemistry. A.V. Hill, a competent mathematician and physiologist, won a Nobel Prize in Physiology or Medicine, not for his studies of mathematics or physiology per se, but for his integrative work with muscle that helped to unravel secrets about the biochemistry of muscular actions.

In the cross-discipline of exercise nutrition, students specialize in neither exercise nor nutrition. Instead, they are trained in aspects of *both* fields. Our concept of an academic discipline agrees with Professor Franklin Henry's ideas

Six Core Areas for Research and Study in the Field of Exercise Nutrition	
Nutritional Enhancement	Optimal nutrition versus optimal nutrition for exercise Environmental stressors Military Spaceflight dynamics
Health and Longevity	Eating patterns Exercise patterns Nutrition–physical activity interactions Reproduction Mortality and morbidity Epidemiology
Energy Balance and Body Composition	Metabolism Exercise dynamics Assessment Weight control/overfatness Body size, shape, and proportion
Peak Physiologic Function	Protein, carbohydrate, and lipid requirements Oxidative stress Fatigue and staleness Tissue repair and growth Micronutrient needs Gender-related effects
Optimal Growth	Normal and abnormal Bone, muscle, and other tissues Life span Effects on cognitive behaviors Effects of chronic exercise Sport-specific interactions
Safety	Disordered eating Ergogenic/ergolytic substances Thermal stress and fluid replacement Nutrient abuse

promoted in the late 1960s.[2] It is an organized body of information collectively embraced in a formal course of instruction worthy of pursuit on its own merits.

Exercise nutrition synthesizes data from biochemistry, bioinformatics, chemistry, epidemiology, epidemiology, health promotion, exercise physiology, medicine, nutrition, and positive psychology. Students of exercise nutrition may not be full-fledged chemists, exercise physiologists, or nutritionists; however, their cross-disciplinary training gives them a broader and more appropriate perspective to advance their discipline. The renal physiologist studies the kidney as an isolated organ to determine its functions, often utilizing exercise as the stressor. The exercise scientist measures the effects of exercise on kidney function. Here the researcher emphasizes exercise physiology more than renal physiology. By contrast, the exercise nutritionist might investigate how combining diet and exercise impact kidney function in general and within circumstances like physical activity under heat stress specifically. Students of the new discipline will pursue graduate education and professional interests in new areas of inquiry, some of which include metabolic regulation of body mass, health management and disease prevention, optimal human growth, peak physiological performance, nutritional assessment/enhancement and environmental effects, personal health/wellness counseling, dietetics, and the role of food and supplements in the diverse aspects of sports medicine. As new markets for the graduates of exercise nutriiton increase, new opportunities of interdisciplinary research and funding will emerge. The intimate interrelationships among food intake, weight control, exercise performance and training responsiveness, and the maintenance of optimal health clearly justify the creation and pursuit of this discipline. We urge the establishment of a separate discipline to unite previously disparate fields. We hope others share our vision.

References

1. Grivetti LE, Applegate EA. From Olympia to Atlanta: a cultural-historical perspective on diet and athletic training. *J Nutr* 1997;127:860S–868S.
2. Henry FM. Physical education: An academic discipline. Proceedings of the 67th Annual Meeting of the National College Physical Education Association for Men, AAHPERD, Washington DC, 1964.

TIMELINE

Key History Makers In Exercise Nutrition Through The Ages, From 1450 To 2000

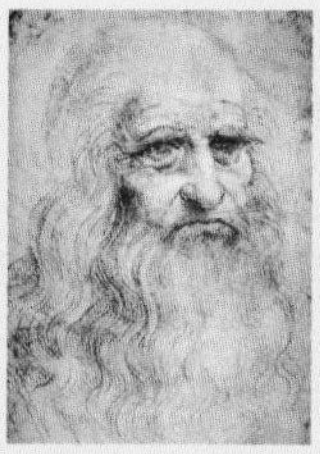

Leonardo da Vinci (1452–1519). Master anatomist produced exquisite drawings of the heart and circulation which showed that air reached pulmonary arteries via bronchi, not directly through the heart as taught by Galenic medicine.

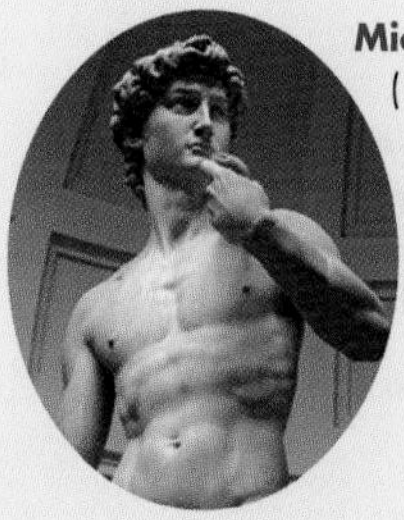

Michelangelo Buonarroti (1475–1564). Realistic sculpture of "David" combined scientific anatomy with ideal body proportions. "David"

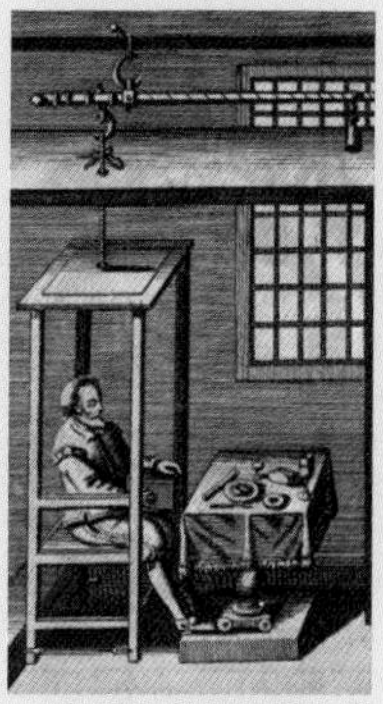

Santorio's scale used to assess his weight.

Santorio (1561–1636). Accurately recorded changes in body weight over a 30-year period to understand metabolism. Published *De Medicina Statica Aphorismi* (Medical Aphorisms), 1614.

1450 **1500** **1600**

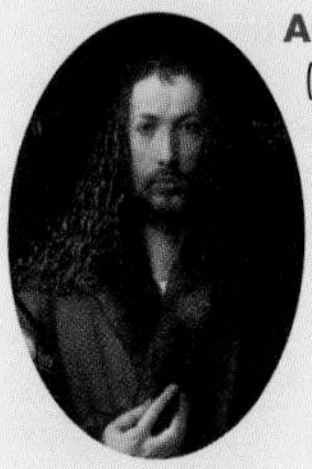

Albrecht Dürer (1471–1528). "Quadrate Man" illustrated age-related differences in body segment ratios.

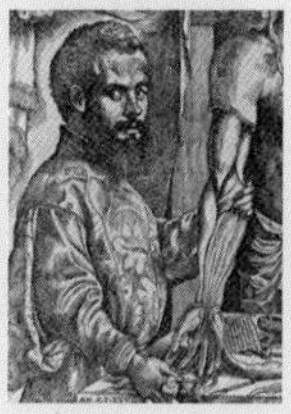

Andreas Vesalius (1514–1564). Incomparable De Humani Corporis Fabrica (On the Composition of the Human Body) and De Fabrica (1543) based on his own dissections demolished traditional Galenic pronouncements about human anatomy.

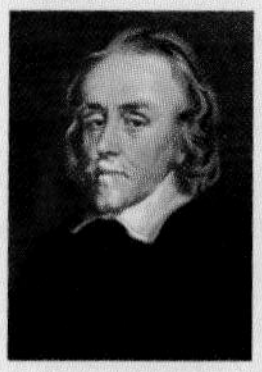

William Harvey (1578–1657). Proved the heart pumped blood one way through a closed circulatory system.

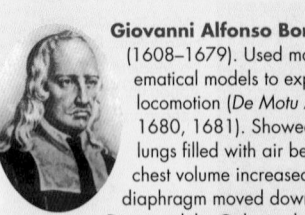

Giovanni Alfonso Borelli (1608–1679). Used mathematical models to explain locomotion (*De Motu Animaliu*, 1680, 1681). Showed that the lungs filled with air because the chest volume increased when diaphragm moved downward. Disproved the Galenic claim that air cooled the heart by showing how respiration, not circulation, required diffusion of air in the alveoli.

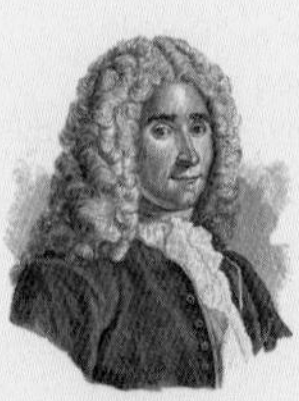

René-Antoine Fercault de Réaumur (1683–1757). Proved by regurgitation experiments that gastric secretions digest foods (*Digestion in Birds*, 1752).

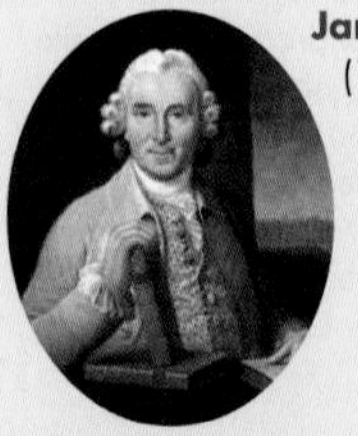

James Lind (1716–1794). Eradicated scurvy by adding citrus fruits to sailors' diets.

1620 **1700** **1735**

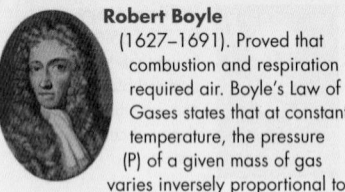

Robert Boyle (1627–1691). Proved that combustion and respiration required air. Boyle's Law of Gases states that at constant temperature, the pressure (P) of a given mass of gas varies inversely proportional to its volume (V): $P_1V_1 = P_2V_2$.

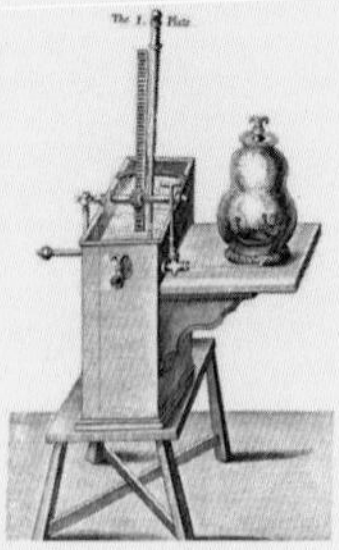

Boyle's "Pneumatical Engine" apparatus

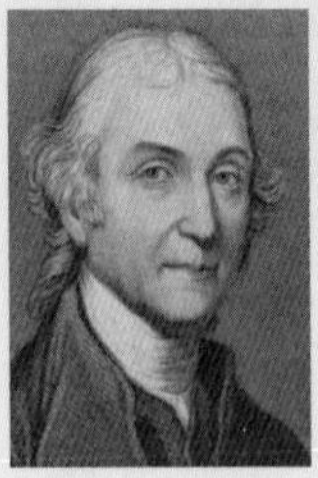

Joseph Priestley (1733–1804). Discovered oxygen by heating red oxide of mercury in a closed vessel (*Observations on Different Kinds of Air*, 1773).

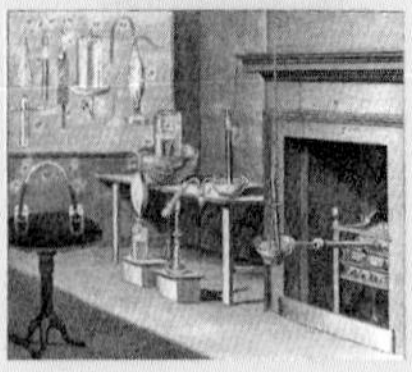

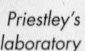

Priestley's laboratory

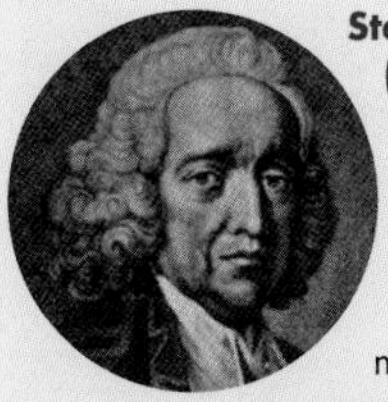

Stephen Hales (1677–1761). *Vegetable Statics* (1727) described how chemical changes occurred in solids and liquids upon calcination (oxidation during combustion), and how the nervous system governed muscular contraction.

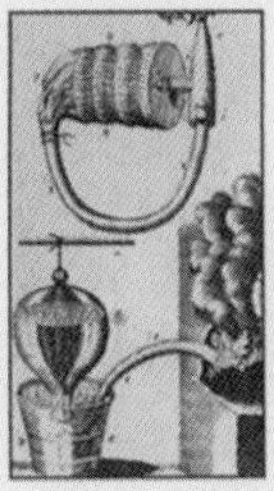

Hale's combustion apparatus

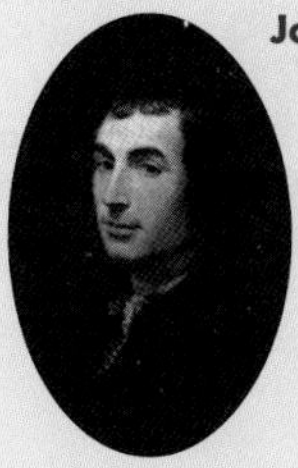

Joseph Black (1728–1799). Isolated carbon dioxide gas in air produced by fermentation (*Experiments Upon Magnesia Alba, Quicklime, And Some Other Alcaline Substances,* 1756).

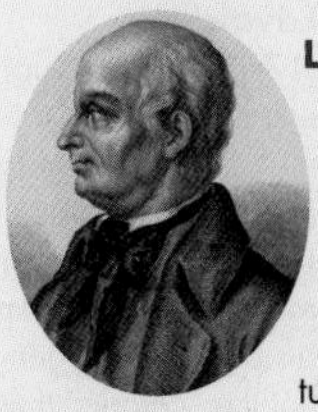

Lazzaro Spallanzani (1729–1799). Proved that tissues of the heart, stomach, and liver consume oxygen and liberate carbon dioxide, even in creatures without lungs.

1620 **1700** **1735**

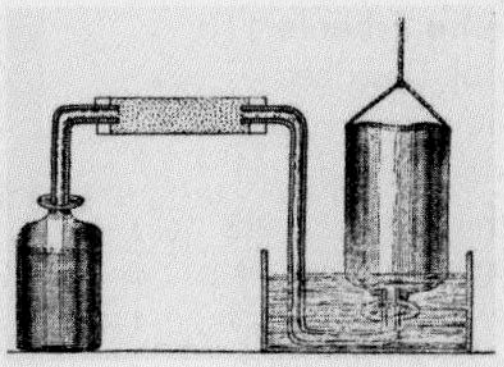

Henry Cavendish (1731–1810). Identified hydrogen produced when acids combined with metals (*On Factitious Air,* 1766). Proved that water formed when "inflammable air" (hydrogen) combined with "deflogisticated air" (oxygen) (*Experiments in Air,* 1784).

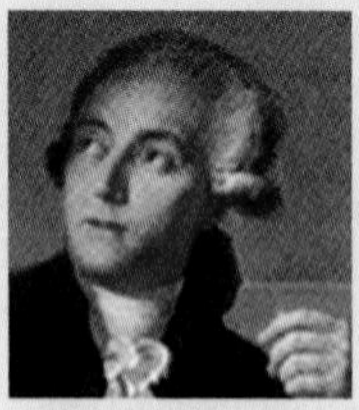

Antoine Laurent Lavoisier
(1743–1794). Quantified effects of muscular work on metabolism by measuring increases in oxygen uptake, pulse rate, and respiration rate. Proved that atmospheric air provides oxygen for animal respiration and that the "caloric" (heat) liberated during respiration is itself the source of the combustion.

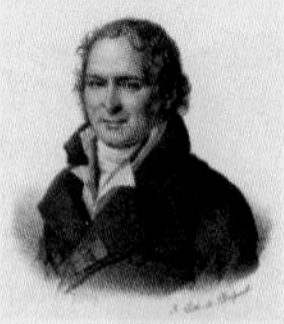

A.F. Fourcroy
(1755–1809). Demonstrated that the same proportions of nitrogen occur in animals and plants.

1740 **1755** **1775**

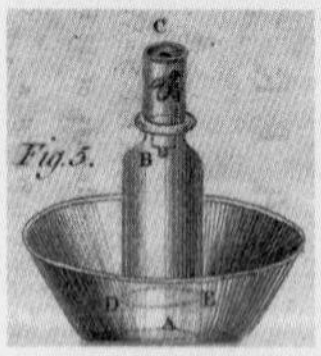

Carl Wilhelm Scheele
(1742–1786). Described oxygen ("fire air") independently of Priestley, and "foul air" (phlogisticated air—later called nitrogen) in a famous experiment with bees (*Chemical Treatise on Air and Fire,* 1777). Scheele's bees living in "fire air" in a closed vessel submerged in limewater.

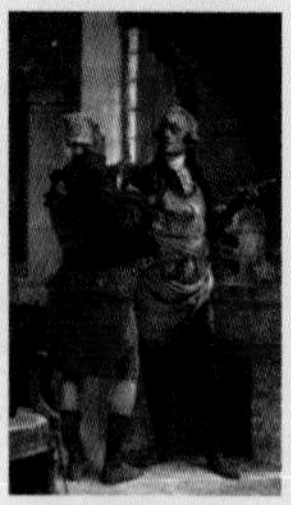

Claude Louis Berthollet
(1748–1822). Proved that animal tissues do not contain ammonia but that hydrogen united with nitrogen during fermentation to produce ammonia. He disagreed with Lavoisier's concept of heat production: "the quantity of heat liberated in the incomplete oxidation of a substance is equal to the difference between the total caloric value of the substance and that of the products formed."

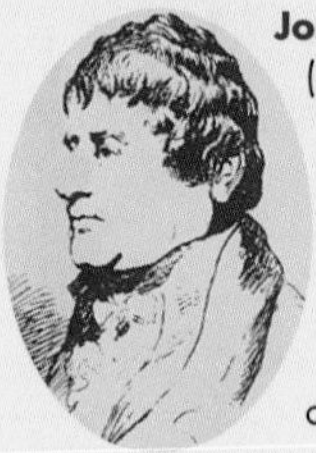

Joseph Louis Proust
(1755–1826). Formulated "Law of Definite Proportions" (chemical constancy of substances permits future analysis of major nutrients, including metabolic assessment by oxygen consumption).

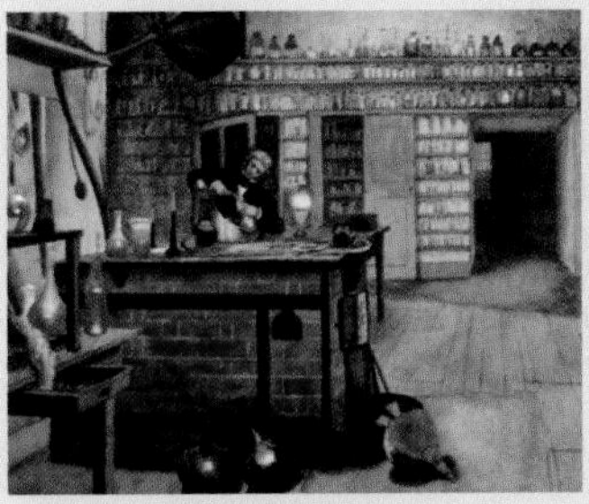

Nineteenth Century Metabolism and Physiology
The untimely death of Lavoisier (1794) did not terminate fruitful research in nutrition and medicine. During the next half century, scientists discovered the chemical composition of carbohydrates, lipids, and proteins, and further clarified the energy balance equation.

Davey's chemistry laboratory where he isolated 47 elements

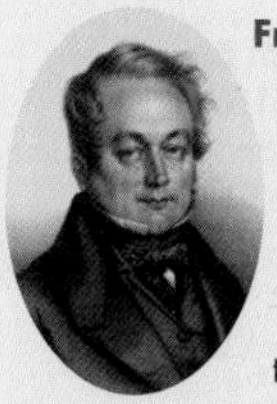

François Magendie
(1783–1855). Established experimental physiology as a science and founded its first journal (*Journal de Physiologie Expérimentale*). Proved that anterior spinal nerve roots control motor activities, while posterior roots control sensory functions. Categorized foods as nitrogenous or non-nitrogenous (*Précis élémentaire de Physiologie,* 1816), arguing that foods, not air, provided nitrogen to tissues.

1778 **1800**

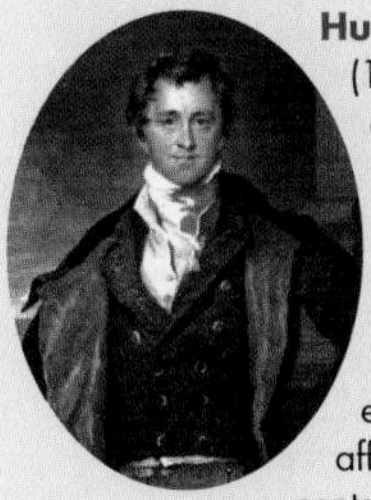

Humphrey Davey
(1778–1829). Consolidated all of the contemporary chemical data related to nutrition, including 47 elements he isolated (*Elements of Agricultural Chemistry,* 1813). Tried to explain how heat and light affect the blood's ability to contain oxygen.

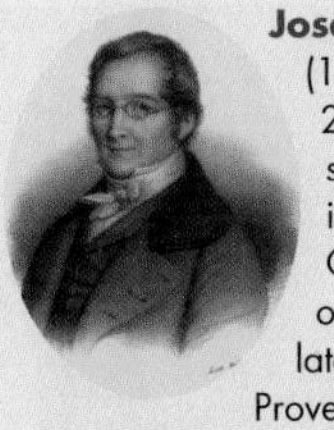

Joseph-Louis Gay-Lussac
(1778–1850). Proved that 20 animal and vegetable substances differed depending on the proportion of H to O atoms. Named one class of compounds ("saccharine") later identified as carbohydrates. Proved the equivalency of oxygen percentage in air at altitude and sea level.

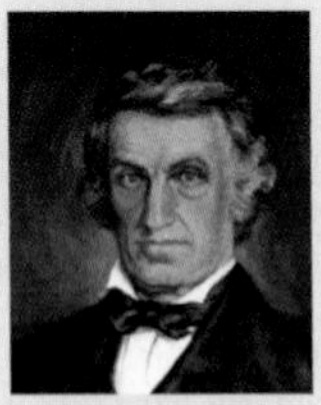

William Beaumont (1785–1853). Explained in vivo and in vitro human digestion.

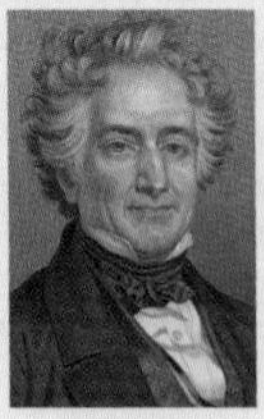

Michel Eugène Chevreul (1786–1889). Explained that fats consist of fatty acids and glycerol (*Chemical Investigations of Fat,* 1823). Coined the term margarine, and showed that lard consists of two main fats he called "stearine and elaine." With Gay-Lussac, patented the manufacture of the stearic acid candle (still used today).

1778 **1800**

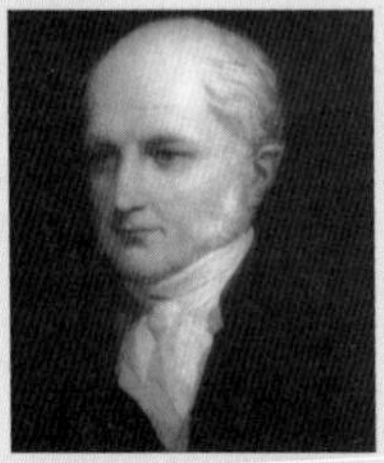

William Prout (1785–1850). First to separate foodstuffs into the modern classification of carbohydrates, fats, and proteins. Measured the carbon dioxide exhaled by men exercising to fatigue (*Annals of Philosophy,* 2: 328, 1813). Showed that walking raised carbon dioxide production to a plateau (ushering in the modern concept of steady-state gas exchange). Proved that free HCl appeared in the stomach's gastric juice. First prepared pure urea. Extolled milk as the perfect food in *Treatise on Chemistry, Meteorology, and the Function of Digestion* (1834).

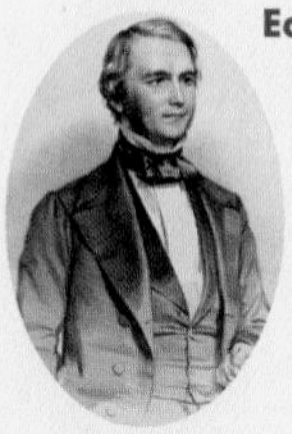

Edward Smith (1819–1874). Used closed-circuit spirometry to assess energy metabolism during forced exercise. Disproved Liebig's claim that protein alone serves as the primary source of muscular power.

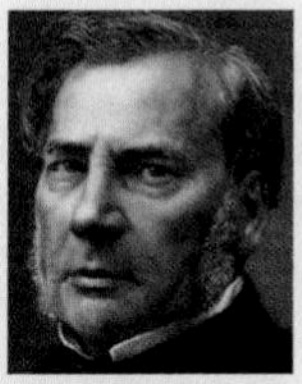

Jean Baptiste Boussingault (1802–1884). Father of "scientific agriculture." Determined the effects of calcium, iron, and nutrient intake (particularly nitrogen) on energy balance in animals and humans.

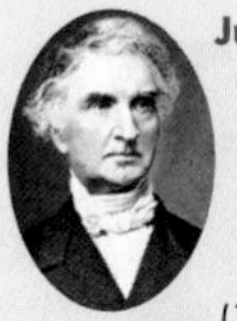

Justus von Liebig (1803–1873). Dominant chemist of his time, yet asserted without evidence that vigorous exercise by humans and animals required a high protein intake (1850s experiments by others disproved his assertions).

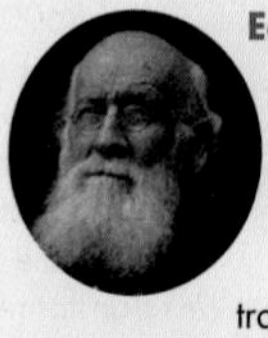

Edward Hitchcock, Jr. (1828–1911). Amherst College professor who pioneered anthropometric assessment of body build and scientific muscular strength training and testing.

1800 **1820** **1835**

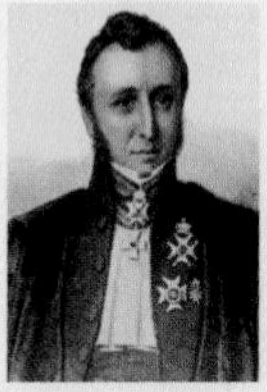

Gerardus Johannis Mulder (1802–1880). Established the field of physiological chemistry (*General Physiological Chemistry*, 1854). Researched albuminous substances he named "proteine." Strongly advocated society's role in promoting quality nutrition. Established minimum standards for protein consumption (laborers 120 g daily, others 60 g).

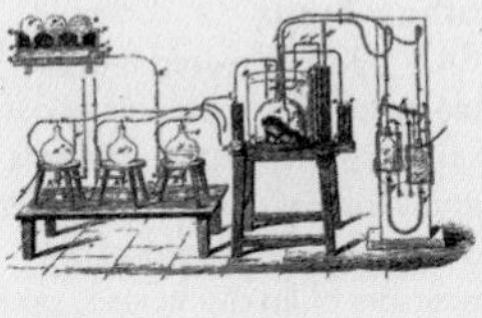

Henri Victor Regnault (1810–1878). Developed closed-circuit spirometry to determine respiratory quotient ($V{\cdot}CO_2/V{\cdot}O_2$). Established relationship between body size and metabolism (heat production). Small animal respiration chamber.

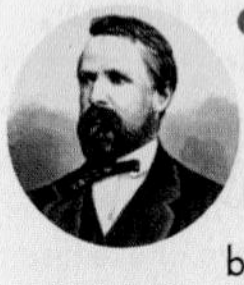

Carl von Voit (1831–1908). Disproved Liebig's assertion about protein as a main energy fuel by demonstrating that protein breakdown does not increase in proportion to exercise intensity or duration.

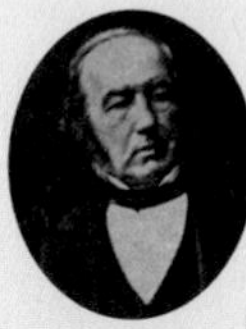

Claude Bernard (1813–1878). Perhaps the greatest experimental physiologist of all time. His discoveries in regulatory physiology helped future scientists understand how metabolism and nutrition affect exercise.

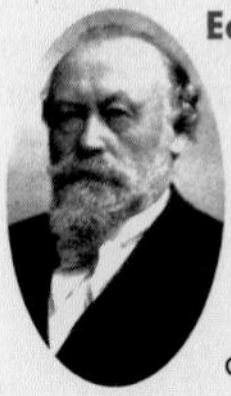

Eduard Pflüger (1829–1910). First demonstrated that minute changes in the partial pressure of gases in blood affects the rate of oxygen release and transport across capillary membranes, thus proving blood flow alone does not govern how tissues use oxygen.

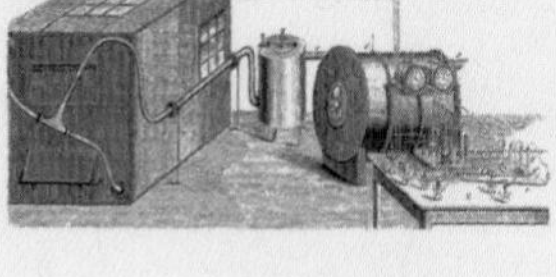

Max Joseph von Pettenkofer (1818–1901). Perfected respiration calorimeter to study human and animal metabolism. Initiated studies of scientific hygiene (air quality, soil composition and ground water, moisture content of structures, building ventilation, functions of clothing, spread of disease, water quality). He discovered creatinine (amino acid in urine), and founded *Zeitschrift für Biologie* (1865 with Voit) and *Zeitschrift für Hygiene* (1885).

Pettenkofer's 1863 respiration chamber. Top image shows the entire apparatus. Image at right is cut-away view showing human experiment. Fresh air was pumped into the sealed chamber and exhausted air sampled for carbon dioxide.

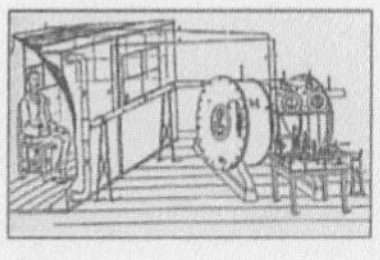

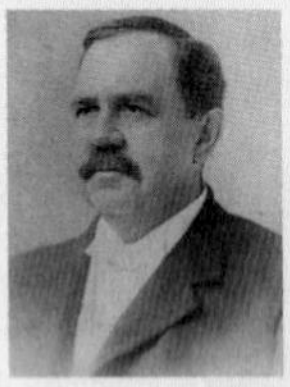

Wilbur Olin Atwater (1844–1907). Published the chemical composition of 2600 American foods (1896) still used in modern databases of food consumption; performed human calorimetric studies. Confirmed that the Law of Conservation of Energy governs transformation of matter in the human body and inanimate world.

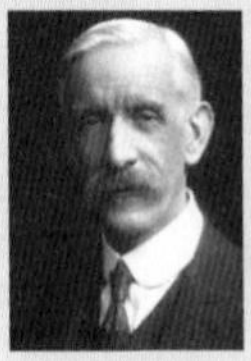

Frederick Gowland Hopkins (1861–1947). Isolated and identified the structure of the amino acid tryptophan (1929 Nobel Prize in Medicine or Physiology).

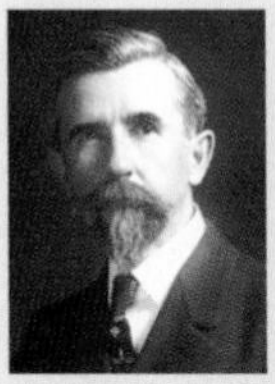

Russel Henry Chittenden (1856–1943). Refocused scientific attention on man's minimal protein requirement while resting or exercising (no debilitation occurred from protein intake less than 1 g · kg^{-1} body mass in either normal and athletic young men (*Physiological Economy In Nutrition, With Special Reference To The Minimal Proteid Requirement Of The Healthy Man. An Experimental Study,* 1897).

1835 **1850** **1860**

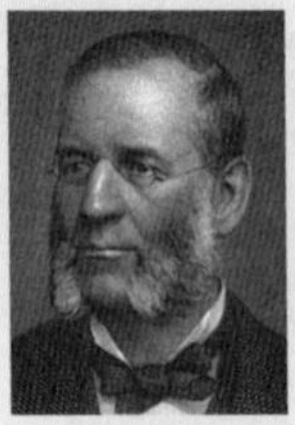

Austin Flint, Jr. (1836–1915). Prolific author and physiology researcher who chronicled topics of importance to the emerging science of exercise physiology and future science of exercise nutrition. His 987-page compendium of five prior textbooks (*The Physiology of Man; Designed to Represent the Existing State of Physiological Science as Applied to the Functions of the Human Body,* 1877) summarized knowledge about exercise, circulation, respiration, and nutrition from French, German, English, and American literature.

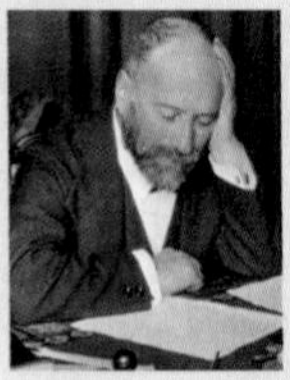

Nathan Zuntz (1847–1920). Devised first portable metabolic apparatus to assess respiratory exchange in animals and humans at different altitudes. Proved that carbohydrates are precursors of lipid synthesis, and that lipids and carbohydrates should not be consumed equally. Zuntz produced 430 articles concerning blood and blood gases, circulation, mechanics and chemistry of respiration, general metabolism and metabolism of specific foods, energy metabolism and heat production, and digestion.

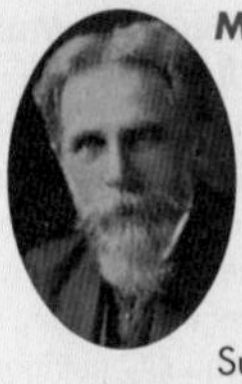

Max Rubner (1854–1932). Discovered the Isodynamic Law and the calorific heat values of foods (4.1 kcal · g^{-1} for protein and carbohydrates, 9.3 kcal · g^{-1} for lipids). Rubner's Surface Area Law states that resting heat production is proportional to body surface area, and that consuming food increases heat production (SDA effect).

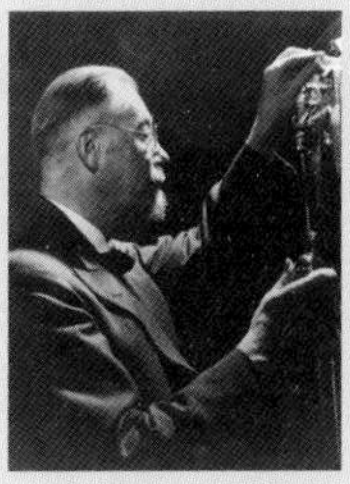

August Krogh (1874–1949). 1920 Nobel Prize in Physiology or Medicine for discovering the mechanism that controls capillary blood flow in resting and active muscle (in frogs). Krogh's 300 published scientific articles link exercise physiology with nutrition and metabolism.

1870 **1900**

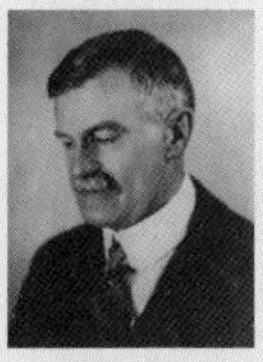

Francis Gano Benedict (1870–1957). Conducted exhaustive studies of energy metabolism in newborn infants, growing children and adolescents, starving people, athletes, and vegetarians. Devised "metabolic standard tables" on sex, age, height, and weight to compare energy metabolism in normals and patients.

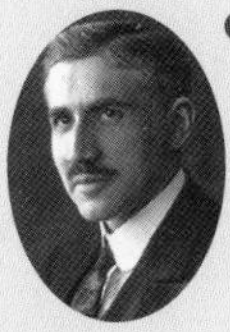

Otto Fritz Meyerhof (1884–1951). 1923 Nobel Prize in Physiology or Medicine with A.V. Hill for elucidating the cyclic characteristics of intermediary cellular energy transformation.

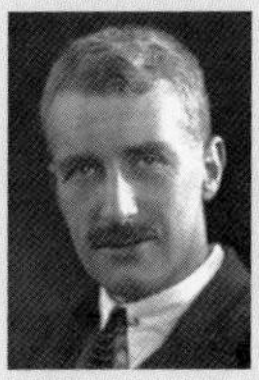

Archibald Vivian (A.V.) Hill (1886–1977). 1922 Nobel Prize in Physiology or Medicine with Meyerhof for discoveries about the chemical and mechanical events in muscle contraction.

Food Nutrients: Structure, Function, and Digestion, Absorption, and Assimilation

PART 1

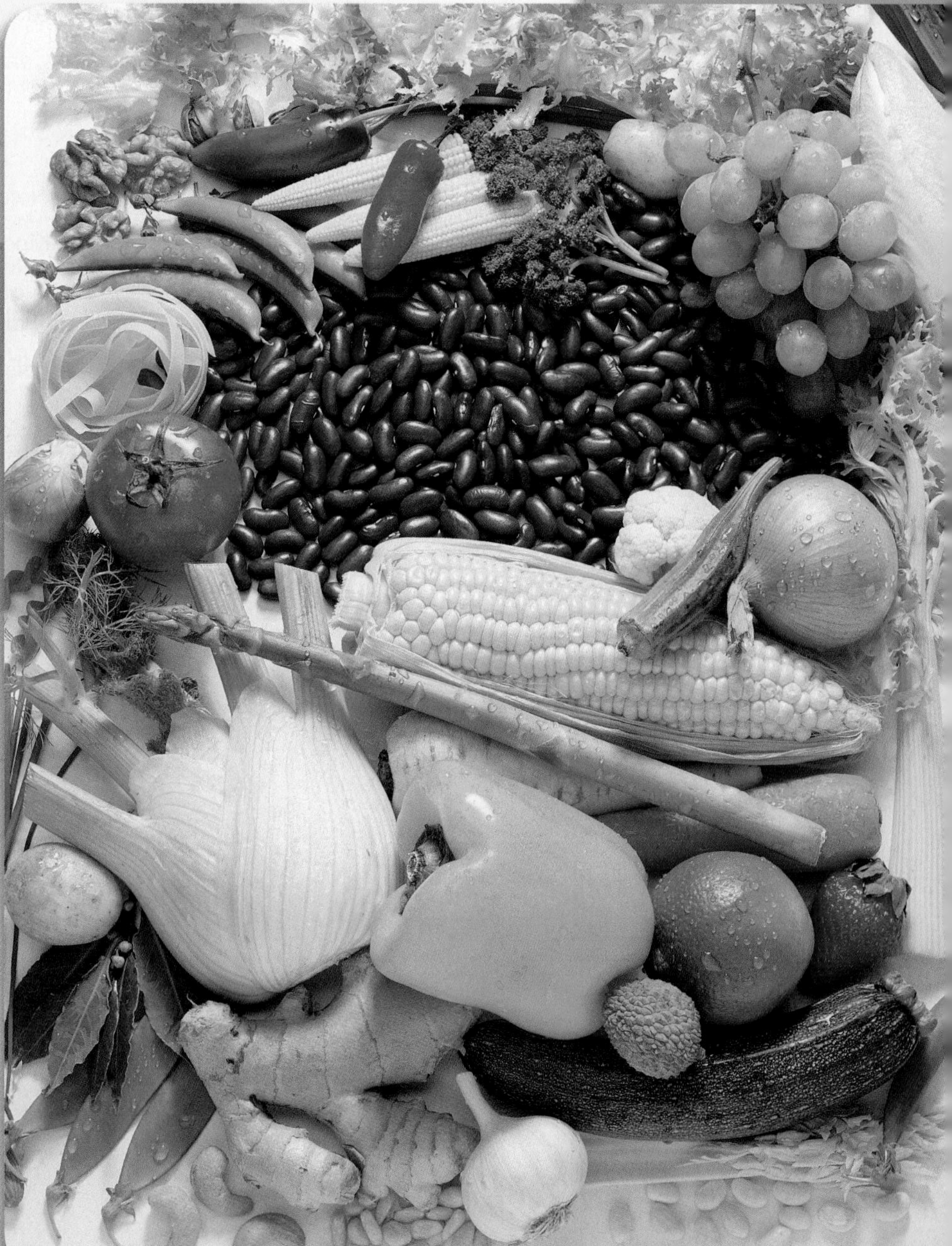

CONTENTS

CHAPTER 1

The Macronutrients

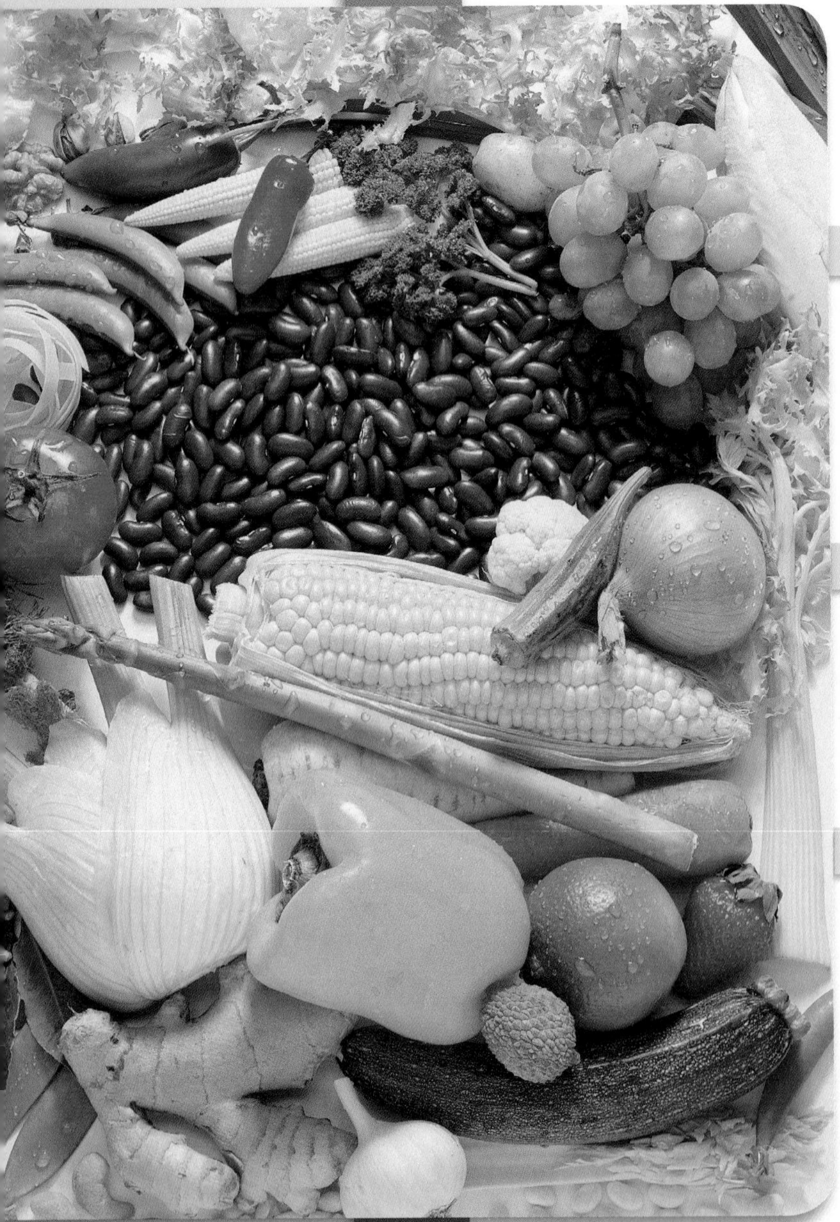

OUTLINE

- Atoms: Nature's Building Blocks
- Carbon: The Versatile Element

Carbohydrates

- Nature of Carbohydrates
- Kinds and Sources of Carbohydrates
- Recommended Dietary Carbohydrate Intake
- Role of Carbohydrate in the Body

Lipids

- Nature of Lipids
- Kinds and Sources of Lipids
- Recommended Dietary Lipid Intake
- Role of Lipid in the Body

Proteins

- Nature of Proteins
- Kinds of Proteins
- Recommended Dietary Protein Intake
- Role of Protein in the Body
- Dynamics of Protein Metabolism

TEST YOUR KNOWLEDGE

Select true or false for the 10 statements below, and then check out the answers at the end of the chapter. Retake the test after you've read the chapter; you should achieve 100%!	True	False
1. Carbohydrates consist of atoms of carbon, oxygen, nitrogen, and hydrogen.	❍	❍
2. Glucose can be synthesized from some amino acids in the body.	❍	❍
3. Dietary fiber's main function is to provide energy for biologic work.	❍	❍
4. Carbohydrate intake for physically active persons should make up about 40% of the total caloric intake.	❍	❍
5. Persons who consume simple carbohydrates run little risk of gaining weight.	❍	❍
6. A given quantity of carbohydrate, lipid, and protein contains about the same amount of energy.	❍	❍
7. Although cholesterol is found predominantly in the animal kingdom, certain plant forms also contain this derived lipid.	❍	❍
8. Vegans are at greater risk for nutrient and energy malnutrition than are persons who consume foods from both plant and animal sources.	❍	❍
9. As a general rule, consuming an extra amount of high-quality protein above recommended levels facilitates increases in muscle mass.	❍	❍
10. Because a male generally has a smaller percentage of body fat than a female counterpart, the protein requirement (per kilogram of body mass) for men is greater than for women.	❍	❍

The carbohydrate, lipid, and protein nutrients ultimately provide energy to maintain body functions during rest and all forms of physical activity. In addition to their role as biologic fuels, these large nutrients called **macronutrients** also maintain the organism's structural and functional integrity. This chapter focuses on each macronutrient's structure, function, and source in the diet.

ATOMS: NATURE'S BUILDING BLOCKS

Of the 103 different atoms or elements identified in nature, the mass of the human organism contains about 3% nitrogen, 10% hydrogen, 18% carbon, and 65% oxygen. These atoms play the major role in chemical composition of nutrients and make up structural units for the body's biologically active substances.

The union of two or more atoms forms a molecule whose particular properties depend on its specific atoms and their arrangement. Glucose is glucose because of the arrangement of three different kinds of 24 atoms within its molecule. Chemical bonding involves a common sharing of electrons between atoms, as occurs when hydrogen and oxygen atoms join to form a water molecule. The force of attraction between positive and negative charges serves as bonding, or "chemical cement," to keep the atoms within a molecule together. A larger aggregate of matter (a substance) forms when two or more molecules bind chemically. The substance can take the form of a gas, liquid, or solid, depending on forces of interaction among molecules. Altering forces by removing, transferring, or exchanging electrons releases energy, some of which powers cellular functions.

CARBON: THE VERSATILE ELEMENT

All nutrients contain carbon except water and minerals. Almost all substances within the body consist of carbon-containing (**organic**) compounds. Carbon atoms share chemical bonds with other carbon atoms and with atoms of other elements to form large carbon-chain molecules. Specific linkages of carbon, hydrogen, and oxygen atoms form lipids and carbohydrates, while addition of nitrogen and certain minerals creates a protein molecule. Carbon atoms linked with hydrogen, oxygen, and nitrogen also serve as atomic building blocks for the body's exquisitely formed structures.

CARBOHYDRATES

NATURE OF CARBOHYDRATES

All living cells contain carbohydrates, a class of organic molecules that includes monosaccharides, disaccharides, and polysaccharides. Except for lactose and a small amount of glycogen from animals, plants provide the major source of carbohydrate in the human diet. As the name suggests, carbohydrates contain carbon and water. Combining atoms of carbon, hydrogen, and oxygen forms a carbohydrate (sugar) molecule with the general formula $(CH_2O)n$, where *n* equals three to seven carbon atoms, with single bonds attaching to hydrogen and oxygen. Carbohydrates with five and six atoms interest nutritionists the most.

FIGURE 1.1 displays the chemical structure of **glucose**, the most typical sugar, along with other carbohydrates synthesized by plants during photosynthesis. Glucose contains six carbon, 12 hydrogen, and six oxygen atoms, having the chemical formula $C_6H_{12}O_6$. Each carbon atom has four bonding sites that link to other atoms, including carbons. Carbon bonds not linked to other carbon atoms remain "free" to accept hydrogen (with only one bond site), oxygen (with two bond sites), or an oxygen–hydrogen combination (OH), termed a hydroxyl. **Fructose** and **galactose**, two other simple sugars, have the same chemical formula as glucose, but with a slightly different carbon-to-hydrogen-to-oxygen linkage. This makes fructose, galactose, and glucose uniquely different in function, each with its own distinctive biochemical characteristics.

KINDS AND SOURCES OF CARBOHYDRATES

Four categories of carbohydrates include **monosaccharides, disaccharides, oligosaccharides,** and **polysaccharides**. The number of simple sugars linked within the molecule distinguishes each carbohydrate type.

Monosaccharides

The monosaccharide molecule represents the basic unit of carbohydrates. More than 200 monosaccharides exist in nature. The number of carbon atoms in their ringed structure determines the category. The Greek word for this number, ending with "ose," indicates they represent sugars. For example, three-carbon monosaccharides are trioses, four-carbon sugars are tetroses, five-carbon sugars are pentoses, six-carbon sugars are hexoses, and seven-carbon sugars are heptoses. The hexose sugars glucose, fructose, and galactose make up the nutritionally important monosaccharides. Glucose, also called dextrose or blood sugar, occurs naturally in food.

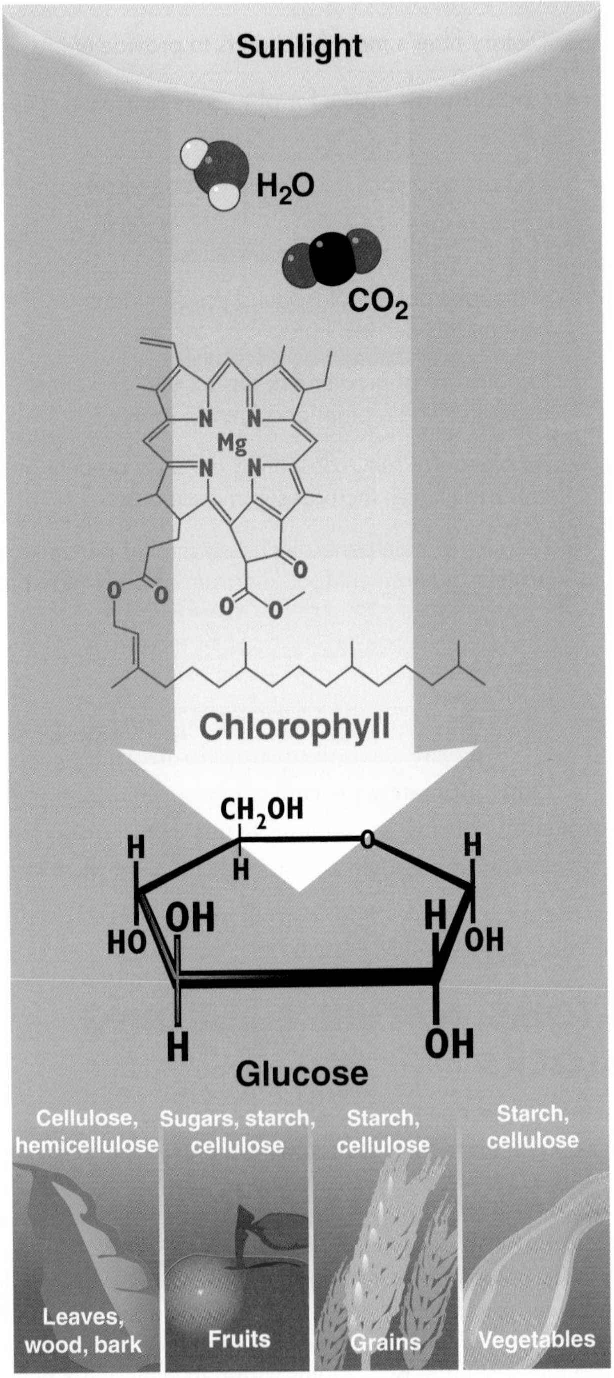

FIGURE 1.1. Three-dimensional ring structure of the simple sugar molecule glucose, formed during photosynthesis when the energy from sunlight interacts with water, carbon dioxide, and the green pigment chlorophyll. The molecule resembles a hexagonal plate to which H and O atoms attach. About 75% of the plant's dry matter consists of carbohydrate.

The digestion of more complex carbohydrates also produces glucose. Furthermore, animals produce glucose by **gluconeogenesis**, synthesizing it (primarily in the liver) from carbon skeletons of specific amino acids and from glycerol, pyruvate, and lactate. The small intestine absorbs glucose, where it then can serve one of three functions:

1. Used directly by cells for energy
2. Stored as glycogen in muscles and liver for later use
3. Converted to fat and stored for energy

Fructose (also called levulose or fruit sugar), the sweetest of the simple sugars, occurs in large amounts in fruits and honey. It accounts for about 9% of the average energy intake in the United States. The small intestine absorbs fructose directly into the blood, and the liver slowly converts it to glucose. Galactose does not occur freely in nature; rather, it forms milk sugar (lactose) in the mammary glands of lactating animals. In the body, galactose converts to glucose for energy metabolism.

Disaccharides and Oligosaccharides

Combining two monosaccharide molecules forms a disaccharide or double sugar. The monosaccharides and disaccharides are collectively called sugars or **simple sugars**.

Each disaccharide includes glucose as a principle component. The three disaccharides of nutritional significance include

1. **Sucrose:** The most common dietary disaccharide; consists of equal parts of glucose and fructose. Sucrose constitutes up to 25% of the total caloric intake in the United States Sucrose occurs naturally in most foods that contain carbohydrates, particularly in beet and cane sugar, brown sugar, sorghum, maple syrup, and honey. Honey, sweeter than table sugar because of its greater fructose content, offers no advantage nutritionally or as an energy source.
2. **Lactose:** Found in natural form only in milk (called milk sugar); consists of glucose plus galactose. The least sweet of the disaccharides, lactose can be artificially processed and is often present in carbohydrate-rich, high-calorie liquid meals. A substantial segment of the world's population is lactose intolerant; these persons lack adequate quantities of the enzyme lactase that splits lactose into glucose and galactose during digestion.
3. **Maltose:** Composed of two glucose molecules; occurs in beer, cereals, and germinating seeds. Also called malt sugar, maltose makes only a small contribution to the carbohydrate content of a person's diet.

Oligosaccharides (*oligo* in Greek, meaning a few) form from combining three to nine monosaccharide residues. The main dietary sources for the oligosaccharides are vegetables, particularly seed legumes (a category that includes peas, beans, and lentils).

Sugar by Any Other Name

Many different terms refer to monosaccharides and disaccharides or to products containing these simple sugars. The box titled "Terms That Denote Sugar" gives names for sugars present either naturally in food products or added during their manufacture. Food labels (see Chapter 9) place all these simple carbohydrates into one category, "sugars."

Sugars Give Flavor and Sweetness to Foods

Receptors in the tongue recognize diverse sugars and even some noncarbohydrate substances. Sugars vary in sweetness

HIGH-FRUCTOSE CORN SYRUP: A NUTRITIONAL HAZARD?

High-fructose corn syrup (HFCS)—also called *glucose-fructose syrup* in the United Kingdom, *glucose/fructose* in Canada, and *high-fructose maize syrup* in other countries—comprises a group of corn syrups that undergo enzymatic processing to convert some of their glucose into fructose for a desired level of sweetness. HFCS is produced by milling corn to produce corn starch, processing that starch to yield corn syrup, which is almost entirely glucose, and then adding enzymes that change some of the glucose into fructose. The most widely used variety of HFCS in the United States is *HFCS 55* (mostly used in soft drinks), which is composed of about 55% fructose and 42% glucose.

Since the introduction of HFCS as a sweetener in the 1970s, concern has been raised about its role in obesity, insulin resistance (type 2 diabetes), and nonalcoholic fatty liver disease. Although HFCS resembles the chemical composition of table sugar (sucrose), the glucose and fructose components in HFCS exist in free solution, whereas in sucrose they are bound together. Consequently, HFCS provides a high glycemic overload without augmenting a corresponding increased insulin response. This is important because without an insulin response after consumption of a high-fructose food, there is no suppression of appetite, which normally induces insulin secretion after a meal. The lack of satiety or suppression of appetite is thought to result in increased food consumption and possible glucose dysregulation. Although many studies link HFCS consumption and obesity, few studies exist to show that higher intakes actually *cause* a body weight increase.

Cummings BP, et al. Dietary fructose accelerates the development of diabetes in UCD-T2DM rats: amelioration by the antioxidant, alpha-lipoic acid. *Am J Physiol Regul Integr Comp Physiol* 2010;298:R1343.

Ngo Sock ET, et al. Effects of a short-term overfeeding with fructose or glucose in healthy young males. *Br J Nutr* 2010;103:939.

Stanhope KL, Havel PJ. Fructose consumption: recent results and their potential implications. *Ann N Y Acad Sci* 2010;1190:15.

Tappy L, Lê KA. Metabolic effects of fructose and the worldwide increase in obesity. *Physiol Rev* 2010;90:23.

Tappy L, et al. Fructose and metabolic diseases: new findings, new questions. *Nutrition* 2010;26:1044.

TERMS THAT DENOTE SUGAR

Sugar	Corn syrup
Sucrose	Natural sweeteners
Brown sugar	High-fructose corn syrup
Confectioner's sugar (powdered sugar)	Date sugar
Turbinado sugar	Molasses
Invert sugar	Maple sugar
Glucose	Dextrin
Sorbitol	Dextrose
Levulose	Fructose
Polydextrose	Maltose
Lactose	Caramel
Mannitol	Fruit sugar
Honey	

on a per gram basis. For example, fructose is almost twice as sweet as sucrose under either acid or cold conditions; sucrose is 30% sweeter than glucose, and lactose is less than half as sweet as sucrose. Sugars are routinely added to many foods to increase sweetness and thus enhance the eating experience.

Polysaccharides

The term *polysaccharide* refers to the linkage of 10 to thousands of monosaccharide residues by **glycosidic bonds**. Polysaccharides classify into plant and animal categories. Cells that store carbohydrate for energy link simple sugar molecules into the more complex polysaccharide form. This reduces the osmotic effect within the cell that would result from storage of an equal energy value of a larger number of simple sugar molecules.

Plant Polysaccharides

Starch and **fiber** represent the two common forms of plant polysaccharides.

STARCH: Starch serves as the storage form of carbohydrate in plants and represents the most familiar form of plant polysaccharide. Starch appears as large granules in the cell's cytoplasm and is plentiful in seeds, corn, and various grains that make bread, cereal, spaghetti, and pastries. Large amounts also exist in peas, beans, potatoes, and roots, where starch serves as an energy store for the plant's future use. Plant starch remains an important source of carbohydrate in the American diet, accounting for approximately 50% of the total carbohydrate intake. Daily starch intake, however, has decreased about 30% since the turn of the 20th century, whereas simple sugar consumption correspondingly has increased from 30 to about 50% of total carbohydrate intake. The term **complex carbohydrate** commonly refers to dietary starch.

The Starch Form Makes a Difference Starch exists in two forms: **amylose**, a long, straight chain of glucose units twisted into a helical coil, and **amylopectin**, a highly branched monosaccharide linkage (**FIG. 1.2**). The relative proportion of each starch form determines the specific characteristics of the starch in a particular plant species. For example, the predominance of one form or the other determines the "digestibility" of a food containing starch. The branching of the amylopectin polymer exposes greater surface area to digestive enzymes than starches whose glucose units link in a straight chain. Chapters 7 and 8 discuss more about the importance of the

Connections to the Past

Frederick Gowland Hopkins (1861–1947)

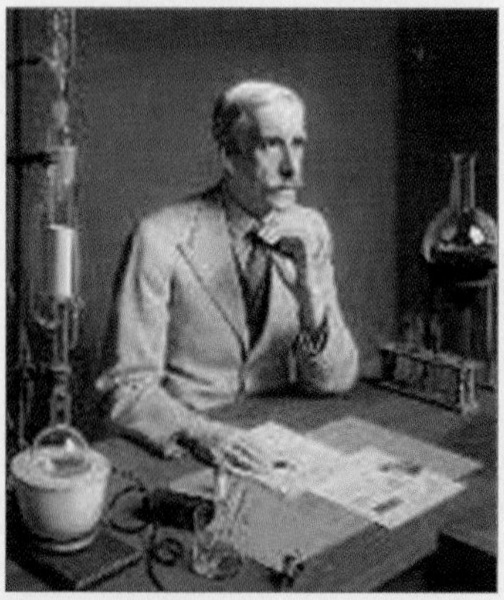

Hopkins did not rise to prominence in the early 20th century by following normal academic channels. He had many interests including invertebrates. At age 17, when he finally left school, he published a paper in *The Entomologist* on the bombardier beetle. Soon after, he began work for an insurance company and then a railroad, and he eventually enrolled in the Royal School of Mines and assisted in a private chemistry laboratory. Hopkins qualified for membership in the Institute of Chemistry by attending lectures at London's University College. Hopkins both produced pioneering studies in nutritional biochemistry and collaborated with physiologist Walter Morley Fletcher (mentor to A.V. Hill) to study muscle chemistry. Their classic 1907 paper in experimental physiology employed new methods to isolate lactic acid in muscle. Prior studies of stimulated muscle showed large concentrations of lactic acid in both stimulated and nonexercised muscle. Fletcher and Hopkins' chemical methods reduced the muscle's enzyme activity prior to analysis to isolate the reactions. They found that a muscle contracting under low oxygen conditions produced lactic acid at the expense of glycogen.

thePoint *Visit* **thePoint.lww.com/MKKSEN4e** *to find more details about how this Nobel Prize recipient pioneered studies in nutritional biochemistry and experimental physiology.*

different carbohydrate forms in feedings before, during, and after strenuous exercise.

Fiber: The Unheralded "Nutrient": Fiber, classified as a nonstarch, structural polysaccharide, includes cellulose, the most abundant organic molecule on earth. Fibrous materials, which contain no nutrients or available calories, resist hydrolysis by human digestive enzymes, although a portion ferments by action of intestinal bacteria and ultimately participates in metabolic reactions following intestinal absorption. *Fibers exist exclusively in plants; they make up the structure of leaves, stems, roots, seeds, and fruit coverings.* Fibers differ widely in physical and chemical characteristics and physiologic action. They are located mostly within the cell wall as cellulose, gums (substances dissolved or dispersed in water that give a gelling or thickening effect), hemicellulose (sugar units containing five or six carbons; insoluble in water but soluble in alkali), pectin (forms gels with sugar and acid and imparts a crispy texture to freshly picked apples), and the noncarbohydrate lignins

DIFFERING STRUCTURE AFFECTS DIGESTION RATE

Starches with a relatively large amount of amylopectin digest and absorb rapidly, whereas starches with high amylose content have a slower rate of chemical breakdown (hydrolysis).

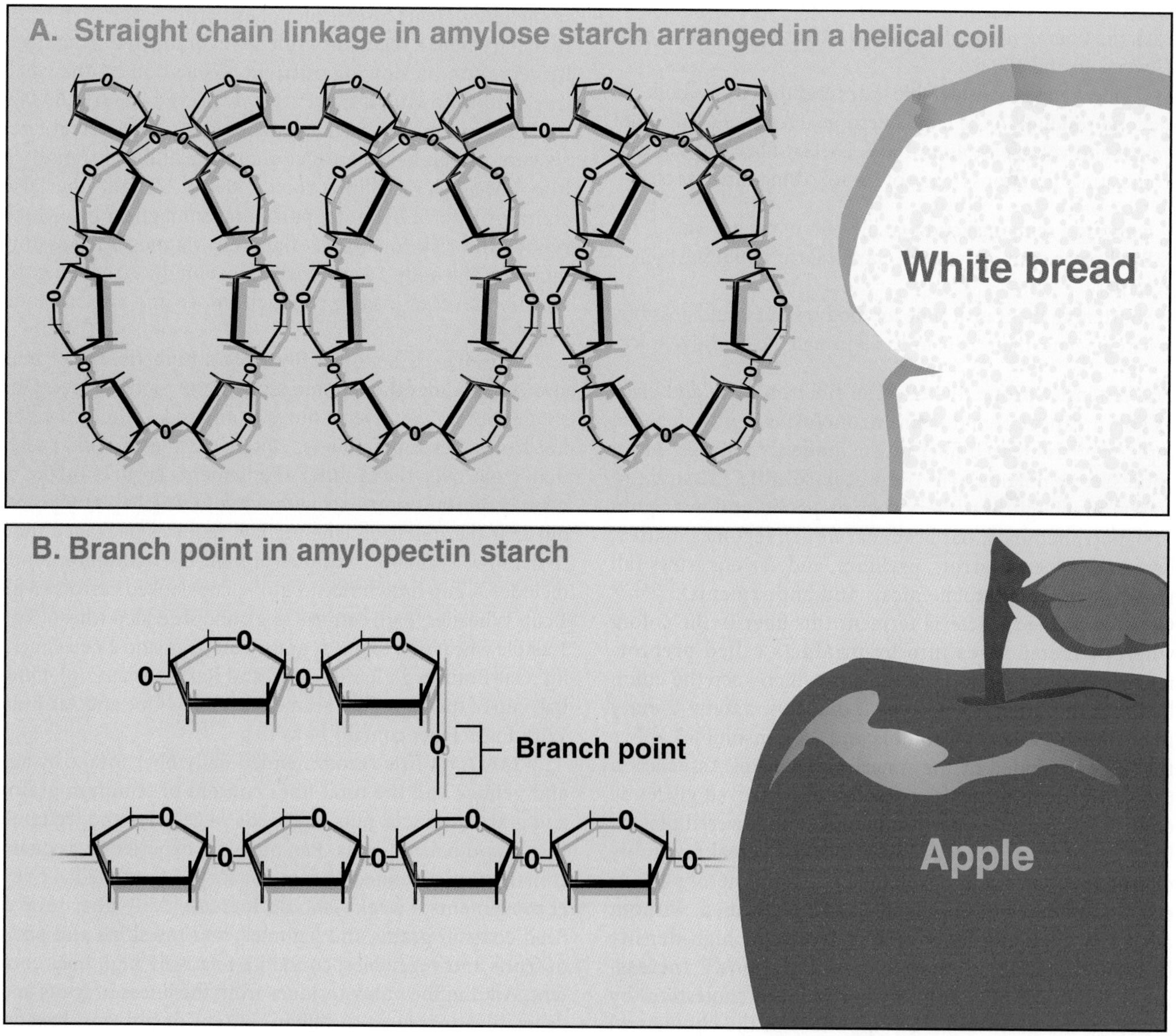

FIGURE 1.2. The two forms of plant starch. **A.** Straight-chain linkage with unbranched bonding of glucose residues (glycosidic linkages) in amylose starch. **B.** Branch point in the highly branched amylopectin starch molecule. The amylopectin structure appears linear, but in reality it exists as a helical coil.

that give rigidity to plant cell walls (increase in content with plant maturity).

Health Implications Dietary fiber has received considerable attention by researchers and the lay press, largely from epidemiologic studies linking high fiber intake (particularly whole grains and beans) with lower occurrence of obesity, insulin resistance, systemic inflammation, the metabolic syndrome, type 2 diabetes, hyperlipidemia, hypertension, intestinal disorders (from constipation to irritable bowel syndrome), heart disease, and overall risk of dying.[22,36,42,55,59,72] The Western diet, high in fiber-free animal foods and low in natural plant fiber lost through processing (refining), contributes to more intestinal disorders in industrialized countries compared with countries that consume a more primitive-type diet high in unrefined, complex carbohydrates. For example, the typical American diet contains a daily fiber intake of about 12 to 15 g. In contrast, the fiber content of diets from Africa and India ranges between 40 and 150 $g \cdot day^{-1}$.

Fiber retains considerable water and thus gives "bulk" to the food residues in the large intestine, often increasing stool weight and volume by 40 to 100%. Dietary fiber may aid gastrointestinal functions in one of the following three ways:

1. Exerting a scraping action on the cells of the gut wall
2. Binding or diluting harmful chemicals or inhibiting their activity
3. Shortening the transit time for food residues (and possibly carcinogenic materials) to pass through the digestive tract

The potential protective effect of fiber on rates and risks of colon cancer remains an inconclusive, hotly debated topic.[9,27,42] Increased fiber intake modestly reduces serum cholesterol, particularly the **water-soluble** (dissolve in water) mucilaginous fibers such as pectin and guar gum in oats (rolled oats, oat bran, oat flour), legumes, barley, brown rice, peas, carrots, psyllium, and various fruits (all rich in diverse phytochemicals and antioxidants).[23,41,92] Once consumed, bacteria ferment this fiber in the colon, where it metabolizes into by-products called prebiotics that feed the bacteria in the gut, which keep the colon healthy. In patients with type 2 diabetes, a daily dietary fiber intake (50 g; 25 g soluble and 25 g insoluble) above that recommended by the American Diabetes Association (24 g; 8 g soluble and 16 g insoluble) improved glycemic control, decreased hyperinsulinemia, and lowered plasma lipid concentrations.[15] A high-fiber oat cereal favorably altered low-density lipoprotein (LDL) cholesterol particle size and number in middle-aged and older men, without adversely changing blood triacylglycerol or high-density lipoprotein (HDL) cholesterol concentrations.[19] Increasing daily intake of guar gum fiber reduced cholesterol by lowering the harmful LDL component of the cholesterol profile.[10,23] In contrast, the **water-insoluble** fibers—the fiber contained in whole-wheat–containing products, cabbage, beets, cauliflower, turnips, and apple skin, which absorb large amounts of water—of cellulose, hemicellulose, lignin, and cellulose-rich wheat bran failed to lower cholesterol.[11] Manufacturers of oatmeal and other oat-based cereals can now claim that their products may reduce heart disease risk, provided the health claim advises one to also eat "diet(s) low in saturated fat and cholesterol."

How dietary fibers favorably affect serum cholesterol remains unknown, although multiple mechanisms likely operate (**FIG. 1.3A**). Perhaps persons who consume the most dietary fiber also lead more healthy overall lifestyles that include engaging in more physical activity, smoking fewer cigarettes, and eating a more nutritious diet. Adding fiber to the diet also replaces cholesterol- and saturated fat-laden food choices. In addition, water-soluble fibers may hinder cholesterol absorption or reduce cholesterol metabolism in the gut. These actions would limit hepatic lipogenesis (less glucose as a substrate and less insulin as an activator) while facilitating excretion of existing cholesterol bound to fiber in the feces. Heart disease and obesity protection may relate to dietary fiber's regulatory role in favorably reducing insulin secretion by slowing nutrient absorption by the small intestine following a meal (**FIG. 1.3B**). For nearly 69,000 middle-aged nurses, each 5-g daily increase in cereal fiber (½ cup of bran flake cereal contains 4 g of fiber) translated into a 37% decrease in coronary risk.[93] Dietary fiber also contains micronutrients, particularly magnesium, which reduce the risk for type 2 diabetes. Magnesium possibly increases the body's sensitivity to insulin, thus reducing the required level of insulin production per unit rise in blood sugar.

The overall health benefits of a high-fiber diet may also come from other components in the food sources. One should obtain the diverse fibers from food in the daily diet, not from fiber supplements. Obtaining fiber in food rather than from over-the-counter supplements ensures intake of other important nutrients within the food. Chapter 9 points out that the nutrition labeling law requires packaged food to list fiber content. Examples of high-fiber common foods include $^2/_3$ cup brown rice (3 g); $^1/_2$ cup cooked carrots (3 g); 1 cup Wheaties (3 g), oatmeal (4 g), and shredded wheat (5 g); 1 whole wheat pita (5 g); $^1/_2$ grapefruit (6 g); and 1 cup Cracklin' Oat Bran (6 g), lentils (7 g), and Raisin Bran (7 g). One-half cup of the high-fiber bran cereals Fiber One and All-Bran With Extra Fiber contain 14 to 15 g.

TABLE 1.1 lists recommended daily fiber intake by age and gender and the total fiber content of common grains and grain products, nuts and seeds, vegetables and legumes, fruits, and baked goods. Persons who experience frequent constipation—defined as three or fewer spontaneous bowel movements a week—should increase daily fiber intake. Seed coats of grains and legumes, and the skins and peels of fruits and vegetables, contain a relatively high fiber content. Adding the pulpy residues from the juices of fruits and vegetables increases the fiber content of biscuits, breads, and other homemade dishes. As a general guideline, recommended fiber intake is 14 g daily per 1000 kcal consumed, which translates to 25 $g \cdot day^{-1}$ for women and 38 g for men.

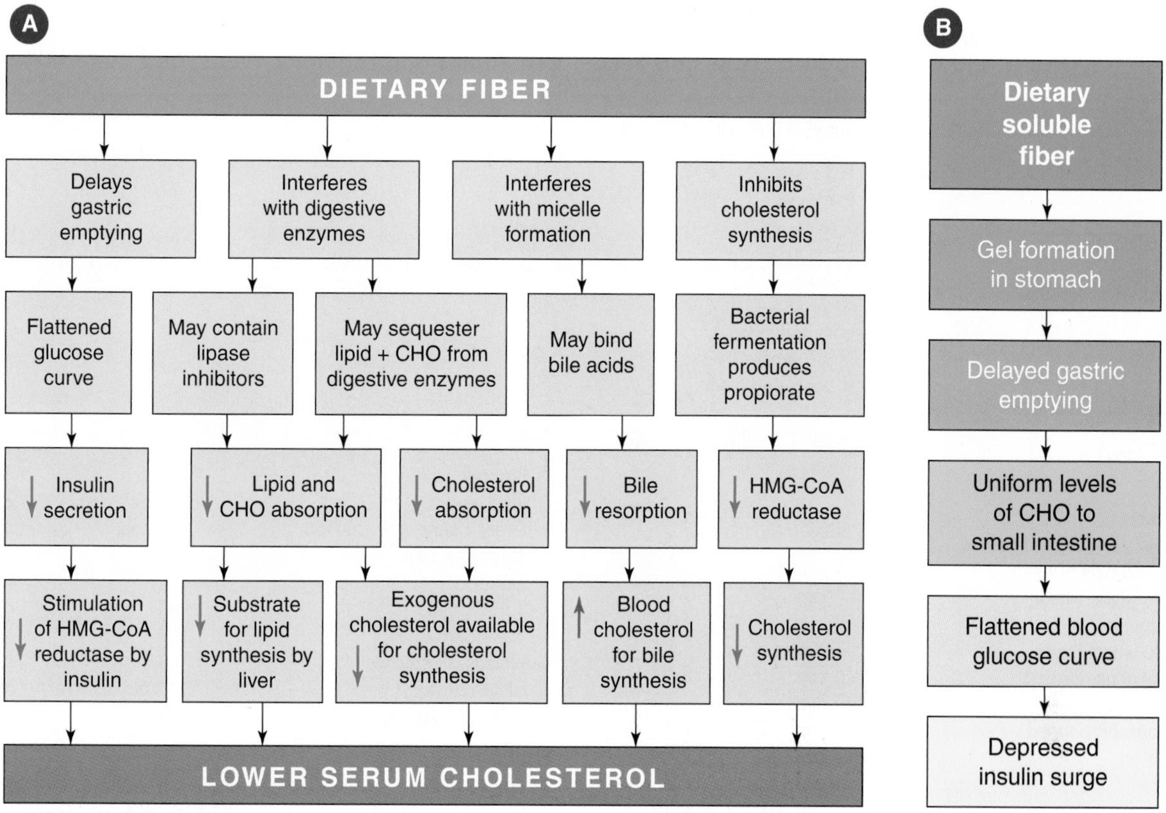

FIGURE 1.3. A. Possible mechanism by which dietary fiber lowers blood cholesterol. (*CHO,* carbohydrate; *HMG-CoA reductase,* hydroxy-3-methylglutaryl–coenzyme A reductase). **B.** Possible mechanisms by which dietary soluble fiber lowers blood glucose. (Modified from McIntosh M, Miller C. A diet containing food rich in soluble and insoluble fiber improves glycemic control and reduces hyperlipidemia among patients with type 2 diabetes. *Nutr Rev* 2001;59:52.)

FIGURE 1.4 shows a sample daily 2200-kcal menu that includes 31 g of fiber (21 g of insoluble fiber). In this meal, lipid calories account for 30% (saturated fat, 10%), protein 16%, and carbohydrate 54% of total caloric intake. Each 10-g increase in a subpar diet's fiber content reduces coronary risk by about 20%. Five daily servings of fruits and vegetables combined with 6 to 11 servings of grains (particularly whole grains) ensures dietary fiber intake at recommended levels. (See Chapter 7 concerning actual serving size, which is smaller than the typical portion size eaten by Americans.) Whole grains provide a nutritional advantage over refined grains because they contain more fiber, vitamins, minerals, and diverse phytochemicals, all of which favorably affect health status. Excessive fiber intake (particularly high-fiber foods with seed coats and thus large amounts of phytates) is ill advised for persons with marginal levels of nutrition; these compounds generally blunt intestinal absorption of the major minerals calcium and phosphorus and some trace minerals, including iron.

Animal Polysaccharides

Glycogen, the storage polysaccharide found in mammalian muscle and liver, consists of an irregularly shaped, branched polysaccharide polymer similar to amylopectin in plant starch. This macromolecule, synthesized from glucose during **glucogenesis**, ranges from a few hundred to thousands of glucose molecules linked together like a chain of sausages, with some branch points for additional glucose linkage. **FIGURE 1.5** shows that glycogen synthesis occurs by adding individual glucose units to an already existing glycogen polymer.

FIGURE 1.6 illustrates that a typical 80-kg person stores approximately 500 g of carbohydrate. Of this, the largest reserve (approximately 400 g) exists as muscle glycogen, 90 to 110 g as liver glycogen (highest concentration that represents 3 to 7% of the liver's weight), and only about 2 to 3 g as blood glucose. Because each gram of either glycogen or glucose contains about 4 kcal of energy, the typical person stores between 1500 and 2000 kcal of carbohydrate energy—enough total energy to power a high-intensity 20-mile run.

Glycogen Dynamics: Several factors determine the rate and quantity of glycogen breakdown and subsequent synthesis. Muscle glycogen serves as the *major source* of carbohydrate energy for active muscles during exercise. In contrast to muscle glycogen, liver glycogen reconverts to glucose (controlled by a specific **phosphatase enzyme**) for transport in the blood to the working muscles. **Glycogenolysis** describes this reconversion process; it provides a rapid extramuscular

TABLE 1.1 Recommended Daily Fiber Intake by Age and Gender and Sources of Total Fiber (g)[a] in Common Grains and Grain Products, Nuts and Seeds, Vegetables and Legumes, Fruits, and Baked Goods

Recommended Daily Fiber Intake (g)	
Children 1–3 years	19
Children 4–8 years	25
Boys 9–13 years	31
Boys 14–18 years	38
Girls 9–18 years	26
Men 19–50 years	38
Men 51 years and older	30
Women 19–50 years	25
Women 51 years and older	21

Food	Serving	Fiber/Serving
Grains		
Oat bran	1 cup	16.4
Refined white flour, bleached	1 cup	3.4
Spaghetti, whole wheat	1 cup	5.0
Penne, whole wheat	1 cup	10.0
Bran muffin	1	4.0
Whole-wheat flour	1 cup	15.1
Wheat germ, toasted	1 cup	15.6
Couscous	1 cup	8.7
Popcorn, air-popped	1 cup	1.3
Rice bran	1 oz	21.7
Millet	1 cup	17.0
Corn grits	1 cup	4.5
Barley, cooked, whole	1 cup	4.6
Bulgur wheat	1 cup	25.6
Rye flour–dark	1 cup	17.7
Wild rice	1 cup	4.0
All-Bran cereal	1/2 cup	8.5
Barley	1 cup	31.8
Oatmeal, cooked	1 cup	4.1
Grape Nuts	1 cup	10.0
Macaroni, cooked enriched	1 cup	2.2
Rice, white	1 oz	1.5
Almonds, dried	1 oz	3.5
Peanut butter	1 tbsp	1.0
Macadamia nuts, dried	1 oz	1.5
Low-fat granola	1 cup	4.5
Cheerios	1 cup	5.0
Nuts and seeds		
Pumpkin seeds, roasted, unsalted	1 oz	10.2
Chestnuts, roasted	1 oz	3.7
Peanuts, dried, unsalted	1 oz	3.5
Sunflower seeds, dry	1 oz	2.0
Walnuts, chopped, black	1 oz	1.6
Vegetables and legumes		
Pinto beans, dry, cooked	1 cup	19.5
Lima beans, fresh, cooked	1 cup	16.0
Black eyed peas, cooked from raw	1 cup	12.2
Mixed vegetables (corn, carrots, beans)	1 cup	7.2
Corn on cob	1	3.2
Broccoli, raw	1 cup	2.9
Black beans	1 oz	2.5
Green beans, raw, cooked	1 cup	2.5
Artichoke, raw	1 oz	2.3
Carrot	1	2.3
Baked potato	1	2.3
Tomato, raw	1	1.8
Onions, sliced, raw	1 cup	1.8
Lentils, stir fry	1 oz	1.1
Chili w/beans	1 oz	0.9
Fruits		
Avocado	1	22.9
Loganberries, fresh	1 cup	9.3
Pear, Bartlett	1	4.6
Figs	2	4.1
Blueberries	1 cup	3.9
Strawberries, fresh	1 cup	3.9
Apple, raw	1	3.5
Orange, navel	1	3.4
Grapefruit, sections, fresh	1	3.0
Banana	1	2.3
Pineapple, chunks	1 cup	2.3
Grapes, Thompson, seedless	1 cup	1.9
Peach, fresh	1	1.5
Plum, small	1	0.6
Baked goods		
Whole-wheat toast	Slice	2.3
Waffle, homemade	1	1.1
Pumpkin pie	Slice	5.4
Oatmeal bread	Slice	1.0
French bread	Slice	0.7
Danish pastry, plain	1	0.7
Fig bar cookie	1	0.6
Chocolate chip cookie, homemade	1	0.2
White bread	Slice	0.6
Pumpernickel bread	Slice	1.7
Rye bread	Slice	1.9
Seven-grain bread	Slice	1.7

Data from the United States Department of Agriculture.

[a] *The crude fiber content of foods reported in food composition tables (including the foods in the above table) refers to the organic portion of the dry, acid, and alkali-extracted residue from the ashing of the food after it is ground up, dried to a constant weight in a low-temperature oven, and had the fat removed with solvents. The fat-free food sample is then boiled in hot sulfuric acid, rinsed in hot water, and then boiled again in dilute sodium hydroxide to yield the food's crude fiber content.*

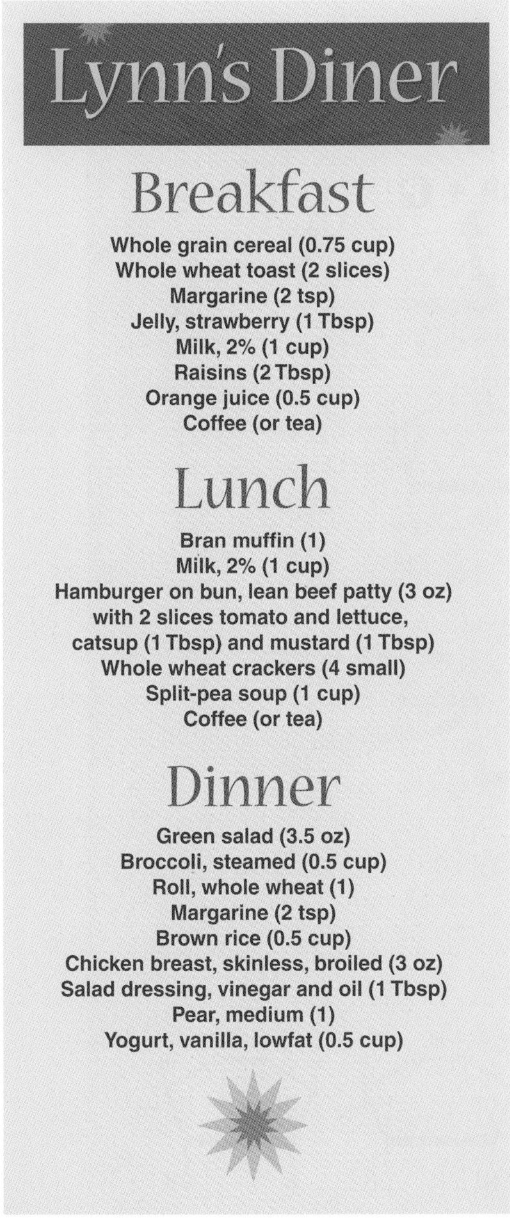

Lynn's Diner
Breakfast
Whole grain cereal (0.75 cup)
Whole wheat toast (2 slices)
Margarine (2 tsp)
Jelly, strawberry (1 Tbsp)
Milk, 2% (1 cup)
Raisins (2 Tbsp)
Orange juice (0.5 cup)
Coffee (or tea)
Lunch
Bran muffin (1)
Milk, 2% (1 cup)
Hamburger on bun, lean beef patty (3 oz)
with 2 slices tomato and lettuce,
catsup (1 Tbsp) and mustard (1 Tbsp)
Whole wheat crackers (4 small)
Split-pea soup (1 cup)
Coffee (or tea)
Dinner
Green salad (3.5 oz)
Broccoli, steamed (0.5 cup)
Roll, whole wheat (1)
Margarine (2 tsp)
Brown rice (0.5 cup)
Chicken breast, skinless, broiled (3 oz)
Salad dressing, vinegar and oil (1 Tbsp)
Pear, medium (1)
Yogurt, vanilla, lowfat (0.5 cup)

FIGURE 1.4. Sample menu for breakfast, lunch, and dinner (2200 kcal) containing 31 g of dietary fiber. The diet's total cholesterol content is less than 200 mg, and total calcium equals 1242 mg.

glucose supply. Depleting liver and muscle glycogen through either dietary restriction or intense exercise stimulates glucose synthesis from the structural components of other nutrients, principally amino acids, through gluconeogenic metabolic pathways.

Hormones control the level of circulating blood glucose and play an important role in regulating liver and muscle glycogen stores. Elevated blood glucose levels cause the beta cells of the pancreas to secrete additional **insulin**, forcing peripheral tissues to take up the excess glucose. This feedback mechanism inhibits further insulin secretion, which maintains blood glucose at an appropriate physiologic concentration. In contrast, when blood glucose falls below the normal range, the pancreas' alpha cells immediately secrete insulin's opposing hormone, **glucagon**, to normalize blood glucose levels. This "insulin antagonist" hormone stimulates liver glycogenolysis and gluconeogenesis to raise the blood glucose concentration.

The body stores comparatively little glycogen, so one's diet profoundly affects the amount available. For example, a 24-hour fast or a low-carbohydrate, normal-calorie (isocaloric) diet greatly reduces glycogen reserves. In contrast, maintaining a carbohydrate-rich isocaloric diet for several days enhances the body's carbohydrate stores to a level almost twice that of a normal, well-balanced diet.

IMPORTANT CARBOHYDRATE CONVERSIONS

Glucogenesis: glycogen synthesis from glucose (glucose → glycogen)

Gluconeogenesis: glucose synthesis largely from structural components of noncarbohydrate nutrients (protein → glucose)

Glycogenolysis: glucose formation from glycogen (glycogen → glucose)

LIMITED STORES OF AN IMPORTANT COMPOUND FOR EXERCISE

The body's upper limit for glycogen storage averages about 15 $g \cdot kg^{-1}$ of body mass, equivalent to 1050 g for an average-sized 70-kg man and 840 g for a typical 56-kg woman.

RECOMMENDED DIETARY CARBOHYDRATE INTAKE

FIGURE 1.7 *(top)* illustrates the carbohydrate content of selected foods. Rich carbohydrate sources include cereals, cookies, candies, breads, and cakes. Fruits and vegetables appear to be less valuable sources because carbohydrate percentage derives from the food's total weight, including water content. The dried portions of these foods, however, exist as almost pure carbohydrate. This makes them an ideal lightweight, "dehydrated" food source during hiking or long treks when one must transport the food supply during the activity. The bottom of the figure lists the amount of carbohydrate in various food categories.

On a worldwide basis, carbohydrates represent the most prevalent source of calories. In Africa, for example, nearly 80% of total caloric intake comes from carbohydrates, while

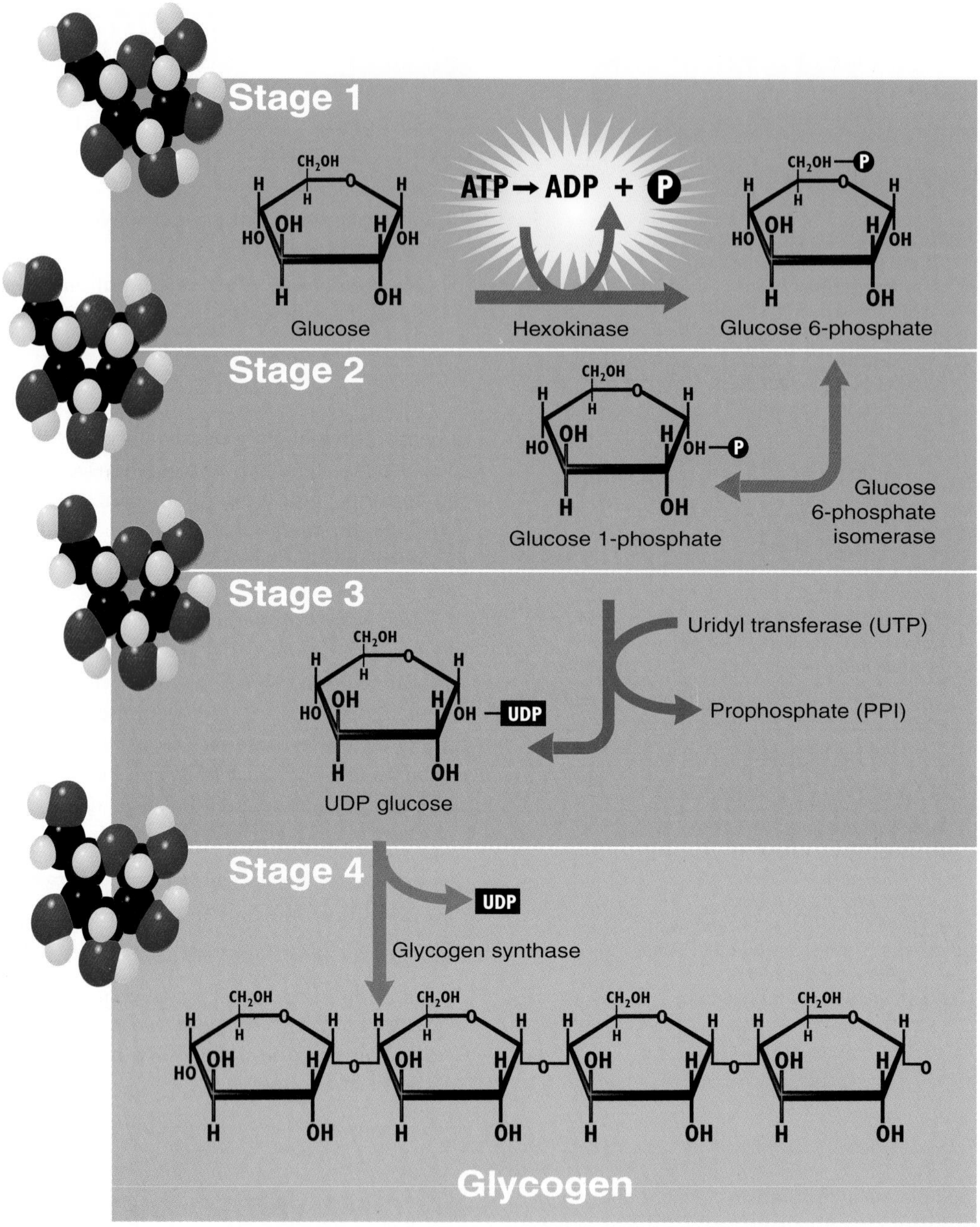

FIGURE 1.5. Glycogen synthesis is a four-step process. *Stage 1,* adenosine triphosphate (ATP) donates a phosphate to glucose to form glucose 6-phosphate. This reaction involves the enzyme hexokinase. *Stage 2,* Glucose 6-phosphate isomerizes to glucose 1-phosphate by the enzyme glucose 6-phosphate isomerase. *Stage 3,* The enzyme uridyl transferase reacts uridyl triphosphate (UTP) with glucose 1-phosphate to form uridine diphosphate (UDP)-glucose (a phosphate is released as UTP → UDP). *Stage 4,* UDP-glucose attaches to one end of an existing glycogen polymer chain. This forms a new bond (known as a glycoside bond) between the adjacent glucose units, with the concomitant release of UDP. For each glucose unit added, 2 moles of ATP convert to adenosine diphosphate (ADP) and phosphate.

in Caribbean countries the value reaches 65%. *Carbohydrates account for between 40 and 50% of the total calories in the typical American diet.* For a sedentary 70-kg person, this translates to a daily carbohydrate intake of about 300 g. For persons who engage in regular physical activity, carbohydrates should supply about 60% (400–600 g) of total daily calories, predominantly as unrefined, fiber-rich fruits, grains, and vegetables. This quantity replenishes, in a nutrient-rich package, the carbohydrate used to power the increased level of physical activity. During intense training, carbohydrate intake should increase to 70% of total calories consumed when in energy balance.[3]

Nutritious dietary carbohydrate sources consist of fruits, grains, and vegetables, but most persons do

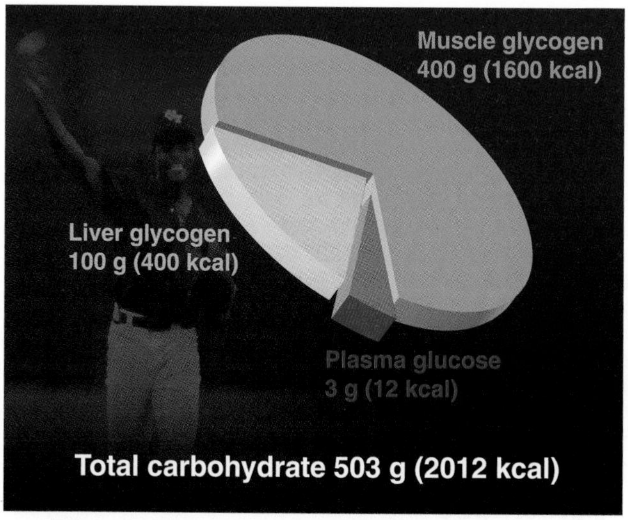

FIGURE 1.6. Distribution of carbohydrate energy for an average 80-kg man.

not consume these foods. In fact, the average American consumes about 50% of carbohydrates as simple sugars (70–100 lb of refined sugars each year), predominantly as table sugar, honey, HFCS, and all other sweeteners with calories. Most of this sugar comes in the form of sugary drinks (soft drinks and juices), candy, cakes, ice cream, and sugars in processed foods. One hundred years ago, the yearly intake of simple sugars averaged only 4 lb per person!

Consuming excessive fermentable carbohydrate (principally sucrose) *causes* tooth decay, but dietary sugar's contributing role to diabetes, obesity, gout, and coronary heart disease still remains an area of controversy (see next section). Substituting fructose for sucrose, a monosaccharide nearly 80% sweeter than table sugar, provides equal sweetness with fewer calories. More is said in Chapter 8 concerning pre-exercise fructose feedings.

Some Confusion Concerning Dietary Carbohydrates

Concern exists about the negative effects of the typical diet that imposes a high **glycemic load**—an index that incorporates both carbohydrate quantity and glycemic index (see Chapter 8)—on risk for obesity, type 2 diabetes, abnormal blood lipids, and coronary heart disease, particularly among sedentary persons.[51,58,77,78,85,86] Frequent and excessive consumption of more rapidly absorbed forms of carbohydrate (i.e., those with high glycemic index) may alter the metabolic profile and increase disease risk, particularly for persons with excess body fat. For example, eating a high-carbohydrate, low-fat meal reduces fat breakdown and increases fat synthesis more in overweight men than in lean men.[54] Women with an increased intake of carbohydrates with the highest glycemic load (rather than the overall quantity of carbohydrates consumed) were 2.24 times more likely to develop heart disease than women with the lowest glycemic load.[74] Dietary patterns of women followed over 6 years showed that those who consumed a high-glycemic starchy diet (potatoes and low-fiber, processed white rice, regular pasta, and white bread, along with nondiet soft drinks) suffered 2.5 times the rate of diabetes of women who consumed less of those foods and more fiber-containing whole-grain cereals, fruits, and vegetables. Participants who became diabetic developed type 2 diabetes, the most common form of the disease that afflicts more than 7.8% of the people in the United States or more than 28 million American adults (diabetes.niddk.nih.gov/). Moreover, more than 70 million have "prediabetes," a condition defined by impaired glucose tolerance or impaired fasting glucose, placing them at increased risk for developing full-blown diabetes. High blood glucose levels in type 2 diabetes can result from these three factors:

1. Decreased effect of insulin on peripheral tissue **(insulin resistance)**
2. Inadequate insulin production by the pancreas to control blood sugar **(relative insulin deficiency)**
3. Combined effect of both factors

FIGURE 1.8 illustrates blood glucose levels for classification as normal, prediabetic, and type 2 diabetic. Insulin, produced by the pancreas, facilitates the transfer of glucose from the blood into the cells of the body. Type 1 diabetes exists when no insulin is produced. If the pancreas produces insulin but your cells are inefficient in removing glucose,

ADDED SUGAR AND THE BLOOD LIPID PROFILE

Researchers divided 6113 participants in the long-running National Health and Nutrition Examination Survey (NHANES) into five groups based on the percentage of total calories consumed as added sugars. Groups ranged in added daily sugar intakes of less than 5% (3 tsp of sugar) to 25% or more (46 tsp of sugar). Sugar intake varied inversely with the healthy HDL cholesterol levels (58.7 $mg \cdot dL^{-1}$ in group consuming the least added sugar to 47.7 $mg \cdot dL^{-1}$ in group consuming the most) and directly with the unhealthy levels of triglycerides (105 $mg \cdot dL^{-1}$ in group consuming the least added sugar to 114 $mg \cdot dL^{-1}$ in group consuming the most). Although the research was not designed to show cause and effect, it does argue for supplanting the empty calories in sugars with foods containing a more nutritious package.

Welsh JA, et al. Caloric sweetener consumption and dyslipidemia among US adults. *JAMA* 2010;303:1490.

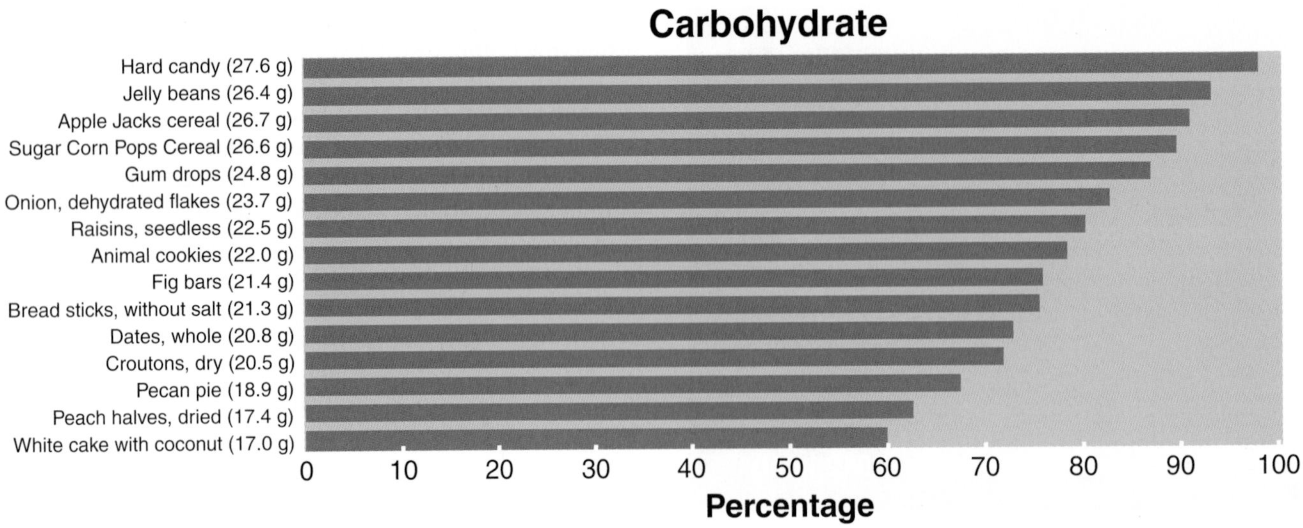

Good food sources of carbohydrates

Food	Amount	CHO (g)
Fruits		
Prunes	10	53
Pear	1 medium	25
Apple	1 medium	20
Orange	1 medium	18
Grapes	1 cup	16
Fruit Roll-ups	1 roll	12
Vegetables		
Potato	1 large	42
Lima beans	1 cup	39
Winter squash	0.5 cup	15
Peas	0.5 cup	12
Carrot	1 medium	10
Breads		
Submarine roll	8-in long	60
Bran muffin	1 large	47
Pancakes	3, (4 in dia)	45
Bagel	1 whole	31
Matzo	1 sheet	28
Whole wheat bread	1 slice	17
Matzo	1 sheet	28
Whole wheat bread	1 slice	17

Food	Amount	CHO (g)
Breakfast cereals		
Oatmeal, instant	1 packet	25
Corn Flakes	0.5 cup	24
Cream of Wheat	1 serving	22
Raisin Bran	0.5 cup	21
Beverages		
Grape juice	8 oz	42
Cola	12 oz	38
Orange juice	8 oz	27
Milk, chocolate	8 oz	26
Milk, skim	8 oz	14
Grains, pastas, starches		50
Rice, cooked	1 cup	46
Spaghetti	2 oz dry	43
Stuffing	1 cup	41
Lentils	1 cup	40
Sweets, snacks, desserts		
Fruit yogurt	1 cup	50
Soft ice cream	1 medium	35
Fig newtons	3	33
Honey	2 Tbsp	30
Maple syrup	2 Tbsp	26
Honey	2 Tbsp	30
Maple syrup	2 Tbsp	26

FIGURE 1.7. *Top.* Percentage of carbohydrate in selected foods arranged by food type. The number in parentheses indicates the number of grams of carbohydrate per ounce (28.4 g) of the food. *Bottom.* The amount of carbohydrate in various foods grouped by category.

AT RISK FOR TYPE 2 DIABETES

You have a higher diabetes risk if you:

- Are age 45 or older
- Are overweight or obese (the strongest risk factor as roughly 80% of people with type 2 diabetes are overweight or obese)
- Are Aftican-American, Hispanic/Latino-American, Asian-American, Pacific Islander, or Native American
- Have a parent, brother, or sister with diabetes
- Have blood pressure above 140 over 90
- Have triglycerides of 250 $mg \cdot dL^{-1}$ or higher
- High levels of visceral fat and fat stored in muscles and liver (closely linked to insulin resistance)
- Had diabetes when pregnant or gave birth to a baby weighing over 9 pounds
- Are physically active fewer than three times a week

Source: Adapted from: www.diabetes.niddk.nih.gov/dm/pubs/riskfortype2/.

LIFESTYLES CHANGES THAT REDUCE DIABETES RISK

A long-term follow-up to the Diabetes Prevention Outcomes Program has identified intensive lifestyle changes that can reduce likelihood of developing type 2 diabetes in the nearly 60 million high-risk Americans. For example:

1. A modest weight loss reduced diabetes risk by 34%.
2. Reducing both dietary fat and calorie intake, walking 150 minutes weekly, and a modest weight loss proved more effective than pharmacologic therapy in prevention of diabetes.
3. Lifestyle changes were particularly effective in people age 60 and older.
4. In addition to reduced diabetes risk, additional long-term health rewards include lower blood pressure and triacylglycerol levels.

Knowler W, et al. 10-year follow-up of diabetes incidence and weight loss in the Diabetes Prevention Program Outcomes Study. *Lancet* 2009;374:1677.

you are insulin resistant or demonstrate poor insulin sensitivity. Persons have prediabetes if fasting blood sugar rises only slightly to between 100 and 125 $mg \cdot dL^{-1}$. The condition becomes type 2 diabetes if blood sugar goes even higher; this accounts for nearly 95% of all diabetes cases. The blood sugar cutoffs depend on whether your blood is tested after a 12-hour fast (fasting blood sugar) or 2 hours after consuming a glucose-laden drink (oral glucose tolerance test). The American Heart Association urges Americans to slash their daily added sugar intake to only 100 calories (6.5 tsp or 25 g) for women and 150 calories (9.5 tsp or 38 g) for men.

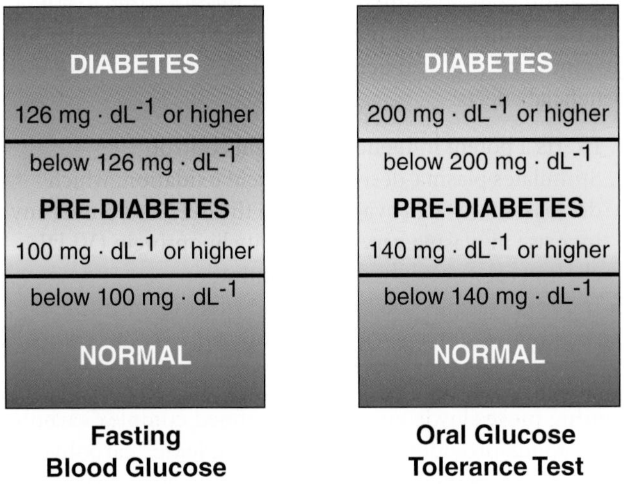

FIGURE 1.8. Classification for normal, prediabetes, and type 2 diabetes based on blood glucose levels in a fasting blood glucose test or an oral glucose tolerance test.

Diet-induced insulin resistance/hyperinsulinemia often precedes manifestations of the **metabolic syndrome**, which is defined as having three or more of the criteria indicated in **TABLE 1.2** and now afflicts more than one in three Americans.[63,76] In essence, the syndrome reflects a concurrence of four factors:

1. Disturbed glucose and insulin metabolism
2. Overweight and abdominal fat distribution
3. Mild dyslipidemia
4. Hypertension

These persons exhibit a high risk of heart attack, stroke, damaging effect on arterial walls with accelerated plaque formation, diabetes, and all-cause mortality, regardless of gender or race.[47] Estimates place the age-adjusted prevalence of the metabolic syndrome in the United States at 25%, or about 47 million men and women. The percentage increases with age and poor levels of cardiovascular fitness[24] and is particularly high among Mexican Americans and African Americans.[17] The syndrome also has emerged among obese children and adolescents.[90]

Not All Carbohydrates Are Physiologically Equal

Digestion rates of different carbohydrate sources possibly explain the carbohydrate intake–diabetes link. Low-fiber processed starches (and simple sugars) digest quickly and enter the blood at a relatively rapid rate (high glycemic index), whereas slow-release forms of high-fiber, unrefined complex carbohydrates minimize surges in blood glucose. The rapid rise in blood glucose with refined, processed

DIABETES CASES DOUBLE WORLDWIDE

The number of adults with diabetes (both type 1 and type 2 diabetes) has doubled world-wide over the last three decades to nearly 350 million from 152 million in 1980 and increased threefold to 28 million in the United States while 70% of this increase links to a growing population and aging, the balance links to changing diets, rising obesity, and growing rates of physical inactivity. Many public health experts view this increase more worrisome than hypertension and high cholesterol levels, which are effectively treated with diverse medications. The total cost of diagnosed diabetes in the United States was estimated at 174 billion according to the latest figures from the American Diabetes Association (www.diabetes.org).

Source: Finucane MM, et al. National, regional, and global trends in fasting plasma glucose and diabetes prevalence since 1980: systematic analysis of health examination surveys and epidemiological studies with 370 country-years and 2.7 million participants. *Lancet.* 2011;378(9785):31.

starch intake increases insulin demand, stimulates overproduction of insulin by the pancreas to accentuate hyperinsulinemia, increases plasma triacylglycerol concentrations, and stimulates fat synthesis. Consuming such foods for prolonged periods may eventually reduce the body's sensitivity to insulin (more insulin resistant), thus requiring progressively greater insulin output to control blood sugar levels. *Type 2 diabetes results when the pancreas cannot produce sufficient insulin to regulate blood glucose.* In contrast, diets with fiber-rich, low-glycemic carbohydrates tend to lower blood glucose and insulin response after eating, improve the blood lipid profile, and increase insulin sensitivity.[28,60,67,88]

Regularly consuming high-glycemic foods can increase cardiovascular risk because elevated blood glucose precipitates oxidative damage and inflammation that elevates blood pressure, stimulates clot formation, and reduces blood flow. For patients with type 1 diabetes who require exogenous insulin, consumption of low–glycemic index foods causes more favorable physiologic adaptations for glycemic control, HDL cholesterol concentrations, serum leptin levels, resting energy expenditure, voluntary food intake, and nitrogen balance.[1,12]

TABLE 1.2 Clinical Identification of the Metabolic Syndrome

Risk Factor	Defining Level
Abdominal obesity[a] (waist circumference)[b]	
Men	>102 cm (>40 in)
Women	>88 cm (>35 in)
Triacylglycerols	$\geq$150 mg·dL^{-1}
HDL cholesterol	
Men	<40 mg·dL^{-1}
Women	<50 mg·dL^{-1}
Blood pressure	$\geq$130/$\geq$85 mm Hg
Fasting blood glucose	$\geq$110 mg·dL^{-1}

[a] *Overweight and obesity associate with insulin resistance and the metabolic syndrome. The abdominal obesity highly correlates more with the metabolic risk factors than an elevated body mass index (BMI). The simple measure of waist circumference is recommended to identify the body weight component of the metabolic syndrome.*

[b] *Some male patients can develop multiple metabolic risk factors when the waist circumference is marginally increased, e.g., 94 to 102 cm (37–40 in). Such patients may have strong genetic contribution to insulin resistance, and they should benefit from changes in life habits, similar to men with categorical increases in waist circumference.*

A Role in Obesity?

About 25% of the population produces excessive insulin from consuming rapidly absorbed carbohydrates. These insulin-resistant persons increase their risk for obesity if they consistently consume such a diet. Weight gain occurs because abnormal quantities of insulin promote glucose penetration into cells and facilitate the liver's conversion of glucose to triacylglycerol, which then becomes stored as body fat in adipose tissue.

The insulin surge in response to a sharp rise in blood glucose following ingestion of high-glycemic carbohydrates often abnormally decreases blood glucose. This **rebound hypoglycemia** sets off hunger signals that cause the person to overeat. This repetitive scenario of high blood sugar followed by low blood sugar exerts the most profound effect on the sedentary obese person who shows the greatest insulin resistance and consequently the greatest insulin surge to a blood glucose challenge. For physically active people, regular low-to-moderate physical activity produces the following three beneficial effects:

1. Exerts a potent influence for weight control
2. Stimulates plasma-derived fatty acid oxidation, which decreases fatty acid availability to the liver and blunts any increase in plasma very low-density lipoprotein (VLDL) cholesterol–triacylglycerol concentrations
3. Improves insulin sensitivity, thus reducing the insulin requirement for a given glucose uptake

To reduce the risks for type 2 diabetes and obesity, consuming more slowly absorbed, unrefined complex carbohydrate foods provides a form of "slow-release" carbohydrate without producing rapid fluctuations in blood sugar. If rice, pasta, and bread remain the carbohydrate sources of choice, they should be consumed in unrefined form as brown rice and whole-grain pastas and breads. The same dietary modification would benefit persons involved in intense physical training and endurance competition. Their daily dietary carbohydrate intake should approach 800 g (8–10 $g \cdot kg^{-1}$ of body mass; refer to Chapter 7).

ROLE OF CARBOHYDRATE IN THE BODY

Carbohydrates serve four important functions related to energy metabolism and exercise performance.

Energy Source

Carbohydrates primarily serve as an energy fuel, particularly during intense exercise. Energy derived from bloodborne glucose and liver and muscle glycogen breakdown ultimately powers the contractile elements of muscle and other forms of more "silent" biologic work.

Carbohydrates exhibit the most dramatic use and depletion in strenuous exercise and intense training, compared with fat and protein. For physically active people, adequate daily carbohydrate intake maintains the body's relatively limited glycogen stores. In contrast, exceeding the cells' capacity to store glycogen triggers conversion and storage of excess dietary carbohydrate calories as fat.

Affects Metabolic Mixture and Spares Protein

Carbohydrate availability affects the metabolic mixture catabolized for energy. **TABLE 1.3** shows the effect of reduced energy intake during a 40-hour fast and 7 days of total food deprivation on plasma glucose and fat breakdown components. After almost 2 days of fasting, blood glucose decreases 35% but does not decrease to a lower level during further prolonged food abstinence. Concurrently, circulating fatty acid and ketone levels (acetoacetate and β-hydroxybutyrate by-products of incomplete fat breakdown) increase rapidly, with plasma ketones rising dramatically after 7 days of starvation.

TABLE 1.3 Changes in the Plasma Concentrations of Glucose, Fatty Acids, and Ketones Following 40 Hours of Fasting and Subsequent 7 Days of Starvation

Nutrient ($mmol \cdot L^{-1}$)	Normal	40 Hours Fasting	7 Days Starvation
Glucose	5.5	3.6	3.5
Fatty acids	0.3	1.15	1.19
Ketones	0.01	2.9	4.5

Adapted from Bender DA. Introduction to Nutrition and Metabolism. London: UCL Press, 1993.

Adequate carbohydrate intake preserves tissue proteins. Normally, protein serves a vital role in tissue maintenance, repair, and growth and, to a lesser degree, as a nutrient energy source. Glycogen reserves readily deplete during these three conditions:

1. Starvation
2. Reduced energy intake and low-carbohydrate diets
3. Prolonged strenuous exercise

Reduced glycogen reserves and plasma glucose levels trigger glucose synthesis from both protein (amino acids) and the glycerol portion of the fat (triacylglycerol) molecule. This gluconeogenic conversion provides a metabolic option to augment carbohydrate availability (and to maintain plasma glucose levels) with depleted glycogen stores. The price paid, however, strains the body's protein components, particularly muscle protein. In the extreme, gluconeogenesis reduces lean tissue mass and produces an accompanying solute load on the kidneys, which must excrete the nitrogen-containing by-products of protein breakdown.

Metabolic Primer/Prevents Ketosis

Components of carbohydrate catabolism serve as "primer" substrate for fat catabolism. Insufficient carbohydrate metabolism—either through limitations in glucose transport into the cell (as in diabetes from too little insulin production or insulin insensitivity) or glycogen depletion through inadequate diet, particularly low-carbohydrate diets, or prolonged exercise—causes more fat mobilization than oxidation. This produces incomplete fat breakdown and the accumulation of acetone like by-products (chiefly acetoacetate and hydroxybutyrate) called **ketone bodies**. Excessive ketone formation increases body fluid acidity, a harmful condition called acidosis, or with regard to fat breakdown, **ketosis**. Chapter 5 continues the discussion of carbohydrate as a primer for fat catabolism.

Fuel for the Central Nervous System

The central nervous system requires carbohydrate to function properly. Under normal conditions, the brain relies on blood glucose almost exclusively as its fuel. In poorly regulated diabetes, during starvation, or with a chronic low carbohydrate intake, the brain adapts after about 8 days by metabolizing relatively large amounts of fat (in the form of ketones) for alternative fuel. Adaptations also occur in skeletal muscle to chronic low-carbohydrate, high-fat diets by increasing fat use during exercise, which spares muscle glycogen.

Liver glycogenolysis primarily maintains normal blood glucose levels at rest and during exercise, usually at 100 $mg \cdot dL^{-1}$ (5.5 mM). In prolonged intense exercise, blood glucose eventually falls below normal levels because liver glycogen

A TIGHTLY REGULATED MACRONUTRIENT

Blood glucose usually remains regulated within narrow limits for two main reasons: (1) it serves as the primary source of energy in nerve tissue functions, and (2) provides the sole energy fuel for red blood cells.

depletes and active muscles continue to use the available blood glucose. Symptoms of an abnormally reduced blood glucose, or **hypoglycemia**, include weakness, hunger, and dizziness. Reduced blood glucose ultimately impairs exercise performance and partially explains "central" fatigue associated with prolonged exercise. Sustained and profound hypoglycemia (e.g., induced by an overdose of exogenous insulin) can trigger loss of consciousness and produce irreversible brain damage.

PERSONAL HEALTH AND EXERCISE NUTRITION 1.1

Diabetes 2011 Facts (www.cdc.gov/diabetes/pubs/pdf/ndfs_2011.pdf)

Each year, at least 1.6 million people in the United States will be added to the number of people diagnosed with diabetes, predominantly of the type 2 variety, the seventh leading cause of death. Diabetes prevalance, expected to double over the next 30 years, makes effective prevention and treatment a public health priority. This segment on Personal Health and Exercise Nutrition is of a general nature that applies to the population rather than to a single person. It reflects the latest statistics about how diabetes—the body's inability to produce sufficient insulin (insulin insufficiency) or use it effectively (insulin resistance) to metabolize sugar—affects this country's millions of adults and children. Slightly more men age 20 and older (12.0 million) than women (11.5 million) have diabetes. About 26.9% of people older than age 65 (10.9 million) had diabetes in 2010. The National Institutes of Health (NIH; www.nih.gov) estimates that 850,000 to 1.7 million Americans have type 1 diabetes. This translates to about one in every 400 to 600 children and adolescents. The remainder have type 2 diabetes, and millions more are not yet diagnosed. In 2005 to 2008, based on fasting glucose or hemoglobin A1c levels (glycated hemoglobin; a form of hemoglobin that identifies average plasma glucose concentration over a prolonged time period), 35% of US adults age 20 years or older had prediabetes (50% of adults age 65 years or older) placing them at increased risk for developing diabetes. Applying this percentage to the entire US population in 2010 yields an estimated 79 million American adults age 20 years or older with prediabetes.

Group	Number or Percentage Who Have Diabetes
Age ≥20 years	25.6 million, or 11.3% of all people, in this age group
Age ≥65 years	10.9 million, or 26.9% of all people, in this age group
Men	13.0 million, or 11.8% of all men aged 20 years or older
Women	12.6 million, or 10.8% of all women aged 20 years or older
Non-Hispanic whites	15.7 million, or 10.2% of all non-Hispanic whites aged 20 years or older
Non-Hispanic blacks	4.9 million, or 18.7% of all non-Hispanic blacks aged 20 years or older

Prediabetes

Prediabetes refers to a condition in which persons have blood glucose or hemoglobin A1c levels higher than normal but not high enough to cross the threshold as diabetes. People with prediabetes have an increased risk of developing type 2 diabetes, heart disease, and stroke.

- Research shows that persons with prediabetes who reduce body weight and increase physical activity can prevent or delay type 2 diabetes and in some cases return their blood glucose levels to normal.
- On the basis of fasting glucose or hemoglobin A1c levels, and after adjusting for population age differences, the percentage of US adults age 20 years or older with prediabetes in 2005 to 2008 was similar for non-Hispanic whites (35%), non-Hispanic blacks (35%), and Mexican Americans (36%).
- Using a different data source than for other race/ethnicity groups, a different age group, and a different definition based on fasting glucose levels only (and adjusting for population age differences), 20% of American Indians age 15 years or older had prediabetes in 2001 to 2004.

If trends continue unchallenged, one of three children born in 2000 will develop diabetes in their lifetime. A chronic elevation in blood glucose level can lead to the following medical complications:

Heart disease and stroke

- In 2004, heart disease was noted on 68% of diabetes-related death certificates among people age 65 years or older.

- In 2004, stroke was noted on 16% of diabetes-related death certificates among people age 65 years or older.
- Adults with diabetes have heart disease death rates about two to four times higher than adults without diabetes.
- The risk for stroke increased two to four times more among people with diabetes.

Hypertension

- In 2005 to 2008 of adults age 20 years or older with self-reported diabetes, 67% had blood pressure greater than or equal to 140/90 mm Hg or used prescription medications for hypertension.

Blindness and eye problems

- Diabetes remains the leading cause of new cases of blindness among adults age 20 to 74 years.
- In 2005 to 2008, 4.2 million people (28.5%) with diabetes age 40 years or older had diabetic retinopathy, and of these, 655,000 (4.4% of those with diabetes) had advanced diabetic retinopathy that could lead to severe vision loss.

Kidney disease

- Diabetes, the leading cause of kidney failure, accounts for 44% of all new cases of kidney failure in 2008.
- In 2008, 48,374 people with diabetes began treatment for end stage kidney disease.
- In 2008, a total of 202,290 people with end stage kidney disease due to diabetes were living on chronic dialysis or with a kidney transplant.

Nervous system disease

- About 60 to 70% of people with diabetes have mild to severe forms of nervous system damage. The results of such damage include impaired sensation or pain in the feet or hands, slowed digestion of food in the stomach, carpal tunnel syndrome, erectile dysfunction, or other nerve problems.
- Almost 30% of people with diabetes age 40 years or older have impaired sensation in the feet (i.e., at least one area that lacks feeling).
- Severe forms of diabetic nerve disease are a major contributing cause of lower extremity amputations.

Amputations

- More than 60% of nontraumatic lower limb amputations occur in people with diabetes.
- In 2006, about 65,700 nontraumatic lower limb amputations were performed in people with diabetes.

Dental disease

- Periodontal (gum) disease is more common in people with diabetes. Among young adults, those with diabetes have about twice the risk of those without diabetes.
- Adults age 45 years or older with poorly controlled diabetes (A1c ≥9%) were 2.9 times more likely to have severe periodontitis than those without diabetes. The likelihood was even greater (4.6 times) among smokers with poorly controlled diabetes.
- About one third of people with diabetes have severe periodontal disease consisting of loss of attachment (5 mm or more) of the gums to the teeth.

Complications of pregnancy

- Poorly controlled diabetes before conception and during the first trimester of pregnancy among women with type 1 diabetes can cause major birth defects in 5 to 10% of pregnancies and spontaneous abortions in 15 to 20% of pregnancies. On the other hand, for a woman with pre-existing diabetes, optimizing blood glucose levels before and during early pregnancy can reduce the risk of birth defects in their infants.
- Poorly controlled diabetes during the second and third trimesters of pregnancy can result in excessively large babies, posing a risk to both mother and child.

Other complications

- Uncontrolled diabetes often leads to biochemical imbalances that can cause acute life-threatening events, such as diabetic ketoacidosis and hyperosmolar (nonketotic) coma.
- People with diabetes are more susceptible to many other illnesses. Once they acquire these illnesses, they often have worse prognoses. For example, they are more likely to die with pneumonia or influenza than people who do not have diabetes.
- People with diabetes age 60 years or older are two to three times more likely to report an inability to walk one quarter of a mile, climb stairs, or do housework compared with people without diabetes in the same age group.
- People with diabetes are twice as likely to have depression, which can complicate diabetes management, than people without diabetes. In addition, depression is associated with a 60% increased risk of developing type 2 diabetes.

Preventing Diabetes Complications

Glucose control

- Studies in the United States and abroad have found that improved glycemic control benefits people with either type 1 or type 2 diabetes. In general, every percentage point drop in A1c blood test results (e.g., from 8.0 to 7.0%) can reduce the risk of microvascular complications (eye, kidney, and nerve diseases) by 40%. The absolute difference in risk may vary for certain subgroups of people.

- In patients with type 1 diabetes, intensive insulin therapy has long-term beneficial effects on the risk of cardiovascular disease.

Blood pressure control

- Among people with diabetes, blood pressure control reduces the risk of cardiovascular disease (heart disease or stroke) by 33 to 50% and the risk of microvascular complications (eye, kidney, and nerve diseases) by approximately 33%.
- In general, for every 10-mm Hg reduction in systolic blood pressure, the risk for any complication related to diabetes is reduced by 12%.
- No benefit of reducing systolic blood pressure below 140 mm Hg has materialized in randomized clinical trials.
- Reducing diastolic blood pressure from 90 mm Hg to 80 mm Hg in people with diabetes reduces the risk of major cardiovascular events by 50%.

Control of blood lipids

- Improved control of LDL cholesterol can reduce cardiovascular complications by 20 to 50%.

Preventive care practices for eyes, feet, and kidneys

- Detecting and treating diabetic eye disease with laser therapy can reduce the development of severe vision loss by an estimated 50 to 60%.
- About 65% of adults with diabetes and poor vision can be helped by appropriate eyeglasses.
- Comprehensive foot care programs (i.e., that include risk assessment, foot care education and preventive therapy, treatment of foot problems, and referral to specialists) can reduce amputation rates by 45 to 85%.
- Detecting and treating early diabetic kidney disease by lowering blood pressure can reduce the decline in kidney function by 30 to 70%. Treatment with particular medications for hypertension called angiotensin-converting enzyme inhibitors (ACEIs) and angiotensin receptor blockers (ARBs) is more effective in reducing the decline in kidney function than is treatment with other blood pressure–lowering drugs.
- In addition to lowering blood pressure, ARBs and ACEIs reduce proteinuria, a risk factor for developing kidney disease, by about 35%.

SUMMARY

1. Atoms provide the basic building blocks of all matter and play the major role in the composition of food nutrients and biologically active substances.
2. Carbon, hydrogen, oxygen, and nitrogen serve as the primary structural units for most of the body's biologically active substances. Specific combinations of carbon with oxygen and hydrogen form carbohydrates and lipids. Proteins consist of combinations of carbon, oxygen, and hydrogen, with nitrogen and minerals.
3. Simple sugars consist of chains of three to seven carbon atoms, with hydrogen and oxygen in the ratio of 2:1. Glucose, the most common simple sugar, contains a six-carbon chain: $C_6H_{12}O_6$.
4. There are three kinds of carbohydrates: monosaccharides (sugars such as glucose and fructose), disaccharides (combinations of two monosaccharides as in sucrose, lactose, and maltose), and oligosaccharides (three to nine glucose residues). Polysaccharides that contain 10 or more simple sugars form starch and fiber in plants and glycogen, the large glucose polymer in animals.
5. Glycogenolysis reconverts glycogen to glucose, whereas gluconeogenesis synthesizes glucose predominantly from the carbon skeletons of amino acids.
6. The two basic starch configurations are (1) amylose, consisting of a long, straight chain of glucose units; and (2) amylopectin, constructed from a highly branched monosaccharide linkage. The "digestibility" of a starch-containing food depends on the predominance of one starch form or the other.
7. Fiber, a nonstarch structural plant polysaccharide, resists human digestive enzymes. Technically not nutrients, water-soluble and water-insoluble dietary fibers confer health benefits for gastrointestinal functioning and reduce cardiovascular disease risks.
8. Heart disease and obesity protection may relate to dietary fiber's regulatory role in favorably reducing insulin secretion by slowing nutrient absorption in the small intestine following a meal.
9. Americans typically consume 40 to 50% of total calories as carbohydrates. Greater sugar intake in the form of sweets (simple sugars) occurs commonly in the population with possibly harmful effects for glucose-insulin regulation, cardiovascular disease, and obesity.
10. Physically active men and women should consume about 60% of daily calories as carbohydrates (400–600 g), predominantly in unrefined complex form. During intense training and prolonged physical activities, carbohydrate intake should increase to 70% of total calories or 8 to 10 $g \cdot kg^{-1}$ body weight.

SUMMARY *(continued)*

11. Frequent and excessive consumption of carbohydrates with a high glycemic index may alter the metabolic profile and increase risk for the metabolic syndrome of obesity, insulin resistance, glucose intolerance, dyslipidemia, and hypertension.
12. Type 2 diabetes, the most common form of the disease, afflicts more than 8% of people in the United States, or more than 28 million American adults. Moreover, more than 70 million have prediabetes, a condition defined by impaired glucose tolerance or impaired fasting glucose, placing them at increased risk for developing diabetes.
13. Carbohydrates stored in limited quantity in liver and muscles (1) serve as a major source of energy, (2) spare protein breakdown for energy, (3) function as a metabolic primer for fat metabolism, and (4) provide fuel for the central nervous system.
14. A carbohydrate-deficient diet rapidly depletes muscle and liver glycogen. This profoundly affects intense anaerobic and long-duration aerobic exercise capacity.

LIPIDS

NATURE OF LIPIDS

Lipid (from the Greek *lipos,* meaning fat), the general term for a heterogeneous group of compounds, includes oils, fats, and waxes and related compounds. Oils become liquid at room temperature, whereas fats remain solid. A lipid molecule contains the same structural elements as carbohydrate except that it differs markedly in its linkage of atoms. Specifically, the lipid's ratio of hydrogen to oxygen considerably exceeds that of carbohydrate. For example, the formula $C_{57}H_{110}O_6$ describes the common lipid stearin, with an H-to-O ratio of 18.3:1; for carbohydrate, the ratio is 2:1. Approximately 98% of dietary lipids exist as triacylglycerols, whereas about 90% of the body's total fat resides in the adipose tissue depots of the subcutaneous tissues.

TABLE 1.4 General Classification of Lipids

Type of Lipid	Example
I. Simple lipids	
Neutral fats	Triglycerides (triacylglycerols)
Waxes	Beeswax
II. Compound lipids	
Phospholipids	Lecithins, cephalins, lipositols,
Glycolipids	Cerebrosides, gangliosides
Lipoproteins	Chylomicrons, VLDLs, LDLs, HDLs
III. Derived lipids	
Fatty acids	Palmitic acid, oleic acid, stearic acid, linoleic acid
Steroids	Cholesterol, ergosterol, cortisol, bile acids, vitamin D, estrogens, progesterone, androgens
Hydrocarbons	Terpenes

KINDS AND SOURCES OF LIPIDS

Plants and animals contain lipids in long hydrocarbon chains. Lipids are generally greasy to touch and remain insoluble in water but soluble in organic solvents such as ether, chloroform, and benzene. According to common classification, lipids belong to one of three main groups: **simple lipids, compound lipids**, and **derived lipids**. **TABLE 1.4** lists the general classification for lipids with specific examples of each form.

Simple Lipids

The simple lipids, or "neutral fats," consist primarily of **triacylglycerols**, the most plentiful fats in the body. They constitute the major storage form of fat in adipose (fat) cells. This molecule consists of two different clusters of atoms. One cluster, **glycerol**, consists of a three-carbon alcohol molecule that by itself does not qualify as a lipid because of its high solubility in water. Three clusters of carbon-chained atoms, usually in even number, termed **fatty acids**, attach to the glycerol molecule. Fatty acids consist of straight hydrocarbon chains with as few as four carbon atoms or more than 20 in their chain, although chain lengths of 16 and 18 carbons prevail.

Three molecules of water form when glycerol and fatty acids join in the synthesis **(condensation)** of the triacylglycerol molecule. Conversely, during hydrolysis, when the fat molecule cleaves into its constituents by the action of **lipase enzymes**, three molecules of water attach at the point where the molecule splits. **FIGURE 1.9** illustrates the basic structure of **saturated fatty acid** and **unsaturated fatty acid** molecules. All lipid-containing foods consist of a mixture of different proportions of saturated and unsaturated fatty acids. Fatty acids get their name because the

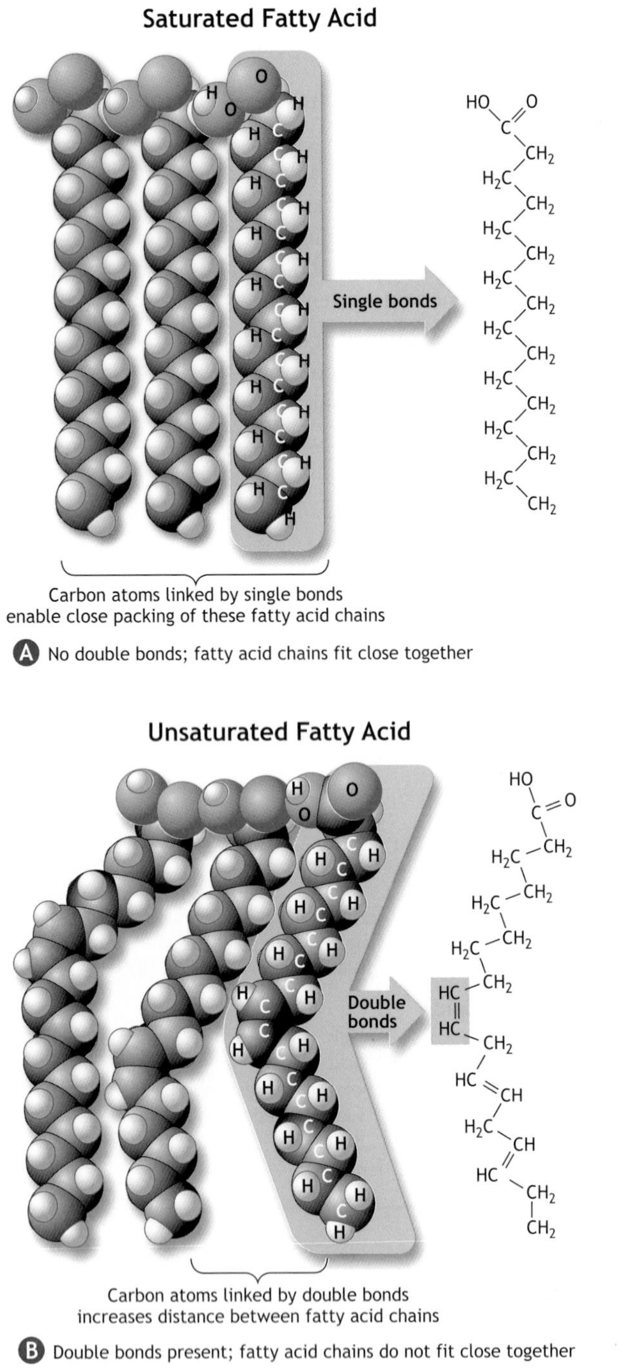
Saturated Fatty Acid
Single bonds
Carbon atoms linked by single bonds enable close packing of these fatty acid chains
A No double bonds; fatty acid chains fit close together
Unsaturated Fatty Acid
Double bonds
Carbon atoms linked by double bonds increases distance between fatty acid chains
B Double bonds present; fatty acid chains do not fit close together

FIGURE 1.9. The presence or absence of double bonds between the carbon atoms is the major structural difference between saturated and unsaturated fatty acids. **A.** The saturated fatty acid palmitic acid has no double bonds in its carbon chain and contains the maximum number of hydrogen atoms. Without double bonds, the three saturated fatty acid chains fit closely together to form a "hard" fat. **B.** The three double bonds in linoleic acid, an unsaturated fatty acid, reduce the number of hydrogen atoms along the carbon chain. Insertion of double bonds into the carbon chain prevents close association of the fatty acids; this produces a "softer" fat, or an oil. (From McArdle WD, et al. *Exercise Physiology: Nutrition, Energy, and Human Performance.* 7th Ed. Baltimore: Lippincott Williams & Wilkins, 2010:20.)

organic acid (COOH) molecule forms part of their chemical structure.

Saturated Fatty Acids

A saturated fatty acid contains only single covalent bonds between carbon atoms; all of the remaining bonds attach to hydrogen. The fatty acid molecule is referred to as saturated because it holds as many hydrogen atoms as chemically possible.

Saturated fatty acids occur primarily in animal products such as beef (52% saturated fatty acids), lamb, pork, chicken, and egg yolk and in dairy fats of cream, milk, butter (62% saturated fatty acids), and cheese. Saturated fatty acids from the plant kingdom include coconut and palm oil (liquid at room temperature because they have short fatty acid chains), vegetable shortening, and hydrogenated margarine; commercially prepared cakes, pies, and cookies also contain plentiful amounts of these fatty acids.

Unsaturated Fatty Acids

Unsaturated fatty acids contain one or more double bonds along the main carbon chain. Each double bond reduces the number of potential hydrogen-binding sites; therefore, the molecule remains unsaturated relative to hydrogen. A **monounsaturated fatty acid** contains one double bond along the main carbon chain. Examples include canola oil, olive oil (77% monounsaturated fatty acids), peanut oil, and the oil in almonds, pecans, and avocados. A **polyunsaturated fatty acid** contains two or more double bonds along the main carbon chain; safflower, sunflower, soybean, and corn oil serve as examples.

Fatty acids from plant sources are generally unsaturated and tend to liquefy at room temperature. Lipids with longer (more carbons in the chain) and more saturated fatty acids remain solid at room temperature, whereas those with shorter and more unsaturated fatty acids stay soft. Oils exist as liquid and contain unsaturated fatty acids. **Hydrogenation** changes oils to semisolid compounds. This chemical process bubbles liquid hydrogen into vegetable oil, which reduces double bonds in the unsaturated fatty acid to single bonds to capture more hydrogen atoms along the carbon chain. This creates firmer fat because adding hydrogen to the carbons increases the lipid's melting temperature. Hydrogenated oil thus behaves as a saturated fat. The most common hydrogenated fats include lard substitutes and margarine.

Triacylglycerol Formation

FIGURE 1.10 outlines the sequence of reactions in triacylglycerol synthesis, a process termed **esterification**. Initially, a fatty acid substrate attached to coenzyme A (CoA) forms fatty acyl-CoA that transfers to glycerol (as glycerol 3-phosphate). In subsequent reactions, two additional fatty acyl-CoAs link to a single glycerol backbone as the composite triacylglycerol

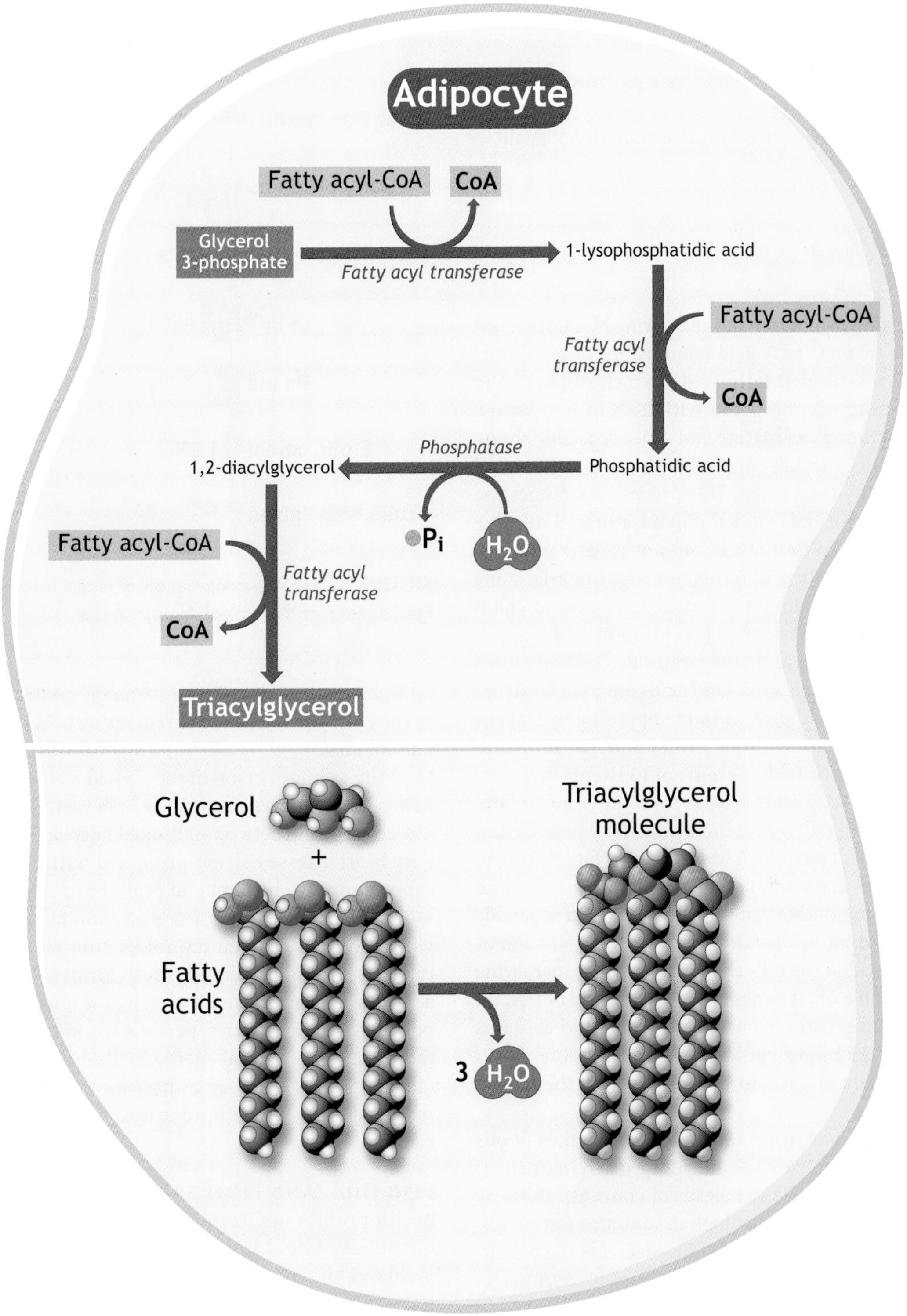

FIGURE 1.10. *Top.* Triacylglycerol formation in adipocytes (and muscle) tissue involves a series of reactions (dehydration synthesis) that link three fatty acid molecules to a single glycerol backbone. The *bottom portion* of the figure summarizes this linkage. (Reprinted with permission from McArdle W, et al. *Exercise Physiology Energy, Nutrition, and Human Performance.* 6th Ed. Baltimore: Lippincott Williams & Wilkins, 2010:22.)

molecule forms. Triacylglycerol synthesis increases following a meal for the following two reasons:

1. Increased blood levels of fatty acids and glucose from food absorption
2. A relatively high level of circulating insulin, which facilitates triacylglycerol synthesis

Butter Versus Margarine: A Health Risk in Trans Fatty Acids

One cannot distinguish butter and margarine by caloric content but rather by their fatty acid composition. Butter contains about 62% saturated fatty acids (which dramatically raise LDL cholesterol) compared with 20% in margarine. During manufacturing, margarine and other vegetable shortenings such as unsaturated corn, soybean, or sunflower oil become partially hydrogenated. This process rearranges the chemical structure of the original polyunsaturated oil. The lipid remains hardened (saturated), but not as hard as butter. A *trans* unsaturated fatty acid forms in margarine when one of the hydrogen atoms along the restructured carbon chain moves from its naturally occurring *cis* position to the opposite side of the double bond that separates two carbon atoms (*trans* position). Although *trans* fatty acids are close in structure to most unsaturated fatty acids, the opposing hydrogens along its carbon chain make the physical properties similar to those of saturated fatty acids. Seventeen to twenty-five percent of margarine's fatty acids exist as *trans* unsaturated fatty acids compared with only 7% in butterfat. Many popular fast foods contain considerably high levels of *trans* fats.[81] A serving of French fries can contain up to 3.6 g of *trans* fat, and doughnuts and pound cake can have 4.3 g. (Liquid vegetable oils normally have no *trans* fatty acids, but they are sometimes added to extend the oil's shelf life.) Because margarine consists of vegetable oil, it contains no cholesterol; butter, on the other hand, originates from a dairy source and contains between 11 and 15 mg of cholesterol per teaspoon. *Trans* fatty acids represent about 5 to 10% of the fat in the typical American diet.

A diet high in margarine and commercial baked goods and deep-fried foods prepared with hydrogenated (hardened) vegetable oils increases LDL cholesterol concentrations by about the same amount as a diet high in saturated fatty acids. Unlike saturated fats, hydrogenated oils decrease the beneficial HDL cholesterol concentration and adversely affect markers of inflammation and endothelial dysfunction.[45,56,61,62] *Trans* fatty acids also elevate plasma levels of triacylglycerols and may impair arterial wall flexibility and function. A prospective study of more than 84,204 healthy middle-aged women demonstrated that diets high in *trans* fatty acids promote resistance to insulin, increasing the risk for type 2 diabetes.[71]

Lipids in the Diet

FIGURE 1.11 shows the approximate percentage contribution of some common food groups to the total lipid content of the typical American diet. Plants generally contribute about 34% to the daily lipid intake; the remaining 66% comes from animal sources.

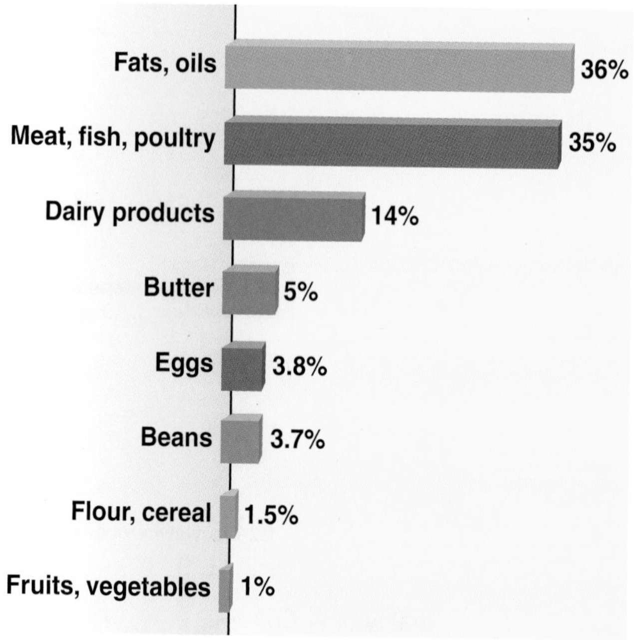

FIGURE 1.11. The contribution of major food sources to the lipid content of the typical American diet.

The average person in the United States consumes about 15% of total calories (more than 50 lb yearly) as saturated fats. The relationship between saturated fatty acid intake and coronary heart disease risk has prompted nutritionists and medical personnel to recommend replacing a large portion of the saturated fatty acids and nearly all *trans* fatty acids in the diet with nonhydrogenated monounsaturated and polyunsaturated fatty acids. Consuming both forms of unsaturated fatty acids lowers coronary risk even below normal levels. From a public health perspective, persons are advised to consume no more than 10% of total energy intake as saturated fatty acids (about 250 kcal or 25–30 $g \cdot day^{-1}$ for the average young adult male) and to keep all lipid intake to less than 30% of total calories.

Fish Oils (and Fish) are Healthful: Studies of the health profiles of Greenland Eskimos, who consume large quantities of lipid from fish, seal, and whale yet have a low incidence of coronary heart disease, indicated the potential for two essential long-chain polyunsaturated fatty acids to confer diverse health benefits. These oils, eicosapentaenoic acid (EPA) and docosahexaenoic acid (DHA), belong to an **omega-3** family of fatty acids (also termed n-3, characterized by a double bond 3 carbons from the n end of the molecule) found primarily in the oils of shellfish and cold-water herring, salmon, sardines, bluefish, and mackerel and sea mammals (**FIG. 1.12**). For non-fish eaters, plant sources for α-linolenic acid, another omega-3 oil and precursor of EPA and DHA, include dark green leafy vegetables and flax, hemp, canola, soy, and walnut oils, which your body

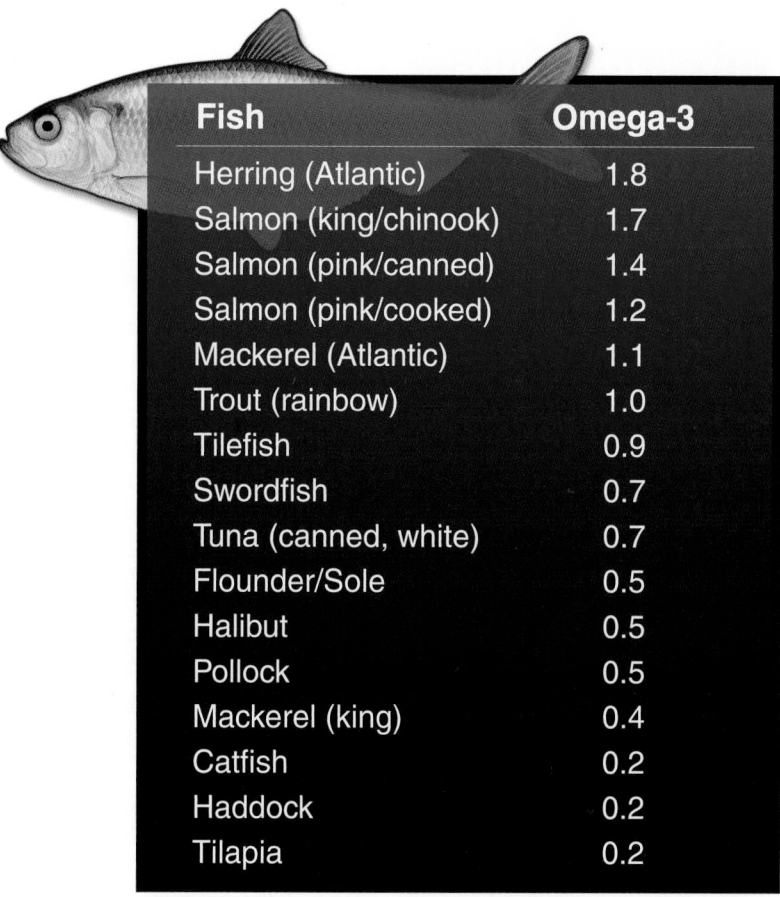

Fish	Omega-3
Herring (Atlantic)	1.8
Salmon (king/chinook)	1.7
Salmon (pink/canned)	1.4
Salmon (pink/cooked)	1.2
Mackerel (Atlantic)	1.1
Trout (rainbow)	1.0
Tilefish	0.9
Swordfish	0.7
Tuna (canned, white)	0.7
Flounder/Sole	0.5
Halibut	0.5
Pollock	0.5
Mackerel (king)	0.4
Catfish	0.2
Haddock	0.2
Tilapia	0.2

FIGURE 1.12. Omega-3 fatty acid content of various types of fish (grams per cooked 3-oz serving).

converts (albeit at a relatively small amount) to EPA and DHA.

Regular fish intake (twice weekly or 8–12 oz of seafood weekly) and fish oil (a minimum daily level of 250 mg for DHA/EPA) exert multiple physiologic effects that protect against coronary artery disease.[21,43] They may benefit one's lipid profile (particularly plasma triacylglycerol),[46,79] overall heart disease risk (particularly risk of ventricular fibrillation and sudden death),[20,37,49,94] inflammatory disease risk,[12] and (for smokers) risk of contracting chronic obstructive pulmonary disease,[73] and may help prevent obesity-related chronic diseases such as diabetes and heart disease.[52] Omega-3 fish oils, particularly DHA, may also prove beneficial in treating diverse psychological disorders and reduce the risk of Alzheimer disease and late-onset dementia but are ineffective in slowing mental and physical decline in older patients with Alzheimer disease.[6,70] The intake of fish and marine fatty acids probably does not reduce cancer risk.[84] It should also be noted that several recent reports raise questions concerning the benefit of seafood and fish oil supplements for all persons, particularly those with documented coronary artery disease.[44,53]

Several mechanisms explain how eating fish—with its additional cardioprotective nutrients of selenium, various natural antioxidants, and protein not present in fish oil—protects against death from heart disease. Fish oil may act as an antithrombogenic agent to prevent blood clot formation on arterial walls. It also may inhibit the growth of atherosclerotic plaques, reduce pulse pressure and total vascular resistance (increase arterial compliance), and stimulate endothelial-derived nitric oxide to facilitate myocardial perfusion. The oil's lowering effect on triacylglycerol also confers protection because plasma triacylglycerol level strongly predicts coronary heart disease risk.

Perhaps the most powerful cardioprotective benefit of fish oils relates to their antiarrhythmic effect on myocardial tissue.[2] This protection against ventricular arrhythmias occurs from the unique effects of dietary n-3 fatty acids on the respective n-3 fatty acid content of the myocardial cell membranes. In the event of severe physiologic stress (e.g., ischemic attack from reduced myocardial blood flow), the n-3 fatty acids in the cell membrane are released and locally protect the myocardium from the development and propagation of a rapid heart rate (tachycardia), which often causes cardiac arrest and sudden death.

All Lipid Intake in Moderation: In the quest for good health and optimal exercise performance, prudent practice entails cooking with and consuming lipids derived primarily from vegetable sources. This approach may be too simp

FISH OIL, REGULAR EXERCISE, AND YOUNGER, HEALTHY CHROMOSOMES

Telomeres, the caps on the end of DNA strands that get snapped when cells divide and replicate, provide a glimpse of biologic aging (as contrasted to chronologic aging) and heart disease risk, with shorter telomeres indicating more rapid aging. It now appears that two modifiable behaviors, regular exercise and consumption of the omega-3 fatty acids in fish, may retard the aging process at the cellular level. For example, maintaining aerobic fitness in middle age and beyond preserves telomere length, which may reflect a molecular mechanism that underlies the anti-aging effects of regular exercise.

From the nutritional perspective, the omega-3 fats in fish oil may also slow biologic aging at the cellular level. In a 5-year longitudinal study of patients with stable coronary heart disease, those with the highest blood levels of omega-3 fatty acids had the least shortening of telomeres, whereas those with the lowest omega-3 levels had the fastest rate of shortening. These findings underscore the American Heart Association's recommendations concerning the benefits of regular exercise and consumption of two or more 3.5-oz weekly servings of fish, particularly those containing high levels of omega-3 fatty acids like salmon (to supply about 500–100 mg of DHA plus EPA daily).

Farzaneh-Far R, et al. Association of marine omega-3 fatty acid levels with telomeric aging in patients with coronary heart disease. *JAMA* 2010;303:25.

LaRocca TJ, et al. Leukocyte telomere length is preserved with aging in endurance-exercise trained adults and related to maximal aerobic capacity. *Mech Ageing Dev* 2010;131:165.

however, because total saturated *and* unsaturated fatty acid intake may constitute a risk for diabetes and heart disease. If so, then one should reduce the intake of all lipids, particularly lipids high in saturated fatty acids and *trans* fatty acids. Concerns also exist over the association of high-fat diets with ovarian, colon, endometrial, and other cancers.

FIGURE 1.13 lists the saturated, monounsaturated, and polyunsaturated fatty acid content of various sources of dietary lipid. All fats contain a mix of each fatty acid type, although different fatty acids predominate in certain lipid sources. In foods, α-linolenic acid is the major omega-3 fatty acid; linoleic acid is the major omega-6 fatty acid; and oleic acid is the major omega-9 fatty acid. These fatty acids provide components for vital body structures, perform important roles in immune function and vision, help form and maintain the integrity of plasma membranes, and produce hormone-like compounds called eicosanoids.

One can obtain omega-3 and omega-6 polyunsaturated fatty acids (abundant in most vegetable oils except tropical ones) only through the diet. Because of their role as precursors of other fatty acids that the body cannot synthesize, they have been termed **essential fatty acids**. About 1 to 2% of the total energy intake should come from linoleic acid. For a 2500-kcal intake, this corresponds to about 1 tbsp of plant oil per day. Mayonnaise, cooking oils, salad dressings, whole grains, vegetables, and other foods readily provide this amount. Fatty fish (salmon, tuna, or sardines) or canola, soybean, safflower, sunflower, sesame, and flax oils provide the best sources for α-linolenic acid or its related omega-3 fatty acids, EPA and DHA.

LIPIDS: THE GOOD, THE BAD, AND THE UGLY

Subjective terms describe the impact of the various forms of fatty acids in the diet. Unsaturated fatty acids, which contain one (monounsaturated) or more (polyunsaturated) double bonds along their main carbon chain, classify as desirable in that they lower blood cholesterol, particularly the harmful LDL cholesterol. In contrast, consumption of saturated fatty acids, which contain only single bonds between carbon atoms, stimulates the liver's production of LDL cholesterol. Even more disturbing, the consumption of partially hydrogenated unsaturated vegetable oils that produce *trans* fatty acids not only increases LDL concentrations but also lowers the beneficial HDL cholesterol.

Compound Lipids

Compound lipids consist of a triacylglycerol molecule combined with other chemicals and represent about 10% of the body's total fat. One group of modified triacylglycerols, the **phospholipids**, contains one or more fatty acid molecules combined with a phosphorus-containing group and a nitrogenous base. These lipids form in all cells, although the liver synthesizes most of them. The phosphorus part of the phospholipids within the plasma membrane bilayer attracts water (hydrophilic), whereas the lipid portion repels water (hydrophobic). Thus, phospholipids interact with water and lipid to modulate fluid movement across cell membranes. Phospholipids also maintain the structural integrity of the cell, play an important role in blood clotting, and provide structural integrity to the insulating sheath around nerve fibers. **Lecithin**, the most widely distributed phospholipid in food sources (liver, egg yolk, wheat germ, nuts, soybeans), functions in fatty acid and cholesterol transport and use. Lecithin does not qualify as an essential nutrient because the body manufactures the required amount.

Other compound lipids include **glycolipids** (fatty acids bound with carbohydrate and nitrogen) and water-soluble **lipoproteins** (formed primarily in the liver when protein joins with either triacylglycerols or phospholipids).

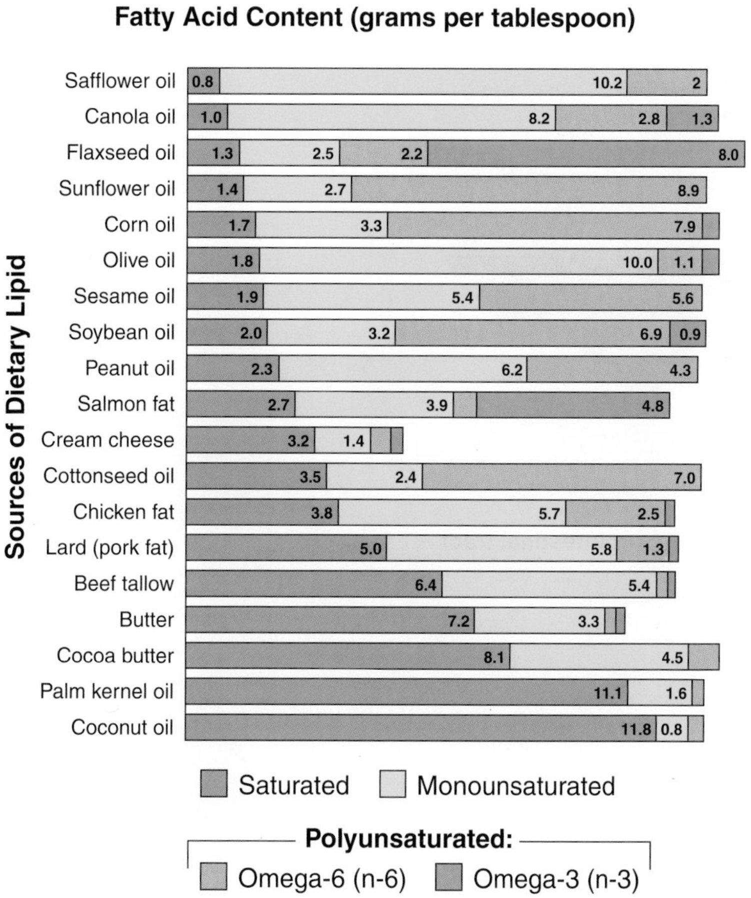

FIGURE 1.13. Saturated, monounsaturated, and polyunsaturated fatty acid content of various sources of dietary lipid.

Lipoproteins provide the major avenue for lipid transport in the blood. If blood lipids did not bind to protein, they literally would float to the top like cream in nonhomogenized fresh milk.

High- and Low-Density Lipoprotein Cholesterol

FIGURE 1.14 illustrates the general dynamics of dietary cholesterol and the lipoproteins, including their transport among the small intestine, liver, and peripheral tissues. Four types of lipoproteins exist according to gravitational density. **Chylomicrons** form when emulsified lipid droplets (including long-chain triacylglycerols, phospholipids, and free fatty acids) leave the intestine and enter the lymphatic vasculature. Under normal conditions, the liver metabolizes chylomicrons and sends them for storage in adipose tissue. Chylomicrons also transport the fat-soluble vitamins A, D, E, and K.

The liver and small intestine produce **HDL**. HDL contains the greatest percentage of protein (about 50%) and the least total lipid (about 20%) and cholesterol (about 20%) compared with the other lipoproteins. Degradation of a **VLDL** produces an **LDL**. VLDL, formed in the liver from fats, carbohydrates, alcohol, and cholesterol, contains the greatest percentage of lipid (95%), of which about 60% consists of triacylglycerol. VLDL transports triacylglycerols to muscle and adipose tissue. Action of the enzyme **lipoprotein lipase** produces

HIGH-DENSITY LIPOPROTEINS AND CANCER RISK

A meta-analysis of 24 randomized controlled trials observed that for every 10 $mg \cdot dL^{-1}$ increase in HDL cholesterol the risk of cancer dropped by 36%, with the relationship becoming even stronger after adjusting for demographics and other cancer risk factors. The researchers speculated that HDL might exhibit anti-inflammatory and antioxidant effects that reduce cancer risk or exert beneficial immune system effects that destroy abnormal cells with potential for tumor growth. It is also possible that healthy lifestyle changes (eating a nutritious diet, regularly exercising, maintaining a healthy body weight, and not smoking) that raise HDL levels also act to reduce the risk of chronic conditions associated with a higher cancer risk.

Karas RH, et al. Baseline and on-treatment high-density lipoprotein cholesterol and the risk of cancer in randomized controlled trials of lipid-altering therapy. *J Am Coll Cardiol* 2010;55:2846.

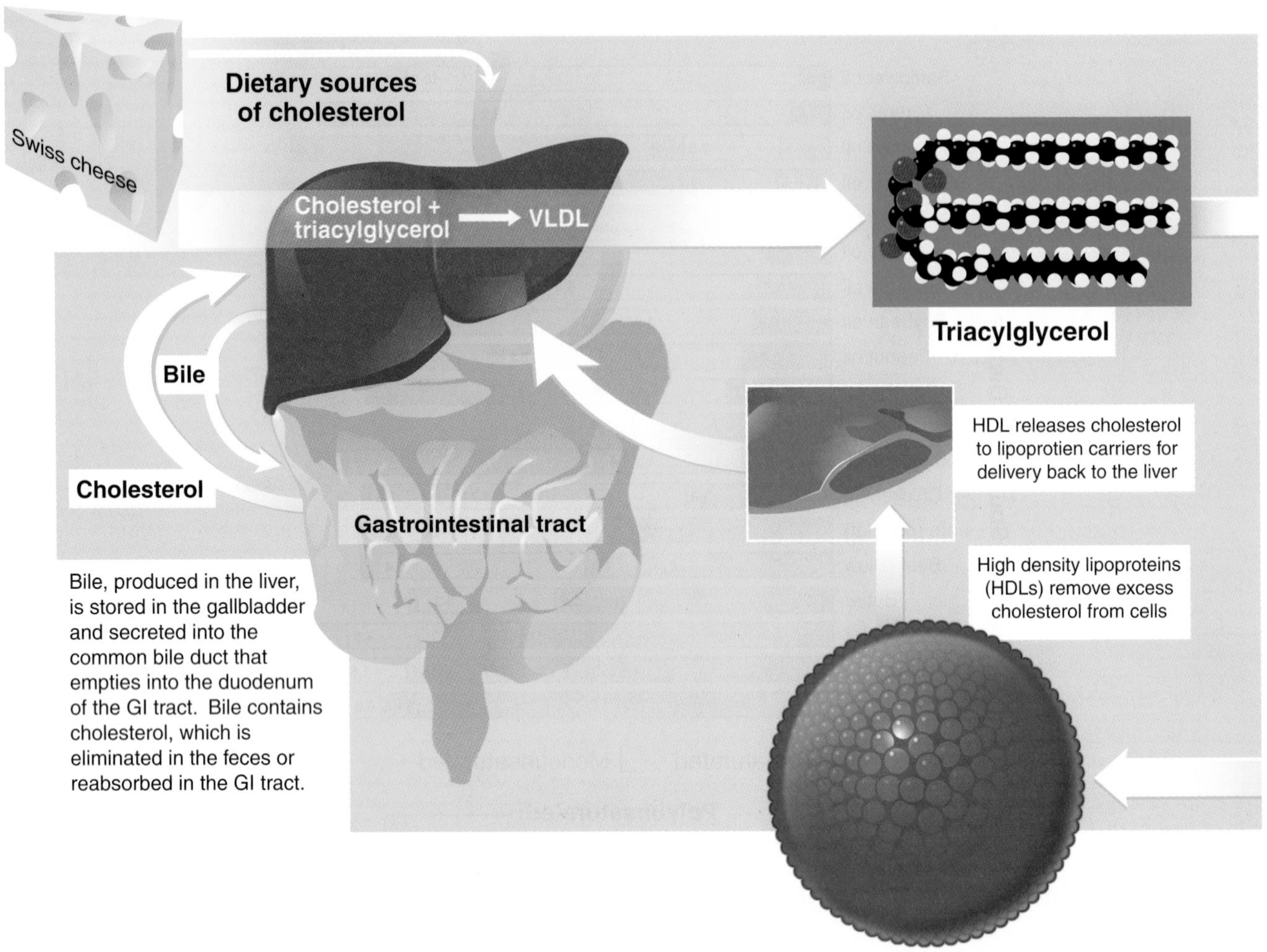
Dietary sources of cholesterol
Swiss cheese
Cholesterol + triacylglycerol → VLDL
Triacylglycerol
Bile
Cholesterol
Gastrointestinal tract
HDL releases cholesterol to lipoprotien carriers for delivery back to the liver
High density lipoproteins (HDLs) remove excess cholesterol from cells
Bile, produced in the liver, is stored in the gallbladder and secreted into the common bile duct that empties into the duodenum of the GI tract. Bile contains cholesterol, which is eliminated in the feces or reabsorbed in the GI tract.

FIGURE 1.14. General interaction between dietary cholesterol and the lipoproteins and their transport among the small intestine, liver, and peripheral tissues.

a denser LDL molecule because now it contains less lipid. LDL and VLDL have the most lipid and least protein components.

"Bad" Cholesterol: Among the lipoproteins, LDL, which normally carries between 60 and 80% of the total serum cholesterol, has the greatest affinity for cells of the arterial wall. LDL delivers cholesterol to arterial tissue, where LDL oxidizes and participates in the proliferation of smooth muscle cells and other unfavorable changes that damage and narrow arteries. According to the US Centers for Disease Control and Prevention, about one third of American adults have elevated LDL, yet only one third have it controlled, and less than one half are treated for it. Regular aerobic exercise, visceral fat accumulation, and the diet's macronutrient composition all impact serum LDL concentrations.

"Good" Cholesterol: Unlike LDL, HDL protects against heart disease. HDL acts as a scavenger in the **reverse transport of cholesterol** by removing cholesterol from the arterial wall. It then delivers it to the liver for incorporation into bile and subsequent excretion via the intestinal tract.

NUTS FOR HEART HEALTH

A cornerstone for the prevention and treatment of heart disease lies in dietary interventions to lower the level of blood cholesterol and favorably modify the lipoprotein concentrations. The consumption of a diverse array of nuts—almonds, hazelnuts, peanuts, pecans, some pine nuts, pistachios, and walnuts—with their rich content of plant proteins, unsaturated fatty acids, dietary fiber, minerals, vitamins, antioxidants, and phytosterols, can play an important role in the dietary armamentarium to achieve these goals. A recent pooled analysis of research studies compared cholesterol levels between groups consuming nuts (nearly 2.4 oz daily) and control groups not consuming nuts over periods ranging from 3 to 8 weeks. Participants who added nuts to their diets averaged a 5.1% decrease in cholesterol, a 7.4% decrease in LDL cholesterol, and a favorable 8.3% improvement in the ratio of LDL to HDL. A 10.2% decline in triglyceride levels was also noted in those persons with high triglyceride levels.

Sabate J, et al. Nut consumption and blood lipid levels: a pooled analysis of 25 intervention trials. *Arch Intern Med* 2010;170:821.

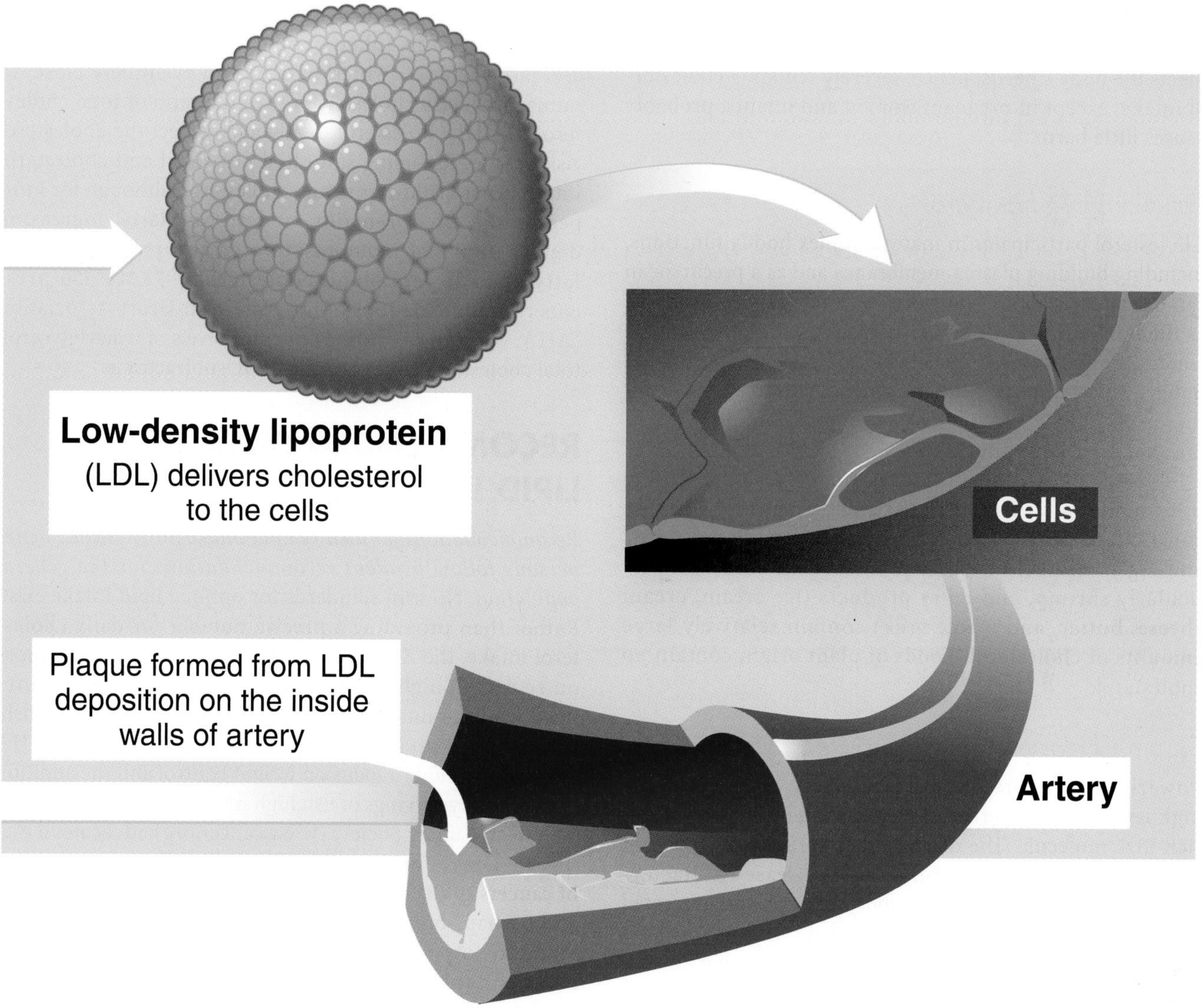
Low-density lipoprotein
(LDL) delivers cholesterol
to the cells
Cells
Plaque formed from LDL
deposition on the inside
walls of artery
Artery

FIGURE 1.14. *Continued*

> **CHECK IT OUT**
>
> An online computer program calculates the risk and the appropriate cholesterol levels for adults (**www.nhlbi.nih.gov/guidelines/cholesterol/index.htm**).

The amount of LDL and HDL cholesterol and their specific ratios (e.g., HDL ÷ total cholesterol) and subfractions provide more meaningful indicators of coronary artery disease risk than does total cholesterol alone. Regular aerobic exercise and abstinence from cigarette smoking increase HDL, lower LDL, and favorably alter the LDL ÷ HDL ratio.[50,80]

Derived Lipids

Derived lipids form from simple and compound lipids. Unlike the neutral fats and phospholipids with hydrocarbon chains, derived lipids contain hydrocarbon rings. **Cholesterol**, *the most widely known derived lipid, exists only in animal tissue.* The chemical structure of cholesterol provides the backbone for synthesizing all of the body's steroid compounds (e.g., bile salts, vitamin D, sex hormones, and adrenocortical hormones). Cholesterol does not contain fatty acids but shares some of the physical and chemical characteristics of lipids. Thus, from a dietary viewpoint, cholesterol is considered a lipid.

Cholesterol, widespread in the plasma membrane of all cells, is obtained either through the diet **(exogenous cholesterol)** or through cellular synthesis **(endogenous cholesterol)**. Even if a person maintains a "cholesterol-free" diet, endogenous cholesterol synthesis varies between 0.5 and 2.0 $g \cdot day^{-1}$. More endogenous cholesterol forms with a diet high in saturated fatty acids, which facilitate cholesterol synthesis by the liver. Although the liver synthesizes about 70% of the body's cholesterol, other tissues—including the walls of the arteries and intestines—also synthesize it. The rate of endogenous synthesis usually meets the body's needs; hence, severely reducing cholesterol intake, except in pregnant women and infants, probably causes little harm.

Functions of Cholesterol

Cholesterol participates in many complex bodily functions, including building plasma membranes and as a precursor in synthesizing vitamin D and adrenal gland hormones, as well as the sex hormones estrogen, androgen, and progesterone. Cholesterol provides a crucial component for the synthesis of bile, which emulsifies lipids during digestion and plays an important role in forming tissues, organs, and body structures during fetal development.

TABLE 1.5 presents the cholesterol content per serving of common foods from meat and dairy sources. Egg yolk contributes a rich source of cholesterol, as do red meats and organ meats (liver, kidney, and brains). Shellfish, particularly shrimp, and dairy products (ice cream, cream cheese, butter, and whole milk) contain relatively large amounts of cholesterol. Foods of plant origin contain *no* cholesterol.

Serum Cholesterol Levels and Heart Disease

Powerful predictors of coronary artery disease include high levels of total serum cholesterol and the cholesterol-rich LDL molecule. The risk becomes particularly apparent when combined with the other heart disease risk factors cigarette smoking, physical inactivity, obesity, and untreated hypertension. A continuous and graded relationship exists between serum cholesterol and death from coronary artery disease; thus, lowering cholesterol appears to offer prudent heart disease protection. For persons with heart disease, coronary blood flow improves (thus reducing myocardial ischemia during daily life) in 6 months or less when drug and diet therapy aggressively lower both total blood cholesterol and LDL cholesterol.[4] For example, drugs called statins reduce cholesterol by up to 60 $mg \cdot dL^{-1}$. Studies with animals show that a diet high in cholesterol and saturated fatty acids raises serum cholesterol in "susceptible" animals. This diet combination eventually produces **atherosclerosis**, a degenerative process that forms cholesterol-rich deposits **(plaque)** on the inner lining of medium and large arteries, which narrow and eventually close. In humans, dietary cholesterol raises the ratio of total cholesterol to HDL cholesterol to adversely affect the cholesterol risk profile. Reducing saturated fatty acid and cholesterol intake generally lowers serum cholesterol, although for most people the effect remains modest. Similarly, increasing dietary intake of monounsaturated and polyunsaturated fatty acids lowers blood cholesterol.[38] **TABLE 1.6** presents recommendations of the American Heart Association (AHA; www.americanheart.org) for levels of triacylglycerol, total cholesterol, and LDL and HDL subfractions.

A SIGNIFICANT DISEASE WITH SOBERING CONSEQUENCES

Cardiovascular disease claims the lives of more US citizens than the next six leading causes of death. More than 600 Americans die each day from heart attacks, of whom nearly one-half are women. Within 6 years of a first heart attack, nearly 20% of men and 35% of women will suffer a second attack.

RECOMMENDED DIETARY LIPID INTAKE

Recommendations for dietary lipid intake for physically active persons follow prudent recommendations for the general population. No firm standards for optimal lipid intake exist. Rather than providing a precise number for daily cholesterol intake, the AHA encourages Americans to focus more on replacing high-fat foods with fruits, vegetables, unrefined whole grains, fat-free and low-fat dairy products, fish, poultry, and lean meat. Other new components of the AHA guidelines include a focus on weight control and the addition of two weekly servings of fish high in omega-3 fatty acids. The American Cancer Society (www.cancer.org) advocates a diet that contains only 20% of its calories from lipid to reduce risk of cancers of the colon and rectum, prostate, endometrium, and perhaps breast. More drastic lowering of total dietary fat intake toward the 10% level may produce even more pronounced cholesterol-lowering effects, accompanied by clinical improvement for patients with established coronary heart disease.[64]

The AHA recommends a cholesterol intake of no more than 300 mg (0.01 oz) daily—almost the amount of cholesterol in an egg yolk—limiting intake to 100 mg per 1000 calories of food consumed. More desirable benefits occur by reducing daily cholesterol intake toward 150 to 200 mg. The main sources of dietary cholesterol include the same animal food sources rich in saturated fatty acids. Reducing intake of these foods not only reduces intake of preformed cholesterol but, more importantly, also reduces intake of saturated fatty acids that stimulate endogenous cholesterol synthesis.

TABLE 1.7 presents three daily menus, each consisting of 2000 kcal but with different percentages of total lipid. *Meal Plan A*, typical of the North American diet, consists of 38% of total calories from lipid. *Meal Plan B* contains 29% lipid, a value recommended by most health professionals. *Meal Plan C*, with 10% lipid, may be desirable from a health perspective but is difficult to maintain, particularly for physically active persons with high daily energy expenditures.

TABLE 1.5 Cholesterol Content of Some Common Foods

Food	Quantity	Cholesterol (mg)	Food	Quantity	Cholesterol (mg)
Meat			**Dairy**		
Brains, pan fried	3 oz	1696	Egg salad	1 cup	629
Liver, chicken	3 oz	537	Custard, baked	1 cup	213
Caviar	3 oz	497	Egg, yolk	1 large	211
Liver, beef, fried	3 oz	410	Ice cream, soft serve, vanilla	1 cup	153
Spare ribs, cooked	6 oz	198	Eggnog	1 cup	149
Shrimp, boiled	3 oz	166	Ice cream, rich	1 cup	88
Tuna, light, water pack	1 can	93	Pizza, cheese	1 slice	47
Chicken breast, fried, no skin	3 oz	91	Milk, whole	1 cup	34
Halibut, smoked	3 oz	86	Cottage cheese, large curd	1 cup	34
Lamb chop, broiled	1	84	Cheese, cheddar	1 oz	30
Abalone, fried	3 oz	80	Milk, low-fat, 2%	1 cup	18
Hamburger patty	3 oz	75	Chocolate milk shake	1 cup	13
Corned beef	3 oz	73	Butter	1 pat	11
Chicken or turkey, light meat	3 oz	70	Cottage cheese, low-fat, 1%	1 cup	10
Lobster, cooked	3 oz	61	Yogurt, low-fat with fruit	1 cup	10
Clams	3 oz	57	Buttermilk (>1% fat)	1 cup	9
Taco, beef	1	57	Milk, skim	1 cup	5
Swordfish, broiled	3 oz	50	Mayonnaise	1 tbsp	5
Bacon strips	3 pieces	36			
Hot dog	1	29			
Hot dog, beef	1	27			
French fries, McDonald's	Regular	13			

TABLE 1.6 American Heart Association Recommendations and Classifications for Total Cholesterol and HDL and LDL Cholesterol and Triacylglycerol

Category	
Total cholesterol level[a]	
≥240	High blood cholesterol. A person with this level has more than twice the risk of heart disease as someone with cholesterol below 200.
200–239	Borderline high.
≤200	Desirable level that puts you at a lower risk for heart disease. Cholesterol level of 200 or higher raises risk.
HDL cholesterol level	
<40	Low HDL cholesterol. A major risk factor for heart disease.
40–59	Higher HDL levels are better.
≥60	High HDL cholesterol. An HDL of 60 $mg \cdot dL^{-1}$ and above is considered protective against heart disease.
LDL cholesterol level	
>190	Very high; cholesterol-lowering drug therapies even if no heart disease and no risk factors.[b]
160–189	High; cholesterol-lowering drug therapies even if there is no heart disease but two or more risk factors are present.
130–159	Borderline high; cholesterol-lowering drug therapies if heart disease is present.
100–129	Near optimal; doctor may consider cholesterol-lowering drug therapies plus dietary modification if heart disease is present.
<100	Optimal; no therapy needed.

(continued)

TABLE 1.6 American Heart Association Recommendations and Classifications for Total Cholesterol and HDL and LDL Cholesterol and Triacylglycerol *(continued)*

Triacylglycerol level	
<150	Normal
150–199	Borderline high
200–499	High
≥500	Very high

[a] *All levels in mg·dL^{-1}.*

[b] *In men younger than age 35 and premenopausal women with LDL cholesterol levels of 190 to 219 mg·dL^{-1}, drug therapy should be delayed except in high-risk patients such as those with diabetes.*

TABLE 1.7 Three Different Daily Meal Plans, Each Consisting of 2000 Calories, but with Different Percentages of Total Fat

Plan A. 38% Fat Diet

Breakfast

1 apple Danish pastry
½ cup orange juice
1 cup whole milk

Lunch

2 slices of wheat bread
2 oz turkey breast
1 oz Swiss cheese
1 teaspoon mayonnaise
1 small banana
1 small bag potato chips (15 chips)

Snack

½ cup vanilla ice cream

Dinner

4 oz T-bone steak
1 large baked potato
1 ½ cup steamed broccoli
1 dinner roll
1 teaspoon margarine
2 tablespoons sour cream
1 ¼ cup fresh strawberries

Snack

15 grapes
2 chocolate chip cookies

Total calories: 1990
Total fat: 84 g; 38% of calories from fat
Saturated fat: less than 10%

Plan B. 29% Fat Diet

Breakfast

1 bagel
1 tablespoon cream cheese
½ cup orange juice
1 cup 1% milk

Lunch

2 slices of wheat bread
2 oz of turkey breast
1 teaspoon of mayonnaise
1 small banana
Lettuce salad with 2 cups of fresh vegetables—broccoli, cauliflower, carrots, cucumbers, cherry tomatoes
3 tablespoons reduced-calorie salad dressing

Snack

1 cup low-fat yogurt
1 fresh peach
6 cups of air-popped popcorn

Dinner

4 oz sirloin (grilled or broiled)
1 large baked potato
1 ½ cup steamed broccoli
1 dinner roll
1 tablespoon reduced-calorie margarine
2 tablespoons sour cream
1 ¼ cup strawberries

Snack

30 grapes

Total calories: 1971
Total fat: 63 g; 29% of calories from fat
Saturated fat: 7% of calories

Plan C. 10% Fat Diet

Breakfast

½ cup bran cereal with raisins
1 bagel
1 tablespoon cream cheese
½ cup orange juice
1 cup skimmed milk
½ grapefruit

Lunch

2 slices of wheat bread
2 oz of turkey breast
1 teaspoon mayonnaise
1 small banana
Lettuce salad with 3 cups of fresh vegetables—broccoli, cauliflower, carrots, cucumbers, cherry tomatoes
3 tablespoons fat-free salad dressing

Snack

1 cup nonfat yogurt
1 fresh peach
6 cups of air-popped popcorn

Dinner

1 large baked potato
1 ½ cup steamed broccoli
2 dinner rolls
1 teaspoon margarine
1 ¼ cup fresh strawberries
1 cup skimmed milk

Snack

30 grapes
1 cup skimmed milk

Total calories: 1990
Total fat: 21 g; 10% of calories from fat
Saturated fat: less than 3%

TABLE 1.8 Examples of Foods High and Low in Saturated Fatty Acids, Foods High in Monounsaturated and Polyunsaturated Fatty Acids, and the Polyunsaturated to Saturated Fatty Acid (P/S) Ratio of Common Fats and Oils

High saturated	**%**
Coconut oil	91
Palm kernel oil	82
Butter	68
Cream cheese	57
Coconut	56
Hollandaise sauce	54
Palm oil	51
Half & half	45
Cheese, Velveeta	43
Cheese, mozzarella	41
Ice cream, vanilla	38
Cheesecake	32
Chocolate almond bar	29
Low saturated	**%**
Popcorn	0
Hard candy	0
Yogurt, nonfat	2
Crackerjacks	3
Milk, skim	4
Cookies, fig bars	4
Graham crackers	5
Chicken breast, roasted	6
Pancakes	8
Cottage cheese, 1%	8
Milk, chocolate, 1%	9
Beef, dried	9
Chocolate, mints	10
High monounsaturated	**%**
Olives, black	80
Olive oil	75
Almond oil	70
Canola oil	61
Almonds, dry	52
Avocados	51
Peanut oil	48
Cashews, dry roasted	42
Peanut butter	39
Bologna	39
Beef, cooked	33
Lamb, roasted	32
Veal, roasted	26
High polyunsaturated	**%**
Safflower oil	77
Sunflower oil	72
Corn oil	58
Walnuts, dry	51
Sunflower seeds	47
Margarine, corn oil	45
Canola oil	32
Sesame seeds	31
Pumpkin seeds	31
Tofu	27
Lard	11
Butter	6
Coconut oil	2
P/S Ratio, Fats and Oils	
Coconut oil	0.2/1.0
Palm oil	0.2/1.0
Butter	0.1/1.0
Olive oil	0.6/1.0
Lard	0.3/1.0
Canola oil	5.3/1.0
Peanut oil	1.9/1.0
Soybean oil	2.5/1.0
Sesame oil	3.0/1.0
Margarine, 100% corn oil	2.5/1.0
Cottonseed oil	2.0/1.0
Mayonnaise	3.7/1.0
Safflower oil	13.3/1.0

Ratio of Polyunsaturated to Saturated Fatty Acids

TABLE 1.8 lists examples of foods high and low in saturated fatty acids, foods high in monounsaturated and polyunsaturated fatty acids, and the ratio of polyunsaturated to saturated fatty acids **(P/S ratio)**. One should attempt to maintain the P/S ratio at least at 1:1 and preferably at 2:1. Based on dietary surveys, the P/S ratio in the United States ranges between 0.43 and 1.0. The P/S ratio has some limitations and should not be used exclusively to guide lipid intake. For example, the ratio does not consider the potential cholesterol-lowering role of monounsaturated fatty acids if they replace the diet's saturated fatty acids. Nevertheless, the P/S ratio provides useful information about the fatty acid content of food, provided the food source lists the fatty acid types.

ROLE OF LIPID IN THE BODY

Four important functions of lipids in the body include:

1. Energy reserve
2. Protection of vital organs
3. Thermal insulation
4. Transport medium for fat-soluble vitamins and hunger suppressor

Additional Insights

Diet Versus Drugs in the Lowering of Cholesterol

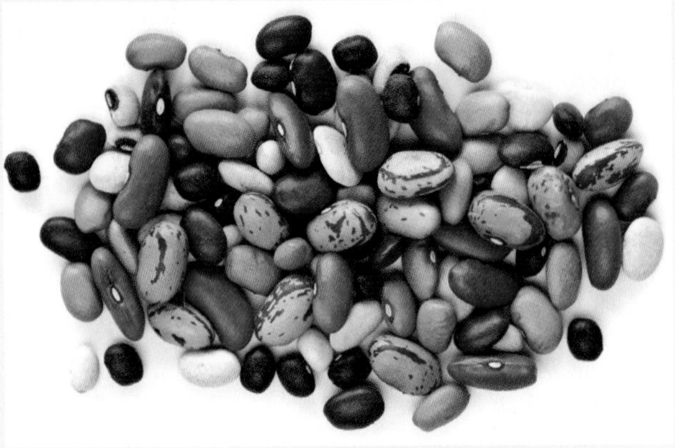

Food *quality* may surpass total fat *quantity* in the battle to lower undesirable blood lipids. That diet can positively impact blood cholesterol and subsequent heart disease risk is well known, but knowledge of the foods that exert the greatest beneficial effect continues to evolve. A recent study systematically examined whether foods considered by the US Food and Drug Administration (FDA; www.fda.org) to lower blood cholesterol could be incorporated into one's diet and produce positive effects in lowering the harmful LDL cholesterol. One diet, a vegetarian-type diet, comprised cholesterol-lowering foods that emphasized nuts, beans, plant sterols, soy protein, and high-viscous fiber grains at two levels of counseling (delivered at different frequencies). The other nonvegetarian low-fat diet focused on low quantities of saturated fat. To evaluate the power of dietary modifications alone on cholesterol lowering, 351 Canadian citizens with elevated cholesterol were placed into one of three groups, all assigned to diets for a 6-month period. Persons on the low–saturated fat (control) diet reduced LDL cholesterol by 8 $mg \cdot dL^{-1}$ compared with decreases of 24 and 26 $mg \cdot dL^{-1}$ on diets composed of plant-based fat and protein—some 13% more than the group eating the low–saturated fat diet.

The cholesterol-lowering effect was large enough to indicate that dietary changes alone could serve as an alternative to statin medications (e.g., Lovastatin, Pravastatin, Atorvastatin, Zocor, Lipitor, Crestor), which have side effects on liver and muscular function.

The new research challenges the notion that simply reducing the diet's content of saturated fat from red meat and dairy product sources is the most effective cholesterol-lowering medical strategy. Evidence now supports the wisdom of consuming a cholesterol-lowering diet of healthful sources of plant-based fat and protein foods from the following four categories:

1. Plant sterol–enriched margarine
2. Peanuts and tree nuts
3. Soy milk, tofu, and soy "meat" products
4. Oats, barley, and other "sticky" or viscous fibers

Source: Jenkins DJ, et al. Effect of a dietary portfolio of cholesterol-lowering foods given at 2 levels of intensity of dietary advice on serum lipids in hyperlipidemia: a randomized controlled diet. *JAMA* 2011;306:831.

Related Literature

Chainani-Wu N, et al. Changes in emerging cardiac biomarkers after an intensive lifestyle intervention. *Am J Cardiol* 2011;108:498.

Krauss RM, et al. AHA dietary guidelines revision 2000: a statement for health care professionals from the Nutrition Committee of the American Heart Association. *Circulation* 2000;102:2284.

Liese AD, et al. Whole-grain intake and insulin sensitivity: the Insulin Resistance Atherosclerosis Study. *Am J Clin Nutr* 2003;78:965.

McIntosh, M, Miller C. A diet containing food rich in soluble and insoluble fiber improves glycemic control and reduces hyperlipidemia among patients with type 2 diabetes. *Nutr Revs* 2001;59:52.

Ornish D, et al. Intensive lifestyle changes for reversal of coronary heart disease. *JAMA* 1998;280:2001.

Energy Source and Reserve

Fat constitutes the ideal cellular fuel because each molecule carries large quantities of energy per unit weight, transports and stores easily, and provides a readily available energy source. In well-nourished persons at rest, fat provides up to 80 to 90% of the energy requirement. One gram of pure lipid contains about 9 kcal (38 kJ) of energy, more than *twice* the energy available to the body in an equal quantity of carbohydrate or protein from the greater quantity of hydrogen in the lipid molecule. Chapter 4 points out that oxidation of hydrogen atoms provides the energy for bodily functions at rest and during exercise. Recall that synthesis of one triacylglycerol molecule from glycerol and three fatty acid molecules creates three water molecules. In contrast, when glucose forms glycogen, 2.7 g of water stores with each gram. *Whereas fat exists as a relatively water-free, concentrated fuel, glycogen becomes hydrated and therefore "heavy" relative to its energy content.*

FIGURE 1.15 illustrates the total mass (and energy content) from fat and various body fat depots in an 80-kg man. Approximately 15% of the body mass for men and 25% for women consists of fat. The potential energy stored in the fat molecules of a typical 80-kg young adult man translates to about 110,700 kcal (12,300 g body fat × 9.0 $kcal \cdot g^{-1}$). Most of this energy—present as adipose tissue and intramuscular triacylglycerols and a small amount of plasma free fatty

PERSONAL HEALTH AND EXERCISE NUTRITION 1.2

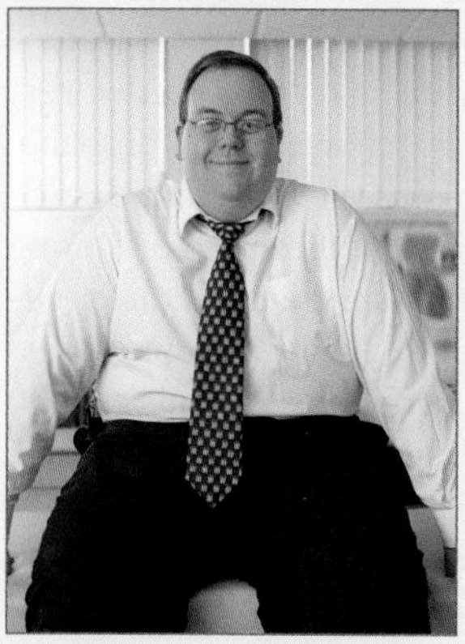

Adult Hyperlipidemia

The following data were obtained on a 58-year-old executive who has not had an annual physical examination in 5 years. He has gained weight and is now concerned about his health status.

Medical History

The patient has no history of chronic diseases or major hospitalization. He does not take medications or dietary supplements and has no known food allergies.

Family History

The patient's father died from a heart attack at age 61; his younger brother has had triple bypass surgery, and his uncle has type 2 diabetes. His mother, physically inactive for most of her adult life, classifies as obese with high serum cholesterol and triacylglycerol levels.

Social History

The patient has been overweight since high school. He has gained 15 lb during the last year, which he attributes to his job and changes in eating habits (eats out more frequently). The patient, J.M., wants to improve his diet but does not know what to do. He typically eats only two meals daily, with at least one meal consumed at a restaurant and several snacks interspersed. He drinks three to five cups of coffee throughout the day and two to three alcoholic drinks every evening. He also smokes one pack of cigarettes daily and reports high stress in his job and at home (two teenage children). Patient states he has little opportunity for exercise or leisure time activities given his present schedule.

Physical Examination/Anthropometric/Laboratory Data

- Blood pressure: 135/90 mm Hg
- Height: 6 ft (182.9 cm)
- Body weight: 215 lb (97.1 kg)
- Body mass index (BMI): 29.0
- Abdominal girth: 40.9 in (104 cm)
- Laboratory data
  - Nonfasting total cholesterol: 267 $mg \cdot dL^{-1}$
  - HDL-C: 34 $mg \cdot dL^{-1}$
  - LDL-C: 141 $mg \cdot dL^{-1}$
  - Blood glucose: 124 $mg \cdot dL^{-1}$
- Dietary intake from 24-hour food recall
  - Calories: 3001 kcal
  - Protein: 110 g (14.7% of total kcal)
  - Lipid: 121 g (36.3% of total kcal)
  - Carbohydrate: 368 g (49% of total kcal)
  - Saturated fatty acids: 18% of total kcal
  - Monounsaturated fatty acids (MUFA): 7% of total kcal
  - Cholesterol: 390 $mg \cdot dL^{-1}$
  - Fiber: 10 g
  - Folic acid: 200 μg
- General impressions: overly fat male with possible metabolic syndrome

Case Questions

1. Provide an overall assessment of the patient's health status.
2. What other laboratory tests could be performed?
3. Interpret the blood lipid profile based on his history, physical examination, and laboratory data.
4. Give recommendations for improving the adequacy of patient's diet.
5. Create the best dietary approach for the patient.
6. What course of action should the patient consider to improve his blood lipid profile?

thePoint *Visit* **thePoint.lww.com/MKKSEN4e** *to review the answers to these case questions.*

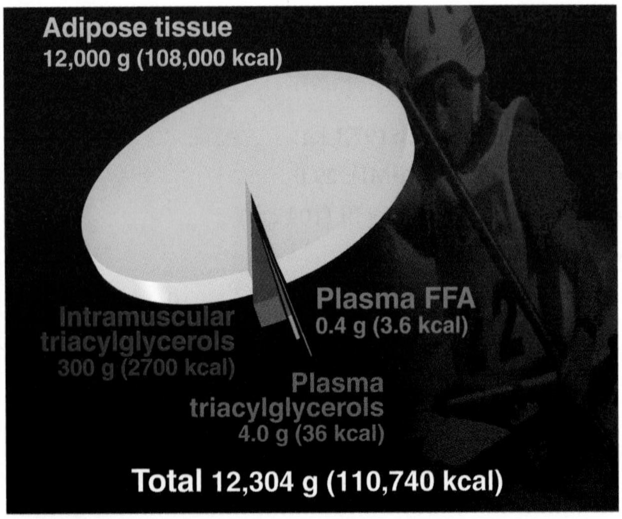

FIGURE 1.15. Distribution of fat energy in an average 80-kg man.

acids—remains available for exercise. This amount of energy would fuel the approximate 950-mile run from Oklahoma City, OK to Tempe, AZ, or Atlanta, GA, to Wichita, KS (assuming an energy expenditure of about 100 kcal a mile). Contrast this fact to the limited 2000-kcal reserve of stored carbohydrate that could only fuel a 20-mile run. Viewed from a different perspective, the body's energy reserves from carbohydrate could power high-intensity running for about 1.6 hours, whereas fat reserves would allow the person to continue for about 120 hours! As is the case for carbohydrate, fat used as a fuel "spares" protein to carry out its important functions of tissue synthesis and repair.

Protection and Insulation

Up to 4% of the body's fat protects against trauma to the heart, liver, kidneys, spleen, brain, and spinal cord. Fats stored just below the skin (subcutaneous fat) provide insulation, determining ability to tolerate extremes of cold exposure. Swimmers who excelled in swimming the English Channel showed only a slight fall in body temperature while resting in cold water and essentially no lowering effect while swimming.[68] In contrast, the body temperature of leaner, non-Channel swimmers decreased markedly under rest and exercise conditions. The insulatory layer of fat probably affords little protection except in cold-related activities such as deep-sea diving or ocean or channel swimming or among Arctic inhabitants. Excess body fat hinders temperature regulation during heat stress, most notably during sustained exercise in air when the body's heat production can increase 20 times above the resting level. The insulation shield from subcutaneous fat retards the flow of heat from the body.

For large football linemen, excess fat storage provides additional cushioning to protect from the sport's normal hazards. Any possible protective benefit, however, must be evaluated against the liability imposed by the "dead weight" of excess fat and its effect on energy expenditure, thermal regulation, and exercise performance.

Vitamin Carrier and Hunger Depressor

Consuming about 20 g of dietary lipid daily provides a sufficient source and transport medium for the fat-soluble vitamins A, D, E, and K. Significantly reducing lipid intake depresses the body's level of these vitamins, which ultimately may lead to vitamin deficiency. Dietary lipid also facilitates absorption of vitamin A precursors from nonlipid plant sources like carrots and apricots. It takes about 3.5 hours after ingesting lipids to empty them from the stomach. Thus, some lipid in the diet can delay the onset of "hunger pangs" and contribute to satiety following the meal. This helps to explain why reducing diets containing a small amount of lipid sometimes prove initially more successful in blunting the immediate urge to eat than do more extreme fat-free diets.

SUMMARY

1. Lipids, like carbohydrates, contain carbon, hydrogen, and oxygen atoms, but with a higher ratio of hydrogen to oxygen. For example, the lipid stearin has the formula $C_{57}H_{110}O_6$. Lipid molecules consist of one glycerol molecule and three fatty acid molecules.
2. Lipids, synthesized by plants and animals, are grouped into one of three categories: (1) simple lipids (glycerol plus three fatty acids), (2) compound lipids (phospholipids, glycolipids, and lipoproteins) composed of simple lipids combined with other chemicals, and (3) derived lipids like cholesterol, synthesized from simple and compound lipids.
3. Saturated fatty acids contain as many hydrogen atoms as chemically possible; thus, "saturated" describes this molecule with respect to hydrogen. Saturated fatty acids exist primarily in animal meat, egg yolk, dairy fats, and cheese. Dietary intakes high in saturated fatty acids elevate blood cholesterol and promote coronary heart disease.
4. Unsaturated fatty acids contain fewer hydrogen atoms attached to the carbon chain. Instead, double bonds connect carbon atoms, and the fatty acid exists as either

SUMMARY *(continued)*

monounsaturated or polyunsaturated with respect to hydrogen. Heart disease protection occurs from increasing the diet's proportion of unsaturated fatty acids.

5. Dietary *trans* fatty acids may account for 30,000 deaths annually from heart disease. High intake of this fatty acid also increases risk for contracting type 2 diabetes.
6. Perhaps the most powerful cardioprotective benefit of fish oils relates to their antiarrhythmic effect on myocardial tissue. The unique effects of these dietary fatty acids on the fatty acid content of the myocardial cell membranes likely provide protection against ventricular arrhythmias and sudden death.
7. Lowering blood cholesterol, especially that carried by LDL, reduces coronary heart disease risk.
8. Dietary lipid currently provides about 36% of total energy intake. Prudent advice recommends a 30% level or lower for dietary lipid, of which 70 to 80% should consist of unsaturated fatty acids.
9. Lipids provide the largest nutrient store of potential energy for biologic work. They also protect vital organs, provide insulation from the cold, and transport the fat-soluble vitamins A, D, E, and K.

PROTEINS

NATURE OF PROTEINS

The body of an average-sized adult contains between 10 and 12 kg of protein, primarily located within skeletal muscle mass. Structurally, proteins (from the Greek word meaning "of prime importance") resemble carbohydrates and lipids because they too contain atoms of carbon, oxygen, and hydrogen. Protein molecules also contain about 16% nitrogen, along with sulfur and occasionally phosphorus, cobalt, and iron. Just as glycogen forms from many simple glucose subunits linked together, the protein molecule polymerizes from its **amino acid** "building-block" constituents in endlessly complex arrays. **Peptide bonds** link amino acids in chains that take on diverse forms and chemical combinations. The hydrogen from the amino acid side chain of one amino acid combines with the hydroxyl group of the carboxylic (organic) acid end of another amino acid. Two joined amino acids produce a **dipeptide**, and linking three amino acids produces a **tripeptide**, and so on. A linear configuration of up to 100 amino acids produces a **polypeptide**, while combining more than 100 amino acids forms a **protein**. Three amino acids make up thyrotropin-releasing hormone, whereas the muscle protein myosin forms from the linkage of 4500 amino acid units. Single cells contain thousands of different protein molecules. In total, approximately 50,000 different protein-containing compounds exist in the body. The biochemical functions and properties of each protein depend on the sequence of specific amino acids.

Each of the 20 different amino acids required by the body has a positively charged amine group at one end and a negatively charged organic acid group at the other end. The amine group consists of two hydrogen atoms attached to nitrogen (NH_2), whereas the organic acid group (technically termed a *carboxylic acid group*) contains one carbon atom, two oxygen atoms, and one hydrogen atom (COOH). The remainder of the amino acid molecule may take several different forms, referred to as the amino acid's functional group, or **side chain**. *The side chain's unique structure dictates the amino acid's particular characteristics.* **FIGURE 1.16 A** shows the structure for the amino acid alanine.

AN UNLIMITED POTENTIAL TO SYNTHESIZE PROTEIN COMPOUNDS

The potential for combining the 20 amino acids creates an almost infinite number of possible proteins. For example, proteins formed from linking just three different amino acids could generate 20^3 or 8000 different proteins, and just six different amino acids could yield 64 million proteins (20^6).

KINDS OF PROTEINS

The body cannot synthesize eight amino acids (nine in children and some older adults), so they must be ingested preformed in foods. Isoleucine, leucine, lysine, methionine, phenylalanine, threonine, tryptophan, and valine make up these essential amino acids. The body also synthesizes cystine from methionine and tyrosine from phenylalanine. Infants cannot synthesize histidine, and children have reduced capability for synthesizing arginine. The body manufactures the

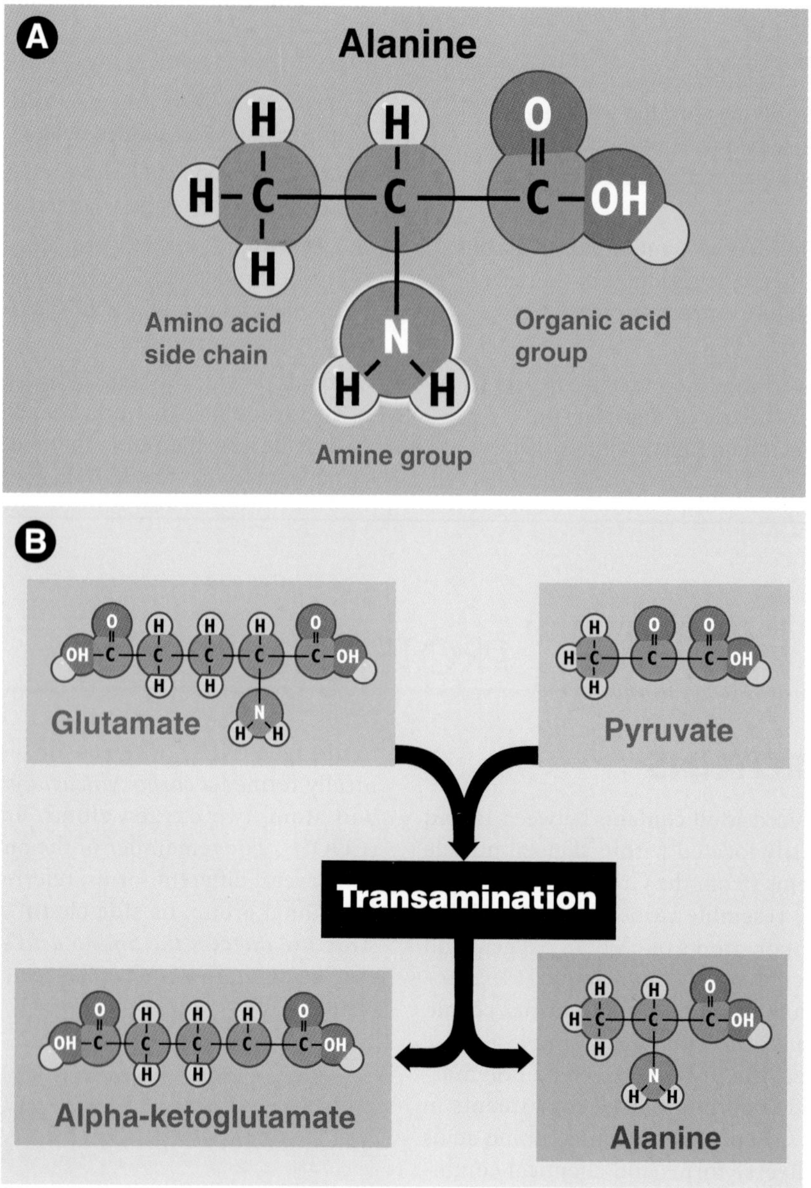

FIGURE 1.16. A. Chemical structure of the amino acid alanine. **B.** Transamination occurs when an amine group from a donor amino acid transfers to an acceptor acid to form a new amino acid.

remaining nine nonessential amino acids. The term nonessential does not mean they are unimportant; rather, they must be synthesized from other compounds already in the body at a rate to meet demands for normal growth and tissue repair.

Fortunately, animals and plants manufacture proteins that contain essential amino acids. No health or physiologic advantage exists from an amino acid derived from an animal compared with the same amino acid from vegetable origin. Plants synthesize amino acids by incorporating nitrogen in the soil along with carbon, oxygen, and hydrogen from air and water. In contrast, animals do not possess broad capability for protein synthesis; they ingest most of their protein.

Synthesizing a specific protein requires the availability of appropriate amino acids. **Complete proteins**, or higher quality proteins, come from foods with all of the essential amino acids in the quantity and the correct ratio to maintain nitrogen balance and allow tissue growth and repair. An **incomplete protein**, or lower quality protein, lacks one or more essential amino acid. Incomplete protein diets eventually lead to protein malnutrition. This occurs whether or not the food sources contain adequate energy or protein quantity.

Protein Sources

Sources of complete protein include eggs, milk, meat, fish, and poultry. Among all food sources, eggs provide the optimal mixture of essential amino acids; hence, eggs receive the highest quality rating of 100 for comparison with other foods. **TABLE 1.9** rates common sources of dietary protein. Presently, animal sources provide almost two thirds of the dietary protein, whereas 85 years ago, protein consumption occurred equally from plant and animal origins. Reliance on animal sources for dietary protein largely accounts for the relatively high intake of cholesterol and saturated fatty acids in the world's major industrialized nations.

The **biologic value** of a food refers to its completeness for supplying essential amino acids. Higher quality protein foods come from animal sources, whereas vegetables (lentils, dried beans and peas, nuts, and cereals) remain incomplete in one or more essential amino acid; thus, these have a relatively lower biologic value. The animal protein collagen remains an exception because it lacks the essential amino acid tryptophan. This protein forms part of the connective tissue of animals. **TABLE 1.10** lists examples of good food sources of protein.

The Vegetarian Approach

Eating various plant foods (grains, fruits, and vegetables) supplies all of the essential amino acids, each providing a different quality and quantity of amino acids. Grains and legumes supply excellent protein content, but neither offers the full complement of essential amino acids. An exception may be well-processed, isolated soybean protein, termed *soy-protein isolates,* whose protein quality matches that of some animal proteins. Grains lack the essential amino acid lysine, whereas legumes contain lysine but lack the sulfur-containing essential amino acid methionine found abundantly in grains. Tortillas and beans, rice and beans, rice and lentils, rice and peas, and peanuts and wheat (bread) serve as staples in many cultures because they provide **complementary protein** sources of all essential amino acids from the plant kingdom. According to the American Dietetic Association (www.eatright.org), "appropriately planned vegetarian diets, including total vegetarian or vegan diets, are healthful, nutritionally adequate, and may provide health benefits in the prevention and treatment of certain diseases. Well-planned vegetarian diets are appropriate for persons during all stages of the life cycle, including pregnancy, lactation, infancy, childhood, and adolescence, and for athletes."[18]

True vegetarians or **vegans** consume nutrients from only two sources—the plant kingdom and dietary supplements. Many physically active vegetarians are at somewhat greater risk for inadequate energy and nutrient intake because they eliminate meat and dairy products from the diet and increasingly rely on foods relatively low in energy, quality protein, and some micronutrients. Vegans make up less than 1% of the US population, although between 5 and 7% of Americans consider themselves "almost" vegetarians. Nutritional diversity remains the key for these men and women. For example, a vegan diet provides all the essential amino acids if the recommended dietary allowance (RDA) for protein contains 60% of protein from grain products, 35% from legumes, and 5% from green leafy vegetables. A 70-kg person obtains all essential amino acids by consuming about 56 g of protein from approximately $1^1/_4$ cups of beans, $^1/_4$ cup of seeds or nuts, 4 slices of whole-grain bread, 2 cups of vegetables (1 cup of leafy green), and $2^1/_2$ cups of grain sources (brown rice, oatmeal, and cracked wheat).

TABLE 1.10 Good Food Sources of Protein

Food	Serving	Protein (g)
Animal		
Tuna	3 oz	22
Turkey, light meat	4 oz	9
Fish	3 oz	17
Hamburger	4 oz	30
Egg, whole	1 large	6
Egg, white	1 large	4
Beef, lean	4 oz	24
Dairy		
Cottage cheese	0.5 cup	15
Yogurt, low fat	8 oz	11
Cheese	1 oz	8
Milk, skim	8 oz	8
Plant		
Peanuts	1 oz	7
Peanut butter	1 tbsp	4
Pasta, dry	2 oz	7
Whole-wheat bread	2 slices	6
Baked beans	1 cup	14
Tofu	3.5 oz	11
Almonds, dried	12	3
Chick peas	0.5 cup	20
Lentils	0.5 cup	9

TABLE 1.9 Rating of Protein Quality of Dietary Sources of Protein

Food	Protein Rating
Eggs	100
Fish	70
Lean beef	69
Cow's milk	60
Brown rice	57
White rice	56
Soybeans	47
Brewer's hash	45
Whole-grain wheat	44
Peanuts	43
Dry beans	34
White potato	34

A POTENTIALLY HEALTHFUL AND NUTRITIOUS WAY FOR ATHLETES TO EAT

Well-balanced vegetarian and vegetarian-type diets provide abundant carbohydrate, crucial during intense, prolonged training. Such diets correlated with reduced body weight and a lower incidence of certain chronic diseases. They contain little or no cholesterol, are high in fiber, and are rich in fruit and vegetable sources of antioxidant vitamins and diverse phytochemicals.

An Increasing Number of Near-Vegetarian Athletes

An increasing number of competitive and champion athletes consume diets composed predominately of nutrients from varied plant sources, including some dairy and meat products. Considering how much time it requires to train and prepare for competition, vegetarian athletes often encounter difficulty in planning, selecting, and preparing nutritious meals from predominantly plant sources without relying on supplementation.[7,87] Approximately two thirds of the world's population subsist on largely vegetarian diets with little reliance on animal protein.

Controlled clinical trials generally conclude that substituting soy protein for animal protein decreases blood pressure, plasma homocysteine levels, triacylglycerol, total cholesterol, and harmful oxidized LDL cholesterol, without reducing beneficial HDL cholesterol.[39,89] For example, daily consumption of as little as 20 g of soy protein instead of animal protein for 6 weeks favorably modified blood lipid profiles.[83] Genistein, a component of soy, also may offer protection against breast cancer.[48]

Obtaining ample higher quality protein becomes the strict vegetarian's main nutritional concern. Children on vegan diets should be monitored to ensure adequate vitamin D and calcium intake, which most Americans obtain from milk products. A **lactovegetarian diet** provides milk and related products such as ice cream, cheese, and yogurt. The lactovegetarian approach minimizes the problem of consuming sufficient higher quality protein and increases the intake of calcium, phosphorus, and vitamin B_{12} (produced by bacteria in the digestive tract of animals). Good meatless sources of iron include fortified ready-to-eat cereals, soybeans, and cooked farina; cereals, wheat germ, and oysters contain high zinc levels. Adding an egg to the diet **(ovolactovegetarian diet)** ensures intake of higher quality protein.

FIGURE 1.17 displays the contribution of various food groups to the protein content of the American diet. By far, the greatest protein intake comes from animal sources, with only about 30% derived from plant sources.

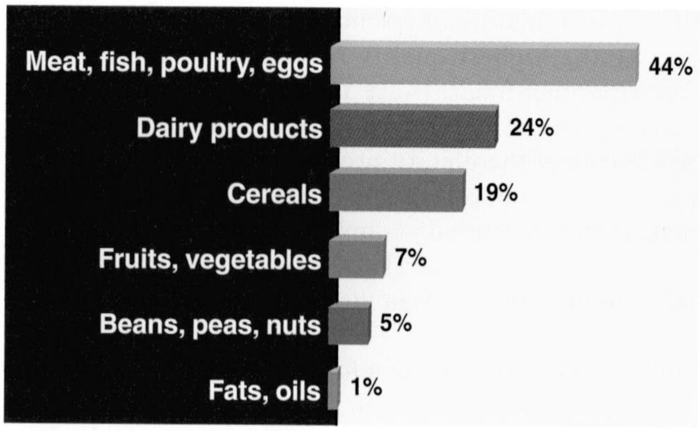

FIGURE 1.17. Contribution from major food groups to the protein content of the typical American diet.

RECOMMENDED DIETARY PROTEIN INTAKE

Despite the beliefs of many coaches, trainers, and athletes, no benefit accrues from eating excessive protein. An intake exceeding three times the recommended level does *not* enhance work capacity during intensive training. *For athletes, muscle mass does not increase simply by eating high-protein foods or special amino acid mixtures.* If lean tissue synthesis resulted from the extra protein consumed by the typical athlete, then muscle mass would increase tremendously. For example, consuming an extra 100 g (400 kcal) of protein daily translates into a daily 500-g (1.1-lb) increase in muscle mass. This obviously does not happen. Excessive dietary protein ultimately is used directly for energy (following deamination) or recycled as components of other molecules, including stored fat in subcutaneous adipose tissue depots. Harmful side effects can occur when dietary protein intake significantly exceeds recommended values. A high protein catabolism strains liver and kidney functions owing to the required elimination of urea and other compounds.

The Recommended Dietary Allowance

The **RDA** for protein, vitamins, and minerals represents a liberal standard for nutrient intake expressed as a daily average. These guidelines were initially developed in May 1942 by the Food and Nutrition Board of the National Research Council/National Academy of Science (www.nas.edu/iom) to evaluate and plan for the nutritional adequacy of groups rather than of individuals. RDA levels represent a liberal yet safe excess to prevent nutritional deficiencies in practically all healthy people. In the 11th edition (1999), RDA recommendations included 19 nutrients, energy intake, and the **Estimated Safe and Adequate Daily Dietary Intakes (ESADDI)** for seven additional vitamins and minerals and three electrolytes. The ESADDI should be viewed as more tentative and evolutionary than the RDA. ESADDI recommendations for certain essential micronutrients (e.g., vitamins biotin and pantothenic acid and trace elements copper, manganese, fluoride, selenium, chromium, and molybdenum) required sufficient scientific data to formulate an intake range considered adequate and safe, yet insufficient for a precise single RDA. Any intake within this range is considered acceptable for maintaining adequate physiologic function and sufficient to prevent underexposure or overexposure. No RDA or ESADDI exists for sodium, potassium, and chlorine; instead, recommendations refer to a minimum requirement for health.

We emphasize that the RDA reflects an ongoing evaluation based on available data for the nutritional needs of a *population* over a prolonged period. Specific individual requirements can be determined only by laboratory measurements. Malnutrition occurs from cumulative weeks, months, and even years of inadequate nutrient intake. Someone who regularly consumes a diet containing nutrients below the RDA standards may not become malnourished. Rather, the RDA represents a probability statement for adequate nutrition; as nutrient intake falls below the RDA, the statistical probability for malnourishment increases for that person. The chance increases progressively with lower nutrient intake. In Chapter 2, we discuss the **Dietary Reference Intakes**, which represent the current set of standards for recommended intake of nutrients and other food components.

TABLE 1.11 lists the protein RDAs for infants, children, adolescents, and adult men and women. On average, 0.83 g of protein per kg of body mass represents the recommended daily intake. To determine protein requirement for men and women ages 18 to 65, multiply body mass in kilograms by 0.83. Thus, for a 90-kg man, total protein requirement equals 75 g (90 × 0.83). The protein RDA holds even for overweight persons; it includes a reserve of about 25% to account for individual differences in protein requirement for about 98% of the population. Generally, the protein RDA (and the quantity of the required essential amino acids) decreases with age. In contrast, the protein RDA for infants and growing children of 2.0 to 4.0 g per kg of body mass facilitates growth and development. Pregnancy requires that daily protein intake increase by 20 g, and nursing mothers should increase intake by 10 g. *A 10% increase in the calculated protein requirement, particularly for a vegetarian-type diet, accounts for dietary fiber's effect in reducing the digestibility of many plant-based protein sources.* Stress, disease, and injury usually increase the protein requirement.

TABLE 1.11 Average Daily Energy Allowance and Recommended Protein Intakes

		Weight[a]		Height[a]		Average Energy Allowance (kcal)[b]		RDA for Protein
Category	Age (years) or Condition	(kg)	(lb)	(cm)	(in)	$kcal \cdot kg^{-1}$	$kcal \cdot d^{-1}$ [c]	$g \cdot d^{-1}$
Infants	0.0–0.5	6	13	60	24	108	650	13
	0.5–1.0	9	20	71	28	89	850	14
Children	1–3	13	29	90	35	102	1300	16
	4–6	20	44	112	44	90	1800	24
	7–10	28	62	132	52	70	2000	28
Males	11–14	45	99	157	62	55	2500	45
	15–18	66	145	176	69	45	3000	59
	19–24	72	160	177	70	40	2900	58
	25–50	79	174	176	70	37	2900	63
	51+	77	170	173	68	30	2300	63
Females	11–14	46	101	157	62	47	2200	46
	15–18	55	120	163	64	40	2200	44
	19–24	58	128	164	65	38	2200	46
	25–50	63	138	163	64	36	2200	50
	51+	65	143	160	63	30	1900	50
Pregnant	First trimester						0	60
	Second trimester						+300	60
	Third trimester						+500	60
Lactating	First 6 months						+500	65
	Second 6 months						+500	62

Source: *National Research Council, Food and Nutrition Board.*

[a] *Weights and heights represent median values.*

[b] *In the range of light-to-moderate activity, the coefficient of variation equals ± 20%.*

[c] *Figure is rounded.*

Some Modifications Required for Recommended Protein Intake for Physically Active Persons

A continuing area of controversy concerns the necessity of a larger than normal protein requirement for still growing adolescent athletes, persons involved in strength development programs that enhance muscle growth and endurance training regimens that increase protein breakdown, and athletes subjected to recurring tissue microtrauma, like wrestlers and football players.[13,29,35,57,65,66,82] Inadequate protein and energy intake can induce a loss of body protein, particularly from skeletal muscle with concomitant performance deterioration. *A definitive answer remains elusive, but protein breakdown above the resting level occurs during intense endurance training and resistance training to a greater degree than previously believed.* Increased protein catabolism occurs to a greater extent when exercising with low carbohydrate reserves and/or low energy intakes. Unfortunately, research has not pinpointed protein requirements for persons who train 4 to 6 hours daily by resistance exercise. Their protein needs may average only slightly more than for sedentary persons. In addition, despite increased protein use for energy during intense training, adaptations may augment the body's efficiency in using dietary protein to enhance amino acid balance. *Until research clarifies this issue, we recommend that athletes who train intensely should consume between 1.2 and 1.8 g of protein/kg of body mass daily.* This protein intake falls within the range typically consumed by physically active men and women, thereby obviating the need to consume supplementary protein.[3,5,29]

With adequate protein intake, consuming animal sources of protein does not facilitate muscle strength or size gains with resistance training compared with protein intake from plant sources.[31] Chapter 7 presents a more complete discussion of protein balance and requirements in exercise and training.

ROLE OF PROTEIN IN THE BODY

Blood plasma, visceral tissue, and muscle represent the three major sources of body protein. No body "reservoirs" of this macronutrient exist. All protein contributes to tissue structures or exists as important constituents of metabolic, transport, and hormonal systems. Protein constitutes between 12 and 15% of the body mass, but the protein content of different cells varies considerably. A brain cell, for example, consists of only about 10% protein, while red blood cells and muscle cells include up to 20% of their total weight as protein. The protein content of skeletal muscle represents about 65% of the body's total protein. This quantity can increase somewhat with exercise training depending on the nature of the training regimen, training duration, type of workout, and other interrelated factors.

Amino acids provide the major building blocks for synthesizing the body's various tissues. They also incorporate nitrogen into RNA and DNA compounds, into the coenzyme electron carriers NAD^+ and FAD (see Chapter 5), into the heme components of the oxygen-binding hemoglobin and myoglobin compounds, into the catecholamine hormones epinephrine and norepinephrine, and into the neurotransmitter serotonin (biochemically derived from tryptophan). Amino acids activate vitamins that play a key role in metabolic and physiologic regulation. **Anabolism** refers to tissue-building processes; the amino acid requirement for anabolism can vary considerably. For example, tissue anabolism accounts for about one third of the protein intake during rapid growth in infancy and childhood. As growth rate declines, so does the percentage of protein retained for anabolic processes. Once a person attains optimal body size and growth stabilizes, a continual turnover still occurs for the tissue's existing protein component.

Proteins serve as primary constituents for plasma membranes and internal cellular material. Proteins in the cell nuclei called nucleoproteins "supervise" cellular protein synthesis and transmission of hereditary characteristics. Collagenous **structural proteins** compose the hair, skin, nails, bones, tendons, and ligaments. Another classification, **globular proteins**, constitutes nearly 2000 different enzymes that modulate the rate of chemical reactions and regulate catabolism of fats, carbohydrates, and proteins for energy release. Blood plasma also contains the specialized proteins thrombin, fibrin, and fibrinogen required for blood clotting. Within red blood cells, the oxygen-carrying compound hemoglobin contains the large globin protein molecule that surrounds and protects the heme molecule.

Proteins play a role in regulating the acid-base quality of the body fluids. Buffering neutralizes excess acid metabolites formed during relatively intense exercise. The structural proteins actin and myosin play an essential role in muscle action; these proteins slide past each other as muscles shorten and lengthen during movement. Even in older adults, the body's protein-containing structures "turn over" on a regular basis; normal protein dynamics require adequate protein intake simply to replace the amino acids continually degraded in the turnover process.

DYNAMICS OF PROTEIN METABOLISM

Dietary protein primarily supplies amino acids for the various anabolic processes. In addition, some catabolism of protein for energy takes place. In well-nourished persons at rest, protein breakdown contributes between 2 and 5% of the body's total energy requirement. During **catabolism**, protein first degrades into its amino acid components. The amino acid molecule then loses its nitrogen (amine group) in the liver by the process of **deamination**. This "freed" nitrogen forms **urea** (H_2NCONH_2), first isolated from urine in 1727 by Dutch scientist Herman Boerhaave (1668–1738). The remaining deaminated carbon compound not excreted by the kidneys can take one of three routes:

1. Synthesized to a new amino acid
2. Converted to carbohydrate or fat
3. Catabolized directly for energy

Urea formed in deamination (including some ammonia) leaves the body in solution as urine. Excessive protein catabolism promotes fluid loss because urea must be dissolved in water for excretion.

In muscle, enzymes facilitate nitrogen removal from certain amino acids and subsequently pass this nitrogen to other compounds in the biochemical reactions of **transamination** (**FIG. 1.16 B**). An amino group shifts from a donor amino acid to an acceptor acid (keto acid), the acceptor thus becoming a new amino acid. A specific transferase enzyme accelerates the transamination reaction. This allows amino acid formation from non–nitrogen-carrying organic compounds formed in metabolism (e.g., pyruvate). In both deamination and transamination, the resulting carbon skeleton of the nonnitrogenous amino acid residue further degrades during energy metabolism.

Fate of Amino Acids After Nitrogen Removal

After deamination, the remaining carbon skeletons of the α-keto acids pyruvate, oxaloacetate, or α-ketoglutarate follow one of three distinct biochemical routes (**FIG. 1.18**):

1. Gluconeogenesis—18 of the 20 amino acids serve as a source for glucose synthesis
2. Energy source—the carbon skeletons oxidize for energy because they form intermediates in citric acid cycle metabolism or related molecules
3. Fat synthesis—all amino acids provide a potential source of acetyl-CoA to furnish substrate to synthesize fatty acids

Nitrogen Balance

Nitrogen balance exists when nitrogen intake from protein equals nitrogen excretion. In **positive nitrogen balance**, nitrogen intake exceeds nitrogen excretion, with the

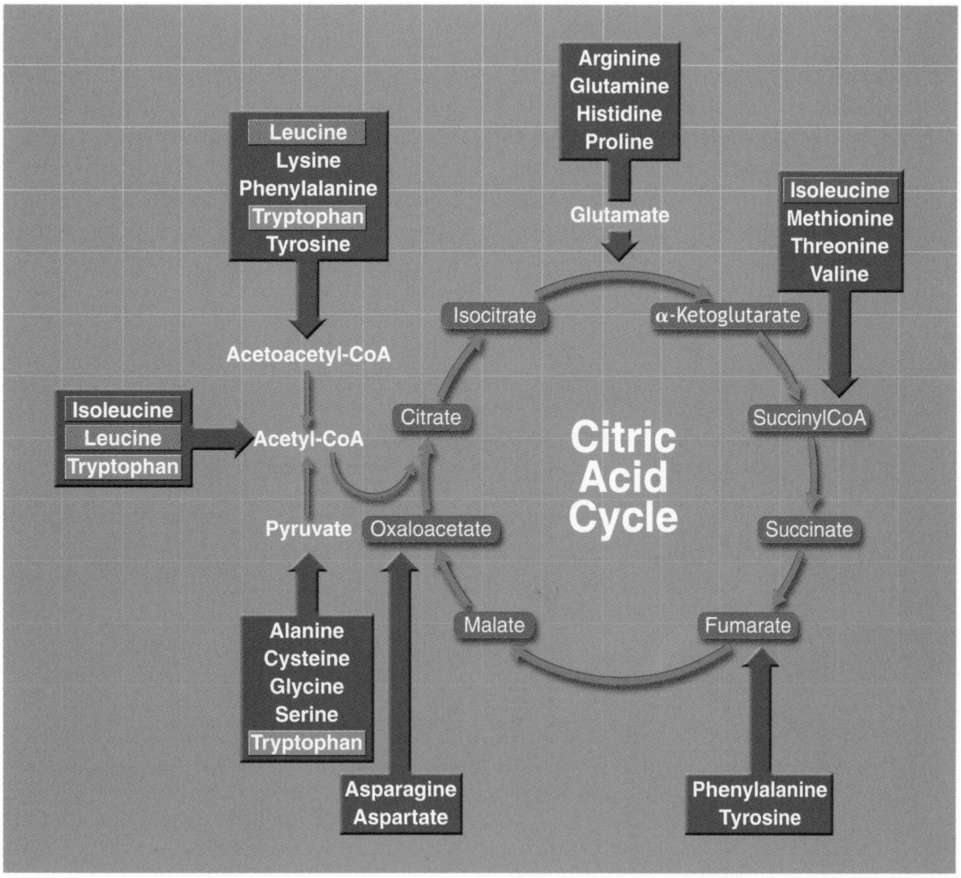

FIGURE 1.18. Major metabolic pathways for amino acids following removal of the nitrogen group by deamination or transamination. Upon removal of their amine group, all amino acids form reactive citric acid cycle intermediates or related compounds. Some of the larger amino acid molecules (e.g., leucine, tryptophan, isoleucine [in colored boxes]) generate carbon-containing compounds that enter metabolic pathways at different sites. (Reprinted with permission from McArdle W, et al. *Exercise Physiology: Nutrition, Energy, and Human Performance.* 7th Ed. Baltimore: Lippincott Williams & Wilkins, 2010:38.)

additional protein used to synthesize new tissues. Positive nitrogen balance occurs in growing children, during pregnancy, in recovery from illness, and during resistance exercise training, in which overloading muscle cells promotes protein synthesis. The body does not develop a protein reserve as it does with fat storage in adipose tissue or as carbohydrate stored as liver and muscle glycogen. Persons who consume adequate protein have a higher content of muscle and liver protein than do persons fed a subpar, low-protein diet. Also, labeling of protein (injecting protein with one or several of its carbon atoms "tagged") shows that some proteins become recruited for energy metabolism. Other proteins in neural and connective tissues remain relatively "fixed" as cellular constituents; they cannot be mobilized without harming tissue functions.

Greater nitrogen output than nitrogen intake (**negative nitrogen balance**) indicates protein use for energy and possible encroachment on amino acid reserves, primarily from skeletal muscle. Interestingly, a negative nitrogen balance occurs even when protein intake exceeds the recommended standard if the body catabolizes protein because it lacks other energy nutrients in the diet. For example, a person engaged in arduous training may consume adequate or excess protein yet be deficient in energy as carbohydrate or lipid. In this scenario, protein becomes a primary energy fuel. This creates a negative protein nitrogen balance that reduces the body's lean tissue mass. The protein-sparing role of dietary lipid and carbohydrate discussed previously becomes important during tissue growth periods and high-energy output requirements of intensive exercise training. Starvation produces the greatest negative nitrogen balance. *Starvation diets, or diets with reduced carbohydrate and/or energy, deplete glycogen reserves, which might trigger a protein deficiency with accompanying lean tissue loss.*

The Alanine–Glucose Cycle

Some body proteins do not readily metabolize for energy, but muscle proteins are more labile. Amino acids participate in energy metabolism when the exercise energy demand increases.[15,16,91] **FIGURE 1.19** shows that alanine release (and possibly glutamine) from active leg muscles increases in proportion to exercise intensity.

A model indicates that alanine *indirectly* serves the energy requirements of exercise. Active skeletal muscle synthesizes alanine during transamination. This occurs from the glucose intermediate pyruvate (with nitrogen derived in part from the amino acid leucine). Alanine deaminates after it leaves the muscle and enters the liver. Gluconeogenesis then converts the remaining carbon skeleton of alanine to glucose, which then enters the blood for use by active muscle. The residual carbon fragment from the amino acid that formed alanine oxidizes for energy within the muscle cell. **FIGURE 1.20** summarizes the sequence of the **alanine–glucose cycle**. After 4 hours of continuous light exercise, the liver's output of alanine-derived glucose accounts for about 45% of the liver's total glucose release. *During prolonged exercise, the alanine–glucose cycle generates from 10 to 15% of the total exercise energy requirement.* Regular exercise training enhances the liver's synthesis of glucose using the carbon skeletons of noncarbohydrate compounds. This facilitates blood glucose homeostasis during prolonged exercise. Chapters 5 and 7 discuss protein's role as a potential energy fuel in exercise and protein requirements of physically active people.

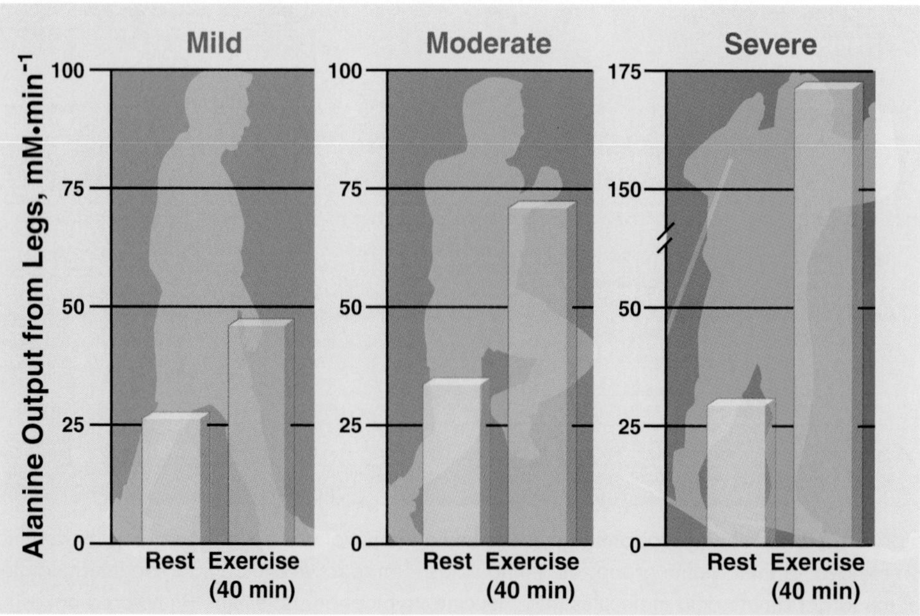

FIGURE 1.19. Dynamics of alanine release from leg muscle during 40 minutes of exercise. Alanine release nearly doubles during mild exercise compared with resting conditions. During the most intense aerobic exercise, the alanine flow from the active legs exceeds the resting value by more than sixfold. (From Felig P, Wahren J. Amino acid metabolism in exercising man. *J Clin Invest* 1971;50:2703.)

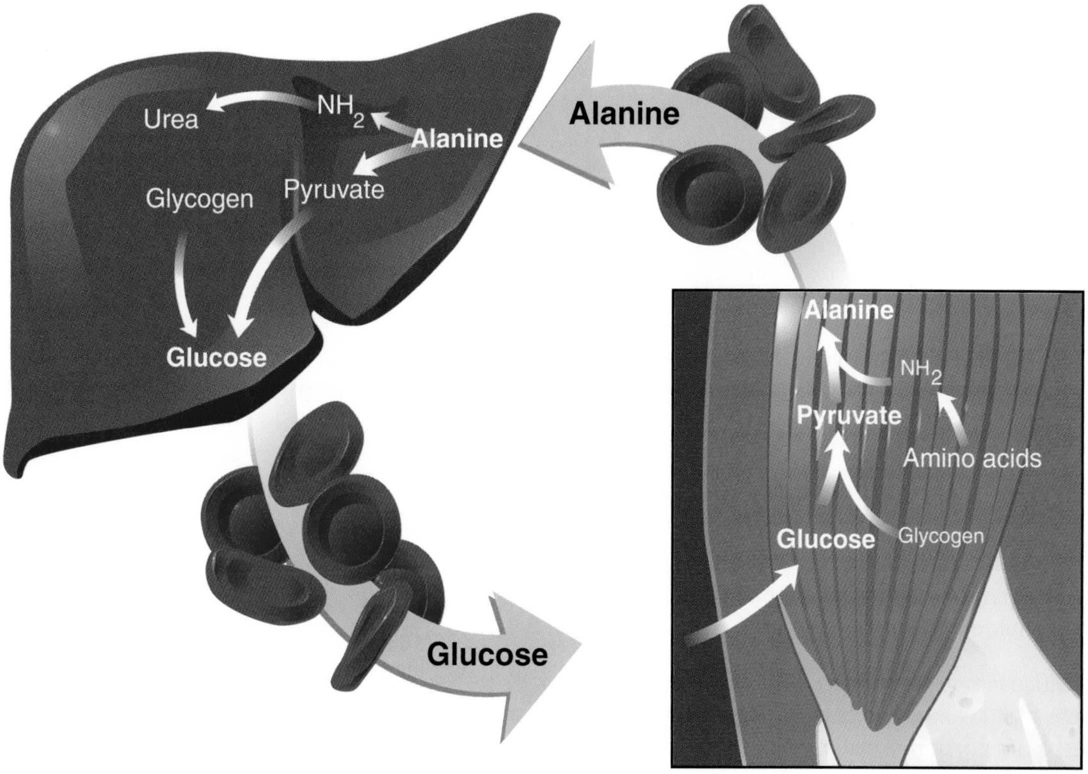

FIGURE 1.20. The alanine–glucose cycle. Alanine, synthesized in muscle from glucose-derived pyruvate via transamination, is released into the blood and converts to glucose and urea in the liver. Glucose release into the blood coincides with its subsequent delivery to the muscle for energy. During exercise, increased production and output of alanine from muscle helps to maintain blood glucose for nervous system and active muscle needs. Exercise training augments processes of hepatic gluconeogenesis. (From Felig P, Wahren J. Amino acid metabolism in exercising man. *J Clin Invest* 1971;50:2703.)

SUMMARY

1. Proteins differ chemically from lipids and carbohydrates because they contain nitrogen in addition to sulfur, phosphorus, and iron.
2. Proteins form from subunits called amino acids. The body requires 20 different amino acids, each containing an amino radical (NH_2) and an organic acid radical called a carboxyl group (COOH). Amino acids contain a side chain that defines the amino acid's particular chemical characteristics.
3. An almost infinite number of possible protein structures can form because of the diverse combinations possible for the 20 different amino acids.
4. The body cannot synthesize eight of the 20 amino acids. These are the essential amino acids that must be consumed in the diet.
5. Animal and plant cells contain protein. Proteins with all the essential amino acids are called complete (higher quality) proteins; the others are called incomplete (lower quality) proteins. Examples of higher quality, complete proteins include animal proteins in eggs, milk, cheese, meat, fish, and poultry.
6. The diets of many physically active persons and competitive athletes consist predominantly of nutrients from plant sources. Consuming various plant foods provides all of the essential amino acids because each food source contains a different quality and quantity of them.
7. Proteins provide the building blocks for synthesizing cellular material during anabolic processes. Amino acids also contribute their "carbon skeletons" for energy metabolism.
8. The RDA, the recommended quantity for nutrient intake, represents a liberal yet safe level of excess to meet the nutritional needs of practically all healthy persons. For adults, the protein RDA equals $0.83\ g \cdot kg^{-1}$ of body mass.
9. Proteins in nervous and connective tissue generally do not participate in energy metabolism. The amino acid alanine, however, plays a key role in providing carbohydrate fuel via gluconeogenesis during prolonged exercise. During strenuous exercise of long duration, the alanine–glucose cycle accounts for up to 40 to 50% of the liver's glucose release.

SUMMARY *(continued)*

10. Protein catabolism accelerates during exercise because carbohydrate reserves deplete. Thus, individuals who train vigorously on a regular basis must maintain optimal levels of muscle and liver glycogen to minimize lean tissue loss and deterioration in performance.

11. Regular exercise training enhances the liver's capacity to synthesize glucose from the carbon skeletons of noncarbohydrate compounds.

thePoint *Visit* **thePoint.lww.com/MKKSEN4e** *to view the following animations related to content presented in Chapter 1:* ***Alanine-glucose cycle; Catabolism; Diabetes; Insulin functions; Glycogen synthesis; Metabolism of amino acids;*** *and* ***Transamination.***

TEST YOUR KNOWLEDGE ANSWERS

1. **False:** Carbohydrates do not contain nitrogen, only carbon, oxygen, and hydrogen atoms. Protein is the only macronutrient to contain nitrogen.

2. **True:** Glucose can be formed by gluconeogenesis, a process that synthesizes glucose (primarily in the liver) from carbon skeletons of specific amino acids including nonprotein glycerol, pyruvate, and lactate.

3. **False:** Fibers exist exclusively in plants; they make up the structure of leaves, stems, roots, seeds, and fruit coverings. Because of its resistance to digestive enzymes, fiber cannot be absorbed by the body and used for energy. However, fiber does retain considerable water as it passes through the digestive tract and thus gives "bulk" to the food residues in the large intestine, often increasing stool weight and volume by 40 to 100%, which aids gastrointestinal function.

4. **False:** For regular exercisers, carbohydrates should supply about 60% of total daily calories (400 to 600 g), predominantly as unrefined, fiber-rich fruits, grains, and vegetables.

5. **False:** About 25% of the population produces excessive insulin in response to an intake of rapidly absorbed carbohydrates (high glycemic rating). These insulin-resistant persons increase their risk for obesity if they consistently eat such a diet. Weight gain occurs because abnormal quantities of insulin (1) promote glucose entry into cells and (2) facilitate the liver's conversion of glucose to triacylglycerol, which then becomes stored as body fat in adipose tissue. Also, excess calories, regardless of dietary source, contribute to obesity.

6. **False:** Carbohydrate and protein each contains 4.0 $kcal \cdot g^{-1}$. In contrast, each gram of lipid contains more than twice that amount at 9.0 kcal.

7. **False:** Cholesterol, the most widely known derived lipid, exists only in animal tissue; it is never found in plants of any origin.

8. **True:** True vegetarians or vegans consume nutrients from only two sources, the plant kingdom and dietary supplements. This places vegans at a somewhat greater risk for inadequate energy and nutrient intake because they eliminate meat and dairy products from the diet and increasingly rely on foods relatively low in energy, quality protein, and certain micronutrients. Nutritional diversity remains the key for these men and women. For example, a vegan diet provides all the essential amino acids if 60% of protein intake comes from grain products, 35% from legumes, and 5% from green, leafy vegetables. Vitamin B_{12}, found only in the animal kingdom, must be obtained in supplement form.

9. **False:** For athletes, muscle mass does not increase simply by eating high-protein foods or special amino acid mixtures. If lean tissue synthesis resulted from extra protein, muscle mass would increase tremendously for persons on the typical Western diet. For example, consuming an extra 100 g (400 kcal) of protein daily theoretically translates into a daily 500-g (1.1-lb) increase in muscle mass. This obviously does not happen. A proper resistance training program combined with a well-balanced diet increases muscle mass. Excessive dietary protein is used directly for energy or recycled as components of other molecules, including fat stored in the subcutaneous adipose tissue depots.

10. **False:** On average, 0.83 g of protein per kg of body mass represents the recommended daily intake for both women and men. For a 90-kg man, the total daily protein requirement equals 75 g (90 × 0.83), whereas a 50-kg woman requires 41.5 g (50 × 0.83). The protein RDA even holds for overweight persons; it includes a reserve of about 25% to account for individual differences in protein requirement for about 98% of the population.

Key References

Agus MS, et al. Dietary composition and physiologic adaptations to energy restriction. *Am J Clin Nutr* 2000;71:901.

American Dietetic Association, et al. American College of Sports Medicine position stand. Nutrition and athletic performance. *Med Sci Sports Exerc* 2009;41:709.

Barr SI, Rideout CA. Nutritional considerations for vegetarian athletes. *Nutrition* 2004;20:696.

Bingham SA, et al. Dietary fibre in food and protection against colorectal cancer in the European Prospective Investigation into Cancer and Nutrition (EPIC): an observational study. *Lancet* 2003;361:1496.

Craig WJ, Mangels AR. Position of the American Dietetic Association: vegetarian diets. *J Am Diet Assoc* 2009;109:1266.

Esmaillzadeh A, Azadbakht L. Whole-grain intake, metabolic syndrome, and mortality in older adults. *Am J Clin Nutr* 2006;83:1439.

Finley CE, et al. Cardiorespiratory fitness, macronutrient intake and the metabolic syndrome: the Aerobics Center Longitudinal Study. *J Am Diet Assoc* 2006;106:673.

Gaine PC, et al. Postexercise whole-body protein turnover response to three levels of protein intake. *Med Sci Sports Exerc* 2007;39:480.

Haub MD, et al. Effect of protein source on resistive-training-induced changes in body composition and muscle size in older men. *Am J Clin Nutr* 2002;76:511.

Hunter JE, et al. Cardiovascular disease risk of dietary stearic acid compared with trans, other saturated and unsaturated fatty acids: a systematic review. *Am J Clin Nutr* 2010;91:46.

Kirkegaard H, et al. Association of adherence to lifestyle recommendations and risk of colorectal cancer: a prospective Danish cohort study. *BMJ* 2010;341:c5407.

Kromhout D, et al. n-3 fatty acids and cardiovascular events after myocardial infarction. *N Engl J Med* 2010;363:2015.

Kummerow FA. The negative effects of hydrogenated trans fats and what to do about them. *Atherosclerosis* 2009;205:458.

Lakka HM, et al. The metabolic syndrome and total and cardiovascular disease mortality in middle-aged men. *JAMA* 2002;288:2709.

Makhoul Z, et al. Associations of obesity with triglycerides and C-reactive protein are attenuated in adults with high red blood cell eicosapentaenoic and docosahexaenoic acids. *Eur J Clin Nutr* 2011;65:808.

Manger MS, et al. Dietary intake of n-3 long-chain polyunsaturated fatty acids and coronary events in Norwegian patients with coronary artery disease. *Am J Clin Nutr* 2010;92:244.

Mozaffarian D, et al. Trans fatty acids and cardiovascular disease. *N Engl J Med* 2006;354:1601.

Ornish D, et al. Intensive lifestyle changes for reversal of coronary heart disease. *JAMA* 1998;280:2001.

Pikosky MA, et al. Increased protein maintains nitrogen balance during exercise-induced energy deficit. *Med Sci Sports Exerc* 2008;40:505.

Qi L, et al. Whole grain, bran, and cereal fiber intakes and markers of systemic inflammation in diabetic women. *Diabetes Care* 2006;29:207.

Quinn J, et al. Docosahexaenoic acid supplementation and cognitive decline in Alzheimer disease. *JAMA* 2010;304:1903.

Seal CJ. Whole grains and CVD risk. *Proc Nutr Soc* 2006;65:24.

Siri-Tarino PW, et al. Meta-analysis of prospective cohort studies evaluating the association of saturated fat with cardiovascular disease. *Am J Clin Nutr* 2010;91:535.

Sluijs I, et al. Carbohydrate quantity and quality and risk of type 2 diabetes in the European Prospective Investigation into Cancer and Nutrition-Netherlands (EPIC-NL) study. *Am J Clin Nutr* 2010;92:676.

Venderley AM, Campbell WW. Vegetarian diets: nutritional considerations for athletes. *Sports Med* 2006;36:293.

thePoint *Visit* **thePoint.lww.com/MKKSEN4e** *for a list of the references cited in this chapter, including additional, relevant references.*

CHAPTER 2

The Micronutrients and Water

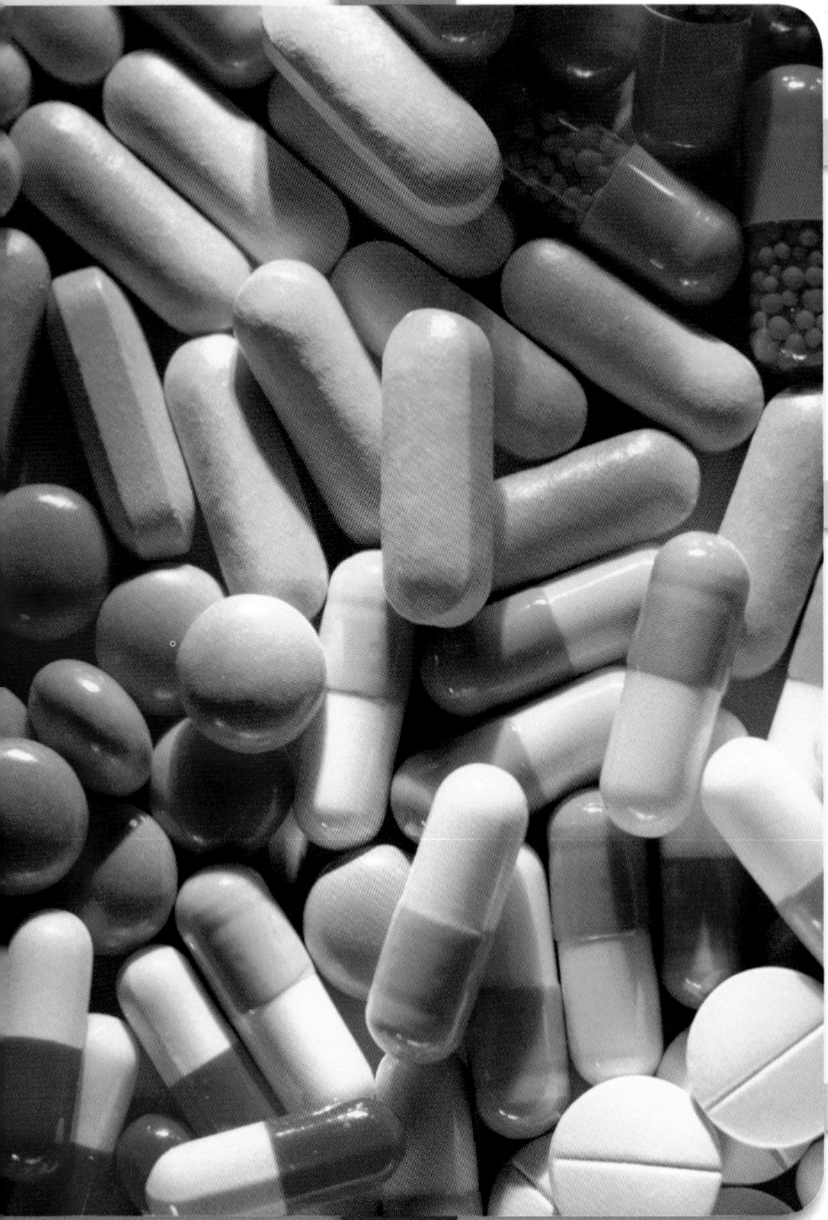

OUTLINE

TEST YOUR KNOWLEDGE

Select true or false for the 10 statements below, then check out the answers at the end of the chapter. Retake the test after you've read the chapter; you should achieve 100%!	True	False
1. Vitamin supplementation above the Recommended Dietary Allowance (RDA) level does not improve exercise performance.	❍	❍
2. From a survival perspective, food is of greater importance than water.	❍	❍
3. Achieving the recommended intake of "major" minerals is more crucial to good health than achieving the recommended intake of "trace" minerals.	❍	❍
4. Plants provide a better source of minerals than do animal sources.	❍	❍
5. Sedentary adults require about 3.785 L (1 gal) of water each day to maintain optimal body functions.	❍	❍
6. Decreasing sodium in the diet represents the only important lifestyle approach to lowering high blood pressure.	❍	❍
7. None of the 13 vitamins required by the body is toxic if consumed in excess.	❍	❍
8. A telltale symptom of iron deficiency anemia is soft and brittle bones.	❍	❍
9. Stationary cycling is one of the best exercises to promote bone health.	❍	❍
10. Pharmacologic approaches to treating borderline hypertension are more effective than dietary approaches.	❍	❍

Effective regulation of all metabolic processes requires a delicate blending of food nutrients in the watery medium of the cell. Of special significance in this regard are the **micronutrients**—the small quantities of vitamins and minerals that facilitate energy transfer and tissue synthesis. For example, the body requires each year only about 350 g (12 oz) of vitamins from the approximate 907 kg (2000 lb) of food consumed annually by the average adult. With proper nutrition from various food sources, the physically active person or competitive athlete need not consume vitamin and mineral supplements; such practices usually prove physiologically and economically wasteful. Some micronutrients consumed in excess can adversely affect health and safety.

VITAMINS

THE NATURE OF VITAMINS

Vitamins achieved importance centuries before scientists isolated and classified them. The Greek physician Hippocrates advocated ingesting liver to cure night blindness. He did not know the reason for the cure, but we now know that vitamin A, which helps to prevent night blindness, occurs plentifully in this organ meat. In 1897, Dutch physician Christiaan Eijkman (1858–1930; shared 1929 Nobel Prize in Physiology or Medicine for discovering the antineuritic vitamin) observed that a regular diet of polished rice caused beriberi in fowl, while adding thiamine-rich rice polishings to table scraps cured the disease. In the early 19th century, adding oranges and lemons to the diet of British sailors on long voyages paved the way for eradicating the dreaded disease scurvy because of the protective effects of the vitamin C contained in the fruits. In 1932, scientific experiments demonstrated that ascorbic acid (technically a liver metabolite) functioned in a manner essentially identical to vitamin C. Interestingly, most animal species synthesize ascorbic acid, except for humans, guinea pigs, and certain monkeys; thus, these species must consume vitamin C in their diet.

The formal discovery of vitamins, initially known as "vital amines," revealed they were organic substances needed by the body in minute amounts. Vitamins, their amine role having been discredited, have no particular chemical structure in common and often are considered accessory nutrients because they neither supply energy nor contribute substantially to body mass. Except for vitamin D, the body cannot manufacture vitamins; hence, foods consumed or supplementation must supply them.

Some foods contain an abundant quantity of vitamins. For example, the green leaves and roots of plants manufacture vitamins during photosynthesis. Animals obtain vitamins from the plants, seeds, grains, and fruits they eat or from the meat of other animals that previously consumed these foods. Several vitamins, notably vitamins A and D, niacin, and folate, become activated from their inactive precursor or **provitamin** form. **Carotenes**, the best known of the provitamins, comprise the yellow and yellow-orange pigment precursors of vitamin A that give color to vegetables (carrots, squash, corn, pumpkins) and fruits (apricots, peaches).

KINDS AND SOURCES OF VITAMINS

Thirteen different vitamins have been isolated, analyzed, classified, and synthesized; and Recommended Dietary Allowance (RDA) levels have been established for these. Vitamins are classified as either **fat soluble** or **water soluble**. The fat-soluble vitamins include vitamins A, D, E, and K. The water-soluble vitamins are vitamin C and the B-complex vitamins (based on their common source distribution and common functional relationships): thiamine (B_1), riboflavin (B_2), pyridoxine (B_6), niacin (nicotinic acid), pantothenic acid, biotin, folic acid (folacin or folate, its active form in the body), and cobalamin (B_{12}).

Fat-Soluble Vitamins

Fat-soluble vitamins dissolve and are stored in the body's fatty tissues without need to consume them daily. Years may elapse before symptoms surface of a fat-soluble vitamin insufficiency. The liver stores vitamins A and D, whereas vitamin E distributes throughout the body's fatty tissues. The liver stores small amounts of vitamin K. Dietary lipid provides the source of fat-soluble vitamins; these vitamins are transported as part of lipoproteins in the lymph and travel to the liver for dispersion to various tissues. Consuming a true "fat-free" diet could certainly accelerate development of a fat-soluble vitamin insufficiency.

Fat-soluble vitamins should not be consumed in excess without medical supervision. Toxic reactions from excessive fat-soluble vitamin intake generally occur at a lower multiple of recommended intakes than for water-soluble vitamins. For example, a daily moderate-to-large excess of vitamin A (as retinol but not in carotene form) and vitamin D produces serious toxic effects. Children are particularly susceptible; excess vitamin D (intakes greater than 10,000 IU daily or blood levels in excess of 50 $ng \cdot mL^{-1}$), for example, can cause excessive calcium deposits and mental retardation and increase the risk of kidney and heart damage and several cancers. Consuming vitamin A in amounts not much greater than recommended values (RDA of 700 $\mu g \cdot d^{-1}$ for women and 900 $\mu g \cdot d^{-1}$ for men) precipitates bone fractures later in life. In addition, high doses consumed early in pregnancy associate with a greater risk of birth defects. In young children, a large vitamin A accumulation in body tissues (called hypervitaminosis A) causes the following four conditions:

1. Irritability
2. Swelling of bones
3. Weight loss
4. Dry, itchy skin

In adults, symptoms can include these six maladies:

1. Nausea
2. Headache
3. Drowsiness
4. Hair loss
5. Diarrhea
6. Loss of calcium from bones, causing osteoporosis and increased risk of fractures

Excess vitamin A inhibits cells that produce new bone, stimulates cells that break down existing bone, and negatively affects the action of vitamin D, which helps the body maintain normal calcium levels and participates in the regulation of as many as 2000 genes. Discontinuing high vitamin A intakes reverses its adverse effects. "Overdoses" from vitamins E and K are rare, but intakes above the recommended levels yield no health benefits.

Water-Soluble Vitamins

The water-soluble vitamins act largely as **coenzymes**—small molecules combined with a larger protein compound (apoenzyme) to form an active enzyme that accelerates the interconversion of chemical compounds. Coenzymes participate directly in chemical reactions; when the reaction runs its course, coenzymes remain intact and participate in further reactions. Water-soluble vitamins, like their fat-soluble counterparts, consist of carbon, hydrogen, and oxygen atoms. They also contain nitrogen and metal ions, including iron, molybdenum, copper, sulfur, and cobalt.

Water-soluble vitamins disperse readily in body fluids without storage in the tissues to any appreciable extent. If the diet regularly contains less than 50% of the recommended values for these vitamins, marginal deficiencies could develop within about 4 weeks. Generally, even an excess intake of water-soluble vitamins becomes voided in the urine. Water-soluble vitamins exert their influence for 8 to 14 hours after ingestion, with their potency decreasing thereafter. For maximum benefit, vitamin C supplements should be consumed at least every 12 hours. Increasing vitamin C intake for healthy

Food Sources

Source (Portion Size)	Vitamin C (mg)
Fruit	
Cantaloupe (1/4 Medium)	60
Fresh grapefruit (1/2 Fruit)	40
Honeydew melon (1/8 Medium)	40
Kiwi (1 Medium)	75
Mango (1 Cup, sliced)	45
Orange (1 Medium)	70
Papaya (1 Cup, cubes)	85
Strawberries (1 Cup, sliced)	95
Tangerines or tangelos (1 Medium)	25
Watermelon (1 Cup)	15
Juice	
Grapefruit (1/2 Cup)	35
Orange (1/2 Cup)	50
Fortified Juice	
Apple (1/2 Cup)	50
Cranberry juice cocktail (1/2 Cup)	45
Grape (1/2 Cup)	120
Vegetables	
Asparagus, cooked (1/2 Cup)	10
Broccoli, cooked (1/2 Cup)	60
Brussels sprouts, cooked (1/2 Cup)	50
Cabbage	
Red, raw, chopped (1/2 Cup)	20
Red, cooked (1/2 Cup)	25
Raw, chopped (1/2 Cup)	10
Cooked (1/2 Cup)	15
Cauliflower, raw or cooked (1/2 Cup)	25
Kale, cooked (1/2 Cup)	55
Mustard greens, cooked (1 Cup)	35
Pepper, red or green	
Raw (1/2 Cup)	65
Cooked (1/2 Cup)	50
Plantains, sliced, cooked (1 Cup)	15
Potato, baked (1 Medium)	25
Snow peas	
Fresh, cooked (1/2 Cup)	40
Frozen, cooked (1/2 Cup)	20
Sweet potato	
Baked (1 Medium)	30
Vacuum can (1 Cup)	50
Canned, syrup-pack (1 Cup)	20
Tomato	
Raw (1/2 Cup)	15
Canned (1/2 Cup)	35
Juice (6 Fluid oz)	35

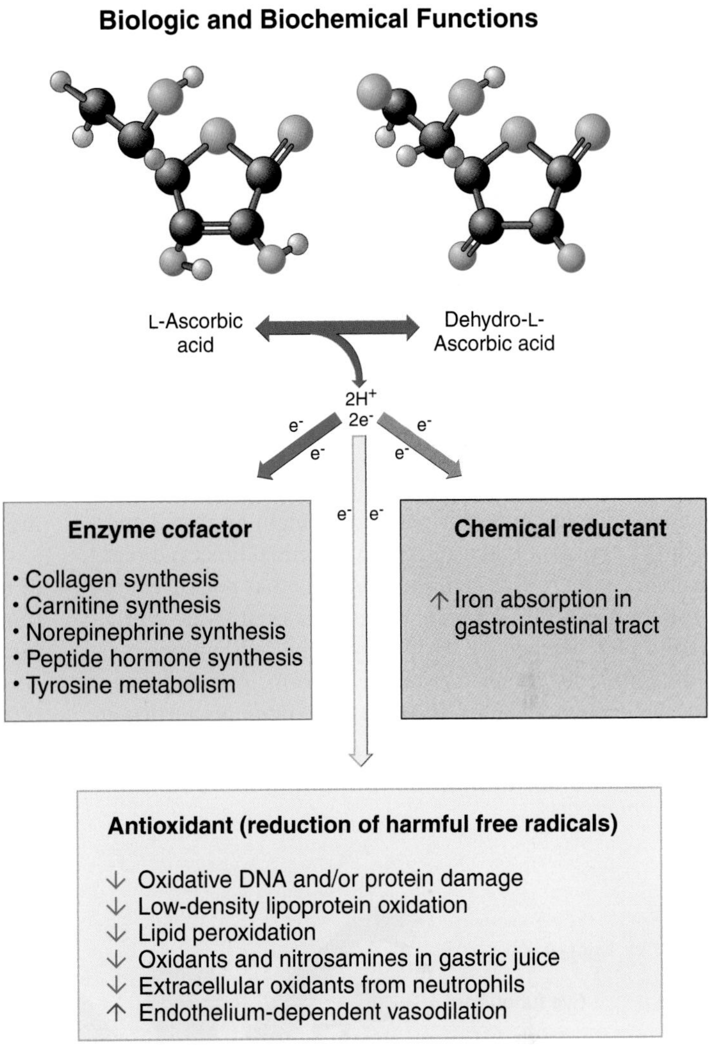

Vitamin C (L-ascorbic acid) oxidation releases donor electrons in pairs for biochemical reactions. The molecular diagrams show carbon atoms in black, oxygen in red, and hydrogen in white. Arrows indicate an increase or decrease in response.

FIGURE 2.1. Various food sources for vitamin C and diverse biologic and biochemical functions. (Modified from Levine M, et al. Criteria and recommendations for vitamin C intake. *JAMA* 1999;281:1415.)

persons from the recommended daily value of 75 mg for women and 90 mg for men to 200 mg (not in supplement form but in two to four daily servings of fruits and three to five servings of vegetables) may ensure optimal cellular saturation. **FIGURE 2.1** illustrates various food sources for vitamin C and its diverse biologic and biochemical functions. These include serving as an electron donor for eight enzymes and as a chemical reducing agent (antioxidant) in intracellular and extracellular reactions. Sweating, even during extreme physical activity in hot and cold environments, produces only a negligible loss of water-soluble vitamins.

Vitamin Storage in the Body

The body does not readily excrete an excess of fat-soluble vitamins. In contrast, water-soluble vitamins continually exit the body because cellular water dissolves these compounds, which the kidneys then excrete. An exception is vitamin B_{12}, which stores more readily than the other water-soluble vitamins. Because of their limited storage, water-soluble vitamins must be consumed regularly to prevent possible deficiency. A wide latitude exists because an average person would require 10 days without consuming thiamine before deficiency symptoms emerge; it takes about 30 to 40 days of lack of vitamin C before symptoms of deficiency appear. A broad array of vitamins is readily available in the foods consumed in a well-balanced diet, so little chance occurs for long-term vitamin deficiency. Exceptions include conditions of starvation, alcoholism (which compromises nutrient intake), or significant deviations from prudent dietary recommendations.

ROLE OF VITAMINS IN THE BODY

FIGURE 2.2 summarizes many of the biologic functions of vitamins. These important nutrients contain no useful energy for the body, but instead serve as essential links and regulators in numerous metabolic reactions that *release* energy from food. Vitamins also control processes of tissue synthesis and help to protect the integrity of the cells' unique plasma membrane. The water-soluble vitamins play important roles in energy metabolism (**TABLE 2.1**). *Vitamins participate repeatedly in metabolic reactions; thus, the vitamin needs of physically active people probably do not exceed those of sedentary counterparts.*

DEFINING NUTRIENT NEEDS

Controversy surrounding the RDAs caused the Food and Nutrition Board and scientific nutrition community to reexamine the usefulness of a single standard. This process, begun in 1997, led the National Academy's Institute of Medicine (in cooperation with Canadian scientists) to develop the **Dietary Reference Intakes** (www.nal.usda.gov/).

Dietary Reference Intakes

Dietary Reference Intakes (DRIs), updated in 2011, represent a radically new and more comprehensive approach to nutritional recommendations for individuals. Think of the DRI as the umbrella term that encompasses the array of new standards—RDAs, Estimated Average Requirement (EAR), Adequate Intake (AI), and the Tolerable Upper Intake Level (UL)—for nutrient recommendations in planning and assessing diets for healthy persons.

Similarities of dietary patterns caused the inclusion of both Canada and the United States in the target population. Recommendations encompass not only daily intakes intended for health maintenance but also upper intake levels that reduce the likelihood of harm from excess nutrient intake. In addition to including values for energy, protein, and the micronutrients, DRIs also provide values for macronutrients and food components of the nutritionally important phytochemicals. Whenever possible, nutrient intakes are

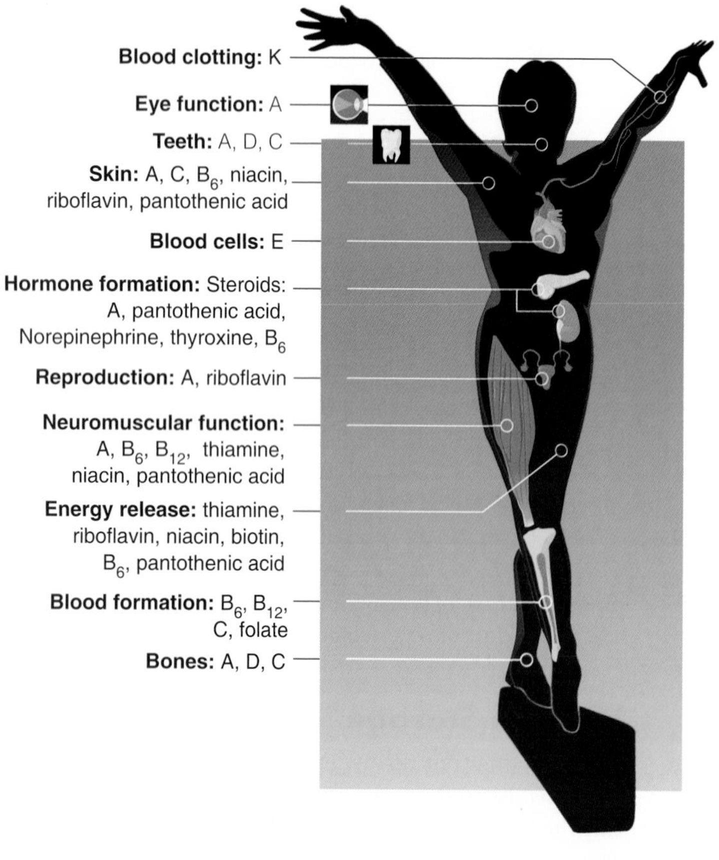

FIGURE 2.2. Biologic functions of vitamins in the body.

TABLE 2.1 Water-Soluble Vitamins and Energy Transfer

Vitamin B_1 (thiamine)	Provides oxidizable substrate in citric acid cycle via oxidative decarboxylation of pyruvate to acetyl-CoA during carbohydrate breakdown; requirement related to total energy expenditure and total carbohydrate breakdown; needs may be somewhat higher in physically active people with large carbohydrate catabolism; membrane and nerve conduction; pentose synthesis; oxidative decarboxylation of α-keto acids in amino acid breakdown
Vitamin B_2 (riboflavin)	Hydrogen (electron) transfer during mitochondrial metabolism in respiratory chain; combines with phosphoric acid to form flavin adenine dinucleotide (FAD) and flavin adenine mononucleotide (FMN)
Vitamin B_6 (pyridoxine)	Important coenzyme in protein synthesis and glycogen metabolism; coenzyme in transamination reactions; formation of precursor compounds for heme in hemoglobin; coenzyme for phosphorylase, which facilitates glycogen release from liver
Vitamin B_{12} (cyanocobalamin)	Important coenzyme in the transfer of single-carbon units in nucleic acid metabolism; influences protein synthesis; role in gastrointestinal, bone, and nervous tissue function
Niacin (nicotinamide and nicotinic acid)	Hydrogen (electron) transfer during glycolysis and mitochondrial metabolism; component of nicotine and nicotine adenine dinucleotide phosphate (NADP); role in fat and glycogen synthesis; amino acid tryptophan converted to niacin; excess niacin may depress fatty acid mobilization, which would facilitate carbohydrate depletion
Pantothenic acid	Component of the citric acid cycle intermediate acetyl-CoA; involved in synthesis of cholesterol, phospholipids, hemoglobin, and steroid hormones
Folate (folic acid, folacin)	Coenzyme in amino acid metabolism and nucleic acid synthesis; essential for normal formation of red and white blood cells; protects against neural tube defects in fetus
Biotin	Essential role in carbohydrate, fat, and amino acid metabolism; involved in carboxyl unit transport and CO_2 fixing in tissues; role in gluconeogenesis and fatty acid synthesis and oxidation
Vitamin C (ascorbic acid)	Antioxidant; may relate to exercise through its role in the synthesis of collagen and carnitine; enhances iron absorption and possibly heat acclimatization; facilitates iron availability; cofactor in some hydroxylation reactions (e.g., dopamine to noradrenaline)

recommended in four categories instead of one. This concept of range places the DRIs more in line with the Estimated Safe and Adequate Daily Dietary Intakes (ESADDIs).

Unlike its RDA predecessor, the DRI value also includes recommendations that apply to gender and life stages of growth and development based on age, pregnancy, and lactation. The goal of a complete revision every 5 years as with the RDAs was abandoned, with the new modification of making immediate changes in the DRI as new scientific data become available. The National Academy Press presents the reports to date on the DRIs (www.nap.edu/; search for "Dietary Reference Intakes").

UNIQUE ASPECTS OF THE DIETARY REFERENCE INTAKES

The DRIs differ from their predecessor RDAs by focusing more on promoting health maintenance and risk reduction for nutrient-dependent diseases (e.g., heart disease, diabetes, hypertension, osteoporosis, various cancers, and age-related macular degeneration), rather than the traditional criterion of preventing the deficiency diseases (e.g., scurvy, beriberi, or rickets).

Connections to the Past

James Lind (1716–1794)

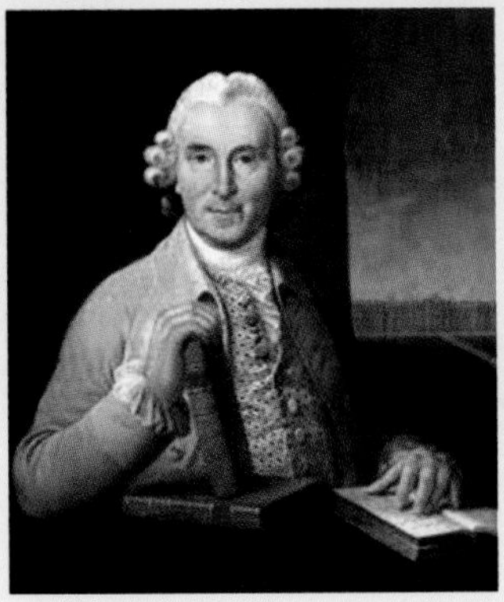

Trained in Edinburgh, Lind entered the British Navy as a surgeon's mate in 1739. During an extended trip in the English Channel in 1747 on the 50-gun, 960-ton *HMS Salisbury*, Lind carried out a decisive experiment (the first planned, controlled clinical trial) that eventually changed the course of naval medicine. Lind knew that scurvy ("the great sea plague") often killed two thirds of a ship's crew. Their diet included 1 lb (0.45 kg) and 4 oz (113.4 g) of cheese biscuits daily, 2 lb (0.90 kg) of salt beef twice weekly, 2 oz (56.7 g) of dried fish and butter thrice weekly, 8 oz (226.8 g) of peas 4 days a week, and 1 gallon (3.79 L) of beer daily. Deprived of vitamin C, sailors fell prey to scurvy. By adding fresh fruit to their diet, Lind fortified their immune systems so that British sailors no longer perished.

thePoint

Visit **thePoint.lww.com/MKKSEN4e** *to find more details about Lind's decisive experiment that changed the course of naval medicine by adding fresh fruit to sailors' diets to fortify their immune systems and defeat scurvy.*

The following definitions apply to the four different sets of values for the intake of nutrients and food components in the DRIs (**FIG. 2.3**):

1. **Estimated Average Requirement:** Average level of daily nutrient intake to meet the requirement of half of the healthy individuals in a particular life-stage and gender group. In addition to assessing nutritional adequacy of intakes of population groups, the EAR provides a useful value for determining the prevalence of inadequate nutrient intake by the proportion of the population with intakes below this value.
2. **Recommended Dietary Allowance:** The average daily nutrient intake level sufficient to meet the requirement of nearly 98% of healthy individuals in a particular life-stage and gender group. For most nutrients, this value represents the EAR plus two standard deviations of the requirement.
3. **Adequate Intake:** The AI provides an assumed adequate nutritional goal when no RDA exists. It represents a recommended average daily nutrient intake level based on observed or experimentally determined approximations or estimates of nutrient intake by a group (or groups) of apparently healthy persons and is used when an RDA cannot be determined. Low risk exists with intakes at or above the AI level.
4. **Tolerable Upper Intake Level:** The highest average daily nutrient intake level likely to pose no risk of adverse health effects to almost all individuals in the specified gender and life-stage group of the general population. As intake increases above the UL, the potential risk of adverse effects increases.

The DRI report indicates that fruits and vegetables yield about one half as much vitamin A as previously believed. Thus, individuals who do not eat vitamin A–rich, animal-derived foods should upgrade their intake of carotene-rich fruits and vegetables. The report also sets a daily maximum intake level for vitamin A in addition to boron, copper, iodine, iron, manganese, molybdenum, nickel, vanadium, and zinc. Specific recommended intakes are provided for vitamins A and K, chromium, copper, iodine, manganese, molybdenum, and zinc. The report concludes that one can meet the daily requirement for the nutrients examined without supplementation. The exception is the mineral iron, for which most pregnant women need supplements to obtain their increased daily requirement.

TABLE 2.2 lists the major bodily functions, dietary sources, and symptoms of a deficiency or excess of the water-soluble and fat-soluble vitamins. **TABLES 2.3** and **2.4** present the RDA, AI, and UL values for these vitamins. Well-balanced meals provide an adequate quantity of all vitamins, regardless of age and physical activity level. *Individuals who expend considerable energy exercising generally need not consume special foods or supplements that increase vitamin intake above recommended levels.* Also, at high levels of daily physical activity, food intake generally increases to sustain the added exercise energy requirements. Additional food through a variety of nutritious meals proportionately increases vitamin and mineral intakes. Chapter 7 summarizes recommendations from

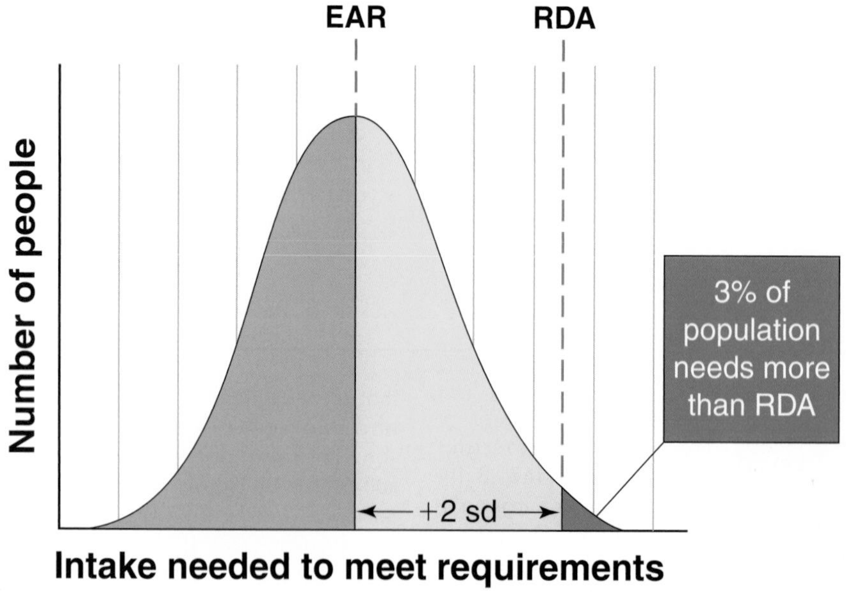

FIGURE 2.3. Theoretical distribution of the number of persons adequately nourished by a given nutrient intake. The RDA is set at an intake level that would meet the nutrient needs of 97 to 98% of the population (2 standard deviations [SD] above the mean). EAR refers to the Estimated Average Requirement, which represents a nutrient intake value estimated to meet the requirement of one half of the healthy individuals in a gender and life-stage group.

TABLE 2.2 Food Sources, Major Bodily Functions, and Symptoms of Deficiency or Excess of the Fat-Soluble and Water-Soluble Vitamins for Healthy Adults (19–50 Years of Age)

Vitamin	Dietary Sources	Major Bodily Functions	Deficiency	Excess
Fat soluble				
Vitamin A (retinol)	Provitamin A (β-carotene) widely distributed in green vegetables. Retinol present in milk, butter, cheese, fortified margarine	Constituent of rhodopsin (visual pigment). Maintenance of epithelial tissues. Role in mucopolysaccharide synthesis.	Xerophthalmia (keratinization of ocular tissue), night blindness, permanent blindness	Headache, vomiting, peeling of skin, anorexia, swelling of long bones
Vitamin D	Cod liver oil, eggs, dairy products, fortified milk, and margarine	Promotes growth and mineralization of bones. Increases absorption of calcium.	Rickets (bone deformities) in children; osteomalacia in adults	Vomiting, diarrhea, loss of weight, kidney damage
Vitamin E (tocopherol)	Seeds, green leafy vegetables, margarines, shortenings	Functions as an antioxidant to prevent cell damage	Possible anemia	Relatively nontoxic
Vitamin K (phylloquinone)	Green leafy vegetables, small amounts in cereals, fruits, and meats	Important in blood clotting (involved in formation of prothrombin)	Conditioned deficiencies associated with severe bleeding; internal hemorrhages	Relatively nontoxic; synthetic forms at high doses may cause jaundice
Water soluble				
Vitamin B_1 (thiamin)	Pork, organ meats, whole grains, nuts, legumes, milk, fruits, and vegetables	Coenzyme (thiamin pyrophosphate) in reactions involving the removal of carbon dioxide	Beriberi (peripheral nerve changes, edema, heart failure)	None reported
Vitamin B_2	Widely distributed in foods: meats, eggs, milk products, whole-grain and enriched cereal products, wheat germ, green leafy vegetables	Constituent of two flavin nucleotide coenzymes involved in energy metabolism (FAD and FMN)	Reddened lips, cracks at mouth corner (cheilosis), eye lesions	None reported
Niacin	Liver, lean meats, poultry, grains, legumes, peanuts (can be formed from tryptophan)	Constituent of two coenzymes in oxidation-reduction reactions (NAD and NADP)	Pellagra (skin and gastrointestinal lesions, nervous mental disorders)	Flushing, burning and tingling around neck, face, and hands
Vitamin B_6	Meats, fish, poultry, vegetables, whole-grain, cereals, seeds	Coenzyme (pyridoxal phosphate) involved in amino acid and glycogen metabolism	Irritability, convulsions, muscular twitching, dermatitis, kidney stones	None reported
Pantothenic acid	Widely distributed in foods: meat, fish, poultry, milk products, legumes, whole grains	Constituent of coenzyme A, which plays a central role in energy metabolism	Fatigue, sleep disturbances, impaired coordination, nausea	None reported
Folate	Legumes, green vegetables, Whole-wheat products, meats, eggs, milk products, liver	Coenzyme (reduced form) involved in transfer of single-carbon units in nucleic acid and amino acid metabolism	Anemia, gastrointestinal disturbances, diarrhea, red tongue	None reported
Vitamin B_{12}	Muscle meats, fish, eggs, dairy products (absent in plant foods)	Coenzyme involved in transfer of single-carbon units in nucleic acid metabolism	Pernicious anemia, neurologic disorders	None reported
Biotin	Legumes, vegetables, meats, liver, egg yolk, nuts	Coenzymes required for fat synthesis, amino acid metabolism, and glycogen (animal starch) formation	Fatigue, depression, nausea, dermatitis, muscular pains	None reported
Vitamin C (ascorbic acid)	Citrus fruits, tomatoes, green peppers, salad greens	Maintains intercellular matrix of cartilage, bone, and dentine; important in collagen synthesis	Scurvy (degeneration of skin, teeth, blood vessels, epithelial hemorrhages)	Relatively nontoxic; possibility of kidney stones

NAD, *nicotine adenine dinucleotide*

TABLE 2.3 DRIs: RDAs and AIs Vitamins

Life-Stage Group	Vitamin A (μg/d)[a]	Vitamin C (mg/d)	Vitamin D (μg/d)[b,c]	Vitamin E (mg/d)[d]	Vitamin K (μg/d)	Thiamin (mg/d)	Riboflavin (mg/d)	Niacin (mg/d)[e]	Vitamin B_6 (mg/d)	Folate (μg/d)[f]	Vitamin B_{12} (μg/d)	Pantothenic Acid (mg/d)	Biotin (μg/d)	Choline (mg/d)[g]
Infants														
0–6 months	400*	40*	10	4*	2.0*	0.2*	0.3*	2*	0.1*	65*	0.4*	1.7*	5*	125*
6–12 months	500*	50*	10	5*	2.5*	0.3*	0.4*	4*	0.3*	80*	0.5*	1.8*	6*	150*
Children														
1–3 years	**300**	**15**	15	**6**	30*	**0.5**	**0.5**	**6**	**0.5**	**150**	**0.9**	2*	8*	200*
4–8 years	**400**	**25**	15	**7**	55*	**0.6**	**0.6**	**8**	**0.6**	**200**	**1.2**	3*	12*	250*
Males														
9–13 years	**600**	**45**	15	**11**	60*	**0.9**	**0.9**	**12**	**1.0**	**300**	**1.8**	4*	20*	375*
14–18 years	**900**	**75**	15	**15**	75*	**1.2**	**1.3**	**16**	**1.3**	**400**	**2.4**	5*	25*	550*
19–30 years	**900**	**90**	15	**15**	120*	**1.2**	**1.3**	**16**	**1.3**	**400**	**2.4**	5*	30*	550*
31–50 years	**900**	**90**	15	**15**	120*	**1.2**	**1.3**	**16**	**1.3**	**400**	**2.4**	5*	30*	550*
51–70 years	**900**	**90**	15	**15**	120*	**1.2**	**1.3**	**16**	**1.7**	**400**	**2.4**[h]	5*	30*	550*
>70 years	**900**	**90**	20	**15**	120*	**1.2**	**1.3**	**16**	**1.7**	**400**	**2.4**[h]	5*	30*	550*
Females														
9–13 years	**600**	**45**	15	**11**	60*	**0.9**	**0.9**	**12**	**1.0**	**300**	**1.8**	4*	20*	375*
14–18 years	**700**	**65**	15	**15**	75*	**1.0**	**1.0**	**14**	**1.2**	**400**[f]	**2.4**	5*	25*	400*
19–30 years	**700**	**75**	15	**15**	90*	**1.1**	**1.1**	**14**	**1.3**	**400**[f]	**2.4**	5*	30*	425*
31–50 years	**700**	**75**	15	**15**	90*	**1.1**	**1.1**	**14**	**1.3**	**400**[f]	**2.4**	5*	30*	425*
51–70 years	**700**	**75**	15	**15**	90*	**1.1**	**1.1**	**14**	**1.5**	**400**	**2.4**[h]	5*	30*	425*
>70 years	**700**	**75**	20	**15**	90*	**1.1**	**1.1**	**14**	**1.5**	**400**	**2.4**[h]	5*	30*	425*
Pregnancy														
14–18 years	**750**	**80**	15	**15**	75*	**1.4**	**1.4**	**18**	**1.9**	**600**[f]	**2.6**	6*	30*	450*
19–30 years	**770**	**85**	15	**15**	90*	**1.4**	**1.4**	**18**	**1.9**	**600**[f]	**2.6**	6*	30*	450*
31–50 years	**770**	**85**	15	**15**	90*	**1.4**	**1.4**	**18**	**1.9**	**600**[f]	**2.6**	6*	30*	450*

Lactation														
14–18 years	**1,200**	**115**	15	**19**	75*	**1.4**	**1.6**	**17**	**2.0**	**500**	**2.8**	7*	35*	550*
19–30 years	**1,300**	**120**	15	**19**	90*	**1.4**	**1.6**	**17**	**2.0**	**500**	**2.8**	7*	35*	550*
31–50 years	**1,300**	**120**	15	**19**	90*	**1.4**	**1.6**	**17**	**2.0**	**500**	**2.8**	7*	35*	550*

Note: *This table (taken from the DRI repons, see* www.nap.edu*) presents RDAs in* **bold type** *and AIs in ordinary type followed by an asterisk (*). An RDA is the average daily dietary intake level; sufficient to meet the nutrient requirements of nearly all (97–98 %) healthy individuals in a group. It is calculated from an EAR. If sufficient scientific evidence is not available to establish an EAR, and thus calculate an RDA, an AI is usually developed. For healthy breastfed infants, an AI is the mean intake. The AI for other life-stage and Lgender groups is believed to cover the needs of all healthy individuals in the groups, but lack of data or uncertainty in the data prevent being able to specify with confidence the percentage of individuals covered by this intake.*

[a]*As retinol activity equivalents (RAEs). 1 RAE = 1 μg retinol, 12 μg α-carotene, 24 μg β-carotene, or 24 μg β-cryptoxanthin. The RAE for dietary provitamin A carotenoids is two fold greater than retinol equivalent (RE), whereas the RAE for preformed vitamin A is the same as RE.*

[b]*As cholecalciferol. 1 μg cholecalciferol = 40 IU vitamin D.*

[c]*Under the assumption of minimal sunlight.*

[d]*As α-tocopherol. α-Tocopherol includes RRR-α-tocopherol, the only form of α-tocopherol that occurs naturally in foods, and the 2R-stereoisomeric forms of α-tocopherol (RRR-, RSR-, RRS-, and RSS-α-tocopherol occur in fortified foods and supplements. It does not include the 2S-stereoisomeric forms of α-tocopherol (SRR-, SSR-, SRS-, and SSS-α-tocopherol), also found in fortified foods and supplements.*

[e]*As niacin equivalents (NE). 1 mg of niacin = 60 mg of tryptophan; 0–6 months = preformed niacin (not NE).*

[f]*As dietary folate equivalents (DFE). 1 DFE = 1 μg food folate = 0.6 μg of folic acid from fortified food or as a supplement consumed with food = 0.5 μg of a supplement taken on an empty stomach.*

[g]*Although AIs have been set for choline, there are few data to assess whether a dietary supply of choline is needed at all stages of the life cycle, and it may be that the choline requirement can be met by endogenous synthesis at some of these stages.*

[h]*Because 10 to 30 % of older people may malabsorb food-bound* B_{12}*, it is advisable for those older than 50 years to meet their RDA mainly by consuming foods fortified with* B_{12} *or a supplement containing* B_{12}.

[i]*In view of evidence linking folate intake with neural tube defects in the fetus, it is recommended that all women capable of becoming pregnant consume 400 μg from supplements or fortified foods in addition to intake food folate from a varied diet.*

[j]*It is assumed that women will continue consuming 400 μg from supplements or fortified food until their pregnancy is confirmed and they enter prenatal care, which ordinarily occurs after the end of the periconceptional period — the critical time for formation of the neural tube.*

Sources: *Dietary Reference Intakes for Calcium, Phosphorous, Magnesium, Vitamin D, and Fluoride* (1997); *Dietary Reference Intakes for Thiamin, Riboflavin, Niacin, Vitamin* B_6*, Folate, Vitamin* B_{12}*. Pantothenic Acid, Biotin, and Choline* (1998); *Dietary Reference Intakes for Vitamin C, Vitamin E, Selenium, and Carotenoids* (2000); *Dietary Reference Intakes for Vitamin A, Vitamin K, Arsenic, Boron, Chromium, Copper, Iodine, Iron, Manganese, Molybdenum, Nickel, Silicon, Vanadium, and Zinc* (2001); *Dietary Reference Intakes for Water, Potassium, Sodium, Chloride, and Sulfate* (2005); and *Dietary Reference Intakes for Calcium and Vitamin D*. These reports may be accessed via www.nap.edu.

TABLE 2.4 DRIs: ULs Vitamins
Food and Nutrition Board, Institute of Medicine, National Academies

Life-Stage Group	Vitamin A (μg/d)[a]	Vitamin C (mg/d)	Vitamin D (μg/d)	Vitamin E (mg/d)[b,c]	Vitamin K	Thiamin	Riboflavin	Niacin (mg/d)[c]	Vitamin B_6 (mg/d)	Folate (μg/d)[c]	Vitamin B_{12}	Pantothenic Acid	Biotin	Choline (g/d)	Carotenoids[d]
Infants															
0–6 months	600	ND[e]	25	ND	ND	ND	ND	ND	ND	ND	ND	ND	ND	ND	ND
6–12 months	600	ND	38	ND	ND	ND	ND	ND	ND	ND	ND	ND	ND	ND	ND
Children															
1–3 years	600	400	63	200	ND	ND	ND	10	30	300	ND	ND	ND	1.0	ND
4–8 years	900	650	75	300	ND	ND	ND	15	40	400	ND	ND	ND	1.0	ND
Males															
9–13 years	1,700	1,200	100	600	ND	ND	ND	20	60	600	ND	ND	ND	2.0	ND
14–18 years	2,800	1,800	100	800	ND	ND	ND	30	80	800	ND	ND	ND	3.0	ND
19–30 years	3,000	2,000	100	1,000	ND	ND	ND	35	100	1,000	ND	ND	ND	3.5	ND
31–50 years	3,000	2,000	100	1,000	ND	ND	ND	35	100	1,000	ND	ND	ND	3.5	ND
51–70 years	3,000	2,000	100	1,000	ND	ND	ND	35	100	1,000	ND	ND	ND	3.5	ND
>70 years	3,000	2,000	100	1,000	ND	ND	ND	35	100	1,000	ND	ND	ND	3.5	ND
Females															
9–13 years	1,700	1,200	100	600	ND	ND	ND	20	60	600	ND	ND	ND	2.0	ND
14–18 years	2,800	1,800	100	800	ND	ND	ND	30	80	800	ND	ND	ND	3.0	ND
19–30 years	3,000	2,000	100	1,000	ND	ND	ND	35	100	1,000	ND	ND	ND	3.5	ND
31–50 years	3,000	2,000	100	1,000	ND	ND	ND	35	100	1,000	ND	ND	ND	3.5	ND
51–70 years	3,000	2,000	100	1,000	ND	ND	ND	35	100	1,000	ND	ND	ND	3.5	ND
>70 years	3,000	2,000	100	1,000	ND	ND	ND	35	100	1,000	ND	ND	ND	3.5	ND

Pregnancy															
14–18 years	2,800	1,800	100	800	ND	ND	ND	30	80	800	ND	ND	ND	3.0	ND
19–30 years	3,000	2000	100	1,000	ND	ND	ND	35	100	1,000	ND	ND	ND	3.5	ND
31–50 years	3,000	2,000	100	1,000	ND	ND	ND	35	100	1,000	ND	ND	ND	3.5	ND
Lactation															
14–18 years	2,800	1,800	100	800	ND	ND	ND	30	80	800	ND	ND	ND	3.0	ND
19–30 years	3,000	2,000	100	1,000	ND	ND	ND	35	100	1000	ND	ND	ND	3.5	ND
31–50 years	3,000	2,000	100	1,000	ND	ND	ND	35	100	1000	ND	ND	ND	3.5	ND

Note: *A UL is the highest level of a daily nutrient intake that is likely to pose no risk of adverse health effects to almost all individuals in the general population. Unless otherwise specified, the UL represents total intake from food, water, and supplements. Due to a lack of suitable data, ULs could not be established for vitamin K, thiamin, riboflavin, vitamin B_{12}, pantothenic acid, biotin, and carotenoids. In the absence of a UL, extra caution may be warranted in consuming levels above recommended intakes. Members of the general population should be advised not to routinely exceed the UL. The UL is not meant to apply to individuals who are treated with the nutrient under medical supervision or to individuals with predisposing conditions that modify their sensitivity to the nutrient.*

[a]*As preformed vitamin A only.*
[b]*As α-tocopherol; applies to any form of supplemental α-tocopherol.*
[c]*The ULs for vitamin E, niacin, and folate apply to synthetic forms obtained from supplements, fortified foods, or a combination of the two.*
[d]*β-Carotene supplements are advised only to serve as a provitamin A source for individuals at risk of vitamin A deficiency.*
[e]*ND = Not determinable due to lack of data of adverse effects in this age group and concern with regard to lack of ability to handle excess amounts. Source of intake should be from food only to prevent high levels of intake.*

Sources: *Dietary Reference Intakes for Calcium, Phosphorous, Magnesium, Vitamin D, and Fluoride* (1997); *Dietary Reference Intakes for Thiamin, Riboflavin, Niacin, Vitamin B_6, Folate, Vitamin B_{12}, Pantothenic Acid, Biotin, and Choline* (1998); *Dietary Reference Intakes for Vitamin C, Vitamin E, Selenium, and Carotenoids* (2000); *and Dietary Reference Intakes for Vitamin A, Vitamin K, Arsenic, Boron, Chromium, Copper, Iodine, Iron, Manganese, Molybdenum, Nickel, Silicon, Vanadium, and Zinc* (2001); *and Dietary Reference Intakes for Calcium and vitamin D* (2011). These reports may be accessed via www.nap.edu.

the DRI report on ranges for macronutrient and fiber intake and daily physical activity to optimize health and reduce chronic illness.

Several possible exceptions exist to the general rule that discounts a need for supplementation if one consumes a well-balanced diet. First, vitamin C and folate exist in foods that usually make up only a small part of most Americans' total caloric intake. The availability of these foods also varies by season. Second, different athletic groups have relatively low intakes of vitamins B_1 and B_6.[39,138] Their AI occurs if the daily diet contains fresh fruit, grains, and uncooked or steamed vegetables. Individuals on meatless diets should consume a small amount of milk, milk products, or eggs because vitamin B_{12} exists only in foods of animal origin. Consuming recommended quantities of folate supports fetal nervous system development in the early stage of pregnancy.

Antioxidant and Disease Protection Role of Specific Vitamins

Most of the oxygen consumed during mitochondrial energy metabolism combines with hydrogen to produce water. Normally, electron "leakage" along the electron transport chain allows about 2 to 5% of oxygen to form the oxygen-containing **free radicals** superoxide (O_2^-), hydrogen peroxide (H_2O_2), and hydroxyl (OH^-) radicals. *A free radical represents a highly chemically reactive atom, molecule, or molecular fragment that contains at least one unpaired electron in its outer orbital or valence shell.* Paired electrons, by way of contrast, represent a far more stable state. These are the same free radicals produced by external factors such as heat and ionizing radiation and carried in cigarette smoke, environmental pollutants, and even some medications. Once formed, free radicals search out other compounds to create new free radical molecules.

When superoxide forms, it dismutates to hydrogen peroxide. Normally, superoxide rapidly converts to O_2 and H_2O by the action of **superoxide dismutase**, an enzyme in the body's first line of antioxidant defense. An accumulation of free radicals increases the potential for cellular damage **(oxidative stress)** to many biologically important substances in processes that add oxygen to cellular components. These substances include the genetic material of DNA and RNA, proteins, and lipid-containing structures, particularly the polyunsaturated fatty acid–rich bilayer membrane that isolates the cell against noxious toxins and carcinogens. Oxygen radicals have strong affinity for the polyunsaturated fatty acids that make up the cell membrane's lipid bilayer.

During unrestrained oxidative stress, the plasma membrane's fatty acids deteriorate. Membrane damage occurs through a chain-reaction series of events termed **lipid peroxidation**. These reactions, which incorporate oxygen into lipids, increase the vulnerability of the cell and its constituents. Free radicals also facilitate low-density lipoprotein (LDL) cholesterol oxidation, thus leading to cytotoxicity and enhanced plaque formation in the coronary arteries.

TOP 15 RICHEST SOURCES OF DIETARY ANTIOXIDANTS

Not all fruits and vegetables are created equal in terms of antioxidant potential. A fascinating study published in 2004 in the *Journal of Agricultural and Food Chemistry* measured the antioxidant capacity of over 100 foods. The following table represents the top 15 antioxidant-rich foods as found in this study.

Rank	Food Item	Serving Size	Total Antioxidant Capacity per Serving
1	Small red bean (dried)	Half cup	13,727
2	Wild blueberry	1 cup	13,427
3	Red kidney bean (dried)	Half cup	13,259
4	Pinto bean	Half cup	11,864
5	Blueberry (cultivated)	1 cup	9019
6	Cranberry	1 cup (whole)	8983
7	Artichoke (cooked)	1 cup (hearts)	7904
8	Blackberry	1 cup	7701
9	Prune	Half cup	7291
10	Raspberry	1 cup	6058
11	Strawberry	1 cup	5938
12	Red Delicious apple	One	5900
13	Granny Smith apple	One	5381
14	Pecan	1 ounce	5095
15	Sweet cherry	1 cup	4873

Antioxidant capacity in micromoles of Trolox (oxygen radical absorbance equivalence) per gram of food.

Wu X, et al. Lipophilic and hydrophilic antioxidant capacities of common foods in the United States. *J Agric Food Chem* 2004;52:4026.

A HARMFUL PROCESS

Oxidative stress ultimately increases the likelihood of cellular deterioration associated with advanced aging, cancer, diabetes, coronary artery disease, exercise-related oxidative damage, and a general decline in central nervous system and immune functions.

No way exists to stop oxygen reduction and subsequent free radical production, but a natural defense against their damaging effects exists within the mitochondria and surrounding extracellular spaces. This defense includes the antioxidant scavenger enzymes catalase, glutathione peroxidase, superoxide dismutase, and metal-binding proteins. In addition, the nonenzymatic nutritive reducing agents vitamins A, C, and E; the vitamin A precursor β-carotene (one of the "carotenoids" in dark green and orange vegetables); the mineral selenium; and a supplement of a mixed fruit and vegetable juice concentrate serve important protective functions.[13,52,84,115,161] These antioxidant chemicals protect the plasma membrane by reacting with and removing free radicals. This quenches the harmful chain reaction. Many of these vitamins and minerals also blunt the damaging effects to cellular constituents of high serum homocysteine levels (see page 63), and appropriate quantities of antioxidant vitamins and other chemoprotective agents reduce the occurrence of cardiovascular disease, diabetes, osteoporosis, cataracts, premature aging, and diverse cancers, including those of the breast, distal colon, prostate, pancreas, ovary, and endometrium.[38,60,71,82,132] A normal to above normal intake of dietary vitamin E (in α- and γ-tocopherol forms[74]) and β-carotene and/or high serum levels of carotenoids may blunt the progression of coronary artery narrowing and reduce risk for heart attack and possibly diabetes in men and women.[48,67] Unfortunately, heart disease protection from vitamin E is not always observed in diverse populations, high-risk patients, and those with congestive heart failure.[77,177,185] For patients with vascular disease or diabetes mellitus, long-term vitamin E supplementation does not prevent cancer or major cardiovascular events and may increase heart failure risk.[98]

Examples of Health Benefits

Maintaining a diet with recommended levels of the antioxidant vitamins (particularly vitamin C) reduces the risk for several types of cancer.[132] Protection against heart disease occurs with relatively high daily intakes from either foods or supplements of the B vitamins folate (400 μg) and vitamin B_6 (3 mg).[131,154] These two vitamins reduce blood levels of homocysteine, an amino acid that increases risk for heart attack and stroke and that may be involved in development of late-onset Alzheimer disease. Good sources of folate include enriched whole-grain cereals, nuts and seeds, dark green, leafy vegetables, beans and peas, and orange juice.

Postmenopausal women whose diets contained the most vitamin E had 62% less chance of dying from coronary heart disease (CHD) than women who consumed the least vitamin E.[85] In elderly men, a high plasma concentration of vitamins C and E and β-carotene associates with a reduced development and progression of early atherosclerotic lesions.[48] One model for heart disease protection proposes that the antioxidant vitamins, particularly vitamin E (recommended intake of 15 $mg \cdot d^{-1}$), inhibit oxidation of LDL cholesterol and its subsequent uptake into foam cells embedded in the arterial wall. The **oxidative modification hypothesis** maintains that the oxidation of LDL cholesterol—a process similar to butter turning rancid—contributes to the plaque-forming, artery-clogging atherosclerotic process. Additional benefits of vitamin E in the diet include protection against prostate cancer (risk reduced by one third and death rate by 40%) and heart disease and stroke, perhaps by preventing blood clot formation from anticoagulant properties of vitamin E quinone, a natural by-product of vitamin E metabolism. All evidence does not support a reduced colorectal cancer risk from increased consumption of vitamin-rich fruits and vegetables.[110,165]

NOT WHAT MOST PEOPLE THINK

Think again if you are counting on your daily multivitamin pill to ward off the killer chronic diseases cancer or heart disease. The largest study to date of multivitamin use in 161,808 postmenopausal women published in February 2009 in the *Archives of Internal Medicine* reported that vitamin supplementation did not affect the risk of cancer, heart disease, or overall mortality, and it made no difference for how long the supplements were taken. This is unfortunate because Americans spend about $23 billion annually on these supplements. The study's lead author offers this advice: "Get nutrients from food. Whole foods are better than dietary supplements."

EAT A VARIETY OF HEALTHFUL FOODS: Several randomized trials of supplements of β-carotene and vitamin A per se did not reveal a reduced incidence of cancer and cardiovascular disease.[65,122] Such findings have caused nutritional guidelines to refocus more on the consumption of a broad array of foods rather than on isolated chemicals within these foods. Disease protection from diet is linked to the myriad of accessory nutrients and substances (e.g., the numerous "chemoprotectant" phytochemicals and zoochemicals) within the vitamin-containing foods in a healthful diet.[68] Nonvitamin plant phytochemicals include isothiocyanates, which are potent stimulators of natural detoxifying enzymes in the body present in broccoli, cabbage, cauliflower, and other cruciferous vegetables. Researchers at the National Eye Institute (**www.nei.nih.gov**) observed that persons with higher intakes of two specific antioxidants, lutein and zeaxanthin (found primarily in green leafy vegetables such as spinach, kale, and collard greens), experienced 70% less age-related macular degeneration than individuals with lower intakes. This disease results from deterioration of the macular cells in the center of the retina, the light-sensitive layer in the back of the eye that enables us to see. Lycopene, a potent antioxidant substance in carotene-rich foods (and what makes tomatoes red) that is released largely by cooking, has been linked to reduced heart disease risk and reduced risk of developing several deadly forms of prostate, colon, and rectal cancers.[9]

KNOW YOUR LEGUMES

Legumes represent a class of vegetables that includes beans, peas, and lentils and are typically low in fat, contain no cholesterol, and are high in folate, potassium, iron, and magnesium. They also contain beneficial fats and soluble and insoluble fiber. A good source of protein, legumes provide a healthful substitute for meat.

	Common Types of Legume	**Common Uses**
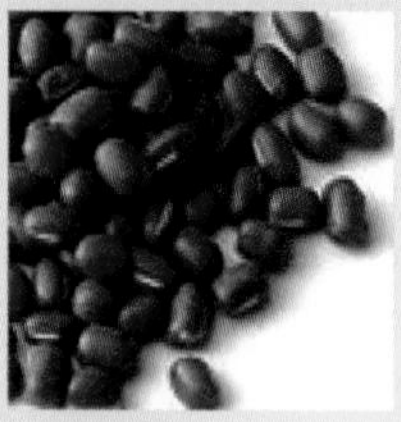	Adzuki beans Also known as azuki beans, asuki beans, field peas, red oriental beans	Rice dishes and Japanese or Chinese cuisine
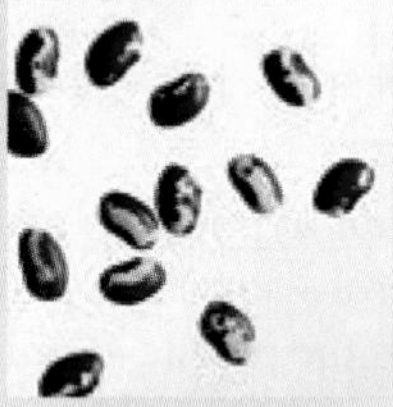	Anasazi beans Also known as Jacob's cattle beans	Homemade refried beans and Southwestern recipes, especially soups
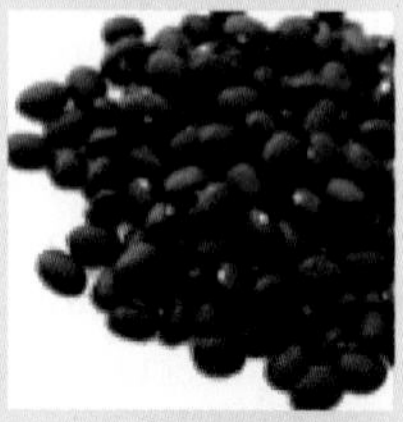	Black beans Also known as turtle beans, black Spanish beans, and Venezuelan beans	Soups, stews, rice and beans, Mexican dishes, and Central and South American cuisine
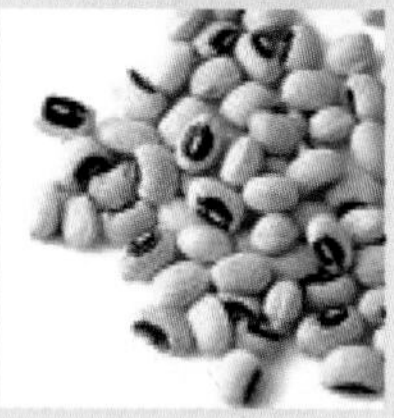	Black-eyed peas Also known as cowpeas, cherry beans, frijoles, China peas, Indian peas	Salads, casseroles, fritters, bean cakes, curry dishes, and Southern dishes with ham and rice
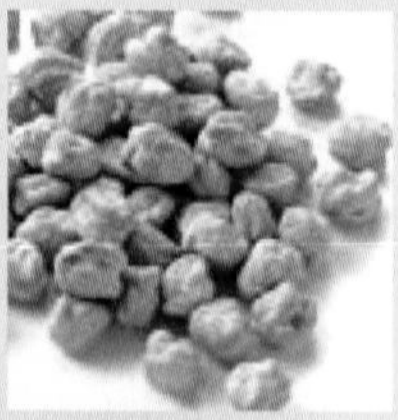	Chickpeas Also known as garbanzos, garbanzo beans, ceci beans	Casseroles, hummus, minestrone soup, Spanish stews, and Indian dishes such as dal
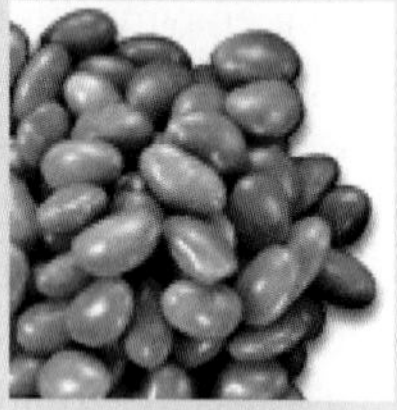	Edamame Also known as green soybeans	Side dishes, snacks, salads, soups, casseroles, and rice or pasta dishes
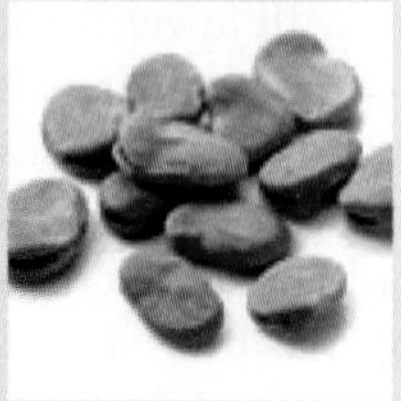	Fava beans Also known as broad beans, faba beans, horse beans	Stews and side dishes

KNOW YOUR LEGUMES

Common Types of Legume		Common Uses
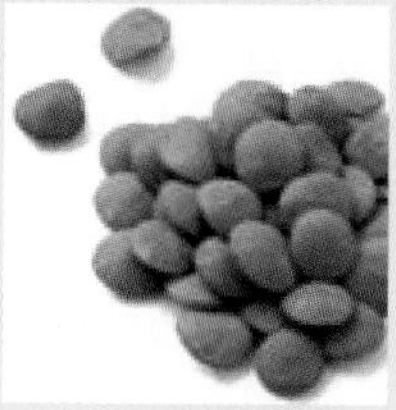	Lentils	Soups, stews, salads, side dishes, and Indian dishes such as dal
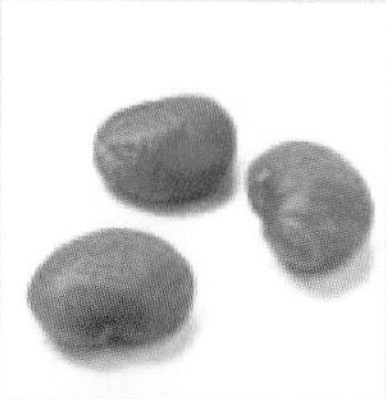	Lima beans Also known as butter beans, Madagascar beans	Succotash, casseroles, soups, and salads
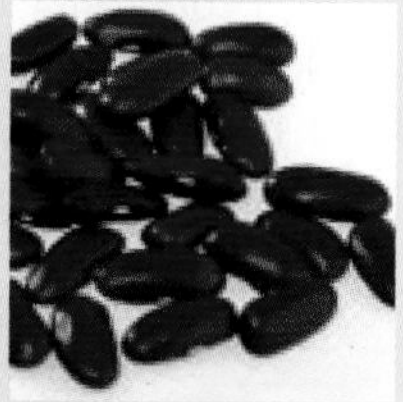	Red kidney beans	Stews, mixed bean salad, chili, and Cajun bean dishes
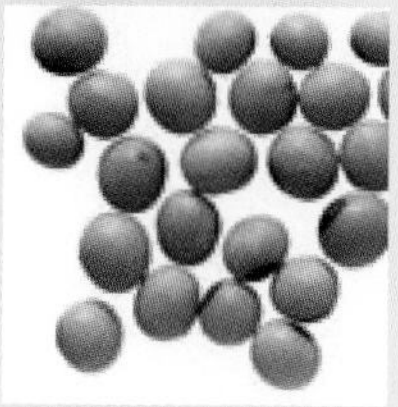	Soy nuts Also known as soybean seeds, roasted soybeans	Snacks or as garnish to salads

Current recommendations advise increased consumption of fruits, vegetables, and whole grains and include lean meat or meat substitutes and low-fat dairy foods to gain substantial health benefits and reduce risk of early mortality. Three potential mechanisms for antioxidant health benefits include:

1. Influencing molecular mechanisms and gene expression
2. Providing enzyme-inducing substances that detoxify carcinogens
3. Blocking uncontrolled growth of cells

Chapter 7 explores the possible interaction of exercise, free radical formation, and antioxidant vitamin requirements.

According to the director of the Division of Cancer Prevention and Control at the National Cancer Institute (NCI; www.cancer.gov/), more than 150 studies have demonstrated that groups of people who consume adequate quantities of fruits and vegetables have less cancer incidence at a number of cancer sites. The NCI encourages consumption of five or more servings (nine recommended for men) of fruits and vegetables daily, while the US Department of Agriculture's (USDA's) *Dietary Guidelines* recommend two to four servings of fruits and three to five servings of vegetables daily. Rich dietary sources of three antioxidant vitamins include:

1. **β-Carotene:** (best known of the pigmented compounds, or carotenoids, that give color to yellow and green leafy vegetables) carrots; dark green leafy vegetables such as spinach, broccoli, turnips, and beet and collard greens; sweet potatoes; winter squash; apricots; cantaloupe; mangos; papaya
2. **Vitamin C**: citrus fruits and juices, cabbage, broccoli, turnip greens, cantaloupe, tomatoes, strawberries, apples with skin
3. **Vitamin E**: vegetable oils, wheat germ, whole-grain bread and cereals, dried beans, green leafy vegetables

BEYOND CHOLESTEROL: HOMOCYSTEINE AND CORONARY HEART DISEASE

In 1969, an 8-year-old boy died of a stroke. Autopsy revealed that his arteries had the sclerotic look of the blood vessels of an elderly man, and his blood contained excess levels of the amino acid **homocysteine**. His rare genetic disorder, homocystinuria, causes premature arterial hardening and early death from heart attack or stroke. In the years following this observation, an impressive number of studies have shown an almost lockstep association between high homocysteine levels and both heart attack and all-cause mortality.[36,59,99,179] In the presence of other conventional CHD risks (e.g., smoking and hypertension), synergistic effects magnify the negative impact of homocysteine.[170,182] Elevated homocysteine levels also associate with increased risk of elevated osteoporotic fracture, cognitive impairment, Alzheimer disease, and adverse outcomes and complications of pregnancy.[107,114,129,173]

All individuals produce homocysteine, but it normally converts to other nondamaging amino acids. Three B vitamins—folate, B_6, and B_{12}—facilitate the conversion. If the conversion slows from a genetic defect or vitamin deficiency, homocysteine levels increase and promote cholesterol's damaging effects on the arterial lumen. **FIGURE 2.4** proposes a mechanism for homocysteine damage. The homocysteine model posits that CHD can mediate through multiple biologic pathways and helps to explain why some people contract heart disease despite low-to-normal LDL cholesterol levels.

Excessive homocysteine associates with the clumping of blood platelets, fostering blood clots, and deterioration of smooth muscle cells that line the arterial wall. Chronic homocysteine exposure can scar and thicken arteries and provides a fertile medium for circulating LDL cholesterol to initiate damage and encourage plaque formation. Persons with elevated homocysteine levels run a greater risk of death from heart disease than individuals with normal levels.

Some Questions About the Strength of the Association

Whether homocysteine behaves more like a marker of the heart disease process rather than a treatment target remains controversial. Blood levels of homocysteine increase as heart disease risk increases, but lowering homocysteine with B vitamin supplements does not reduce heart disease risk. A report analyzed the data from 30 studies of almost 17,000 people who collectively suffered 5073 heart attacks and 1113 strokes.[166] After controlling for high blood pressure and stroke, a person who lowered homocysteine level by 25% reduced the heart attack risk by a modest 11%

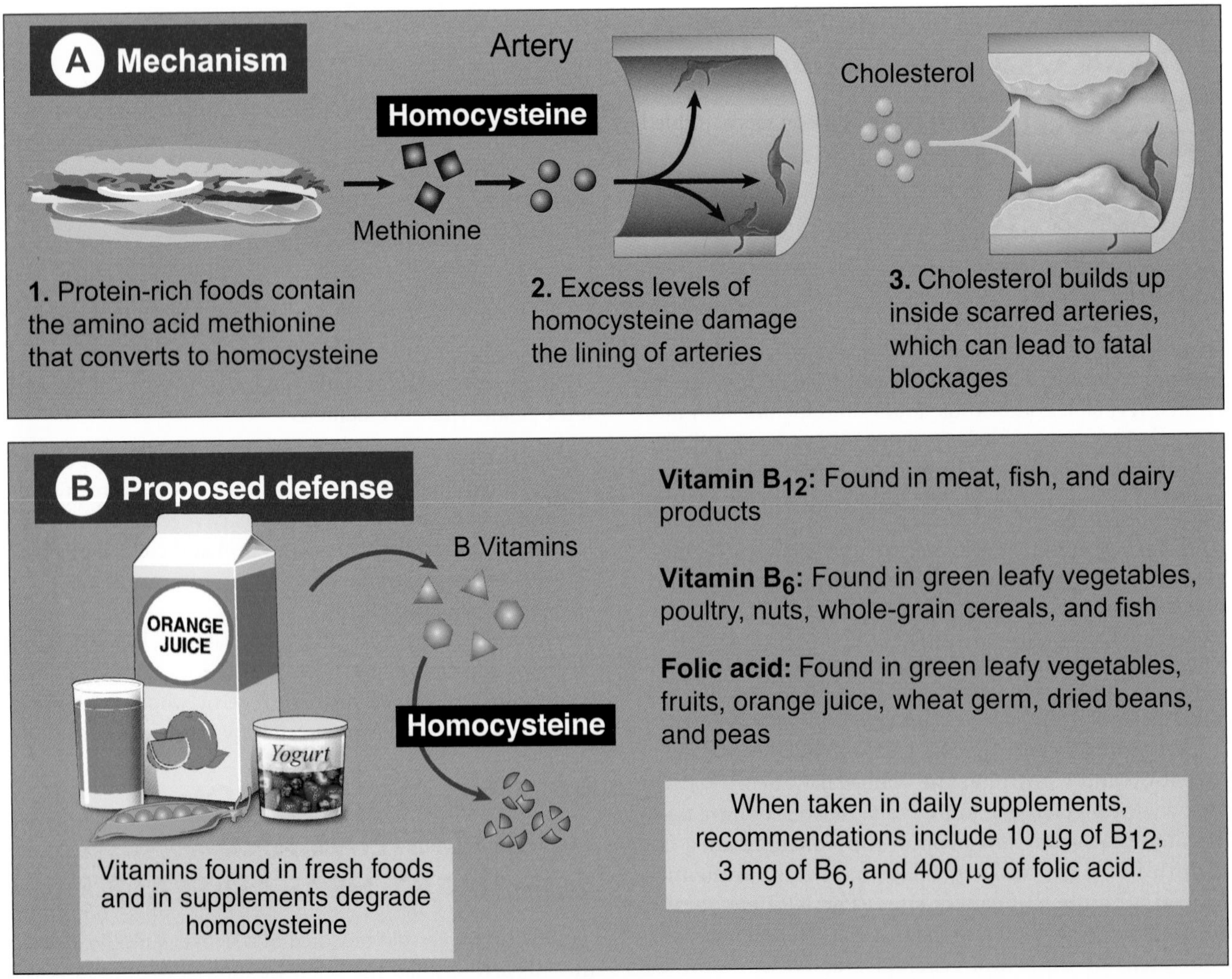
A Mechanism
Artery
Homocysteine
Methionine
Cholesterol
1. Protein-rich foods contain the amino acid methionine that converts to homocysteine
2. Excess levels of homocysteine damage the lining of arteries
3. Cholesterol builds up inside scarred arteries, which can lead to fatal blockages
B Proposed defense
B Vitamins
ORANGE JUICE
Yogurt
Homocysteine
Vitamins found in fresh foods and in supplements degrade homocysteine
Vitamin B12: Found in meat, fish, and dairy products
Vitamin B6: Found in green leafy vegetables, poultry, nuts, whole-grain cereals, and fish
Folic acid: Found in green leafy vegetables, fruits, orange juice, wheat germ, dried beans, and peas
When taken in daily supplements, recommendations include 10 μg of B12, 3 mg of B6, and 400 μg of folic acid.

FIGURE 2.4. A. Proposed mechanism for how the amino acid homocysteine damages the lining of arteries and sets the stage for cholesterol infiltration into a blood vessel. **B.** Proposed defense against the possible harmful effects of elevated homocysteine levels.

PERSONAL COMMITMENTS TO GOOD NUTRITION

1. Eat cereals high in bran and whole grains to maximize fiber intake to lower heart disease risk and produce less weight gain.
2. Go meatless or at least reduce processed meat intake; instead, replace with fish, poultry, or beans to reduce risk of colon, stomach, pancreatic, and possibly prostate cancer.
3. Eat at least three cups of legumes each day to optimize potassium, folate, iron, and protein intake and perhaps reduce risk of colon cancer.
4. Decrease the intake of cheese to lower intake of cholesterol-raising saturated fatty acids.
5. Smarten up on snacks and cut calories from muffins, chips, candies, scones, and assorted pastries. Switch to lower calorie density, nutrient-rich snacks such as fresh fruits and veggies.
6. Eat fish at least two times a week to reduce intake of saturated fat and increase omega-3 fats that may lower heart disease risk.

and stroke risk by 19%. More definitive assessments of homocysteine and cardiovascular disease risk will emerge from prospective, randomized clinical trials currently under way that involve administering vitamins B_6 and B_{12} and folate to healthy persons and evaluating disease outcome over at least 5 years.

It remains uncertain what causes some persons to accumulate homocysteine, but evidence points to deficiency of B vitamins and lifestyle factors such as cigarette smoking, alcohol and coffee consumption, and high meat intake.[49,108,146,162] No clear standard for normal or desirable homocysteine levels currently exists. Research must show that normalizing homocysteine actually reduces risk of heart attack and stroke. In this regard, homocysteine-lowering therapy with the combination of folate and vitamins B_{12} and B_6 improved the outcome for heart disease patients undergoing coronary angioplasty.[148] Sufficient evidence supports a beneficial effect of consuming adequate B vitamins, particularly folate. Even minute amounts of this vitamin (plentiful in enriched whole-grain cereals, nuts and seeds, dark green, leafy vegetables, beans and peas, and orange juice) provide a cost-efficient means of lowering homocysteine levels (**FIG. 2.4**).[168] All white flour, breads, pasta, grits, white rice, and cornmeal are fortified with folate. The current recommended daily folate intake is between 300 and 400 μg.

SUMMARY

1. Vitamins are organic substances that neither supply energy nor contribute to body mass. Vitamins serve crucial functions in almost all bodily processes; they must be obtained from food or dietary supplementation.
2. Plants manufacture vitamins during photosynthesis. Animals obtain vitamins from the plants they eat or from the meat of other animals that previously consumed these foods. Animals also produce some vitamins from precursor substances known as provitamins.
3. Thirteen known vitamins are classified as either water soluble or fat soluble. The fat-soluble vitamins are vitamins A, D, E, and K; vitamin C and the B-complex vitamins compose the water-soluble vitamins.
4. Excess fat-soluble vitamins accumulate in body tissues and can increase to toxic concentrations. Except in relatively rare instances, excess water-soluble vitamins generally remain nontoxic and eventually are excreted in the urine. Their maximum potency for the body occurs within 8 to 14 hours following ingestion.
5. The DRIs differ from their predecessor RDAs by focusing more on promoting health maintenance and risk reduction for nutrient-dependent diseases rather than the traditional criterion of preventing deficiency diseases.
6. Think of the DRI as the umbrella term that encompasses the new standards—the RDAs, EARs, AIs, and the ULs—for nutrient recommendations for use in planning and assessing diets for healthy people. DRI values include recommendations that apply to gender and life stages of growth and development based on age and, when appropriate, pregnancy and lactation.
7. Vitamins regulate metabolism, facilitate energy release, and serve important functions in bone and tissue synthesis.
8. Consuming vitamin supplements above the RDA does not improve exercise performance or the potential for sustaining intense physical training. In fact, serious illness occurs from regularly consuming an excess of fat-soluble and, in some instances, water-soluble vitamins.
9. Vitamins A, C, and E and β-carotene serve important protective functions as antioxidants. A diet containing foods with appropriate levels of these micronutrients can reduce the potential for free radical damage (oxidative stress) and may protect against heart disease and cancer.
10. All individuals produce homocysteine, but it normally converts to other nondamaging amino acids. Three B vitamins—folate, B_6, and B_{12}—facilitate the conversion. If the conversion slows due to a genetic defect or vitamin deficiency, homocysteine levels increase and promote cholesterol's damaging effects on the arterial lumen.

MINERALS

THE NATURE OF MINERALS

Approximately 4% of the body's mass (about 2 kg for a 50-kg woman) consists of a group of 22 mostly metallic elements collectively called **minerals**. Minerals serve as constituents of enzymes, hormones, and vitamins; they combine with other chemicals (e.g., calcium phosphate in bone, iron in the heme of hemoglobin) or exist singularly (free calcium in body fluids).

The minerals essential to life include seven **major minerals** (required in amounts >100 mg daily) and 14 minor or **trace minerals** (required in amounts <100 mg daily). Trace minerals account for less than 15 g (approximately 0.5 oz) or 0.02% of the total body mass, a truly minuscule amount. *Like excess vitamins, excess minerals serve no useful physiologic purpose and can produce toxic effects.* RDAs and recommended ranges of intakes have been established for many minerals; if the diet supplies these recommended levels, this ensures an AI of the remaining minerals.

AVAILABLE AT NO EXTRA COST

Most major and trace minerals occur freely in nature, mainly in the waters of rivers, lakes, and oceans, in topsoil, and beneath the earth's surface. Minerals exist in the root systems of plants and in the body structure of animals that consume plants and water containing minerals.

KINDS AND SOURCES OF MINERALS

TABLE 2.5 lists the major bodily functions, dietary sources, and symptoms of deficiency or excess of the minerals. **TABLES 2.6** and **2.7** present the RDA, AI, and UL values for these elements. Mineral supplements, like vitamin supplements, generally confer little benefit because the required minerals occur readily in food and water. Some supplementation may be necessary in geographic regions where the soil or water supply lacks a particular mineral. Iodine is required by the thyroid gland to synthesize thyroxine and triiodothyronine, two hormones that accelerate resting metabolism. Adding iodine to the water supply or to table salt (iodized salt) easily prevents iodine deficiency. A common mineral deficiency in the United States results from iron deficiency in the diet. Between 30 and 50% of American women of child-bearing age suffer some form of dietary iron insufficiency. As discussed on page 84, upgrading one's diet with iron-rich foods or prudent use of iron supplements alleviates this problem.

ROLE OF MINERALS IN THE BODY

In contrast to vitamins that activate chemical processes without becoming part of the by-products of the reactions they catalyze, minerals often become incorporated within the body's structures and existing chemicals. Minerals serve three broad roles in the body:

1. Provide structure in forming bones and teeth
2. Maintain normal heart rhythm, muscle contractility, neural conductivity, and acid-base balance
3. Regulate metabolism by becoming constituents of enzymes and hormones that modulate cellular activity

FIGURE 2.5 lists minerals that participate in catabolic and anabolic cellular processes. Minerals activate reactions that release energy during carbohydrate, fat, and protein breakdown. In addition, minerals are essential for synthesizing biologic nutrients: glycogen from glucose, triacylglycerol from fatty acids and glycerol, and protein from amino acids. A lack of essential minerals disrupts the fine balance between catabolism and anabolism. Minerals also form important components of hormones. Inadequate thyroxine production from iodine deficiency slows the body's resting metabolism. In extreme cases, this predisposes a person to develop obesity. The synthesis of insulin (first discovered in 1921 by Canadian scientists Fredrick Banting, Charles Best, J.J.R. Macleod, and James Collip), the hormone that facilitates glucose uptake by cells, requires zinc (as do approximately 100 other enzymes), whereas the mineral chlorine forms the digestive acid hydrochloric acid.

Mineral Bioavailability

The body varies considerably in its capacity to absorb and use the minerals in food. For example, spinach contains considerable calcium, but only about 5% of this calcium becomes absorbed. The same holds true for dietary iron, which the small intestine absorbs with an efficiency averaging 5 to 10%. Four factors affect the **bioavailability** of minerals in food:

1. **Type of food**: The small intestine readily absorbs minerals in animal products because plant binders and dietary fibers are unavailable to hinder digestion and absorption. Also, foods from the animal kingdom generally contain a high mineral concentration (except for magnesium, which has a higher concentration in plants).
2. **Mineral–mineral interaction**: Many minerals have the same molecular weight and thus compete for intestinal absorption. This makes it unwise to consume an excess of

TABLE 2.5 The Important Major and Minor (Trace) Minerals for Healthy Adults (19–50 Years of Age) and Their Dietary Requirements, Food Sources, Functions, and the Effects of Deficiencies and Excesses

Mineral	Dietary Sources	Major Bodily Functions	Deficiency	Excess
Major				
Calcium	Milk, cheese, dark green vegetables, dried legumes	Bone and tooth formation, blood clotting, nerve transmission	Stunted growth, rickets, osteoporosis, convulsions	Not reported in humans
Phosphorus	Milk, cheese, yogurt, meat, poultry, grains, fish	Bone and tooth formation, acid-base balance, helps prevent loss of calcium from bone	Weakness, demineralization	Erosion of jaw (phossy jaw)
Potassium	Leafy vegetables, cantaloupe, lima beans, potatoes, bananas, milk, meats, coffee, tea	Fluid balance, nerve transmission, acid-base balance	Muscle cramps, irregular cardiac rhythm, mental confusion, loss of appetite, can be life-threatening	None if kidneys function normally; poor kidney function causes potassium buildup and cardiac arrhythmias
Sulfur	Obtained as part of dietary protein and is present in food preservatives	Acid-base balance, liver function	Unlikely to occur if dietary intake is adequate	Unknown
Sodium	Common salt	Acid-base balance, body water balance, nerve function	Muscle cramps, mental apathy, reduced appetite	High blood pressure
Chlorine (chloride)	Chloride is part of salt-containing food; some vegetables and fruits	Important part of extracellular fluids	Unlikely to occur if dietary intake is adequate	Along with sodium contributes to high blood pressure
Magnesium	Whole grains, green leafy vegetables	Activates enzymes involved in protein synthesis	Growth failure, behavioral disturbances	Diarrhea
Minor				
Iron	Eggs, lean meats, legumes, whole grains, green leafy vegetables	Constituent of hemoglobin and enzymes involved in energy metabolism	Iron deficiency anemia (weakness, reduced resistance to infection)	Siderosis; cirrhosis of the liver
Fluorine	Drinking water, tea, seafood	May be important in maintenance of bone structure	Higher frequency of tooth decay	Mottling of teeth, increased bone density
Zinc	Widely distributed in foods	Constituent of enzymes involved in digestion	Growth failure, small sex glands	Fever, nausea, vomiting, diarrhea
Copper	Meats, drinking water	Constituent of enzymes associated with iron metabolism	Anemia, bone changes (rare)	Rare metabolic condition (Wilson disease)
Selenium	Seafood, meats, grains	Functions in close association with vitamin E	Anemia (rare)	Gastrointestinal disorders, lung irritations
Iodine (iodide)	Marine fish and shellfish, dairy products, vegetables, iodized salt	Constituent of thyroid hormones	Goiter (enlarged thyroid)	Very high intakes depress thyroid activity
Chromium	Legumes, cereals, organ meats, fats, vegetable oils, meats, whole grains	Constituent of some enzymes; involved in glucose and energy metabolism	Rarely reported in humans; impaired ability to metabolize glucose	Inhibition of enzymes Occupational exposures: skin and kidney damage

any one mineral because it can retard another mineral's absorption.

3. **Vitamin–mineral interaction**: Various vitamins interact with minerals in a manner that affects mineral bioavailability. From a positive perspective, vitamin D facilitates calcium absorption and vitamin C improves iron absorption.
4. **Fiber–mineral interaction**: High fiber intake blunts the absorption of some minerals (e.g., calcium, iron, magnesium, phosphorus) by binding to them, causing them to pass unabsorbed through the digestive tract.

In the subsequent sections, we describe specific functions of the more important minerals related to physical activity.

TABLE 2.6 DRIs: RDAs and AIs Elements
Food and Nutrition Board, Institute of Medicine, National Academies

Life-Stage Group	Calcium (mg/d)	Chromium (μg/d)	Copper (μg/d)	Flouride (mg/d)	Iodine (mg/d)	Iron (mg/d)	Magnesium (mg/d)	Maganese (mg/d)	Molybdenum (μg/d)	Phosphorus (mg/d)	Selenium (μg/d)	Zinc (mg/d)	Potassium (mg/d)	Sodium (mg/d)	Chloride (g/d)
Infants															
0–6 months	200*	0.2*	200*	0.01*	110*	0.27*	30*	0.003*	2*	100*	15*	2*	0.4*	0.12*	0.18*
6–12 months	260*	5.5*	220*	0.5*	130*	11*	75*	0.6*	3*	275*	20*	3	0.7*	0.37*	0.57*
Children															
1–3 years	700	11*	340	0.7*	90	7	80	1.2*	17	460	20	3	3.0*	1.0*	1.5*
4–8 years	1000	15*	440	1*	90	10	130	1.5*	22	500	30	5	3.8*	1.2*	1.9*
Males															
9–13 years	1300	25*	700	2*	120	8	240	1.9*	34	1250	40	8	4.5*	1.5*	2.3*
14–18 years	1300	35*	890	3*	150	11	410	2.2*	43	1250	55	11	4.7*	1.5*	2.3*
19–30 years	1000	35*	900	4*	150	8	400	2.3*	45	700	55	11	4.7*	1.5*	2.3*
31–50 years	1000	35*	900	4*	150	8	420	2.3*	45	700	55	11	4.7*	1.5*	2.3*
51–70 years	1000	30*	900	4*	150	8	420	2.3*	45	700	55	11	4.7*	1.3*	2.0*
>70 years	1200	30*	900	4*	150	8	420	2.3*	45	700	55	11	4.7*	1.2*	1.8*
Females															
9–13 years	1300	21*	700	2*	120	8	240	1.6*	34	1250	40	8	4.5	1.5*	2.3*
14–18 years	1300	24*	890	3*	150	15	360	1.6*	43	1250	55	9	4.7*	1.5*	2.3*
19–30 years	1000	25*	900	3*	150	18	310	1.8*	45	700	55	8	4.7*	1.5*	2.3*
31–50 years	1000	25*	900	3*	150	18	320	1.8*	45	700	55	8	4.7*	1.5*	2.3*
51–70 years	1200	20*	900	3*	150	8	320	1.8*	45	700	55	8	4.7*	1.3*	2.0*
>70 years	1200	20*	900	3*	150	8	320	1.8*	45	700	55	8	4.7*	1.2*	1.8*
Pregnancy															
14–18 years	1300	29*	1,000	3*	220	27	400	2.0*	50	1250	60	12	4.7*	1.5*	2.3*
19–30 years	1000	30*	1,000	3*	220	27	350	2.0*	50	700	60	11	4.7*	1.5*	2.3*
31–50 years	1000	30*	1,000	3*	220	27	360	2.0*	50	700	60	11	4.7*	1.5*	2.3*
Lactation															
14–18 years	1300	44*	1,300	3*	290	10	360	2.6*	50	1250	70	13	5.1*	1.5*	2.3*
19–30 years	1000	45*	1,300	3*	290	9	310	2.6*	50	700	70	12	5.1*	1.5*	2.3*
31–50 years	1000	45*	1,300	3*	290	9	320	2.6*	50	700	70	12	5.1*	1.5*	2.3*

Note: *This table (taken from the DRI reports, see www.nap.edu) presents RDAs in* **bold type** *and AIs in ordinary type followed by an asterisk (*). An RDA is the average daily dietary intake level; sufficient to meet the nutrient requirements of nearly all (97–98%) healthy individuals in a group. It is calculated from an EAR. If sufficient scientific evidence is not available to establish an EAR, and thus calculate an RDA, an AI is usually developed. For healthy breastfed infants, the AI is the mean intake. The AI for other life-stage and gender groups is believed to cover needs of all healthy individuals in the groups, but lack of data or uncertainty in the data prevent being able to specify with confidence the percentage of individuals covered by this intake.*

Sources: *Dietary Reference Intakes for Calcium, Phosphorous, Magnesium, Vitamin D and Fluoride* (1997); *Dietary Reference Intakes for Thiamin, Riboflavin, Niacin, Vitamin B_6 Folate, Vitamin B_{12}, Pantothenic Acid, Biotin, and Choline* (1998); *Dietary Reference Intakes for Vitamin C, Vitamin E, Selenium, and Carotenoids* (2000); and *Dietary Reference Intakes for Vitamin A, Vitamin K, Arsenic, Boron, Chromium, Copper, Iodine, Iron, Manganese, Molybdenum, Nickel, Silicon, Vanadium, and Zinc* (2001). *Dietary Reference Intakes for Water, Potassium, Chloride, and Sulfate* (2005); and *Dietary Reference Intakes for Calcium and Vitamin D* (2011). These reports may be accessed via www.nap.edu.

TABLE 2.7 DRIs: ULs, Elements
Food and Nutrition Board, Institute of Medicine, National Academies

Life-Stage Group	Arsenic[a]	Boron (mg/d)	Calcium (mg/d)	Chromium	Copper (μg/d)	Flouride (mg/d)	Iodine (μg/d)	Iron (mg/d)	Magnesium (mg/d)	Manganese (mg/d)	Molybdenum (μg/d)	Nickel (mg/d)	Phosphorus (g/d)	Selenium (μg/d)	Silicon[c]	Vanadium (mg/d)[d]	Zinc (mg/d)	Sodium (g/d)
0–6 months	ND[e]	ND	1000	ND	ND	0.7	ND	40	ND	ND	ND	ND	ND	45	ND	ND	4	ND
6–12 months	ND	ND	1500	ND	ND	0.9	ND	40	ND	ND	ND	ND	ND	60	ND	ND	5	ND
Children																		
1–3 years	ND	3	2500	ND	1000	1.3	200	40	65	2	300	0.2	3	90	ND	ND	7	1.5
4–8 years	ND	6	2500	ND	3000	2.2	300	40	110	3	600	0.3	3	150	ND	ND	12	1.9
Males																		
9–13 years	ND	11	3000	ND	5000	10	600	40	350	6	1100	0.6	4	280	ND	ND	23	2.2
14–18 years	ND	17	3000	ND	8000	10	900	45	350	9	1700	1.0	4	400	ND	ND	34	2.3
19–30 years	ND	20	2500	ND	10000	10	1,100	45	350	11	2000	1.0	4	400	ND	1.8	40	2.3
31–50 years	ND	20	2500	ND	10000	10	1,100	45	350	11	2000	1.0	4	400	ND	1.8	40	2.3
51–70 years	ND	20	2000	ND	10000	10	1,100	45	350	11	2000	1.0	4	400	ND	1.8	40	2.3
>70 years	ND	20	2000	ND	10000	10	1,100	45	350	11	2000	1.0	3	400	ND	1.8	40	2.3
Females																		
9–13 years	ND	11	3000	ND	5000	10	600	40	350	6	1100	0.6	4	280	ND	ND	23	2.2
14–18 years	ND	17	3000	ND	8000	10	900	45	350	9	1700	1.0	4	400	ND	ND	34	2.3
19–30 years	ND	20	2500	ND	10000	10	1,100	45	350	11	2000	1.0	4	400	ND	1.8	40	2.3
31–50 years	ND	20	2500	ND	10000	10	1,100	45	350	11	2000	1.0	4	400	ND	1.8	40	2.3
51–70 years	ND	20	2000	ND	10000	10	1,100	45	350	11	2000	1.0	4	400	ND	1.8	40	2.3
>70 years	ND	20	2000	ND	10000	10	1,100	45	350	11	2000	1.0	3	400	ND	1.8	40	2.3
Pregnancy																		
14–18 years	ND	17	3000	ND	8000	10	900	45	350	9	1700	1.0	3.5	400	ND	ND	34	2.3
19–30 years	ND	20	2500	ND	10000	10	1,100	45	350	11	2000	1.0	3.5	400	ND	ND	40	2.3
61–50 years	ND	20	2500	ND	10000	10	1,100	45	350	11	2000	1.0	3.5	400	ND	ND	40	2.3

(continued)

TABLE 2.7 DRIs: TULs Elements *(Continued)*
Food and Nutrition Board, Institute of Medicine, National Academies

Life-Stage Group	Arsenic[a]	Boron (mg/d)	Calcium (mg/d)	Chromium	Copper (μg/d)	Flouride (mg/d)	Iodine (μg/d)	Iron (mg/d)	Magnesium (mg/d)	Manganese (mg/d)	Molybdenum (μg/d)	Nickel (mg/d)	Phosphorus (g/d)	Selenium (μg/d)	Silicon[c]	Vanadium (mg/d)[d]	Zinc (mg/d)	Sodium (g/d)
Lactation																		
14–18 years	ND	17	3000	ND	8000	10	900	45	350	9	1700	1.0	4	400	ND	ND	34	2.3
19–30 years	ND	20	2500	ND	10000	10	1,100	45	350	11	2000	1.0	4	400	ND	ND	40	2.3
31–50 years	ND	20	2500	ND	10000	10	1,100	45	350	11	2000	1.0	4	400	ND	ND	40	2.3

Note: *A UL is the highest level of daily nutrient intake that is likely to pose no risk of adverse health effects to almost all individuals in the general population. Unless otherwise specified, the UL represents total intake from food, water, and supplements. Due to a lack of suitable data, ULs could not be established for vitamin K, thiamin, riboflavin, vitamin B_{12}, pantothenic acid, biotin, and carotenoids. In the absence of a UL, extra caution may be warranted in consuming levels above recommended intakes. Members of the general population should be advised not to routinely exceed the UL. The UL is not meant to apply to individuals who are treated with the nutrient under medical supervision or to individuals with predisposing conditions that modify their sensitivity to the nutrient.*

[a] *Although the UL was not determined for arsenic, there is no justification for adding arsenic to food or supplements.*
[b] *The ULs for magnesium represent intake from a pharmacologic agent only and do not include intake from food and water.*
[c] *Although silicon has not been shown to cause adverse effects in humans, there is no justification for adding silicon to supplements.*
[d] *Although vanadium in food has not been shown to cause adverse effects in humans, there is no justification for adding vanadium to food and vanadium supplements should be used with caution. The UL is based on adverse effects in laboratory animals and this data could be used to set a UL for adults but not children and adolescents.*
[e] *ND = not determinable due to lack of data of adverse effects in this age group and concern with regard to lack of ability to handle excess amounts. Source of intake should be from food only to prevent high levels of intake.*

Sources: *Dietary Reference Intakes for Calcium, Phosphorous, Magnesium, Vitamin D and Fluoride* (1997); *Dietary Reference Intakes for Thiamin, Riboflavin, Niacin, Vitamin B_6, Folate, Vitamin B_{12}, Pantothenic Acid, Biotin, and Choline* (1998); *Dietary Reference Intakes for Vitamin C, Vitamin E, Selenium, and Carotenoids* (2000); and *Dietary Reference Intakes for Vitamin A, Vitamin K, Arsenic, Boron, Chromium, Copper, Iodine, Iron, Manganese, Molybdenum, Nickel, Silicon, Vanadium, and Zinc* (2001). *Dietary Reference Intakes for Water, Potassium, Sodium, Chloride, and Sulfate* (2005); and *Dietary Reference Intakes for Calcium and Vitamin D* (2011). These reports may be accessed via www.nap.edu.

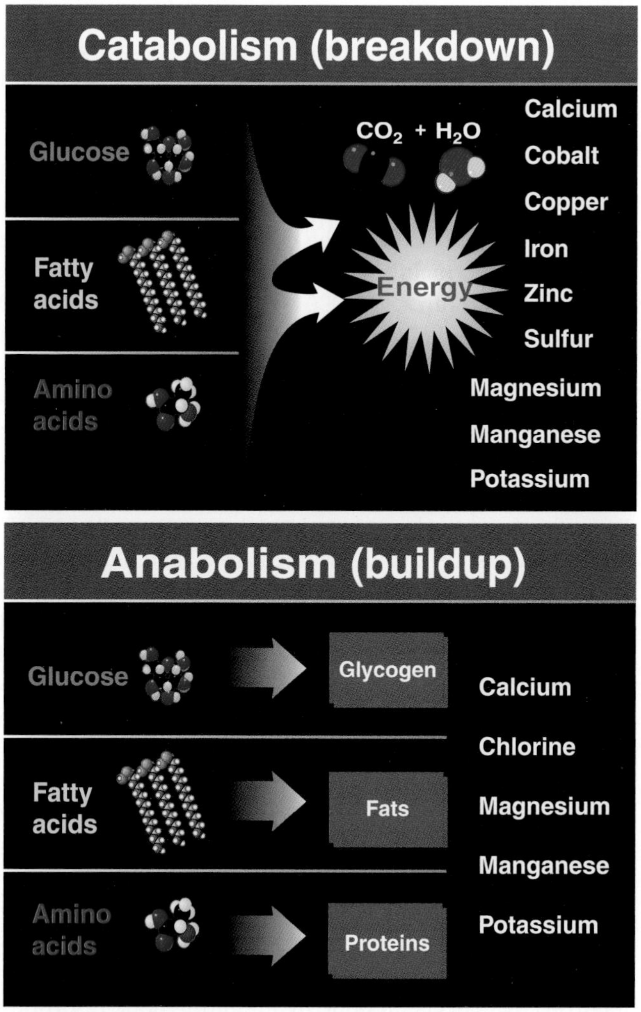

FIGURE 2.5. Minerals function in the catabolism and anabolism of macronutrients.

CALCIUM

Calcium, the body's most abundant mineral, combines with phosphorus to form bones and teeth. These two minerals represent about 75% of the body's total mineral content or about 2.5% of body mass. In its ionized form (about 1% of the body's 1200 mg), calcium plays an important role in muscle action, blood clotting, nerve transmission, activation of several enzymes, synthesis of calcitriol (active form of vitamin D), and transport of fluids across cell membranes. Calcium also may contribute to the following[2,72]:

1. Premenstrual syndrome
2. Easing polycystic ovary syndrome
3. Preventing colon cancer
4. Optimizing blood pressure regulation

Osteoporosis: Calcium, Estrogen, and Exercise

Bone represents a dynamic tissue matrix of collagen, minerals, and about 50% water. **Bone modeling** promotes continual increases in skeletal size and shape during youth. Bone also exists in a continual state of flux called **bone remodeling**. In this process, bone-destroying cells called osteoclasts cause the breakdown or resorption of bone while bone-forming osteoblast cells synthesize bone. An array of growth factors, gonadal hormones, and pituitary hormones governs bone remodeling. Calcium availability combined with regular physical activity affects the dynamics of bone remodeling. Calcium from food or calcium derived from the resorption of the bone mass maintains the plasma calcium level (regulated by hormonal action). Two broad categories of bone include:

1. **Cortical bone**: dense, hard outer layer of bone such as the shafts of the long bones of the arms and legs
2. **Trabecular bone**: spongy, less dense, and relatively weaker bone most prevalent in the vertebrae and ball of the femur

A Mineral Whose Requirement Is Often Not Met

Growing children require more calcium per unit body mass than do adults, yet many adults remain deficient in calcium intake. Based on guidelines from the Institute of Medicine (IOM; www.iom.edu), children age 1 to 3 years require 700 mg daily, and women age 51 and older require up to 1200 mg daily. The main change from the IOM's 1997 recommendations was to lower the level for men age 50 to 70 to 1000 mg from 1200 mg, or about as much calcium as in four to five 8-oz glasses of milk. Unfortunately, calcium remains one of the most frequent nutrients lacking in the diet of sedentary and physically active individuals, particularly adolescent girls. For an average adult, daily calcium intake ranges between 500 and 700 mg. *Female dancers, gymnasts, and endurance athletes are most prone to calcium dietary insufficiency.*

More than 75% of adults consume less than the RDA; about 25% of women in the United States consume less than 300 mg of calcium daily. Inadequate calcium intake forces the body to draw on its bone calcium "reserves" to restore the deficit. Prolonging this restorative imbalance, either from inadequate calcium intake or low levels of calcium-regulating hormones, promotes one of two conditions:

1. **Osteopenia**: from the Greek words *osteo,* meaning bone, and *penia,* meaning poverty—a midway condition of depletion whereby bones weaken with increased fracture risk

NATIONAL ACADEMY OF SCIENCES RECOMMENDED DAILY CALCIUM INTAKE

Age (years)	Amount (mg)
1–3	500
4–8	800
9–18	1300
19–50	1000
51 and older	1200

2. **Osteoporosis**: literally meaning "porous bones," with bone density more than 2.5 standard deviations below normal for age and sex

Osteoporosis develops progressively as bone loses its calcium mass (bone mineral content) and calcium concentration (bone mineral density) and progressively becomes porous and brittle (**FIG. 2.6**). The stresses of normal living often cause bone to break.

Currently, osteoporosis afflicts more than 28 million Americans, with 80 to 90% women and another 18 million individuals having low bone mass (**www.nof.org**). Fifty percent of all women eventually develop osteoporosis. Men are not immune to osteoporosis, with about two million men in the Unites States currently suffering from this affliction. In fact, one in two women and one in four men over age 50 will break a bone because of osteoporosis. Among older individuals, particularly women above age 60, this disease has reached near-epidemic proportions. Osteoporosis accounts for more than 1.5 million fractures (the clinical manifestation of the disease) yearly, including about 600,000 spinal fractures, 300,000 hip fractures, 200,000 wrist fractures, and 300,000 fractures of other body parts. Nearly 15% of postmenopausal women will fracture a hip, and about 33% will suffer spine-shortening and often painful and debilitating vertebral fractures. Only 15% of patients who suffer a hip fracture can walk unassisted across a room 6 months later. Of the women who suffer a bone fracture after age 85, 25% die within 1 year. Estimates from the largest study to date indicate that nearly one half of postmenopausal women age 50 and older with no previous osteoporosis diagnosis have low bone mineral density, including 7% with osteoporosis.[153] This indicates that one of two women (lower risk among African American and Hispanic women) and one of four men over age 50 will experience an osteoporosis-related fracture in their lifetime. In 1990, researchers estimated that by the year 2040, the number of yearly hip fractures would exceed 500,000. However, since 2000, the annual number of hip fractures has remained relatively unchanged (**www.cdc.gov/HomeandRecreationalSafety/Falls/adulthipfx.html**).

Increased susceptibility to osteoporosis among older women coincides with the marked decrease in estrogen secretion that accompanies menopause. Whether estrogen exerts its protective effects on bone by inhibiting bone resorption or decreasing bone turnover remains unknown (see page 80 for estrogen's possible actions). Men normally produce some estrogen, which largely explains their relatively low prevalence of osteoporosis. A portion of circulating testosterone converts to estradiol (an estrogen form), which also promotes positive calcium balance. Most men maintain adequate testosterone levels throughout life. Risk factors for men include low testosterone levels, cigarette smoking, and use of steroid medications.

DEFICIENCY BEGINS AT AN EARLY AGE

Inadequate dietary calcium affects about 50% of American children under age 5, 65% of teenage boys, and 85% of teenage girls. This inadequate intake of calcium partly occurs because Americans now drink far less milk than soft drinks—about 23 gallons of milk a year versus 49 gallons of soft drinks.

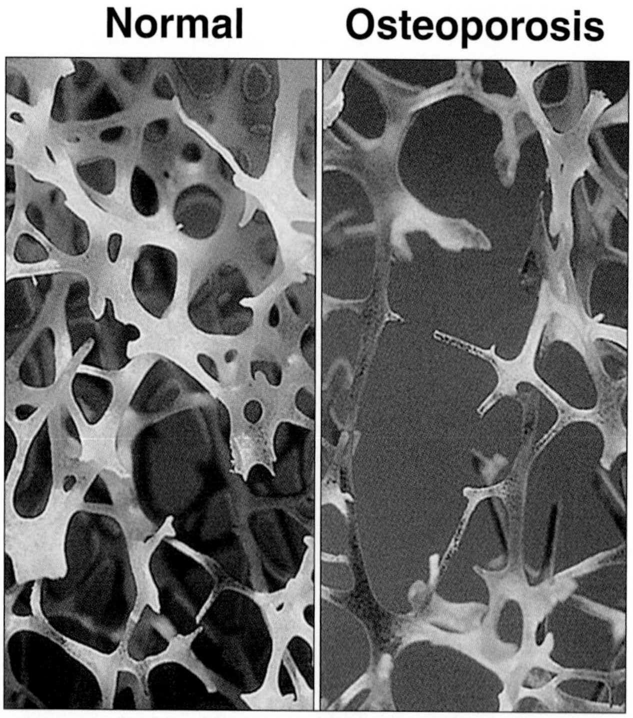

FIGURE 2.6. Micrograph of normal bone (*left*) and osteoporotic bone (*right*). Osteoporotic bone shows the following characteristics: loss of mineral matter, brittleness, cortex thinning (concomitant medullary diameter increase), increased porosity, imbalance between bone formation and resorption, disrupted bone architecture and cross-sectional geometry, microfracture accumulation, loss of mechanical integrity, and less tolerance to bending stress and thus more susceptibility to fracture.

BONE HEALTH DIAGNOSTIC CRITERIA BASED ON VARIATION (STANDARD DEVIATION [SD]) OF OBSERVED BONE DENSITY; VALUES COMPARED WITH VALUES FOR SEX-MATCHED YOUNG ADULT POPULATION

Normal	<1.0 SD below mean
Osteopenia	1.0–2.5 SD below mean
Osteoporosis	>2.5 SD below mean
Severe osteoporosis	>2.5 SD below mean plus one or more fragility fractures

A Progressive Disease

Between 60 and 80% of an individual's susceptibility to osteoporosis links to genetic factors, while 20 to 40% remains lifestyle related. Women normally show gains in bone mass throughout the third decade of life with proper nutrition and regular moderate physical activity. Particularly important nutrients are adequate calcium and vitamin D, which increases efficiency of calcium absorption. Vitamin D also may upgrade the body's immune responses, protect against cognitive decline as adults age, and provide protection against diverse cardiovascular complications, while its protective effects against cancer incidence and related mortality remains equivocal.[89,102,142,167,175] Adolescence serves as the prime bone-building years to maximize bone mass; 90% of bone mass accumulates by about age 17.[7,112] In reality, osteoporosis for many women begins early in life because the average teenager consumes suboptimal calcium to support growing bones. This imbalance worsens into adulthood, particularly among women with a genetic predisposition that limits their ability to compensate for low calcium intake by increasing calcium absorption.[43,50,97] By middle age, adult women generally consume only one third of the calcium required for optimal bone maintenance.

Beginning around age 50, the average man experiences a bone loss of about 0.4% each year, whereas the female begins to lose twice this amount at age 35. For men, the normal rate of bone mineral loss does not usually pose a problem until their eighth decade. Menopause makes women highly susceptible to osteoporosis because little or no estrogen release occurs from the ovaries. Muscle, adipose tissue, and connective tissue continue to produce estrogen, but only in limited quantities. The dramatic fall in estrogen production at menopause coincides with reduced intestinal calcium absorption, less calcitonin production (a hormone that inhibits bone resorption), and increased bone resorption as bone loss accelerates to 3 to 6% a year in the 5 years following menopause. The rate then drops to approximately 1% yearly. At this rate, the typical woman loses 15 to 20% of her bone mass in the first decade following menopause, with some women losing 30% by age 70. Women can augment their genetically determined bone mass through purposeful increases in weight-bearing exercise (e.g., walking and running, not swimming or bicycling) and adequate calcium intake throughout life.

IMPORTANT RISK FACTORS FOR OSTEOPOROSIS

1. Advanced age
2. White or Asian female
3. Slight build or tendency to be underweight
4. Anorexia nervosa or bulimia nervosa
5. Sedentary lifestyle
6. Postmenopause including early or surgically induced menopause
7. Low testosterone levels in men
8. High protein intake
9. Excess sodium intake
10. Cigarette smoking
11. Excessive alcohol use
12. Abnormal absence of menstrual periods (amenorrhea)
13. Calcium-deficient diet in years before and after menopause
14. Family history (genetic predisposition) of osteoporosis
15. High caffeine intake (possible)
16. Vitamin D deficiency, either through inadequate exposure to sunlight or dietary insufficiency (prevalent in about 40% of adults); aging skin loses much of its ability to synthesize vitamin D, even when exposed to sunlight

Prevention Through Diet

FIGURE 2.7 illustrates that variation in bone mass within a population results from a complex interaction among various factors that affect bone mass rather than the distinct effect of each factor.[158,172] Because of this lack of independence among factors that influence bone mass, the portion of bone mass variation attributable to diet within a group may actually reflect how diet interacts with genetic factors, physical activity patterns, body weight, and drug or medication use (e.g., estrogen therapy). *Adequate calcium intake throughout life remains a prime defense against bone loss with aging.* In fact, milk intake during childhood and adolescence associates with increased bone mass and bone density in adulthood and reduced fracture risk, independent of current milk or calcium intake.[75,143] Increasing the calcium intake of adolescent girls from their typical 80% of the RDA level to the 110% level through supplementation increased total body calcium and spinal bone mineral density. A National Institutes of Health consensus panel in 2000 recommended that adolescent girls consume 1500 mg of calcium daily, an intake level that does not adversely affect zinc balance.[105] Increasing daily calcium intake for middle-aged women, particularly for estrogen-deprived women after menopause, to between 1200 and 1500 mg (preferably from the diet) improves the body's calcium balance and slows the rate of bone loss. A positive link also exists between consuming diverse fruits and vegetables and bone health.[118] The association between carbonated beverage intake and increased bone fracture risk most likely results from the beverage displacing milk consumption rather than the effects on urinary calcium excretion of one or more of the beverage's constituents.[62] Conversely, drinking tea may protect against osteoporosis. Although tea contains caffeine (about one half to one-third less than the same volume of coffee), it also contains flavonoids that positively influence bone accretion.[63]

TABLE 2.8 *(top)* indicates that good dietary calcium sources include milk and milk products, calcium-fortified orange juice, canned sardines and canned salmon with bones, almonds, and dark green, leafy vegetables.

Calcium supplements can correct dietary deficiencies regardless of whether extra calcium comes from fortified

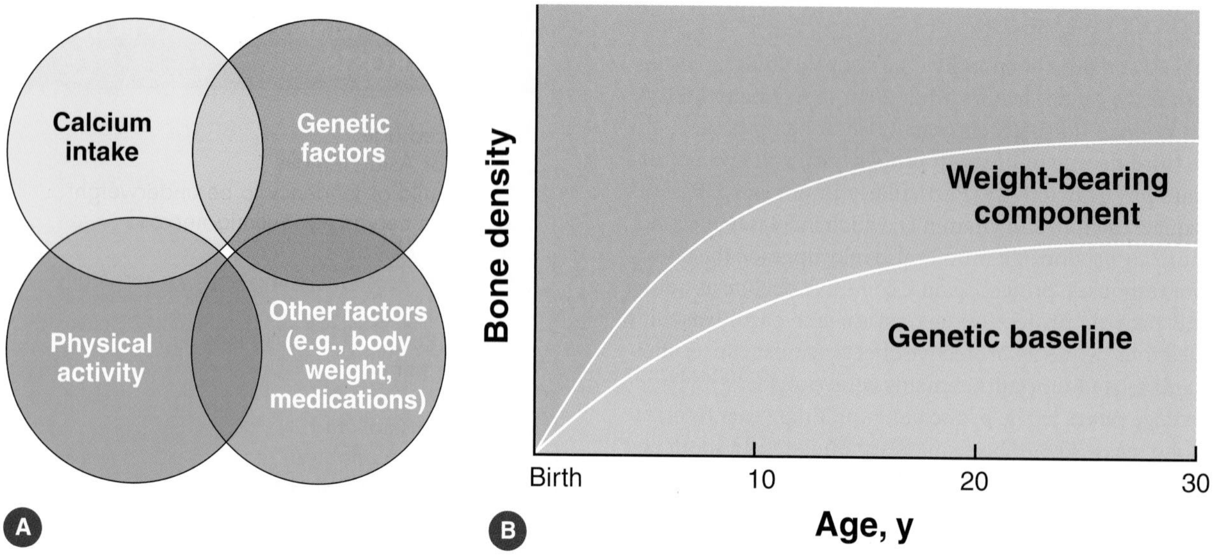

FIGURE 2.7. A. The variation in bone mass within the population is likely a function of how the different factors that affect bone mass interact with each other. (Modified from Specker BL. Should there be dietary guidelines for calcium intake? *Am J Clin Nutr* 2000;71:663.) **B.** Weight-bearing exercise augments skeletal mass during growth above the genetic baseline. The degree of augmentation depends largely on the amount of mechanical loading to which a particular bone is subjected. (Modified from Turner CH. Site-specific effects of exercise: importance of interstitial fluid pressure. *Bone* 1999;24:161.)

COMPLIANCE REMAINS CRITICAL TO PROVIDE BONE-PROTECTIVE BENEFITS OF EXTRA CALCIUM

Regular intake of calcium is crucial in providing bone-protective benefits. Several studies have cast doubts on the benefits of supplemental calcium for bone health. On further analysis of the data, it turned out that nearly 60% of the subjects failed to regularly take the supplements. For the 40% who consistently took calcium, a 30 to 40% reduction occurred in fracture risk. In essence, use of supplemental calcium does reduce fracture risk for aging women, but it must be taken regularly.

foods or commercial supplements (calcium citrate [less likely to cause stomach upset than other forms and also enhances iron absorption], calcium gluconate, calcium carbonate [can be constipating, especially for older people with low levels of stomach acid], or commercial products such as Tums). We strongly recommend checking the label for the amount of calcium, not the combined chemical per dose. Calcium carbonate contains about 40% per dose, whereas calcium citrate contains 21% and calcium gluconate contains 9%. Unfortunately, many calcium supplements, including those from refined sources, contain measurable lead. One should seek out brands that have been labeled as "tested for lead."[140] In addition, adequate vitamin D (600 IU a day for infants through adults age 70 and 800 IU after age 71 based on recommendations from the IOM) should be obtained from food or supplements. The most effective absorption of supplements occurs when taken with the largest meal of the day; this facilitates calcium uptake, whereas excessive meat, salt, coffee, and alcohol consumption inhibits its absorption. The IOM also raised the acceptable upper limit of daily intake of vitamin D to 4000 IU for adults. Assessment of vitamin D sufficiency is generally measured through the quantitative determination of 25-hydroxy vitamin D (calcidiol) in the blood. It reflects vitamin D produced in the skin and obtained in the diet. The kidney changes this into the active vitamin D form. The bottom of Table 2.8 indicates the calcium and vitamin D content of selected dietary supplements.

BENEFICIAL SUPPLEMENT WHEN SUNLIGHT IS SCARCE

A daily vitamin D supplement of 200 IU is recommended for individuals who live and train in northern latitudes, primarily gymnasts and figure skaters who train indoors.[5]

In postmenopausal women, estrogen supplements or low-dose, slow-release fluoride-plus-calcium supplements can treat severe osteoporosis. Estrogen therapy increases bone density of the spine and hip during the first several

TABLE 2.8 (Top) Calcium Content in Common Foods; *(Bottom)* Calcium Content and Vitamin D Content in Selected Supplements

Food	Amount	Calcium Content (mg)
Yogurt, plain, nonfat	8 oz	450
Yogurt, plain, low fat	8 oz	350–415
Yogurt, low fat with fruit	8 oz	250–350
Milk, skim	1 cup	302–316
Milk, 2%	1 cup	313
Cheddar cheese	1 oz	204
Provolone	1 oz	214
Mozzarella cheese, part skim	1 oz	207
Ricotta cheese, part skim	1 cup	337
Swiss cheese	1 oz	272
Almonds	1/2 cup	173
Figs, dried	10	269
Orange juice, calcium fortified	1 cup	250
Orange	1 medium	56
Rhubarb, cooked with sugar	1/2 cup	174
Collards, turnip greens, spinach, cooked	1 cup	200–270
Broccoli, cooked	1 cup	178
Oatmeal with milk	1 cup	313
Salmon, canned with bones	3 1/2 oz	230
Sardines, canned with bones	3 1/2 oz	350
Halibut	One half	95
Elemental Supplement	**Calcium per Tablet (mg)**	**Vitamin D per Tablet (IU)**
Calcium carbonate (generic)	600	200
Tums	200	0
Tums 500	500	0
Viactiv Soft Calcium chews	500	100
Citracal Caplets + D	315	200

years of hormone treatment in both middle-aged and frail elderly women.[20,95,176] However, this treatment is not without risk, as discussed later in the Personal Health and Exercise Nutrition 2.1.

More is Not Necessarily Better: The National Academy of Sciences (**www.nationalacademies.org**) has established an upper level intake of 2500 mg of calcium per day—the equivalent of about eight glasses of milk—for all age groups. Indiscriminate use of calcium supplements, particularly calcium carbonate antacids, in excess of twice the recommended amount places an individual at risk for developing kidney stones. Another possible downside from excessively high calcium intakes concerns reduced zinc absorption and zinc balance.[183] Individuals with high calcium intake should monitor the adequacy of dietary zinc intake (red meats and poultry contain the most readily available form of zinc).

Exercise Is Helpful

Regular dynamic weight-bearing exercise helps to build bone mass and bone strength and slow the rate of skeletal aging. Children and adults, regardless of age, who maintain an active lifestyle show greater bone mass and bone density with substantial improvements in mechanical strength of bone than sedentary counterparts.[40,58,61,92,121,123,159] Benefits of regular exercise and everyday physical activity on bone mass accretion (and perhaps bone shape and size) are greatest during childhood and adolescent years when peak bone mass can increase to the greatest extent (**FIG. 2.7B**).[5,28,73,93,94,96] For example, long-term soccer participation, starting at prepubertal age, relates to markedly increased bone mineral content and bone density at the femoral neck and lumbar spine region.[19] Collegiate female gymnasts demonstrate greater whole-body, spine, femur, and upper limb bone mineral density and bone mineral content than inactive controls.[127] These differences appear to reflect gymnastics activity rather than self-selection because the athletes showed similar bone density values between dominant and nondominant arms in contrast to controls. For these athletes, bone mineral density increases during the competitive season and decreases in the off season.[156] The benefits of regular exercise often accrue into the seventh and even eighth decades of life.[12,83,155,164,178]

REGULAR EXERCISE AND INCREASED MUSCLE STRENGTH SLOW SKELETAL AGING

Moderate-to-intense aerobic exercise (weight-bearing) performed for 50 to 60 minutes 3 days a week builds bone and retards its rate of loss. Muscle-strengthening exercises also benefit bone mass. Individuals with greater back strength and those who train regularly with resistance exercise have a greater spinal bone mineral content than weaker and untrained individuals.

The decline in vigorous physical activity typically observed in advancing age closely parallels the age-related bone mass loss. In this regard, moderate levels of physical activity, including walking, associate with substantially lower risk of hip fracture in postmenopausal women.[41] Even prior exercise and sports experience provides a residual effect on an adult's bone mineral density. For example, former female gymnasts had greater bone mass as adults than females with no previous athletic experience.[79] Consciously restricting food intake blunts the bone-building benefits of regular physical activity.[106]

The osteogenic effect of exercise becomes particularly effective during the growth periods of childhood and

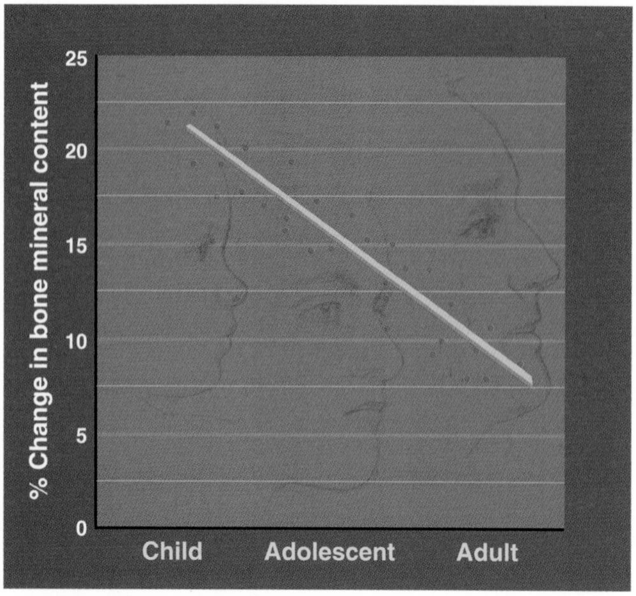

FIGURE 2.8. Generalized curve for the association between age and the effects of regular bouts of intermittent, dynamic exercise on bone mass accretion.

adolescence (**FIG. 2.8**) and may reduce fracture risk later in life.[76] **FIGURE 2.9** illustrates the beneficial effects of weight-bearing exercise. *Short intense bouts of mechanical loading of bone through dynamic exercise performed three to five times a week provide a potent stimulus to maintain or increase bone mass.* This form of exercise includes walking, running, dancing, rope skipping, high-impact jumping, winter sports, basketball, and gymnastics; intense resistance exercises and circuit resistance training also exert a positive effect. These exercises generate considerable impact load and/or intermittent force against the body's long bones.[33,96,109] Activities providing relatively high impact on the skeletal mass (e.g., volleyball, basketball, gymnastics, judo, and karate) induce the greatest increases in bone mass, particularly at weight-bearing sites.[25,153] Even walking 1 mile daily benefits bone mass during and following menopause.

Mechanism of action: Intermittent muscle forces acting on bones during physical activity modify bone metabolism at the point of stress.[57,78,88,90] For example, the lower limb bones of older cross-country runners have greater bone mineral content than the bones of less active counterparts. Likewise, the playing arm of tennis players and the throwing arm of baseball players show greater bone thickness than their less-used, nondominant arm.

Prevailing theory considers that dynamic loading creates hydrostatic pressure gradients within a bone's fluid-filled network. Fluid movement within this network in response to pressure changes from dynamic exercise generates fluid shear stress on bone cells that initiates a cascade of cellular events to ultimately stimulate the production of bone matrix protein.[172] The mechanosensitivity of bone and its subsequent buildup of calcium depends on two main factors:

1. Magnitude of the applied force (strain magnitude)
2. Frequency or number of cycles of force application

Owing to the transient sensitivity of bone cells to mechanical stimuli, shorter, more frequent periods of mechanical strain facilitate bone mass accretion.[26,87,136,137] As the applied force and strain increase, the number of cycles required to initiate

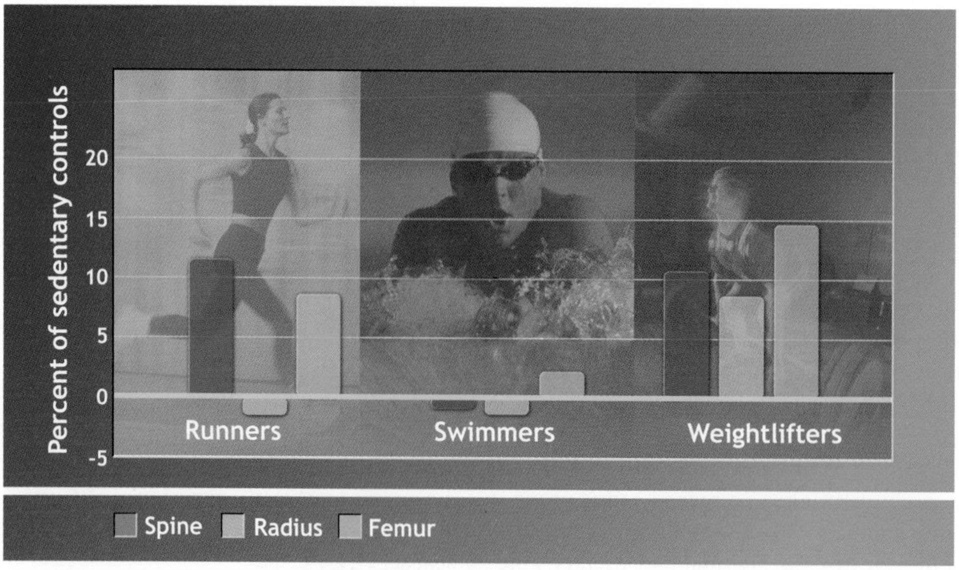

FIGURE 2.9. Bone mineral density expressed as a percentage of sedentary control values at three skeletal sites for weightlifters, swimmers, and runners. (From Drinkwater BL. Physical activity, fitness, and osteoporosis. In: Bouchard C, et al., eds. *Physical Activity, Fitness, and Health*. Champaign, IL: Human Kinetics, 1994.)

bone formation decreases. Chemicals produced in bone itself also may contribute to bone formation. Alterations in bone's geometric configuration to long-term exercise enhance its mechanical properties.[10] **FIGURE 2.10** illustrates the anatomic structure and cross-sectional view of a typical long bone and depicts the dynamics of bone growth and remodeling.

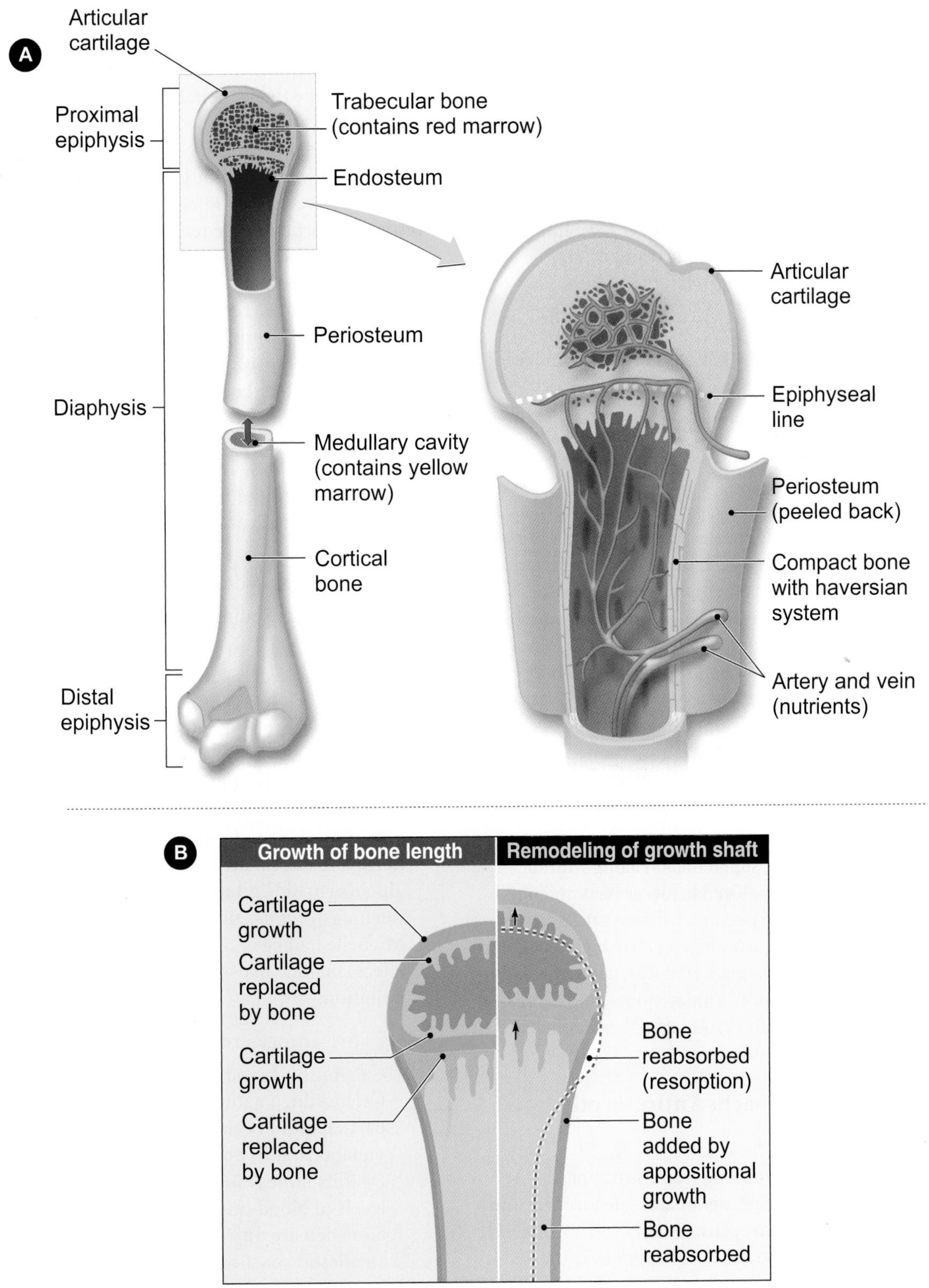

FIGURE 2.10. **A.** Anatomic structure and longitudinal view of a typical long bone. **B.** Bone dynamics during growth and continual remodeling.

PERSONAL HEALTH AND EXERCISE NUTRITION 2.1

Bone Health: Nutrition and Pharmacologic Therapy

Michelle became a near-vegan (consumes some fish) at age 12 years when she stopped eating meat and dairy products on urging from her mother, who had been a vegan throughout her adult life. Now in her 20s and running regularly, Michelle remains a strict vegetarian. She plans to start a family in a year or so but is concerned that her diet may be inadequate in vitamins and minerals, particularly calcium, to ensure her and her baby's health. She also expresses concern she may be at high risk for osteoporosis because both her mother and grandmother have this disease. Michelle takes prednisone (a glucocorticoid drug) for psoriasis; she has normal estrogen levels.

Case Questions

1. What bone assessment tests should Michelle undergo?
2. Review possible treatments options for Michelle.
3. Give the long-term outlook for Michelle's bone health status.

Dietary Approach

Michelle needs to ensure adequate calcium intake. The 1000 $mg \cdot d^{-1}$AI level for calcium (see Table 2.6 in text) for a person of Michelle's age is based on an estimated 40% total for calcium absorption. However, calcium absorption efficiency varies among persons; individuals who absorb calcium with poor efficiency should consume more. In all likelihood, Michelle falls into the category of a "poor absorber" because her diet contains adequate calcium from such foods as cooked spinach (1 cup = 280 mg calcium), canned sardines (2 oz = 220 mg calcium), cooked turnip greens (1 cup = 200 mg calcium), and canned salmon (3 oz = 180 mg calcium).

Michelle should increase her calcium intake to at least 1500 $mg \cdot d^{-1}$ (food and/or supplements) along with the pharmacologic intervention listed below as recommended by her physician. For some persons, calcium intake in excess of 2000 $mg \cdot day^{-1}$ causes inordinately high blood and urinary calcium concentrations, irritability, headache, kidney failure, soft tissue calcification, kidney stones, and decreased absorption of other minerals (2500 $mg \cdot d^{-1}$ represents the Tolerable Upper Intake value).

Pharmacologic Approach: Antiresorptive Medications

Currently, the US Food and Drug Administration (FDA; www.fda.gov) approves bisphosphonates (alendronate and risedronate), calcitonin, estrogens, parathyroid hormone, and raloxifene to prevent and treat osteoporosis. These substances affect the bone remodeling cycle; they classify as antiresorptive medications. Bone remodeling progresses in two distinct stages: bone resorption and bone formation. During resorption, special osteoclast cells on the bone's surface dissolve bone tissue to create small cavities. During the formation stage, osteoblast cells fill the cavities with new bone tissue. Usually, bone resorption and bone formation occur in close sequence and remain balanced. A chronic negative balance in the bone-remodeling cycle causes bone loss that eventually leads to osteoporosis. Antiresorptive medications slow or stop the bone-resorbing portion of the remodeling cycle but do not slow the bone-forming stage. New bone formation occurs at a greater rate than resorption, and bone density may increase over time. Teriparatide (a form of parathyroid hormone) is an approved osteoporosis medication. It is the first osteoporosis medication to increase the rate of bone formation in the bone-remodeling cycle.

Possible medications for Michelle include:

a. Bisphosphonates. These compounds incorporate into the bone matrix to inhibit cells that break down bone. Only these medications have been shown to reduce hip fracture risk.

- Alendronate sodium (brand name Fosamax)
- Risedronate sodium (brand name Actonel)

Both drugs are approved for prevention (5 $mg \cdot d^{-1}$ or 35 mg once weekly) and treatment (10 $mg \cdot d^{-1}$ or 70 mg once weekly) of postmenopausal osteoporosis in women and for treatment in men. The drug is taken on an empty stomach, first thing in the morning, with 8 oz of water (no other liquid) at least 30 minutes before eating or drinking. The patient must remain upright during this 30-minute period. Alendronate sodium also is approved to treat glucocorticoid-induced osteoporosis as occurs with the long-term use of prednisone and cortisone, which Michelle had been taking for her psoriasis. Major side effects include nausea, heartburn, and esophageal irritation.

b. Selective estrogen receptor modulators (SERMs)

- Calcitonin (brand names Miacalcin and Calcimar). Calcitonin, a naturally occurring hormone, participates in calcium regulation and bone metabolism. In postmenopausal women, calcitonin inhibits bone resorption in the presence of high levels of blood calcium and increases spinal bone density. Injectable calcitonin may cause an allergic reaction and flushing of the face and hands, increase urinary frequency, promote nausea, and produce a rash. Side effects for nasal administration of this drug are uncommon but may include nasal irritation, backache, nosebleed, and headaches.

- Raloxifene (brand name Evista). Raloxifene is used for prevention and treatment of osteoporosis in women and increases bone density at the spine, hip, and neck and reduces spinal fractures. Common side effects include hot flashes and leg cramps. Blood clots are a rare side effect.

c. Estrogen replacement therapy (ERT) and hormone replacement therapy (HRT) (multiple brand names). ERT and HRT are approved to treat postmenopausal women. *Their use is not approved for premenopausal women with normal estrogen levels. Side effects may include vaginal bleeding, breast tenderness, mood disturbances, and gallbladder disease.*

A Word of Caution

An 8.5-year study of 16,808 healthy women age 50 to 79 years showed that although combined estrogen and progestin therapy reduced incidence of bone fractures and colorectal cancer, dramatic increases occurred in blood clots, strokes, heart attacks, and breast cancer.[184] These findings caused researchers to halt the study 3 years early. Consequently, hormone treatment for osteoporosis should be viewed as a more dramatic approach requiring medical consultation and appropriate supervision.

thePoint *Visit* **thePoint.lww.com/MKKSEN4e** *to review answers to the Case Questions, as well as further information about Michelle's dietary and pharmacologic approaches.*

The Female Triad: An Unexpected Problem for Women Who Train Intensely

A paradox exists between exercise and bone dynamics for highly active premenopausal women, particularly young athletes who have yet to attain peak bone mass. Women who train intensely and emphasize weight loss often exhibit **disordered eating behaviors**—a serious ailment that in the extreme causes diverse and life-threatening complications (see Chapter 15).[21,86,125] This further decreases energy availability, reducing body mass and body fat to a point at which significant alterations occur in secretion of the pituitary gonadotropic hormones. This, in turn, alters ovarian secretions, triggering irregular cycles (**oligomenorrhea**; six to nine menstrual cycles per year; 35–90 days between cycles) or cessation, a condition termed **secondary amenorrhea**. Chapter 13 more fully discusses the interactions between leanness, exercise, and menstrual irregularity.

The interacting, tightly bound continuum that generally begins with disordered eating (and a resultant energy drain) and leads to amenorrhea and then osteoporosis reflects the clinical entity labeled the **female athlete triad** (**FIG. 2.11**). Some researchers and physicians prefer the term **female triad** because this syndrome of disorders also afflicts physically active women in the general population who do not fit the typical competitive athlete profile.

Limited data exist about the prevalence of the triad, mainly because of a disagreement about how to define the disorder. The combined prevalence of disordered eating, menstrual dysfunction, and low bone mineral density remains small among high school and collegiate athletes.[6,11,100,120,130] Many young women who play sports, particularly sports that emphasize leanness, likely suffer from at least one of the triad's irregularities, particularly disordered eating behaviors, which occur in 15 to 70% of female athletes based on informal surveys and detailed questionnaires.[11,81] **FIGURE 2.12** illustrates the contributing factors associated with exercise-related amenorrhea, which is considered the "red flag" or most recognizable symptom for the triad's presence. Female athletes of the 1970s and 1980s believed that the loss of normal menstruation reflected appropriately hard training and an inevitable consequence of athletic success. The prevalence of amenorrhea among female athletes in body weight-related distance running, gymnastics, ballet, cheerleading, figure skating, and body building probably

A CLINICAL DEFINITION

Clinicians define secondary amenorrhea as the cessation of monthly menstrual cycles for at least three consecutive months after establishing regular cycles.

EXCELLENT WEB RESOURCES

Some colleges and universities maintain web pages that deal directly with the female triad:

- www.bc.edu/bc_org/svp/uhs/eating/eating-femaleathletes.htm
- www.celebrate.uchc.edu/girls/body/triad.htlml
- www.vanderbilt.edu/AnS/psychology/health_psychology/AthleteTriad.htm

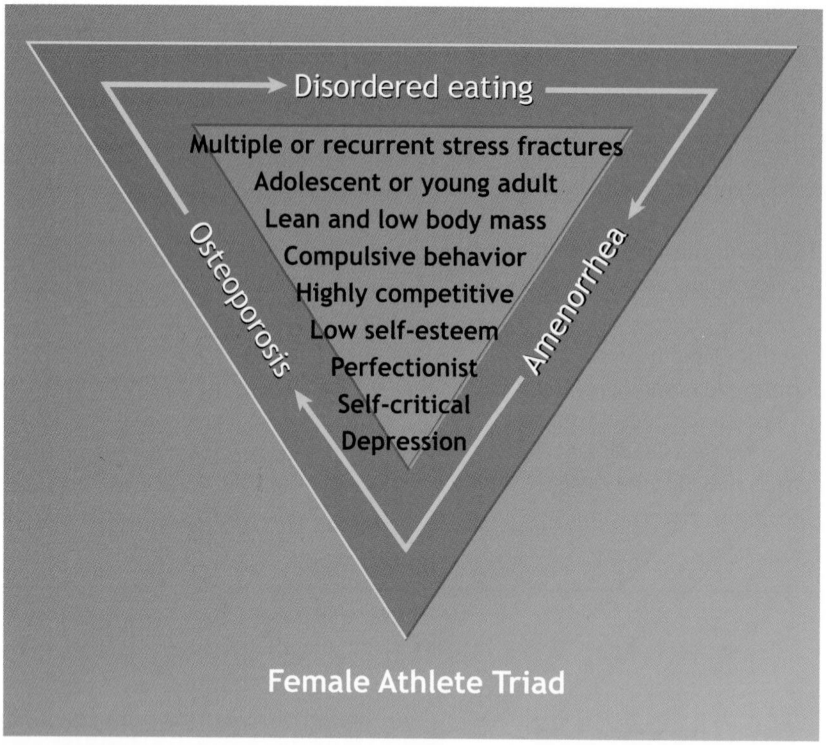

FIGURE 2.11. The female athlete triad: disordered eating, amenorrhea, and osteoporosis.

ranges between 25 and 75%, whereas no more than 5% of nonathletic women of menstruating age experience this condition.

In general, bone density relates closely to menstrual regularity and total number of menstrual cycles. Cessation of menstruation removes estrogen's protective effect on bone, making calcium loss more prevalent with concomitant decreases in bone mass. The most severe menstrual disorders exert the greatest negative effect on bone mass. Lowered bone density from extended amenorrhea often occurs at multiple sites, including the lumbar spine and bone areas subjected to increased force and impact loading during exercise. Concurrently, the problem worsens in individuals undergoing an energy deficit and accompanying low protein, lipid, and energy intakes.[186] In such cases, a poor diet also provides inadequate calcium intake. Persistent amenorrhea that begins at an early age diminishes the benefits of exercise on bone mass and increases risk for musculoskeletal injuries (particularly repeated stress fractures) during exercise.[53,55] For example, a 5% bone mass loss increases stress fracture risk by nearly 40%. Re-establishing normal menses causes some regain in bone mass, but it does *not* reach levels achieved with normal menstruation.

Once lost, bone mass is not easily regained. When a young adult loses bone mass, it may permanently remain at suboptimal levels throughout adult life, leaving women at increased risk for osteoporosis and stress fractures even years after competitive athletic participation.[31,111]

SIX PRINCIPLES FOR PROMOTING BONE HEALTH THROUGH EXERCISE

1. **Specificity:** Exercise provides a local osteogenic effect.
2. **Overload:** Progressively increasing exercise intensity promotes continued improvement.
3. **Initial values:** Individuals with the smallest total bone mass have the greatest potential for improvement.
4. **Diminishing returns:** As one approaches the biologic ceiling for bone density, further gains require greater effort.
5. **More not necessarily better:** Bone cells become desensitized in response to prolonged mechanical-loading sessions.
6. **Reversibility:** Discontinuing exercise overload reverses the positive osteogenic effects of exercise.

ESTROGEN'S THREE ROLES IN BONE HEALTH

1. Increases intestinal calcium absorption
2. Reduces urinary calcium excretion
3. Facilitates calcium retention by bone

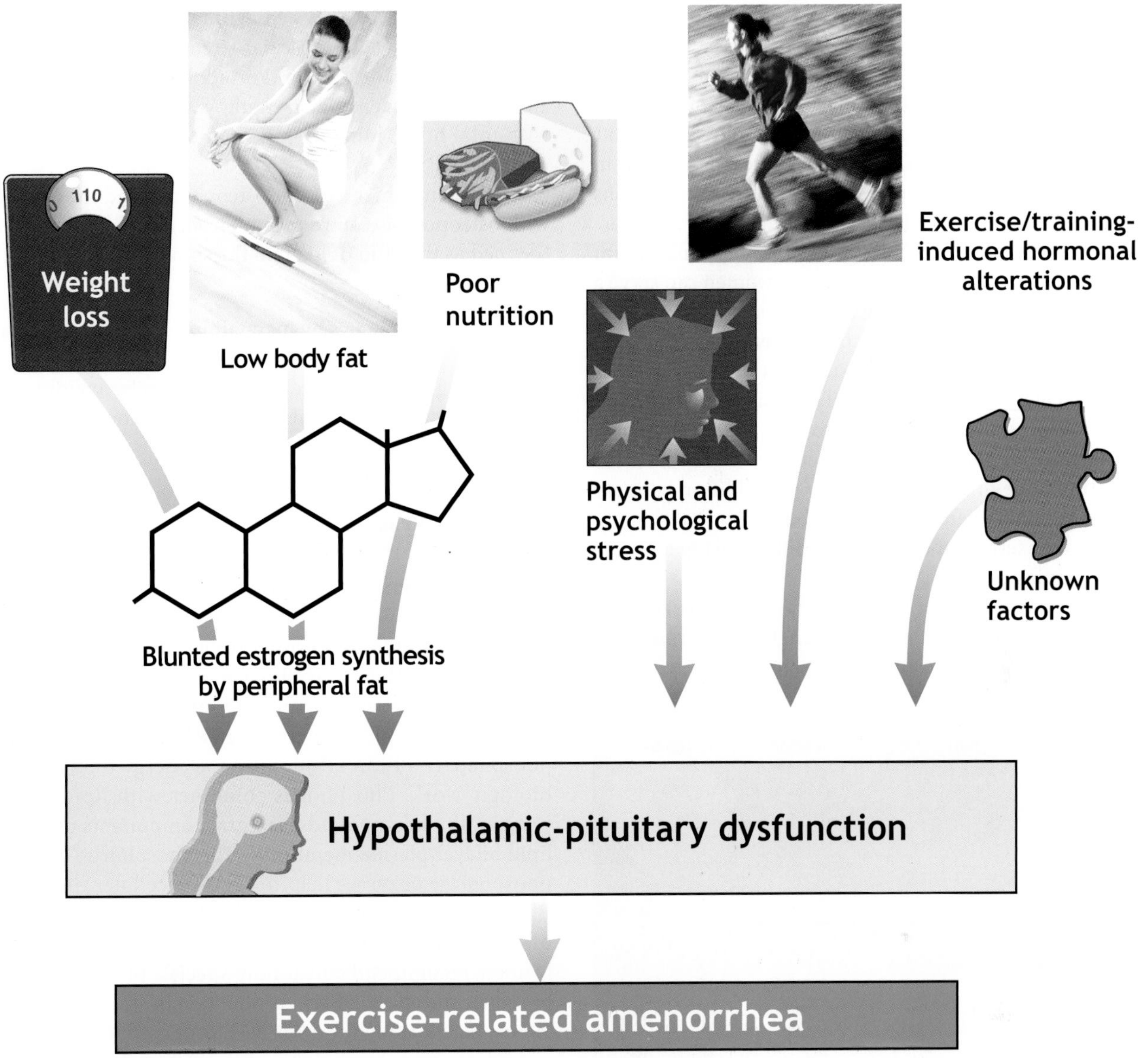

FIGURE 2.12. Factors contributing to the development of exercise-related amenorrhea.

Professional organizations recommend that intervention begin within 3 months of the onset of amenorrhea. Successful treatment of athletic amenorrhea requires a nonpharmacologic, behavioral approach that includes the following four factors[3]:

1. Reduce training level by 10 to 20%
2. Gradually increase total energy intake
3. Increase body weight by 2 to 3%
4. Maintain 1500 mg daily calcium intake

As with most medical ailments, prevention offers the most effective treatment for the female triad. Ideally, screening for the triad should begin in junior high school and high school at the preparticipation medical exam and subsequent evaluations. Such screenings provide insight about behaviors and symptoms related to disordered eating and menstrual irregularity. In addition, coaches and athletic trainers should routinely monitor athletes for changes in menstrual patterns and eating behaviors. *The identification of any one ailment in the triad requires prompt screening for the other two disorders.* Chapter 15 discusses various eating disorders with emphasis on athletes and physically active individuals.

DOES MUSCLE STRENGTH RELATE TO BONE DENSITY?

Men and women who participate in strength and power activities have as much or more total bone mass than endurance athletes.[135] Such findings have caused some speculation about the possible relationship between muscular strength and bone mass. Laboratory experiments have documented greater maximum flexion and extension dynamic strength in postmenopausal women without osteoporosis than in osteoporotic counterparts. **FIGURE 2.13** displays unequivocal chest flexion and extension strength results in normal and osteoporotic women. Women with normal lumbar spine and femur neck bone mineral density exhibited 20% greater strength in 11 of 12 test comparisons for flexion; four of 12 comparisons for extension showed 13% higher values for women with normal bone density. Quite possibly, differences in maximum dynamic strength among postmenopausal women can serve a clinically useful role in screening for osteoporosis and risk of stress fractures.[45,126] Other data complement these findings; they indicate that regional lean tissue mass (often an indication of muscular strength) accurately predicts bone mineral density.[119] The lumbar spine and proximal femur bone mass of elite teenage weightlifters exceeds representative values for fully mature bone of reference adults.[24] In addition, a linear relation exists between increases in bone mineral density and total and exercise-specific weight lifted during a 1-year strength-training program.[27]

For female gymnasts, bone mineral density correlated moderately with maximal muscle strength and serum progesterone.[64] Many of these athletes exhibited oligomenorrhea and amenorrhea, yet they can maintain bone mineral density levels that correlate to muscular strength in the axial (L2–L4) and appendicular skeleton. For adolescent female athletes, absolute knee extension strength was moderately associated with total body, lumbar spine, femoral neck, and leg bone mineral density.[33]

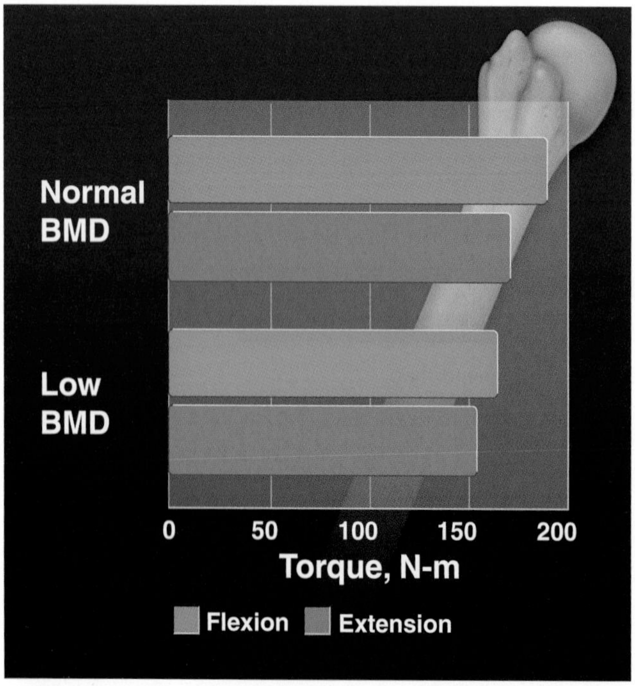

FIGURE 2.13. Comparison of chest press extension and flexion strength in age- and weight-matched postmenopausal women with normal and low bone mineral density (BMD). Women with low BMD scored significantly lower on each measure of muscular strength than the reference group. (From Stock JL, et al. Dynamic muscle strength is decreased in postmenopausal women with low bone density. *J Bone Miner Res* 1987;2:338; Janey C, et al. Maximum muscular strength differs in postmenopausal women with and without osteoporosis. *Med Sci Sports Exerc* 1987;19:S61.)

Women at high risk for osteoporosis and those afflicted with osteoporosis can reduce their *factor of risk* for fracture (defined as the ratio of load on the spine to the bone's failure load) in two ways:

1. Strengthening bones by maintaining or increasing their density
2. Reducing the magnitude of spinal forces by avoiding higher risk activities that increase spinal compression such as heavy lifting activities

PHOSPHORUS

Phosphorus combines with calcium to form hydroxyapatite and calcium phosphate—two compounds that provide rigidity to bones and teeth. Phosphorus also serves as an essential component of the intracellular mediator, cyclic adenosine monophosphate (AMP), and the intramuscular high-energy compounds phosphocreatine (PCr) and adenosine triphosphate (ATP). ATP supplies the energy for all forms of biologic work. Phosphorus combines with lipids to form phospholipid compounds, integral components of the cells' lipid bilayer plasma membrane. The phosphorus-containing phosphatase enzymes help to regulate cellular metabolism. Phosphorus also participates in buffering acid end products of energy metabolism. For this reason, some coaches and trainers recommend consuming special "phosphate drinks" to reduce the effects of acid production in strenuous exercise. "Phosphate loading" also has been proposed to facilitate oxygen release from hemoglobin at the cellular level. In Chapter 11, we discuss the usefulness of specific buffering drinks to augment intense exercise performance. Most studies confirm that the phosphorus intake of athletes generally attains recommended levels, with the possible exception of female dancers and gymnasts. Rich dietary sources of phosphorus include milk products (8 oz skim milk = 247 mg; 8 oz plan nonfat yogurt = 385 mg); cooked halibut and salmon (3 oz = 250 mg); cooked beef, chicken, and turkey (3 oz = 165 mg); cooked lentils (½ cup = 178 mg); and almonds (1 oz, or about 23 almonds = 134 mg).

MAGNESIUM

About 400 enzymes that regulate metabolism contain magnesium. Magnesium plays a vital role in glucose metabolism by helping to form muscle and liver glycogen from blood-borne glucose. The 20 to 30 g of magnesium in the body also participates as a cofactor to degrade glucose, fatty acids, and amino acids during energy metabolism. Magnesium affects lipid and protein synthesis and contributes to proper functioning of the neuromuscular system. Magnesium also acts as an electrolyte that, along with potassium and sodium, helps to stabilize blood pressure within the normal range. By regulating DNA and RNA synthesis and structure, magnesium regulates cell growth, reproduction, and the structure of plasma membranes. As its role as a Ca^{2+} channel blocker, a depressed magnesium concentration could lead to hypertension and cardiac arrhythmias. Intense sweating generally produces only small magnesium losses.

Conflicting data exist concerning the possible effects of magnesium supplements on exercise performance and the training response. In one study, magnesium supplementation did not affect quadriceps muscle strength or measures of fatigue in the 6-week period following a marathon.[169] Subsequent research showed that 4 weeks of 212 $mg \cdot d^{-1}$ of a magnesium oxide supplement increased resting magnesium levels but did not affect anaerobic or aerobic exercise performance compared with a placebo.[42] In contrast, untrained men and women who supplemented with magnesium increased quadriceps power compared with a placebo treatment during 7 weeks of resistance training.[15]

The magnesium intake of athletes generally attains recommended levels, although female dancers and gymnasts have low intakes.[113] Green leafy vegetables, legumes, nuts, bananas, mushrooms, and whole grains are rich sources of magnesium. We do not recommend taking magnesium supplements because these often are mixed with dolomite ($CaMg[CO_3]_2$), an extract from dolomitic limestone and marble, which often contains the toxic elements mercury and lead.

IRON

The body normally contains between 3 and 5 g (about 1/6 oz) of the trace mineral iron. Approximately 80% of this amount exists in functionally active compounds, predominantly combined with **hemoglobin** in red blood cells. This iron–protein compound increases the oxygen-carrying capacity of blood approximately 65 times. **FIGURE 2.14** displays the percentage composition of centrifuged whole blood for plasma and concentration of red blood cells (called the **hematocrit**), including average hemoglobin values for men and women.

Iron serves other important exercise-related functions besides its role in oxygen transport in blood. It serves as a structural component of **myoglobin** (about 5% of total iron), a compound with some similarities to hemoglobin that aids in oxygen storage and transport within the muscle cell. Small amounts of iron also exist in **cytochromes**, the specialized substances that facilitate energy transfer within the cell. About 20% of the body's iron does not combine in functionally active compounds but exists as **hemosiderin** and **ferritin** stored in the liver, spleen, and bone marrow. These stores replenish iron lost from the functional compounds and provide the iron reserve during periods of insufficient dietary iron intake. Another plasma protein, **transferrin**, transports iron from ingested food and damaged red blood cells for delivery to tissues in need. *Plasma levels of transferrin generally reflect the adequacy of current iron intake*

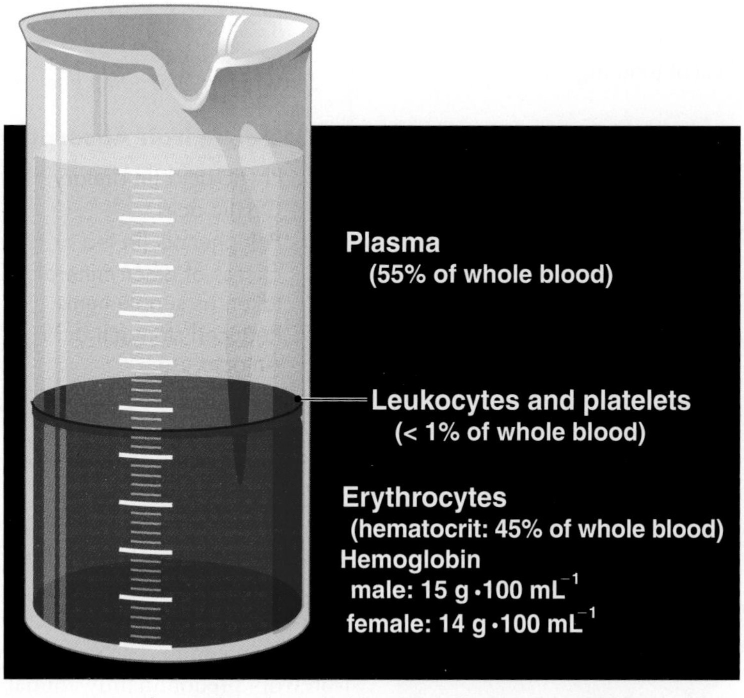

FIGURE 2.14. Percentage composition of centrifuged whole blood for plasma and red blood cell concentration (hematocrit). Also included are average values for hemoglobin for men and women per 100 mL of blood.

Physically active individuals should include normal amounts of iron-rich foods in their daily diet. Persons with inadequate iron intake or with limited rates of iron absorption or high rates of iron loss often develop a reduced concentration of hemoglobin in red blood cells. This extreme condition of iron insufficiency, called **iron deficiency anemia**, produces general sluggishness, loss of appetite, and reduced capacity to sustain even mild exercise. "Iron therapy" with this condition normalizes the hemoglobin content of the blood and improves exercise capacity. **TABLE 2.9** lists recommendations for iron intake for children and adults.

Women: A Population at Risk

Insufficient iron intake represents the most common micronutrient insufficiency, affecting between 20 and 50% of the world's population. In the United States, estimates place between 10 and 13% of premenopausal women as deficient in iron intake, and between 3 and 5% are anemic by conventional diagnostic criteria.[35] Inadequate iron intake frequently occurs among young children, teenagers, and women of child-bearing age, including many physically active women. In addition, pregnancy can trigger a moderate iron deficiency anemia from the increased iron demand for both mother and fetus.

Iron loss from the 30 to 60 mL of blood lost during a menstrual cycle ranges between 15 and 30 mg. This loss requires an additional 5-mg of dietary iron daily for premenopausal females, which increases the average monthly iron requirement by about 150 mg. Thus, an additional 20 to 25 mg of iron becomes available to females each month (assuming typical iron absorption) for synthesizing red blood cells lost during menstruation. Dietary iron insufficiencies of the large number of American premenopausal women relate to a limited supply of iron in the typical diet, which averages about 6 mg of iron per 1000 kcal of food ingested.

TABLE 2.9 Recommended Dietary Allowances for Iron

	Age (years)	Iron (mg)
Children	1–10	10
Males	11–18	12
	191	10
Females	11–50	15
	51+	10
	Pregnant	30[a]
	Lactating	15[a]

[a]Generally, this increased requirement cannot be met by ordinary diets; therefore, the use of 30 to 60 mg of supplemental iron is recommended.

Food and Nutrition Board, National Academy of Sciences-National Research Council, Washington, DC. Recommended dietary allowances, revised 2001.

Iron Source Is Important

Intestinal absorption of iron varies closely with iron need, yet considerable variation in bioavailability occurs because of diet composition. For example, the intestine usually absorbs between 2 and 10% of iron from plants (trivalent ferric or **nonheme** elemental **iron**), whereas iron absorption from animal sources (divalent ferrous or **heme iron**) increases to between 10 and 35%. The body absorbs about 15% of ingested iron, depending on iron status, form of iron ingested, and meal composition. For example, intestinal absorption of nonheme (but not heme) iron increases when consuming diets with low iron bioavailability.[69] Conversely, iron supplementation reduces nonheme iron but not heme iron absorption from food.[141] Despite this partial adaptation in iron absorption, iron stores remain greater after supplementation than after placebo treatment. The presence of heme iron in food also increases iron absorption from nonheme sources. Consuming more meat maintains iron status more effectively in exercising women than supplementing with commercial iron preparations.[101]

FACTORS THAT INCREASE AND DECREASE IRON ABSORPTION

Increase Iron Absorption

1. Stomach acid
2. Dietary iron in heme form
3. High body demand for red blood cells (blood loss, high altitude exposure, exercise training, pregnancy)
4. Presence of meat protein factor (MPF), a substance in meat, poultry, and fish that aids in nonheme iron absorption
5. Vitamin C in small intestine

Decrease Iron Absorption

1. Phytic acid (in dietary fiber)
2. Oaxlic acid
3. Polyphenols (in tea or coffee)
4. Excess of other minerals (Zn, Mg, Ca), particularly taken as supplements
5. Reduced stomach acid
6. Antacid use

Concern to Vegetarians

The relatively low bioavailability of nonheme iron places women on vegetarian-type diets at increased risk for developing iron insufficiency. Female vegetarian runners have a poorer iron status than counterparts who consume the same quantity of iron from predominantly animal sources.[157] Including foods rich in vitamin C in the diet (see Fig. 2.1) upgrades the bioavailability of dietary iron. This occurs because ascorbic acid increases the solubility of nonheme iron, making it available for absorption at the alkaline pH of the small intestine. The ascorbic acid in a glass of orange juice, for example, significantly increases nonheme iron absorption from a breakfast meal.

The *top* panel of **FIGURE 2.15** clearly illustrates the effect of exogenous vitamin C on nonheme iron absorption. Eight healthy men without iron deficiency were studied at rest after taking either 100 mg of ferric sodium citrate complex, 100 mg of ferric sodium citrate complex with 200 mg ascorbic acid, or no exogenous iron. The iron supplement alone caused an 18.4% increase in serum iron concentration compared with the control, no iron condition. Combining iron and vitamin C induced a peak 72% increase in serum iron. Furthermore, taking the iron-only supplement followed by 1 hour of moderate exercise produced a 48.2% increase in serum iron concentration compared with only an 8.3% increase at rest (**FIG. 2.15**, *bottom*). Combining exercise and iron supplementation plus vitamin C did not augment physical activity's effect on iron absorption. These data convincingly indicate that moderate exercise does not impair the body's absorption of supplemental iron; instead, it facilitates iron uptake to the same amount as vitamin C supplementation without exercise. These findings also provide a nutrition-based justification for moderate exercise following eating.

Heme iron sources include tuna (3 oz = 1.6 mg), chicken (4.0 oz breast = 1.8 mg), clams (3 oz = 2.6 mg), beef (3 oz = 2.7 mg), oysters (3 oz = 5.9 mg), and beef liver (3 oz = 6.6 mg); **nonheme iron sources** include oatmeal (1 cup nonfortified = 1.6 mg; fortified with nutrient added = 6.3 mg), spinach (½ cup cooked = 2.0 mg), soy protein (tofu, piece 2 ½ × 2 ¾ × 1 inch = 2.3 mg), dried figs (4 figs = 2.3 mg), beans (½ cup refried = 2.3 mg), raisins (½ cup = 2.5 mg), lima beans (½ cup = 2.5 mg), prune juice (1 cup = 3.0 mg), peaches (½ cup dried = 3.3 mg), and apricots (1 cup dried = 6.1 mg). Fiber-rich foods, coffee, and tea contain compounds that interfere with the intestinal absorption of iron (and zinc).

Are Physically Active Individuals at Greater Risk for Iron Insufficiency?

Interest in endurance sports, combined with increased participation of women in these activities, has focused research on the influence of strenuous training on the body's iron status. The term **sports anemia** frequently describes reduced hemoglobin levels approaching clinical anemia (12 $g \cdot dL^{-1}$ of blood for women and 14 $g \cdot dL^{-1}$ for men) attributable to intense training.

Some researchers maintain that exercise training creates an added demand for iron that often exceeds its intake. This would tax iron reserves and eventually depress hemoglobin synthesis and/or reduce iron-containing compounds within the cell's energy transfer system. Individuals susceptible to an "iron drain" could experience reduced exercise capacity because of iron's crucial role in oxygen transport and use.

Intense training theoretically increases iron demand from iron loss in sweat; it also increases demand from hemoglobin loss in urine from red blood cell destruction with increased temperature, spleen activity, circulation rates, and mechanical trauma from runners' feet pounding on the running surface (foot-strike hemolysis).[149] Gastrointestinal

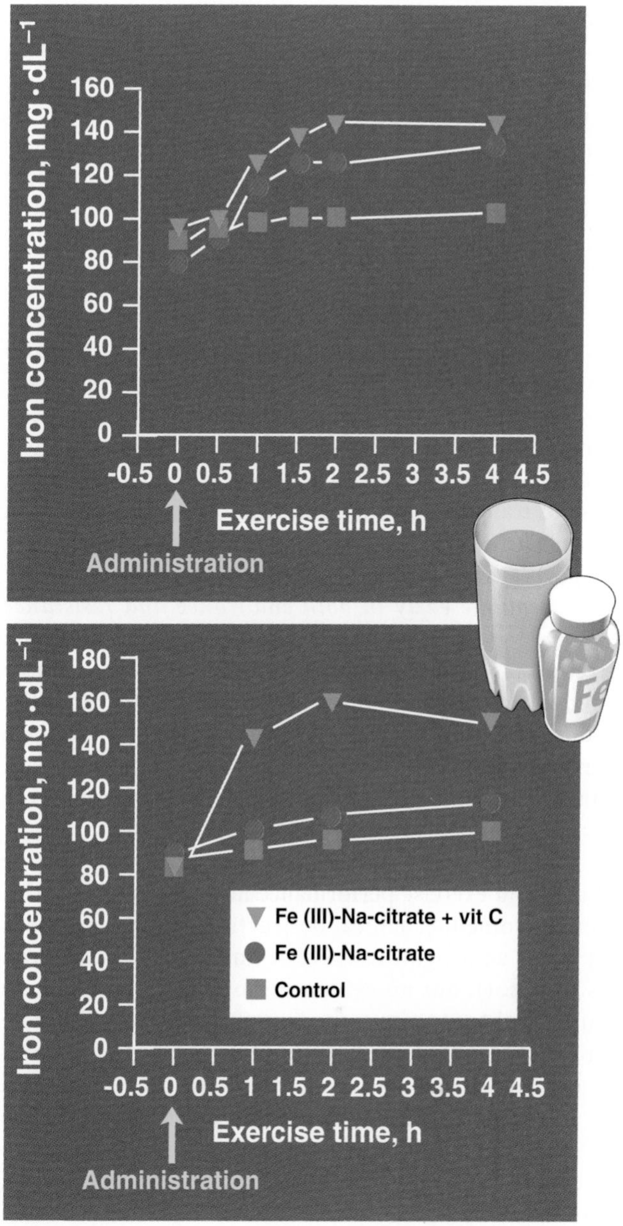

FIGURE 2.15. *Top.* Serum iron concentrations following administration of a single dose of 100 mg of ferric sodium citrate complex (Fe [III]-Na-citrate) or 100 mg of sodium citrate complex with 200 mg of ascorbic acid (Fe [III]-Na-citrate + vit C) compared with controls at rest. *Bottom.* Serum iron concentrations following administration of a single dose of 100 mg of ferric sodium citrate complex (Fe [III]-Na-citrate) or 100 mg of sodium citrate complex with 200 mg of ascorbic acid (Fe [III]-Na-citrate + vit C) compared with controls during moderate (60% $\dot{V}O_{2max}$) exercise. (From Schmid A, et al. Effect of physical exercise and vitamin C on absorption of ferric sodium citrate. *Med Sci Sports Exerc* 1996;28:1470.)

bleeding unrelated to age, sex, or performance time also can occur with long-distance running.[104,116,134] Such iron loss would stress the body's iron reserves required to synthesize 260 billion new red blood cells generated daily in the bone marrow of the skull, upper arm, sternum, ribs, spine, pelvis, and upper leg. Iron loss poses an additional burden to premenopausal women with a greater iron requirement yet lower iron intake than men.

AN OBJECTIVE MEASURE OF IRON RESERVES

Measuring serum ferritin concentration provides useful information about iron reserves. Depleted iron reserves occur when values are below 20 $\mu g \cdot L^{-1}$ for women and 30 $\mu g \cdot L^{-1}$ for men.

Real Anemia or Pseudoanemia?

Apparent suboptimal hemoglobin concentrations and hematocrits occur more frequently among endurance athletes, supporting the possibility of an exercise-induced anemia. On closer scrutiny, reductions in hemoglobin concentration appear transient, occurring in the early phase of training and then returning toward pretraining values. *The decrease in hemoglobin concentration generally parallels the disproportionately large expansion in plasma volume early in both endurance and resistance training.*[30,157,149] For example, just several days of training increases plasma volume by 20%, while the total volume of red blood cells remains unchanged.[54] Consequently, **total hemoglobin** (an important factor in endurance performance) remains the same or increases somewhat with training, yet hemoglobin *concentration* decreases in the expanding plasma volume.

Despite hemoglobin's apparent dilution, aerobic capacity and exercise performance normally improve with training. Some mechanical destruction of red blood cells may occur with vigorous exercise (including minimal iron loss in sweat), but no evidence shows that these factors strain an athlete's iron reserves sufficiently to precipitate clinical anemia as long as iron intake remains at recommended levels. Applying stringent criteria for both anemia and insufficient iron reserves makes sports anemia much less prevalent among highly trained athletes than generally believed.[180] For male collegiate runners and swimmers, no indications of the early stages of anemia were noted despite large changes in training volume and intensity during different phases of the competitive season.[124] Data from female athletes indicate the prevalence of iron deficiency anemia did *not* differ in comparisons among specific athletic groups or with a nonathletic control group.[133] A relatively high prevalence of nonanemic iron depletion exists among athletes in diverse sports and recreationally active men and women.[34,56,151]

Should Physically Active Individuals Supplement with Iron?

Depleting iron with exercise training (coupled with poor dietary habits) in adolescent and premenopausal females, particularly among those in the low-weight or body-appearance sports, could strain an already limited iron reserve. This does not mean that all physically active individuals should take supplementary iron or that all indications of sports anemia result from dietary iron deficiency or iron loss caused by exercise. It does suggest, however, the importance of monitoring an athlete's iron status by periodic evaluation of hematologic characteristics and iron reserves, particularly athletes who choose to supplement with iron. This is important because reversal of full-blown iron deficiency anemia can require up to 6 months of iron therapy.

Hemoglobin concentration of 12 $g \cdot dl^{-1}$ for women represents the cutoff for the clinical classification of anemia. Low values within the "normal" range could reflect **functional anemia** or **marginal iron deficiency**. Depleted iron stores, reduced iron-dependent protein production (e.g., oxidative enzymes), but relatively *normal* hemoglobin concentrations characterize this condition. The ergogenic effects of iron supplementation on aerobic exercise performance and training responsiveness have been noted for such groups of iron-deficient athletes.[16,17,46] For example, physically active but untrained women classified as iron depleted (serum ferritin, $\leq 16\ \mu g \cdot L^{-1}$) but not anemic (hemoglobin $\geq 12\ g \cdot dL^{-1}$) received either iron therapy (50 mg ferrous sulfate) or a placebo twice daily for 2 weeks.[66] All subjects then completed 4 weeks of aerobic training. The iron-supplemented group increased serum ferritin levels with only a small (nonsignificant) increase in hemoglobin concentration. The supplemented group also had twice the improvement in 15-km endurance cycling time (3.4 vs 1.6 minutes faster) than the women who consumed the placebo. The researchers concluded that women with low serum ferritin levels but hemoglobin concentrations above 12 $g \cdot dL^{-1}$, although not clinically anemic, might still be functionally anemic and thus benefit from iron supplementation to help exercise performance. Similarly, iron-depleted but nonanemic women received either a placebo or 20 mg of elemental iron as ferrous sulfate twice daily for 6 weeks.[18] **FIGURE 2.16** shows that the iron supplement attenuated the rate of decrease in maximal force measured sequentially during approximately 8 minutes of dynamic knee extension exercise.

These findings support current recommendations to use an iron supplement for physically active women with low serum ferritin levels. Iron supplementation exerts little effect on hemoglobin concentration and red blood cell volume in iron-deficient but nonanemic groups. Any improved exercise capacity most likely occurs from increased muscle oxidative capacity, not the blood's oxygen transport capacity.

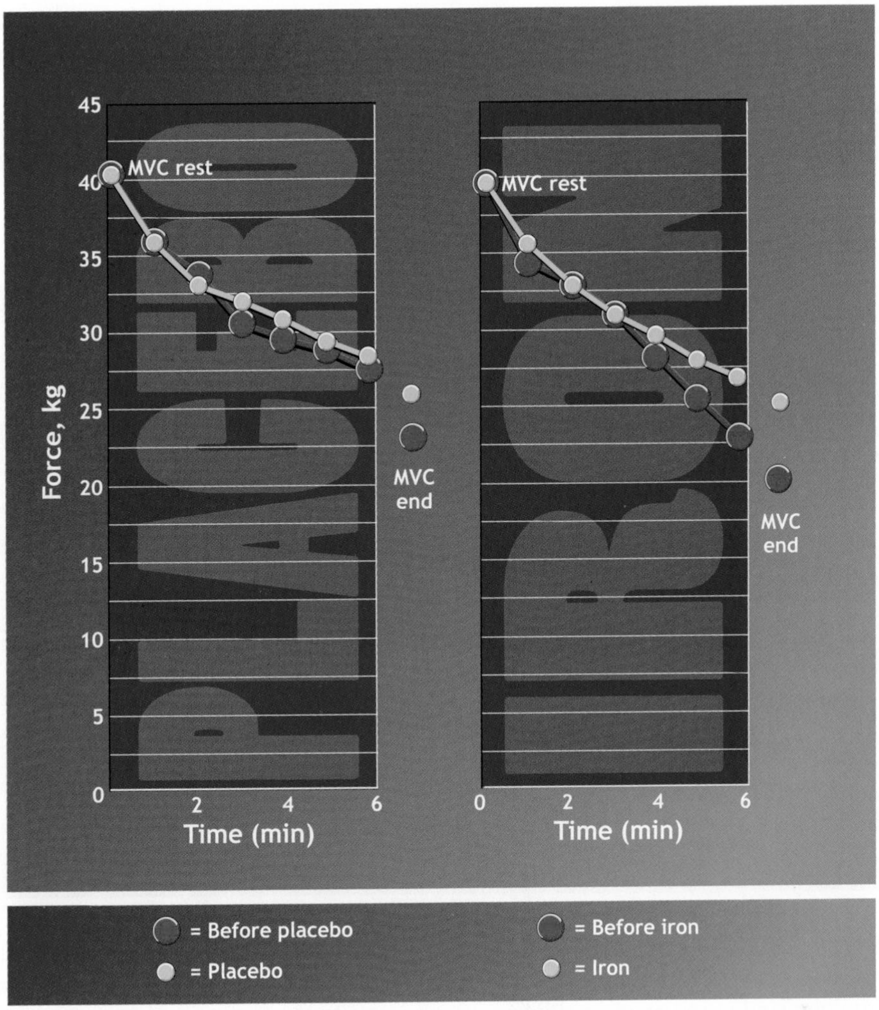

FIGURE 2.16. Maximal voluntary static contractions (MVCs) over the first 6 minutes of a progressive fatigue test of dynamic knee extensions before (●) and after (●) supplementation with either a placebo or iron. MVC end represents the last MVC of the protocol and occurred at different times (average ~ 8 minutes) for each subject. (From Brutsaert TD, et al. Iron supplementation improves progressive fatigue resistance during dynamic knee extensor exercise in iron-depleted, nonanemic women. *Am J Clin Nutr* 2003;77:441.)

Steer Clear of Iron Supplements Unless an Insufficiency Exists

For healthy individuals whose diets contain the recommended iron intake, excess iron either through diet or supplementation does not increase hemoglobin, hematocrit, or other measures of iron status or exercise performance.[171] Potential harm exists from the overconsumption or overabsorption of iron, particularly with an excessive consumption of red meat and ready availability of iron and vitamin C supplements, which facilitate iron absorption.[44] Supplements should not be used indiscriminately because excessive iron can accumulate to toxic levels and contribute to diabetes, liver disease, and heart and joint damage. Excess iron intake may even augment the growth of latent cancers (e.g., colorectal cancer) and infectious organisms.[117] Controversy exists as to whether individuals with high levels of body iron stores have a higher CHD risk than individuals with iron levels in the low-to-normal range.[29,80,128] If risk exists, one explanation postulates that high serum iron catalyzes free radical formation, which augments the oxidation of LDL cholesterol, thus promoting atherosclerosis. Currently, the evidence supporting this hypothesis remains inconsistent and inconclusive.[150]

Approximately 1.5 million Americans have a genetic abnormality called **hereditary hemochromatosis**. This condition represents the most common genetic disorder in the United States that affects approximately 1 of every 200 to 300 Americans. Hereditary hemochromatosis predisposes individuals to accumulate iron in body tissues. If undetected, this genetic abnormality produces excessive iron absorption and accumulation with early symptoms of chronic fatigue,

DIETARY MODIFICATIONS TO REDUCE COLORECTAL CANCER RISK

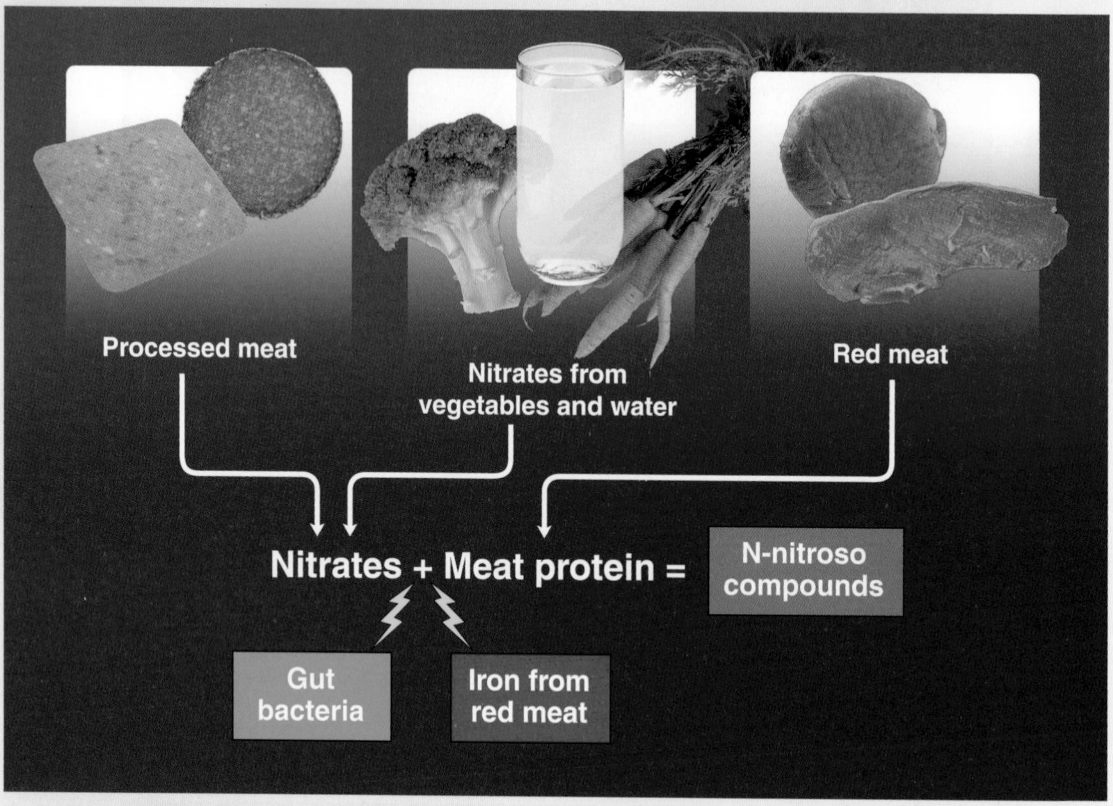

What scientists call *N-nitroso compounds* can be cancer forming. These compounds seem to form in the digestive tract when heme iron (the kind in red meat) and intestinal bacteria trigger meat protein to combine with the nitrites that are added to processed meats of with the nitrites that the body makes from the nit*rates* in water and in some vegetables (such as spinach and carrots).

Three strategies to reduce this risk:

1. Cut back on red and processed meats. Aim for only about one serving weekly.
2. Replace red meat with poultry, fish, beans, nuts, and soy-based veggie meats. Buy deli meats that are free of nitrates.
3. Aim for adequate calcium intake: 1000 mg a day for those age 50 or younger and 1200 mg for those older than age 50.

Source: Nutrition Action Health Letter, June 2009.

abdominal pain, and menstrual dysfunction in females. In the extreme, hemochromatosis leads to cirrhosis or liver cancer, heart and thyroid disease, diabetes, arthritis, and infertility. Early diagnosis and treatment can prevent the serious complications of hemochromatosis.

SODIUM, POTASSIUM, AND CHLORINE

Sodium, potassium, and chlorine, collectively termed **electrolytes**, remain dissolved in the watery medium of the body's cells as electrically charged particles called ions. Sodium and chlorine represent the chief minerals contained in blood plasma and extracellular fluid. Electrolytes modulate fluid exchange within the body's fluid compartments, allowing a well-regulated exchange of nutrients and waste products between the cell and its external fluid environment. Potassium is the chief intracellular mineral. Adequate potassium intake also may provide health benefits, particularly in countering the elevation in blood pressure caused by excess sodium intake. This beneficial effect of potassium may reside in making the larger blood vessels more flexible and dilating the smaller blood vessels to reduce peripheral resistance to blood flow. The relatively high potassium content of the Dietary Approaches to Stop Hypertension (DASH) diet see p. 91—rich in fruits and vegetables, with two servings of low-fat dairy foods, and a low content of saturated fat, added sugars, and refined flour—may contribute to this diet's blood pressure–lowering effect.

The most important function of sodium and potassium ions concerns their role in establishing the proper electrical gradient across cell membranes. This difference in electrical balance between the cell's interior and exterior membranes allows the transmission of nerve impulses, the stimulation and action of muscle, and proper gland functioning. Electrolytes also maintain plasma membrane permeability and regulate acid and base qualities of body fluids, particularly the blood. **TABLE 2.10** lists values considered normal for electrolyte concentrations in serum and sweat, and electrolyte and carbohydrate concentrations of common oral rehydration beverages.

How Much Sodium Is Enough?

With low-to-moderate sodium intake, the hormone **aldosterone** acts on the kidneys to conserve sodium. Conversely, high dietary sodium inhibits aldosterone release. Any excess sodium becomes excreted in the urine. Consequently, salt balance generally remains normal throughout a wide range of intakes. This does not occur in individuals who cannot adequately regulate excessive sodium intake. Abnormal sodium accumulation in body fluids increases fluid volume and elevates blood pressure to levels that pose a health risk. **Sodium-induced hypertension** occurs in about one third of individuals with hypertension.

Sodium, widely distributed naturally in foods, allows one to readily obtain the daily requirement without adding "extra" salt to foods. Sodium intake in the United States (about 1.5 tsp of salt daily) regularly exceeds the 1500-mg daily recommended maximum for adults, or the amount of sodium in less than two thirds of a teaspoon of table salt (sodium makes up about 40% of salt). This amounts to 60% of the daily allotment in one serving of vegetable soup, which contains 900 mg of sodium. The typical Western diet contains nearly 4000 mg of sodium (7–12 g of salt) each day with three quarters hidden inside processed foods and restaurant meals. This represents 10 times the 500 mg of sodium the body actually

LESS MAY EVEN BE MORE BENEFICIAL

The Centers for Disease Control and Prevention (www.cdc.gov) state that nearly 70% of adult Americans should follow a low-salt diet that cuts the recommended daily sodium intake of 2300 mg to 1500 mg, about the amount found in two-thirds of a teaspoon of salt. The three groups at special risk for sodium sensitivity include (1) people with existing hypertension (30.5% of the adult population), (2) those age 40 and older without hypertension (34.4%), and (3) African Americans age 20 to 39 without hypertension (4.2%). In addition, reducing sodium intake may have health benefits beyond lowering blood pressure; it may improve flow-mediated dilation, the measure of a blood vessel's healthy ability to relax. As of 2010, the federal *Dietary Guidelines for Americans* has now extended this 1500-mg recommendation to all Americans regardless of health status.

SOME SODIUM CULPRITS

Burger King's Country Pork Sandwich (3310 mg)
Canadian bacon, 3.5 oz (2500 mg)
Wendy's Hot & Spicy Boneless Wings (2490 mg)
Jack in the Box Deli Trio Grilled Sandwich (2460 mg)
Subway's Footlong Black Forest Ham Sub (2400 mg)
McDonald's Big Breakfast with Hotcakes and Large Size Biscuit (2260 mg)
Taco Bell's Chicken Grilled Stuffed Burrito (2180 mg)
Corned beef, 3.5 oz (1740 mg)
Seasoned rice mixes (1000 mg)
Canned soups (400–900 mg)
Ham, bacon, sausages, and luncheon meats (423 mg)
Store-bought salad dressing (300–600 mg)

TABLE 2.10 Electrolyte Concentrations in Blood Serum and Sweat, and Carbohydrate and Electrolyte Concentrations of Some Common Beverages

	Na^+ ($mEq \cdot L^{-1}$)	K^+ ($mEq \cdot L^{-1}$)	Ca^{2+} ($mEq \cdot L^{-1}$)	Mg^{2+} ($mEq \cdot L^{-1}$)	Cl^- ($mEq \cdot L^{-1}$)	Osmolality ($mOsm \cdot L^{-1}$)	CHO ($g \cdot L^{-1}$)
Blood serum	140	4.5	2.5	1.5–2.1	110	300	–
Sweat	60–80	4.5	1.5	3.3	40–90	170–220	–
Coca Cola	3.0	–	–	–	1.0	650	107
Gatorade	23.0	3.0	–	–	14.0	280	62
Fruit juice	0.5	58.0	–	–	–	690	118
Pepsi Cola	1.7	Trace	–	–	Trace	568	81
Water	Trace	Trace	–	–	Trace	10–20	–

Additional Insights

Is Excess Salt Really That Harmful?

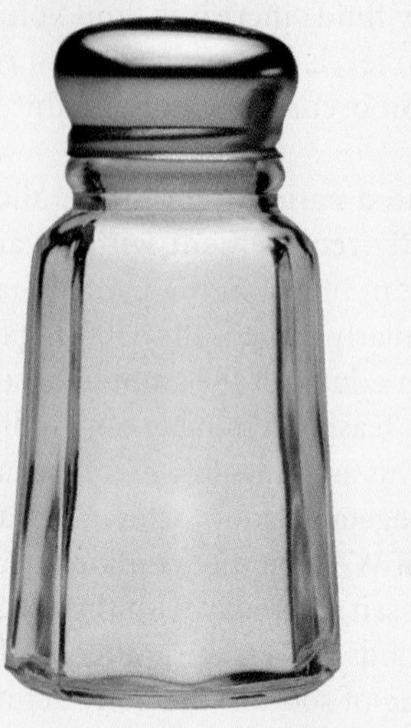

The 2010 federal *Dietary Guidelines for Americans* recommend limiting daily sodium intake to 2300 mg with a lower 1500-mg ceiling for African- Americans, people older than 51, and those with hypertension, diabetes, and chronic kidney disease. Now, Belgian researchers have challenged the conventional wisdom that just about any reduction in salt intake provides beneficial effects to blood pressure and overall cardiovascular health. Their research examined the incidence of death, hypertension, and overall cardiovascular illness related to a single 24-hour urinary sodium excretion as the salt intake baseline marker. Approximately 4000 participants initially without cardiovascular disease (n = 2096 with normal blood pressure at the start) were followed over an 8-year period. Individuals with the highest sodium excretion levels had the fewest deaths from cardiovascular disease. No association emerged between sodium levels and disease risk among those with normal blood pressure at the start of the study. The expected link between high sodium intake and increasing blood pressure occurred only among a cohort of 1499 individuals without hypertension medication, and this relationship emerged only for systolic blood pressure. The researchers concluded: "Our findings do also not support the current recommendations of a generalized and indiscriminate reduction of salt intake at the population level."

Criticism of these findings was quick to follow and negative. A member of the US Centers for Disease Control and Prevention criticized the study for using relatively young subjects (initial average age about 40) who experienced few cardiovascular deaths. In addition, only a single urinary excretion measure was provided—at the start of the study—with no follow-up samples as the study progressed and at the study end point. The president of the American Heart Association said that while the study raises some interesting questions, the "bulk of the evidence" supports the potential health benefits of a reduced sodium intake, and the Association would stand by its recently updated advice for all individuals to limit sodium intake to 1500 mg daily. Until subsequent research clarifies the issue, the prudent advice is to follow the recommendations of either the *Dietary Guidelines* or American Heart Association.

Source: Stolarz-Skrzypek K, et al. Fatal and nonfatal outcomes, incidence of hypertension, and blood pressure changes in relation to urinary sodium excretion. *JAMA* 2011;305:1777.

Related References

Bray GA, et al. A further subgroup analysis of the effect of the DASH diet and three sodium levels on blood pressure; results of the Dash-Sodium Trial. *Am J Cardiol* 2004;94:222.

Fung TT, et al. Adherence to a DASH-style diet and risk of coronary heart disease and stroke in women. *Arch Intern Med* 2008;168:713.

Kajantie E, et al. The association between salt intake and adult systolic blood pressure is modified by birth weight. *Am J Clin Nutr* 2011;93:422.

Kesteloot H, et al. Relation of urinary calcium and magnesium excretion to blood pressure: The International Study of Macro- and Micro-nutrients and Blood Pressure and The International Cooperative Study on Salt, Other Factors, and Blood Pressure. *Am J Epidemiol* 2011;174:44.

Madero M, et al. Dietary fructose and hypertension. *Curr Hypertens Rep* 2011;13:29.

Ohta Y, et al. Relationship between blood pressure control status and lifestyle in hypertensive outpatients. *Intern Med* 2011;50:2107.

Oliveira LP, Lawless CE. Hypertension update and cardiovascular risk reduction in physically active individuals and athlevtes. *Phys Sportsmed* 2010;38:11.

needs. Reliance on table salt in processing, curing, cooking, seasoning, and preserving common foods accounts for the large sodium intake. Aside from table salt, common sodium-rich dietary sources include monosodium glutamate (MSG), soy sauce, condiments, canned foods, baking soda, most luncheon meats, and baking powder.

For decades, one low-risk, first line of defense in treating high blood pressure has been to eliminate excess sodium from the diet. Reducing sodium intake possibly lowers sodium and body fluid, thereby lowering blood pressure. This effect is particularly apparent for "salt-sensitive" individuals; reducing dietary sodium decreases their blood pressure.[70,160] Debate concerns the magnitude of this reduction for most hypertensives.[1,3,8,22] If dietary constraints prove ineffective in lowering blood pressure, drugs that induce a water loss called diuretics become the next line of defense. Unfortunately, diuretics also produce losses in other minerals, particularly potassium. A potassium-rich diet (potatoes, bananas, oranges, tomatoes, and meat) becomes a necessity for a patient using diuretics. Recent research indicates that lowering salt intake reduces risk of cardiovascular disease and stroke. For example, a reduction of intake of 5 g of salt daily (about one half the daily intake in the American diet of about 10 g) is associated with a 23% lower rate of strokes and a 17% lower risk of cardiovascular disease.[163]

HEART DISEASE RISKS AFFECT NEARLY 50% OF US ADULTS

According to the national Centers for Disease Control and Prevention, nearly half of all adult Americans have high cholesterol, hypertension, or diabetes, with one in eight having at least two of the conditions and one in 33 having all three. African Americans had the highest proportion of hypertension (42%), whereas whites were more likely to have elevated cholesterol and Mexican Americans were more likely to have diabetes. The encouraging news is that all of these conditions are treatable with either lifestyle changes or medications.

THE DASH EATING PLAN

One in three adults in the Unites States has hypertension; among those older than age 65, the figure increases to two out of three, with current estimates indicating that hypertension accounts for one in six deaths. Nearly 75 million adults have hypertension, a condition that, if left untreated, increases the risk of stroke, heart attack, arterial wall stiffness, congestive heart failure, and kidney disease. Fifty percent actually seek treatment, and only about one half of these individuals achieve long-term success. One reason for the lack of compliance concerns possible side effects of readily available antihypertensive medications. For example, fatigue and impotence often discourage patients from maintaining a chronic medication schedule required by pharmacologic hypertension treatment.

Research on the **DASH** (**www.nhlbi.nih.gov/health/public/heart/hbp/dash/**) diet to treat hypertension shows that this diet lowers blood pressure in the general population, in the obese, and in persons with stage 1 hypertension to the same extent as pharmacologic therapy and often more than other lifestyle changes.[4,23,144] Two months of the diet reduced systolic pressure by an average of 11.4 mm Hg; diastolic pressure decreased by 5.5 mm Hg. Every 2-mm Hg reduction in systolic pressure lowers heart disease risk by 5% and stroke risk by 8%.

TABLE 2.11 shows the specifics of the DASH diet with its high content of fruits, vegetables, and dairy products and low-fat composition. Further good news emerges from the latest research from the DASH group indicating that the standard DASH diet combined with a daily salt intake of 1150 mg—called the DASH-sodium diet—produced greater blood pressure reductions than achieved with only the DASH diet.[14,47,145]

Blood pressure declined for both normotensive and hypertensive subjects, with the greatest benefits for subjects with high blood pressure. The DASH diet alone and sodium restriction alone both lowered blood pressure, but the greatest reductions emerged with the DASH–low sodium combination. The best scientific information currently recommends the following five lifestyle approaches to prevent hypertension[37,181]:

1. Regularly engage in moderate physical activity
2. Maintain normal body weight
3. Limit alcohol consumption
4. Reduce sodium intake and maintain an AI of potassium
5. Consume a diet rich in fruits, vegetables, and low-fat dairy products and reduced in saturated fatty acids and total fat

TABLE 2.12 shows a sample DASH diet consisting of approximately 2100 kcal. This level of energy intake provides a stable body weight for a typical 70-kg person. More physically active and heavier individuals should boost portion size or number of individual items to maintain weight. Individuals desiring to lose weight or who are lighter and/or sedentary

SIGNIFICANT BENEFITS IN CUTTING SALT INTAKE

Reducing the typical daily sodium intake of 3000 mg for American women and 4000 mg for American men to 1500 mg daily for those who are middle-aged or older, black, or already hypertensive or to 2300 mg for all others could achieve the following four health benefits:

1. Prevent up to 92,000 deaths and 66,000 strokes yearly
2. Prevent nearly 100,000 Americans from having a heart attack and nearly 120,000 others from acquiring heart disease yearly. It can reduce the risk of heart failure, which afflicts 5.8 million Americans, as well as the risk of abnormal function of the kidneys, brain, and heart and arterial system in general
3. Save between $10 and $25 billion in healthcare costs yearly
4. Counter the average 5-year, 5-mm Hg average rise in systolic blood pressure in individuals age 45 to 64 years

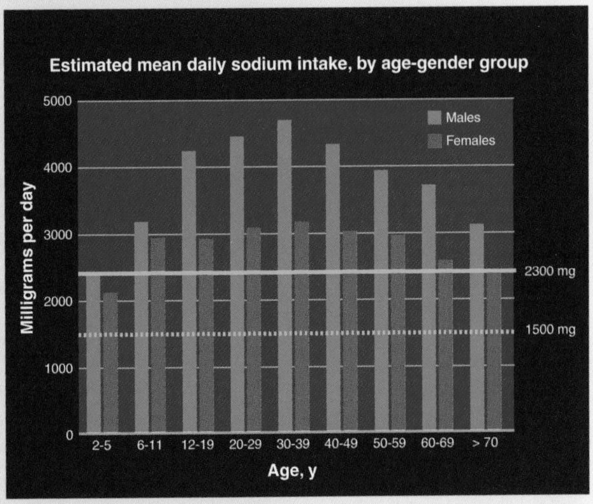

TABLE 2.11 Daily Nutrient Goals Used in the DASH Studies (for a 2100-Calorie Eating Plan)

Total fat	27% of calories
Saturated fat	6% of calories
Protein	18% of calories
Carbohydrate	55% of calories
Cholesterol	150mg
Sodium	2300mg[a]
Potassium	4700mg
Calcium	1250mg
Magnesium	500mg
Fiber	30g

[a]1500 mg sodium was a lower goal tested and found to be even better for lowering blood pressure. It was particularly effective for middle-aged and older individuals, African Americans, and those who already had high blood pressure.

From US Department of Health and Human Services, National Institutes of Health, National Heart, Lung, and Blood Institute. Your Guide to Lowering Your Blood Pressure With DASH. 2006. Available at: http://www.nhlbi.nih.gov/health/public/heart/hbp/dash/new_dash.pdf.

should eat less, but not less than the minimum serving number for each food group listed in Table 2.11.

Can Sodium Intake Be Too Low?

A low-sodium diet in conjunction with excessive perspiration, persistent vomiting, or diarrhea creates the potential to deplete the body's sodium content to critical levels in a condition termed **hyponatremia**. This potential medical emergency causes a broad array of symptoms ranging from muscle cramps, nausea, vomiting, and dizziness to, in the extreme, shock, coma, and death.[139] A minimal likelihood of hyponatremia exists for most persons because responses by the kidneys to low sodium status trigger sodium conservation. In addition, sodium availability in so many foods makes it improbable that sodium levels would fall to critically low levels.

Even when body weight loss from perspiration reaches 2 to 3% of body weight (about 5–7 lb), adding a pinch of table salt to food usually restores sodium for most persons. Endurance athletes and basketball, baseball, soccer, and football players who routinely lose more than 4% of body weight following competition should consume salt-containing drinks before and after heavy sweating to ensure adequate sodium concentrations in the body. Chapter 10 discusses exercise, fluid intake, and risks of hyponatremia in greater detail.

A BREAKFAST DRINK TO LOWER BLOOD PRESSURE

Researchers investigated the effect of orange juice consumption and its major flavonoid, hesperiden, on microvascular reactivity, blood pressure, and cardiovascular risk biomarkers. Twenty-four healthy, overweight middle-aged men participated in a randomized, controlled, crossover study. For three 4-week periods, the men consumed 500 mL (17 oz) of either orange juice (which contains about 300 mg of hesperidin), a control drink plus 300 mg of hesperidin, or a control drink plus an inert placebo. At the end of both the orange juice and hesperidin test periods, diastolic blood pressure was significantly lower and endothelium-dependent microvascular reactivity (ability of blood vessels to dilate) was greater than after the placebo period, suggesting that hesperidin could be causally linked to the beneficial effect of orange juice. The fact that orange juice produced greater improvements in blood vessel activity than hesperidin alone suggests that the juice, which contains numerous polyphenols and phytochemicals, in addition to vitamin C, folate, calcium, and potassium, may act both in an additive and synergistic fashion compared to the action of a single flavonoid. A decrease of several points in diastolic blood pressure could translate to a 20% reduction in CHD risk.

Morand C, et al. Hesperidin contributes to the vascular protective effects of orange juice: a randomized crossover study in healthy volunteers. *Am J Clin Nutr* 2011;93:73.

TABLE 2.12 Sample DASH diet (including recommended substitutions to reduce sodium to 1500 mg daily) consisting of approximately 2100 kcal

2300 mg Sodium Menu	Sodium (mg)	Substitution To Reduce Sodium to 1500 mg	Sodium (mg)
Breakfast			
¾ cup bran flakes cereal:	220	¾ cup shredded wheat cereal	1
1 medium banama	1		
1 cup low-fat milk	107		
1 slice whole wheat bread	149		
1 tsp soft (tub) margarine	26	1 tsp unsalted soft (tub) margarine	0
1 cup orange juice	5		

(continued)

TABLE 2.12 Sample DASH diet (including recommended substitutions to reduce sodium to 1500 mg daily) consisting of approximately 2100 kcal *(continued)*

2300 mg Sodium Menu	Sodium (mg)	Substitution To Reduce Sodium to 1500 mg	Sodium (mg)
Lunch			
¾ cup chicken salad:	179	Remove salt from the recipe	120
2 slices whole wheat bread	299		
1 Tbsp Dijon mustard	373	1 tbsp regular mustard	175
Salad:			
½ cup fresh cucumber slices	1		
½ cup tomato wedges	5		
1 tbsp sunflower seeds	0		
1 tsp Italian dressing, low calorie	43		
½ cup fruit cocktail, juice pack	5		
Dinner			
3 oz beef, eye of the round:	35		
2 tbsp beef gravy, fat-free	165		
1 cup green beans, sautéed with:	12		
½ tsp canola oil	0		
1 small baked potato:	14		
1 tbsp sour cream, fat-free	21		
1 tbsp grated natural cheddar chesse, reduced fat	67	1 tbsp natural cheddar cheese, reduced fat, low sodium	1
1 tbsp chopped scallions	1		
1 small whole wheat roll:	148		
1 tsp soft (tub) margarine	26	1 tsp unsalted soft (tub) margarine	0
1 small apple	1		
1 cup low-fat milk	107		
Snacks			
¼ cup almonds, unsalted	0		
¼ cup raisins	4		
½ cup fruit yogurt, fat-free, no sugar added	86		
Totals	**2101**		**1507**

From US Department of Health and Human Services, National Institutes of Health, National Heart, Lung, and Blood Institute. Your Guide to Lowering Your Blood Pressure With DASH. Available at: http://www.nhlbi.nih.gov/health/public/heart/hbp/dash/new_dash.pdf.

SUMMARY

1. Approximately 4% of the body mass consists of 22 elements called minerals. Minerals become distributed in all body tissues and fluids.
2. Minerals occur freely in nature, in the waters of rivers, lakes, and oceans and in soil. The root system of plants absorbs minerals; they eventually become incorporated into the tissues of animals that consume plants.
3. Minerals function primarily in metabolism as constituents of enzymes. Minerals provide structure in the formation of bones and teeth and synthesize the biologic macronutrients glycogen, fat, and protein.
4. A balanced diet generally provides adequate mineral intake, except in some geographic locations lacking specific minerals (e.g., iodine).
5. Osteoporosis has reached almost epidemic proportions among older individuals, particularly women. Adequate calcium intake and regular weight-bearing exercise and/or resistance training provide an effective defense against bone loss at any age.

SUMMARY *(continued)*

6. Paradoxically, women who train intensely but cannot match energy intake to energy output reduce body weight and body fat to the point that may adversely affect menstruation. These women often show advanced bone loss at an early age. Restoration of normal menstruation does not totally restore bone mass.
7. The association between muscular strength and bone density raises the likelihood of using strength testing of postmenopausal women as a clinically useful tool to screen for osteoporosis.
8. About 40% of American women of child-bearing age suffer from dietary iron insufficiency that could lead to iron deficiency anemia. This condition negatively affects aerobic exercise performance and the ability to perform intense training.
9. For women on vegetarian-type diets, the relatively low bioavailability of nonheme iron increases the risk for developing iron insufficiency. Vitamin C (in food or supplement form) and moderate physical activity increase intestinal absorption of nonheme iron.
10. Regular physical activity generally does not create a significant drain on the body's iron reserves. If it does, women with the greatest iron requirement and lowest iron intake could increase their risk for anemia. Assessment of the body's iron status should evaluate hematologic characteristics and iron reserves.
11. The DASH eating plan lowers blood pressure in some individuals to the same extent as pharmacologic therapy and often more than other lifestyle changes.

WATER

WATER IN THE BODY

Water makes up from 40 to 70% of an individual's body mass depending on age, sex, and body composition; it constitutes 65 to 75% of the weight of muscle and about 50% of the weight of body fat (adipose tissue). Consequently, differences in the relative percentage of total body water among individuals result largely from variations in body composition (i.e., differences in lean vs fat tissue).

FIGURE 2.17 depicts the fluid compartments of the body, the normal daily body water variation, and specific terminology to describe the various states of human hydration. The body contains two fluid "compartments." The first compartment, **intracellular**, refers to inside the cells; the second, **extracellular**, indicates fluids surrounding the cells. Extracellular fluid includes the blood plasma and interstitial fluids, which primarily comprise the fluid that flows in the microscopic spaces among the cells. Also included as interstitial fluid are lymph, saliva, and fluid in the eyes; fluids secreted by glands and the digestive tract; fluids that bathe the nerves of the spinal cord; and fluids excreted from the skin and kidneys. Blood plasma accounts for 20% of the extracellular fluid (3–4 L). Of the total body water, an average of 62% (26 L of the body's 42 L of water for an average-sized man) represents intracellular water and 38% comes from extracellular sources. These volumes do not remain static but represent averages from a dynamic exchange of fluid between compartments, particularly in physically active individuals.[103,147,174] Exercise training often increases the percentage of water distributed within the intracellular compartment from increases in muscle mass and its accompanying large water content. In contrast, an acute bout of exercise temporarily shifts fluid from the plasma to the interstitial and intracellular spaces from the increased hydrostatic (fluid) pressure within the active circulatory system.

> **EXCESSIVE SWEATING SHRINKS PLASMA VOLUME**
>
> The extracellular fluid lost through sweating comes predominantly from blood plasma.

FUNCTIONS OF BODY WATER

Water is a ubiquitous, remarkable nutrient. Without water, death usually occurs within 7 days. It serves as the body's transport and reactive medium; diffusion of gases always takes place across surfaces moistened by water. Nutrients and gases travel in aqueous solution; waste products leave the body through the water in urine and feces. Water, in conjunction with various proteins, lubricates joints and protects a variety of "moving" organs like the heart, lungs, intestines, and eyes. Because it is noncompressible, water gives structure and form to the body through the turgor provided for body tissues. Water has tremendous heat-stabilizing qualities because it absorbs considerable heat with only minor changes in temperature. This quality, combined with water's high heat of vaporization (energy required to change 1 g of a liquid into the gaseous state at the boiling point), facilitates maintenance of a relatively constant body temperature during environmental heat stress and the large increase in internal heat generated by exercise.

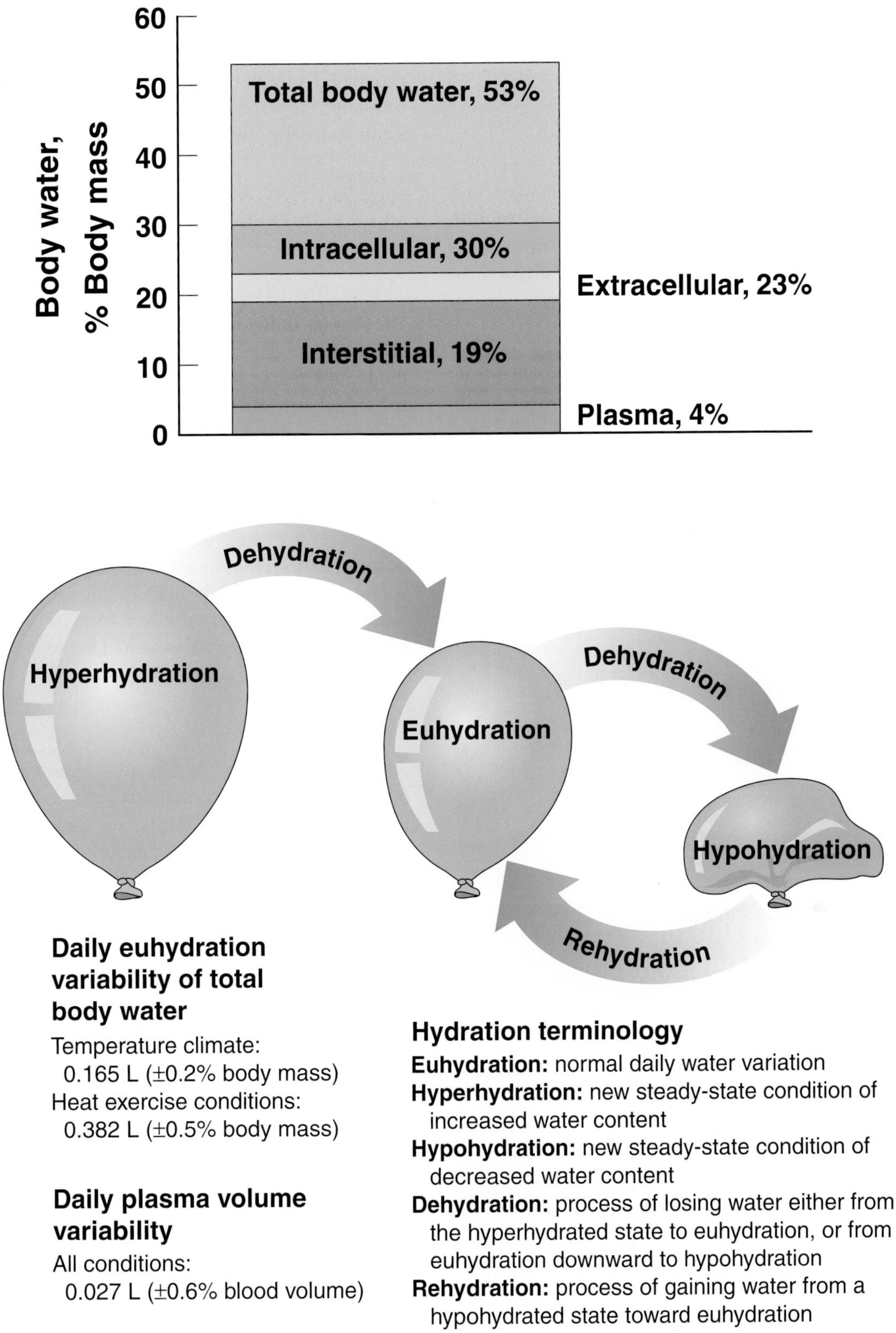

FIGURE 2.17. Fluid compartments, average volumes and variability, and hydration terminology. Volumes represent those for an 80-kg man. Approximately 60% of the body mass consists of water in striated muscle (80% water), skeleton (32% water), and adipose tissue (50% water). For a man and woman of similar body mass, the woman contains less total water because of her larger ratio of adipose tissue to lean body mass (striated muscle + skeleton). (Adapted from Greenleaf JE. Problem: thirst, drinking behavior, and involuntary dehydration. *Med Sci Sports Exerc* 1992;24:645.)

Chapter 10 more fully discusses the dynamics of thermoregulation during heat stress, particularly water's important role.

WATER BALANCE: INTAKE VERSUS OUTPUT

The body's water content remains relatively stable over time. Considerable water output occurs in physically active individuals, while appropriate fluid intake usually restores any imbalance in the body's fluid level. **FIGURE 2.18** displays the sources of water intake and output.

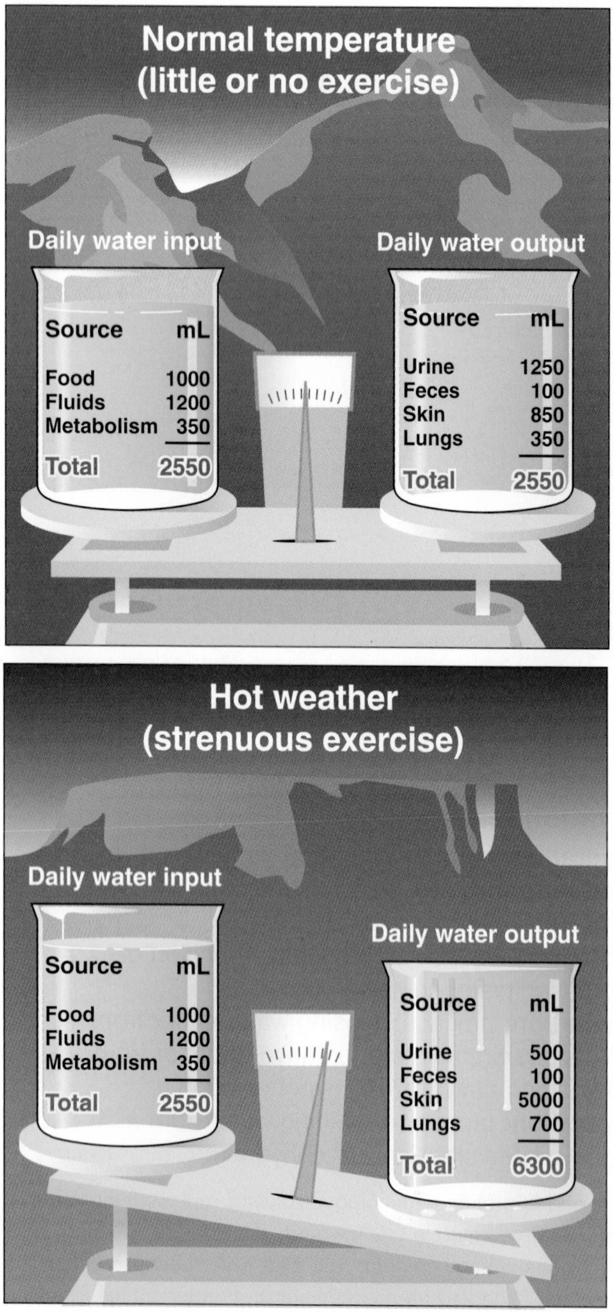

FIGURE 2.18. Water balance in the body. *Top.* Little or no exercise in normal ambient temperature and humidity. *Bottom.* Moderate to intense exercise in a hot, humid environment.

Water Intake

A sedentary adult in a thermoneutral environment requires about 2.5 L of water daily. For an active person in a hot environment, the water requirement often increases to between 5 and 10 L daily. Three sources provide this water:

1. Liquids
2. Foods
3. Metabolic processes

Water from Liquids

The average individual normally consumes 1200 mL or 41 oz of water each day. Exercise and thermal stress can increase fluid intake five or six times above normal. At the extreme, an individual lost 13.6 kg (30 lb) of water weight during a 2-day, 17-hour, 55-mile run across Death Valley, California (lowest point in the Western Hemisphere at almost 300 feet below sea level; recognized as one of the hottest places on earth with the second highest recorded temperature of 134°F; highest was 136°F in Al'Aziziyah, Libya; temperatures above 120°F occur in 22 different locations, mainly in Africa). However, with proper fluid ingestion, including salt supplements, body weight loss amounted to only 1.4 kg. In this example, fluid loss and replenishment represented between 3.5 and 4 gallons of liquid!

Water in Foods

Fruits and vegetables contain considerable water, up to 90% or more (e.g., lettuce, cantaloupe, and watermelon); in contrast, butter, oils, dried meats, and chocolate, cookies, and cakes have a relatively low water content of under 20%.

Metabolic Water

Carbon dioxide and water form when food molecules catabolize for energy. Termed **metabolic water**, this fluid provides about 14% of a sedentary person's daily water requirement. The complete breakdown of 100 g of carbohydrate, protein, and fat yields 55, 100, and 107 g of metabolic water, respectively. Additionally, each gram of glycogen joins with 2.7 g of water as its glucose units link together; subsequently, glycogen liberates this bound water during its catabolism for energy.

Water Output

Water loss from the body occurs in one of four ways:

1. In urine
2. Through skin
3. Water vapor in expired air
4. In feces

Water Loss in Urine

Under normal conditions, the kidneys reabsorb about 99% of the 140 to 160 L of filtrate formed each day; consequently, the volume of urine excreted daily by the kidneys ranges from 1000 to 1500 mL or about 1.5 quarts.

Elimination of 1 g of solute by the kidneys requires about 15 mL of water. A portion of water in urine becomes "obligated" to rid the body of metabolic by-products like urea, an end product of protein breakdown. Catabolizing large quantities of protein for energy (as occurs with a high-protein diet) actually accelerates the body's dehydration during exercise.

Water Loss Through the Skin

A small quantity of water, perhaps 350 mL, termed **insensible perspiration**, continually seeps from the deeper tissues through the skin to the body's surface. Water loss through the skin also occurs as sweat produced by specialized sweat glands beneath the skin's surface. Evaporation of sweat's water component provides the refrigeration mechanism to cool the body. Daily sweat rate under normal conditions amounts to between 500 and 700 mL. This by no means reflects sweating capacity; the well-acclimatized person can produce up to 12 L of sweat (equivalent of 12 kg) at a rate of 1 L per hour during prolonged exercise in a hot environment.

TRAVELERS' DIARRHEA IN ATHLETES

Taking Precautions Can Make a Huge Difference

Athletes travel for sports competition to different geographic regions, often to third-world countries or to regions with different sanitary standards compared to their own country. All members of the Team England squad who participated in the Youth 2008 Commonwealth Games in India followed evidence-based guidelines to prevent and manage travelers' diarrhea (TD) and record the incidence of TD during an elite sporting trip. Hygiene guidelines included only drinking bottled water, eating hot food, and regular hand washing with alcohol gel. Ciprofloxacin (a drug used to prevent certain infections caused by bacteria) was offered to nonathlete team members as prophylaxis but not to athletes because of its possible association with tendon disease. After implementation of these guidelines, the incidence of TD in the whole squad was 24 of 122 (20%) compared with 7 of 14 (50%) during the travel trip before guidelines were implemented. In those taking prophylactic ciprofloxacin, the incidence was 4 of 33 (12%) compared with 20 of 89 (23%) in those not taking the drug. No athlete missed an event because of TD. The authors concluded that TD incidence was less during the event when athletes followed the guidelines than when they did not follow the guidelines. Prophylactic ciprofloxacin also reduced the incidence of TD, but its use is probably inappropriate for elite athletes.

Source: Tillett E, Loosemore M. Setting standards for the prevention and management of travellers' diarrhoea in elite athletes: an audit of one team during the Youth Commonwealth Games in India. *Br J Sports Med* 2009;43:1045.

Water Loss as Water Vapor

Insensible water loss through small water droplets in exhaled air amounts to 250 to 350 mL daily. The complete moistening of all inspired air as it passes down the pulmonary airways accounts for this avenue of water loss. Exercise affects this source of water loss because inspired air requires humidification. For physically active persons, the respiratory passages release 2 to 5 mL of water each minute during strenuous exercise depending on climatic conditions. Ventilatory water loss is least in hot, humid weather and greatest in cold temperatures (inspired cold air contains little moisture) or at altitude because inspired air volumes exceed those at sea-level conditions.

Water Loss in Feces

Intestinal elimination produces between 100 and 200 mL of water loss because water constitutes approximately 75% of fecal matter. The remainder comprises nondigestible material including bacteria from the digestive process and the residues of digestive juices from the intestine, stomach, and pancreas. With diarrhea or vomiting, water loss increases to between 1500 and 5000 mL.

PHYSICAL ACTIVITY AND ENVIRONMENTAL FACTORS PLAY AN IMPORTANT ROLE

The loss of body water represents the most serious consequence of profuse sweating. The severity of physical activity, environmental temperature, and humidity determine the amount of water lost through sweating. Exercise-induced increases in sweating also occur in the water environment through activities such as vigorous swimming or water polo.[91] Relative humidity (water content of the ambient air) affects the efficiency of the sweating mechanism for temperature regulation. Ambient air becomes completely saturated with water vapor at 100% relative humidity. This blocks evaporation of fluid from the skin surface to the air, thus negating this important avenue for body cooling. Under such conditions, sweat beads on the skin and eventually rolls off without providing an evaporative cooling effect. On a dry day, air can hold considerable moisture and fluid rapidly evaporates from the skin. Thus, the sweat mechanism functions at optimal efficiency, and body temperature remains regulated within a narrow range. Importantly, plasma volume begins to

AN EASY YET EFFECTIVE METHOD

Monitoring changes in body weight provides a convenient way to assess fluid loss during exercise and/or heat stress. Each 0.45 kg (1 lb) of body weight loss corresponds to 450 mL of dehydration.

decrease when sweating causes a fluid loss equal to 2 or 3% of body mass. Fluid loss from the vascular compartment strains circulatory function, which ultimately impairs exercise capacity and thermoregulation.

SUMMARY

1. Water constitutes 40 to 70% of the total body mass; muscle contains 72% water by weight, whereas water represents only about 50% of the weight of body fat (adipose tissue).
2. Of the total body water, roughly 62% exists intracellularly (inside the cells) and 38% occurs extracellularly in the plasma, lymph, and other fluids outside the cell.
3. The normal average daily water intake of 2.5 L comes from liquid (1.2 L) and food (1.0 L) intake and metabolic water produced during energy-yielding reactions (0.3 L).
4. Daily water loss occurs in urine (1–1.5 L), through the skin as insensible perspiration (0.50–0.70 L), as water vapor in expired air (0.25–0.30 L), and in feces (0.10 L).
5. Food and oxygen exist in the body in aqueous solution, whereas nongaseous waste products always leave in a watery medium. Water also provides structure and form to the body and plays a crucial role in temperature regulation.
6. Exercise in hot weather greatly increases the body's water requirement. In extreme conditions, fluid needs increase five or six times above normal.

thePoint *Visit* **thePoint.lww.com/MKKSEN4e** *to view the following animations related to content presented in Chapter 2:* ***Biological function of vitamins; Calcium in muscles; Cardiac cycle; Catabolism; Congestive heart failure; Hypertension; Myocardial blood flow; Stroke; Vitamin C as an antioxidant;*** *and* ***Water balance.***

TEST YOUR KNOWLEDGE ANSWERS

1. **True:** Vitamin intake above the RDA does not improve exercise performance or the potential to sustain physical training. In fact, serious illness occurs from regularly consuming excess fat-soluble vitamins and, in some instances, water-soluble vitamins.

2. **False:** Although the body can conserve water, there is some loss every day. After only a few days, severe dehydration can result in death. In contrast, death from starvation takes much longer, perhaps 60 days or more.

3. **False:** The terms *major* and *trace* do not reflect nutritional importance; rather, these classifications refer to the amount needed for daily functioning. In essence, each of the major or trace micronutrients remains critical to maintenance of optimal physiologic functioning and good health.

4. **False:** Most major and trace minerals occur freely in nature, mainly in the waters of rivers, lakes, and oceans, in topsoil, and beneath the earth's surface. Minerals exist in the root systems of plants and in the body structure of animals that consume plants and water containing minerals. Neither plant nor animal kingdom provides a "better" source for these micronutrients.

5. **False:** Adults need about 1 mL of water per kcal of energy expended each day. If the average woman expends 2400 kcal per day, she then requires about 2400 mL (2.4 L) of water on a daily basis. This volume transposes to about 0.63 gallons (2.4 L ÷ 3.785).

6. **False:** While sodium is an important contributor to increased blood pressure in some hypertensive individuals, weight (fat) loss, regular exercise, and a well-balanced diet are also important changes a person can make to lower blood pressure.

7. **False:** Fat-soluble vitamins should not be consumed in excess without medical supervision. Toxic reactions from excessive fat-soluble vitamin intake generally occur at a lower multiple of recommended intakes than water-soluble vitamins. An excess intake of certain water-soluble vitamins also causes untoward effects in certain individuals.

8. **False:** Iron deficiency anemia impairs the body's ability to transport oxygen and process it in energy transfer reactions. This conditi`on produces general sluggishness, loss of appetite, and reduced capacity to sustain even mild exercise.

9. **False:** Short intense bouts of mechanical loading of bone through weight-bearing exercise performed three to five times a week provides a potent stimulus

to maintain or increase bone mass. This form of exercise includes walking, running, dancing, and rope skipping; high-intensity resistance exercises and circuit resistance training also exert a positive effect. Sport activities providing relatively high impact on the skeletal mass (e.g., volleyball, basketball, gymnastics, judo, and karate) also induce increases in bone mass, particularly at weight-bearing sites.

10. **False:** Research on the DASH diet to treat hypertension demonstrates this type of diet lowers blood pressure in the general population and in people with stage 1 hypertension to the same extent as pharmacologic therapy, and often more than other lifestyle changes.

Key References

Al-Solaiman Y, et al. DASH lowers blood pressure in obese hypertensives beyond potassium, magnesium and fiber. *J Hum Hypertens* 2010;24:237.

American College of Sports Medicine. Position stand on physical activity and bone health. *Med Sci Sports Exerc* 2004;36:1985.

American College of Sports Medicine position stand. Nutrition and athletic performance. American Dietetic Association; Dietitians of Canada; American College of Sports Medicine, *Med Sci Sports Exerc* 2009;41:709. Review.

Beals KA, Hill AK. The prevalence of disordered eating, menstrual dysfunction, and low bone mineral density among US collegiate athletes. *Int J Sport Nutr Exerc Metab* 2006;16:1.

Bergland A, et al. Effect of exercise on mobility, balance, and health-related quality of life in osteoporotic women with a history of vertebral fracture: a randomized, controlled trial. *Osteoporos Int* 2010 (In Press)

Bloomer RJ, et al. Oxidative stress response to aerobic exercise: comparison of antioxidant supplements. *Med Sci Sports Exerc* 2006;38:1098.

Brownlie IV T, et al. Tissue iron deficiency without anemia impairs adaptation in endurance capacity after aerobic training in previously untrained women. *Am J Clin Nutr* 2004;79:437.

Cussler EC, et al. Weight lifted in strength training predicts bone change in postmenopausal women. *Med Sci Sports Exerc* 2003;35:10.

Drinkwater BL, et al. Menstrual history as a determinant of current bone density in young athletes. *JAMA* 1990;263:545.

Elmer PJ, et al. Effects of comprehensive lifestyle modification on diet, weight, physical fitness and blood pressure control: 18-month results of a randomized trial. *Ann Intern Med* 2006;144:127.

Frank AW, et al. J Muscle cross sectional area and grip torque contraction types are similarly related to pQCT derived bone strength indices in the radii of older healthy adults. *Musculoskelet Neuronal Interact.* 2010;10:136.

Fung TT, et al. Adherence to a DASH-style diet and risk of coronary heart disease and stroke in women. *Arch Intern Med* 2008;168:713.

Goldfarb AH, et el. Combined antioxidant treatment affects blood oxidative stress after eccentric exercise. *Med Sci Sports Exerc* 2005;37:234.

Gropper SS, et al. Iron status of female collegiate athletes involved in different sports. *Biol Trace Elem Res* 2006;109:1.

Guadalupe-Grau A, et al. Exercise and bone mass in adults. *Sports Med* 2009;39: 439.

Hamilton KL. Antioxidants and cardioprotection. *Med Sci Sports Exerc* 2007;39:1544,

Klungland Torstveit M, Sundgot-Borgen J. The female athlete triad: are elite athletes at increased risk? *Med Sci Sports Exerc* 2005;237:184.

Korpelainen R, et al. Long-term outcomes of exercise: follow-up of a randomized trial in older women with osteopenia. *Arch Intern Med* 2010;170:1548.

Lambrinoudaki I, Papadimitriou D. Pathophysiology of bone loss in the female athlete. *Ann N Y Acad Sci.* 2010;1205:45.

LaMothe JM, Zernicke RF. Rest-insertion combined with high-frequency loading enhances osteogenesis. *J Appl Physiol* 2004;96:1788.

Li WC, et al. Effects of exercise programs on quality of life in osteoporotic and osteopenic postmenopausal women: a systematic review and meta-analysis. *Clin Rehabil.* 2009;23:888.

Maughan RJ, Shirreffs SM. Development of individual hydration strategies for athletes. *Int J Sport Nutr Exerc Metab* 2008;18:457. Review.

Pollock N, et al. Bone-mineral density and other features of the female athlete triad in elite endurance runners: a longitudinal and cross-sectional observational study. *Int J Sport Nutr Exerc Metab.* 2010; 20:418.

Rosner MH. Exercise-associated hyponatremia. *Semin Nephrol.* 2009;29:271. Review.

Strazzullo P, et al. Salt intake, stroke, and cardiovascular disease: meta-analysis of prospective studies. *Brit Med J* 2009;339:b4980.

thePoint *Visit* **thePoint.lww.com/MKKSEN4e** *for a list of the references cited in this chapter, including additional, relevant references.*

CHAPTER 3

Digestion and Absorption of the Food Nutrients

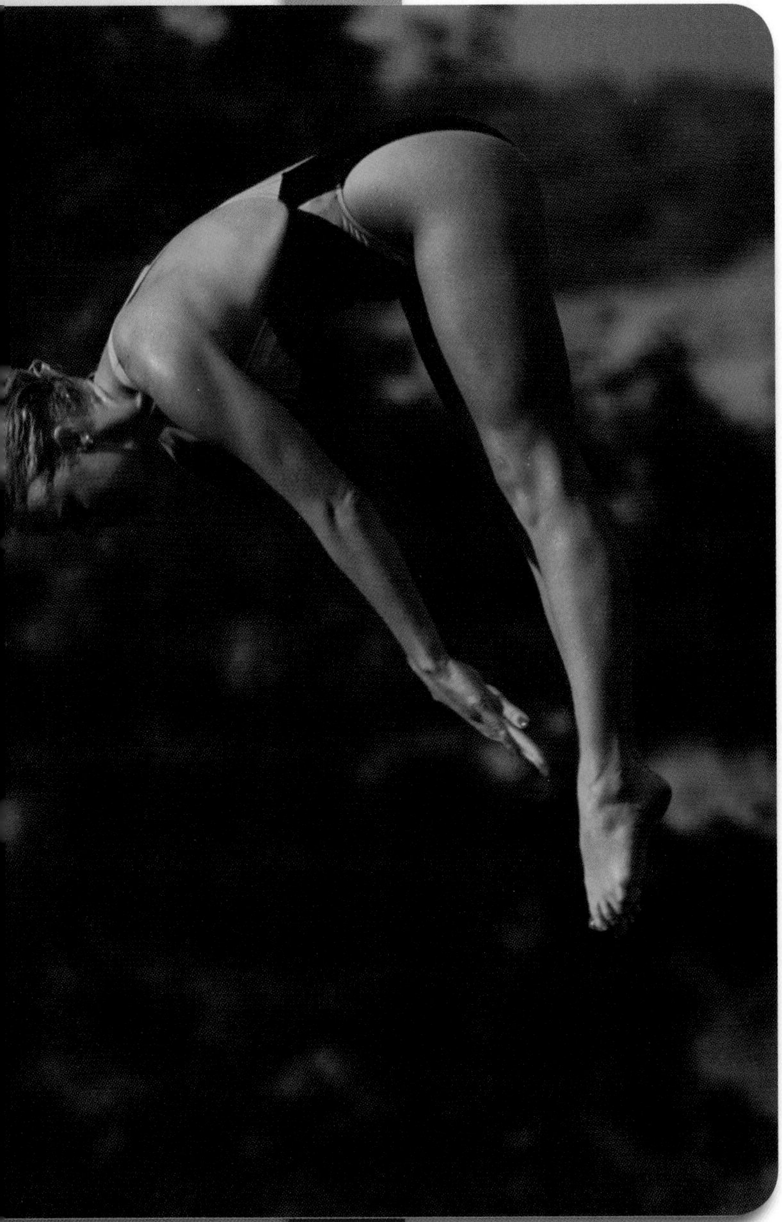

OUTLINE

- Digestion and Absorption of Food Nutrients
- Anatomy of the Gastrointestinal Tract
- Digestion of Food Nutrients
- Exercise Effects on Gastrointestinal Functions
- Health Status, Emotional State, and Gastrointestinal Tract Disorders
- Acute Gastroenteritis: Bacterial and Viral Induced

TEST YOUR KNOWLEDGE

Select true or false for the 10 statements below, and then check out the answers at the end of the chapter. Retake the test after you've read the chapter; you should achieve 100%!	True	False
1. The digestion of food begins in the stomach.	❍	❍
2. The colon is another name for the large intestine.	❍	❍
3. The liver, gallbladder, and pancreas are all organs through which food nutrients must pass during digestion.	❍	❍
4. Glucose absorption requires energy, while the absorption of dietary fat occurs passively without expenditure of energy.	❍	❍
5. Active transport of a nutrient across the plasma membrane occurs by electrostatic transfer that does not require energy.	❍	❍
6. The main absorption of lipids takes place in the stomach's distal portion.	❍	❍
7. Almost all nutrient digestion and absorption takes place in the small intestine.	❍	❍
8. Glucose absorption takes place predominantly in the large intestine.	❍	❍
9. When amino acids reach the liver, they immediately release into the blood.	❍	❍
10. The caloric content of ingested food is the most important factor affecting gastric emptying.	❍	❍

Proper food intake provides a steady supply of energy and tissue-building chemicals to sustain life. For exercise and sports participants, the ready availability of specific food nutrients takes on added importance because physical activity increases energy expenditure and need for additional tissue repair and synthesis. Nutrient uptake by the body involves complex physiologic and metabolic processes that usually progress unnoticed for a lifetime. Hormones and enzymes work nonstop in concert throughout the digestive tract at proper levels of acidity–alkalinity to enhance the breakdown of complex nutrient molecules into simpler subunits. The razor-thin lining of the small intestine absorbs substances produced during digestion, which then pass into the blood and lymph. Self-regulating processes within the digestive tract usually move food along at a slow enough rate to allow its complete absorption, yet rapid enough to ensure timely delivery of its nutrient components. Fibrous materials that resist digestion pass unabsorbed from one end of the body to the other.

The sections that follow outline the digestion and absorption of the various nutrients consumed in the diet. We also discuss the different relationships among nutrition, exercise, and gastrointestinal tract disorders.

DIGESTION AND ABSORPTION OF FOOD NUTRIENTS

The digestive process, essential to the body's nourishment, represents the mechanical and chemical breakdown of food into smaller components or individual nutrients. These nutrients from the diet are then absorbed across the intestinal mucosa into the blood for storage or further chemical change. For the healthy person the process of digestion, absorption, and elimination usually requires between 24 and 72 h.

The Digestive Process

Digestion occurs almost entirely under involuntary control in harmony with exquisite neural and hormonal regulation to continually stabilize the cell's internal environment. Polypeptides and polysaccharides degrade into simpler subunits to enter the epithelial cells of the intestinal villi for absorption into the blood. Fats, emulsified by bile, hydrolyze or break down into their fatty acid and monoglyceride subunits where intestinal villi absorb them. Within the epithelial cells of the villi, triacylglycerols resynthesize and combine with protein for secretion into the lymphatic fluid. The autonomic nervous system controls the entire gastrointestinal (GI) tract: The parasympathetic nervous system generally increases gut activity, while the sympathetic nervous system exerts an inhibitory effect. Even without neural control, intrinsic autoregulatory mechanisms eventually return gut function to near-normal levels.

Beginning of Digestion: Smell, Taste, Teeth, and Tongue

Digestion begins with smell and taste. Different foods emit various odors. Interestingly, the sense of smell has evolved over time to recognize more than 10,000 different odors. Approximately 1000 genes that "control" olfactory receptors decode human smells. The smell of baking biscuits or the aroma of vanilla bean coffee, for example, stimulates specialized nerve cells within the olfactory passages. In the mouth, taste (including texture and temperature) combines with the odors to produce a *perception* of flavor. It is flavor, sensed mainly through smell, that tells us whether we are eating an onion or an apple, or garlic or a fudge brownie. Holding your nose while eating a Belgian chocolate, for example, makes it difficult to identify this substance, even though one can distinguish the food's sweetness or bitterness. In fact, familiar flavors are sensed largely by odor, and the combination of two aromatic substances could create a third odor sensation unlike the odor of either of the original ones. In 2004, Linda B. Buck (1947–) of the Fred Hutchinson Cancer Research Center, Seattle, WA, shared the Nobel Prize in Physiology or Medicine for her pioneering research that explained the odorant receptors and olfactory system organization. The research identified approximately 1000 different genes that promote an equivalent number of olfactory receptor types (**www.nobelprize.org/nobel_prizes/medicine/laureates/**). In essence, the research provided the molecular details about the sense of smell. The sight, smell, thought, and taste of food, and perhaps the sounds made by chewing different foods such as crunching or smashing, trigger responses that prepare the digestive tract to receive the food—the mouth begins to salivate, and stomach secretions begin to flow.

Digestive enzymes can act only on the surface of food particles. This makes chewing important because it mechanically breaks food progressively into smaller particles, thereby increasing the surface area that contacts the salivary enzymes. Most adults have 32 teeth, each specialized for one of four functions—biting, tearing, grinding, and crushing. The tongue also plays a major role in digestion, helping to move and position food between the different teeth. Tongue movements also mix food with saliva and help form the food into a bolus—a ball of chewed food mixed with saliva. Chewing also breaks apart the fiber that traps nutrients in some foods. For example, raisins need to be thoroughly chewed to break the fiber and release their nutrient contents for passage to the stomach and then absorption in the small intestine.

Hormones and Digestive Secretions that Control Digestion

Gastrin, secretin, cholecystokinin (CCK), and gastric inhibitory peptide (GIP) represent the four hormones that regulate digestion (**TABLE 3.1**). Hormone-like compounds, many of which occur in the small intestine and brain (e.g., vasoactive intestinal peptide, bombesin [BBS], substance P, and somatostatin), control other important aspects of GI function. These compounds diffuse from cells or nerve endings throughout the GI tract to exert their influence on nearby cells.

Connections to the Past

William Beaumont (1785–1853)

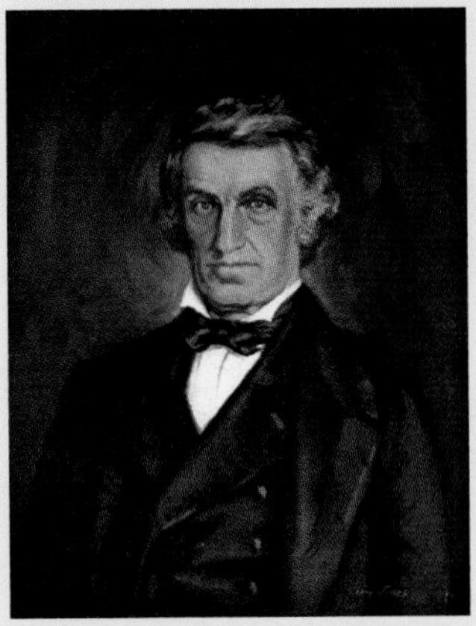

One of the most fortuitous experiments in medicine began on June 6, 1822, at Fort Mackinac on the upper Michigan peninsula. Beaumont tended the accidental shotgun wound that perforated the abdominal wall and stomach of Alexis St. Martin, a 19-year-old voyageur for the American Fur Company. Part of the wound formed a small natural "valve" that led directly into the stomach. Beaumont turned St. Martin on his left side, depressing the valve, and then inserted a tube the size of a large quill 5 or 6 inches into the stomach. Beaumont performed two kinds of experiments on the digestive processes from 1825 to 1833. First, he observed the fluids discharged by the stomach when different foods were eaten (*in vivo*). Second, he extracted samples of the stomach's content and put them into glass tubes to determine the time required for "external" digestion (*in vitro*). For centuries, the stomach was thought to produce heat that somehow cooked foods. Alternatively, the stomach was imaged as a mill, a fermenting vat, or a stew pan. Through his experiments, Beaumont revolutionized concepts about digestion.

thePoint *Visit* **thePoint.lww.com/MKKSEN4e** *to find more details about Beaumont's fortuitous experiments with the digestive process.*

TABLE 3.1 Hormones That Regulate Digestion

Hormone	Origin	Secretion Stimulus	Action
Gastrin	Pyloric areas of stomach and upper duodenum	Food in stomach (protein, caffeine, spices, alcohol); nerve input sphincter; slows gastric emptying	Stimulates flow of stomach enzymes and acid; stimulates action of lower esophageal
GIP	Duodenum, jejunum	Lipids; proteins	Inhibits secretion of stomach acid and enzymes; slows gastric emptying
CCK	Duodenum, jejunum	Lipids and proteins in duodenum	Contraction of gallbladder and flow of bile to duodenum; causes secretion of enzyme-rich pancreatic juice and bicarbonate-rich pancreatic fluid; slows gastric emptying
Secretin	Duodenum, jejunum	Acid chyme; peptones	Secretion of bicarbonate-rich pancreatic fluid and slows gastric emptying

Secretions from the salivary glands, stomach, pancreas, liver via the gallbladder, and small intestine also deliver fluids and digestive enzymes to degrade food particles to prepare them for absorption. **TABLE 3.2** lists these digestive secretions and their major actions.

Transport of Nutrients Across Cell Membranes

Literally thousands of chemicals, including ions, vitamins, minerals, acids, salts, water, gases, hormones, and carbohydrate, protein, and lipid components, continually traverse the cell's bilayer plasma membrane during exchange between the cell and its surroundings. Plasma membranes remain highly permeable to some substances but not others. Such selective permeability allows cells to maintain reasonable consistency in chemical composition. Disrupting the equilibrium triggers immediate adjustments to restore constancy in the cell's "internal milieu." This occurs by two processes:

1. **Passive transport** of substances through the plasma membrane achieved without an energy requirement
2. **Active transport** through the plasma membrane, which requires metabolic energy to "power" the exchange of materials

Passive Transport Processes

Simple diffusion, facilitated diffusion, osmosis, and filtration represent the four types of passive transport. **FIGURE 3.1** shows an example of each.

Simple Diffusion

In the cellular environment, **simple diffusion** involves the free and continuous net movement of molecules in aqueous solution across the plasma membrane. **FIGURE 3.1** depicts that molecules of water, small lipids, and gases move unimpeded from outside the cell through the lipid bilayer into the intracellular fluid. In simple diffusion, a substance moves from an area of higher concentration to lower concentration until it evenly disperses. Only the kinetic energy of the molecules themselves, without expenditure of stored cellular energy,

TABLE 3.2 Digestive Secretions and Their Actions

Organ	Target Organ	Secretion	Action
Salivary glands	Mouth	Saliva	Breaks down carbohydrate
Gastric glands	Stomach	Gastric juice	Mixes with food bolus; hydrochloric acid and enzymes break down proteins
Pancreas	Small intestine	Pancreatic juice	Bicarbonate neutralizes acidic gastric juices; pancreatic enzymes break down carbohydrates, fats, and proteins
Liver	Gallbladder	Bile	Bile stored until needed
Gallbladder	Small intestine	Bile	Bile emulsifies fat to facilitate breakdown by enzymes
Intestinal glands	Small intestine	Intestinal juice	Intestinal enzymes break down carbohydrates, fat, and protein

Digestive enzymes, proteins found in digestive juices, act on food to degrade it to simpler components. Most enzymes end with –ase (pronounced ace), with the beginning of the word identifying the compounds the enzyme works on. For example, carbohydrase hydrolyzes carbohydrates, lipase hydrolyzes lipids, and protease enzymes hydrolyze proteins. Hydrolysis represents a chemical process where a major reactant splits into two end products, with the addition of a hydrogen atom (H^+) to one product and a hydroxyl group (OH^-) to the other.

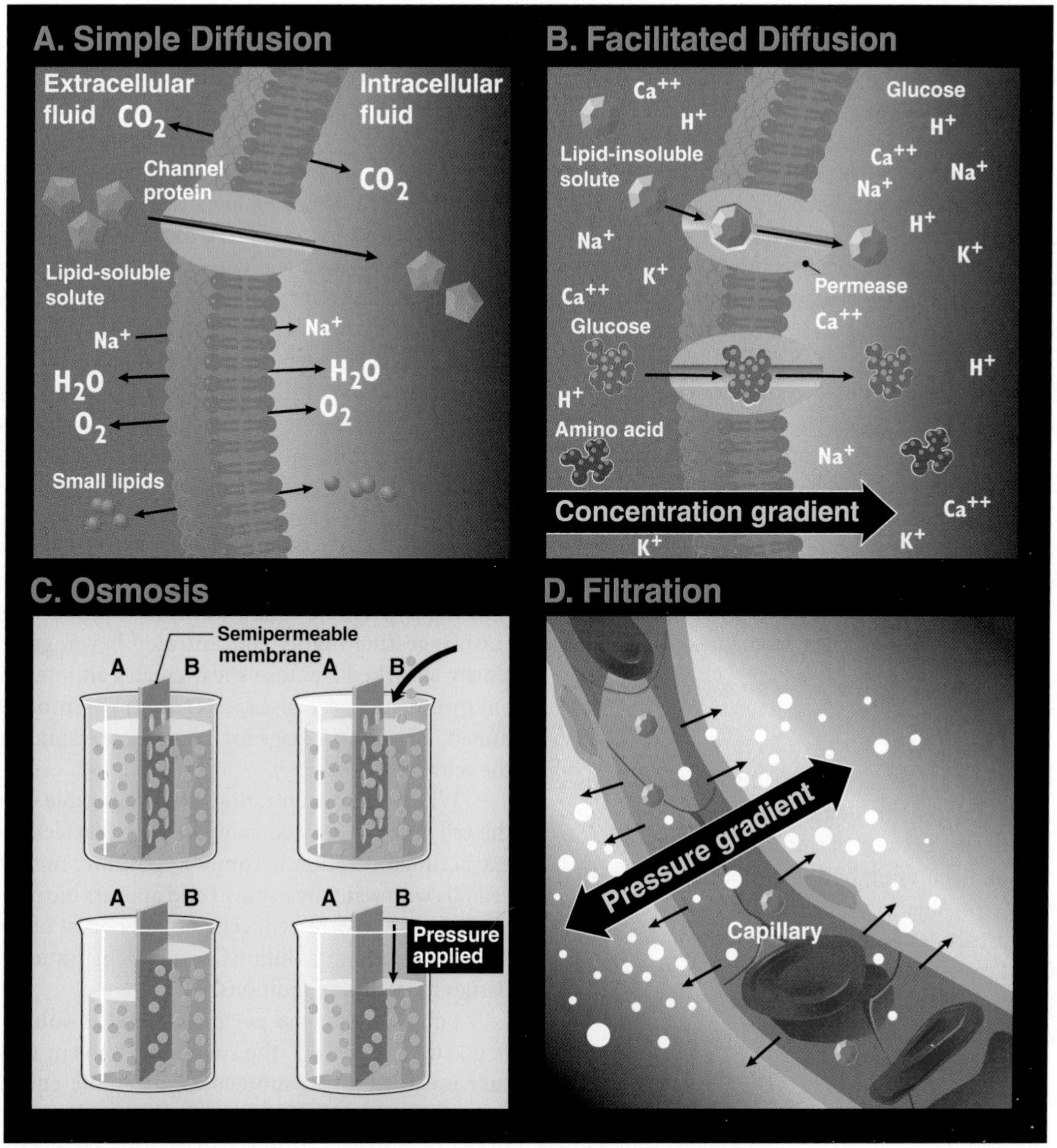

FIGURE 3.1. **A.** Simple diffusion. **B.** Facilitated diffusion. **C.** Osmosis. **D.** Filtration.

powers this passive process. When sugar and water mix, for example, the sugar molecules dissolve and evenly disperse by their continuous, random movement. Hot water speeds diffusion because higher temperature increases molecular movement and thus diffusion rate. When particles remain within a closed system, they eventually distribute evenly without further particle movement.

Simple diffusion across plasma membranes occurs for water molecules; the dissolved gases oxygen, carbon dioxide, and nitrogen; the small uncharged polar molecules urea and alcohol; and various lipid-soluble molecules. These substances diffuse quickly because the plasma membrane consists of sheetlike, fluid structures mainly composed of lipids. These structures allow relatively small, uncomplicated molecules to easily traverse the membrane. For example, when a molecule of oxygen diffuses from its normal higher concentration outside the cell toward a lower concentration on the cell's inside, it moves down or along its concentration gradient. This gradient determines the direction and magnitude of molecular movement. This explains how oxygen molecules continuously diffuse into cells. In contrast, the higher concentration of carbon dioxide within the cell causes this gaseous end product of energy metabolism to move down its concentration gradient and continually diffuse from the cell into the blood.

Facilitated Diffusion

Facilitated diffusion involves the passive, highly selective binding of lipid-insoluble molecules and other large molecules to a lipid-soluble carrier molecule. This contrasts with simple diffusion where molecules pass unaided through the semipermeable plasma membrane. The carrier molecule, a protein called a transporter or **permease**, spans the plasma membrane. Its function facilitates the transfer of the membrane-insoluble chemicals hydrogen, sodium, calcium, and potassium ions and glucose and amino acid molecules down their concentration gradients across the cell's plasma membrane consisting of a phospholipid bilayer with embedded proteins.

Glucose transport into the cell provides an excellent example of facilitated diffusion. Glucose, a large lipid-insoluble, uncharged molecule would not pass readily into the cell without its specific permease. More specifically, if simple diffusion were the only means by which glucose enters a cell, its maximum rate of uptake would be nearly 500 times slower than glucose transport by facilitated diffusion. Facilitated diffusion allows glucose molecules to first attach to a binding site on a specific permease in the plasma membrane. A structural change then occurs in the permease that creates a "passageway" so the glucose molecule penetrates the permease to enter the cytoplasm. Fortunately, facilitated diffusion of glucose keeps this important energy fuel readily available. Also, glucose transport does not require cellular energy. Consequently, facilitated diffusion serves as an energy-conserving mechanism that spares cellular energy for other vital cellular functions.

Osmosis

Osmosis represents a special case of diffusion. Osmosis moves water (the solvent) through a selectively permeable membrane. This occurs because of a difference in the concentration of water molecules on both sides of the membrane, which is more permeable to water than to the solute. This passive process distributes water throughout the intracellular, extracellular, and plasma fluid body compartments.

In the example in **FIGURE 3.1C**, a semipermeable membrane separates compartments A and B. When an equal number of solute particles appears on sides A and B, the same water volume exists in both compartments. By adding a solute to an aqueous solution, the concentration of the solution increases by the amount of solute added. Adding more solute increases the concentration of particles while correspondingly decreasing the concentration of water molecules. In the example, adding nondiffusable solute to side B forces water from side A to move through the semipermeable membrane to side B. This makes the volume of water greater on side B than side A. More water flows into an area containing more particles, leaving less water on the side with fewer solute particles. Eventually, by osmotic action, the concentration of solute particles equalizes on sides A and B.

Osmolality refers to the concentration of particles in solution, expressed as osmolal units of particles or ions formed when a solute dissociates. In living tissue, a difference always exists in the osmolality of the various fluid compartments because the semipermeable membrane retards the passage of ions and intracellular proteins. Selective permeability maintains a difference in solute concentration on both sides of the membrane. Water diffuses freely through the plasma membrane so a net movement of water occurs as the system attempts to equalize osmolality on both sides of the membrane. This can produce dramatic volume changes in the two fluid compartments. At some point, water no longer enters the cell because the hydrostatic pressure of water on one side of the cell balances the pressure tending to draw water through the membrane. A solution's **osmotic pressure** refers to the physical pressure on one side of a membrane required to prevent the osmotic movement of water from the other side.

Altering the water volume inside a cell changes its shape or "tone," a characteristic referred to as tonicity. When a cell neither loses nor gains water when placed in a solution, the solution becomes **isotonic** relative to the cell. In isotonic solutions, the concentration of a nonpenetrating solute such as sodium chloride equalizes on the inside and outside of the cell without net water movement. The body's extracellular fluid under normal conditions provides an example of an isotonic solution.

A **hypertonic** solution contains a higher concentration of nonpenetrating solutes outside rather than inside the cell membrane. When this occurs, water migrates out of the cell by osmosis, causing the cell to shrink in size. Edema, an excess accumulation of water in body tissues, can be countered by infusing hypertonic solutions into the bloodstream. In contrast, ingesting highly concentrated beverages with salt or slowly absorbed fructose sugar creates an intestinal osmotic environment that causes water to move into the intestinal lumen. This sets the stage for intestinal cramping and impedes the rehydration process.

When the concentration of nondiffusible solutes outside the cell becomes diluted compared with the cell's interior, the extracellular solution becomes **hypotonic**. In such cases, the cell fills with water by osmosis and appears bloated. If the condition goes uncorrected, cells actually burst or lyse. Administering hypotonic solutions during dehydration restores the tissues to isotonic conditions.

For a membrane permeable to the solute and water (e.g., sugar in water), the solute and solvent molecules diffuse until the sugar molecules distribute equally. In contrast, for a membrane impermeable to the solute, osmotic pressure draws water in the direction that equalizes the solute concentration on both sides of the membrane. Water movement continues until solute concentration equalizes or until the hydrostatic pressure on one side of the membrane counteracts the force exerted by osmotic pressure. **FIGURE 3.2** illustrates the osmotic effect on cells placed in isotonic, hypertonic, and hypotonic solutions.

Filtration

In **filtration**, water and its solutes flow passively from a region of higher hydrostatic pressure to one of lower pressure. The filtration mechanism allows plasma fluid and its solutes to glide across the capillary membrane to literally bathe the tissues. Filtration moves the plasma filtrate (the fluid portion of the blood with no significant concentration of proteins) through the kidney tubules during urine production.

Active Transport Processes

Energy-requiring **active transport** comes into play when a substance cannot move across the cell membrane by one of

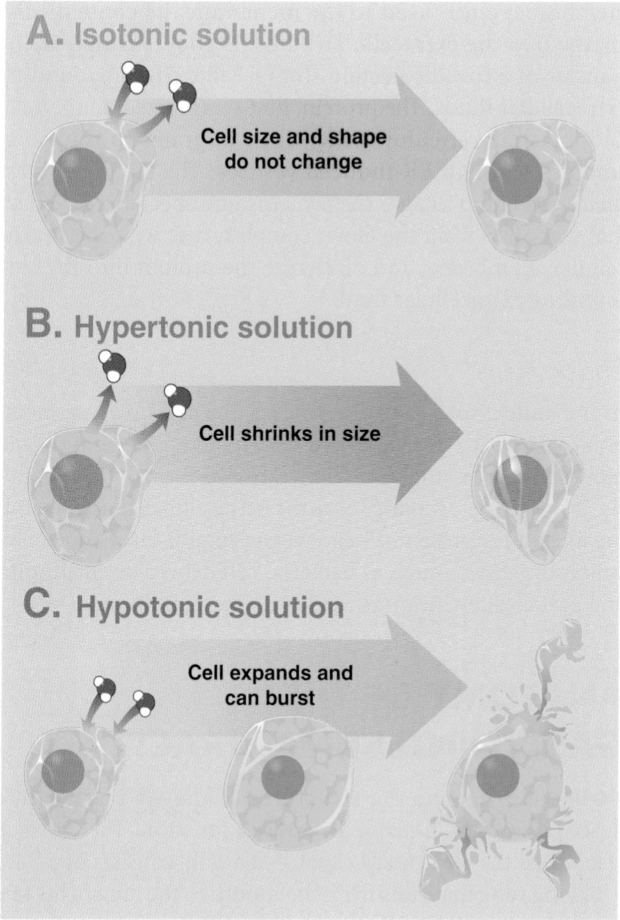

FIGURE 3.2. **A.** *Isotonic solution.* The cell retains its shape because of equal concentrations of solute inside and outside the cell. **B.** *Hypertonic solution.* The cell shrinks (crenates) because the outside of the cell has a higher concentration of nondiffusible solutes than the inside. **C.** *Hypotonic solution.* The concentration of nondiffusible solutes outside the cell is diluted compared to the concentration within the cell. The cell takes on water by osmosis, which can burst (lyse) the cell.

the four passive transport processes. Each active transport process requires the expenditure of cellular energy from adenosine triphosphate (ATP).

Sodium–Potassium Pump

FIGURE 3.3 illustrates the operation of the **sodium–potassium pump**, one of the main active transport mechanisms for moving substances through semipermeable membranes. Energy from ATP "pumps" ions "uphill" against their electrochemical gradients through the membrane by a specialized carrier enzyme called sodium–potassium ATPase that serves as the pumping mechanism. Recall that substances usually diffuse along their concentration gradients from an area of higher to lower concentration. In the living cell, diffusion alone cannot provide optimal distribution of cellular chemicals. Instead, charged sodium and potassium ions and large amino acid molecules insoluble in the lipid bilayer must move against their concentration gradients to fulfill normal functions. Sodium ions, for example, exist in relatively low concentration inside the cell; thus, extracellular Na^+ tends to continually diffuse into the cell. In contrast, potassium ions exist in higher concentration inside the cell, and intracellular K^+ tends to diffuse toward the extracellular space. Consequently, to achieve proper Na^+ and K^+ concentrations about the plasma membrane for normal nerve and muscle functions, both ions continually move against their normal concentration gradients. This concentrates Na^+ extracellularly, whereas K^+ builds up within the cell. Countering the normal tendency of solutes to diffuse by the sodium–potassium pump provides the biologic way to establish normal electrochemical gradients for proper nerve and muscle stimulation.

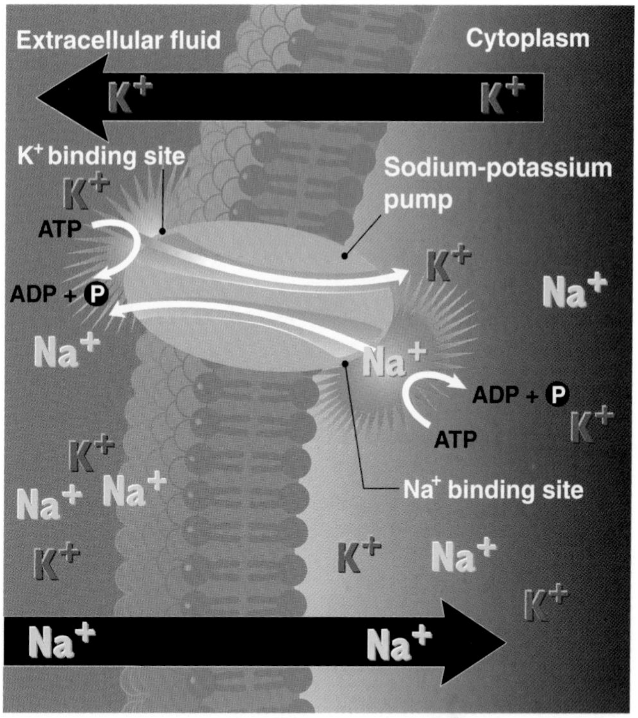

FIGURE 3.3. The dynamics of the sodium–potassium pump. (ATP, adenosine triphosphate; ADP, adenosine diphosphate; P, phosphate.)

Coupled Transport

Active transport absorbs nutrients through the digestive tract's epithelial cells and reabsorbs important plasma chemicals filtered by the kidneys. Absorption of intestinal glucose, for example, takes place by a form of active transport called **coupled transport**. **FIGURE 3.4** shows glucose and Na^+ molecules coupling together before they enter an intestinal villus; they move in the same direction when "pumped" through the plasma membrane to the cell's inside and subsequently into the bloodstream. Amino acids also join with Na^+ for active absorption through the small intestine. A cotransporter or **symport** refers to the simultaneous transport of two chemicals in the same direction; each symport has its own specialized permease with a specific binding site for each substance.

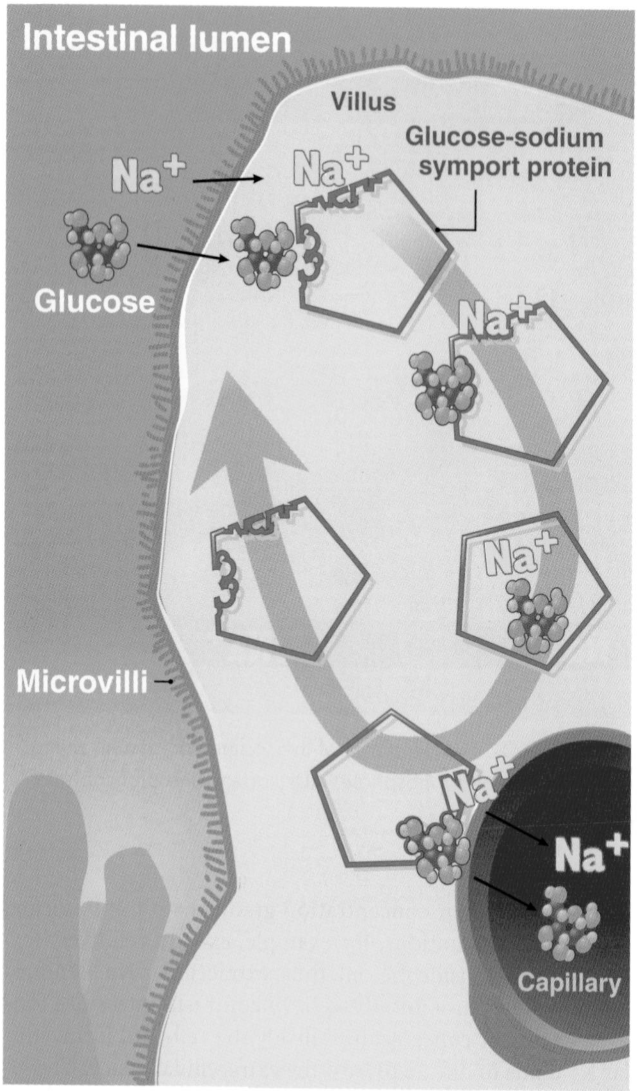

FIGURE 3.4. Coupled transport. A molecule of glucose and a sodium ion move together in the same direction through the plasma membrane in a symport protein.

Coupled transport occurs in one direction only. When the glucose–sodium and amino acid–sodium symports move from the intestine to the blood, they cannot move back and re-enter the intestine.

Bulk Transport

Bulk transport moves a large number of particles and macromolecules through cell membranes by an energy-requiring process. Bulk transport occurs by exocytosis and endocytosis.

Exocytosis

Exocytosis transfers hormones, neurotransmitters, and mucous secretions from intracellular to extracellular fluids. Exocytosis involves several distinct phases. First, the substance for transfer encloses within a membranous, saclike pouch, with the pouch then migrating to the plasma membrane; once fused to the membrane, its contents discharge *into* the extracellular fluids. A good example is the transfer of a specific protein from a cell to the surrounding extracellular fluids. The protein, first synthesized on the cell's endoplasmic reticulum (ER), then migrates to the Golgi complex through ER-induced vesicles. The Golgi complex then sorts and packages the proteins into specialized vesicles that tear away from the Golgi complex, fuse with the nearby cellular membrane, and discharge the protein into the surrounding extracellular fluid.

Endocytosis

In the **endocytosis** transfer process, the cell's plasma membrane surrounds the substance, which then pinches away and moves *into* the cytoplasm. There are two forms of endocytosis. Pinocytosis primarily absorbs extracellular fluids including all solutes present. Phagocytosis engulfs large molecules (microorganisms such as bacteria, cell debris, or small mineral particles) by means of vesicular internalization.

ANATOMY OF THE GASTROINTESTINAL TRACT

FIGURE 3.5 depicts the structures of the **GI tract** with a description of each major structure's function. The GI tract, also called the alimentary canal, essentially consists of a 7- to 9-m long tube that runs from the mouth to the anus. This serpentlike tube supplies the body with water and nutrients.

Mouth and Esophagus

The journey of a bite of food begins in the mouth. Crushing forces of up to 90 kg cut, grind, mash, and soften the food. **Mechanical digestion** increases the food particles' surface area, making them easier to swallow and more accessible to enzymes and other digestive substances that start the degradation process. With swallowing, the bolus of food moves past the pharynx at the back of the mouth and enters the **esophagus**, the 25-cm portion of the GI tract that connects the pharynx and stomach. Two layers of muscle tissue encircle the length of the esophagus; the inner layer consists of circular bands of muscle, while the outer tissue layer runs longitudinally. The esophagus constricts when the circular muscles reflexly contract and the longitudinal muscles relax; the reverse causes the esophagus to bulge. These powerful waves of rhythmic contraction and relaxation called **peristalsis** propel the small round food mass down the esophagus (**FIG. 3.6A**).

Peristalsis involves progressive and recurring waves of smooth muscle contractions that compress the alimentary tube in a squeezing action, causing its contents to mix and move forward. This intrinsic means of food propulsion can occur in the microgravity of space flight and even when a person turns upside down. The end of the esophagus contains a one-way ring or valve of smooth muscle called the **esophageal**

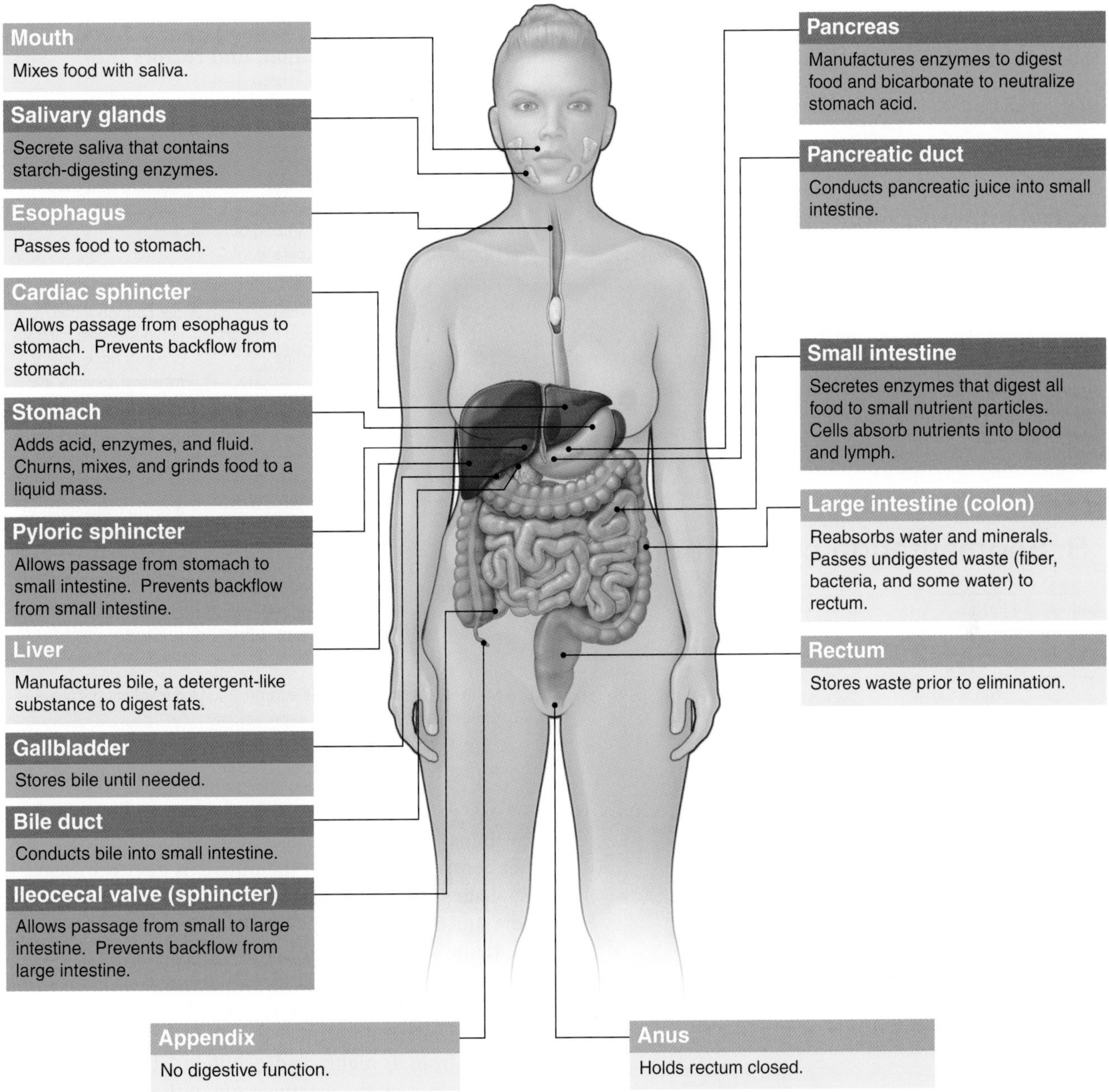
Mouth
Mixes food with saliva.
Salivary glands
Secrete saliva that contains starch-digesting enzymes.
Esophagus
Passes food to stomach.
Cardiac sphincter
Allows passage from esophagus to stomach. Prevents backflow from stomach.
Stomach
Adds acid, enzymes, and fluid. Churns, mixes, and grinds food to a liquid mass.
Pyloric sphincter
Allows passage from stomach to small intestine. Prevents backflow from small intestine.
Liver
Manufactures bile, a detergent-like substance to digest fats.
Gallbladder
Stores bile until needed.
Bile duct
Conducts bile into small intestine.
Ileocecal valve (sphincter)
Allows passage from small to large intestine. Prevents backflow from large intestine.
Appendix
No digestive function.
Pancreas
Manufactures enzymes to digest food and bicarbonate to neutralize stomach acid.
Pancreatic duct
Conducts pancreatic juice into small intestine.
Small intestine
Secretes enzymes that digest all food to small nutrient particles. Cells absorb nutrients into blood and lymph.
Large intestine (colon)
Reabsorbs water and minerals. Passes undigested waste (fiber, bacteria, and some water) to rectum.
Rectum
Stores waste prior to elimination.
Anus
Holds rectum closed.

FIGURE 3.5. Structures of the gastrointenstinal tract including each structure's digestive function.

sphincter, which relaxes to allow the food mass entry into the **stomach**—the next section of the GI tract. This sphincter then constricts to help prevent the stomach contents from regurgitating back into the esophagus termed *gastric reflux*. The stomach serves as a temporary "storage tank" for the partially digested food before moving it into the small intestine.

Sphincters That Control Food Passage

A sphincter, a circular muscle arrangement acting as a one-way valve, regulates the flow of material through the GI tract. Several sphincters exist throughout the length of the GI tract; they respond to stimuli from nerves, hormones, and hormonelike substances and increases in pressure around them. **TABLE 3.3** lists the important sphincters, their location in the digestive tract, and the factors that control them.

Stomach

FIGURE 3.7 shows structural details of the approximately 25-cm long, J-shaped stomach, the most distensible portion of the GI tract; the inset details the stomach wall showing the gastric glands. The **parietal cells** of the gastric glands secrete hydrochloric acid—stimulated by gastrin, acetylcholine, and

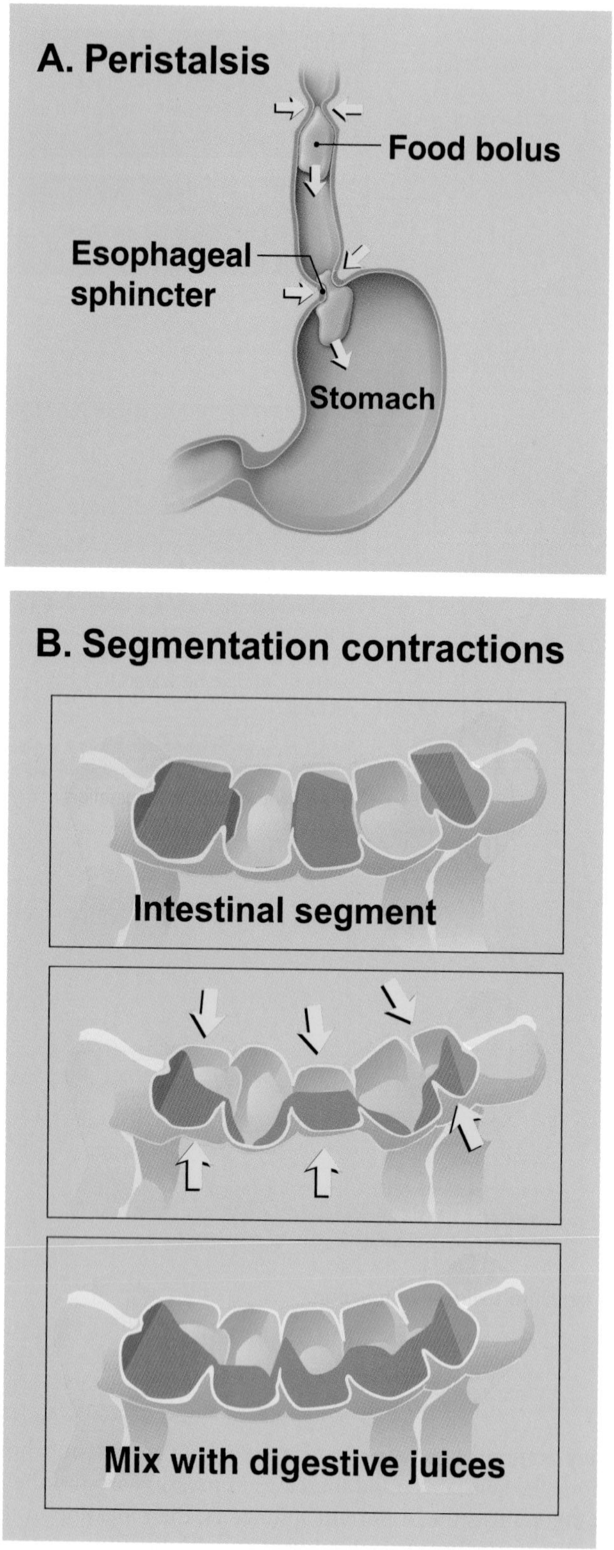

FIGURE 3.6. Propulsion of nutrients through the GI tract. **A.** Peristalsis involves the reflex-controlled alternate contraction and relaxation of adjacent segments of the GI tract, which causes one-directional flow of food with some mixing. **B.** Segmentation contractions involve the alternate contraction and relaxation of nonadjacent segments of the intestine. This localized intestinal rhythmicity propels food forward and then backward, causing food to mix with digestive juices.

TABLE 3.3 Sphincters in the Digestive Tract, Their Location, and Factors That Influence Them

Sphincter	Location	Comments
Esophageal (upper and lower cardiac sphincter)	Junction between esophagus and stomach; prevents back flow (reflux) of stomach contents into the esophagus	Opens only when esophageal muscles contract
Pyloric	Junction between stomach and first part of the intestine	Under hormonal and nervous system control; prevents back flow of intestinal contents into stomach
Oddi	End of common bile duct	When hormone CCK stimulates gallbladder to contract during digestion, this sphincter relaxes to allow bile to flow down the common bile duct and enter the intestinal duodenum
Ileocecal	Terminus of the small intestine	Opens in the presence of intestinal contents
Anal (two sphincters)	Terminus of the large intestine	Under voluntary control

histamine—and powerful enzyme-containing digestive juices that continually degrade the nutrients after they leave the esophagus and enter the stomach. Alkaline mucus, secreted from mucous neck cells, protects the mucosal lining of gastric tissues. The buffering action of bicarbonate in alkaline pancreatic juice and alkaline secretions from glands in the submucosa of the duodenum (the first portion of the small intestine) normally protect the duodenum portion of the stomach from its highly acidic contents. The chief cells produce pepsinogen, the inactive form of the protein-digesting enzyme pepsin. Simple sugars are the easiest nutrients to digest, followed by proteins and then lipids. With the exception of alcohol and aspirin, little absorption takes place in the stomach.

The stomach's volume averages about 1.5 L; however, it can hold a volume ranging from only 50 mL, or about 1.5 oz when nearly "empty," to about 6 L (6000 mL) when fully distended following a large meal. Regardless of its volume, the stomach contents mix with chemical substances to produce **chyme**, a slushy, acidic mixture of food and digestive juices.

After eating, the stomach usually takes 1 to 4 h to empty depending on the relative concentration of each nutrient and the meal's volume. A large meal takes longer to clear the stomach than a smaller one. When eaten singularly, carbohydrates leave the stomach most rapidly, followed by proteins and then lipids. The stomach may retain a high-fat meal for up to 6 h before its chyme empties into the **small intestine**.

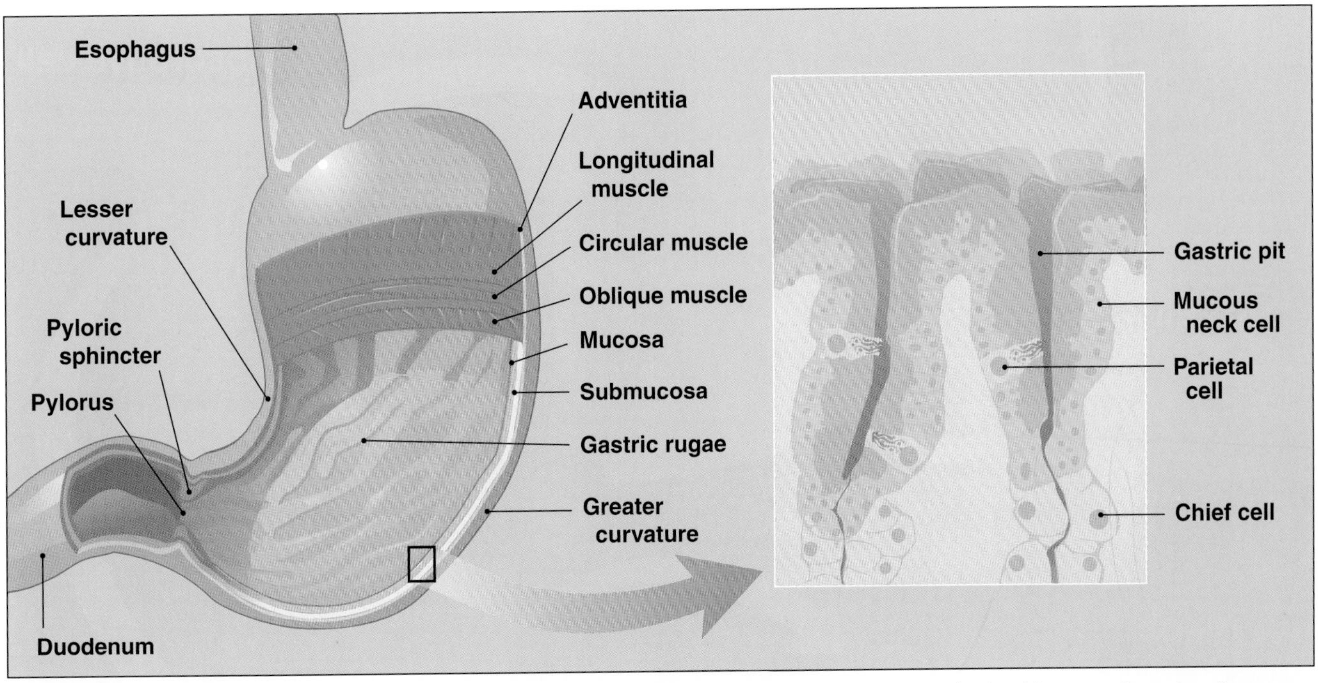

FIGURE 3.7. Structure of the stomach and gastric glands. The parietal cells primarily secrete hydrochloric acid, neck cells secrete mucus, and chief cells produce pepsinogen.

Furthermore, food in liquefied form and fluids per se pass from the stomach most rapidly, whereas solids undergo a liquefaction phase. The nervous system, through hormonal regulation, largely controls the time and rate of stomach emptying via peristaltic waves that traverse the stomach toward the opening of the small intestine. A self-regulating feedback control also occurs between the stomach and small intestine. Excessive stomach distension from volume overload transmits signals that cause the sphincter at the intestinal entrance to relax to allow more chyme to enter. Gastric emptying reflexly slows when the first portion of the small intestine distends, or when in the presence of excessive protein, lipid, or highly concentrated or acidic solutions. A unique life-sustaining stomach function is its secretion of **intrinsic factor**, a polypeptide required for vitamin B_{12} absorption by the small intestine's terminal portion.

Small Intestine

Approximately 90% of digestion and essentially all lipid digestion occur in the first two sections of the 3-m long small intestine. This coiled structure consists of three sections: the **duodenum** (first 0.3 m), **jejunum** (next 1–2 m, where most digestion occurs), and **ileum** (last 1.5 m). Absorption takes place through millions of specialized protruding structures of the intestinal mucosa. These fingerlike protrusions called **villi** move in wavelike fashion. Most nutrient absorption through villi occurs by active transport that uses a carrier molecule and expends ATP energy. **FIGURE 3.8** shows that highly vascularized surfaces of villi contain small projections known as **microvilli**. These structures contain the digestive enzymes embedded within its cell membranes; they absorb the smaller digested units of carbohydrates, proteins, and lipids, electrolytes (80% absorbed), alcohol, vitamins, and minerals.

Villi increase the absorptive surface of the intestine by up to 600-fold compared with a flat-surfaced tube of the same dimensions. If spread out, the small intestine's 300 m^2 surface area would cover the area of a tennis court or about 150 times the body's external surface! This large surface greatly augments the speed and capacity for nutrient absorption. Each villus contains small lymphatic vessels called **lacteals** that absorb most digested lipids from the intestine. They transport via the lymphatic vessels that drain into the large veins near the heart.

Intestinal Contractions

It usually takes 1 to 3 days after consuming food before the GI tract eliminates its residues. The movement of chyme through the small intestine takes 3 to 10 h. Peristaltic contractions are much weaker in the small intestine than in the esophagus and stomach. The intestine's major contractile activity occurs by segmentation contractions. These intermittent oscillating contractions and relaxations of the intestinal wall's circular smooth muscle augment mechanical mixing of intestinal chyme with bile, pancreatic juice, and intestinal juice. **FIGURE 3.6B** shows that segmentation contractions give the small intestine section of the GI tract a "sausage-link" look because the alternating contraction and relaxation occur in nonadjacent segments of this structure. Thus, instead of propelling food directly forward as in peristalsis (**FIG. 3.6A**), the food moves slightly backward before advancing. This gives the digestive juices additional time to blend with the

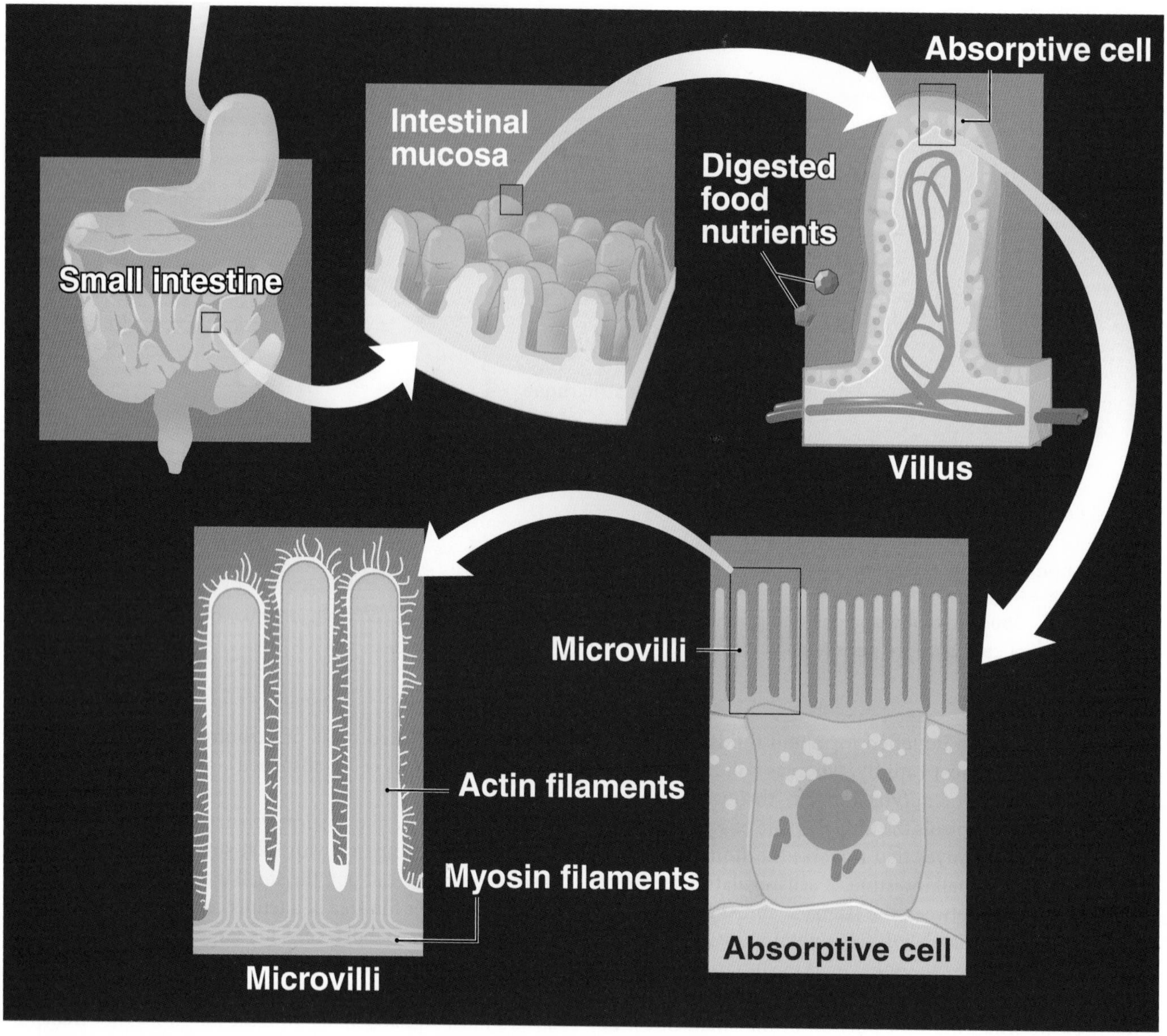

FIGURE 3.8. Microscopic structure of the small intestine. Tiny villi and microvilli projections (termed *brush border*) greatly increase the surface area of the mucosal cell's plasma membrane for nutrient absorption.

food mass before it reaches the large intestine. The propulsive movements of segmentation contractions continue to churn and mix the chyme before it passes the pyloric sphincter and enters the large intestine.

During digestion, **bile** produced in the liver and stored and secreted by the **gallbladder** increases the lipid droplets' solubility and digestibility through **emulsification**. The lipid content of the intestinal chyme stimulates the gallbladder's pulsatile release of bile into the duodenum. In a manner similar to the action of many household detergents, bile salts separate fat into numerous smaller droplets that do not coalesce. This renders fatty acid end products insoluble in water so the small intestine can absorb them. Some bile components are excreted in the feces, but the intestinal mucosa reabsorbs most of the bile salts. They then return in the hepatic portal blood to the liver as components in the resynthesis of new bile.

The **pancreas** secretes between 1.2 and 1.6 L of alkali-containing juice (digestive enzymes in an inactive form plus sodium bicarbonate) to help buffer the hydrochloric acid from the stomach that remains in the intestinal chyme. At a higher pH, pancreatic enzymes released by neural and hormonal mechanisms degrade the larger protein, carbohydrate, and lipid nutrients into smaller subunits for further digestion and absorption. The intestinal lining cannot withstand the highly acidic gastric juices from the stomach. Neutralizing this acid provides crucial protection against duodenal damage, which in extreme form triggers tissue ulceration or ulcers.

Large Intestine

FIGURE 3.9 depicts the components of the **large intestine**, the final digestive structure for absorbing water and

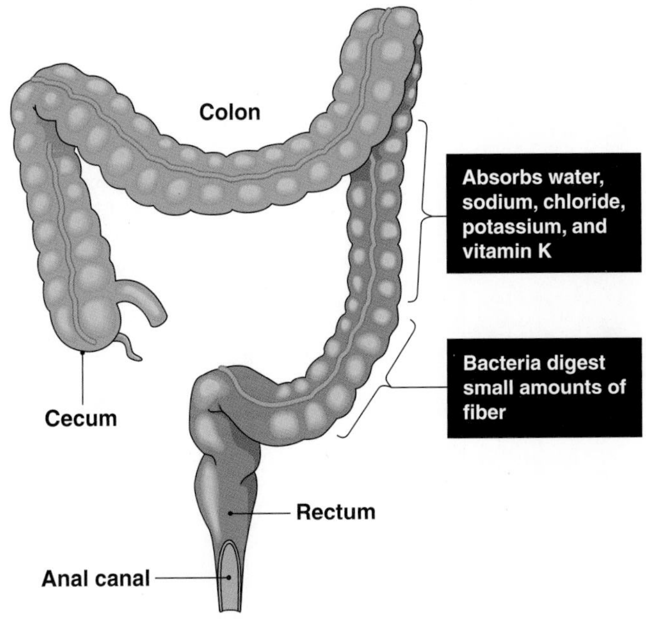

FIGURE 3.9. The large intestine, a 5-ft long tube, includes the cecum, colon, rectum, and anal canal. As chyme fills the cecum, a local reflex signals the ileocecal valve to close, preventing material from re-entering the ileum and small intestine.

electrolytes from the chyme it receives and storing digestive residues as fecal matter. This terminal 1.2-m (4-ft) portion of the GI tract, also known as the **colon**, or **bowel**, has no villi. Its major anatomic sections include the ascending colon, transverse colon, descending colon, sigmoid colon, rectum, and anal canal. Of the 8- to 12-L volume of food, fluid, and gastric secretions that enter the GI tract daily, only about 750 mL pass into the large intestine. There are trillions of bacteria, yeasts, and parasites (more than 400 species) living mostly in the colon. Here, bacteria ferment the remaining undigested food residue, which is devoid of all but about 5% of useful nutrients. Intestinal bacteria, through their own metabolism, synthesize small amounts of vitamins B_{12}, K, and biotin, which then become absorbed. Bacterial fermentation also produces about 500 mL of gas (flatus) each day. This gas consists of hydrogen, nitrogen, methane, hydrogen sulfide, and carbon dioxide. A small amount produces no outward effects, but excessive flatus can trigger severe abdominal distress as usually occurs from consuming large quantities of beans or dairy products. These foods leave partially digested sugars that contribute to larger than normal intestinal gas production. Mucus, the only significant secretion of the large intestine, protects the intestinal wall and helps to bind fecal matter together.

DIGESTION OF FOOD NUTRIENTS

FIGURE 3.10 presents an overview of digestive processes throughout the GI tract for the three food macronutrients. The diagram also lists the major enzymes and hormones that act on proteins, lipids, and carbohydrates during their convoluted journey from the mouth through the GI tract.

Carbohydrate Digestion and Absorption

Starch hydrolysis begins once food enters the mouth. The **salivary glands** located along the underside of the jaw continually secrete lubricating mucous substances that combine with food particles during chewing. The salivary gland's enzyme **salivary α-amylase** or ptyalin attacks starch and reduces it to smaller linked glucose molecules and the simpler disaccharide form maltose. When the food–saliva mixture enters the more acidic stomach, some additional starch breakdown occurs, but this quickly ceases because salivary amylase deactivates at the acidic low pH of gastric juice.

Food entering the alkaline environment of the small intestine's duodenum encounters **pancreatic amylase**, a powerful pancreatic enzyme. This enzyme, in conjunction with other enzymes, completes the hydrolysis of starch into smaller branched chains of glucose molecules (4–10 glucose linkages called dextrins and oligosaccharides); the disaccharides cleave into simple monosaccharides. Enzyme action on the surface of the cells of the intestinal lumen's brush border completes the final stage of carbohydrate digestion to simple monosaccharide form. For example, **maltase** breaks down maltose to its glucose components, **sucrase** reduces sucrose to the simple sugars glucose and fructose, and **lactase** degrades lactose to glucose and galactose. Active transport by common protein carriers in the intestinal villi and microvilli absorbs the monosaccharides (see **FIG. 3.3**). Glucose and galactose absorption occurs by a sodium-dependent, carrier-mediated active transport process (see **FIG. 3.4**). The electrochemical gradient created with sodium transport augments the absorption of these monosaccharides.

The maximum rate of glucose absorption from the small intestine ranges between 50 and 80 $g{\cdot}h^{-1}$ for a person who weighs 70 kg. If we assume that intense aerobic exercise (20 $kcal{\cdot}min^{-1}$) derives 80% of its energy from carbohydrate breakdown, then roughly 4 g of carbohydrate (1 g carbohydrate = 4.0 kcal) are catabolized each minute (or 240 $g{\cdot}h^{-1}$). Even under optimal conditions for intestinal absorption, carbohydrate intake during prolonged intense exercise cannot balance its utilization rate.[10] Fructose does not absorb via active transport; instead, it occurs in combination with a carrier protein by the much slower method of facilitated diffusion.

If disease affects intestinal enzymes or the villi themselves, the GI tract can become "upset" and take several weeks to resume normal functioning.[3] For example, carbohydrates cannot completely degrade with altered digestive enzyme levels. A person recovering from diarrhea or intestinal infection often experiences transient **lactose intolerance** and should avoid milk products that contain lactose. Re-establishing appropriate lactase concentration allows a person to consume this sugar once again without undesirable consequences. About 70% of the world's population suffers from reduced

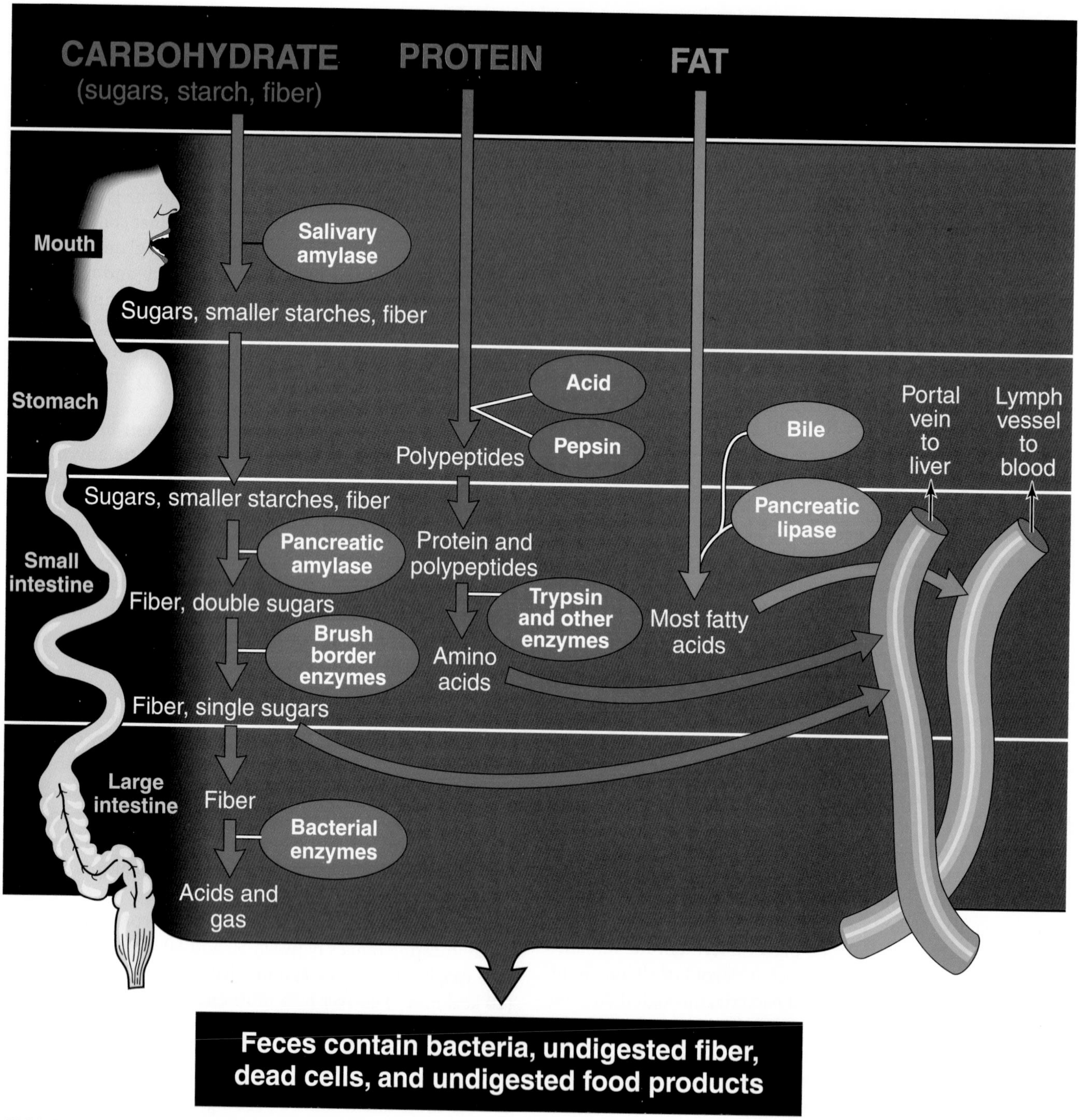

FIGURE 3.10. Overview of human digestion.

intestinal lactase levels to the point that it affects milk sugar digestion.

The small intestine's epithelial cells secrete monosaccharides into the bloodstream for transport by capillaries to the hepatic portal vein, which then empties directly to the liver. The liver removes the greatest portion of glucose and essentially all of the absorbed fructose and galactose. Peripheral tissues under the influence of insulin absorb any remaining blood glucose.

Circulatory transport from the GI tract occurs via the **hepatic portal circulation**. Blood drained from the small intestine does not pass directly to the heart. Instead, intestinal blood travels to the liver, which processes its nutrients before they finally enter the general circulation. The hepatic portal circulation also drains blood from the stomach and pancreas.

The colon provides the "end of the line" for undigested carbohydrates including fibrous substances. Further digestion and water reabsorption occur here; then peristaltic and segmentation actions push the remaining semisolid stool contents into the rectum for expulsion through the anus.

HEMORRHOIDS

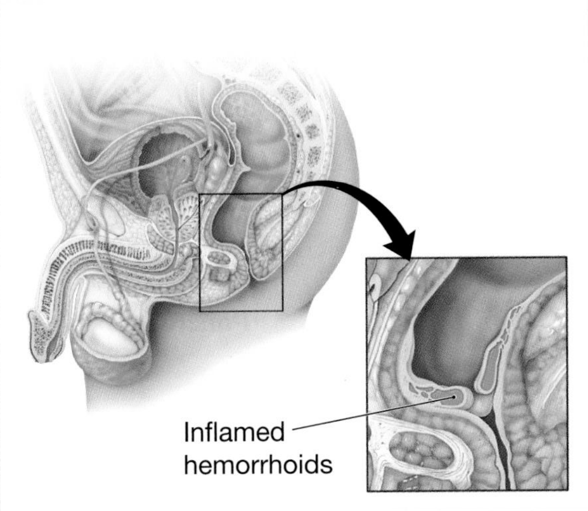

(Asset provided by Anatomical Chart Co.)

Hemorrhoids are painful, swollen veins in the lower portion of the rectum or anus. They result from increased pressure in the veins of the anus, which causes the veins to bulge and expand, making them painful, particularly when sitting.

Hemorrhoids occur equally in men and women; the most common cause results from straining during bowel movements. They also result from chronic constipation in endurance athletes who routinely train for long durations and experience repeated bouts of relative dehydration that leads to constipation. Hemorrhoids also commonly occur during pregnancy. About one half of the population has hemorrhoids by age 50. Internal hemorrhoids occur just inside the anus and the beginning of the rectum. External hemorrhoids occur at the anal opening and may hang outside the anus.

Five common hemorrhoidal symptoms include:

1. Anal itching
2. Anal ache or pain, especially while sitting
3. Bright red blood on toilet tissue, stool, or in the toilet bowl
4. Pain during bowel movements
5. One or more hard tender lumps near the anus

Home treatment includes over-the-counter corticosteroid creams that reduce pain and swelling. For cases that do not respond to home remedies, a rectal surgeon or gastroenterologist can apply nonsurgical heat treatment, called infrared coagulation, to shrink internal hemorrhoids. Surgical treatments include rubber band ligation and surgical hemorrhoidectomy and are only used for patients with severe pain or bleeding who do not respond to other conventional therapies.

Consuming too much dietary fiber usually produces an overly soft stool, whereas inadequate fiber intake has the opposite effect of compacting the stool. The pressure exerted during a bowel movement expels the stool. Excessive pressure during defecation can damage supporting tissues and cause the rectal blood vessels to balloon, a condition called **hemorrhoids**. In severe cases, hemorrhoidal bleeding requires surgery. Gradually increasing the diet's fiber content often relieves constipation and hemorrhoidal symptoms.

Lipid Digestion and Absorption

FIGURE 3.11 illustrates that lipid digestion begins in the mouth and stomach by the action of acid-stable **lingual lipase**, an enzyme secreted in the mouth. This enzyme, which operates effectively in the stomach's acid environment, primarily digests short-chain (4–6 carbons) and medium-chain (8–10 carbons) saturated fatty acids such as those in coconut and palm oil. Chewing food mixes lipase with the food and reduces particle size; this increases the exposed surface to facilitate digestive juice action.

The stomach secretes **gastric lipase**, its own lipid-digesting enzyme. This enzyme works with lingual lipase to continue hydrolysis of a small amount of triacylglycerol that contains short- and medium-chain fatty acids. The major breakdown of lipids, particularly triacylglycerols containing long-chain 12- to 18-carbon fatty acids, occurs in the small intestine. When chyme enters the small intestine, mechanical mixing with bile acts on the triacylglycerols bound together as large lipid globules and emulsifies them into a fine immersion of oil droplets in an aqueous suspension. Bile contains no digestive enzymes; its action breaks up the fat droplets and thereby increases surface contact between lipid molecules and the water-soluble enzyme **pancreatic lipase**. Pancreatic lipase exerts a strong effect on the surface of the fat droplets to hydrolyze some triacylglycerol molecules further to one fatty acid connected to glycerol called a monoglyceride plus free fatty acids. These simpler fats, which have greater polarity than unhydrolyzed lipids, pass through the microvilli membrane to enter intestinal epithelial cells. Pancreatic lipase effectively digests long-chain fatty acids common in animal fats and plant oils.

The peptide hormone **CCK**, released from the wall of the duodenum, controls the release of enzymes into the stomach and small intestine. CCK regulates the following four GI functions:

1. Stomach motility
2. Stomach secretion
3. Gallbladder contraction and bile flow
4. Enzyme secretion by the pancreas

A high lipid content in the stomach reduces gastric motility from the action of the peptide hormones **GIP** and **secretin**. Slowing of gut movement retains chyme in the stomach and explains why a high-fat meal prolongs the digestive process; one positive effect for dieters is a temporary feeling of fullness compared with a meal of lower lipid content.

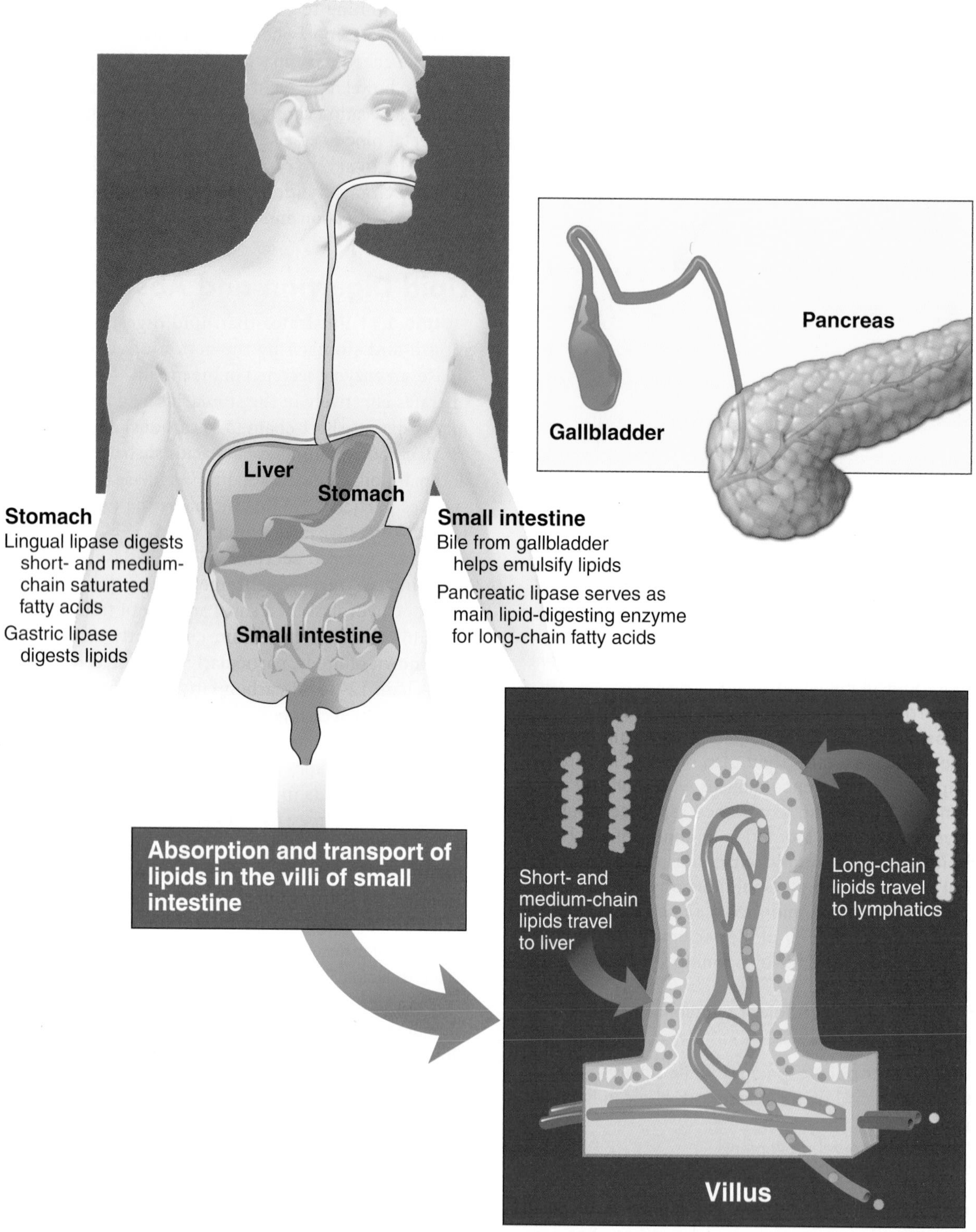

FIGURE 3.11. Digestion of dietary lipids.

Micelles, fat–bile salt clusters, form when water-insoluble monoglyceride and free fatty acid end products from lipid hydrolysis bind with bile salts. The outer brush border of intestinal villi absorbs the micelles by diffusion. The micelles then split, bile returns to the liver, and triacylglycerol synthesis occurs within intestinal epithelial cells from fatty acids and monoglycerides.

Fatty Acid Carbon Chain Length Affects Digestive and Metabolic Processes

Triacylglycerols synthesized within the intestinal epithelium take one of two routes (hepatic portal system or lymphatic system) depending on their chain length. Most **medium-chain triacylglycerols (MCTs)** absorb directly into the portal vein of the hepatic portal system bound to albumin as glycerol and medium-chain free fatty acids. MCTs bypass the lymphatic system by entering the bloodstream rapidly for transport to the liver for subsequent tissue use in energy metabolism. MCT supplementation has clinical application for patients with tissue-wasting disease or with intestinal malabsorption difficulties. Chapter 12 discusses the proposed use of MCTs as an energy aid to enhance endurance exercise performance.

Once absorbed inside epithelial cells, long-chain fatty acids (more than 12 carbons in the fatty acid chain) reform into triacylglycerols. These combine with a small amount of phospholipid, protein, and cholesterol to form small fatty droplets called **chylomicrons**. These molecules move slowly upward via the second route—the lymphatic system. They eventually empty into the venous circulation in the neck region via the thoracic duct. Through the action of the enzyme **lipoprotein lipase**, which lines capillary walls, the chylomicrons in the bloodstream readily hydrolyze to provide free fatty acids and glycerol for use by peripheral tissues. The liver then takes up the remaining cholesterol-containing remnant chylomicron particles. It generally takes 3 to 4 h before ingested long-chain triacylglycerols enter the blood.

Protein Digestion and Absorption

The digestive efficiency for protein, particularly animal protein, normally remains high, with less than 3% appearing in the feces. Indigestible components of this macronutrient include meat's fibrous connective tissue, some grain coverings, and particles of nuts that escape digestive enzymes. In essence, protein digestion liberates the building blocks of ingested proteins to produce the final end products—simple amino acids and dipeptides and tripeptides—for absorption across the intestinal mucosa. Selective enzymes within the stomach and small intestine promote protein hydrolysis.

The powerful enzyme **pepsin** initiates protein digestion chiefly to short-chain polypeptides in the stomach (see **FIG. 3.10**). Pepsin, a group of protein-digesting enzymes, represents the active form of its precursor pepsinogen. The peptide hormone **gastrin** controls pepsin's release from stomach cells of the wall. Gastrin is secreted in response to external environmental cues (sight and smell of food) or internal cues (thought of food or stomach distension by food contents). Gastrin also stimulates gastric hydrochloric acid secretion, a harsh acid that lowers the pH of gastric contents to about 2.0. The acidification of ingested food achieves the following five objectives:

1. Activates pepsin
2. Kills pathogenic organisms
3. Improves iron and calcium absorption
4. Inactivates hormones of plant and animal origin
5. Denatures food proteins, making them more vulnerable to enzyme action

Pepsin, particularly effective in the stomach's acidic medium, easily degrades meat's collagenous connective tissue fibers. Once dismantled, other enzymes digest the remaining animal protein material.

Stomach enzymes and acids attack the long, complex protein strands to hydrolyze about 15% of the ingested proteins. Uncoiling the three-dimensional shape of protein breaks it into smaller polypeptide and peptide units. Pepsin inactivates at the relatively high pH of the duodenum as the chyme passes into the small intestine.

The final steps in protein digestion occur in the small intestine. Here the peptide fragments dismantle further by alkaline enzyme action from the pancreas—most notably **trypsin** from its inactive precursor **trypsinogen**—into tripeptides, dipeptides, and single, free amino acids. Free amino acid absorption occurs by active transport by coupling to the transport of sodium for delivery to the liver via the hepatic portal vein. In contrast, dipeptides and tripeptides move into the intestinal epithelial cells by a single membrane carrier that uses an H^+ gradient for active transport. The dipeptides and tripeptides once inside the cytoplasm hydrolyze into their amino acid constituents and flow into the bloodstream.

One important function of the small intestine is to absorb amino acids and protein in more complex form. When amino acids reach the liver, one of three events occurs:

1. Conversion to glucose (glucogenic amino acids)
2. Conversion to fat (ketogenic amino acids)
3. Direct release into the bloodstream as plasma proteins such as albumin or as free amino acids

Free amino acids synthesize into biologically important proteins, peptides (e.g., hormones), and amino acid derivatives such as phosphocreatine and choline (the essential component of the neurotransmitter acetylcholine).

Vitamin Absorption

Vitamin absorption occurs mainly by the passive process of diffusion in the small intestine's jejunum and ileum regions. Absorption and storage by the body stores constitute a major difference between the fat-soluble and water-soluble forms.

Fat-Soluble Vitamins

Up to 90% of fat-soluble vitamins are absorbed with dietary lipids as part of dietary fat containing micelles in the small intestine. Once absorbed, chylomicrons and lipoproteins transport these vitamins to the liver and body's fatty tissues.

Water-Soluble Vitamins

Diffusion absorbs water-soluble vitamins except for vitamin B_{12}. This vitamin combines with intrinsic factor that the stomach produces, which the intestine absorbs by endocytosis. Water-soluble vitamins do not remain in tissues to any great extent. Instead, they pass into urine when their concentration in plasma exceeds renal capacity for reabsorption. Consequently, food intake must regularly replenish water-soluble vitamins. Ingested B vitamins in food exist as part of coenzymes; digestion then releases them to their free vitamin

Additional Insights
Multivitamins and Heart Attack Protection

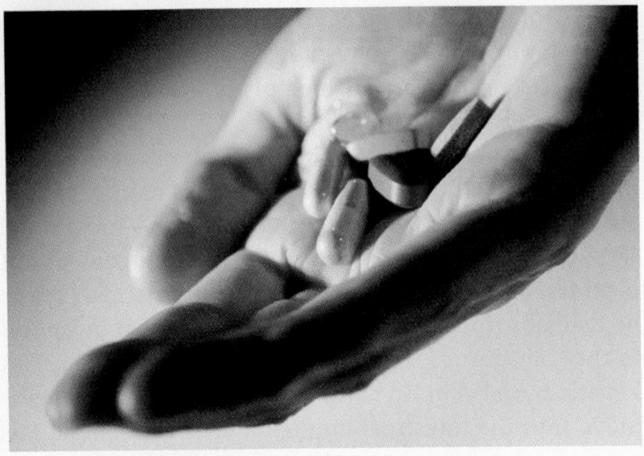

Headlines claiming that "Multivitamins Shield from Heart Attack" and "Multivitamin Use Lowers Heart Attack Risk" often tempt one to join the ranks of the more than 75 million Americans who routinely consume daily multivitamin supplements in pill and powder form at a cost that can reach $75 monthly. Much of the recent media hype comes from a 10-year follow-up study of 31,671 healthy women and 2262 women with documented cardiovascular disease (that included metabolic syndrome, hypertension, and stroke risk factors) who consumed multivitamins on a daily basis. The multivitamins were estimated to contain nutrients close to recommended daily allowances for vitamin A (0.9 mg), vitamin C (60 mg), vitamin D (5 μg), vitamin E (9 mg), thiamine (1.2 mg), riboflavin (1.4 mg), vitamin B_6 (1.8 mg), vitamin B_{12} (3 μg), and folic acid (400 μg). For the healthy women, taking multivitamins for 10 or more years coincided with a 42% lower likelihood of heart attack. Less positive results emerged for the women with heart disease, as no significant difference in heart attack incidence was associated with multivitamin and supplement use. It is important to note that this study did not *prove* that multivitamin and supplement use protects against heart attacks because this retrospective, observational study was not a randomized experiment designed to tease out cause and effect. To do so, an equal number of women with and without heart disease would be randomly assigned to a control or experimental group. The experimental group would receive supplements while the control group would not take supplements. At the end of the treatment period (e.g., 10 years), the number of deaths between the two groups would be compared. If the supplements "worked," then significantly fewer deaths would occur in the supplemented group compared to the nonsupplemented counterparts.

A plausible explanation of the current observational study maintains that persons who regularly use vitamin supplements usually live healthier overall lifestyles than nonsupplement users—they smoke less, pay more attention to their weight, remain more physically active, and generally eat a more healthful diet. The plausible reality is that multivitamin supplement use may actually be a surrogate measure of a healthy lifestyle, which in itself provides considerable heart disease protection. The bottom line is that well-controlled experiments find little or no long-lasting benefit from taking a daily multivitamin/mineral supplement on longevity; breast, ovarian, colorectal, or other cancers; coronary heart disease or stroke; viral infections; or performance on memory and cognitive tests. The best advice is to maintain a healthy lifestyle and obtain daily nutrients in a well-balanced dietary regimen and not from store-bought supplements.

Source: Rautiainen S, et al. Multivitamin use and the risk of myocardial infarction: a population-based cohort of Swedish women. *Am J Clin Nutr* 2011;93:674.

Related References

Chlebowski RT, et al. Calcium plus vitamin D supplementation and the risk of breast cancer. *J Natl Cancer Inst* 2008;100:1581.

deVogel S, et al. Dietary folate, methionine, riboflavin, and vitamin B-6 and risk of sporadic colorectal cancer. *J Nutr* 2008;138:2372.

Park SY, et al. Multivitamin use and the risk of mortality and cancer: the multiethnic cohort study. *Am J Epidemiol* 2011;173:906.

Sesso HD, et al. Vitamins E and C in the prevention of cardiovascular disease in men. The Physicians' Health Study II Randomized Controlled Trial. *JAMA* 2008;300:2123.

LET NATURE DO IT

The normal process for protein digestion and absorption that provides amino acids in readily available form argues against the widespread practice advocated in body building and strength training magazines of ingesting a "predigested," hydrolyzed simple amino acid supplement to facilitate amino acid availability. The advertising hype does not justify the purchase of these products.

form. This coenzyme breakdown occurs first in the stomach and then along sections of small intestine where absorption proceeds. Effective vitamin nutrition for healthy men and women depends mainly on *consuming* various vitamin-laden nutrients, not on limitations in their *absorption.*

Mineral Absorption

Both extrinsic (dietary) and intrinsic (cellular) factors control the eventual fate of ingested minerals. Overall, the body does not absorb minerals well. Intestinal absorption

ABSORPTION SITES FOR WATER-SOLUBLE VITAMINS

- **Vitamin C**: Approximately 90% of absorption takes place in the distal portion of the small intestine. Excess vitamin C intake above about 1500 mg daily decreases kidney reabsorption efficiency, with large amounts voided in the urine.
- **Thiamine**: Absorption occurs mainly in the jejunum of the small intestine. Alcoholics, persons on extremely low-calorie diets, and the confined elderly often show symptoms of thiamine deficiency (beriberi, depression, mental confusion, loss of muscle coordination). Symptoms often become evident within 10 days because of the body's small thiamine reserve.
- **Riboflavin:** Absorption occurs mainly in the proximal portion of the small intestine.
- **Niacin:** Some absorption takes place in the stomach, but most occurs in the small intestine.
- **Pantothenic acid:** This vitamin exists as part of coenzyme A. Absorption occurs readily throughout the small intestine when the vitamin releases from its coenzyme.
- **Biotin:** Absorption occurs mainly in the upper one third to one half of the small intestine.
- **Folate:** Absorption occurs in the small intestine with the help of a specialized intestinal enzyme system (conjugase).
- **Vitamin B_6 (pyridoxine):** Absorption occurs mainly in the intestinal jejunum.
- **Vitamin B_{12}:** A salivary enzyme initially acts on this vitamin in the stomach. The vitamin then combines with intrinsic factor, a glycoprotein secreted by the gastric glands, before it enters the small intestine. The pancreatic enzyme trypsin then liberates vitamin B_{12} from the intrinsic factor. The small intestine absorbs up to 70% in the ileum.

increases to preserve the small micronutrient quantities when dietary intake of a particular mineral falls below the required level. The converse holds when mineral supplies exceed their limit, allowing little need for further increased absorption. For most persons, minerals exist in more than adequate amounts if they consume a well-balanced diet consisting of various foods from the main food groups. This means the body has little need to stockpile minerals. A possible exception exists for iron and calcium, two minerals that tend to be insufficient in the typical diet of American females (see Chapter 2).

The body's mineral availability depends on its chemical form. For example, heme iron has an absorptive capacity of about 15% compared with nonheme iron absorption, which ranges between 2 and 10%. Variation in mineral absorption also exists between the sexes. Men absorb calcium better than women, yet total calcium absorption rarely exceeds 35% of the amount ingested, with the remaining two thirds excreted in the feces. Of the calcium absorbed, one half is voided in the urine. For phosphorus, about two thirds is excreted daily in the urine. Poor absorption also occurs for magnesium (20–30%) and the trace minerals zinc (14–40%) and chromium (less than 2%). Future research needs to determine the absorption rates for the other minerals. **FIGURE 3.12** presents a generalized schema for major and trace mineral absorption, including the common pathways for their excretion.

Calcium, phosphorus, magnesium, and trace mineral absorption occurs mainly in the small intestine. Six factors affect mineral absorption:

1. Bioavailability
2. Transit time from the source in the diet to the absorption site
3. Quantity of digestive juices
4. pH of intestinal lumen contents
5. Receptor sites in the intestine's mucosal lining and brush border
6. Availability of substances that combine with the minerals during movement from the gut (via diffusion, facilitated diffusion, and/or active transport) and across cell membranes

Metallic minerals combine with a specific protein transporter (e.g., iron binds with transferrin) or a general protein carrier such as albumin (which binds with many minerals). Peptide and amino acid complexes also carry a small amount of each mineral in the blood. Excessive dietary fiber negatively affects absorption of certain minerals, so consuming the recommended 30 to 40 g of fiber daily generally eliminates this concern.

Water Absorption

The passive process of osmosis in the small intestine determines the major absorption of ingested water and water contained in foods. **FIGURE 3.13** shows that in addition to the 2 L of water ingested daily by the typical sedentary adult, saliva, gastric secretions, bile, and pancreatic and intestinal secretions contribute an additional 7 L. This means that the intestinal tract absorbs about 9 L of water each day. Seventy-two percent of this water becomes absorbed in the proximal small intestine and 20% from its distal segment—the large intestine absorbs the remaining 8%.

The continuous secretion and absorption of water within the GI tract makes it difficult to quantify the body's net water uptake. The intestinal mucosa absorbs electrolytes and components of macronutrient hydrolysis. This makes the intestinal medium progressively more hypotonic than the opposite side of the lumen membrane. Such a difference creates an osmotic gradient that forces water to move from the intestine to maintain isotonicity between the two fluid "compartments." In contrast, ingesting fluid hypertonic to plasma greater than 280 $mOsm \cdot L^{-1}$ causes water secretion into the intestinal lumen. This retards net water absorption and increases the potential for GI distress. This can occur when consuming salt tablets, concentrated mixtures of simple amino acids, or

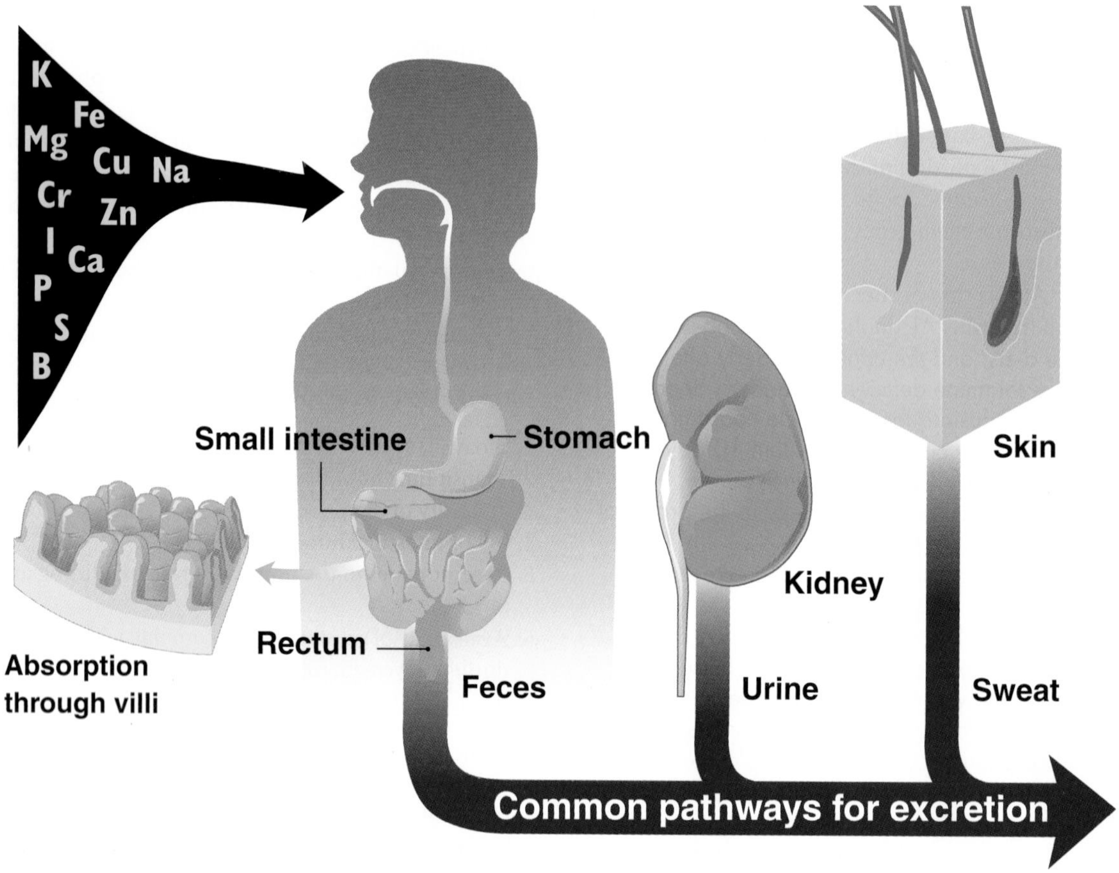

FIGURE 3.12. Absorption of minerals and their common excretion pathways.

a "sports drink" with a high percentage of simple sugars and minerals (see Chapter 10).

EXERCISE EFFECTS ON GASTROINTESTINAL FUNCTIONS

Exercise alters blood flow dynamics to body organs. It therefore follows that different modes, intensities, and durations of exercise *acutely* affect GI functions. Also, intense exercise training alters *chronic* GI function.[2–4,7,8,10,11,13–16]

After a meal, food passes from the stomach to the small intestine for complete digestion and subsequent absorption into the blood. While in the stomach, the food mixes in solution with different gastric secretions, digestive enzymes, and hydrochloric acid, and then empties into the small intestine. Five important factors affect gastric emptying rate (GER):

1. Solution volume: Larger food volume solutions increase GER.
2. Caloric content: Larger calorie food solutions decrease GER.
3. Meal osmolality: Higher food-solution osmolality decreases GER.
4. Temperature: Cooler compared to warmer food solutions increase GER.
5. pH: Higher acidic food solutions decrease GER.

Emotional state, caffeine, environmental conditions, menstrual cycle stage, and fitness status also exert an effect on GER.

Exercise Intensity

Gastric emptying of carbohydrate drinks or water moderately increases during light and moderate exercise at 20 to 60% $\dot{V}O_{2max}$ compared to rest, and decreases at exercise intensities equal to or above 75% $\dot{V}O_{2max}$. GER increases observed during moderate-intensity treadmill exercise may relate to associated increases in intragastric pressure induced by contractile activity of the abdominal muscles in exercise. Also, segmental colonic transit in the descending colon accelerates during light and moderate exercise compared to rest.[6,9,12]

Wide variability in individual GER exists, particularly at less than maximum exercise intensities. This variation relates to exercise type, training status, timing of fluid and meal ingestion, and even measurement issues. An overlooked factor relates to a person's variability in GER. In unpublished data from one of our laboratories, test-retest reliability of only $r = 0.51$ occurred between gastric emptying for water at different exercise intensities. This level of inconsistency in response within a person may explain a large part of the inherent variability among different exercise intensities and GER.

Exercise Mode

Not all exercise affects GI functions similarly. For example, 20 min of light- to moderate-intensity running results in a faster fluid GER (water and water plus carbohydrate) than cycling.

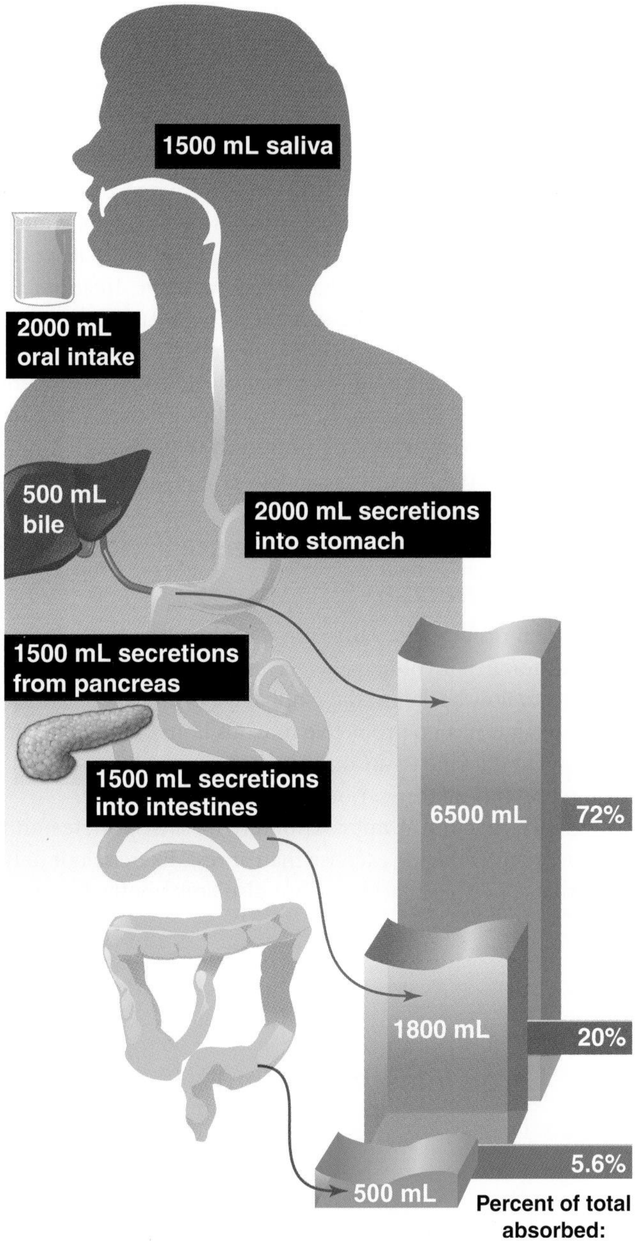

FIGURE 3.13. Estimated daily volumes of water that enter the small and large intestines of a sedentary adult and the volumes absorbed by each component of the intestinal tract. (From Gisolfi CV, Lamb DR, eds. *Perspectives in Exercise and Sports Medicine: Fluid Homeostasis During Exercise.* Indianapolis: Benchmark Press, 1990.)

Exercise Duration

Limited data exist on the effect of exercise duration on GER. One of the more interesting studies showed no difference in gastric emptying at various intervals throughout 2 h of cycling exercise at an intensity less than 80% $\dot{V}O_{2max}$.[14]

Exercise and Nutrient Absorption

Researchers generally agree that GI blood flow decreases as exercise intensity increases; thus, it should follow that intestinal absorption should correspondingly decrease. An early study showed that exercise at 75% $\dot{V}O_{2max}$ did not impair intestinal fluid absorption. In more recent research of intense exercise training, small bowel transit time increased without changes in GER, and stool frequency increased while stool composition tended to remain looser during the training period compared with no physical activity. Additional research indicates high incidences of GI distress including diarrhea and abdominal cramps, which suggests interruptions in oxygen supply (and blood flow) including increased parasympathetic nervous system activity during exercise.[15] Both diarrhea and abdominal cramping indicate abnormal intestinal absorption of water from the food residues. Three factors help to explain exercise-related alterations in nutrient and fluid absorption:

1. Exercise mode
2. Environmental temperature
3. Type of food/liquid ingested

HEALTH STATUS, EMOTIONAL STATE, AND GASTROINTESTINAL TRACT DISORDERS

Many factors influence GI function. The brain exerts a strong influence through diverse neurochemical connections with different digestive organs. Emotional state affects to some degree nearly the entire GI tract. For example, many persons experience intestinal cramping or a queasy stomach before an important event including athletic competition. Top athletes in almost every sport, whether an individual event such as a golf tournament or gymnastics routine or team sports like baseball, football, basketball, or soccer, experience such discomfort just prior to the event. This effect magnifies in front of small or large crowds, especially with family members or significant others present. Some persons complain of an "upset stomach" at the sight of their own blood (or blood of others), and that chronic emotional stress produces gastric mucosal abnormalities. In contrast, other GI tract disorders originally linked to emotional distress such as peptic ulcer disease are probably caused by infection and other physical ailments (see p. 123). Fortunately a healthful diet, regular exercise, and maintaining a healthy body weight resolve most GI tract problems.

A physically active lifestyle promotes two positive health benefits for the GI tract:

1. Enhances gut emptying
2. Reduce incidence of liver disease, gallstones, colon disorders, and constipation

Conversely, persons who frequently engage in intense exercise report GI symptoms such as self-limited food poisoning, gastroesophageal reflux disease (GERD), hiatal hernia, irritable bowel syndrome (IBS), and viral gastroenteritis. These symptoms, reported by between 20 and 50% of high-performance athletes, occur (1) more frequently in women than men,

(2) more commonly in younger athletes, and (3) less frequently among athletes in sports that incorporate gliding movements such as cycling.

Sedentary persons experience the following five more serious GI conditions:

1. Crohn disease (ongoing inflammation of the ileum)
2. Ulcerative colitis (inflammatory bowel disease that affects the large intestine and rectum)
3. Appendicitis (inflammation of the appendix, a small pouch attached to the beginning of the large intestine)
4. Mesenteric adenitis (self-limited inflammatory process that affects the mesenteric lymph nodes in the large intestine's right lower quadrant)
5. Invasive diarrhea (frequent passing of small amounts of "mucous" stool caused by bacterial enteropathogens and accompanied mainly by fever, irritability, loss of appetite, cramps, and abdominal pain)

Constipation

Constipation reflects a delay in stool movement through the colon because the large intestine absorbs excessive water, producing hard, dry stools. Diets high in fat and low in water and fiber represent the most common cause. Some fibers such as pectin in fruits and gums in beans dissolve easily in water and take on a soft, gel-like texture in the colon. Other fibers such as the cellulose in wheat bran pass essentially unchanged as they move through the colon to increase stool size. The combined softer texture and bulking action of water-soluble and water-insoluble fibers help to prevent the hardening of undigested stool material.

Diarrhea (Lower Intestinal Motility Disorder)

Loose, watery stools more than three times a day occur because digestive products move through the large intestine too rapidly for sufficient water reabsorption. The condition termed **diarrhea** often represents a symptom of increased peristalsis, intestinal irritation or damage, medication side effects, intolerance to gluten (a protein in some wheat products), and perhaps stress.

From an exercise perspective, distance runners and female athletes are most susceptible to diarrhea and IBS (see p. 123). Possible causative factors include fluid and electrolyte imbalance and altered colonic motility. Fortunately, acute exercise-induced diarrhea (also known as "runner's trots") is considered physiologic diarrhea that does not produce dehydration or electrolyte imbalance and tends to improve as fitness level improves. In healthy athletes, acute diarrhea is typically of limited duration and is induced by running, food poisoning, traveler's diarrhea, or viral gastroenteritis.

Prolonged diarrhea can produce dehydration, particularly in children and those of small body size. In general, recovery improves with a diet of broth, tea, toast, and other low-fiber and potassium-rich foods, including the avoidance of lactose, fructose, caffeine, and sugar alcohols.

Diverticulosis

Common among older persons, the colon develops small pouches that bulge outward through tissue weak spots, a condition known as **diverticulosis** (FIG. 3.14). This condition afflicts about one half of all Americans age 60 to 80 years and almost everyone older than 80 years of age. In about 10 to 25% of people with this disorder, the pouches become infected or inflamed (diverticulitis). Diverticulosis and diverticulitis are more common in industrialized countries where persons typically consume low-fiber diets; it rarely occurs in Asia and Africa where people routinely eat high-fiber, plant-based diets.

Heartburn and Gastroesophageal Reflux Disease

Heartburn occurs when the sphincter between the esophagus and stomach involuntarily relaxes, allowing the stomach's contents to flow back into the esophagus. Unlike the stomach, the esophagus has no protective mucous lining, allowing acid backflow to damage tissue and produce pain. Chronic heartburn represents a more serious disorder called **GERD.**

GERD occurs in approximately 60% of athletes and more frequently during exercise than at rest. Exercise not only exacerbates GERD in athletes, but also contributes to reflux

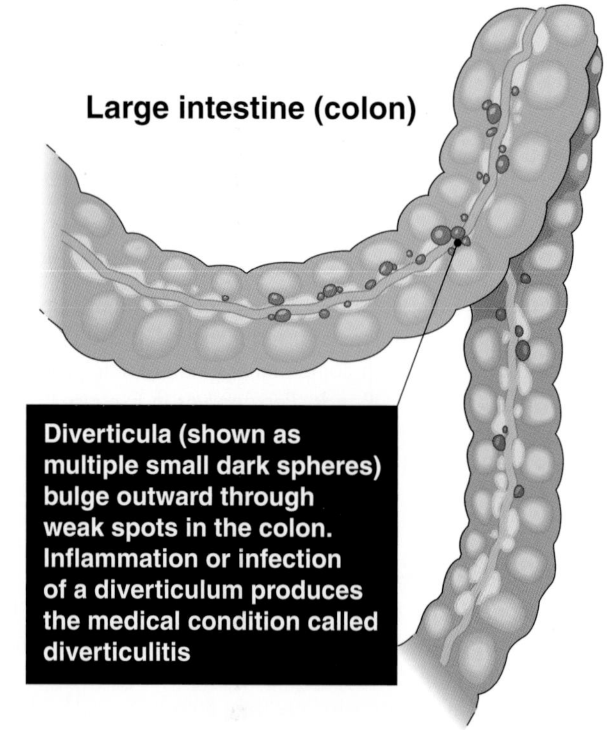

Large intestine (colon)
Diverticula (shown as multiple small dark spheres) bulge outward through weak spots in the colon. Inflammation or infection of a diverticulum produces the medical condition called diverticulitis

FIGURE 3.14. Diverticulosis is common among older people, particularly those who consume a diet with inadequate fiber.

in healthy volunteers. The precise causative mechanisms of exercise-induced reflux are not well defined. Suggested mechanisms, either singularly or in combination, include the following six factors:

1. Gastric dysmotility from the relaxation of the lower esophageal sphincter
2. Enhanced pressure gradient between the stomach and esophagus
3. Gastric distension
4. Delayed gastric emptying, especially in a dehydrated state
5. Enhanced intra-abdominal pressure in sports like football, weightlifting, and cycling
6. Increased mechanical stress by the bouncing of organs related to GI function

Athletes involved in predominantly anaerobic sports such as weightlifting experience the most frequent heartburn and gastric reflux; in contrast, runners have mild symptoms and moderate reflux, whereas cyclists have mild symptoms and mild reflux.

Six exercise-related GERD symptoms include the following:

1. Substernal chest pressure
2. Pain or burning that mimics angina
3. Sour taste
4. Eructation (the voiding through the mouth of gas or a small quantity of acid fluid from the stomach)
5. Nausea
6. Vomiting

A subset of athletes may present with atypical cough, hoarseness, and wheezing—symptoms that mimic either exercise-induced bronchospasm or vocal cord dysfunction.

Effective lifestyle modifications remain the treatment of choice for athletes with GERD. These include avoidance of the following three factors:

1. Attempting sleep within 4 h after the evening meal
2. Postprandial exercise
3. Excessive consumption of foods that relax the lower esophageal sphincter such as chocolate, peppermint, onions, high-fat foods, alcohol, tobacco, coffee, and citrus products

Sleeping on two pillows to enhance gravity-associated esophageal clearance often reduces GERD symptoms. Athletes treated with calcium channel blockers for migraine headaches or to control hypertension should be counseled on the propensity for these drugs to worsen GERD symptoms. GERD and obesity represent key risk factors for esophageal cancer.

Irritable Bowel Syndrome

IBS represents a functional GI tract disorder devoid of structural, biomechanical, radiologic, or laboratory abnormalities. The condition afflicts up to 20% of the adult population. The two IBS forms include "diarrhea-predominant" and "constipation-predominant" syndromes. IBS, twice as common in women than men, typically presents in the second or third decade of life. Approximately 50% of patients with IBS also report depression and anxiety.

Eight factors can cause IBS:

1. Increased GI motor reactivity to various stimuli such as stress
2. Foods high in fat, insoluble fiber, caffeine, coffee (including decaf), carbonation, or alcohol
3. Dysfunction of the CCK release system (a peptide hormone responsible for stimulating fat and protein digestion)
4. Impaired transit of bowel gas
5. Visceral hypersensitivity
6. Impaired reflex control that delays gas transit
7. Autonomic dysfunction
8. Altered immune activation.

The four most common symptoms of IBS include

1. Cramping abdominal pain relieved by defecation
2. Altered stool frequency

HELICOBACTER PYLORI BACTERIUM: HALF OF THE WORLD INFECTED

More than half of the world's population is infected with a type of bacterium, *Helicobacter pylori*, that causes ulcers in the stomach and esophagus, a long-term condition that associates with gastric cancer development. The end result of *H. pylori* infection promotes the rise in destructive superoxide radicals that attack cells of the stomach's protective mucosal lining. Within a few days of infection, gastritis and eventually peptic ulcer occur. The classic sign of a peptic ulcer is a gnawing, burning pain in the upper abdomen. Other symptoms include a dull, persistent ache that comes and goes over several days and pain that occurs 2 to 3 h following a meal (previously relieved by eating) and responds to antacid medications. Other symptoms can include weight loss, poor appetite, excessive burping, bloating, and vomiting. It may not be *H. pylori* itself that causes peptic ulcer, but inflammation of the mucosal lining in peptic ulcer that represents a response to *H. pylori*. Researchers believe that *H. pylori* is transmitted orally by means of fecal matter contained in tainted food or water. Possible transmission could also occur from the stomach to the mouth through gastroesophageal reflux (a small amount of the stomach's contents is involuntarily forced into the esophagus) or belching—common symptoms of gastritis. The bacterium can then be transmitted through oral contact.

3. Altered stool form (mucous, watery, hard, or loose) and passage (strain, urgency, or a sense of incomplete evacuation)
4. Abdominal distension especially following meals

Athletes with IBS rarely experience nocturnal symptoms and do not manifest systemic signs of illness. The IBS diagnosis includes diarrhea secondary to celiac sprue (a genetic, inherited autoimmune disease of the small bowel that afflicts nearly 5000 Americans) or lactose intolerance, thyroid dysfunction, laxative abuse, diabetes, and psychiatric illness.

Four lifestyle and dietary modifications effectively counter IBS:

1. Stress reduction
2. Consumption of daily small meals
3. Consumption of a high-fiber diet
4. Avoidance of foods that contain lactose and candy that contains sorbitol (six-carbon sugar alcohol formed by reducing the carbonyl group of naturally occurring glucose in fruits)

Participating in regular physical activity also plays a positive role in treating IBS. Antidiarrheal and antispasmodic drugs effectively treat diarrhea-predominant IBS. For constipation-predominant IBS, dietary fiber, bulk laxatives, and stool softeners are often used, but their efficacy varies and sometimes can worsen symptoms.

Gastrointestinal Gas

Swallowing air while eating or drinking commonly produces stomach **gas**. A person can take in an excess of air while eating or drinking rapidly, chewing gum, or smoking. Burping or belching is the most common means that swallowed air leaves the stomach. Any remainin g gas moves into the small intestine and becomes partially absorbed. A small amount of this air travels into the large intestine for release through the rectum. Rectal gas seldom signifies serious disease.

Flatus (lower tract intestinal gas) composition depends to a great extent on nutrient intake (carbohydrates produce the most gas, fats and proteins the least) and the colon's bacterial population. In the large intestine, bacteria partially break down undigested carbohydrate to produce hydrogen, carbon dioxide, and in about 30% of the population, methane gas. These gases eventually exit through the rectum. The amount and type of GI bacteria largely determine variation in the quantity of colonic gas production among persons.

Carbohydrates that commonly cause gas production include raffinose and stachyose (found in beans), fructose (found in soft drinks and fruit drinks), lactose, and the artificial sweetener sorbitol. Other gas-producing starches include potatoes, onions, carrots, celery, cucumbers, cruciferous vegetables (broccoli, cabbage, cauliflower), corn, noodles, and wheat products. Rice contains the only starch that does not cause abdominal or colonic gas. The fiber in oat bran, beans, peas, and most fruits causes gas. In contrast, fiber in wheat bran and in some vegetables passes essentially unchanged through the intestinal tract and produces little if any abdominal gas.

PROBIOTICS, PREBIOTICS, SYNBIOTICS

Probiotics are live microorganisms—microscopic organisms such as bacteria, viruses, and yeasts—when administered in adequate amounts, confer a health benefit on the host. **Prebiotics** are nondigestible food ingredients that selectively stimulate the growth and/or activity of beneficial existing microorganisms in the colon. When probiotics and prebiotics mix together, they form a **synbiotic**.

Probiotics are available in foods and as dietary supplements mainly in capsules, tablets, and powders. Yogurt, fermented and unfermented milk, miso (Japanese fermented soybean paste), tempeh (Indonesian soy product), and some juices and soy beverages are examples of probiotic-containing foods. In probiotic foods and supplements, the bacteria may have been present originally or added during commercial preparation.

Most probiotics are bacteria similar to those naturally found in the gut, especially in those of breastfed infants (who have natural protection against many diseases). Most often, the bacteria come from the *Lactobacillus* or *Bifidobacterium* groups. Different species exist within each group (e.g., *Lactobacillus acidophilus* and *Bifidobacterium bifidus*). Also, different strains or varieties exist within each species. The common probiotics *Saccharomyces boulardii* are yeasts, which differ from bacteria.

Researchers are now exploring whether probiotics can treat infectious diarrhea, IBS, inflammatory bowel disease (e.g., ulcerative colitis and Crohn disease), infection with *H. pylori*, tooth decay and periodontal disease, vaginal infections, stomach and respiratory infections, skin infections, and immune dysfunction.

Encouraging evidence exists of the effectiveness of specific probiotic formulations to treat diarrhea (the strongest area of evidence, especially for diarrhea from rotavirus); to prevent and treat infections of the urinary tract or female genital tract; to treat IBS; to reduce recurrence of bladder cancer; to shorten the duration of intestinal infection; to prevent and treat pouchitis (a condition that can follow surgery to remove the colon); and to prevent and manage atopic dermatitis (eczema) in children.

In studies that use probiotics as cures, any beneficial effect is usually low with evidence of a strong placebo effect. Large, carefully designed clinical trials are needed to draw firmer conclusions.[1,5,17]

Functional Dyspepsia

Functional dyspepsia refers to chronic pain in the upper abdomen without obvious physical cause. It produces vague GI symptoms that include gnawing or burning in the stomach, epigastric pain, nausea, vomiting, belching, bloating, indigestion, and generalized abdominal discomfort. The three most common causes for dyspepsia include:

1. Peptic ulcer disease
2. GERD
3. Gastritis (inflammation of the lining of the stomach that leads to pain)

Other less common causes include diabetes, thyroid disease, lactose intolerance, frequent dehydration, repeated stress of sports competition, excessive use of nonsteroidal anti-inflammatory drugs (NSAIDs), and alcohol and caffeine products. Dietary supplements with amino acids and creatine may further exacerbate mucosal injury and eventually lead to blood loss and anemia.

Lifestyle modifications to treat GERD represent the treatment of choice for dyspepsia. Also, avoidance of NSAIDs, caffeine, tobacco, gas-producing foods, and dairy products in persons with lactose intolerance generally helps to alleviate most symptoms.

ACUTE GASTROENTERITIS: BACTERIAL AND VIRAL INDUCED

Only a few GI illnesses associate with travel, yet athletes show particular susceptibility to travel-induced **acute gastroenteritis** from bacterial and viral causes. Acute gastroenteritis typically presents with fever, nausea, vomiting, diarrhea, and cramping. Outbreaks have occurred in athletic populations during competitions where athletes from different countries congregate and share food, bathroom facilities, and sleeping quarters. Athletes with acute gastroenteritis, particularly those involved in contact sports, should not participate in practices and competition unless they receive adequate treatment, present without fever, and are hemodynamically stable. To prevent contamination and spread of the illness, the fundamental importance of good hygiene (especially frequent washing of hands with hot water and soap) must be practiced.

PERSONAL HEALTH AND EXERCISE NUTRITION 3.1

Fundamentals of Nutritional Assement: Applying Analysis Skills

Nutritional assessment evaluates a person's nutritional status and nutrient requirements on the basis of interpretation of clinical information from different sources. Examples include diet history, medical history, review of symptoms, and physical examination that includes anthropometric and laboratory data. The nutritional assessment should include defining current nutritional status, determining levels of nutritional support, and monitoring changes in nutrient intake from a particular intervention program.

Nutritional deficiency usually develops over time, starting at a young age and progressing in stages. An overt deficiency often remains unrecognized until the condition passes the person's "clinical horizon" and moves into a disease state or becomes manifested by acute trauma (e.g., heart attack or type 2 diabetes complications). Nutritional assessment during any developmental stage of deficiency provides the basis for identifying a problem area and planning a prudent intervention.

Assessing Dietary Intake

Four common methods provide dietary information.

Method 1: 24-H Dietary Recall

This approach, usually a qualitative assessment by the individual or another person, involves informal oral questioning about food and beverage intake during the previous 24 h. The person recalls all foods and beverages consumed starting from the last meal and includes the approximate portion size and specifics of food preparation. This method is relatively easy, particularly when administered by a registered dietitian. Particular problems involve inaccuracy in quantity assessment and method of food preparation. This frequently produces gross underestimation of hidden fats (and hence calories) in such foods as sauces and dressings. Repeat 24-h recalls that span several days provide a more accurate and reliable estimate of a typical day.

Method 2: Food Diary

With the food diary method, the person records all foods and beverages at the time consumed or as close to the time as possible. This approach enables the recording of food by brand, weight, and portion size. Typically, the person maintains a food diary for 2 to 7 days. Assessment includes at least 1 weekend day because most people eat differently on the weekend than during a typical school day or work day. The method can, however, become tedious; when confronted with having to record everything eaten, persons often change what they eat or eat nothing to avoid the hassle.

Method 3: Food Frequency Assessment

A food frequency questionnaire lists various foods, and the person estimates the frequency of consuming each item. This method does not itemize a specific day's intake;

instead, it provides a general picture of the typical food consumption pattern.

Method 4: Diet History

A diet history yields general information about a person's dietary patterns. Factors include eating habits (number of meals per day, who prepares meals, and patterns of food preparation), food preferences, eating locations, and typical food choices in different situations.

Analyzing Dietary Intake

A combination of methods proves more valid than a single method in developing a comprehensive dietary assessment. For a general picture of the adequacy of a person's dietary intake, compare the food record with an established guide for diet planning such as MyPlate and the *Dietary Guidelines for Americans* discussed in Chapter 7. Evaluate the energy and macronutrient and micronutrient content of the diet through food labels and food composition tables. The most comprehensive food database is the US Department of Agriculture Nutrient Database for Standard Reference Release 13 available at **www.nal.usda.gov/fnic/foodcomp/Data/SR13/sr13.html**. With most computer programs for diet analysis, one enters each food and the exact size of the portion consumed. Based on the input data, the program calculates the nutrients consumed for each day or provides an average over several days. In essence, a dietary analysis program compares nutrient intake to "average" recommended values based on large-scale nutrition surveys for a particular population.

Medical History

Personal Medical History

A medical history includes immunizations, hospitalizations, surgeries, and acute and chronic injuries and illness—each of these has nutritional implications. History of prescriptions and the use of vitamin and mineral supplements, laxatives, topical medications, and herbal remedies (herbs and other supplements not typically identified as medications) also provides valuable information.

Family Medical and Social History

Medical histories that include information about the health/nutrition/exercise status of parents, siblings, children, and spouse can reveal risk for chronic diseases related to a genetic or social connection. Sociocultural relationships regarding food choices help to understand individual eating patterns and practices. Information about duration and frequency of use of alcohol, tobacco, illicit drugs, and caffeine helps to formulate a more effective treatment plan and assess risk for chronic diseases.

Physical Examination

Nutrition-oriented aspects of the physical examination focus on the mouth, skin, head, hair, eyes, fingernails, extremities, abdomen, skeletal musculature, and fat stores. Dry skin, cracked lips, or lethargy may indicate nutritional deficiencies. The accompanying table lists specific signs of vitamin or mineral deficiencies. Malnutrition often results from low calorie intake and protein deficiency. This produces a condition known as *marasmus*, which is characterized by severe tissue wasting, loss of subcutaneous fat, and usually dehydration. Marasmus typically occurs in patients with anorexia nervosa (see Chapter 15).

Anthropometric Data

Use of anthropometric data permits nutritional classification of individuals by categories ranging from undernourished to obese. Interpreting nutritional status involves comparing a person with reference data from large numbers of healthy people of similar age and gender.

A typical nutritional assessment collects the following anthropometric data:

1. Height
2. Body weight
3. Body mass index (BMI; body weight, kg ÷ height^2, m)
4. Waist girth above 102 cm (40 in) in men and 88 cm (35 in) in women indicates increased disease risk
5. Percentage weight change over several months or longer should be computed as follows: percentage weight change = (usual weight − current weight ÷ usual weight) × 100
6. Triceps skinfold (triceps skinfold above the 95th percentile for age and gender indicates excess energy stored as subcutaneous fat)

Laboratory Data

Measures of nutrients or their by-products in body cells or blood or urine often detect nutrient deficiencies or excesses. Typical laboratory measures include serum albumin to indicate total body protein status and liver and renal disease; serum transferrin to assess protein balance and iron status; serum prealbumin to show protein status and liver disease; and concentrations of sodium, potassium, chloride, phosphorus, and magnesium to reflect overall mineral status. Other valuable laboratory tests that diagnose selected clinical conditions related to nutrition include iron and hemoglobin, glucose, zinc, cholesterol, and the different lipid subfractions high-density lipoprotein, low-density lipoprotein, and very low-density lipoprotein.

Clinical Signs and Symptoms of Nutritional Inadequacy

Organ	Sign/Symptom	Probable Cause
Skin	Pallor	Iron folate, vitamin B_{12} deficiency
	Ecchymosis (purplish patch)	Vitamin K deficiency
	Pressure ulcers/delayed healing	Protein malnutrition
	Hair hyperkeratosis (excess eruption)	Vitamin A deficiency
	Petechiae (minute hemorrhagic spots)	Vitamin A, C, or K deficiency
	Purpura (hemorrhage into skin)	Vitamin C or K deficiency
	Rash/eczema/scaling	Zinc deficiency
Hair	Dyspigmentation, easy pluckability	Protein malnutrition
Head	Temporal muscle wasting	Protein-energy malnutrition
Eyes	Night blindness, xerosis	Vitamin A deficiency (pathologic dryness)
Mouth	Bleeding gum	Vitamin C, riboflavin deficiency
	Tongue fissuring (splitting), raw tongue, tongue atrophy (wasting)	Niacin, riboflavin deficiency
Heart	Tachycardia	Thiamin deficiency
Genital/urinary	Delayed puberty	Protein-energy malnutrition
Extremities	Bone softening	Vitamin D, calcium, phosphorous deficiency
	Bone/joint aches	Vitamin C deficiency
	Edema	Protein deficiency
	Muscle wasting	Protein-energy malnutrition
	Ataxia	Vitamin B_{12} deficiency
Neurologic deficiency	Tetany (muscle twitches, cramps)	Calcium, magnesium
	Paresthesia (abnormal sensation)	Thiamin deficiency
	Loss of reflexes, wrist/foot drop	Thiamin, vitamin B_{12} deficiency
	Dementia	Niacin deficiency

Applying Critical Analysis Skills

1. Keep a food diary of everything consumed for 3 days including 1 weekend day. Prepare a form that contains the following headings:

Food or Beverage	Kind/How Prepared	Amount
____________	______________	__________
____________	______________	__________

2. Record food as eaten without relying on memory at a later time. Accuracy increases by adhering to the following guidelines:
   a. Be specific when recording food intake; record size, type (chicken leg vs thigh), and amount (oz, tsp).
   b. Record the method of preparation (i.e., baked vs fried; peeled vs not peeled; skinless vs with skin).
   c. Include items like butter, ketchup, and salad dressing.
   d. Include all deserts and toppings.
   e. If you eat out, indicate where.
   f. If you eat mixed dishes, break them down into component ingredients. For example, a chicken sandwich might be listed as 2 slices of white bread, 1 tbsp of mayonnaise, and 3 oz of skinless chicken breast.
3. Answer the following questions:
   a. Compare and contrast your nutrient intake with Dietary Reference Intakes for your age and sex on pages 55-59 and 68-70.

b. Suppose you consumed two plain doughnuts extra each day (about 200 kcal each) above your current energy balance. How much extra weight would you gain in 6 months? How much in 12 months? 36 months? What specific additional energy expenditure with specific exercise examples would you need to offset this weight gain for each time period?

c. List and discuss specific changes you need to make in your energy and nutrient intake to improve your personal health profile.

Evans-Stoner N. Nutritional assessment: a practical approach. *Nurs Clin North Am* 1997;32:637.

Johansson L, et al. Under- and over-reporting of energy intake related to weight status and lifestyle in a nationwide sample. *Am J Clin Nutr* 1998;68:266.

Mascarenas MR, et al. Nutritional assessment in pediatrics. *Nutrition* 1998;14:105.

SUMMARY

1. Digestion hydrolyzes complex molecules into simpler substances for absorption. Self-regulating processes within the digestive tract largely control the liquidity, mixing, and transit time of the digestive mixture.
2. Physically altering food in the mouth makes it easier to swallow, while at the same time increasing its accessibility to enzymes and other digestive substances. Swallowing transfers the food mixture to the esophagus, where peristaltic action forces it into the stomach.
3. In the stomach, hydrochloric acid and enzymes continue the breakdown process of the food mixture. Little absorption occurs in the stomach except for some water and alcohol and aspirin.
4. The enzyme salivary α-amylase degrades starch to smaller linked glucose molecules and simpler disaccharides in the mouth. In the duodenum of the small intestine, pancreatic amylase continues carbohydrate hydrolysis into smaller chains of glucose molecules and simple monosaccharides.
5. Enzyme action on the surfaces of the intestinal lumen's brush border completes the final stage of carbohydrate digestion to simple monosaccharides.
6. Lipid digestion begins in the mouth by lingual lipase and in the stomach by gastric lipase. The major lipid breakdown occurs in the small intestine by the emulsifying action of bile and the hydrolytic action of pancreatic lipase.
7. Medium-chain triacylglycerol rapidly absorbs into the portal vein bound to glycerol and medium-chain free fatty acids.
8. Once absorbed by the intestinal mucosa, long-chain fatty acids reform into triacylglycerols. They then form small fatty droplets called chylomicrons. These substances move slowly through the lymphatic system to eventually empty into the venous blood of the systemic circulation.
9. The enzyme pepsin initiates protein digestion in the stomach. The final steps in protein digestion occur in the small intestine, most notably under the action of the enzyme trypsin.
10. Vitamin absorption occurs mainly by the passive process of diffusion in the jejunum and ileum portions of the small intestine.
11. The large intestine serves as the final path for water and electrolyte absorption, including storage of undigested food residue (feces).
12. Gastric emptying of carbohydrate drinks or water moderately increases during light and moderate exercise (20–60% $\dot{V}O_{2max}$) compared to rest and decreases at exercise intensities equal to 75% $\dot{V}O_{2max}$ or higher.
13. Increases in gastric emptying during moderate-intensity treadmill exercise may relate to increases in intragastric pressure from contractile activity of the abdominal muscles.
14. Many factors influence GI function. The brain exerts a strong influence on the GI tract through diverse neurochemical connections with digestive organs.
15. Persons who engage in frequent, high-intensity exercise report GI symptoms that include self-limited food poisoning, GERD, hiatal hernia, IBS, and viral gastroenteritis.
16. The most common GI tract disorders include constipation, diarrhea, diverticulosis, GERD, IBS, and excessive gas production.

thePoint *Visit* thePoint.lww.com/MKKSEN4e *to view the following animations related to content presented in Chapter 3:* ***Condensation****;* ***Digestion of carbohydrate****;* ***Hormonal control****;* ***Hydrolysis****; and* ***Renal function****.*

TEST YOUR KNOWLEDGE ANSWERS

1. **False:** For many foods, digestion begins during cooking when protein structures degrade, starch granules swell, and vegetables fibers soften. For the most part, food breakdown begins in the mouth, where mechanical digestion increases the surface area of the food particles, making them easier to swallow and more accessible to enzymes and other digestive substances that start the breakdown process. For example, the enzyme salivary α-amylase (ptyalin) attacks starch and reduces it to smaller linked glucose molecules and the simpler disaccharide form maltose. Lipid digestion also begins in the mouth by the action of lingual lipase.

2. **True:** The colon represents the division of the large intestine that extends from the cecum to the rectum. It comprises the ascending colon (portion between the ileocecal orifice and the right colic flexure), descending colon (portion that extends from the left colic flexure to the pelvic brim), transverse colon (portion between the right and left colic flexures), and sigmoid colon (S-shaped final portion of colon that is continuous with the rectum).

3. **False:** The liver, pancreas, and gallbladder play key roles in the process of digesting and assimilating food nutrients, but they are not structures through which the nutrients pass directly during the digestive process.

4. **True:** The small intestine absorbs glucose and galactose into the blood against a concentration gradient; thus energy must be expended to power additional glucose absorption across the intestinal mucosa. Absorption occurs by a sodium-dependent, carrier-mediated active transport process. The electrochemical gradient created with sodium transport augments absorption of these monosaccharides. In contrast, the low concentration of fat in intestinal cells allows for passive absorption of these substances.

5. **False:** Active transport of nutrients across cell membranes requires the expenditure of cellular energy from ATP. This process occurs when a substance cannot be transported by one of the four passive transport processes.

6. **False:** With the exception of some water and alcohol and aspirin, no nutrient absorption takes place in any portion of the stomach.

7. **True:** Approximately 90% of digestion (and essentially all lipid digestion) and absorption occurs in the first two sections of the 3-m long small intestine. This coiled structure consists of three sections: the duodenum (first 0.3 m), jejunum (next 1–2 m, where most of digestion occurs), and ileum (last 1.5 m).

8. **False:** Starch hydrolysis begins when food enters the mouth. The salivary glands continually secrete lubricating mucous substances that combine with food particles during chewing. The enzyme salivary α-amylase (ptyalin) attacks starch and reduces it to smaller linked glucose molecules and the disaccharide maltose. When the food–saliva mixture enters the more acidic stomach, some additional starch breakdown occurs but quickly ceases because salivary amylase deactivates under the low pH of the stomach's gastric juices.

9. **False:** When amino acids reach the liver, one of three events occurs:

    1. Conversion to glucose (glucogenic amino acids)
    2. Conversion to fat (ketogenic amino acids)
    3. Direct release into the bloodstream as plasma proteins such as albumin or as free amino acids

    Free amino acids are synthesized into biologically important proteins, peptides (e.g., hormones), and the amino acid derivatives phosphocreatine and choline, the essential component of the neurotransmitter acetylcholine.

10. **False:** The following five important factors affect GER:

    1. Solution volume: Larger food volume solutions increase GER.
    2. Caloric content: Larger calorie food solutions decrease GER.
    3. Meal osmolality: Higher food solution osmolality decreases GER.
    4. Temperature: Cooler compared to warmer food solutions increase GER.
    5. pH: Higher acidic food solutions decrease GER.

    Other factors like emotional state, caffeine, environmental conditions, menstrual cycle stage, and fitness status also exert an effect on GER.

Key References

Aureli P, et al. Probiotics and health: An evidence-based review. *Pharmacol Res* 2011;63:366.

Bi L, Triadafilopoulos G. Exercise and gastrointestinal function and disease: an evidence-based review of risks and benefits. *Clin Gastroenterol Hepatol* 2003;1:345.

Casey E, et al. Training room management of medical conditions: sports gastroenterology. *Clin Sports Med* 2005;24:525.

Collings KL, et al. Esophageal reflux in conditioned runners, cyclists, and weightlifters. *Med Sci Sports Exerc* 2003;35:730.

Hill C. Probiotics and pharmabiotics: alternative medicine or an evidence-based alternative? *Bioeng Bugs* 2010;1:79.

Lancaster GI, et al. Effect of pre-exercise carbohydrate ingestion on plasma cytokine, stress hormone, and neutrophil degranulation responses to continuous, high-intensity exercise. *Int J Sport Nutr Exerc Metab* 2003;13:436.

Lustyk MK, et al. Does a physically active lifestyle improve symptoms in women with irritable bowel syndrome? *Gastroenterol Nurs* 2001;24:129.

Moses FM. The effect of exercise on the gastrointestinal tract. *Sports Med* 1990;9:159.

Neufer PD, et al. Gastric emptying during walking and running: effects of varied exercise intensity. *Eur J Appl Physiol Occup Physiol* 1989;58:440.

Packer N, et al. Does physical activity affect quality of life, disease symptoms and immune measure in patients with inflammatory bowel disease? A systematic review. *J Sports Med Phys Fitness* 2010;50:1.

Peters HP, et al. Potential benefits and hazards of physical activity and exercise on the gastrointestinal tract. *Gut* 2001;48:435.

Rao KA, et al. Objective evaluation of small bowel and colonic transit time using pH telemetry in athletes with gastrointestinal symptoms. *Br J Sports Med* 2004;38:482.

Sanchez LD, et al. Ischemic colitis in marathon runners: a case-based review. *J Emerg Med* 2006;30:321.

Strid H, et al. Effects of heavy exercise on gastrointestinal transit in endurance athletes. *Scan J Gastroenterol* 2011;46:673.

Van Nieuwenhoven MA, et al. Gastrointestinal profile of symptomatic athletes at rest and during physical exercise. *Eur J Appl Physiol* 2004;91:429.

Wade TJ, et al. Rapidly measured indicators of recreational water quality are predictive of swimming-associated gastrointestinal illness. *Environ Health Perspect* 2006;114:24.

West NP, et al. Probiotics, immunity and exercise: a review. *Exerc Immunol Rev* 2009;15:107.

thePoint *Visit* **thePoint.lww.com/MKKSEN4e** *for a list of the references cited in this chapter, including additional, relevant references.*

Nutrient Bioenergetics in Exercise and Training

PART 2

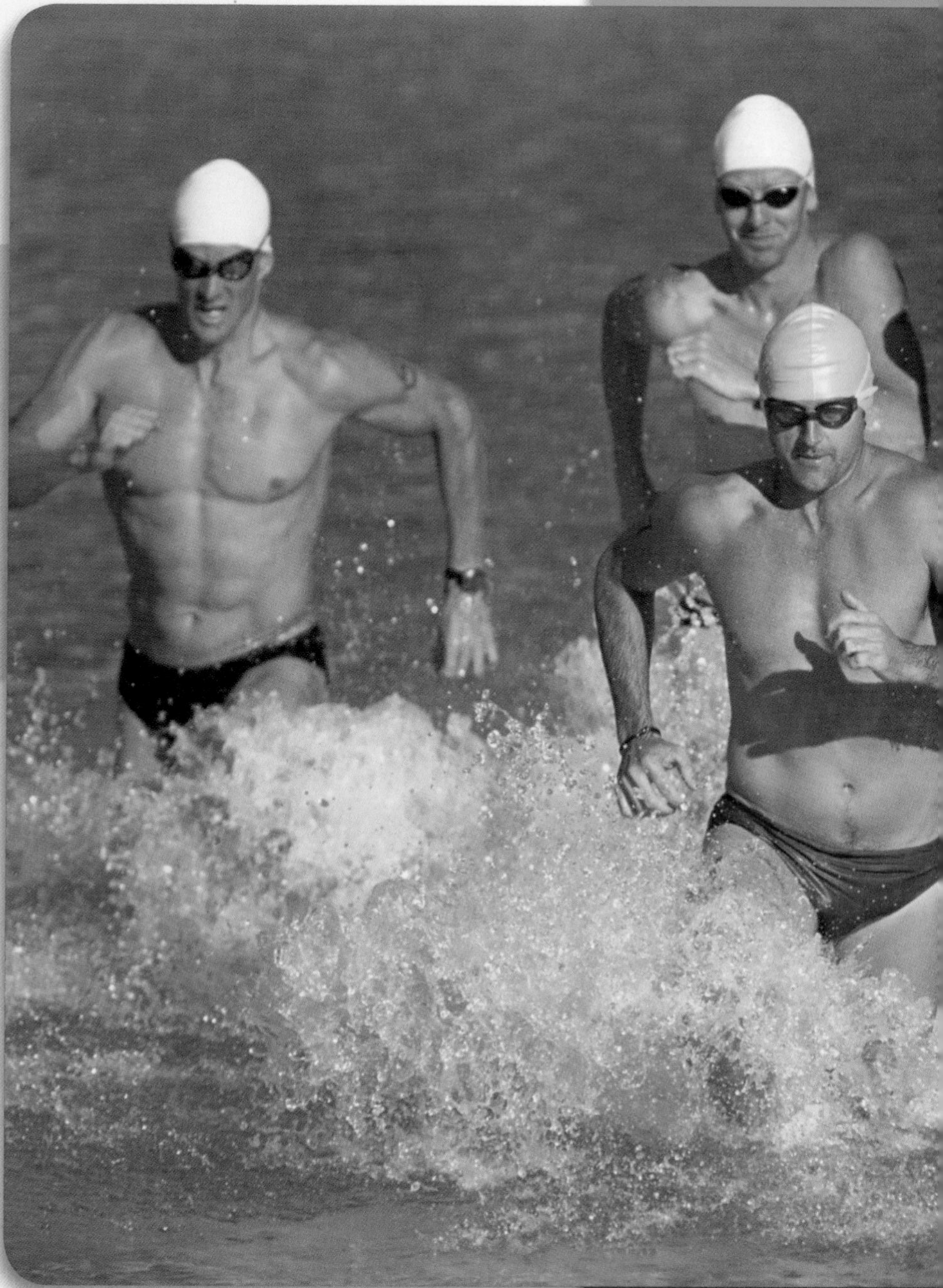

CONTENTS

CHAPTER 4

Nutrient Role in Bioenergetics

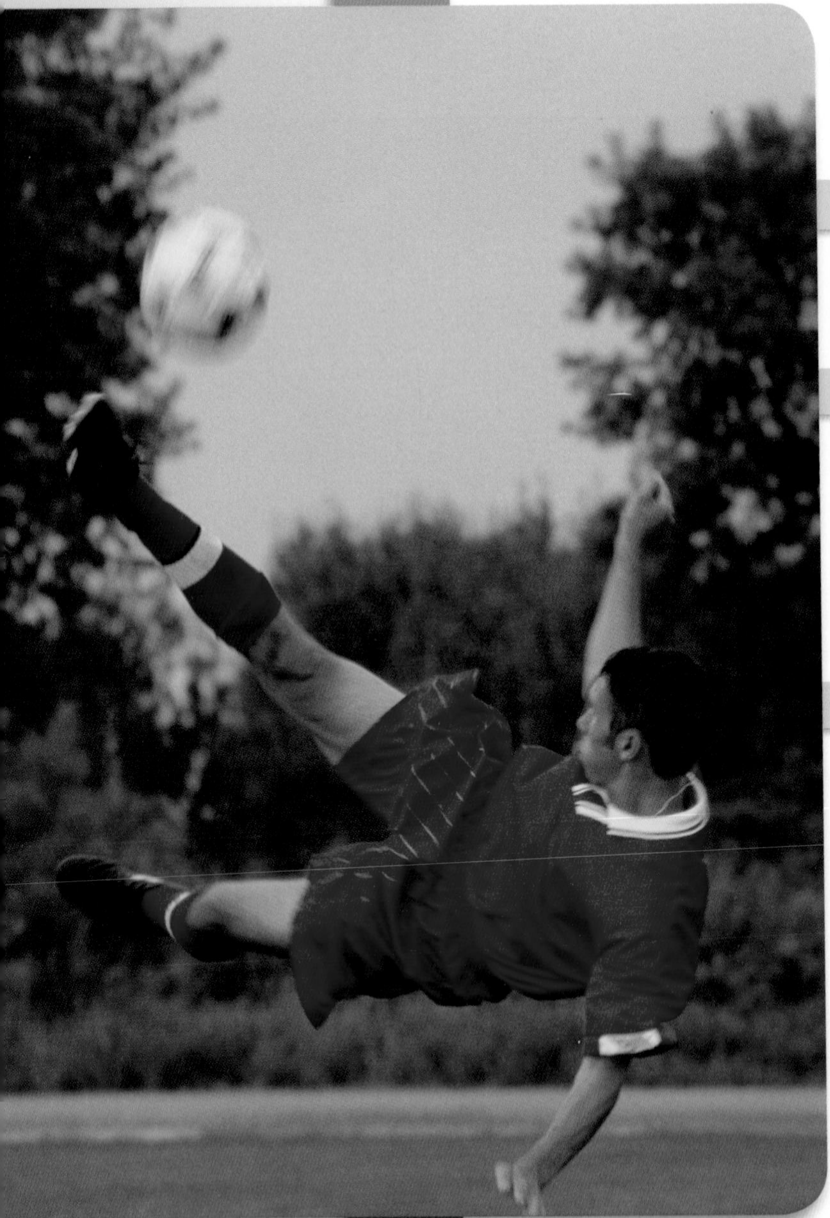

OUTLINE

- Nutrition–Energy Interaction

Introduction to Energy Transfer

- Energy: The Capacity for Work
- Oxidation and Reduction

Phosphate Bond Energy

- Adenosine Triphosphate: The Energy Currency
- Phosphocreatine: The Energy Reservoir
- Cellular Oxidation
- Role of Oxygen in Energy Metabolism

Energy Release from Macronutrients

- Energy Release from Carbohydrate
- Energy Release from Fat
- Fats Burn in a Carbohydrate Flame
- Lipogenesis
- Energy Release from Protein
- The Metabolic Mill
- Regulation of Energy Metabolism

TEST YOUR KNOWLEDGE

Select true or false for the 10 statements below, then check out the answers at the end of the chapter. Retake the test after you've read the chapter; you should achieve 100%!

	True	False
1. Carbohydrates are used for energy and stored as glycogen in the liver and muscles. They also readily convert to fat for storage in adipose tissue.	❍	❍
2. Lipids are used for energy and stored as fat. Fatty acids also readily convert to carbohydrate.	❍	❍
3. An enzyme is an inorganic, nonprotein compound that catalyzes the body's chemical reactions.	❍	❍
4. Excessive protein intake does not contribute to body fat accumulation because of the enzyme lack to facilitate this conversion.	❍	❍
5. ATP forms only from the breakdown of the glycerol and fatty acid components of the triacylglycerol molecule.	❍	❍
6. The first law of thermodynamics refers specifically to the process of photosynthesis.	❍	❍
7. Oxidation and reduction refer to the conversion of oxygen into useful energy.	❍	❍
8. Energy is defined as ability to perform work.	❍	❍
9. The main role for oxygen in the body is to combine with ADP in the synthesis of ATP.	❍	❍
10. The total net energy yield from the complete breakdown of a glucose molecule is 40 ATPs.	❍	❍

Understanding each macronutrient's role in energy metabolism becomes crucial to optimize the interaction between food intake and storage and exercise performance. No nutritional "magic bullets" exist per se, yet the quantity and blend of the daily diet's macronutrients profoundly affect exercise capacity, training response, and overall health.

A useful analogy shows how a car and the human body both obtain energy to make them "go." In an automobile engine, igniting an optimal mixture of gasoline fuel with oxygen provides the energy required to drive the pistons. Gears and linkages harness the energy to turn the wheels, and increasing or decreasing energy release either speeds up or slows down the engine. Similarly, the human body continuously extracts the energy from its fuel nutrients and harnesses it to perform its many complex biologic functions. The body expends considerable energy for muscle action during physical activity, including energy for four other "quieter" forms of biologic work:

1. Digestion, absorption, and assimilation of food nutrients
2. Glandular function that secretes hormones at rest and exercise
3. Maintenance of electrochemical gradients along cell membranes for proper neuromuscular function
4. Synthesis of new chemical compounds such as thick and thin protein structures in skeletal muscle tissue that enlarge with resistance training

NUTRITION–ENERGY INTERACTION

Bioenergetics refers to the flow of energy within a living system. The body's capacity to extract energy from food nutrients and transfer it to the contractile elements in skeletal muscle determines capacity to swim, run, bicycle, and ski long distances at high intensity. Energy transfer occurs through thousands of complex chemical reactions using a balanced mixture of macro- and micronutrients and a continual supply and use of oxygen. The term **aerobic** describes such oxygen-requiring energy reactions. In contrast, **anaerobic** chemical reactions generate energy rapidly for short durations without oxygen. Rapid anaerobic energy transfer maintains a high standard of performance in maximal short-term efforts such as sprinting in track and swimming or repeated stop-and-go sports like soccer, basketball, lacrosse, water polo, volleyball, field hockey, and football, including the high power outputs generated during resistance training. The following point requires emphasis: *Anaerobic and aerobic breakdown of ingested food nutrients provides the energy source for synthesizing the chemical fuel that powers all forms of biologic work.*

INTRODUCTION TO ENERGY TRANSFER

ENERGY: THE CAPACITY FOR WORK

Extracting energy from the stored macronutrients and ultimately transferring it to skeletal muscle's contractile proteins greatly influences exercise performance. But unlike the physical properties of matter, energy cannot be defined in concrete terms of size, shape, or mass. Rather, motion plays a part in all forms of energy. This suggests a dynamic state related to change; thus, the presence of energy emerges only when a change occurs. Within this context, energy relates to the performance of work—as work increases so does energy transfer.

The First Law of Thermodynamics

The **first law of thermodynamics** describes one of the most important principles related to work within biologic systems. The basic tenet states that energy is neither created nor destroyed, but instead transforms from one state to another without being used up. In essence, this law describes the immutable principle of the **conservation of energy** that applies to both living and nonliving systems first validated by English, French, and German chemists in the 19th century. For example, the large amount of chemical energy "trapped" within the structure of fuel oil readily converts to heat energy in the home oil burner. In the body, chemical energy stored within the macronutrients' bonds does not immediately dissipate as heat. Rather, a large portion is conserved as chemical energy before changing into mechanical energy (and then ultimately to heat energy) by the musculoskeletal system. **FIGURE 4.1** illustrates the interconversions for the six different forms of energy.

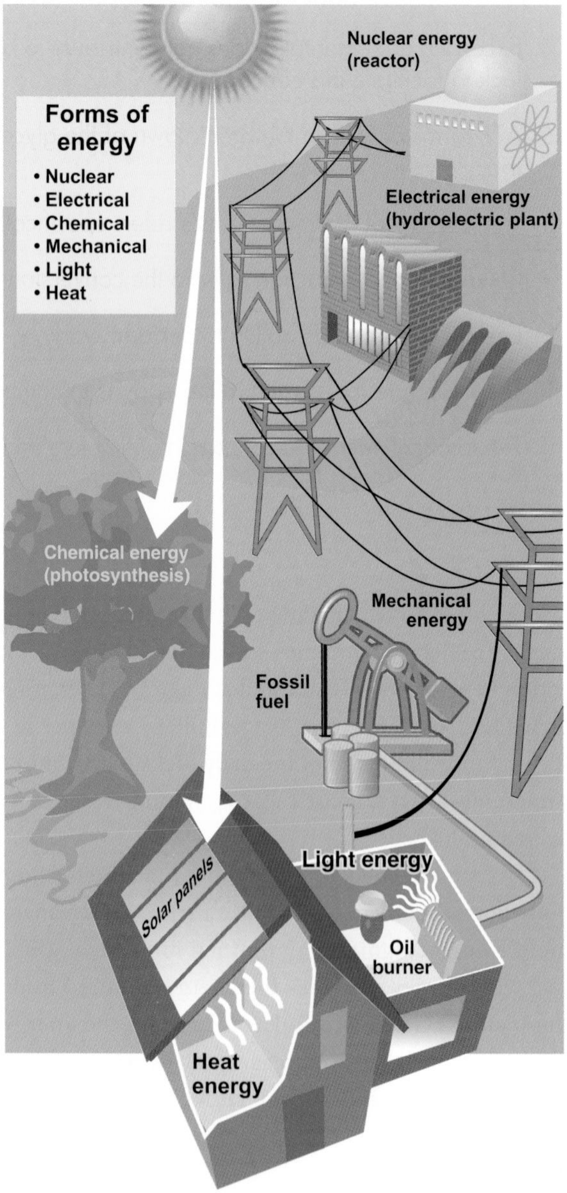

FIGURE 4.1. Interconversions of the six forms of energy.

THE BODY DOES NOT PRODUCE ENERGY

The first law of thermodynamics dictates that the body does not produce, consume, or use up energy; it merely transforms energy from one state to another as physiologic systems undergo continual change.

Photosynthesis and Respiration

Photosynthesis and respiration provide the most fundamental examples of energy conversion in living cells.

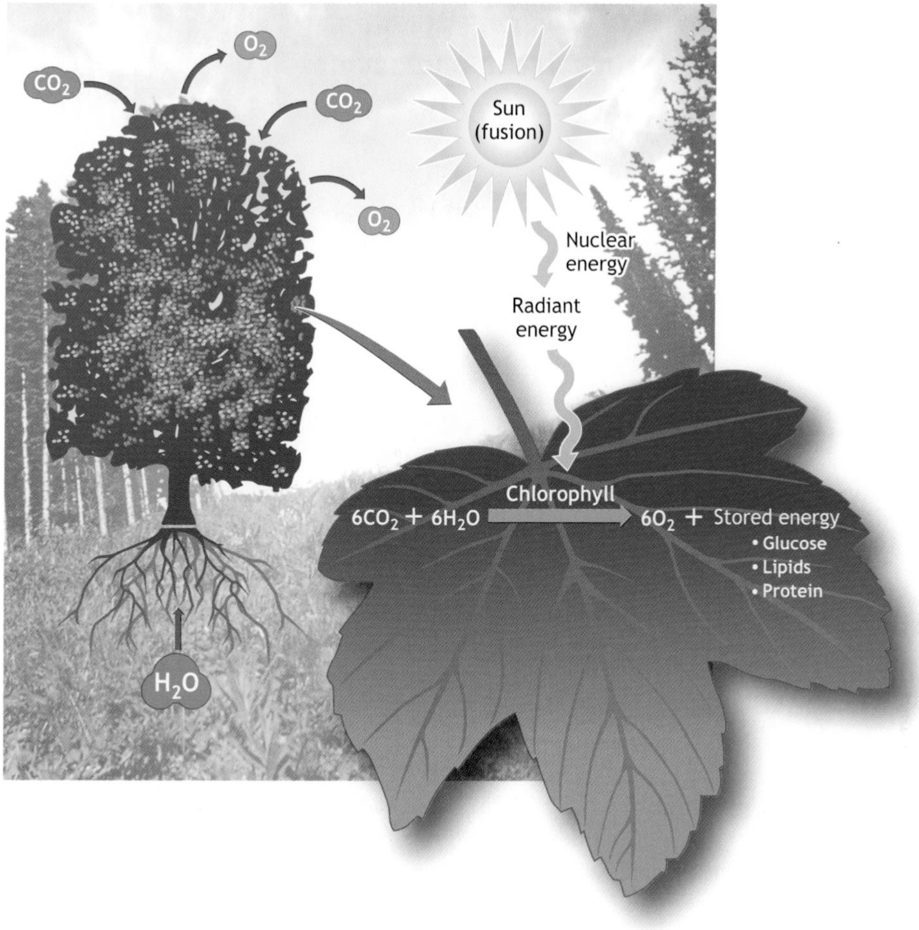

FIGURE 4.2. Photosynthesis serves as the plant's mechanism for synthesizing carbohydrates, lipids, and proteins. In this example, a glucose molecule forms from the union of carbon dioxide and water.

Photosynthesis

In the sun, nuclear fusion releases part of the potential energy stored in the nucleus of the hydrogen atom. This energy, in the form of gamma radiation, converts to radiant energy.

FIGURE 4.2 depicts the process of **photosynthesis**. The plant pigment chlorophyll contained in chloroplasts and large organelles located in the leaf's cells, absorbs radiant (solar) energy to synthesize glucose from carbon dioxide and water with oxygen escaping to the environment. Animals subsequently use glucose and oxygen during respiration. Plants also convert carbohydrates to lipids and proteins. Animals then ingest plant nutrients to serve their own energy needs. In essence, solar energy coupled with photosynthesis powers the animal world with food and oxygen.

Cellular Respiration

FIGURE 4.3 shows that the reactions of **respiration** are the reverse of photosynthesis, as animals recover the plant's stored energy for their use in biologic work. During respiration, extraction of chemical energy stored in glucose, lipid, or protein molecules occurs in the presence of oxygen. A portion of energy remains in other chemical compounds that the body uses in diverse energy-requiring processes; the remaining energy flows as heat to the environment.

Biologic Work in Humans

FIGURE 4.3 also illustrates that biologic work takes one of three forms:

1. **Mechanical work** of muscle contraction
2. **Chemical work** for synthesizing cellular molecules
3. **Transport work** that concentrates diverse substances in the intracellular and extracellular fluids

Mechanical Work

Mechanical work generated by muscle contraction provides the most obvious example of energy transformation. A muscle fiber's protein filaments directly convert chemical energy into mechanical energy of muscle action. However, this does not represent the only form of mechanical work. In the cell

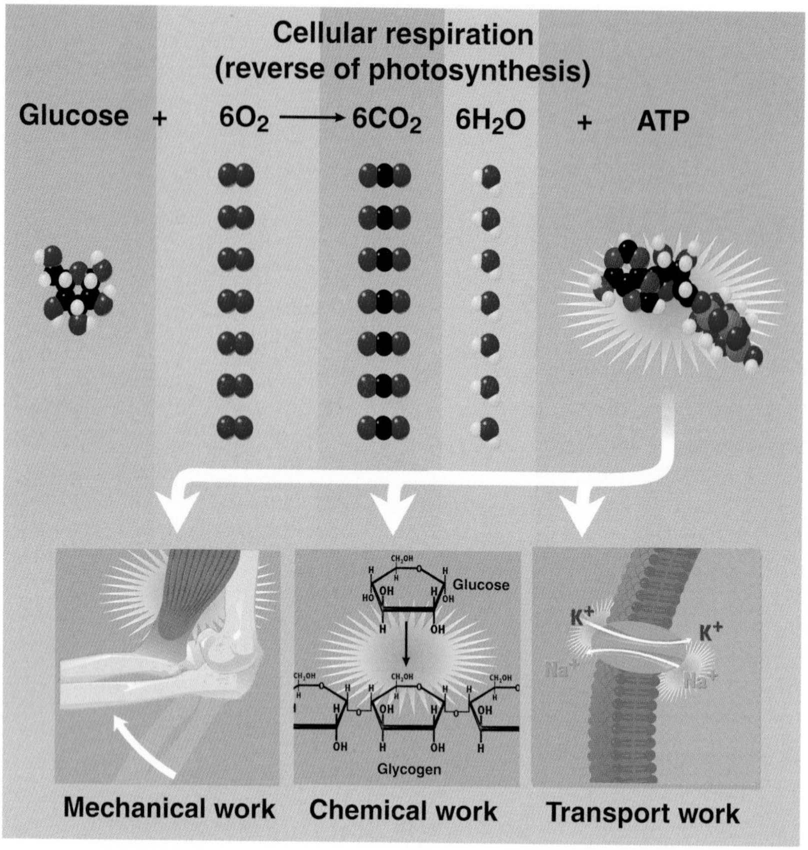

FIGURE 4.3. Respiration harvests the potential energy in food to form adenosine triphosphate (ATP). The energy in ATP powers all forms of biologic work.

nucleus, for example, contractile elements literally tug at the chromosomes to facilitate cell division. Specialized structures such as cilia also perform mechanical work in many cells.

Chemical Work

All cells perform chemical work for maintenance and growth. Continuous synthesis of cellular components occurs as other components break down. The extreme of muscle tissue synthesis from chronic overload in resistance training vividly illustrates this form of biologic work.

Transport Work

The biologic work of concentrating substances in the body referred to as transport work progresses much less conspicuously than mechanical or chemical work. Cellular materials normally flow from an area of high concentration to one of lower concentration. This passive process of diffusion requires no energy. For proper physiologic functioning, certain chemicals require transport uphill against their normal concentration gradients from an area of lower to one of higher concentration. Active transport describes this energy-requiring process (see Chapter 3). Secretion and reabsorption in the kidney tubules use active transport mechanisms, as does neural tissue in establishing the proper electrochemical gradients about its plasma membranes. These "quiet" forms of biologic work require continual expenditure of stored chemical energy.

Potential and Kinetic Energy

Potential energy and kinetic energy constitute the total energy of any system. **FIGURE 4.4** shows potential energy as energy of position similar to water at the top of a hill before it flows downstream.

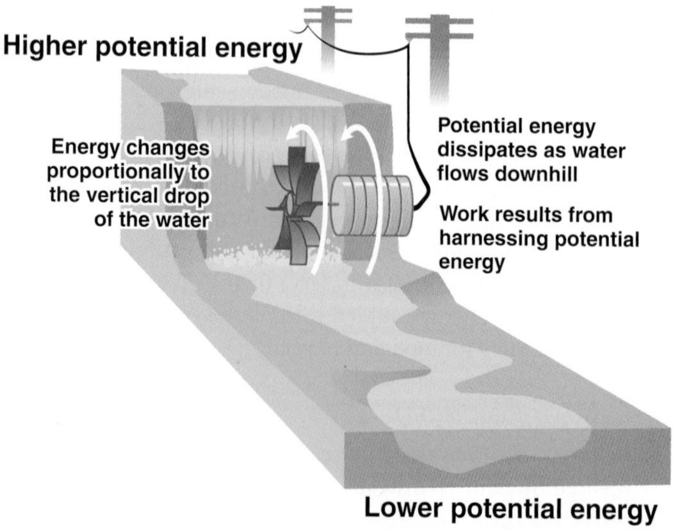

FIGURE 4.4. Potential energy to perform work transforms into kinetic energy.

In this example, energy changes proportionally to the water's vertical drop—the greater the vertical drop, the greater the potential energy at the top. Other examples of potential energy include bound energy within the internal structure of a battery, a stick of dynamite, or a macronutrient before release of its stored energy through metabolism. *Releasing potential energy transforms it into kinetic energy of motion.* In some cases, bound energy in one substance directly transfers to other substances to increase their potential energy. Energy transfers of this type provide the necessary energy for the body's chemical work of biosynthesis. Specific building-block atoms of carbon, hydrogen, oxygen, and nitrogen join other atoms and molecules to synthesize important biologic compounds (e.g., cholesterol, enzymes, and hormones). Some newly created compounds serve structural needs of bone or the lipid-containing plasma bilayer membrane that encapsulates each cell. Other synthesized compounds such as ATP and phosphocreatine (PCr) serve the cell's energy needs.

OXIDATION AND REDUCTION

Literally thousands of simultaneous chemical reactions occur in the body that involve transfer of electrons from one substance to another. ***Oxidation reactions** transfer oxygen atoms, hydrogen atoms, or electrons.* A loss of electrons occurs in oxidation reactions, with a corresponding gain in valence. For example, removing hydrogen from a substance yields a net gain of valence electrons. ***Reduction reactions** involve any process in which the atoms in an element gain electrons with a corresponding decrease in valence.*

Oxidation and reduction reactions are always characteristically **coupled**, so that any energy released by one reaction incorporates into the products of another reaction. In essence, energy-liberating reactions couple to energy-requiring reactions. The term **reducing agent** describes the substance that donates or loses electrons as it oxidizes. The substance being reduced or gaining electrons is called the electron acceptor or **oxidizing agent**. The term ***redox reaction*** describes a coupled oxidation–reduction reaction.

An excellent example of an oxidation reaction involves electron transfer within the mitochondria. Here, special carrier molecules transfer oxidized hydrogen atoms and their removed electrons for delivery to oxygen, which becomes reduced. The carbohydrate, lipid, and protein nutrient substrates provide the source of hydrogen. Dehydrogenase (oxidase) enzymes tremendously speed up redox reactions. Two hydrogen-accepting dehydrogenase coenzymes are the vitamin B–containing nicotinamide adenine dinucleotide (NAD^+), derived from the B vitamin niacin, and flavin adenine dinucleotide (FAD), derived from another B vitamin, riboflavin. Transferring electrons from NADH and $FADH_2$ harnesses energy in the form of ATP (see p. 142).

*The transport of electrons by specific carrier molecules constitutes the **respiratory chain**.* Electron transport represents the final common pathway in aerobic (oxidative) metabolism. For each pair of hydrogen atoms, two electrons flow down the chain and reduce one atom of oxygen. The process ends when oxygen accepts hydrogen and forms water. The coupled redox process constitutes hydrogen oxidation coupled to subsequent oxygen reduction. Chemical energy trapped or conserved in cellular oxidation–reduction reactions powers multiple forms of biologic work.

FIGURE 4.5 illustrates a redox reaction during vigorous physical activity. As exercise intensifies, hydrogen atoms strip from the carbohydrate substrate at a greater rate than their oxidation in the respiratory chain. To continue energy metabolism, the nonoxidized excess hydrogens must be "accepted" by a chemical other than oxygen. A molecule of pyruvate, an intermediate compound formed in the initial phase of carbohydrate catabolism, temporarily accepts a pair of hydrogens (electrons). A new compound called **lactic acid** (in the body as **lactate**) forms when reduced pyruvate accepts additional hydrogens. In other words, adding two hydrogens to pyruvate changes the molecule into lactic acid. As illustrated in the figure, more intense exercise produces a greater flow of excess hydrogens to pyruvate, and lactate concentration rises rapidly within the active muscle. During recovery, excess hydrogens in lactate oxidize (electrons removed and passed to NAD^+) to reform a pyruvate molecule. The enzyme lactate dehydrogenase (LDH) facilitates this reaction.

SUMMARY

1. Energy, defined as the ability to perform work, appears only when a change occurs.
2. Energy exists in either potential or kinetic form. Potential energy refers to energy associated with a substance's structure or position; kinetic energy refers to energy of motion. Potential energy can be measured when it transforms to kinetic energy.
3. There are six forms of interchangeable energy states—chemical, mechanical, heat, light, electrical, and nuclear—and each can convert or transform to another form.
4. In photosynthesis, plants transfer the energy of light into the potential energy of carbohydrates, lipids, and proteins. Respiration releases stored energy in plants and couples it to other chemical compounds for biologic work.
5. Biologic work takes one of three forms: chemical (biosynthesis of cellular molecules), mechanical (muscle contraction), or transport (transfer of substances among cells).
6. Oxidation–reduction (redox) reactions couple so oxidation (a substance loses electrons) coincides with the reverse reaction of reduction (a substance gains electrons). Redox reactions power the body's energy transfer processes.

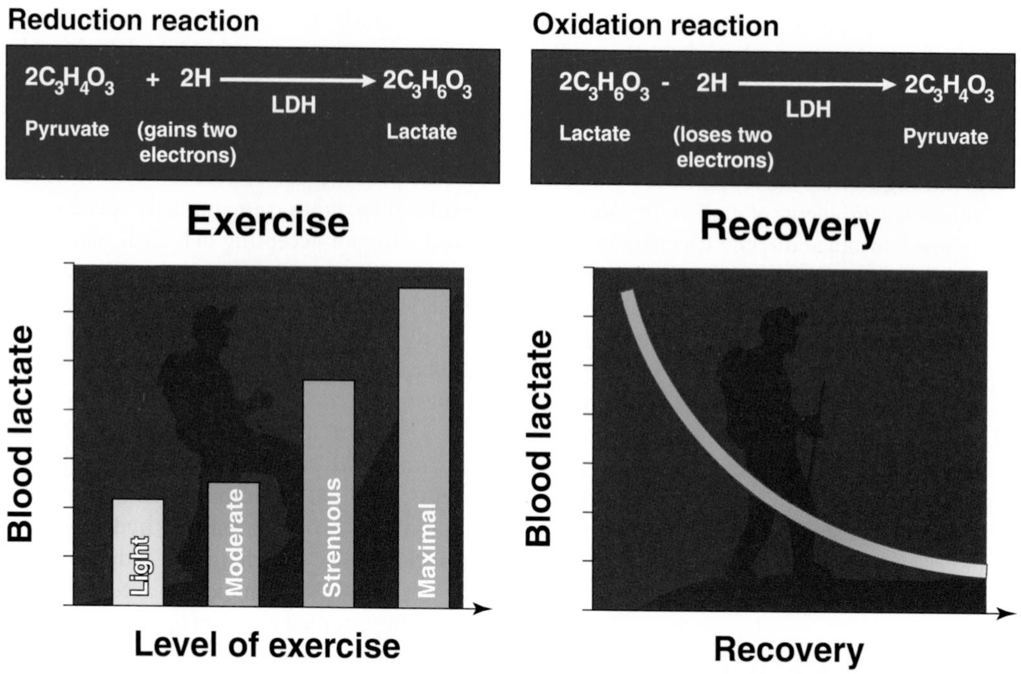

FIGURE 4.5. Example of a redox (oxidation–reduction) reaction. During progressively strenuous exercise when the oxygen supply becomes inadequate, some pyruvate formed in energy metabolism gains two hydrogens (gains two electrons) and becomes *reduced* to a new compound, lactate. In recovery, when oxygen supply becomes adequate, lactate loses two hydrogens (two electrons) and *oxidizes* back to pyruvate.

PHOSPHATE BOND ENERGY

The body demands a continual supply of chemical energy to perform its many complex functions. Energy transformations in the body largely depend on two factors:

1. Oxidation–reduction reactions
2. Chemical reactions that conserve and liberate the energy in ATP

Energy derived from the oxidation of food does not release suddenly at some kindling temperature (**FIG. 4.6A**) because the body, unlike a mechanical engine, cannot use heat energy. If it did, the body fluids would actually boil and tissues would burst into flames. Instead, extraction of chemical energy trapped within the bonds of the macronutrients releases in relatively small quantities during complex, enzymatically controlled reactions within the cell's relatively cool, watery environment. This temporarily conserves some energy that otherwise would dissipate as heat and provides greater efficiency in energy transformations. In a sense, the cells receive energy as needed.

The story of how the body maintains its continuous energy supply begins with **ATP**, the body's special carrier for free energy.

ADENOSINE TRIPHOSPHATE: THE ENERGY CURRENCY

The energy in food does not transfer directly to the cells for biologic work. Instead, "macronutrient energy" funnels through the energy-rich ATP compound. The potential energy within this molecule provides for *all* of the cell's energy-requiring processes. In essence, this energy receiver–energy donor role of ATP represents the cells' two major energy-transforming activities:

1. Extract potential energy from food and conserve it within the bonds of ATP
2. Extract and transfer the chemical energy in ATP to power biologic work

FIGURE 4.7 shows how ATP forms from a molecule of adenine and ribose (called adenosine) linked to three phosphate molecules. The bonds linking the two outermost phosphates are termed **high-energy bonds** because they represent a considerable quantity of potential energy trapped within the ATP molecule.

During hydrolysis, adenosine triphosphatase catalyzes the reaction when ATP joins with water. In the degradation of 1 mole of ATP to **adenosine diphosphate (ADP)**, the

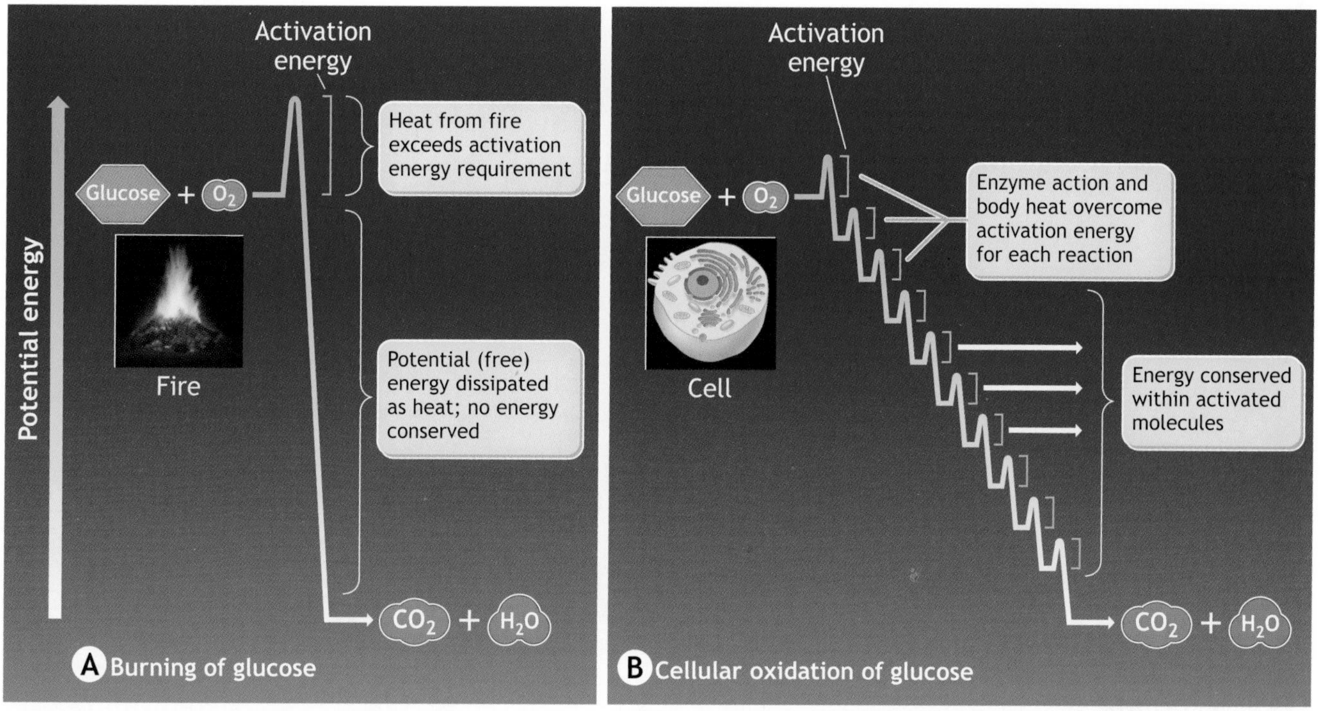

FIGURE 4.6. **A.** The heat generated by fire exceeds the activation energy requirement of a macronutrient (e.g., glucose), causing all of the molecule's potential energy to release suddenly at kindling temperature and dissipate as heat. **B.** Human energy dynamics involve release of the same amount of potential energy from carbohydrate in small quantities when bonds split during enzymatically controlled reactions. The formation of new molecules conserves energy.

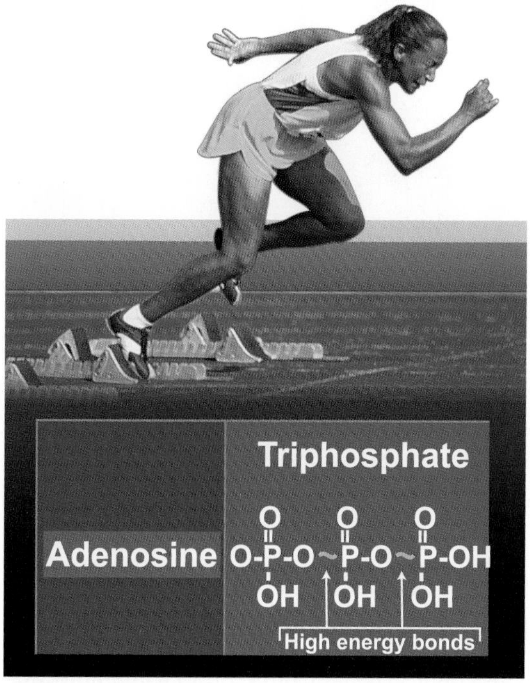

FIGURE 4.7. Simplified illustration of ATP, the energy currency of the cell. The symbol ▪ represents the high-energy bonds.

outermost phosphate bond splits and liberates approximately 7.3 kilocalories (kcal) of free energy (i.e., energy available for work).

$$ATP + H_2O \xrightarrow{ATPase} ADP + P - 7.3\ kcal{\cdot}mole^{-1}$$

The free energy liberated in ATP hydrolysis reflects the energy difference between the reactant and end products. This reaction generates considerable energy, so we refer to ATP as a **high-energy phosphate** compound. Infrequently, additional energy releases when another phosphate splits from ADP. In some reactions of biosynthesis, ATP donates its two terminal phosphates simultaneously to synthesize cellular material. Adenosine monophosphate (AMP) becomes the new molecule with a single phosphate group.

The energy liberated during ATP breakdown transfers directly to other energy-requiring molecules. In muscle, for example, this energy activates specific sites on the contractile elements, causing the muscle fiber to shorten. *Because energy from ATP powers all forms of biologic work, ATP constitutes the cell's "energy currency."* **FIGURE 4.8** illustrates the general role of ATP as energy currency.

The splitting of an ATP molecule takes place immediately and without oxygen. The cell's capability for ATP breakdown generates energy for rapid use; this would not occur if energy

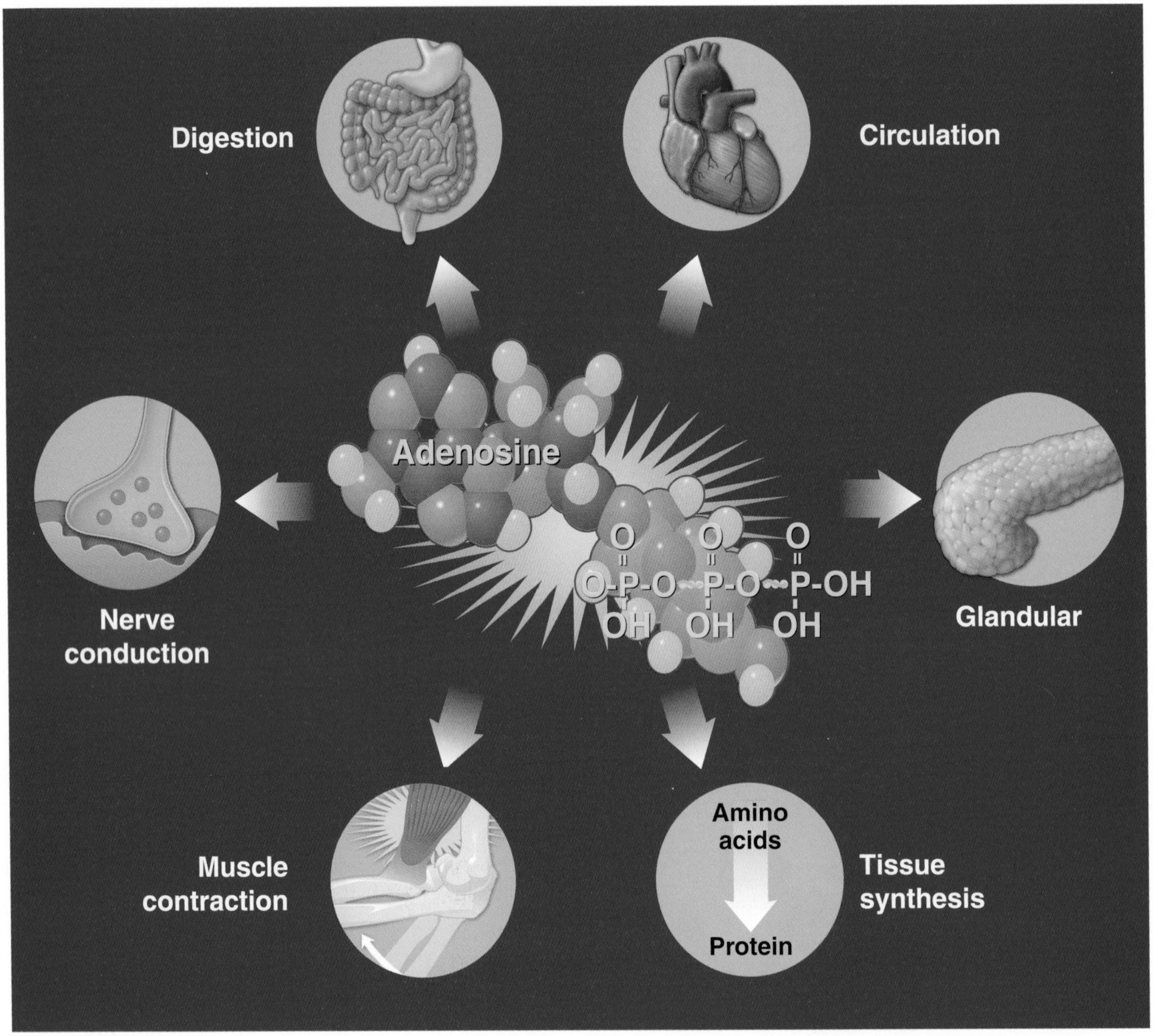

FIGURE 4.8. ATP, the energy currency, powers all forms of biologic work. The symbol ■ represents the high-energy bonds.

metabolism always required oxygen. Anaerobic energy release can be thought of as a back-up power source called upon when the body requires energy in excess of what can be generated aerobically. For this reason, any form of physical activity can take place immediately without instantaneously consuming oxygen; examples include sprinting for a bus, lifting a weight, driving a golf ball, spiking a volleyball, doing a pushup, or jumping up in the air. The well-known practice of holding one's breath during a short sprint swim or run provides a clear example of ATP splitting without reliance on atmospheric oxygen. Withholding air (oxygen), although inadvisable, can be done during a 60-yard sprint on the track, lifting a barbell, opening and closing your hand as fast as possible for 20 seconds (we recommend trying this to demonstrate the basic principle), or dashing up multiple flights of stairs. In each case, energy metabolism proceeds uninterrupted because the energy for performing the activity comes almost exclusively from intramuscular anaerobic sources, not the ability to take in a breath of air and deliver its oxygen to the active muscles and other tissues.

PHOSPHOCREATINE: THE ENERGY RESERVOIR

Cells store only a small quantity of ATP and must therefore continually resynthesize it at its rate of use. This provides a biologically useful mechanism to regulate energy metabolism. By maintaining only a small amount of ATP, its relative concentration (and corresponding ADP concentration) changes rapidly, increasing a cell's energy demands. Any increase in energy

DIVERSE WAYS TO PRODUCE ATP

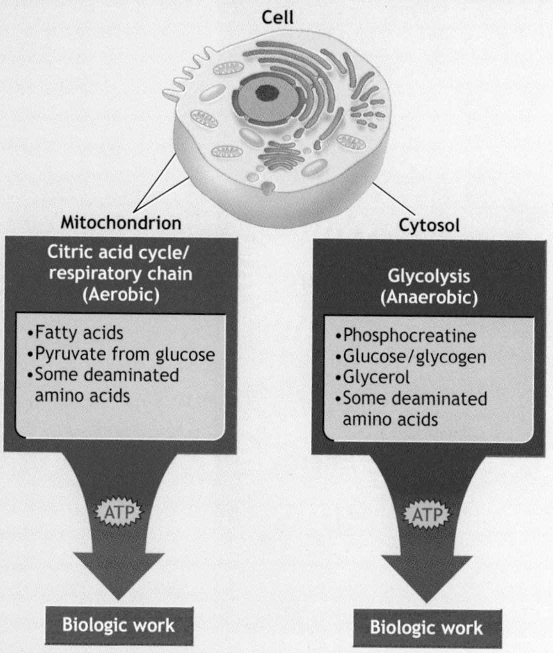

The body maintains a continuous ATP supply through different metabolic pathways: Some are located in the cell's cytosol, whereas others operate within the mitochondria. For example, the cytosol contains pathways for ATP synthesis from the anaerobic breakdown of PCr, glucose, glycerol, and the carbon skeletons of deaminated amino acids. Reactions that harness cellular energy to generate ATP aerobically—the citric acid cycle, β-oxidation, and respiratory chain—reside within the mitochondria.

requirement that disturbs the cell's current state immediately disrupts the ATP to ADP balance. An imbalance immediately stimulates breakdown of other stored energy-containing compounds to resynthesize ATP. This helps to explain why energy transfer increases rapidly when exercise begins. As one might expect, increases in energy transfer depend on exercise intensity. Energy transfer increases about fourfold in the transition from sitting in a chair to walking. In contrast, changing from a walk to an all-out sprint almost immediately accelerates the rate of energy transfer about 120 times!

As pointed out earlier, a limited quantity of ATP serves as the energy currency for all cells. In fact, the body stores only 80 to 100 g (about 3.0 oz) of ATP at any one time. This provides enough intramuscular stored energy for several seconds of explosive, all-out muscular exertion. To overcome this storage limitation, ATP resynthesis occurs continually to supply energy for biologic work. Fatty acids and glycogen represent the major energy sources to maintain continual ATP resynthesis. Some energy for ATP resynthesis, however, comes directly from the anaerobic splitting of a phosphate from another intracellular high-energy phosphate compound **PCr**, also known as creatine phosphate or CP. PCr, similar to ATP, releases a large amount of energy when the bond splits between creatine and phosphate molecules. **FIGURE 4.9** schematically illustrates the release and use of phosphate-bond energy in ATP and PCr. The terms **high-energy phosphates** and **phosphagens** describe these stored intramuscular compounds.

In each reaction, the arrow points in both directions to indicate a reversible reaction. In other words, phosphate (P) and creatine (Cr) join again to re-form PCr. This also applies to ATP as ADP plus P re-forms ATP. Cells store approximately four to six times more PCr than ATP. *The onset of intense exercise triggers PCr hydrolysis for energy; it does not require oxygen and reaches a maximum in about 10 seconds.*[39] Thus, PCr serves as a "reservoir" of high-energy phosphate bonds. PCr's speed for ADP phosphorylation considerably exceeds anaerobic energy transfer from stored muscle glycogen owing to the high activity rate of the creatine phosphokinase reaction.[16] If maximal effort continues beyond 10 seconds, the energy for continual ATP resynthesis must originate from the less rapid catabolism of the stored macronutrients.[11] Chapter 12 discusses the potential for exogenous creatine supplementation to increase intracellular levels of PCr and enhance short-term, all-out exercise performance.

Intramuscular High-Energy Phosphates

Energy release from the intramuscular energy-rich phosphates ATP and PCr sustains all-out exercise for approximately 5 to 8 seconds. Thus, for example, in the 100-m sprint in world record time of 9.58 s set by Jamaican Usain Bolt (August 16, 2009), the runner could not maintain maximum speed throughout this duration. During the last few seconds of the race, the competitors actually slow down, with the winner often slowing down least! If all-out muscular effort continues beyond 8 seconds or if moderate exercise continues for much longer periods, ATP resynthesis requires an additional energy source other than PCr. If resynthesis does not happen, the "fuel" supply diminishes, and high-intensity movement ceases. As we discuss later, the foods we eat and store for ready access provide chemical energy to continually recharge cellular supplies of ATP and PCr.

TRAINING THE IMMEDIATE ENERGY SYSTEM

Exercise training increases the muscles' quantity of high-energy phosphates. The most effective training to increase the intramuscular phosphagens uses repeat 6- to 10-second intervals of maximal exercise in the specific activity requiring improved power-output capacity from this energy transfer system.

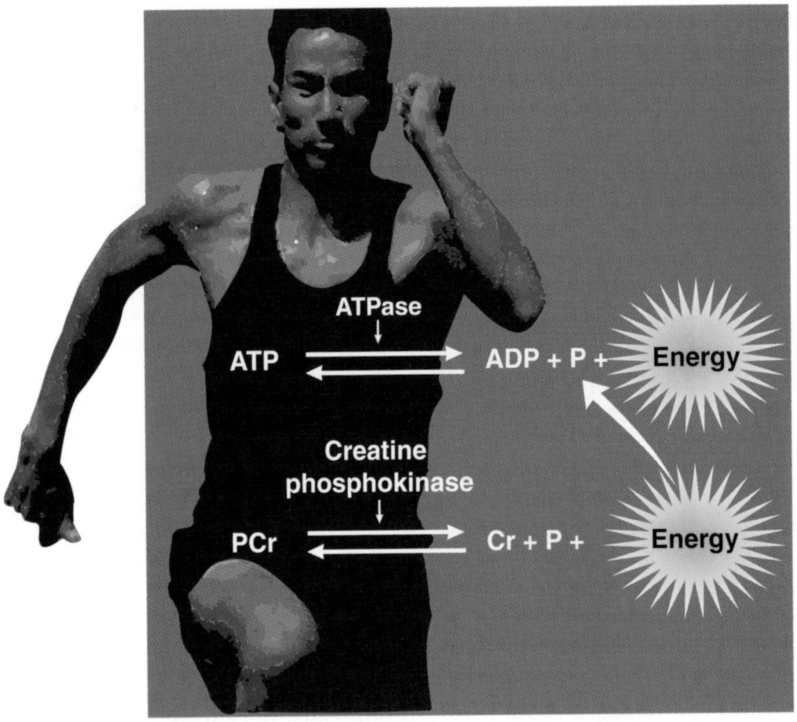

FIGURE 4.9. ATP and PCr provide anaerobic sources of phosphate-bond energy. The energy liberated from the hydrolysis (splitting) of PCr rebonds ADP and phosphate (P) to form ATP.

Transfer of Energy by Chemical Bonds

Human energy dynamics involve the transfer of energy by means of chemical bonds. Potential energy releases by the splitting of bonds and is conserved by the formation of new bonds. Some energy lost by one molecule transfers to the chemical structure of other molecules without appearing as heat. In the body, biologic work occurs when compounds relatively low in potential energy become "juiced up" from transfer of energy via high-energy phosphate bonds.

ATP serves as the ideal energy transfer agent. In one respect, phosphate bonds of ATP "trap" a relatively large portion of the original food molecule's potential energy. ATP also transfers this energy to other compounds to raise them to a higher activation level. **Phosphorylation** refers to energy transfer through phosphate bonds.

HIGH-ENERGY PHOSPHATES IN EXERCISE

To appreciate the importance of the intramuscular high-energy phosphates in exercise, consider activities in which success requires short, intense bursts of energy transfer. Football, tennis, track and field, golf, volleyball, field hockey, baseball, weightlifting, and wood chopping often require bursts of maximal effort for only up to 8 seconds.

CELLULAR OXIDATION

Most of the energy for ATP phosphorylation comes from oxidation ("biologic burning") of the carbohydrate, lipid, and protein macronutrients consumed in the diet. Recall that a molecule reduces when it accepts electrons from an electron donor. In turn, the molecule that gives up electrons is oxidized. Oxidation reactions (donating electrons) and reduction reactions (accepting electrons) remain coupled because every oxidation coincides with a reduction. *In essence, cellular oxidation–reduction constitutes the mechanism for energy metabolism.* This process often involves the transfer of hydrogen atoms (contains one electron and one proton in its nucleus) rather than free electrons. Thus, a molecule that loses hydrogen oxidizes and one that gains hydrogen reduces. For example, the stored carbohydrate, fat, and protein molecules continually provide hydrogen atoms from their degradation. The mitochondria, the cell's "energy factories," contain carrier molecules that remove electrons from hydrogen (oxidation) and eventually pass them to oxygen (reduction). Synthesis of the high-energy phosphate ATP occurs during oxidation–reduction reactions.

Electron Transport

FIGURE 4.10 illustrates the general scheme for hydrogen oxidation and accompanying electron transport to oxygen. During cellular oxidation, hydrogen atoms are not merely turned loose in the cell fluid. Rather, highly specific **dehydrogenase coenzymes** catalyze hydrogen's release from the nutrient substrate. The

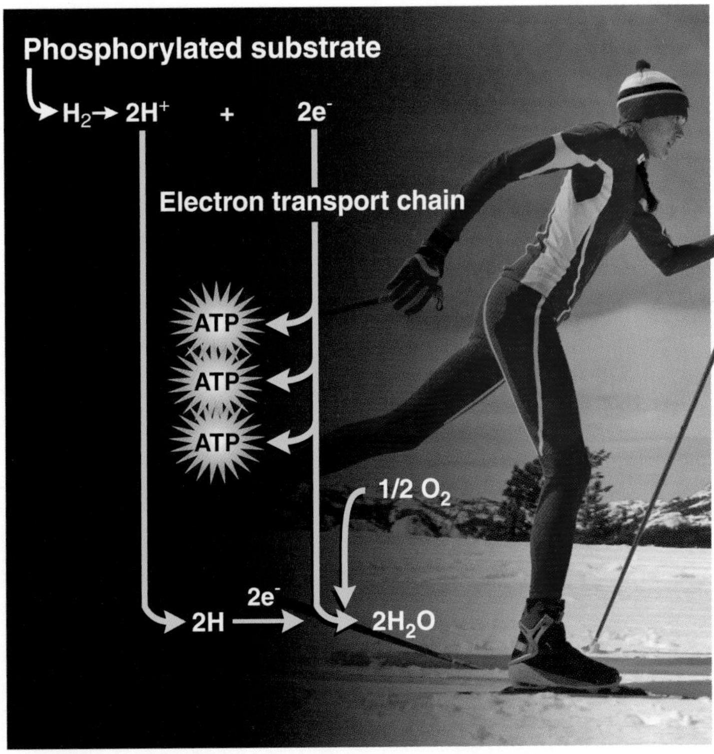

FIGURE 4.10. General scheme for oxidation (removing electrons) of hydrogen and accompanying electron transport. In this process, oxygen becomes reduced (gain of electrons) and water forms.

MISLEADING INFORMATION FROM THE SUPPLEMENT PURVEYORS

The coenzymes NAD^+ and FAD are derived from the water-soluble vitamins niacin and riboflavin, respectively. Unfortunately, vitamin manufacturers often misleadingly link the over-consumption of these vitamins to increased energy capacity. To the contrary, once sufficient amounts of these coenzymes are available in the body, any excess vitamins are voided in the urine.

LINKS IN ENERGY AND TRANSFER

NAD^+ and FAD represent crucial oxidizing agents (electron acceptors) in energy metabolism. Oxidation reactions couple to reduction reactions, allowing electrons (hydrogens) picked up by NAD^+ and FAD to transfer to other compounds (reducing agents) during energy metabolism.

coenzyme part of the dehydrogenase (usually the niacin-containing coenzyme **NAD^+**) accepts pairs of electrons (energy) from hydrogen. While the substrate oxidizes and loses hydrogen (electrons), NAD^+ gains one hydrogen and two electrons and reduces to NADH; the other hydrogen appears as H^+ in the cell fluid.

The riboflavin-containing coenzyme **FAD** serves as the other important electron acceptor in oxidizing food fragments. FAD catalyzes dehydrogenations and accepts pairs of electrons. Unlike NAD^+, however, FAD, by accepting both hydrogens, becomes the new molecule $FADH_2$. *The NADH and $FADH_2$ formed in the breakdown of food are energy-rich molecules that carry electrons with a high energy transfer potential.*

The **cytochromes**, a series of iron–protein electron carriers, then pass in "bucket brigade" fashion pairs of electrons carried by NADH and $FADH_2$ on the inner membranes of mitochondria. The iron portion of each cytochrome exists in either its oxidized (ferric or Fe^{3+}) or reduced (ferrous or Fe^{2+}) ionic state. By accepting an electron, the ferric portion of a specific cytochrome reduces to its ferrous form. In turn, ferrous iron donates its electron to the next cytochrome, and so on down the line. By shuttling between these two iron forms, the cytochromes transfer electrons to their ultimate destination, where they reduce oxygen to form water. The NAD^+ and FAD then recycle for subsequent use in energy metabolism.

Electron transport by specific carrier molecules constitutes the respiratory chain; this serves as the final common pathway where the electrons extracted from hydrogen pass to oxygen. For each pair of hydrogen atoms, two electrons flow down the chain and reduce one atom of oxygen to form water. Of the five specific cytochromes, only the last one, cytochrome oxidase (cytochrome aa_3, with a strong affinity for oxygen), discharges its electron directly to oxygen. The right panel of **FIGURE 4.11** shows the route in the respiratory chain for hydrogen oxidation, electron transport, and energy transfer. The respiratory

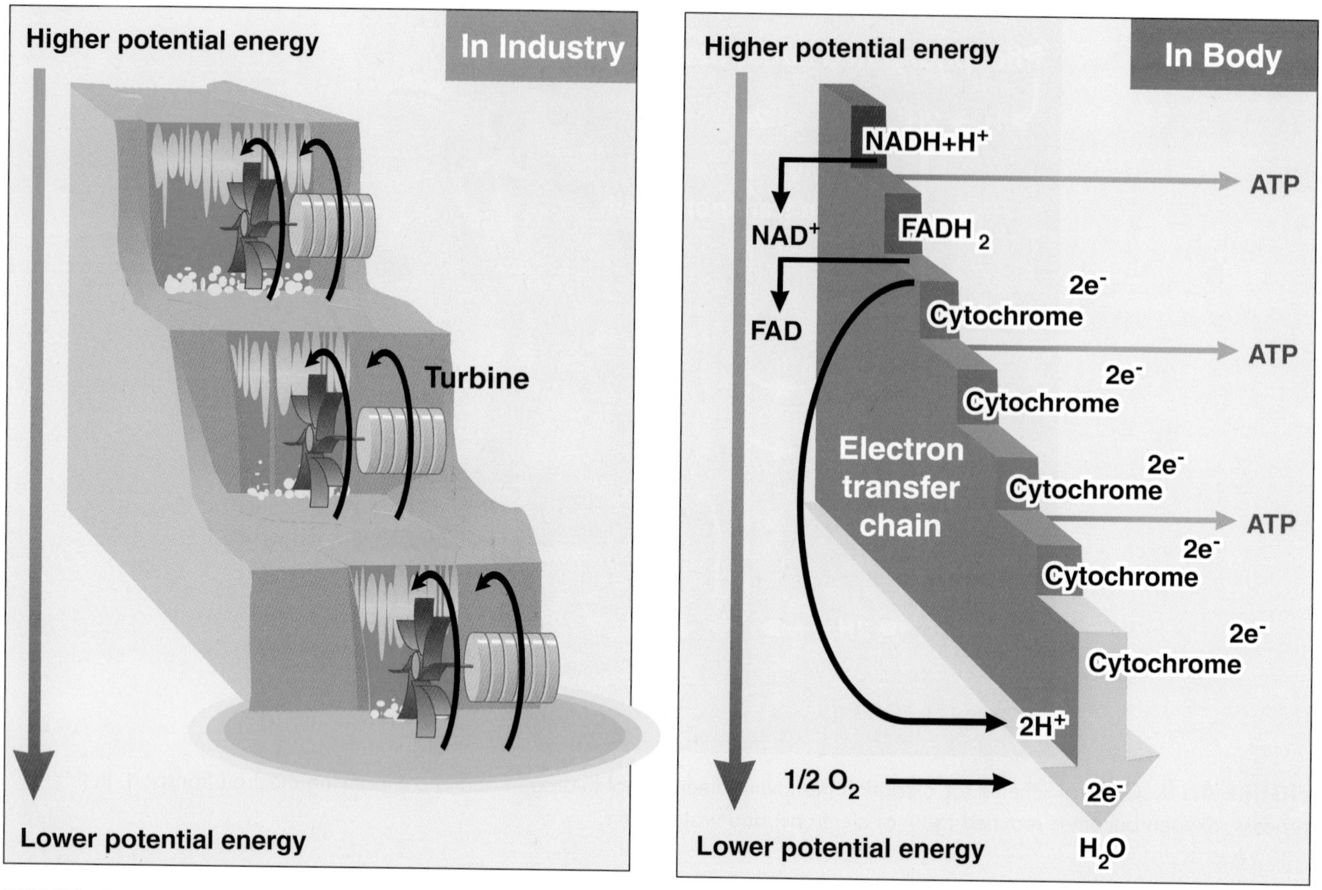

FIGURE 4.11. Examples of harnessing potential energy. *Left.* In industry, energy from falling water becomes harnessed to turn the waterwheel, which in turn performs mechanical work. *Right.* In the body, the electron transfer chain removes electrons from hydrogens for ultimate delivery to oxygen. In oxidation–reduction, much of the chemical energy stored within the hydrogen atom does not dissipate to kinetic energy, but instead is conserved within ATP.

chain releases free energy in relatively small amounts. In several of the electron transfers, energy conservation occurs by forming high-energy phosphate bonds.

Oxidative Phosphorylation

Oxidative phosphorylation synthesizes ATP by transferring electrons from NADH and $FADH_2$ to oxygen. This primary process represents the cell's way of extracting and trapping chemical energy in the high-energy phosphates. *More than 90% of ATP synthesis takes place in the respiratory chain by oxidative reactions coupled with phosphorylation.*

In a way, oxidative phosphorylation can be likened to a waterfall divided into several separate cascades by the intervention of water wheels at different heights. The left panel of **FIGURE 4.11** depicts water wheels harnessing the energy of falling water. Similarly, electrochemical energy generated via electron transport in the respiratory chain is harnessed and transferred (or coupled) to ADP. Three distinct coupling sites during electron transport transfer the energy in NADH to ADP to re-form ATP (**FIG. 4.11**, *right panel*). The theoretical value for ATP production from the oxidation of hydrogen and subsequent phosphorylation is as follows:

$$NADH + H^+ + 3\ ADP + 3\ P + \frac{1}{2}\ O_2 \rightarrow NAD^+ + H_2O + 3\ ATP$$

Note in the above reaction that three ATP molecules form for each NADH plus H^+ oxidized. Biochemists have recently adjusted their accounting transpositions regarding conservation of energy in the resynthesis of an ATP molecule in aerobic pathways. Energy provided by oxidation of NADH and $FADH_2$ resynthesizes ADP to ATP within the mitochondria. However, additional energy (H^+) also is required to transport the newly formed ATP molecule out across the mitochondrial membrane into the cell's cytoplasm. This occurs in exchange for ADP and P, which then move from the cytoplasm into the mitochondria. This added energy of transport reduces the *net* ATP yield for glucose metabolism. Actually, on average, only 2.5 ATP molecules form from oxidation of one NADH molecule. This decimal value for ATP does not indicate formation of one-half ATP molecule but rather indicates the average number of ATP produced per NADH oxidation with the energy for mitochondrial transport subtracted. When $FADH_2$ donates hydrogen, then on average only 1.5 molecules of ATP form for each hydrogen pair oxidized.

Efficiency of Electron Transport and Oxidative Phosphorylation

The formation of each mole of ATP from ADP conserves approximately 7 kcal of energy. Because 2.5 moles of ATP come

FREE RADICALS FORMED DURING AEROBIC METABOLISM

The passage of electrons along the electron transport chain sometimes forms free radicals, molecules with an unpaired electron in their outer orbit making them highly reactive. These reactive, free radicals bind quickly to other molecules that promote potential damage to the combining molecule. Free radical formation in muscle, for example, might contribute to muscle fatigue or soreness or a potential reduction in metabolic potential.

from oxidizing 1 mole of NADH, about 18 kcal (7 kcal·mole^{-1} × 2.5) are conserved as chemical energy. A relative efficiency of 34% occurs for harnessing chemical energy by electron transport–oxidative phosphorylation, since the oxidation of 1 mole of NADH liberates a total of 52 kcal (18 kcal ÷ 52 kcal × 100). The 66% remaining energy dissipates as heat. Considering that a steam engine transforms its fuel into useful energy at only about 30% efficiency, the value of 34% for the human body represents a remarkably high efficiency rate.

ROLE OF OXYGEN IN ENERGY METABOLISM

Three prerequisites exist for continual resynthesis of ATP during coupled oxidative phosphorylation from macronutrient catabolism. Satisfying the following three conditions causes hydrogen and electrons to shuttle uninterrupted down the respiratory chain to oxygen during energy metabolism:

Condition 1. Availability of the reducing agent NADH (or $FADH_2$) in the tissues

Condition 2. Presence of an oxidizing agent (oxygen) in the tissues

Condition 3. Sufficient concentration of enzymes and mitochondria in the tissues to ensure that energy transfer reactions proceed at their appropriate rate

In strenuous exercise, inadequate oxygen delivery (condition 2) or its rate of use (condition 3) creates a relative imbalance between hydrogen release and its final acceptance by oxygen. If either of these conditions occurs, electron flow down the respiratory chain "backs up" and hydrogens accumulate bound to NAD^+ and FAD. A subsequent section (see page 149) provides the details on how lactate forms when the compound pyruvate temporarily binds these excess hydrogens (electrons); lactate formation allows continuation of electron transport–oxidative phosphorylation.

Aerobic metabolism refers to energy-generating catabolic reactions. In this scenario, oxygen serves as the final electron acceptor in the respiratory chain and combines with hydrogen to form water. In one sense, the term *aerobic* is misleading because oxygen does not participate directly in ATP synthesis. On the other hand, oxygen's presence at the "end of the line" largely determines one's capacity for ATP production and ability to sustain intense, endurance exercise.

PERSONAL HEALTH AND EXERCISE NUTRITION 4.1

Overuse Injuries and Subsequent Pain

Bill, a former collegiate football athlete, has remained generally sedentary for the past 10 years. One weekend a month, he participates in vigorous competitive sports such as tennis, touch football, and skiing on consecutive days. He then complains of soreness and pain in his knees, back, shoulders, feet, and ankles. He stretches daily periodically to help "loosen" his back. The stretching does not relieve the aches and pains of his skeletal maladies.

Medical History

Bill does not smoke, has no history of major disease, and maintains desirable body weight (although he weighs 10 pounds more than in college) and normal blood pressure. All blood work done yearly at a local hospital falls within normal range. He is healthy, but more sedentary than he desires.

Diagnosis

Weekend warrior with signs and symptoms of overuse injuries.

Case Questions

1. Track progression of an overuse injury.
2. Give immediate first aid procedures for treating an overuse injury.
3. Describe how to prevent overuse injuries.

thePoint *Visit* **thePoint.lww.com/MKKSEN4e** *to find suggested answers to these Case Questions.*

SUMMARY

1. Energy within the chemical structure of carbohydrate, fat, and protein molecules does not suddenly release in the body at some kindling temperature. Rather, energy release occurs slowly in small amounts during complex enzymatically controlled reactions, thus enabling more efficient energy transfer and conservation.
2. About 34% of the potential energy in food nutrients transfers to the high-energy compound ATP.
3. Splitting the terminal phosphate bond of ATP liberates free energy to power all forms of biologic work.
4. ATP serves as the body's energy currency, although its quantity amounts to only about 3.0 oz.
5. PCr interacts with ADP to form ATP. This nonaerobic, high-energy reservoir replenishes ATP rapidly.
6. Phosphorylation refers to energy transfer by phosphate bonds, in which ADP and creatine continually recycle into ATP and PCr.
7. Cellular oxidation occurs on the inner lining of the mitochondrial membranes; it involves transferring electrons from NADH and $FADH_2$ to oxygen. This process results in the release and coupled transfer of chemical energy to form ATP from ADP plus a phosphate ion.
8. During aerobic ATP resynthesis, oxygen serves as the final electron acceptor in the respiratory chain and combines with hydrogen to form water.

ENERGY RELEASE FROM MACRONUTRIENTS

The energy released in macronutrient breakdown serves one crucial purpose—to phosphorylate ADP to reform the energy-rich compound ATP (**FIG. 4.12**). Macronutrient catabolism favors the generation of phosphate-bond energy, yet the specific pathways of degradation differ depending on the nutrients metabolized. In the sections that follow, we show how ATP resynthesis occurs from extraction of potential energy in the food macronutrients.

FIGURE 4.13 outlines the basic macronutrient fuel sources that supply substrate for oxidation and subsequent ATP formation. These four sources consist of the following:

1. Glucose derived from liver glycogen
2. Triacylglycerol and glycogen molecules stored within muscle cells
3. Free fatty acids (FFAs) derived from triacylglycerol (in liver and adipocytes) that enter the bloodstream for delivery to active muscle
4. Intramuscular and liver-derived carbon skeletons of amino acids

A small amount of ATP also forms from these two sources:

1. Anaerobic reactions in the cytosol in the initial phase of glucose or glycogen breakdown
2. Phosphorylation of ADP by PCr under enzymatic control by creatine phosphokinase

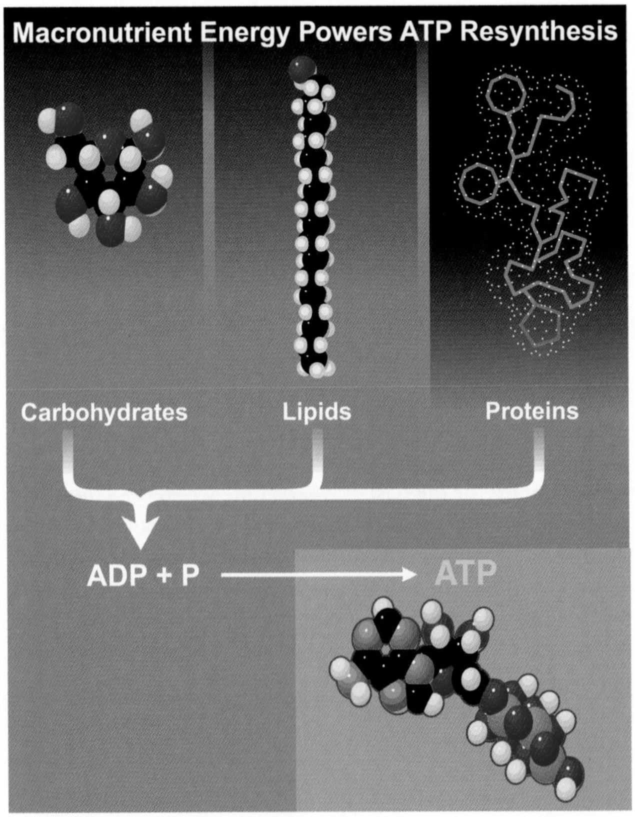

FIGURE 4.12. The potential energy in the macronutrients powers adenosine triphosphate (ATP) resynthesis. ADP, adenosine diphosphate, P, and phosphate.

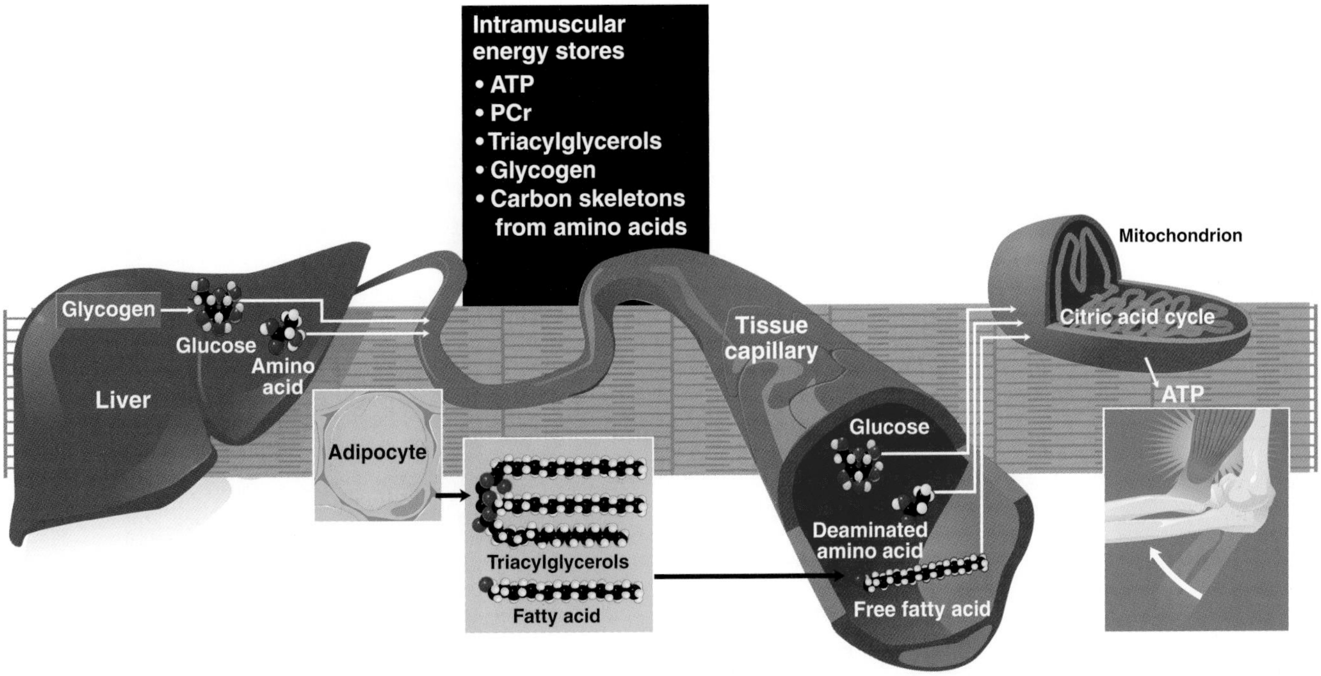

FIGURE 4.13. Basic macronutrient fuel sources that supply substrates for regenerating ATP. The liver provides a rich source of amino acid and glucose, whereas adipocytes generate large quantities of energy-rich fatty acid molecules. Once released, the bloodstream delivers these compounds to the muscle cell. Most of the cells' energy transfer takes place within the mitochondria. Mitochondrial proteins carry out oxidative phosphorylation in the inner membranous walls of this architecturally elegant complex. The intramuscular energy sources consist of the high-energy phosphates ATP and PCr and triacylglycerols, glycogen, and amino acids.

ENERGY RELEASE FROM CARBOHYDRATE

The primary function of carbohydrate is to supply energy for cellular work. The complete breakdown of 1 mole of glucose (180 g) to carbon dioxide and water yields a maximum of 686 kcal of chemical free energy available for work. In the body, complete glucose breakdown conserves only some of this energy in the form of ATP.

$$C_6H_{12}O_6 + 6O_2 \rightarrow 6CO_2 + 6H_2O + 686\ \text{kcal}\cdot\text{mole}^{-1}$$

Synthesizing 1 mole of ATP from ADP and phosphate ion requires 7.3 kcal of energy. Therefore, coupling all of the energy in glucose oxidation to phosphorylation could theoretically form 94 moles of ATP per mole of glucose (686 kcal ÷ 7.3 kcal·mole^{-1}). In muscle, however, the phosphate bonds conserve only 34%, or 233 kcal, of energy, with the remainder dissipated as heat. Consequently, glucose breakdown regenerates 32 moles of ATP (233 kcal ÷ 7.3 kcal·mole^{-1}), with an accompanying free energy gain of 233 kcal.

Anaerobic Versus Aerobic

Glucose degradation occurs in two stages.

Stage One: Glucose breaks down relatively rapidly to two molecules of pyruvate. Energy transfers occur without oxygen (anaerobic).

Stage Two: Pyruvate degrades further to carbon dioxide and water. Energy transfers from these reactions require electron transport and accompanying oxidative phosphorylation (aerobic).

Glycolysis: Anaerobic Energy from Glucose Catabolism

The first stage of glucose degradation within cells involves a series of chemical reactions collectively termed **glycolysis** (also termed the Embden-Meyerhof pathway for its two biochemist discoverers). This series of reactions, summarized in **FIGURE 4.14**, occurs in the cell's watery medium outside of the mitochondrion. In a sense, the reactions represent a more primitive form of energy transfer well developed in amphibians, reptiles, fish, and marine mammals. In humans, the cells' capacity for glycolysis becomes crucial during physical activities that require maximal muscular effort for up to 90 seconds.

In the first reaction of **FIGURE 4.14**, ATP acts as a phosphate donor to phosphorylate glucose to glucose 6-phosphate. In most body tissues, phosphorylation "traps" the glucose molecule in the cell. In the presence of **glycogen synthase**, glucose polymerizes (joins) with other glucose molecules to form glycogen. In energy metabolism, glucose 6-phosphate changes to fructose 6-phosphate. At this stage, no energy extraction occurs, yet energy incorporates into

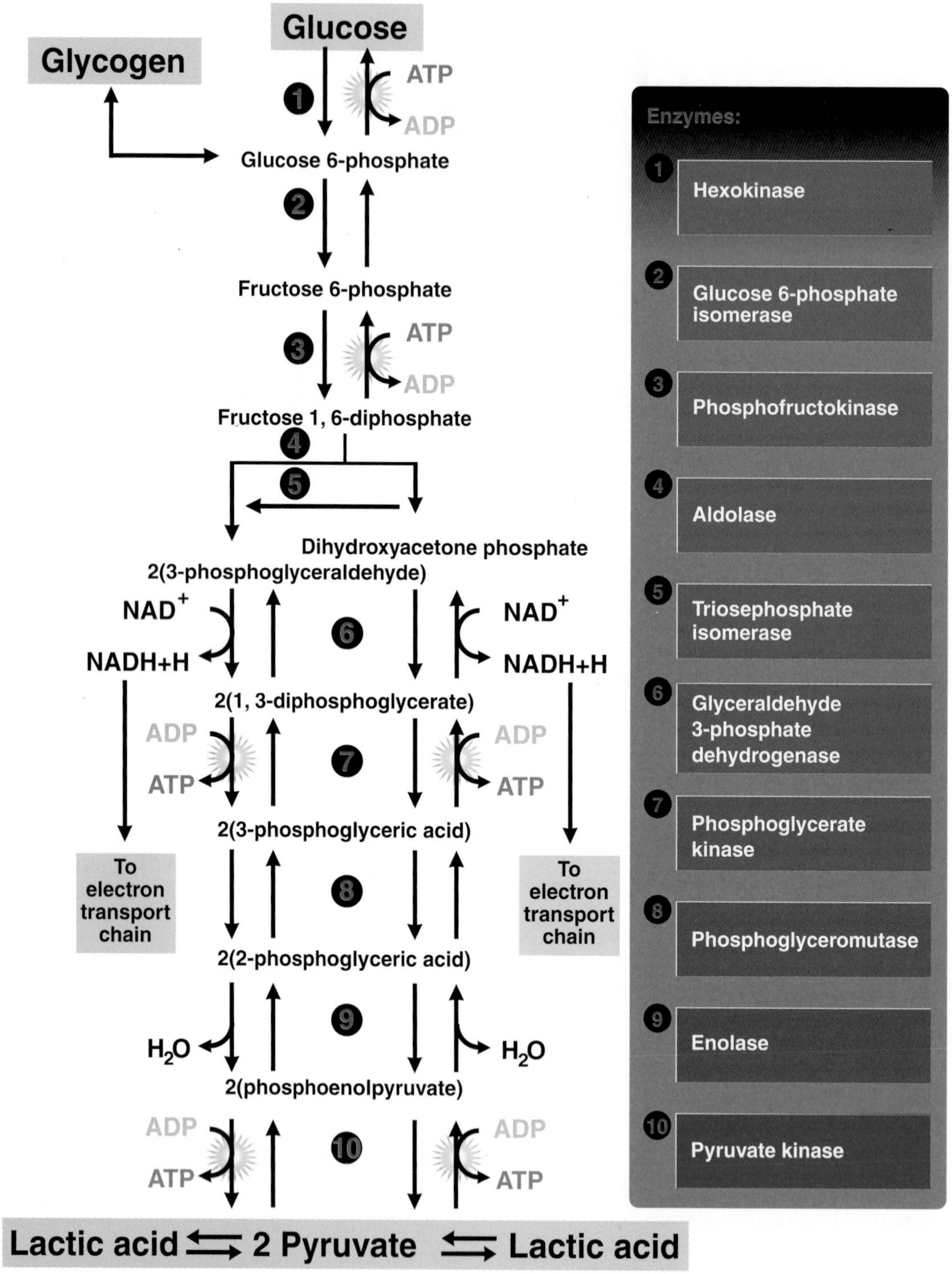

FIGURE 4.14. Glycolysis, a series of 10 enzymatically controlled chemical reactions, creates two molecules of pyruvate from the anaerobic breakdown of glucose. Lactic acid (lactate in the body) forms when NADH oxidation does not keep pace with its formation in glycolysis.

the original glucose molecule at the expense of one ATP molecule. In a sense, phosphorylation "primes the pump" for energy metabolism to proceed. The fructose 6-phosphate molecule gains an additional phosphate from ATP and changes to fructose 1,6-diphosphate under control of **phosphofructokinase (PFK).** The activity level of PFK probably places a limit on the rate of glycolysis during maximum-effort exercise. Fructose 1,6-diphosphate then splits into two

IMPORTANCE OF CARBOHYDRATES IN ENERGY METABOLISM

1. Carbohydrates are the only macronutrient whose stored energy generates ATP anaerobically. This becomes important in maximal exercise that requires rapid energy release above levels supplied by aerobic metabolic reactions. In this case, most of the energy for ATP resynthesis comes from stored intramuscular glycogen.
2. During light and moderate aerobic exercise, carbohydrates supply about one third of the body's energy requirements.
3. Processing fat through the metabolic mill for energy requires some carbohydrate catabolism.
4. Aerobic breakdown of carbohydrate for energy occurs more rapidly than energy generation from fatty acid breakdown. Thus, depleting glycogen reserves significantly reduces exercise power output. In prolonged intense aerobic exercise such as marathon running, athletes often experience nutrient-related fatigue—a state associated with muscle and liver glycogen depletion.
5. The central nervous system requires an uninterrupted stream of carbohydrate to function properly. Under normal conditions, the brain uses blood glucose almost exclusively as its fuel. In poorly regulated diabetes, during starvation, or with a prolonged low carbohydrate intake, the brain adapts after about 8 days and metabolizes relatively large amounts of fat (as ketones) for alternative fuel.

phosphorylated molecules, each with three carbon chains; these further decompose to pyruvate in five successive reactions. Fast-twitch muscle fibers contain relatively large quantities of PFK; this makes them ideally suited to generate rapid anaerobic energy from glycolysis.

Glycogen Catabolism

Glycogenolysis describes the cleavage of glucose from stored glycogen (glycogen → glucose). The **glycogen phosphorylase** enzyme in skeletal muscle regulates and limits glycogen's breakdown for energy. **Epinephrine**, a sympathetic nervous system hormone, influences the activity of this enzyme to separate one glucose component at a time from the glycogen molecule.[4,10] The glucose residue then reacts with a phosphate ion to produce glucose 6-phosphate, bypassing step 1 of the glycolytic pathway. Thus, when glycogen provides a glucose molecule for glycolysis, a net gain of three ATP molecules occurs rather than the two ATP molecules that occur during this first phase of glucose breakdown (see next section).

Substrate-Level Phosphorylation in Glycolysis

Most of the energy generated in the cytoplasmic reactions of glycolysis does not result in ATP resynthesis but instead dissipates as heat. In reactions 7 and 10, the energy released from the glucose intermediates stimulates the direct transfer of phosphate groups to ADPs while generating four ATP molecules. *Because two molecules of ATP were lost in the initial phosphorylation of the glucose molecule, glycolysis generates a net gain of two ATP molecules.* These specific energy transfers from substrate to ADP by phosphorylation do not require oxygen. Rather, energy transfers directly via phosphate bonds in the anaerobic reactions called **substrate-level phosphorylation.** Energy conservation during glycolysis operates at an efficiency of about 30%.

Glycolysis generates only about 5% of the total ATP formed during the glucose molecule's complete breakdown. However, the high concentration of glycolytic enzymes and the speed of these reactions provide significant energy for intense muscle action. The following represent examples of activities that rely heavily on ATP generated by glycolysis: sprinting at the end of the mile run, performing all-out from start to finish in the 50- and 100-m swim, routines on gymnastics apparatus, and sprint running races up to 200 m.

Hydrogen Release in Glycolysis

During glycolysis, two pairs of hydrogen atoms are stripped from the substrate (glucose), and their electrons pass to NAD^+ to form NADH (**FIG. 4.14**). *Because two molecules of NADH form in glycolysis, five molecules of ATP (2.5 per NADH) generate aerobically by subsequent electron transport–oxidative phosphorylation.*

Lactate Formation

Sufficient oxygen bathes the cells during light-to-moderate levels of energy metabolism. Consequently, the hydrogens (electrons) stripped from the substrate and carried by NADH oxidize within the mitochondria to form water when they join with oxygen. In a biochemical sense, a "steady state," or more precisely a "steady rate," exists because hydrogen oxidizes at about the same *rate* that it becomes available. Biochemists frequently refer to this relatively steady dynamic condition as **aerobic glycolysis**, with pyruvate the end product.

In strenuous exercise, when energy demands exceed either the oxygen supply or its rate of use, the respiratory chain cannot process all of the hydrogen joined to NADH. Continued release of anaerobic energy in glycolysis depends on NAD^+ availability for oxidizing 3-phosphoglyceraldehyde (see reaction 6 in **FIG. 4.14**); otherwise, the rapid rate of glycolysis "grinds to a halt." Under **anaerobic glycolysis**, NAD^+ reforms as pairs of "excess" nonoxidized hydrogens combine temporarily with pyruvate to form lactate in an additional

Connections to the Past

Otto Fritz Meyerhof (1884–1951)

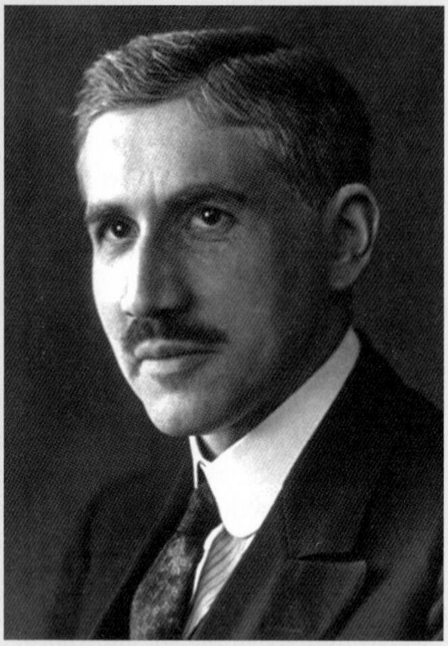

The distinguished German physician-biochemist Otto Fritz Meyerhof contributed significantly to muscle physiology, muscle chemistry, and exercise nutrition. His early research investigated metabolism in sea urchins, blood corpuscles, and bacteria's nitrifying respiratory processes. These studies eventually led to discoveries about intermediary cellular events during muscular activity. Meyerhof chose muscle as the experimental tissue because he believed muscle offered the best opportunity to explain chemical transformations by heat production and mechanical work. Meyerhof and his student's discovery that some phosphorylated compounds were rich in energy led to a shift in the way physiologists viewed intermediary metabolism and changed the biochemical explanation of muscle contraction. Meyerhof also realized that many enzymatic reactions and compounds (including the high-energy bonds of adenosine triphosphate, which became known as the universal energy donor) supplied the energy for endergonic reactions of biosynthesis. Meyerhof's research described the glycolytic enzyme–mediated energy transfer system in muscle, similar to the functioning of an isolated pathway system prevalent in yeast. This insight provided a decisive step to understand the inner workings of the anaerobic reactions of glycolysis. Meyerhof reconstructed in vitro the main steps of the interrelated chain of reactions from the breakdown of glycogen to lactic acid. In 1932, he verified parts of the chemical reaction scheme proposed by the German physiologic chemist Gustav Embden (1874–1933). Embden had developed a chemical perfusion technique to prevent tissue damage in the liver, thereby discovering the liver's important role in metabolism and normal sugar metabolism. Meyerhof built upon this work by recognizing that oxidative deamination was a way to catabolize amino acids, synthesize sugar from lactic acid, and in connection with the β-oxidation of fatty acids, create acetoacetic acid and acetone as end products of pathologic sugar metabolism. The steps by which glycogen is converted to lactic acid are now often known as the Embden-Meyerhof pathway, after Meyerhof and his coworker.

thePoint *Visit* **thePoint.lww.com/MKKSEN4e** *for more details on Meyerhof's contributions that led to his 1922 Nobel Prize in Physiology or Medicine with A.V. Hill for elucidating the cyclic characteristics of intermediary cellular energy transformation processes.*

step, catalyzed by **LDH**, in the reversible reaction shown in **FIGURE 4.15**.

The temporary storage of hydrogen with pyruvate represents a unique aspect of energy metabolism because it provides a ready "reservoir" to temporarily store the end products of anaerobic glycolysis. Also, once lactic acid forms in the muscle, it diffuses into the blood for buffering to sodium lactate and removal from the site of energy metabolism. In this way, glycolysis continues to supply additional anaerobic energy for ATP resynthesis. This avenue for extra energy remains temporary; blood and muscle lactate levels increase, and ATP regeneration cannot keep pace with its utilization rate. Fatigue soon sets in, and exercise performance diminishes. Increased acidity from lactate accumulation (and perhaps the effect of the lactate anion itself) mediates fatigue by inactivating various enzymes involved in energy transfer and inhibiting some aspect of the muscle's contractile machinery.[3,15,21,27]

Do not view lactate as a metabolic "waste product."[2,13] To the contrary, it provides a valuable source of chemical energy that accumulates in the body during intense exercise. When sufficient oxygen once again becomes available during recovery, or when exercise pace slows, NAD^+ scavenges hydrogens attached to lactate; these hydrogens subsequently oxidize to synthesize ATP. Consequently, considerable circulating blood lactate becomes an energy source that readily reconverts to pyruvate. In addition, the liver cells conserve the potential energy in the lactate and pyruvate molecules formed during exercise as the carbon skeletons of these molecules become synthesized to glucose in the

SOME BLOOD LACTATE AT REST

Even at rest, energy metabolism in red blood cells forms some lactate. This occurs because the red blood cells contain no mitochondria and thus must derive their energy from anaerobic glycolysis.

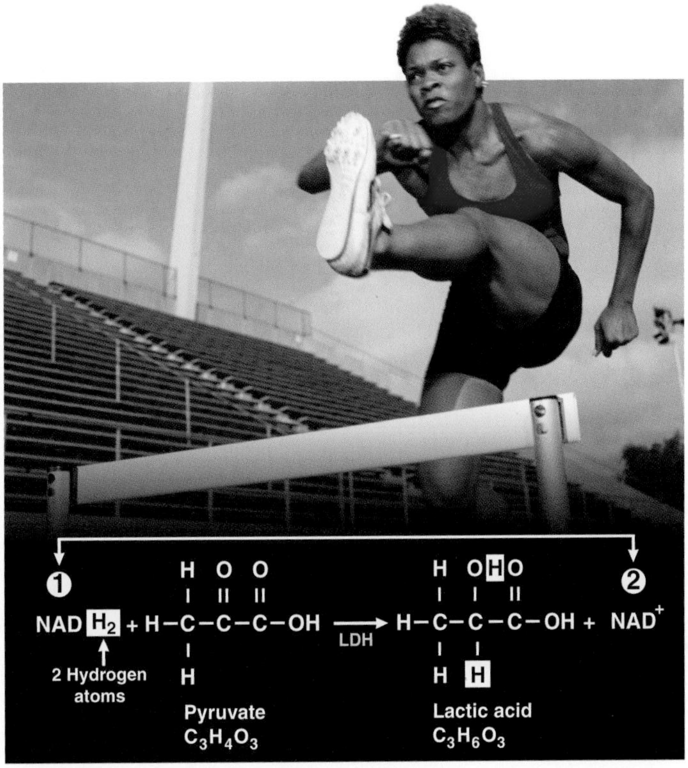

FIGURE 4.15. *(1)* Lactic acid forms when excess hydrogens from NADH combine temporarily with pyruvate. *(2)* This frees up NAD^+ to accept additional hydrogens generated in glycolysis.

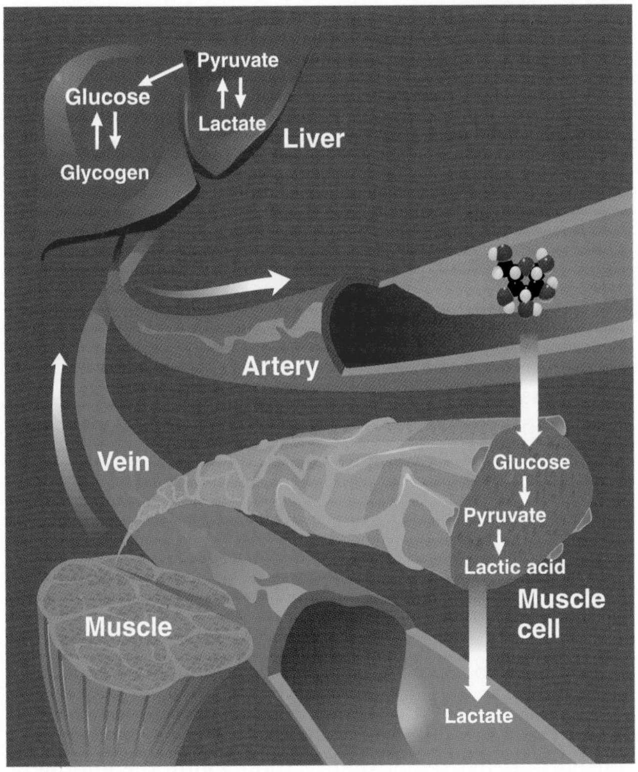

FIGURE 4.16. In the Cori cycle, lactic acid from muscle enters the venous system and converts to lactate. Lactate then enters the liver for conversion to pyruvate and synthesis to glucose for subsequent delivery to muscle. This gluconeogenic process helps to maintain carbohydrate reserves.

Cori cycle (**FIG. 4.16**). The Cori cycle not only removes lactate, but it also uses the lactate substrate to resynthesize blood glucose and muscle glycogen (via gluconeogenesis in the liver) depleted in intense exercise.[37]

Citric Acid Cycle: Aerobic Energy from Glucose Catabolism

Anaerobic glycolysis releases only about 10% of the energy within the original glucose molecule. Thus, extracting the remaining energy requires an additional metabolic pathway. This occurs when pyruvate irreversibly converts to acetyl-coenzyme A (CoA), a form of acetic acid. Acetyl-CoA enters the second stage of carbohydrate breakdown termed the citric acid cycle, also known as the Krebs cycle in honor of chemist Hans Krebs (1900–1981), who shared the 1953 Nobel Prize in Physiology or Medicine for his discovery of the citric acid cycle.

As shown schematically in **FIGURE 4.17**, the citric acid cycle degrades the acetyl-CoA substrate to carbon dioxide and hydrogen atoms within the mitochondria. Hydrogen atoms then oxidize during electron transport–oxidative phosphorylation with subsequent ATP regeneration. **FIGURE 4.18** shows pyruvate preparing to enter the citric acid cycle by joining with the vitamin B (pantothenic acid) derivative coenzyme A (A stands for acetic acid) to form the two-carbon compound acetyl-CoA. This process releases two hydrogens and transfers their electrons

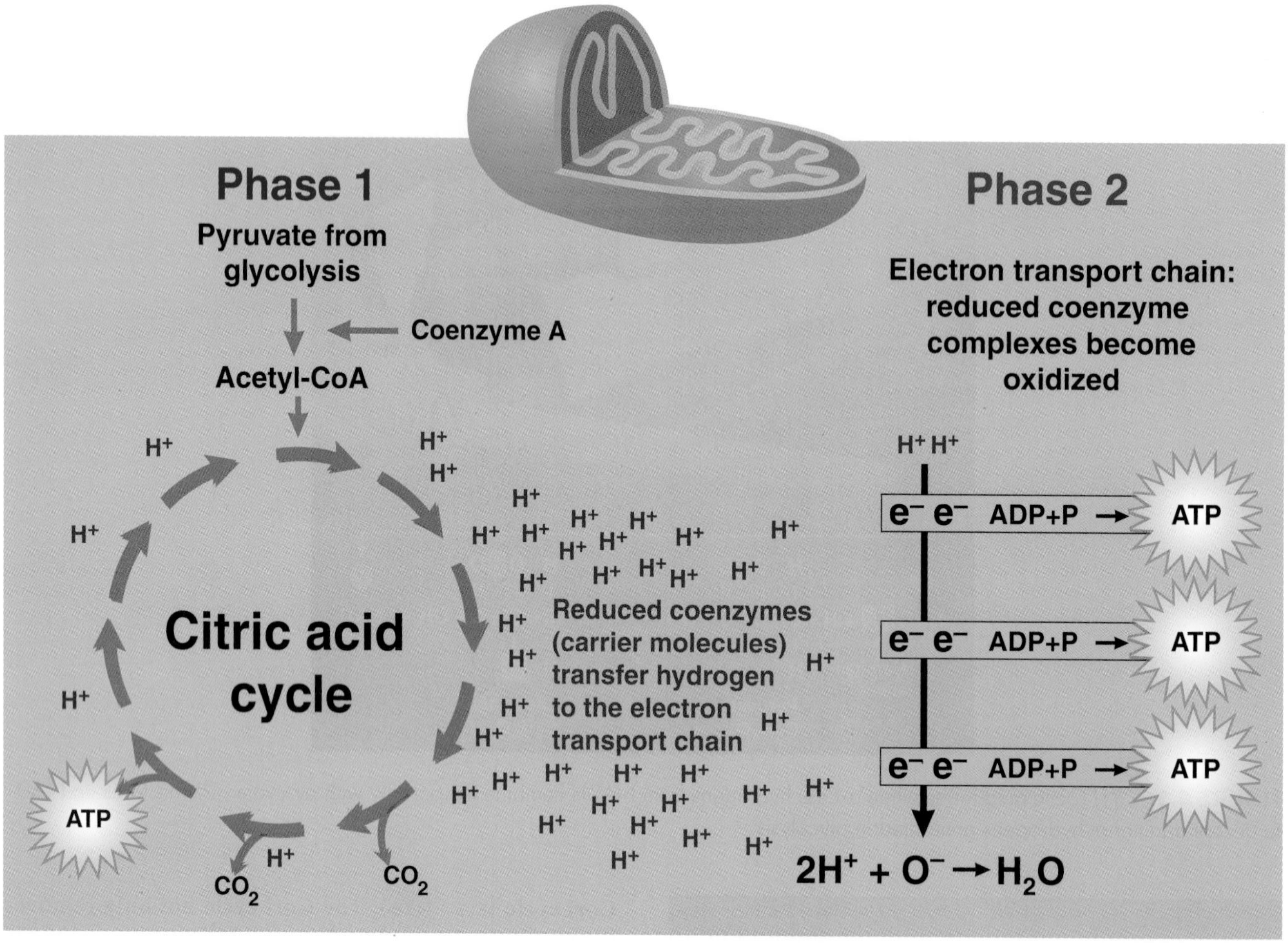

FIGURE 4.17. Hydrogen formation and subsequent oxidation during aerobic energy metabolism. *Phase 1.* In the mitochondria, the citric acid cycle generates hydrogen atoms during acetyl-CoA breakdown. *Phase 2.* Significant quantities of ATP regenerate when these hydrogens oxidize via the aerobic process of electron transport–oxidative phosphorylation (electron transport chain). P, phosphate.

to NAD^+. This forms one molecule of carbon dioxide as follows:

$$\text{Pyruvate} + NAD^+ + \text{CoA} \rightarrow \text{Acetyl-CoA} + CO_2 + NADH + H^+$$

The acetyl portion of acetyl-CoA joins with oxaloacetate to form citrate (citric acid), the same six-carbon compound found in citrus fruits, which then proceeds through the citric acid cycle. The citric acid cycle continues its operations because it retains the original oxaloacetate molecule to join with a new acetyl fragment that then enters the cycle.

Each acetyl-CoA molecule entering the citric acid cycle releases two carbon dioxide molecules and four pairs of hydrogen atoms. One molecule of ATP also regenerates directly by substrate-level phosphorylation from citric acid cycle reactions (see reaction 7 in **FIG. 4.18**). As summarized at the bottom of **FIGURE 4.18**, four hydrogens release when acetyl-CoA forms from the two pyruvate molecules created in glycolysis, and 16 hydrogens release in the citric acid cycle. The most important function of the citric acid cycle generates electrons (H^+) for passage in the respiratory chain to NAD^+ and FAD.

CARBOHYDRATE DEPLETION REDUCES EXERCISE POWER OUTPUT

Carbohydrate depletion depresses exercise capacity (expressed as a percentage of maximum). This capacity progressively decreases after 2 hours to 50% of the initial exercise intensity. Reduced power directly results from the relatively slow rate of aerobic energy release from fat oxidation, which now becomes the major energy pathway.

Oxygen does not participate directly in citric acid cycle reactions. The major portion of the chemical energy in pyruvate transfers to ADP through the aerobic process of electron transport–oxidative phosphorylation within the folding or cristae of the inner mitochondrial membrane. With adequate oxygen, including enzymes and substrate, NAD^+ and FAD regeneration takes place and citric acid cycle metabolism proceeds unimpeded.

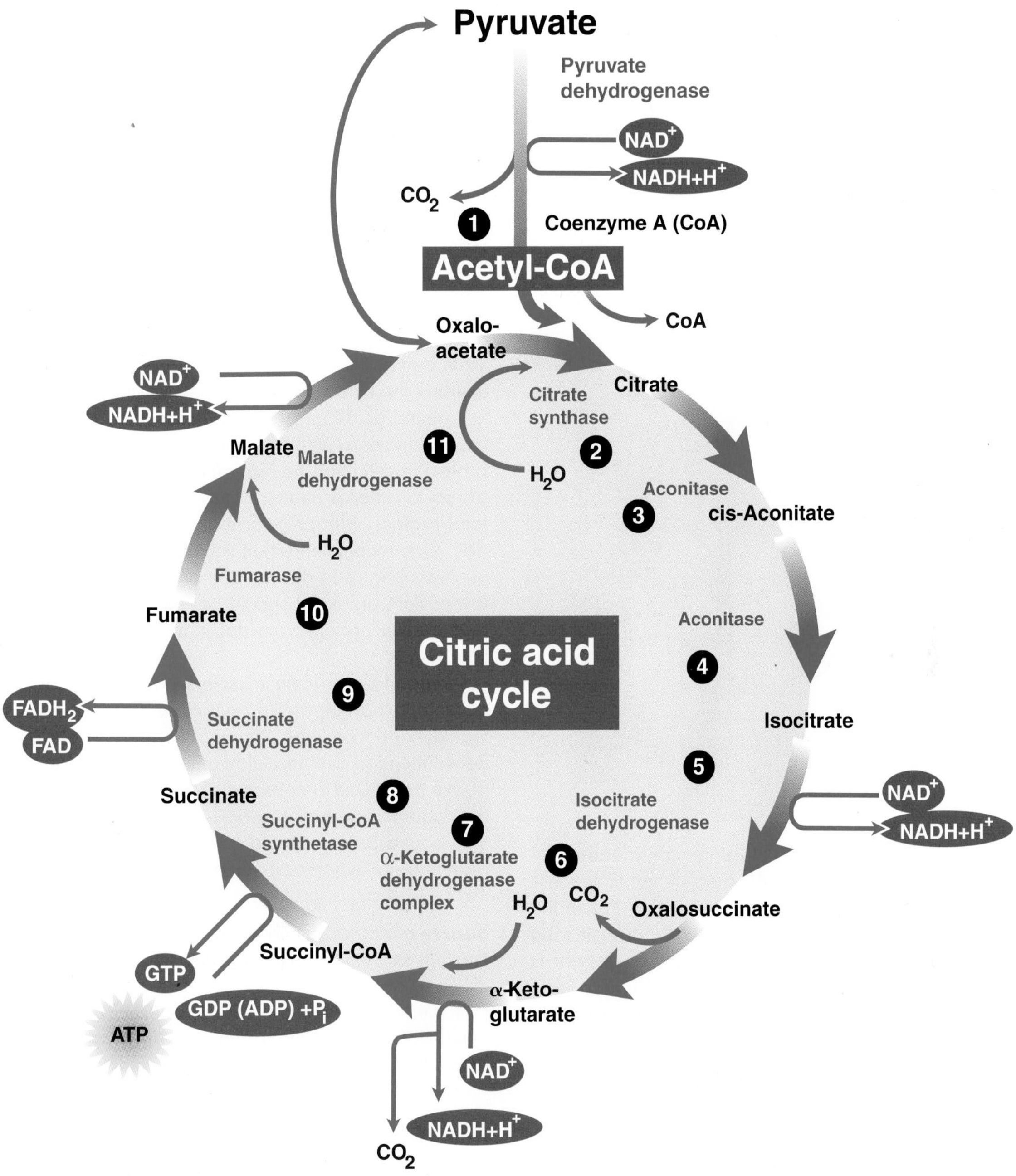

Net reaction: two pyruvate molecules form 20 hydrogen atoms

$$2 \text{ pyruvate} + 6\ H_2O \longrightarrow 6\ CO_2 + 2\ OH + 2\ CoA$$

	CO_2	H
2 pyruvate molecules	2	4
2 acetyl-CoA molecules	4	16
Total:	6	20

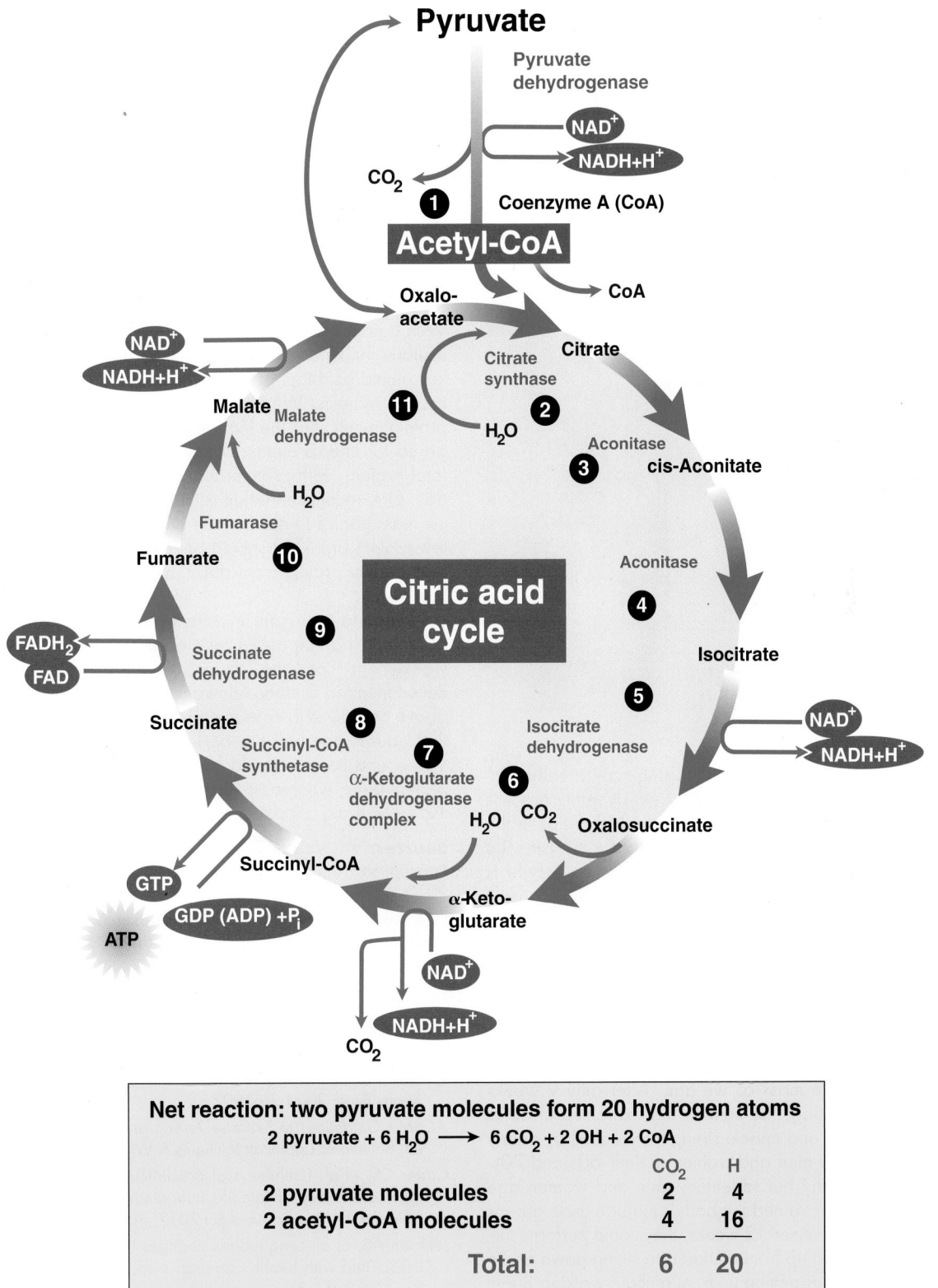

FIGURE 4.18. Schematic illustration and quantification for hydrogen (H) and carbon dioxide (CO_2) release in the mitochondrion during the breakdown of one pyruvate molecule. All values have been doubled when computing the net gain of H and CO_2 from pyruvate breakdown because glycolysis produces two molecules of pyruvate from one molecule of glucose. Note the formation of guanosine triphosphate (GTP), a molecule similar to ATP, from guanosine diphosphate (GDP) by substrate-level phosphorylation in reaction 8. P_i, phosphate.

Additional Insights

Can Exercise and Diet Preserve Muscle Mass as We Age?

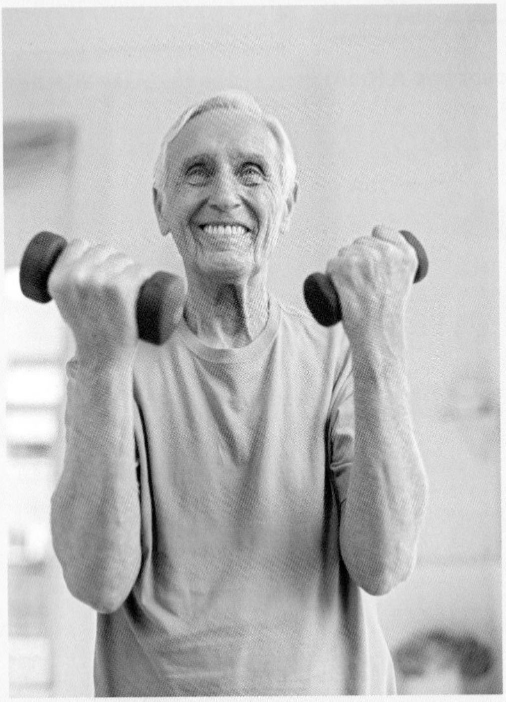

Sarcopenia, or muscle loss with aging, continually progresses beginning at about age 40 as a dynamic process of muscle breakdown, repair, and synthesis that tips in the direction of greater protein breakdown than synthesis. The current question that scientists are attempting to answer is the role that resistance training plays in building muscle or stemming muscle loss with aging. Also of interest is the role that dietary protein plays in retarding the sarcopenia of aging.

Exercise

A modest program of regular resistance training represents the exercise intervention of choice to build new muscle or conserve muscle mass as we age. After only 9 weeks of resistance training, the size of the exercised muscles increased by 12% and muscle strength increased by nearly 30% in 23 healthy men and women in their 60s and 70s. Recently, 50 healthy but sedentary men and women age 65 to 85 resistance trained the body's major muscle groups three times a week. After 12 weeks, they could perform simple tasks like getting up from a chair and sitting down again five times in a row or getting up from a chair, walking 8 feet around a cone, and then sitting down again at a faster rate than they could when the study began. And the good news is that in addition to building or at least maintaining muscle mass in the elderly, resistance training also provides stimulus to maintain or possibly improve bone mineral density and help to control blood sugar in individuals with type 2 diabetes. The American Heart Association and the American College of Sports Medicine recommend that all healthy adults do 8 to 10 strength-training exercises at least twice weekly that incorporate six of the major muscle groups—chest, shoulders, arms, back, abdomen, and legs.

Diet

With aging, the body appears to require more protein, particularly the kind rich in the essential amino acid leucine, a key amino acid that provides the building blocks for muscle tissue synthesis. Whey protein, which constitutes 20% of protein in milk, has the highest concentration of leucine compared to other proteins. Many older people require more total protein, with protein intake distributed throughout the day. One recommendation is that in middle age, when muscle mass begins to decline, the protein content of the typical low-protein breakfast should be upgraded to 20 to 30 g of high-quality protein from dairy, meat, poultry, fish, or egg sources.

To maintain or gain muscle with aging, most individuals should participate in resistance training at least twice weekly and consume 25 to 50% more protein than the Recommended Dietary Allowance. The goal for individuals above age 50 is to consume an amount of protein in grams that equals one half the body weight in pounds. Thus, a 154-pound person should consume about 72 g (2.5 oz) of protein daily, whereas a 250-pound person should consume 125 g (4.4 oz) of protein.

Sources: *ACSM's Guidelines to Exercise Testing and Prescription.* 10th ed. Baltimore: Lippincott Williams & Wilkins, 2010.

Peterson MD, Gordon PM. Resistance exercise for the aging adult: clinical implications and prescription guidelines. *Am J Med* 2011;124:194.

Related References

ACSM best practices statement: physical activity programs and behavior counseling in older adult populations. *Med Sci Sports Exerc* 2004;36:1997.

ACSM's Guidelines to Exercise Testing and Prescription. 10th ed. Baltimore: Lippincott Williams & Wilkins, 2010.

Carter CS, et al. Usefulness of preclinical models for assessing the efficacy of late-life interventions for sarcopenia. *J Gerontol A Biol Sci Med Sci* 2012; in press.

Jackson AS, et al. Longitudinal changes in body composition associated with healthy ageing: men, aged 20-96 years. *Br J Nutr* 2011;3:1.

Leiter JR, et al. Exercise-induced muscle growth is muscle-specific and age-dependent. *Muscle Nerve* 2011;43:828.

Walker DK, et al. Exercise, amino acids and aging in the control of human muscle protein synthesis. *Med Sci Sports Exerc* 2011; 43:2249.

AN IMPORTANT MACRONUTRIENT COMPONENT OF BLOOD

Blood sugar usually remains regulated within narrow limits for two main reasons: (1) glucose serves as a primary fuel for nerve tissue metabolism and (2) glucose represents the sole energy source for red blood cells, which contain no mitochondria. At rest and during exercise, liver glycogenolysis maintains normal blood glucose levels, usually at 100 $mg \cdot dL^{-1}$ (5.5 mM). In prolonged, intense exercise such as marathon running, blood glucose concentration eventually falls below normal levels because liver glycogen depletes, and active muscle continues to catabolize the available blood glucose. Symptoms of significantly reduced blood glucose (hypoglycemia: <45 $mg \cdot dL^{-1}$) include weakness, hunger, and dizziness. This ultimately impairs exercise performance and can contribute to central nervous system fatigue associated with prolonged exercise. Sustained and profound hypoglycemia triggers unconsciousness and produces irreversible brain damage.

Net Energy Transfer from Glucose Catabolism

FIGURE 4.19 summarizes the five pathways for energy transfer during glucose breakdown in skeletal muscle that culminate in the production of 32 moles of ATP. Two ATPs (net gain) are formed from substrate-level phosphorylation in glycolysis. The remaining ATPs are accounted for as follows:

1. Four extramitochondrial hydrogens (two NADH) generated in glycolysis yield five ATPs during oxidative phosphorylation.
2. Four hydrogens (two NADH) released in the mitochondrion as pyruvate degrades to acetyl-CoA yield five ATPs.
3. Two GTPs (a molecule similar to ATP) are produced in the citric acid cycle via substrate-level phosphorylation.
4. Twelve of the sixteen hydrogens (six NADH) released in the citric acid cycle yield fifteen ATPs (6 NADH × 2.5 ATP per NADH = 15 ATP).
5. Four hydrogens joined to FAD (two $FADH_2$) in the citric acid cycle yield three ATPs.

Thirty-four ATPs represent the total ATP yield from the complete breakdown of glucose. *Because two ATP molecules initially phosphorylate glucose, 32 ATP molecules equal the net ATP yield from complete glucose breakdown in skeletal muscle. Four ATP molecules form directly from substrate-level phosphorylation (glycolysis and citric acid cycle), whereas 28 ATP molecules regenerate during oxidative phosphorylation.* Chapter 5 explains the specifics of carbohydrate's role in energy release under anaerobic and aerobic exercise conditions.

ENERGY RELEASE FROM FAT

Stored fat represents the body's most plentiful source of potential energy. Relative to carbohydrate and protein, stored fat provides almost unlimited energy. The fuel reserves in a typical young adult male equal between 60,000 and 100,000 kcal from triacylglycerol in fat cells **(adipocytes)** and about 3000 kcal from intramuscular triacylglycerol (12 $mmol \cdot kg^{-1}$ muscle). In contrast, the carbohydrate energy reserve generally amounts to less than 2000 kcal. Three energy sources for fat catabolism include:

1. Triacylglycerol stored directly within the muscle fiber in close proximity to the mitochondria (more in slow-twitch than fast-twitch muscle fibers)
2. Circulating triacylglycerol in lipoprotein complexes that hydrolyze on the surface of a tissue's capillary endothelium catalyzed by lipoprotein lipase
3. Circulating FFAs mobilized from triacylglycerol in adipose tissue that serve as bloodborne energy carriers

Before energy release from fat, hydrolysis (**lipolysis** or fat breakdown) splits the triacylglycerol molecule into glycerol and three water-insoluble fatty acid molecules. The enzyme **hormone-sensitive lipase** catalyzes triacylglycerol breakdown as follows:

$$\text{Triacylglycerol} + 3\ H_2O \xrightarrow{\text{lipase}} \text{Glycerol} + 3\ \text{Fatty acids}$$

An intracellular mediator, **adenosine 3',5'-cyclic monophosphate**, or **cyclic AMP**, activates hormone-sensitive lipase and thus regulates fat breakdown.[34] The various fat-mobilizing hormones—epinephrine, norepinephrine, glucagon, and growth hormone—activate cyclic AMP in both adipocytes and muscle cells, which themselves cannot enter the cell.[35] Lactate, ketones, and insulin inhibit cyclic AMP activation.[7]

Adipocytes: Site of Fat Storage and Mobilization

FIGURE 4.20 outlines the dynamics of fat storage and fat mobilization. All cells store some fat; however, adipose tissue serves as an active and major supplier of fatty acid molecules. Adipocytes specialize in synthesizing and storing triacylglycerol. Triacylglycerol fat droplets occupy up to 95% of the adipocyte cell's volume. Once hormone-sensitive lipase stimulates fatty acids to diffuse from the adipocyte into the circulation, nearly all bind to plasma albumin for transport as **FFAs** to active tissues.[8,32] Hence, FFAs are not truly "free" entities. At the muscle site, FFAs release from the albumin–FFA complex for transport across the plasma membrane (by diffusion and/or a protein-mediated carrier system). Once inside the muscle cell, FFAs either re-esterify to form intracellular triacylglycerols or they bind with intramuscular proteins and enter the mitochondria for energy metabolism by action of **carnitine–acyl-CoA transferase.** Medium- and short-chain fatty acids do not depend on carnitine–acyl-CoA

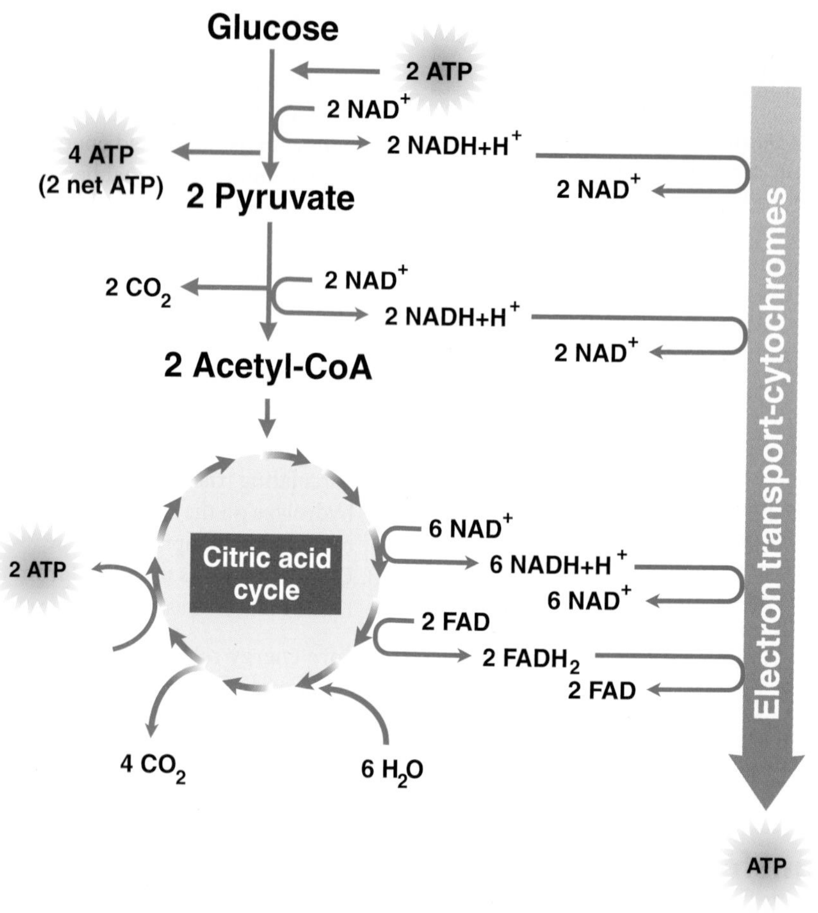

Net ATP from glucose metabolism

Source	Reaction	Net ATP
Substrate phosphorylation	Glycolysis	2
2 H_2 (4 H^+)	Glycolysis	5
2 H_2 (4 H^+)	Pyruvate → Acetyl-CoA	5
Substrate phosphorylation	Citric acid cycle	2
6 H_2 (12 H^+)	Citric acid cycle	15
2 H_2 (H H^+)	Citric acid cycle	3
	Total:	32 ATP

FIGURE 4.19. Net yield of 32 ATP molecules from energy transfer during the complete oxidation of one glucose molecule through glycolysis, the citric acid cycle, and electron transport.

transferase transport, as most diffuse freely into the mitochondrion.

The water-soluble glycerol molecule formed during lipolysis readily diffuses from the adipocyte into the circulation. As a result, plasma glycerol levels often reflect the level of the body's triacylglycerol breakdown.[29] When delivered to the liver, glycerol serves as a gluconeogenic precursor for glucose synthesis. This relatively slow process explains why glycerol supplementation contributes little as an energy substrate during exercise.[24]

Hormonal Effects

Epinephrine, norepinephrine, glucagon, and growth hormone augment lipase activation and subsequent lipolysis and FFA mobilization from adipose tissue. Plasma concentrations of these lipogenic hormones increase during exercise to continually supply active muscles with energy-rich substrate. The intracellular mediator, cyclic AMP, activates hormone-sensitive lipase and thus regulates fat breakdown. The various lipid-mobilizing hormones, which themselves do not enter

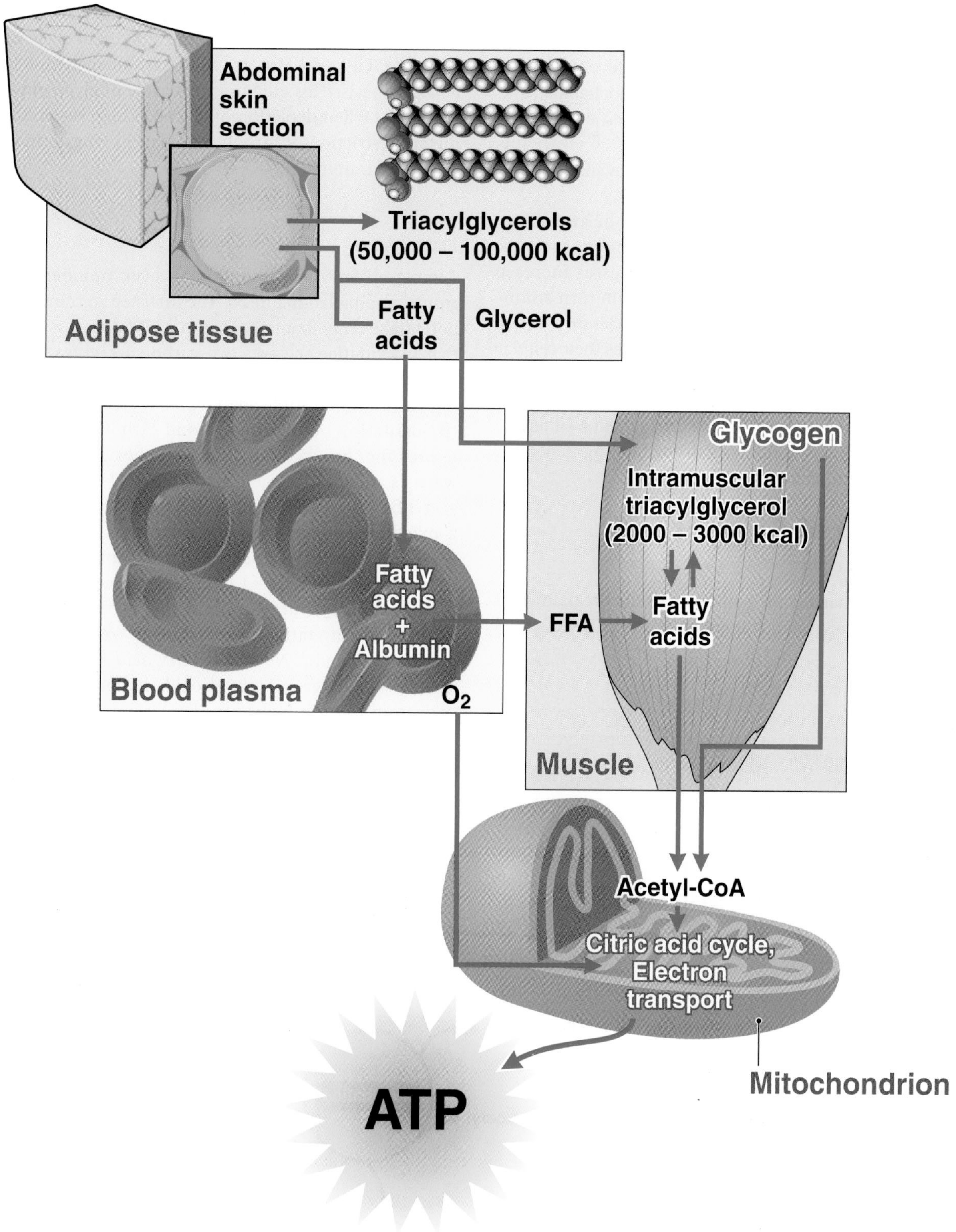

FIGURE 4.20. Dynamics of fat mobilization and storage. Hormone-sensitive lipase stimulates triacylglycerol breakdown into glycerol and fatty acid components. After their release from adipocytes, the blood transports FFAs bound to plasma albumin. Fats stored within the muscle fiber also degrade to glycerol and fatty acids to provide energy.

the cell, activate cyclic AMP.[33] Circulating lactate, ketones, and particularly insulin inhibit cyclic AMP activation.[9] Exercise training–induced increases in the activity level of skeletal muscle and adipose tissue lipases, including biochemical and vascular adaptations in the muscles themselves, enhance fat use for energy during moderate exercise.[6,8,18–20,22,28] Paradoxically, excess body fat decreases fatty acid availability and oxidation during exercise.[23]

Fat breakdown or synthesis depends on the availability of fatty acid molecules. After a meal, when energy metabolism remains relatively low, digestive processes increase FFA and triacylglycerol delivery to cells; this in turn stimulates triacylglycerol synthesis. In contrast, moderate exercise increases fatty acid use of energy, which reduces their cellular concentration. The decrease in intracellular FFAs stimulates triacylglycerol breakdown into glycerol and fatty acid components. Concurrently, hormonal release triggered by exercise stimulates adipose tissue lipolysis to further augment FFA delivery to active muscle.

Breakdown of Glycerol and Fatty Acids

FIGURE 4.21 summarizes the pathways for the breakdown of the glycerol and fatty acid fragments of the triacylglycerol molecule.

Glycerol

The anaerobic reactions of glycolysis accept glycerol as 3-phosphoglyceraldehyde, which then degrades to pyruvate to form ATP by substrate-level phosphorylation. Hydrogen atoms pass to NAD^+, and the citric acid cycle oxidizes pyruvate. Glycerol also provides carbon skeletons for glucose synthesis. This gluconeogenic role of glycerol becomes important when depletion of glycogen reserves occurs from dietary restriction of carbohydrates or in long-term exercise or intense training.

Fatty Acids

Almost all fatty acids contain an even number of carbon atoms ranging from 2 to 26. The first step in transferring the potential energy in a fatty acid to ATP (a process termed *fatty acid oxidation*) cleaves two-carbon acetyl fragments split from the long chain of the fatty acid. The process of converting an FFA to multiple acetyl-CoA molecules is called **beta (β)-oxidation** because the second carbon on a fatty acid is termed the "beta carbon." ATP phosphorylates the reactions, water is added, hydrogens pass to NAD^+ and FAD, and the acetyl fragment joins with coenzyme A to form acetyl-CoA. *β-oxidation provides the same two-carbon acetyl unit as acetyl generated from glucose breakdown.* β-oxidation continues until the entire fatty acid molecule degrades to acetyl-CoA for direct entry into the citric acid cycle. The hydrogens released during fatty acid catabolism oxidize through the respiratory chain. *Note that fatty acid breakdown relates directly with oxygen uptake.* β-oxidation proceeds only when oxygen joins with hydrogen. Under anaerobic conditions, hydrogen remains with NAD^+ and FAD, bringing a halt to fat catabolism.

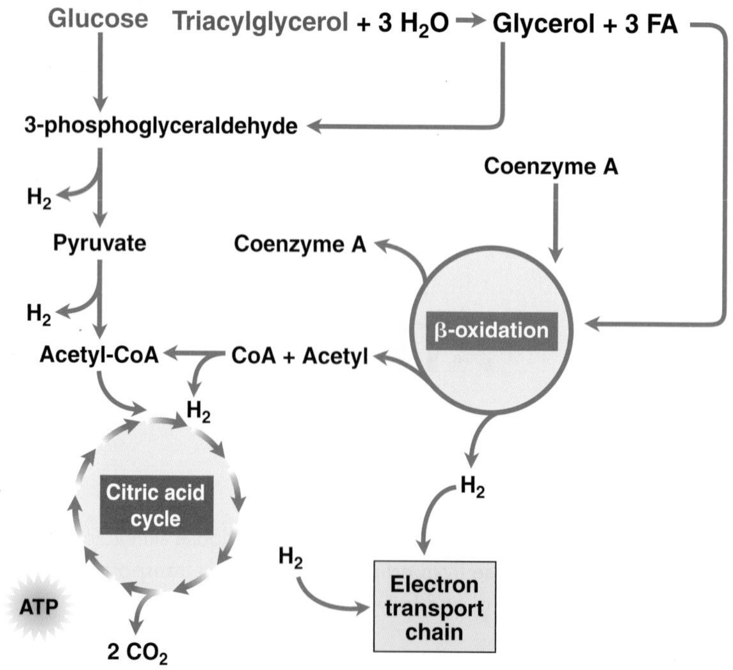

FIGURE 4.21. General scheme for the breakdown of the glycerol and fatty acid fragments of triacylglycerol. Glycerol enters the energy pathways during glycolysis. The fatty acid fragments prepare to enter the citric acid cycle through β-oxidation. The electron transport chain accepts hydrogens released during glycolysis, β-oxidation, and citric acid cycle metabolism. FA, fatty acids.

GLUCOSE IS NOT RETRIEVABLE FROM FATTY ACIDS

Cells can synthesize glucose from pyruvate and other three carbon compounds. However, glucose cannot form from the two-carbon acetyl fragments of the β-oxidation of fatty acids. Consequently, fatty acids cannot readily provide energy for tissues that use glucose almost exclusively for fuel (e.g., brain, blood, and nerve tissues). Just about all dietary lipid occurs in triacylglycerol form. Triacylglycerol's glycerol component can yield glucose, but the glycerol molecule contains only three (6%) of the 57 carbon atoms in the molecule. Thus, fat from dietary sources or stored in adipocytes does not provide an adequate potential glucose source; about 95% of the fat molecule *cannot* be converted to glucose.

Energy Transfer from Fat Catabolism

The breakdown of a fatty acid molecule progresses in three stages as follows:

Stage 1. β-oxidation produces NADH and $FADH_2$ by cleaving the fatty acid molecule into two-carbon acetyl fragments.

Stage 2. Citric acid cycle degrades acetyl-CoA into carbon dioxide and hydrogen atoms.

Stage 3. Hydrogen atoms oxidize by electron transport–oxidative phosphorylation.

The rich hydrogen content of each of the triacylglycerol's three fatty acid molecules allows the complete oxidation of one triacylglycerol molecule to generate about 12 times more ATPs compared with the oxidation of one glucose molecule. Depending on a person's state of nutrition, level of training, and intensity and duration of physical activity, intra- and extracellular lipid molecules usually supply between 30 and 80% of the energy for biologic work.[29,38,41]

EXERCISE INTENSITY AND DURATION AFFECT LEVEL OF FAT OXIDATION

Considerable fatty acid oxidation occurs during low-intensity exercise. For example, fat combustion almost totally powers exercise at 25% of aerobic capacity. Carbohydrate and fat contribute energy equally during more moderate-intensity exercise. Fat oxidation then gradually increases as exercise extends to an hour or more and glycogen depletes. Toward the end of prolonged exercise (with glycogen reserves low), circulating FFAs supply nearly 80% of the total energy required.

When intense, long-duration exercise depletes glycogen reserves, fat serves as the *primary* fuel for exercise and recovery.[20]

FATS BURN IN A CARBOHYDRATE FLAME

Interestingly, fatty acid breakdown depends in part on a continual background level of carbohydrate breakdown. Recall that acetyl-CoA enters the citric acid cycle by combining with oxaloacetate to form citrate. This oxaloacetate is generated from pyruvate during carbohydrate breakdown (under the control of pyruvate carboxylase), which adds a carboxyl group to the pyruvate molecule. Carbohydrate depletion decreases pyruvate production during glycolysis. Diminished pyruvate reduces levels of citric acid cycle intermediates (oxaloacetate and malate), which slows citric acid cycle activity (see **FIGS. 4.18 and 4.23**).[27,31,35,40] Citric acid cycle degradation of fatty acids depends on sufficient oxaloacetate availability to combine with the acetyl-CoA formed during β-oxidation. When the carbohydrate level decreases, the oxaloacetate level may become inadequate. In this sense, "fats burn in a carbohydrate flame."

A Slower Rate of Energy Release from Fat

A rate limit exists for fatty acid use by active muscle.[42] Aerobic training enhances this limit, but the power generated solely by fat breakdown still represents only about one-half that achieved with carbohydrate as the chief aerobic energy source. Thus, depleting muscle glycogen decreases a muscle's maximum aerobic power output. Just as the hypoglycemic condition coincides with a "central" or neural fatigue, muscle glycogen depletion probably causes "peripheral" or local muscle fatigue during exercise.[26]

EXCESS MACRONUTRIENTS (REGARDLESS OF SOURCE) CONVERT TO FAT

Excess energy intake from any fuel source can be counterproductive because this excess, regardless of source, converts to fatty acids and then accumulates as body fat. Surplus dietary carbohydrate first fills the glycogen reserves. Once these reserves fill, excess carbohydrate converts to triacylglycerols for storage in adipose tissue. Excess dietary fat calories move readily into the body's fat depots. Athletes and others who believe that taking protein supplements builds muscle beware. Extra protein consumed above the body's requirement (normally achieved with a well-balanced diet) ends up either catabolized for energy or converted to body fat!

Gluconeogenesis provides a metabolic option to synthesize glucose from noncarbohydrate sources; it cannot, however, replenish or even maintain glycogen stores unless one regularly consumes carbohydrates. Appreciably reducing carbohydrate availability seriously limits energy transfer capacity. Glycogen depletion could occur in prolonged marathon running, consecutive days of heavy training, inadequate energy intake, dietary elimination of carbohydrates (as advocated with high-fat, low-carbohydrate "ketogenic" diets), or diabetes. Diminished aerobic exercise intensity occurs even though large amounts of fatty acid substrate circulate to muscle. During extreme carbohydrate depletion, the acetate fragments produced in β-oxidation accumulate in the extracellular fluids because they cannot readily enter the citric acid cycle. The liver converts these compounds to ketone bodies (four-carbon long acidic derivatives, acetoacetic acid and β-hydroxybutyric acid together with acetone), some of which pass in the urine. If ketosis persists, the acid quality of the body fluids can increase to potentially toxic levels.

LIPOGENESIS

Lipogenesis describes the formation of fat that mostly occurs in the cytoplasm of liver cells. It occurs as follows: Ingested excess glucose or protein not used immediately to sustain metabolism converts into stored triacylglycerol. For example, when muscle and liver glycogen stores fill, as they do following a large carbohydrate-containing meal, insulin release from the pancreas causes a 30-fold increase in glucose transport into adipocytes. Insulin initiates the translocation of a latent pool of GLUT4 transporters from the adipocyte cytosol to the plasma membrane. GLUT4 action facilitates glucose transport into the cytosol for synthesis to triacylglycerols and subsequent storage within the adipocyte.[5] This lipogenic process requires ATP energy and the B vitamins biotin, niacin, and pantothenic acid.

POTENTIAL FOR GLUCOSE SYNTHESIS FROM TRIACYLGLYCEROL COMPONENTS

Although humans cannot convert fatty acids to glucose, the glycerol component of triacylglycerol breakdown supplies the liver with substrate for glucose synthesis. This provides the body with an important, albeit limited, option for maintaining blood glucose for neural and red blood cell functions. It also helps to minimize the muscle-wasting effects of low blood glucose in stimulating excessive muscle protein degradation to gluconeogenic constituents to sustain plasma glucose levels.

Lipogenesis begins with carbons from glucose and the carbon skeletons from amino acid molecules that metabolize to acetyl-CoA (see section on protein metabolism). Liver cells bond the acetate parts of the acetyl-CoA molecules in a series of steps to form the 16-carbon saturated fatty acid palmitic acid. Palmitic acid can then lengthen to an 18- or 20-carbon chain fatty acid in either the cytosol or the mitochondria. Ultimately, three fatty acid molecules join or esterify with one glycerol molecule produced during glycolysis to yield one triacylglycerol molecule. Triacylglycerol releases into the circulation as a very low-density lipoprotein (VLDL); cells may use VLDL for ATP production or store it in adipocytes along with other fats from dietary sources.

ENERGY RELEASE FROM PROTEIN

Chapter 1 emphasized that protein plays a role as an energy substrate during endurance-type activities and intense training. The amino acids, primarily the branched-chain amino acids leucine, isoleucine, valine, glutamine, and aspartate, first convert to a form that readily enters pathways for energy release. This conversion requires nitrogen (amine) removal from the amino acid molecule. The liver serves as the main site for **deamination**, but skeletal muscle also contains enzymes that remove nitrogen from an amine group of an amino acid and pass it to other compounds during **transamination**. In this way, the "carbon skeleton" by-products of donor amino acids participate directly in energy metabolism within muscle. Enzyme levels for transamination increase with exercise training to further facilitate protein's use as an energy substrate.

Once an amino acid loses its nitrogen-containing amine group, the remaining compound (usually a component of the citric acid cycle's reactive compounds) contributes to ATP formation. Some amino acids are **glucogenic** and when deaminated yield intermediate products for glucose synthesis via gluconeogenesis (**FIG. 4.22**). For example, pyruvate forms in the liver as alanine loses its amine group and gains a double-bond oxygen. This makes it possible for pyruvate to synthesize to glucose. This gluconeogenic method serves as an important adjunct to the Cori cycle to provide glucose during prolonged exercise. Regular exercise training enhances the liver's capacity for gluconeogenesis from alanine.[36,37] Other amino acids (such as glycine) are **ketogenic** and when deaminated yield the intermediate acetyl-CoA or acetoacetate. These compounds cannot be synthesized to glucose, but instead are synthesized to fat or catabolized for energy in the citric acid cycle.

Protein Conversion to Fat

Surplus dietary protein (like excess carbohydrate) can readily convert to fat. The amino acids absorbed by the small intestine after protein's digestion are transported in the circulation to the liver. **FIGURE 4.23** illustrates that carbon skeletons derived from these amino acids after deamination

WHEY PROTEIN—THE MOST POPULAR PROTEIN SUPPLEMENT

Whey protein, a mixture of globular proteins derived from milk proteins as part of the cheese manufacturing process, represents the most popular protein supplement sold in powder format. Remember the nursery rhyme *"Little Miss Muffet sat on a tuffet, Eating her curds and whey"*? For decades, whey was used as animal feed. Veterinarians noticed how healthy the animals became when fed whey, which led to research into the benefits of whey protein for humans. By 1992, a process was developed to extract the pure amino acids from milk proteins leaving behind all the remaining sugar (lactose), fat, and cholesterol. What the nutritional scientists came up with is the purest and most biologically available (most easily absorbed) source of protein. Whey protein isolate is a rich source of the eight essential amino acids (including branched-chain amino acids) that the body needs for tissue synthesis, energy, and health.

Whey protein is currently marketed as a dietary supplement and as an aid to facilitate muscular development in response to resistance training. Due to its rapid rate of digestion, it provides a rapid source of amino acids, which are taken up by the muscles to ultimately repair and rebuild muscle tissue. It is most commonly supplemented immediately after resistance training workouts. Recent *Consumer Reports* testing found that due to contamination, some bodybuilding whey-containing protein shakes purchased online exceeded standards for exposure to heavy metals when three servings a day were consumed. Depending on each product's individual serving size recommendations, some three-serving samples involved as much as 210 g (7.4 oz) of powder being tested.

Alert: protein drinks. You don't need the extra protein or the heavy metals our tests found. *Consumer Reports*, July 2010, p. 24–27.

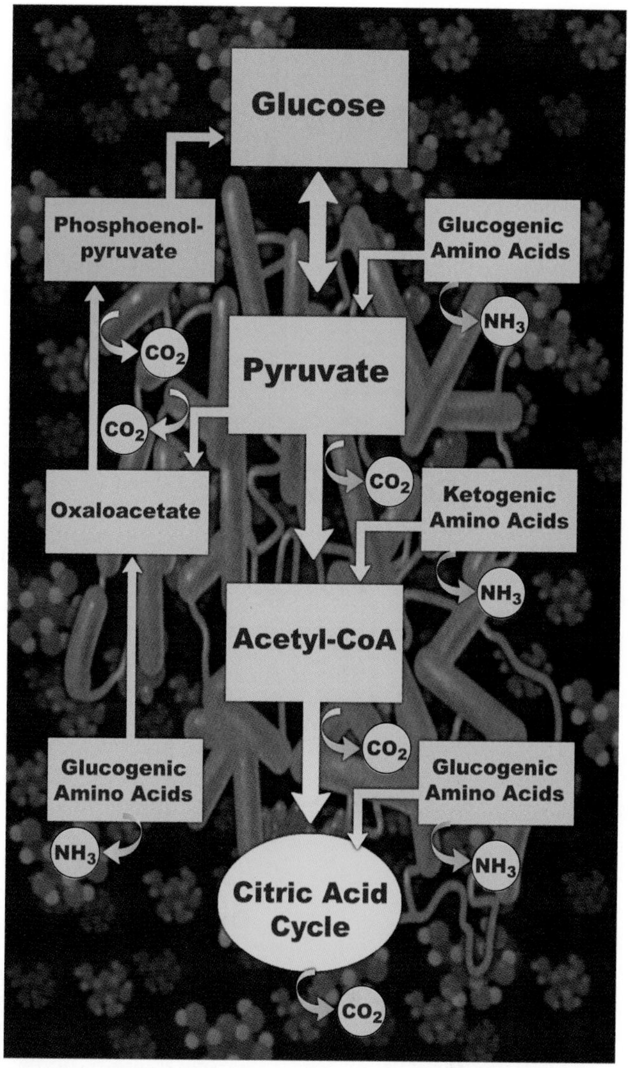

FIGURE 4.22. Glucogenic and ketogenic amino acids. Carbon skeletons from amino acids that form pyruvate or directly enter the citric acid cycle are glucogenic because these carbon compounds can form glucose. Carbon skeletons that form acetyl-CoA are ketogenic because they cannot form glucose molecules but rather synthesize fat.

convert to pyruvate. Pyruvate then enters the mitochondrion for conversion to acetyl-CoA for one of the following functions:

1. Catabolism in the citric acid cycle
2. Fatty acid synthesis

Protein Breakdown Facilitates Water Loss

When protein provides energy, the body must eliminate the nitrogen-containing amine group and other solutes from protein breakdown. This requires excretion of "obligatory" water because the waste products of protein catabolism leave the body dissolved in fluid as urine. For this reason, excessive protein catabolism increases the body's water needs.

THE METABOLIC MILL

The citric acid cycle plays a much more important role than simply degrading pyruvate produced during glucose catabolism. Fragments from other organic compounds formed from fat and protein breakdown provide energy during citric acid cycle metabolism. **FIGURE 4.23** illustrates that deaminated residues of excess amino acids enter the citric acid cycle at various intermediate stages. In contrast, the glycerol fragment of triacylglycerol catabolism gains entrance

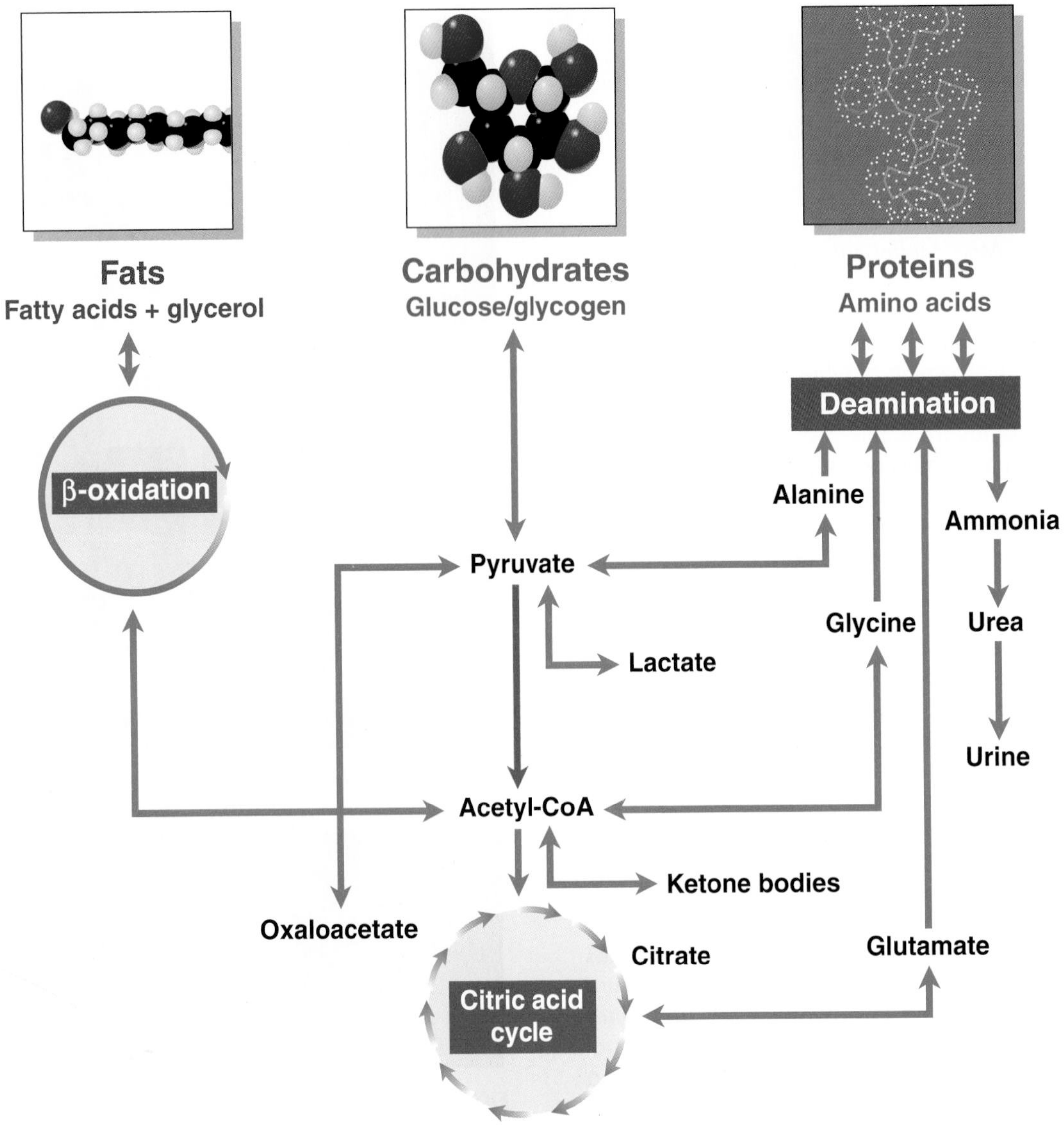

Predominant interconversions	
Carbohydrates	Fats or nonessential amino acids
Fats	Nonessential amino acids
Proteins	Carbohydrates or fats

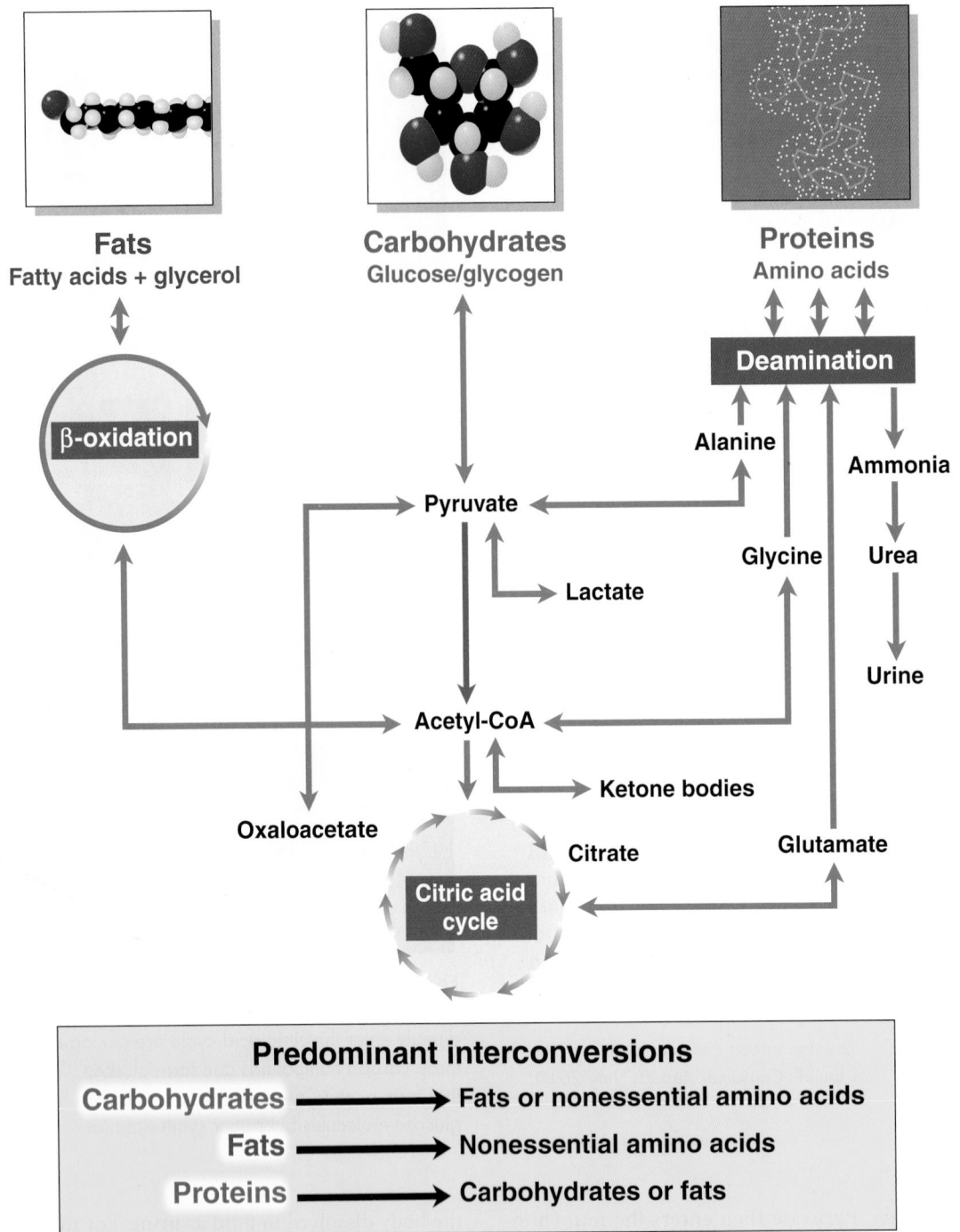

FIGURE 4.23. The "metabolic mill" shows important interconversions among carbohydrates, fats, and proteins. Note that all interconversions are possible except that fatty acids cannot contribute to glucose synthesis (note one-way *red arrow*).

via the glycolytic pathway. Fatty acids become oxidized in β-oxidation to acetyl-CoA. This compound then enters the cycle directly.

The "metabolic mill" depicts the citric acid cycle as the vital link between food (macronutrient) energy and the chemical energy of ATP. The citric acid cycle also serves as a "metabolic hub" to provide intermediates that cross the mitochondrial membrane into the cytosol to synthesize bionutrients for maintenance and growth. For example, excess carbohydrates provide glycerol and acetyl fragments to synthesize triacylglycerol. Acetyl-CoA also functions as the branch point for synthesizing cholesterol, bile, and many hormones, including ketone bodies and fatty acids. Fatty acids *cannot* contribute to glucose synthesis because the conversion of pyruvate to acetyl-CoA does not reverse (notice the one-way arrow in **FIG. 4.23**). Many of the carbon compounds generated in citric cycle reactions also provide the organic starting points for synthesizing nonessential amino acids.

REGULATION OF ENERGY METABOLISM

Under normal conditions, electron transfer and subsequent energy release tightly couple to ADP phosphorylation. In general, without the availability of ADP for phosphorylation to ATP, electrons do not shuttle down the respiratory chain to oxygen. Compounds that either inhibit or activate enzymes at key control points in the oxidative pathways modulate regulatory control of glycolysis and the citric acid cycle.[1,12,14,17,25] Each pathway has at least one enzyme considered "rate limiting" because it controls the speed of that pathway's reactions. By far, cellular ADP concentration exerts the greatest effect on the rate-limiting enzymes that control the energy metabolism of carbohydrates, fats, and proteins. This mechanism for respiratory control makes sense because any increase in ADP signals a need for energy to restore ATP levels. Conversely, high levels of cellular ATP indicate a relatively low energy requirement. From a broader perspective, ADP concentrations function as a cellular feedback mechanism to maintain a relatively constant or homeostatic level of energy currency available for biologic work. Other rate-limiting modulators include cellular levels of phosphate, cyclic AMP, calcium, NAD^+, citrate, and pH.

SUMMARY

1. Food macronutrients provide the major sources of potential energy to rejoin ADP and phosphate ion to form ATP.
2. The complete breakdown of 1 mole of glucose liberates 689 kcal of energy. Of this, ATP bonds conserve about 224 kcal (34%), with the remainder dissipated as heat.
3. During glycolytic reactions in the cell's cytosol, a net of two ATP molecules forms during anaerobic substrate-level phosphorylation.
4. Pyruvate converts to acetyl-CoA during the second stage of carbohydrate breakdown within the mitochondrion. Acetyl-CoA then progresses through the citric acid cycle.
5. Hydrogen atoms released during glucose breakdown oxidize via the respiratory chain; the energy generated couples to ADP phosphorylation.
6. The complete breakdown of a glucose molecule in skeletal muscle theoretically yields a net total of 32 ATP molecules.
7. A biochemical "steady state" or "steady rate" exists when hydrogen atoms oxidize at their rate of formation.
8. During intense exercise, when hydrogen oxidation does not keep pace with its production, lactate forms as pyruvate temporarily binds hydrogen. This allows progression of anaerobic glycolysis for an additional time period.
9. The complete breakdown of a triacylglycerol molecule yields about 460 molecules of ATP. Fatty acid catabolism requires oxygen; the term *aerobic* describes such reactions.
10. Protein serves as a potentially important energy substrate. After nitrogen removal from the amino acid molecule during deamination, the remaining carbon skeletons enter various metabolic pathways to produce ATP aerobically.
11. Numerous interconversions take place among the food nutrients. Fatty acids represent a noteworthy exception because they cannot be synthesized to glucose.
12. Fats require a certain level of carbohydrate breakdown for their continual catabolism for energy in the metabolic mill. To this extent, "fats burn in a carbohydrate flame."
13. Compounds that either inhibit or activate enzymes at key control points in the oxidative pathways modulate control of glycolysis and the citric acid cycle. Cellular ADP concentration exerts the greatest effect on the rate-limiting enzymes that control energy metabolism.

thePoint *Visit* **thePoint.lww.com/MKKSEN4e** *to view the following animations related to content presented in Chapter 4:* ***Biomechanical reactions of the Cori Cycle; Triacylglycerol breakdown; Chemical reactions of mitochondrion; Citric acid cycle; Electron transport; Electron transport chain; Fat mobilization and use; Glycogen synthesis; Glycolysis; Metabolism of amino acids;*** *and* ***Transamination.***

TEST YOUR KNOWLEDGE ANSWERS

1. **True:** Carbohydrates provide 4 $kcal \cdot g^{-1}$ for the body to resynthesize ATP. They convert to glycogen in glycogenesis for storage in muscle and liver. Once the glycogen reserves become filled, any excess energy from carbohydrate readily converts to stored body fat primarily in adipose tissue.

2. **False:** Lipids provide 9 $kcal \cdot g^{-1}$ for ATP resynthesis. They store as fat in adipose tissue for future energy needs. Fatty acids cannot contribute to glucose formation because of the unavailability of the enzyme to convert acetyl-CoA (from fatty acid breakdown) to pyruvate for glucose synthesis.

3. **False:** An enzyme is a highly specific and large organic protein catalyst that accelerates the rate of chemical reactions without being consumed or changed in the reactions.

4. **False:** As for carbohydrates and lipids, excess energy from dietary protein readily converts to fat for storage in adipose tissue. Thus, high-protein diets, if they constitute excess caloric intake, result in positive energy balance and a gain in body fat.

5. **False:** The catabolism of carbohydrates, lipids, and proteins results in ATP formation. On a relative basis, fat and carbohydrate provide their carbon skeletons for ATP synthesis more readily than protein, which primarily serves an anabolic role.

6. **False:** The first law of thermodynamics states that energy is neither created nor destroyed but instead transforms from one form to another without being used up. In essence, the law dictates that the body does not produce, consume, or use up energy; it merely transforms energy from one form into another as physiologic systems undergo continual change.

7. **False:** Oxidation reactions transfer oxygen atoms, hydrogen atoms, or electrons. A loss of electrons occurs in oxidation reactions with a corresponding gain in valence. Reduction reactions involve any process in which atoms gain electrons with a corresponding decrease in valence. Oxidation and reduction reactions always couple, so the energy released by one reaction becomes incorporated into the products of the other reaction.

8. **True:** The term *energy* suggests a dynamic state related to change; thus energy emerges only when a change occurs. Potential energy and kinetic energy constitute the total energy of a system. Potential energy refers to energy associated with a substance's structure or position, while kinetic energy refers to energy of motion. Potential energy can be measured when it transforms to kinetic energy. There are six forms of energy—chemical, mechanical, heat, light, electrical, and nuclear—and each can convert or transform to another form.

9. **False:** In essence, cellular oxidation–reduction constitutes the biochemical mechanism that underlies energy metabolism. The mitochondria, the cell's "energy factories," contain carrier molecules that remove electrons from hydrogen (oxidation) and eventually pass them to oxygen (reduction). ATP synthesis occurs during oxidation–reduction reactions. Aerobic metabolism refers to energy-generating catabolic reactions in which oxygen serves as the final electron acceptor in the respiratory chain and combines with hydrogen to form water. In one sense, the term *aerobic* seems misleading because oxygen does not participate directly in ATP synthesis. On the other hand, oxygen's presence at the end of the line largely determines the capacity for ATP production.

10. **False:** Thirty-four ATP molecules represent the total (gross) ATP yield from the complete breakdown of a glucose molecule. Because two ATP molecules initially phosphorylate glucose, 32 ATP molecules equal the net ATP yield from glucose breakdown in skeletal muscle. Four ATP molecules form directly from substrate-level phosphorylation (glycolysis and citric acid cycle), whereas 28 ATP molecules regenerate during oxidative phosphorylation.

Key References

Balban RS. Regulation of oxidative phosphorylation in the mammalian cell. *Am J Physiol* 1990;258:C377.

Brooks GA. Cell-cell and intracellular lactate shuttles. *J Physiol* 2009;1;587 (Pt 23):5591.

Carins SP, et al. Role of extracellular [Ca2+] in fatigue of isolated mammalian skeletal muscle. *J Appl Physiol* 1998;84:1395.

DiPietro L. Exercise training and fat metabolism after menopause: implications for improved metabolic flexibility in aging. *J Appl Physiol* 2010;109:1569.

Donsmark M, et al. Hormone-sensitive lipase as mediator of lipolysis in contracting skeletal muscle. *Exerc Sport Sci Rev* 2005;33:127.

Febbario MA, et al. Effect of epinephrine on muscle glycogenolysis during exercise in trained men. *J Appl Physiol* 1998;84:465.

Greehnaff PL, Timmons JA. Interaction between aerobic and anaerobic metabolism during intense muscle contraction. *Exerc Sport Sci Rev* 1998;26:1.

Hardie DG. AMP-activated protein kinase: a key system mediating metabolic responses to exercise. *Med Sci Sports Med* 2004;36:28.

Hashimoto T, Brooks GA. Mitochondrial lactate oxidation complex and an adaptive role for lactate production *Med Sci Sports Exerc* 2008;40:486.

Hawley JA, Zierath JR. Integration of metabolic and mitogenic signal transduction in skeletal muscle. *Exerc Sport Sci Rev* 2004;32:4.

Johnson ML, et al. Twelve weeks of endurance training increases FFA mobilization and reesterfication in postmenopausal women. *J Appl Physiol* 2010;109:1573.

Jorgensen SB, et al. Role of AMPK in skeletal muscle metabolic regulation and adaptation in relation to exercise. *J Physiol* 2006;574(pt 1):17.

Kiens B. Skeletal muscle lipid metabolism in exercise and insulin resistance. *Physiol Rev* 2006;86:205.

Messonnierl L, et al. Are the effects of training on fat metabolism involved in the improvement of performance during high intensity exercise? *Eur J Appl Physiol* 2005;94:434.

Mittendorfer B, et al. Excess body fat in men decreases plasma fatty acid availability and oxidation during endurance exercise. *Am J Physiol Endocrinol Metab* 2004;286:E354.

Myburgh KH. Can any metabolites partially alleviate fatigue manifestations at the cross-bridge? *Med Sci Sports Exerc* 2004;36:20.

Nybo L. CNS fatigue and prolonged exercise: effect of glucose supplementation. *Med Sci Sports Exerc* 2003;35:589.

Romijn JA, et al. Regulations of endogenous fat and carbohydrate metabolism in relation to exercise intensity and duration. *Am J Physiol* 1993;265:E380.

Rose AJ, Richter EA. Skeletal muscle glucose uptake during exercise: how is it regulated? *Physiology* 2005;20:260.

Seip RL, Semenkovich CF. Skeletal muscle lipoprotein lipase: molecular regulation and physiological effects in relation to exercise. *Exerc Sport Sci Rev* 1998;26:191.

Sumida KD, Donovan CM. Enhanced hepatic gluconeogenic capacity for selected precursors after endurance training. *J Appl Physiol* 1995;79:1883.

Thompson DL, et al. Substrate use during and following moderate- and low-intensity exercise: implications for weight control. *Eur J Appl Physiol* 1998;78:43.

Trump ME, et al. Importance of muscle phosphocreatine during intermittent maximal cycling. *J Appl Physiol* 1996;80:1574.

Venables MC, et al. Determinants of fat oxidation during exercise in healthy men and women: a cross-sectional study. *J Appl Physiol* 2005;98:160.

Vusse van der GJ, et al. Section 12: Exercise—regulation and integration of multiple systems. In: *Lipid Metabolism in Muscle: Handbook of Physiology.* New York: Oxford Press, 1996.

thePoint *Visit* **thePoint.lww.com/MKKSEN4e** *for a list of the references cited in this chapter, including additional, relevant references.*

CHAPTER 5

Macronutrient Metabolism in Exercise and Training

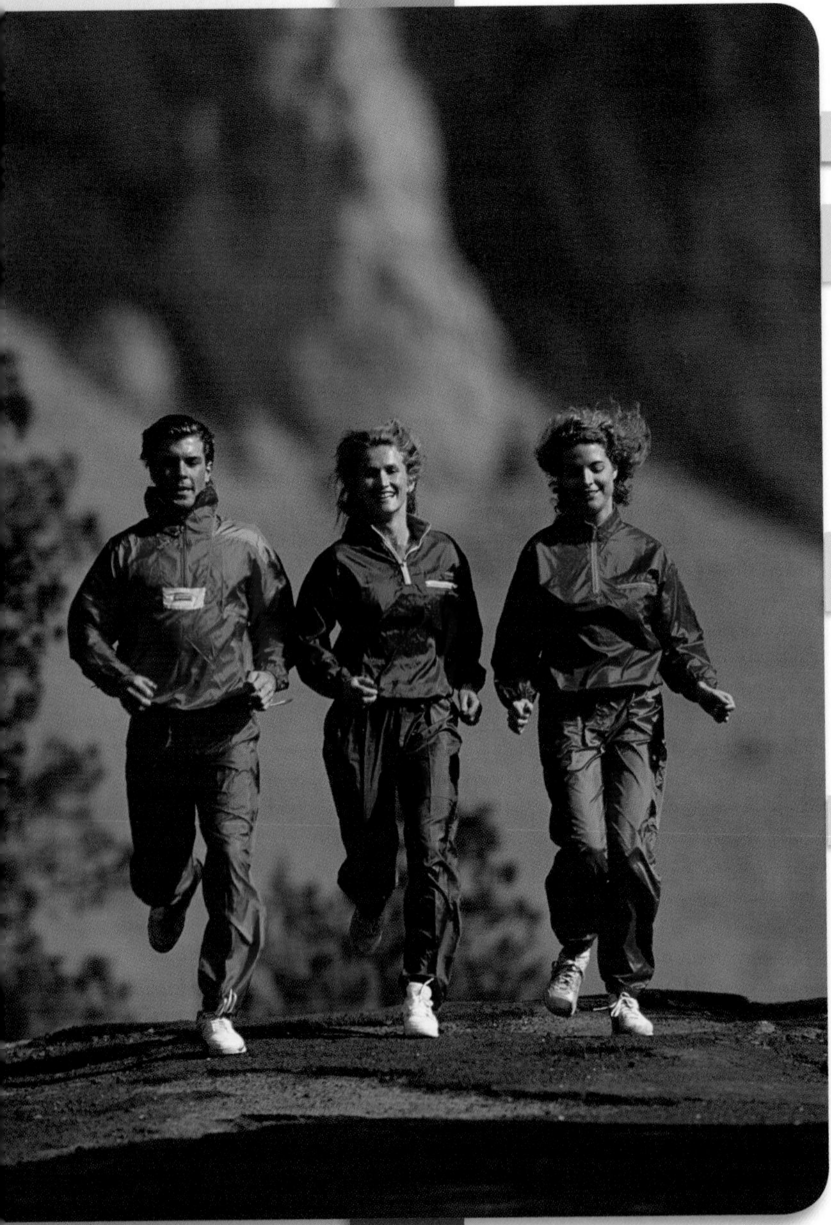

OUTLINE

TEST YOUR KNOWLEDGE

Select true or false for the 10 statements below, then check out the answers at the end of the chapter. Retake the test after you've read the chapter; you should achieve 100%!

	True	False
1. Anaerobic sources supply the predominant energy for short-term, powerful movement activities.	❍	❍
2. Lipid provides the primary energy macronutrient for ATP resynthesis during intense aerobic exercise.	❍	❍
3. As blood flow increases with light and moderate exercise, more free fatty acids leave adipose tissue depots for delivery to active muscle.	❍	❍
4. Carbohydrate provides the preferential energy fuel during intense anaerobic exercise.	❍	❍
5. Severely lowered liver and muscle glycogen levels during prolonged exercise induce fatigue, despite sufficient oxygen availability to muscles and an almost unlimited potential energy from stored fat.	❍	❍
6. A diet low in lipid content reduces fatty acid availability, which negatively affects endurance capacity in intense aerobic exercise.	❍	❍
7. A decrease in blood sugar during prolonged exercise concomitantly increases fat catabolism for energy.	❍	❍
8. Aerobic exercise training enhances the ability to oxidize carbohydrate but not fat during exercise.	❍	❍
9. Because protein provides the building block molecules for tissue synthesis, its catabolism occurs only minimally (<2% of total energy) during exercise.	❍	❍
10. Consuming a high-fat diet in the 7- to 10-day period before a bout of intense exercise significantly improves exercise performance.	❍	❍

Gas exchange in the lungs along with biochemical and biopsy techniques, magnetic resonance imaging, and labeled nutrient tracers provide insight into contributions of the stored macronutrients and high-energy phosphates to exercise bioenergetics. The needle biopsy technique samples small quantities of active muscle to assess intramuscular nutrient kinetics throughout exercise. Such data provide an objective basis for recommending meal plans during exercise training and specific nutritional modifications before, during, and in recovery from strenuous competition. *The fuel mixture that powers exercise generally depends on the intensity and duration of effort and the exerciser's fitness and nutritional status.*

THE ENERGY SPECTRUM OF EXERCISE

FIGURE 5.1 depicts the relative contributions of anaerobic and aerobic energy sources during various durations of maximal exercise. In addition, **TABLE 5.1** lists the approximate percentage of total energy for adenosine triphosphate (ATP) resynthesis from each energy transfer system for different competition running events. The data represent estimates from all-out running experiments in the laboratory, but they can relate to other activities by drawing the appropriate time relationships. A 100-m sprint run equates to any all-out activity lasting about 10 seconds, whereas an

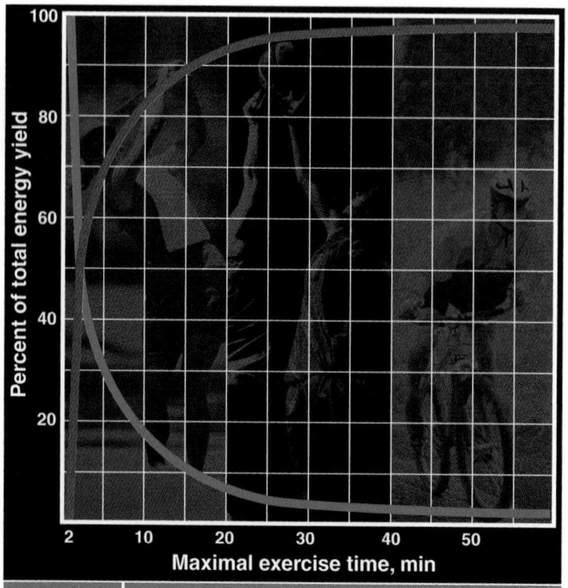

	Duration of maximal exercise									
	seconds			minutes						
	10	30	60	2	4	10	30	60	120	
Percent anaerobic	90	80	70	50	35	15	5	2	1	
Percent aerobic	10	20	30	50	65	85	95	98	99	

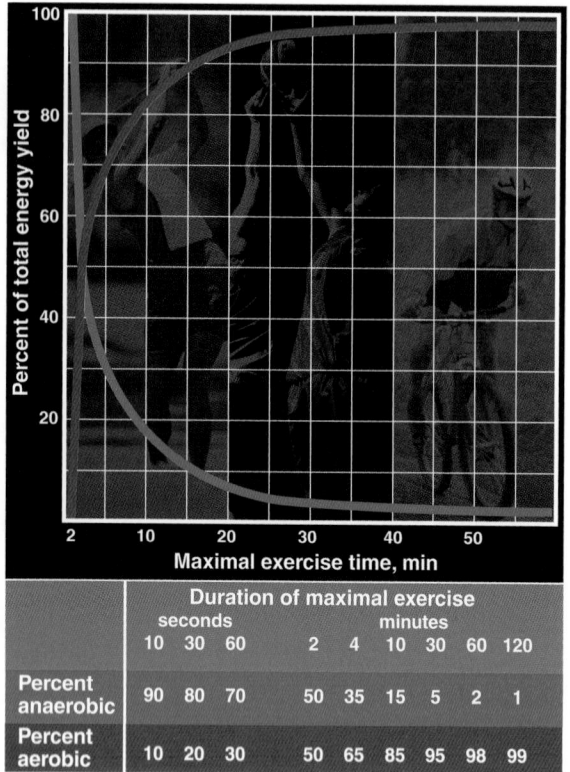

FIGURE 5.1. Relative contributions of aerobic (*red*) and anaerobic (*blue*) energy metabolism during maximal physical effort of varying durations. Note that 2 minutes of maximal effort require about 50% of the energy from both aerobic and anaerobic processes. At a world-class 4-minute per mile pace, approximately 65% of the energy comes from aerobic metabolism, with the remainder generated from anaerobic processes. For a marathon, on the other hand, the energy derived from aerobic processes almost totally powers the run.

800-m run lasts approximately 2 minutes. Maximal exercise for 1 minute includes the 400-m dash in track, the 100-m swim, and multiple full-court presses at the end of a basketball game.

The sources for energy transfer exist along a continuum. At one extreme, intramuscular high-energy phosphates ATP and phosphocreatine (PCr) supply most energy for exercise. The ATP–PCr and lactic acid systems provide about half of the energy required for intense exercise lasting 2 minutes; aerobic reactions provide the remainder. For top performance in all-out 2-minute exercise, a person must possess a well-developed capacity for *both* aerobic and anaerobic metabolism. Intense exercise of intermediate duration performed for 5 to 10 minutes, like middle-distance running and swimming or basketball, requires a greater demand for aerobic energy transfer. Performances of longer duration—marathon running, distance swimming and cycling, recreational jogging, and hiking and backpacking—require a fairly steady energy supply derived aerobically without reliance on lactate formation.

Generally, anaerobic sources supply most of the energy for fast movements or during increased resistance to movement at a given speed. When movement begins at either fast or slow speed, the intramuscular high-energy phosphates provide immediate anaerobic energy for muscle action. After a few seconds, the glycolytic pathway (intramuscular glycogen breakdown in glycolysis) generates an increasingly greater proportion of energy for ATP resynthesis. Intense exercise continued beyond 30 seconds places a progressively greater demand on the relatively slower aerobic energy metabolism of the stored macronutrients. For example, power output during 30 seconds of maximal exercise (e.g., sprint cycling or running) is about twice the power output generated exercising all-out for 5 minutes at one's maximal

TABLE 5.1 Estimated Percentage Contribution of Different Fuels to ATP Generation in Various Running Events

	Percentage contribution to ATP generation				
		Glycogen			
Event	Phosphocreatine	Anaerobic	Aerobic	Blood glucose (Liver glycogen)	Triacylglycerol (Fatty acids)
100 m	50	50	—	—	—
200 m	25	65	10	—	—
400 m	12.5	65.5	25	—	—
800 m	6	50	44	—	—
1500 m	[a]	25	75	—	—
5000 m	[a]	12.5	87.5	—	—
10,000 m	[a]	3	97	—	—
Marathon	—	—	75	5	20
Ultramarathon (80 km)	—	—	35	5	60
24-hour race	—	—	10	2	88

From Newsholme EA, et al. Physical and mental fatigue. Br Med Bull 1992;48:477.

[a] *In such events, phosphocreatine will be used for the first few seconds and, if it has been resynthesized during the race, in the sprint to the finish.*

oxygen uptake. Some activities rely predominantly on a single energy transfer system, whereas more than one energy system powers most physical activities, depending on their intensity and duration. Higher intensity and shorter duration activities place greater demand on anaerobic energy transfer.

LACTIC ACID AND PH

Hydrogen ions (H^+) dissociating from lactic acid, rather than undissociated lactate (La^-), present the primary problem to the body. At normal pH levels, lactic acid almost immediately completely dissociates to H^+ and La^- ($C_3H_5O_3^-$). There are few problems if the amount of free H^+ does not exceed the body's ability to buffer them and maintain the pH at a relatively stable level. The pH decreases when excessive lactic acid (H^+) exceeds the body's immediate buffering capacity. Discomfort occurs and performance decreases as the blood becomes more acidic.

Two main macronutrient sources provide energy for ATP resynthesis during exercise: (1) liver and muscle glycogen and (2) triacylglycerols within adipose tissue and active muscle. To a lesser degree, amino acids within skeletal muscle donate carbon skeletons (minus nitrogen) to processes of energy metabolism. **FIGURE 5.2** provides a generalized overview of the relative contribution to energy metabolism of carbohydrate, fat, and protein for adequately nourished individuals during rest and various exercise intensities. This illustration does not depict the considerable alterations in metabolic mixture (increases in fat and protein breakdown) during prolonged, intense exercise with accompanying depletion of liver and muscle glycogen. The following sections discuss the specific energy contribution of each macronutrient during exercise and the adaptations in substrate use with training.

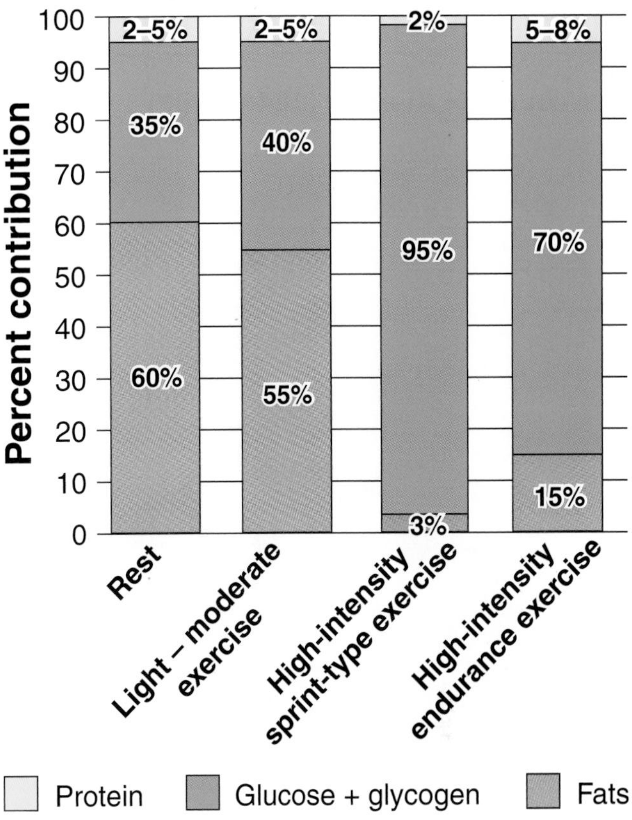

FIGURE 5.2. Generalized illustration of the contribution of the carbohydrate (green), fat (orange), and protein (yellow) macronutrients to energy metabolism at rest and during various intensities of exercise.

CARBOHYDRATE MOBILIZATION AND USE DURING EXERCISE

The liver markedly increases its release of glucose for use by active muscle as exercise progresses from low to high intensity.[9,58] Simultaneously, glycogen stored within muscle serves as the predominant carbohydrate energy source during the early stages of exercise and as exercise intensity increases.[21,43,50,53] Compared with fat and protein catabolism, carbohydrate remains the preferential fuel during intense aerobic exercise because it rapidly supplies ATP during oxidative processes. In anaerobic effort (reactions of glycolysis), carbohydrate becomes the *sole* contributor of ATP.

Carbohydrate availability in the metabolic mixture during exercise helps regulate fat mobilization and its use for energy.[14,15] For example, increasing carbohydrate oxidation by ingesting rapidly absorbed (high-glycemic) carbohydrates before exercise (with associated hyperglycemia and hyperinsulinemia) blunts long-chain fatty acid oxidation by skeletal muscle and free fatty acid (FFA) liberation from adipose tissue during exercise. Perhaps increased carbohydrate availability (and resulting increased catabolism) inhibits long-chain fatty acid transport into the mitochondria, thus controlling the metabolic mixture in exercise. It also appears that the concentration of blood glucose provides feedback regulation of the liver's glucose output; an increase in blood glucose inhibits hepatic glucose release during exercise.[24]

Connections to the Past

Wilbur Olin Atwater (1844–1907)

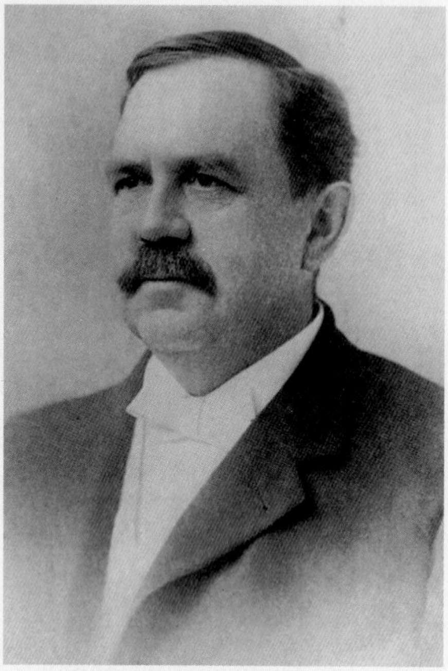

Wilbur O. Atwater received his Ph.D. from Yale University in 1869 for studies on the chemical composition of corn. Studying in Berlin and Leipzig, he became familiar with well-known scientists Voit, Rubner, and Zuntz. As Professor of Chemistry at Wesleyan University, he studied the effects of fertilizers in farming and established the first agricultural experimental station in the United States at Wesleyan in 1875, (which in 1877 became part of the famous Sheffield Scientific School at Yale. From 1879 to 1882, Atwater determined the chemical composition and nutritive values of fish and animal tissues. Returning to Germany in 1882–1883, he studied the metabolism of mammals in Voit's laboratory. Atwater's familiarity with German techniques for measuring respiration and metabolism helped him to conduct human nutrition studies—food analysis, dietary evaluations, energy requirements for work, digestibility of foods, and economics of food production. He helped to convince the United States Government to fund studies of human nutrition. Atwater directed various studies at agricultural experiment stations throughout the country that resulted in the 1896 publication of 2600 chemical analyses of American foodstuffs. An additional 4000 analyses were completed in 1899, including another 1000 analyses done under Atwater's supervision.

thePoint *Visit* **thePoint.lww.com/MKKSEN4e** *for more details about Atwater's pioneering metabolic studies that helped shape the emerging science of human nutrition and exercise physiology.*

INTENSE EXERCISE

With strenuous exercise, neural–humoral factors increase hormonal output of epinephrine, norepinephrine, and glucagon and decrease insulin release. These actions stimulate **glycogen phosphorylase** to augment glycogen breakdown (glycogenolysis) in the liver and active muscles. In the early minutes of exercise when oxygen use fails to meet energy demands, stored muscle glycogen becomes the primary energy contributor because it provides energy without oxygen. As exercise duration progresses, bloodborne glucose from the liver increases its contribution as a metabolic fuel. Blood glucose, for example, can supply 30% of the total energy required by active muscle, with *most* of the remaining carbohydrate energy supplied by intramuscular glycogen.[17,45] *Carbohydrate availability in the metabolic mixture controls its use. In turn, carbohydrate intake dramatically affects its availability.*

One hour of intense exercise decreases liver glycogen by about 55%, and a 2-hour strenuous workout just about depletes glycogen in the liver and specifically exercised muscles. **FIGURE 5.3** illustrates that muscle uptake of circulating blood glucose increases sharply during the initial stage of exercise and continues to increase as exercise progresses. By the 40-minute mark, glucose uptake rises to between 7 and 20 times the resting uptake, depending on exercise intensity. Carbohydrate breakdown predominates when oxygen supply or use does not meet a muscle's needs, as in intense anaerobic exercise.[7] *During intense aerobic exercise, the advantage of selective dependence on carbohydrate metabolism lies in its two times more rapid energy transfer compared with that of fat or protein.* Furthermore, compared with fat, carbohydrate generates about 6% more energy per unit of oxygen consumed.

Moderate and Prolonged Exercise

Glycogen stored in active muscle supplies almost all of the energy in the transition from rest to moderate exercise, just as it does in intense exercise. During the next 20 minutes or so of exercise, liver and muscle glycogen supply between 40 and 50% of the energy requirement; the remainder is provided by fat breakdown (intramuscular triacylglycerols, which may contribute up to 20% of the total exercise energy expenditure,[41] including a small use of protein). (The nutrient energy mixture depends on the relative intensity of submaximal exercise. In light exercise, fat remains the main energy substrate [see **FIG. 5.9**]). As exercise continues and muscle glycogen stores diminish, blood glucose from the liver becomes the major supplier of carbohydrate energy. Still, fat provides an

Additional Insights

Can Sudden Strenuous Exercise Be Harmful to the Heart?

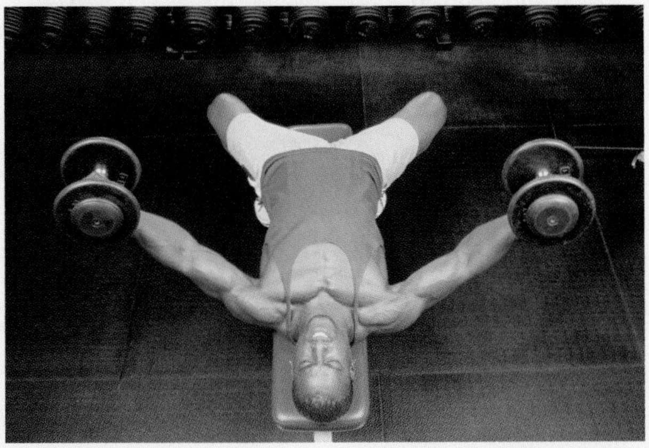

A person running along the roadside, swimming laps in the pool, or shoveling snow from the walkway on a winter day projects the image of health along the wellness spectrum. Yet, is there any truth to those reports about poorly conditioned people suffering a heart attack or sudden death during an uncharacteristic sudden burst of strenuous physical activity—including a broad range of sexual activity. Recent research analyzed 14 studies of "episodic physical activity" and concluded it related to a more than a three fold increased risk of heart attack and a five fold increase in sudden death risk brought on by a confluence of hemodynamic and electrophysiologic maladjustments to exercise in susceptible individuals. Of those studies reviewed, 10 assessed heart attacks, 3 evaluated sudden cardiac death (with fatal arrhythmia the most common mechanism of death), and considered the risk of acute coronary syndrome. Overall, the absolute increased risk for heart attack associated with 1 hour of sporadic physical activity weekly was only two to three additional coronary events per 10,000 person-years and one per 10,000 person-years for sudden cardiac death, with the risk greatest for those unaccustomed to regular physical activity.

The takeaway message is to enhance one's physical activity profile so it changes to more regular rather than sporadic. Individuals with the highest levels of regular exercise had a smaller risk increase, if any at all. For every additional time per week an individual was habitually exposed to physical activity, the relative risk for myocardial infarction decreased by 45% and sudden cardiac death risk decreased by 30%.

Source: Dahabreh IJ, Paulus JK. Association of episodic physical and sexual activity with triggering of acute cardiac events: systematic review and meta-analysis. *JAMA* 2011;305:1225.

Related References

American College of Sports Medicine and American Heart Association: Joint position statement. Exercise and acute cardiovascular events: placing the risks into perspective. *Med Sci Sports Exerc* 2007;9:886.

Chiuve SE, et al. Adherence to a low-risk, healthy lifestyle and risk of sudden cardiac death among women. *JAMA* 2011;306:62.

Čulić V. Association between episodic physical and sexual activity and acute cardiac events. *JAMA* 2011;306:265.

Smith DL. Firefighter fitness: improving performance and preventing injuries and fatalities. *Curr Sports Med Rep* 2011;10:167.

increasingly larger percentage of the total energy metabolism. Eventually, plasma glucose concentration decreases because the liver's glucose output fails to keep pace with its use by muscles. During 90 minutes of strenuous exercise, blood glucose may actually decrease to **hypoglycemic levels** (<45 mg · dL^{-1} blood).[18]

FIGURE 5.4 depicts the metabolic profile during prolonged exercise in the glycogen-depleted and glycogen-loaded states. With glycogen depletion, blood glucose levels fall as submaximal exercise progresses. Concurrently, the level of fatty acids circulating in the blood increases dramatically compared with the same exercise with adequate glycogen reserves. Protein also provides an increased contribution to the energy pool. With carbohydrate depletion, exercise intensity (expressed as a percentage of maximum) progressively decreases after 2 hours to about 50% of the starting exercise intensity. The reduced power output level comes directly from the relatively slow rate of aerobic energy release from fat oxidation, which now becomes the primary energy source.[22,54]

Carbohydrate and fat breakdown use identical pathways for acetyl-coenzyme A (CoA) oxidation. Thus, metabolic processes that precede the citric acid cycle (e.g., β-oxidation, fatty acid activation, and intracellular and mitochondrial transport) most likely account for the relatively slow rate of fat versus carbohydrate oxidation. **FIGURE 5.5** lists these possible rate-limiting factors.

Nutrient-Related Fatigue

Severely lowered levels of liver and muscle glycogen during exercise induce fatigue, despite sufficient oxygen availability to muscles and almost unlimited potential energy from stored fat. Endurance athletes commonly refer to this extreme sensation of fatigue as "bonking" or "hitting the wall." The image of hitting the wall suggests an inability to continue exercising, which in reality is not the case, although pain becomes apparent in the active muscles and exercise intensity decreases markedly. Because of the absence of the phosphatase enzyme in skeletal muscle (which releases glucose from liver cells), the relatively inactive muscles retain all of their glycogen. Controversy exists about

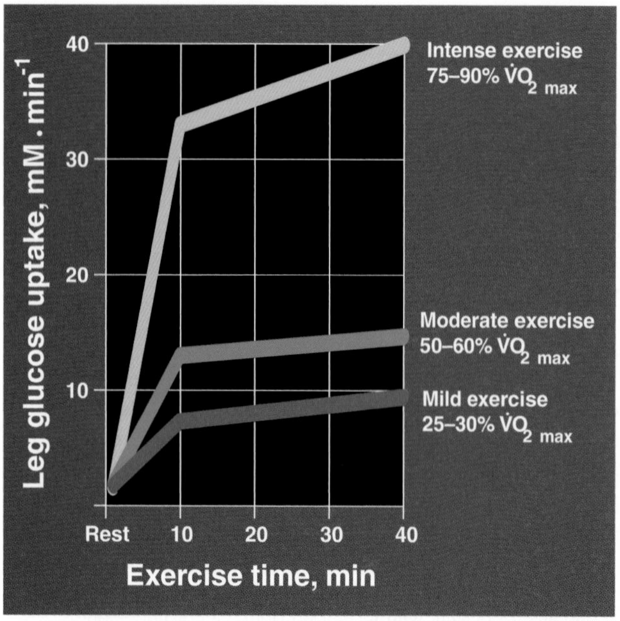

FIGURE 5.3. Exercise duration and intensity affect blood glucose uptake by the leg muscles. Exercise intensity is expressed as a percentage of an individual's $\dot{V}O_{2max}$. (From Felig P, Wahren J. Fuel homeostasis in exercise. *N Engl J Med* 1975;293:1078.)

why carbohydrate depletion during prolonged exercise coincides with reduced exercise capacity. Part of the answer relates to three factors:

1. Use of blood glucose as energy for the central nervous system
2. Muscle glycogen's role as a "primer" in fat metabolism
3. Slower rate of energy release from fat catabolism than from carbohydrate breakdown

REGULAR EXERCISE IMPROVES CAPACITY FOR CARBOHYDRATE METABOLISM

Aerobically trained muscle exhibits a greater capacity to oxidize carbohydrate than untrained muscle. Consequently, considerable amounts of pyruvate move through the aerobic energy pathways during intense endurance exercise following training.[20] A trained muscle's augmented mitochondrial oxidative capacity and increased glycogen storage helps to explain its enhanced capacity for carbohydrate breakdown. During submaximal exercise, the endurance-trained muscle exhibits *decreased* reliance on muscle glycogen and blood glucose as fuel sources and *greater*

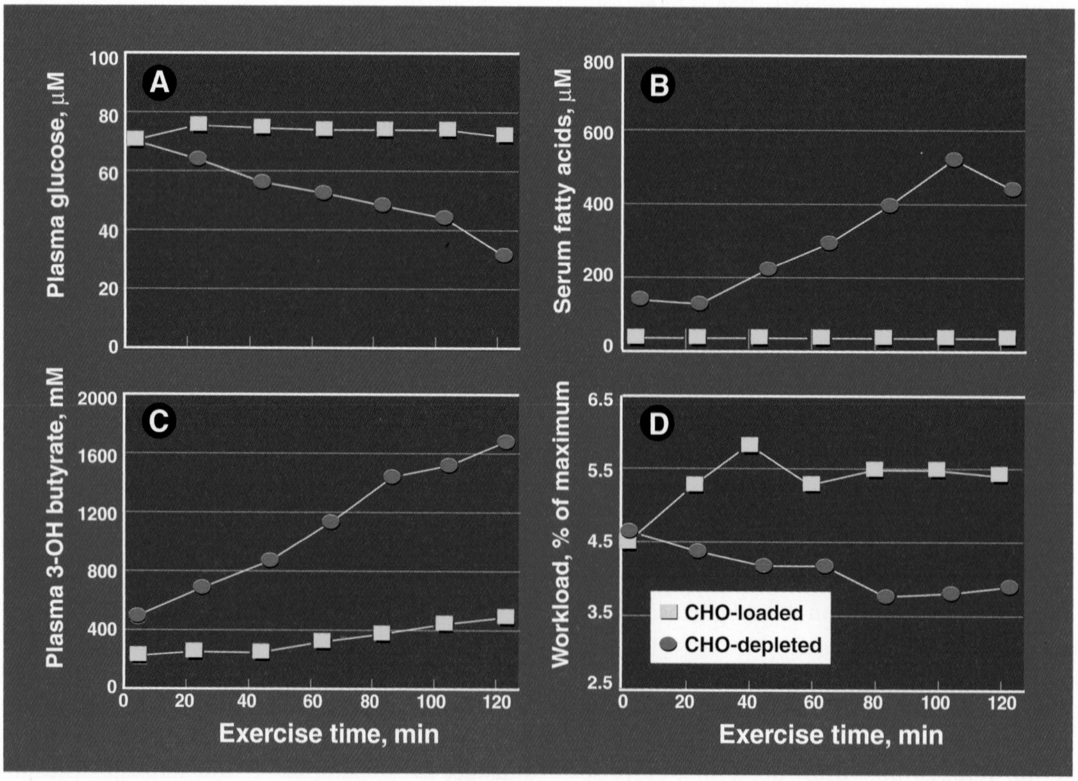

FIGURE 5.4. Dynamics of nutrient metabolism in the glycogen-loaded and glycogen-depleted states. During exercise with limited carbohydrate (CHO) availability, blood glucose levels **(A)** progressively decrease, while fat metabolism **(B)** progressively increases compared with similar exercise when glycogen loaded. In addition, protein use for energy **(C),** as indicated by plasma levels of 3-OH butyrate, remains considerably higher with glycogen depletion. After 2 hours, exercise capacity **(D)** decreases to about 50% of maximum in exercise begun in the glycogen-depleted state. (From Wagenmakers AJM, et al. Carbohydrate supplementation, glycogen depletion, and amino acid metabolism. *Am J Physiol* 1991;260:E883.)

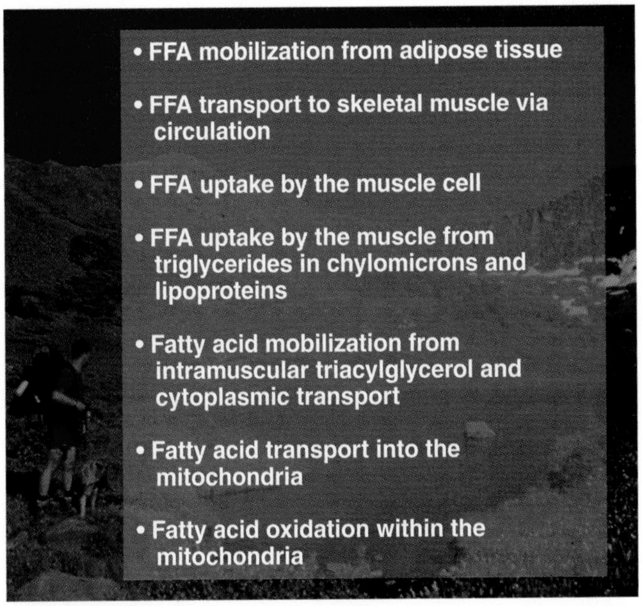
• FFA mobilization from adipose tissue
• FFA transport to skeletal muscle via circulation
• FFA uptake by the muscle cell
• FFA uptake by the muscle from triglycerides in chylomicrons and lipoproteins
• Fatty acid mobilization from intramuscular triacylglycerol and cytoplasmic transport
• Fatty acid transport into the mitochondria
• Fatty acid oxidation within the mitochondria

FIGURE 5.5. Processes that potentially limit the magnitude of fat oxidation during aerobic exercise.

fat use. This training adaptation represents a desirable response because it conserves the body's limited glycogen reserves.

Gender Differences in Substrate Use During Exercise

Available data support the notion of gender differences in carbohydrate metabolism in exercise. During submaximal exercise at equivalent percentages of $\dot{V}O_{2max}$ (i.e., same relative workload), women derive a *smaller* proportion of total energy from carbohydrate oxidation than men; this gender difference in substrate oxidation does not persist into recovery.[23,25]

Gender Differences in Training Effects on Substrate Use

With similar endurance training protocols, both women and men show a decrease in glucose flux for a given submaximal power output.[10,19] At the same relative workload after training, women display an exaggerated shift toward fat catabolism, whereas men do not.[26] This suggests that endurance training induces greater glycogen sparing at a given relative submaximal exercise intensity for women than for men. This gender difference in substrate metabolism's response to training may reflect differences in sympathetic nervous system adaptation to regular exercise (i.e., a more blunted catecholamine response for women). The sex hormones estrogen and progesterone may affect metabolic mixture indirectly via interactions with the catecholamines or directly by augmenting lipolysis and/or constraining glycolysis.[6] Five potential sites for endocrine regulation of substrate use include:

1. Substrate availability (via effects on nutrient storage)
2. Substrate mobilization from body tissue stores
3. Substrate uptake at tissue site of use
4. Substrate uptake within tissue itself
5. Substrate trafficking among storage, oxidation, and recycling

Any glycogen-sparing metabolic adaptations to training could benefit a woman's performance during intense endurance competition.

EFFECT OF DIET ON GLYCOGEN STORES AND ENDURANCE CAPACITY

We emphasized earlier that active muscle relies on ingested carbohydrate as a readily available energy nutrient. Diet composition profoundly affects glycogen reserves. **FIGURE 5.6** shows the results from a classic experiment in which dietary

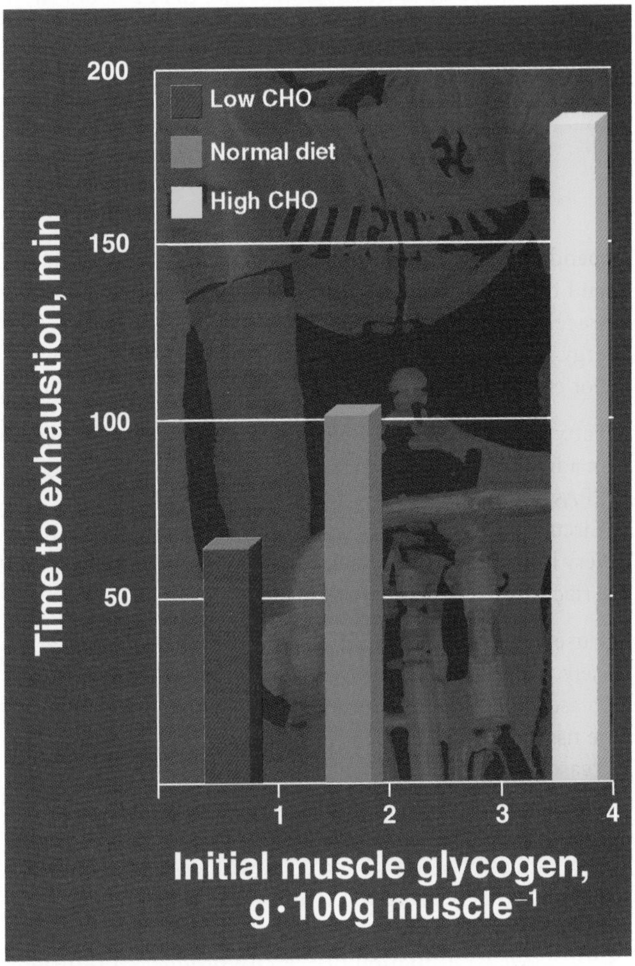

FIGURE 5.6. Effects of a low-carbohydrate (CHO) diet, mixed diet, and high-CHO diet on glycogen content of the quadriceps femoris muscle and duration of endurance exercise on a bicycle ergometer. With a high-CHO diet, endurance time increases three times more than with a low-CHO diet. (Adapted from Bergstrom J, et al. Diet, muscle glycogen and physical performance. *Acta Physiol Scand* 1967;71:140.)

manipulation varied muscle glycogen concentration. In one condition, caloric intake remained normal in six subjects for 3 days when lipid supplied most ingested calories (<5% as carbohydrate). In the second condition, the 3-day diet contained the recommended daily percentages of carbohydrate, lipid, and protein. With the third diet, carbohydrates supplied 82% of the calories. The needle biopsy technique determined glycogen content of the quadriceps femoris muscle; it averaged 0.63 g of glycogen per 100 g wet muscle with the high-fat diet, 1.75 g for the normal diet, and 3.75 g for the high-carbohydrate diet.

Endurance capacity during cycling exercise varied considerably depending on each person's diet for the 3 days before the exercise test. With the normal diet, exercise lasted an average of 114 minutes, but only 57 minutes with the high-fat diet. Endurance capacity of subjects fed the high-carbohydrate diet averaged more than three times greater than that with the high-fat diet. In all instances, the point of fatigue coincided with the same low level of muscle glycogen. This clearly demonstrated the importance of muscle glycogen to maintain intense exercise lasting more than 1 hour. These results emphasize the important role that diet plays in establishing appropriate energy reserves for long-term exercise and strenuous training.

A carbohydrate-deficient diet rapidly depletes muscle and liver glycogen; it subsequently affects performance in all-out, short-term (anaerobic) exercise and in prolonged intense endurance (aerobic) activities. These observations pertain to both athletes and physically active individuals who modify their diets by reducing carbohydrate intake below recommended levels (see Chapter 1). Reliance on starvation diets or potentially harmful low-carbohydrate, high-fat diets or low-carbohydrate, high-protein diets remains counterproductive for weight control, exercise performance, optimal nutrition, and good health. A low-carbohydrate diet makes it extremely difficult from the standpoint of energy supply to engage in vigorous physical activity.[3,13,34,41] Because of carbohydrate's important role in central nervous system function and neuromuscular coordination, training and competing under conditions of low glycogen reserves also increases the likelihood of injury. More is said in Chapter 8 concerning optimizing carbohydrate availability before, during, and in recovery from intense exercise training and competition.

FAT MOBILIZATION AND USE DURING EXERCISE

Depending on nutritional and fitness status of the individual and the exercise intensity and duration, intracellular and extracellular fat supplies between 30 and 80% of exercise energy requirement.[4,30,46,57] Three lipid sources supply the major energy for light-to-moderate exercise:

1. Fatty acids released from the triacylglycerol storage sites in adipocytes and delivered relatively slowly to muscles as FFAs bound to plasma albumin
2. Circulating plasma triacylglycerol bound to lipoproteins as very low-density lipoproteins and chylomicrons
3. Triacylglycerol within the active muscle itself

Fat use for energy in light and moderate exercise varies closely with blood flow through adipose tissue (a threefold increase is not uncommon) and through active muscle. Adipose tissue releases more FFAs to active muscle as blood flow increases with exercise. Hence, somewhat greater quantities of fat from adipose tissue depots participate in energy metabolism. The energy contribution from intramuscular triacylglycerol ranges between 15 and 35%, with endurance-trained men and women using the largest quantity, and substantial impairment in use among the obese and type 2 diabetics.[16,29,30,32,42,51] Initiation of exercise produces a transient initial drop in plasma FFA concentration from the increased uptake by active muscles and the time lag in the release and delivery from adipocytes. Subsequently, increased FFA release from adipose tissue (and concomitant suppression of triacylglycerol formation) occurs through hormonal–enzymatic stimulation by sympathetic nervous system activation and decreased insulin levels. Subcutaneous abdominal adipocytes represent a particularly lively area for lipolysis compared with fat cells in the gluteal–femoral region. When exercise transitions to a high intensity, FFA release from adipose tissue fails to increase much above resting levels, which eventually produces a decrease in plasma FFAs. This, in turn, increases muscle glycogen usage, with a concurrent large increase in intramuscular triacylglycerol oxidation (see **FIG. 5.9**).[44]

On a relative basis, considerable fatty acid oxidation occurs during low-intensity exercise. For example, fat combustion almost totally powers light exercise at 25% of aerobic capacity. Carbohydrate and fat combustion contribute energy equally during moderate exercise. Fat oxidation gradually increases as exercise extends to an hour or more and glycogen depletes. Toward the end of prolonged exercise (with glycogen reserves low), circulating FFAs supply nearly 80% of the total energy required. **FIGURE 5.7** shows this phenomenon for a subject who exercised continuously for 6 hours. A steady decline occurred in carbohydrate combustion (reflected by the respiratory quotient [RQ]; see Chapter 6) during exercise with an accompanying increase in fat combustion. Toward the end of exercise, 84% of the total energy for exercise came from fat breakdown! This experiment, conducted nearly 75 years ago, illustrates fat oxidation's important contribution in prolonged exercise with glycogen depletion.

The hormones epinephrine, norepinephrine, glucagon, and growth hormone activate hormone-sensitive lipase. This causes lipolysis and mobilization of FFAs from adipose tissue. Exercise increases plasma levels of lipogenic hormones, so the active

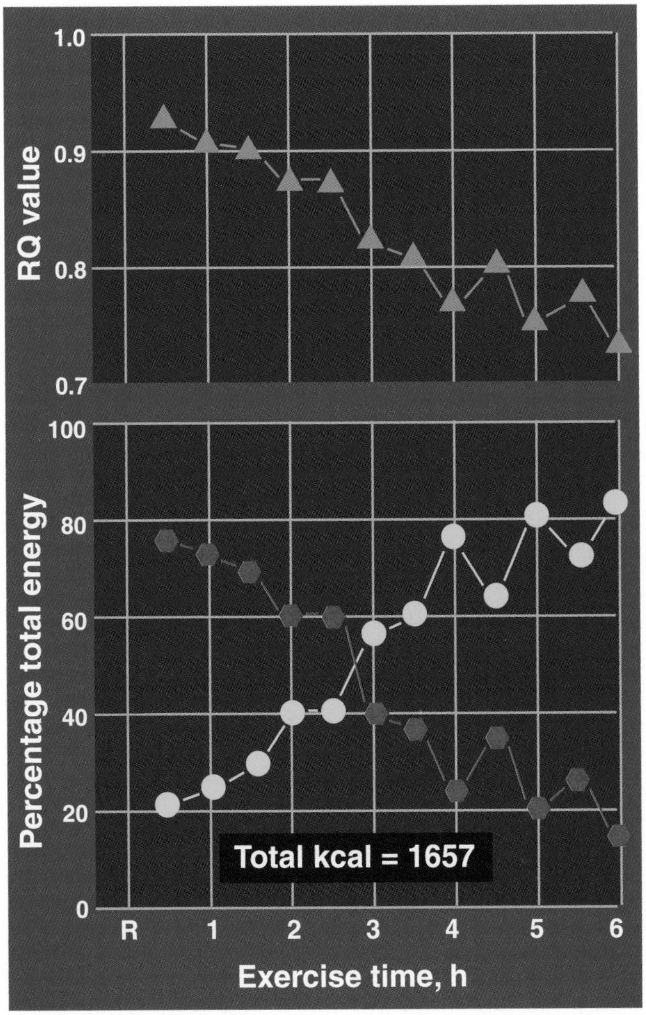

FIGURE 5.7. *Top:* Reduction in *RQ* at an oxygen uptake of 2.36 L·min^{-1} during 6 hours of continuous exercise. *Bottom:* Percentage of energy derived from carbohydrate (CHO) *(red)* and fat *(yellow)* (1 kcal = 5 4.2 kJ; R, rest). (Modified from Edwards HT, et al. Metabolic rate, blood sugar and utilization of carbohydrate. *Am J Physiol* 1934;108:203.)

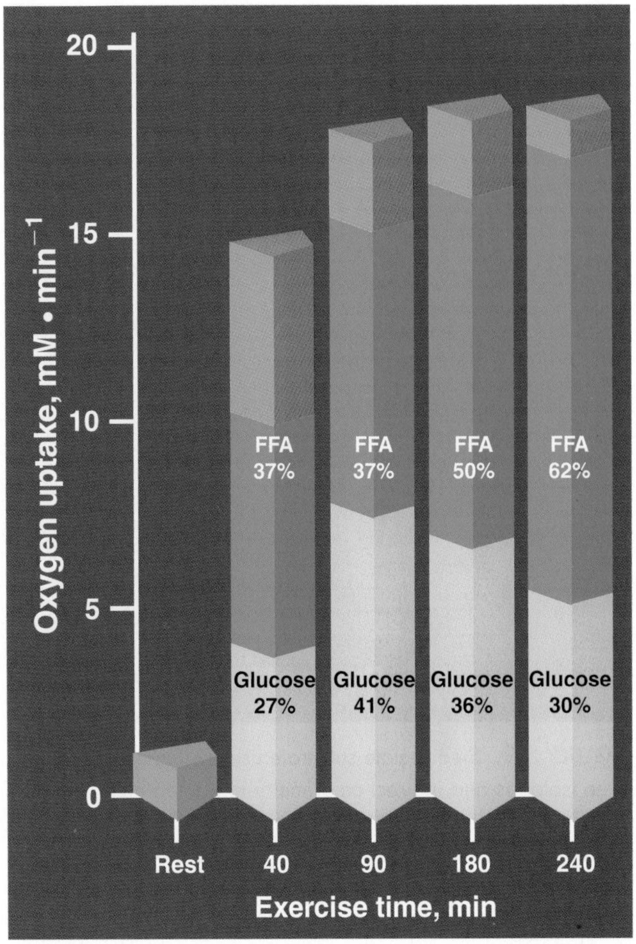

FIGURE 5.8. Uptake of oxygen and nutrients by the legs during prolonged exercise. *Green* and *yellow* areas represent the proportion of total oxygen uptake caused by oxidation of FFAs and blood glucose oxidation, respectively. *Orange* areas indicate the oxidation of nonbloodborne fuels (muscle glycogen and intramuscular fat and proteins). (From Ahlborg G, et al. Substrate turnover during prolonged exercise in man. *J Clin Invest* 1974;53:1080.)

muscles receive a continual supply of energy-rich fatty acid substrate. Increased activity of skeletal muscle and adipose tissue lipases, including biochemical and vascular adaptations within the muscle, help to explain the training-induced enhanced use of fats for energy during moderate-intensity exercise.[11,12,28,36,37,47]

Augmented fat metabolism in prolonged exercise probably results from a small drop in blood sugar, accompanied by a decrease in insulin (a potent inhibitor of lipolysis) and increased glucagon output by the pancreas as exercise progresses. These changes ultimately reduce glucose metabolism to further stimulate FFA liberation for energy. **FIGURE 5.8** shows that FFA uptake by working muscle rises during 1 to 4 hours of moderate exercise. In the first hour, fat supplies about 50% of the energy, whereas in the third hour, fat contributes up to 70% of the total energy requirement. *With carbohydrate depletion, exercise intensity decreases to a level governed by the body's ability to mobilize and oxidize fat.* Interestingly, prior exercise also partitions the trafficking of dietary fat fed in recovery toward a direction that favors its oxidation rather than storage. This may partly explain the protection against weight gain offered by regular physical activity.[31,56]

Consuming a high-fat diet for a protracted period produces enzymatic adaptations that enhance capacity for fat oxidation during exercise.[33,38,48,59] We discuss the effectiveness of this dietary manipulation to improve endurance performance in Chapter 8.

EXERCISE INTENSITY MAKES A DIFFERENCE

The contribution of fat to the metabolic mixture in exercise differs depending on exercise intensity. For moderately

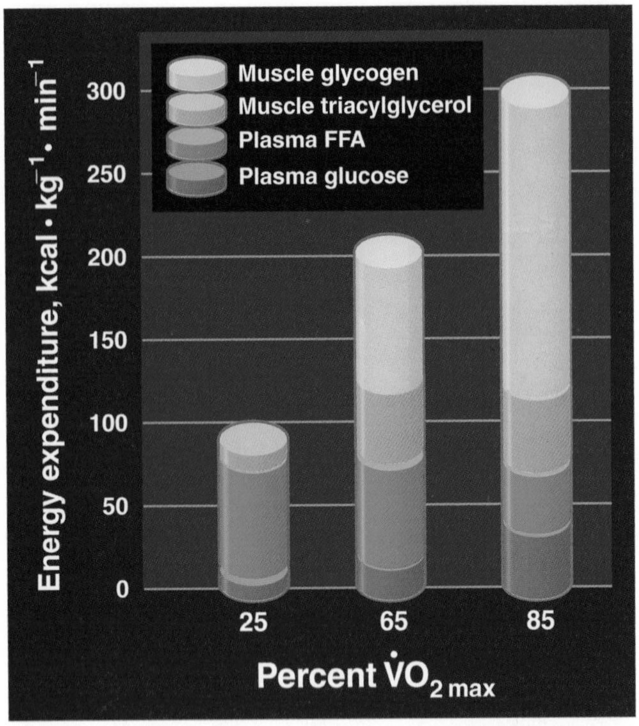

FIGURE 5.9. Steady-state substrate use calculated using three isotopes and indirect calorimetry in trained men performing cycle ergometer exercise at 25, 65, and 85% of $\dot{V}O_{2max}$. As exercise intensity increases, absolute use of glucose and muscle glycogen increases, whereas muscle triacylglycerol and plasma FFA use decreases. (From Romijn JA, et al. Regulation of endogenous fat and carbohydrate metabolism in relation to exercise intensity and duration. *Am J Physiol* 1993;265:E380.)

trained subjects, the exercise intensity that maximizes fat burning ranges between 55 and 72% of $\dot{V}O_{2max}$.[1,2] **FIGURE 5.9** illustrates the dynamics of fat use by trained men who cycled at 25 to 85% of their aerobic capacity. During light-to-mild exercise (40% of maximum or less), fat provided the main energy source, predominantly as plasma FFAs from adipose tissue depots. Increasing exercise intensity produced an eventual *crossover* in the balance of fuel use. The total energy from fat breakdown (from all sources) remained essentially unchanged, while blood glucose and muscle glycogen supplied the added energy for more intense exercise.

MORE FAT BURNED DURING SUBMAXIMAL EFFORT

Adaptations producing enhanced responsiveness of adipocytes to lipolysis allow the trained person to exercise at a higher absolute level of submaximal exercise before experiencing the fatiguing effects of glycogen depletion.

No difference existed in total energy from fats during exercise at 85% of maximum and exercise at 25% of maximum. *Such data highlight the important role that carbohydrate, particularly muscle glycogen, plays as the major fuel source during intense aerobic exercise.*

NUTRITIONAL STATUS PLAYS A ROLE

The dynamics of fat breakdown or its synthesis depend on the availability of the "building block" fatty acid molecules. After a meal, when energy metabolism is low, digestive processes increase FFA and triacylglycerol delivery to cells. Increased fat delivery, in turn, promotes triacylglycerol synthesis through esterification. In contrast, with moderate exercise, increased use of fatty acids for energy reduces their concentration in the active cells, thus stimulating triacylglycerol breakdown into its glycerol and fatty acid components. Concurrently, hormonal release in exercise stimulates adipose tissue lipolysis, which further augments FFA delivery to active muscle. Prolonged exercise in the fasted or glycogen-depleted state places heavy demands on FFA metabolism and enhances fat use as an exercise energy substrate.[35,52]

EXERCISE TRAINING AND FAT METABOLISM

Regular aerobic exercise profoundly improves ability to oxidize long-chain fatty acids, particularly from triacylglycerol stored within active muscle, during mild- to moderate-intensity exercise.[27–29,36,39,40] **FIGURE 5.10** shows the increase in fat catabolism during submaximal exercise following aerobic training, with a corresponding decrease in carbohydrate

SIX FAT-BURNING ADAPTATIONS WITH AEROBIC TRAINING

1. Facilitated rate of lipolysis and re-esterification within adipocytes.
2. Proliferation of capillaries in trained muscle to create a greater total number and density of these microvessels.
3. Improved transport of FFAs through the plasma membrane (sarcolemma) of the muscle fiber.
4. Augmented transport of fatty acids within the muscle cell by the action of carnitine and carnitine acyltransferase.
5. Increased size and number of muscle mitochondria.
6. Increased quantity of enzymes involved in β-oxidation, citric acid cycle metabolism, and the electron transport chain within specifically trained muscle fibers.

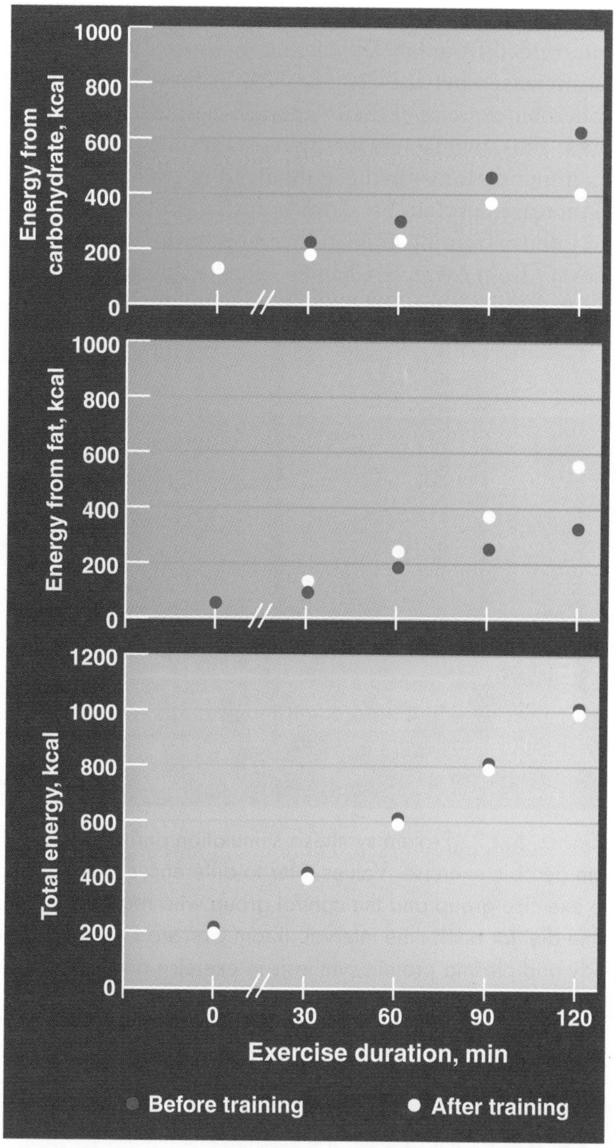

FIGURE 5.10. Training enhances catabolism of fat. During constant-load prolonged exercise, energy from fat oxidation significantly increases following aerobic training, while corresponding decreases occur in carbohydrate breakdown. Carbohydrate-sparing adaptations can occur in two ways: *(a)* release of fatty acids from adipose tissue depots (augmented by a reduced level of blood lactate) and *(b)* greater intramuscular fat stores in the endurance-trained muscle. (From Hurley BF, et al. Muscle triglyceride utilization during exercise: effect of training. *J Appl Physiol* 1986;60:562.)

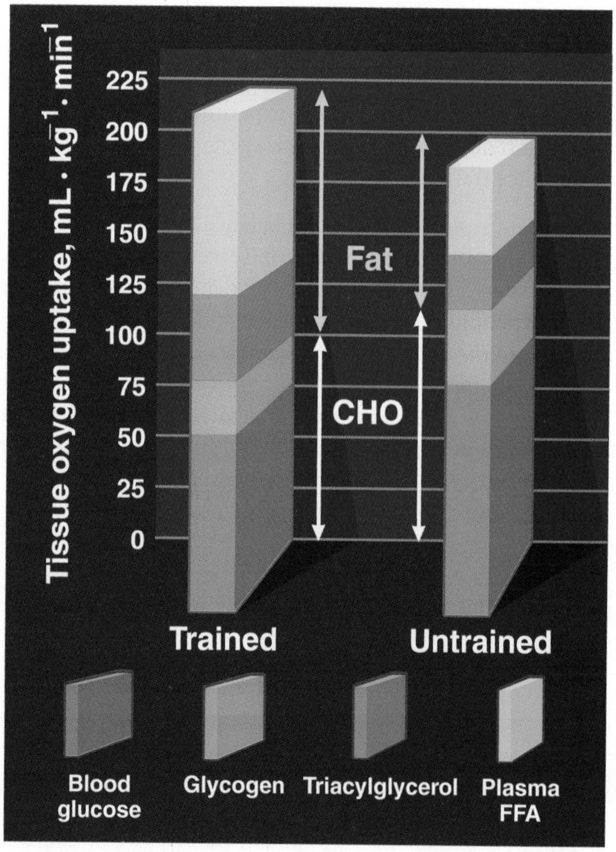

FIGURE 5.11. Estimated contribution of various substrates to energy metabolism in trained and untrained limb muscles. (From Saltin B, Åstrand P-O. Free fatty acids and exercise. *Am J Clin Nutr* 1993;57[Suppl]:752S.)

breakdown. Even for endurance athletes, the improved capacity for fat oxidation cannot sustain the level of aerobic metabolism generated when oxidizing glycogen for energy. Consequently, well-nourished endurance athletes rely almost totally on oxidation of stored glycogen in near-maximal, sustained aerobic effort.

FIGURE 5.11 displays the contribution of various energy substrates to exercise metabolism of trained and untrained limb muscles. The important point concerns the greater uptake of FFAs (and concurrent conservation of limited glycogen reserves) by the trained limb during moderate exercise through the six mechanisms shown in the box (on page 176) "Six Fat-Burning Adaptations with Aerobic Training."

PROTEIN USE DURING EXERCISE

Nutritionists and exercise physiologists have long maintained that the protein Recommended Dietary Allowance (RDA) represents a liberal "margin of safety" to account for amino acids catabolized during exercise and amino acids required for protein synthesis following exercise. For the past 100 years, three reasons stand out as to why protein constitutes a limited fuel in exercise:

1. Protein's primary role provides amino acid building blocks for tissue synthesis

2. Early studies show only minimal protein breakdown during endurance exercise as reflected by urinary nitrogen excretion
3. Theoretical computations and experimental evidence of protein requirements for muscle tissue synthesis with resistance training

More recent research on protein balance in exercise presents a compelling argument that protein serves as energy fuel to a much greater extent than previously believed, depending on energy expenditure and nutritional status.[5,8,49,55] *This applies primarily to the branched-chain amino acids (for the way the side chain branches from the molecule's amine core) leucine, valine, and isoleucine oxidized in skeletal muscle rather than in the liver.* As was shown in **FIGURE 5.4**, endurance exercise in a carbohydrate-depleted state caused considerably more protein catabolism than protein breakdown with ample carbohydrate reserves.

Whereas protein breakdown generally increases only modestly with exercise, muscle protein synthesis rises markedly following both endurance and resistance-type exercise.

ENERGY INTAKE MUST BALANCE ENERGY OUTPUT

If energy intake does not match energy expenditure in intense training, even twice the protein RDA intake may not maintain nitrogen balance. Thus, dieting could negatively affect training regimens geared to increase muscle mass or maintain muscular strength and power.

FIGURE 5.12 shows that the rate of muscle protein synthesis (determined from labeled leucine incorporation into muscle) increased between 10 and 80% in the 4 hours following aerobic exercise. It then remained elevated for at least 24 hours. Thus, two factors justify re-examining protein intake recommendations for those involved in exercise training: (1) increased protein breakdown during prolonged exercise and intense training and (2) increased protein synthesis in recovery from exercise. Chapter 7 further discusses the adequacy of the protein RDA for those who undertake intense training.

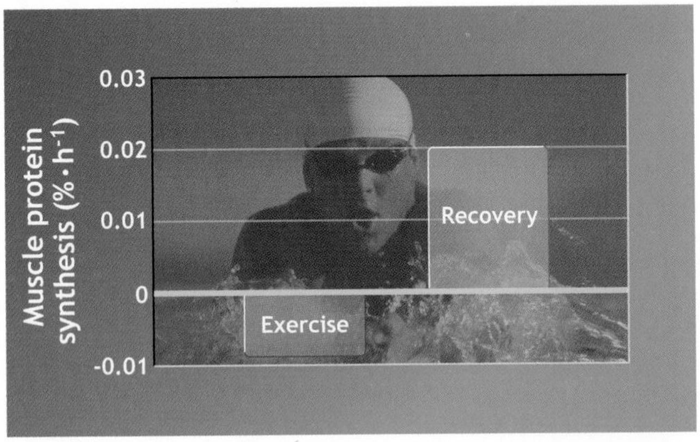

FIGURE 5.12. Protein synthesis stimulation during recovery from aerobic exercise. Values refer to differences between the exercise group and the control group who received the same diet for each time interval. (From Carraro F, et al. Whole body and plasma protein synthesis in exercise and recovery in human subjects. *Am J Physiol* 1990;258:E821.)

PERSONAL HEALTH AND EXERCISE NUTRITION 5.1

Know What You Eat: Benefits of Phytochemicals

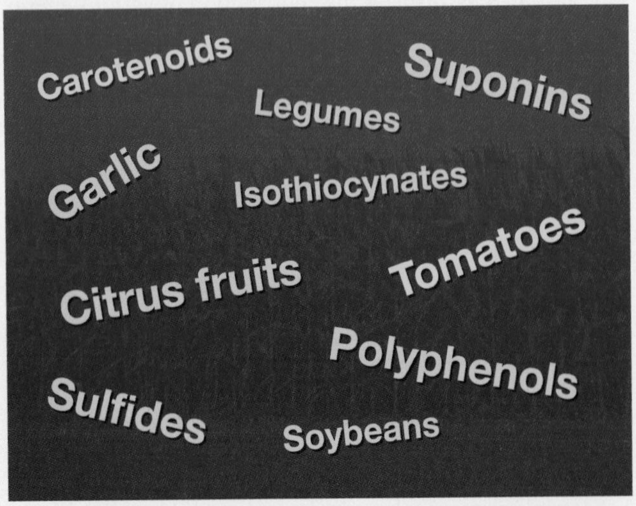

Background

Based on years of research in the field of nutrition, current consensus suggests that an optimum diet should:

1. Supply an individual's needs for energy (calories) and macronutrients and micronutrients
2. Support health and promote successful aging
3. Provide pleasure, both individual and social, and reinforce personal and cultural identity

Within this framework, the following represent five major characteristics of an optimum diet that most scientists from diverse disciplines would agree with:

1. Contain foods of sufficient variety from all the major food groups

2. Contain as much fresh food as possible
3. Contain as few processed foods as possible
4. Contain an abundance of fruits and vegetables
5. Contain foods that provide health benefits beyond basic nutrition

Foods that provide health benefits beyond basic nutrition have been termed *functional foods*. Beneficial substances in these foods include both *zoochemicals* (health-promoting compounds from the animal kingdom) and *phytochemicals* (health-promoting compounds from the plant kingdom). Much research has focused on phytochemicals because of their protective role in fighting chronic disease. Foods such as garlic, soybeans, cruciferous vegetables, legumes, onions, citrus fruits, tomatoes, whole grains, and diverse herbs and spices are excellent sources of chemoprotective phytochemicals. Specific phytochemicals with health benefits include allium compounds, isoflavones, saponins, indoles, isothiocyanates, dithiolthione, ellagic acid, polyacetylenes, flavonoids, carotenoids, phytates, lignins, glucarates, phthalides, and terpenoids.

Student Activity

List 10 different foods you would include in a "phytochemical rich" dinner salad:

1. ______________________
2. ______________________
3. ______________________
4. ______________________
5. ______________________
6. ______________________
7. ______________________
8. ______________________
9. ______________________
10. ______________________

Know Your Phytochemicals

Many different plants contain healthful phytochemicals. For example, carotenoids, polyphenols, and saponins exert strong antioxidant effects; sulfides and isothiocyanates stimulate enzymes that deactivate carcinogens; phytosterols and saponins alter the harmful effects of excess cholesterol; phytoestrogens possess a chemical structure similar to that of hormones and act by blocking deleterious effects of excessive hormone production. The accompanying table lists the more important phytochemicals, their biologic activity, and food sources.

Phytochemical	Activity and Effects	Food Sources
Carotenoids (α-carotene, β-carotene, β-cryptoxanthin, luten, lycopene, zeaxanthin)	Vitamin-A precursors; antioxidants; increase cell-to-cell communication; decrease risk of macular degeneration	Yellow-orange fruits and vegetable (e.g., apricots, carrots, cantaloupe, broccoli, tomatoes, sweet potatoes); leafy greens such as spinach; dairy products, eggs, and margarine
Flavonoids (quercetin, kaempferol, myricetin), flavones (apigenin), flavonols (catechins)	Decrease capillary fragility and permeability; block carcinogens and slow growth of cancer cells	Fruits, vegetables, berries, citrus fruits, onions, purple grapes, tea, red wine
Phytoestrogens (isoflavones—genistein, biochanin A, daidzein, and lignins)	Metabolized to estrogen-like compounds in the GI tract; induce cancer cell death (apoptosis); slow cancer cell growth; reduce risk of breast, ovarian, colon, and prostate cancer; inhibit cholesterol synthesis; may reduce risk of osteoporosis	Isoflavones in soybeans and soy products; lignins in flax, rye, some berries, and some vegetables
Phytosterols (β-sitosterol, stigmasterol, campesterol)	Decrease cholesterol absorption; inhibit proliferation of colonic cells	Vegetable oils, nuts, seeds, cereals, legumes
Saponins (soyasaponins, soyasapogenols)	Bind bile acids and cholesterol in the GI tract to reduce absorption; toxic to tumor cells; antioxidant effects	Soybeans, modified margarines
Glucosinolates (glucobrassicin, isothiocyanates [sulphorophane], indoles [indole-3-carbinol])	Increase enzyme activity that deactivates carcinogens; favorably alter estrogen metabolism; affect regulation of gene expression	Cruciferous vegetables (broccoli, Brussels sprouts, cabbage), horseradish, mustard greens
Sulfides and thiols (dithiolthiones and allium compounds like diallyl sulfides, allyl methyl trisulfides)	Increase activity of enzymes that deactivate carcinogens; decrease conversion of nitrates to nitrites in intestines; may lower cholesterol, prevent blood clotting, and normalize blood pressure	Sulfides in onions, garlic, leeks, scallions; dithiolthiones in cruciferous vegetables
Inositol phosphates (phytate, inositol, pentaphosphate)	Bind metal ions and prevent them from generating free radicals; protect against cancer	Cereals, soybeans, soy-based foods, cereal grains, nuts, and seeds (especially abundant in sesame seeds and soybeans)

Phytochemical	Activity and Effects	Food Sources
Phenolic acids (caffeic and ferulic acids, ellagic acid)	Anticancer properties; prevent formation of stomach carcinogens	Blueberries, cherries, apples, oranges, pears, potatoes
Protease inhibitors	Bind to trypsin and chymotrypsin; decrease cancer cell growth and inhibit malignant changes in cells; inhibit hormone binding; may aid DNA repair to slow cancer cell division; prevent tumors from releasing proteases that destroy neighboring cells	Soybeans; other legumes, cereals, vegetables
Tannins	Antioxidant effects; may inhibit activation of carcinogens and slow cancer promotion	Grapes, tea, lentils, red and white wine, black-eyed peas
Capsaicin	Modulates blood clotting	Hot peppers
Coumarin (phenolic)	Promotes enzyme function to protect against cancer	Citrus fruits
Curcumin (phenolic)	Inhibits enzymes that activate carcinogens; antiinflammatory and antioxidant properties	Turmeric, mustard
Monoterpene (limonene)	Triggers enzyme production to detoxify carcinogens; inhibits cancer promotion and cell proliferation; favorably affects blood clotting and cholesterol levels	Citrus fruit peels and oils, garlic

From Grosvenor MB, Smolin LA. Nutrition. From Science to Life. Philadelphia: Harcourt College Publishers, 2002.

SUMMARY

1. The major pathway for ATP production differs depending on exercise intensity and duration.
2. For all-out, short-duration efforts (100-m dash, lifting heavy weights), the intramuscular stores of ATP and PCr (immediate energy system) provide the required energy for exercise.
3. For intense exercise of longer duration (1–2 min), the anaerobic reactions of glycolysis (short-term energy system) provide the majority of energy.
4. When exercise progresses beyond several minutes, the aerobic system predominates with oxygen uptake capacity becoming the important factor (long-term energy system).
5. Muscle glycogen and blood glucose serve as primary fuels during intense anaerobic exercise beyond 10-seconds in duration. Glycogen stores also play an important energy metabolism role in sustained high levels of aerobic exercise such as marathon running, distance cycling, and endurance swimming.
6. Trained muscle exhibits an augmented capacity to catabolize carbohydrate aerobically for energy because of increased oxidative capacity of the mitochondria and increased glycogen storage.
7. Women derive a smaller proportion of the total energy from carbohydrate oxidation than do men during submaximal exercise at equivalent percentages of aerobic capacity. Following aerobic exercise training, women show a more exaggerated shift toward fat catabolism than men.
8. A carbohydrate-deficient diet rapidly depletes muscle and liver glycogen and profoundly affects both anaerobic capacity and prolonged, intense aerobic physical effort.
9. Fat contributes about 50% of the energy requirement during light and moderate exercise. The role of stored fat (intramuscular and derived from adipocytes) becomes even more important at the latter stages of prolonged exercise. In this situation, the fatty acid molecules (mainly as circulating FFAs) provide more than 80% of the exercise energy requirements.
10. With carbohydrate depletion, exercise intensity decreases to a level determined by how well the body mobilizes and oxidizes fat.
11. Aerobic training increases long-chain fatty acid oxidation, particularly the fatty acids derived from triacylglycerols within active muscle during mild- to moderate-intensity exercise.
12. Enhanced fat oxidation spares glycogen, permitting trained individuals to exercise at a higher absolute level of submaximal exercise before experiencing the fatiguing effects of glycogen depletion.
13. A high-fat diet stimulates adaptations that augment fat use, yet reliable research has not yet demonstrated consistent exercise or training benefits from such dietary modifications.
14. Protein serves as an energy fuel to a much greater extent than previously thought, depending on nutritional status and the intensity of exercise training or competition. This applies particularly to branched-chain amino acids that oxidize within skeletal muscle rather than within the liver.
15. Re-examining the current protein RDA seems justified for those who engage in intense exercise training. Protein intake must account for the increased protein breakdown during exercise and the augmented protein synthesis in recovery.

thePoint *Visit* **thePoint.lww.com/MKKSEN4e** *to view the following animations related to content presented in Chapter 5:* ***Triacylglycerol breakdown****;* ***Fat mobilization and use****;* ***Glycolysis****;* ***Oxygen consumption****; and* ***Oxygen transport****.*

TEST YOUR KNOWLEDGE ANSWERS

1. **True:** Anaerobic sources supply most of the energy for fast, powerful movements, or during increased resistance to movement at a given speed. When movement begins at either fast or slow speed, the intramuscular high-energy phosphates (ATP and PCr) provide immediate anaerobic energy for muscle action. After a few seconds, the glycolytic pathway (intramuscular glycogen breakdown via glycolysis) generates an increasingly greater proportion of energy for ATP resynthesis.

2. **False:** Liver and muscle glycogen provide the main macronutrient energy sources for ATP resynthesis during intense aerobic exercise. The liver markedly increases its release of glucose as exercise progresses from low to high intensity. Concurrently, glycogen stored within the active muscles serves as the predominant energy source during the early stages of exercise and in intense aerobic exercise. Compared with fat and protein catabolism, carbohydrate remains the preferential fuel during intense aerobic exercise because it more rapidly supplies ATP in oxidative processes. More specifically, dependence on carbohydrate during intense aerobic exercise lies in its two-times more rapid rate of energy transfer than with fat and protein. Furthermore, carbohydrate generates about 6% more energy per unit of oxygen consumed than fat.

3. **True:** Depending on the nutritional and fitness status of the individual and exercise intensity and duration, fat supplies between 30 and 80% of the exercise energy requirement. Fat use in light and moderate exercise varies closely with blood flow through adipose tissue and blood flow through active muscle. Adipose tissue releases more FFAs for delivery to active muscle as blood flow increases with exercise. Hence, somewhat greater quantities of fat from adipose tissue depots participate in energy metabolism.

4. **True:** In predominantly anaerobic effort, carbohydrate becomes the sole macronutrient contributor of energy for ATP resynthesis. Carbohydrate breakdown in glycolysis provides the only available means for rapid anaerobic energy. This anaerobic energy is unavailable via the breakdown of fatty acids and amino acids, which provide energy only through aerobic metabolism.

5. **True:** Controversy exists as to why carbohydrate depletion during prolonged exercise coincides with a reduced exercise capacity, commonly termed "bonking" or "hitting the wall." Part of the answer relates to the use of blood glucose as energy for the central nervous system, muscle glycogen's role as a "primer" in fat metabolism, and the slower rate of energy release from fat than from carbohydrate breakdown. In essence, with carbohydrate depletion, exercise intensity decreases to a level governed by the body's ability to mobilize and oxidize fat.

6. **False:** A carbohydrate-deficient diet, not a diet deficient in fat, rapidly depletes muscle and liver glycogen. This diet subsequently impairs performance in all-out, short-term (anaerobic) exercise and in prolonged intense endurance (aerobic) activities. These observations pertain to both athletes and physically active individuals who modify their diets by reducing carbohydrate intake below recommended levels.

7. **True:** Carbohydrate availability during exercise helps to regulate fat mobilization and its use for energy. Augmented fat metabolism in prolonged exercise probably results from a small drop in blood sugar, accompanied by a decrease in insulin (a potent inhibitor of lipolysis) and increased glucagon output by the pancreas as exercise progresses. These changes ultimately reduce glucose metabolism to further stimulate FFA liberation for energy. Toward the end of prolonged exercise (with glycogen reserves low), circulating FFAs supply nearly 80% of the total energy requirement.

8. **False:** Regular aerobic exercise profoundly improves the ability to oxidize long-chain fatty acids, particularly from triacylglycerol stored within active muscle, during mild- to moderate-intensity exercise. These adaptations allow the trained person to exercise at a higher absolute level of submaximal exercise before experiencing the fatiguing effects of glycogen depletion. Even for endurance athletes, however, improved capacity for fat oxidation cannot sustain the high level of aerobic metabolism generated when oxidizing glycogen for energy.

9. **False:** Protein serves as an energy fuel to a much greater extent than previously thought, depending on nutritional status and exercise intensity. This applies particularly to branched-chain amino acids that oxidize within skeletal muscle rather than within the liver. The use of protein for energy most frequently occurs in a glycogen-depleted state as amino acids donate their carbon skeletons for the synthesis of glucose by the liver.

10. **False:** Individuals consuming a high-carbohydrate diet perform significantly better after 7 weeks of training than individuals consuming a high-fat diet.

A high-fat diet stimulates adaptive responses that augment fat use, but reliable research has yet to demonstrate consistent exercise or training benefits from such dietary modifications. Furthermore, one should carefully consider recommending a diet consisting of up to 60% total calories from lipid in terms of detrimental health risks, particularly those associated with cardiovascular disease.

Key References

Achten J, et al. Determination of the exercise intensity that elicits maximal fat oxidation. *Med Sci Sports Exerc* 2002;34:92.

Achten J, Jeukendrup AE. Optimizing fat oxidation through exercise and diet. *Nutrition* 2004;20:716.

Bowtell JL, et al. Modulation of whole body protein metabolism, during and after exercise, by variation of dietary protein. *J Appl Physiol* 1998;85:1744.

Carraro F, et al. Alanine kinetics in humans during low-intensity exercise. *Med Sci Sports Exerc* 1994;26:48.

Coggan AR. Plasma glucose metabolism during exercise: effect of endurance training in humans. *Med Sci Sports Exerc* 1997;29:620.

Coyle EF, et al. Fatty acid oxidation is directly regulated by carbohydrate metabolism during exercise. *Am J Physiol* 1997;273:E268.

DiPietro L. Exercise training and fat metabolism after menopouse: implications for improved metabolic flexibility in aging. *J Appl Physiol* 2010;109:1569.

Friellander AL, et al. Training induced alterations in carbohydrate metabolism in women: women respond differently than men. *J Appl Physiol* 1998;85:1175.

Hargreaves M. Interactions between muscle glycogen and blood glucose during exercise. *Exerc Sport Sci Rev* 1997;25:21.

Horton TJ, et al. Fuel metabolism in men and women during and after long-duration exercise. *J Appl Physiol* 1998;85:1823.

Jeukendrup AE, et al. Exogenous glucose oxidation during exercise in endurance-trained and untrained subjects. *J Appl Physiol* 1997;83:835.

Johnson ML, et al. Twelve weeks of endurance training increases FFA mobilization and reesterfication in postmenopausal women *J Appl Physiol* 2010;109:1573.

Kiens B. Skeletal muscle lipid metabolism in exercise and insulin resistance. *Physiol Rev* 2006;86:205.

Martin WH. Effect of acute and chronic exercise on fat metabolism. *Exerc Sport Sci Rev* 1996;24:203.

Nicklas BJ. Effects of endurance exercise on adipose tissue metabolism. *Exerc Sport Sci Rev* 1997;25:77.

Pendergast DR, et al. Influence of exercise on nutritional requirements. *Eur J Appl Physiol* 2011;111:379.

Roepstorff C, et al. Intramuscular triacylglycerol in energy metabolism during exercise in humans. *Exer Sport Sci Rev* 2005;33:182.

Romijn JA, et al. Relationship between fatty acid delivery and fatty acid oxidation during strenuous exercise. *J Appl Physiol* 1995;79:1939.

Sherman WM. Metabolism of sugars and physical performance. *Am J Clin Nutr* 1995;62(Suppl):228S.

Stellingwerff T, et al. Decreased PDH activation and glycogenolysis during exercise following fat adaption with carbohydrate restoration. *Am J Physiol Endocrinol Metab* 2006;298:E380.

Van Proeyen K, et al. Beneficial metabolic adaptations due to endurance exercise training in the fasted state. *J Appl Physiol.* 2011;110:236.

Venables MC, et al. Determinants of maximal fat oxidation during exercise in healthy men and women. *J Appl Physiol* 2005;98:160.

Wagenmakers AJM. Muscle amino acid metabolism at rest and during exercise: role in human physiology and metabolism. *Exerc Sport Sci Rev* 1998;26:287.

Winder WW. Malonyl-CoA: regulator of fatty acid oxidation in muscle during exercise. *Exerc Sport Sci Rev* 1998;26:117.

Zderic TW, et al. High-fat diet elevates resting intramuscular triglyceride concentration and whole body lipolysis during exercise. *Am J Physiol Endocrinol Metab* 2004;286:E217.

thePoint *Visit* **thePoint.lww.com/MKKSEN4e** *for a list of the references cited in this chapter, including additional, relevant references.*

CHAPTER 6

Measurement of Energy in Food and During Physical Activity

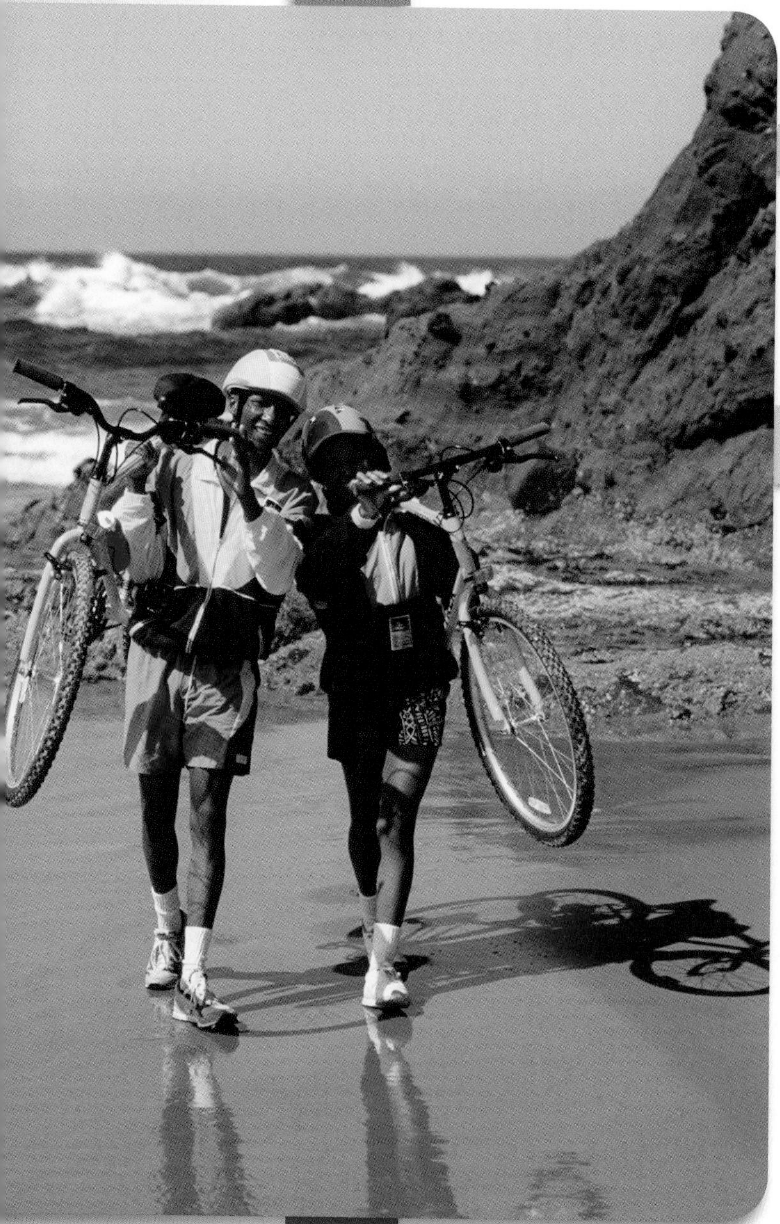

OUTLINE

TEST YOUR KNOWLEDGE

Select true or false for the 10 statements below and then check out the answers at the end of the chapter. Retake the test after you've read the chapter; you should achieve 100%!

	True	False
1. The calorie is a unit of energy measurement.	❍	❍
2. The bomb calorimeter operates on the principle of indirect calorimetry by measuring the oxygen consumed as the food burns completely.	❍	❍
3. Heat of combustion refers to a food's ability to release carbon dioxide in relation to oxygen consumed as the food burns completely.	❍	❍
4. The heat of combustion for all carbohydrates averages 5.0 $kcal \cdot g^{-1}$.	❍	❍
5. The heat of combustion for lipid averages 6.0 $kcal \cdot g^{-1}$.	❍	❍
6. The heat of combustion for protein averages 7.0 $kcal \cdot g^{-1}$.	❍	❍
7. The doubly labeled water technique provides a means to evaluate sweat loss during intense exercise.	❍	❍
8. In terms of net energy release in the body, each of the three macronutrients releases about 4.0 $kcal \cdot g^{-1}$.	❍	❍
9. Celery would become a "fattening" food if consumed in excess.	❍	❍
10. The respiratory quotient (RQ) for carbohydrate equals 1.00.	❍	❍

All biologic functions require energy. The carbohydrate, lipid, and protein macronutrients contain the energy that ultimately powers biologic work, making energy the common denominator for classifying both food and physical activity.

MEASUREMENT OF FOOD ENERGY

THE CALORIE—A UNIT OF ENERGY MEASUREMENT

In nutritional terms, 1 calorie expresses the quantity of heat necessary to raise the temperature of 1 kg (1 L) of water 1°C (from 14.5 to 15.5°C). Thus, **kilogram calorie** or kilocalorie **(kcal)** more accurately defines calorie. (Note the use of the letter k to designate a kilocalorie, as compared to a small calorie [c], which indicates the quantity of heat necessary to raise the temperature of 1 g of water 1°C.) For example, if a particular food contains 300 kcal, then releasing the potential energy trapped within this food's chemical structure increases the temperature of 300 L of water 1°C.

Different foods contain different amounts of potential energy. One-half cup of peanut butter with a caloric value of 759 kcal contains the equivalent heat energy to increase the temperature of 759 L of water 1°C. A corresponding unit of heat using Fahrenheit degrees is the British thermal unit or BTU. One BTU represents the quantity of heat necessary to raise the temperature of 1 lb (weight) of water 1°F from 63 to 64°F. *A clear distinction exists between temperature and heat. Temperature reflects a quantitative measure of an object's hotness or coldness. Heat describes energy transfer or exchange from one body or system to another.* The following conversions apply:

$$1 \text{ cal} = 4.184 \text{ J}$$
$$1 \text{ kcal} = 1000 \text{ cal} = 4186 \text{ J} = 4.184 \text{ kJ}$$
$$1 \text{ BTU} = 778 \text{ ft lb} = 252 \text{ cal} = 1055 \text{ J}$$

The joule (J), or **kilojoule (kJ),** reflects the standard international unit (SI unit) for expressing energy. To convert kilocalories to kilojoules, multiply the kilocalorie value by 4.184. The kilojoule value for 1/2 cup of peanut butter, for example, would equal 759 kcal × 4.184 or 3176 kJ. The **megajoule (MJ)** equals 1000 kJ; its use avoids unmanageably large numbers. The name **joule** honors British scientist Sir Prescott Joule (1818–1889) who studied how vigorous stirring of a paddle-wheel warmed water. Joule determined that the movement of the paddle-wheel added energy to the water, raising the water temperature in direct proportion to the work done.

GROSS ENERGY VALUE OF FOODS

Laboratories use **bomb calorimeters** similar to the one illustrated in **FIGURE 6.1** to measure the total heats of combustion values of the various food macronutrients. Bomb calorimeters operate on the principle of **direct calorimetry** by measuring the heat liberated as the food burns completely.

Figure 6.1 shows food within a sealed chamber charged with oxygen at high pressure. An electrical current moving through the fuse at the tip ignites the food–oxygen mixture. As the food burns, a water jacket surrounding the bomb absorbs the heat or energy liberated. The calorimeter is fully insulated from the outside environment, so the increase in water temperature *directly* reflects the heat released during a food's oxidation or "burning."

Heat of combustion refers to the heat liberated by oxidizing a specific food; it represents the food's total energy value. For example, 1 tsp of margarine releases 100 kcal of heat energy when burned completely in a bomb calorimeter. This equals the energy required to raise 1.0 kg (2.205 lb) of ice water to its boiling point. The oxidation pathways of food in the intact organism and the bomb calorimeter differ, but the energy liberated in the complete breakdown of a food remains the same regardless of the combustion pathway.

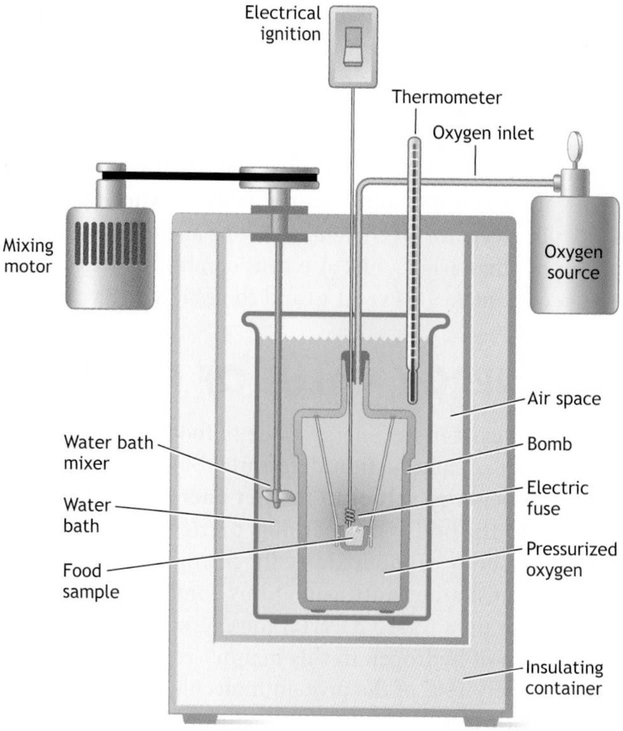

FIGURE 6.1. A bomb calorimeter directly measures the energy value of food.

Carbohydrates

The heat of combustion for carbohydrate varies depending on the arrangement of atoms in the particular carbohydrate molecule. For glucose, heat of combustion equals 3.74 kcal $\cdot$ g^{-1}, about 12% less than for glycogen (4.19 kcal) and starch (4.20 kcal). *A value of 4.2 kcal generally represents the average heat of combustion for 1 g of carbohydrate.*

Lipids

The heat of combustion for lipid varies with the structural composition of the triacylglycerol molecule's fatty acid components. For example, 1 g of either beef or pork fat yields 9.50 kcal, whereas oxidizing 1 g of butterfat liberates 9.27 kcal. The average energy value for 1 g of lipid in meat, fish, and eggs equals 9.50 kcal. The energy equivalent amounts to 9.25 kcal $\cdot$ g^{-1} in dairy products and 9.30 kcal in vegetables and fruits. *The average heat of combustion for lipid equals 9.4 kcal $\cdot$ g^{-1}.*

Proteins

Two factors affect energy release from protein combustion:

1. Type of protein in the food
2. Relative nitrogen content of the protein

Common proteins in eggs, meat, corn (maize), and beans (jack, lima, navy, soy) contain approximately 16% nitrogen and have a corresponding heat of combustion that averages 5.7 kcal $\cdot$ g^{-1}. Proteins in other foods have a somewhat higher nitrogen content; most nuts and seeds contain 18.9% nitrogen, and whole-kernel wheat, rye, millets, and barley contain 17.2% nitrogen. Other foods contain a slightly lower nitrogen percentage; for example, whole milk has 15.7% and bran has 15.8%. *The heat of combustion for protein averages 5.65 kcal $\cdot$ g^{-1}* (assuming an average nitrogen content of 16%).

Comparing Macronutrient Energy Values

The average heats of combustion for the three macronutrients (carbohydrate, 4.2 kcal $\cdot$ g^{-1}; lipid, 9.4 kcal $\cdot$ g^{-1}; protein, 5.65 kcal $\cdot$ g^{-1}) demonstrate that the complete oxidation of lipid in the bomb calorimeter liberates about 65% more energy per gram than protein oxidation and 120% more energy than carbohydrate oxidation. Recall from Chapter 1 that a lipid molecule contains more hydrogen atoms than either carbohydrate or protein molecules. The common fatty acid palmitic acid, for example, has the structural formula $C_{16}H_{32}O_2$. The ratio of hydrogen atoms to oxygen atoms in fatty acids always greatly exceeds the 2:1 ratio found in carbohydrates. Simply

Connections to the Past

Antoine Laurent Lavoisier (1743–1794)

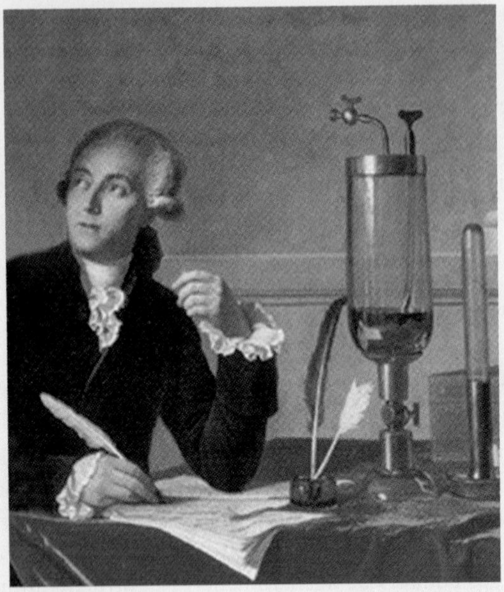

Lavoisier and his wife, Marie-Anne Paulze (1758–1836), who shared Lavoisier's passion for chemistry. She took painting lessons from the famous French artist David who painted this commissioned work for 7000 pounds in 1788, an extraordinary sum at that time. The Metropolitan Museum of Art, New York, encapsulates the essence of the chemistry aspect of the painting: "The laboratory instruments share this quietly shimmering quality. The distillation flask on the right has the transparency and brilliance of the finest glass, while the test tubes on the table have the flat, dense look of thick glass; each instrument has its own distinct texture and reflections play off their surfaces with a marvelous lightness. They are in the picture to bear witness to the Lavoisiers' experiments and their sole object is to serve as symbols and emblems. They are, above all, still-life masterpieces."

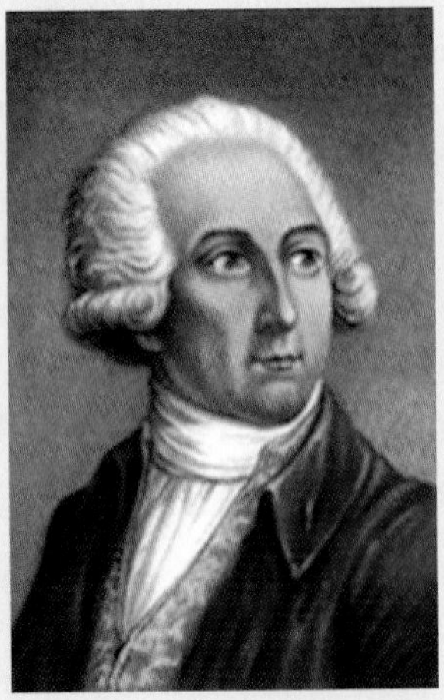

Antoine Lavoisier ushered in modern concepts in chemistry, metabolism, and nutrition, with application to exercise physiology and exercise and sport nutrition. His contributions include analysis and synthesis of air, composition of oxides and acids, composition of water, theory of combustion, respiration and animal heat, permanence of weight of matter and simple substances, and the imponderable nature of heat and its role in chemistry. The accomplishments most germane to sports and exercise nutrition pertain to respiratory chemistry and exercise metabolism. Lavoisier used accurate balance scales to determine what his contemporaries could not explain: An animal in a closed chamber consumed "air eminently respirable" (oxygéne) and produced "aëriform calcic acid" (carbon dioxide).

thePoint *Visit* **thePoint.lww.com/MKKSEN4e** *to find more details about Lavoisier's experiments with respiration and metabolism.*

stated, lipid molecules have more hydrogen atoms available for cleavage and subsequent oxidation for energy than carbohydrates and proteins.

Clearly, lipid-rich foods have higher energy contents than foods relatively fat free. One cup of whole milk contains 160 kcal, for example, whereas the same quantity of skim milk contains only 90 kcal. If a person who normally consumes 1 quart of whole milk each day switches to skim milk, the total calories ingested each year would decrease by the equivalent calories in 25 lb of fat! In 3 years, all other things remaining constant, body fat loss would approximate 75 pounds. Such a theoretical comparison merits serious consideration because of the almost identical nutritional composition between whole milk and skim milk except for fat content. Drinking an 8-oz glass of skim milk rather than whole milk also considerably reduces saturated fatty acid intake (0.4 vs 5.1 g) and cholesterol (0.3 vs 33 mg).

INTERCHANGEABLE EXPRESSION FOR ENERGY AND WORK

1 foot-pound (ft-lb) = 0.13825 kilogram-meters (kg-m)

1 kg-m = 7.233 ft-lb = 9.8066 joules

1 kilocalorie (kcal) = 3.0874 ft-lb = 426.85 kg-m = 4.186 kilojoules (kJ)

1 joule (J) = 1 Newton-meter (Nm)

1 kilojoule (kJ) = 1000 J = 0.23889 kcal

NET ENERGY VALUE OF FOODS

Differences exist in the energy value of foods when comparing the heat of combustion determined by direct calorimetry (**gross energy value**) to the **net energy value** actually available to the body. This pertains particularly to proteins because the body cannot oxidize the nitrogen component of this nutrient. Rather, nitrogen atoms combine with hydrogen to form urea (NH_2CONH_2) for excretion in the urine. Elimination of hydrogen in this manner represents a loss of approximately 19% of the protein molecule's potential energy. This hydrogen loss reduces protein's heat of combustion in the body to approximately 4.6 $kcal \cdot g^{-1}$ instead of the 5.65 $kcal \cdot g^{-1}$ released during oxidation in the bomb calorimeter.

In contrast, *identical* physiologic fuel values exist for carbohydrates and lipids (which contain no nitrogen) compared with their respective heats of combustion in the bomb calorimeter.

Coefficient of Digestibility

The efficiency of the digestive process influences the ultimate caloric yield from macronutrients. Numerically defined as the **coefficient of digestibility**, digestive efficiency represents the percentage of food digested and absorbed to serve the body's metabolic needs. The food remaining unabsorbed in the intestinal tract becomes voided in the feces. Dietary fiber reduces the coefficient of digestibility: A high-fiber meal has less total energy absorbed than does a fiber-free meal of equivalent caloric content. This difference occurs because fiber moves food more rapidly through the intestine, thereby reducing absorption time. Fiber also may cause mechanical erosion of the intestinal mucosa, which then becomes resynthesized through energy-requiring processes.

TABLE 6.1 shows different digestibility coefficients, heats of combustion, and net energy values for nutrients in the various food groups. *The relative percentage of macronutrients completely digested and absorbed averages 97% for carbohydrate, 95% for lipid, and 92% for protein.* Little difference exists in digestive efficiency between obese and lean persons. Considerable variability, however, exists in efficiency percentages for any food within a particular category. Proteins in particular have variable digestive efficiencies; they range from a low of about 78% for high-fiber legumes to a high of 97% for protein from animal sources. Some advocates promote the use of vegetables in weight loss diets because of plant protein's relatively low coefficient of digestibility. Those on a vegetarian-type diet should consume adequate and diverse protein food sources to obtain all essential amino acids (see Chapter 1).

From the data in Table 6.1, the average net energy values can be rounded to simple whole numbers referred to as **Atwater general factors** (www.sportsci.org/news/history/atwater/atwater.html).

These values, named for Wilbur Olin Atwater (1844–1907; profiled in Chapter 5), the 19th century chemist who pioneered human nutrition and energy balance studies, represent the energy available to the body from ingested foods. Except when requiring exact energy values for experimental or therapeutic diets, the Atwater general factors accurately estimate the *net metabolizable energy* of typically consumed foods. For alcohol, 7 kcal (29.4 kJ) represents each gram (milliliter) of pure (200 proof) alcohol ingested. For metabolizable energy available to the body, alcohol's efficiency of use equals that of other carbohydrates.[17]

TABLE 6.1 Factors for Digestibility, Heats of Combustion, and Net Physiologic Energy Values[a] of Dietary Protein, Lipid, and Carbohydrate

Food Group	Digestibility (%)	Heat of Combustion ($kcal \cdot g^{-1}$)	Net Energy ($kcal \cdot g^{-1}$)
Protein			
Meats, fish	97	5.65	4.27
Eggs	97	5.75	4.37
Dairy products	97	5.65	4.27
Animal food (Average)	97	5.65	4.27
Cereals	85	5.80	3.87
Legumes	78	5.70	3.47
Vegetables	83	5.00	3.11
Fruits	85	5.20	3.36
Vegetable food (Average)	85	5.65	3.74
Total protein, Average	**92**	**5.65**	**4.05**
Lipid			
Meat and eggs	95	9.50	9.03
Dairy products	95	9.25	8.79
Animal food	95	9.40	8.93
Vegetable food	90	9.30	8.37
Total lipid, Average	**95**	**9.40**	**8.93**
Carbohydrate			
Animal food	98	3.90	3.82
Cereals	98	4.20	3.11
Legumes	97	4.20	4.07
Vegetables	95	4.20	3.99
Fruits	90	4.00	3.60
Sugars	98	3.95	3.87
Vegetable food	97	4.15	4.03
Total carbohydrate, Average	**97**	**4.15**	**4.03**

From Merrill AL, Watt BK. Energy Values of Foods: Basis and Derivation. Agricultural Handbook No. 74, Washington, DC: US Department of Agriculture, 1973.

[a]Net physiologic energy values computed as the coefficient of digestibility times the heat of combustion adjusted for energy loss in urine.

ATWATER GENERAL FACTORS

- 4 $kcal \cdot g^{-1}$ for carbohydrate
- 9 $kcal \cdot g^{-1}$ for lipid
- 4 $kcal \cdot g^{-1}$ for protein

ENERGY VALUE OF A MEAL

The Atwater general factors can determine the caloric content of any portion of food (or an entire meal) from the food's composition and weight. **TABLE 6.2** illustrates the method for calculating the kilocalorie value of 100 g (3.5 oz) of chocolate chip ice cream. Based on laboratory analysis, this ice cream mixture contains approximately 3% protein, 18% lipid, and 23% carbohydrate, with the remaining 56% being essentially

TABLE 6.2 Method to Calculate the Caloric Value of a Food from Its Composition of Macronutrients

Food: ice cream (chocolate with chocolate chips)
Weight: 3/4 cup = 100 g

	Composition		
	Protein	Lipid	Carbohydrate
Percentage	3%	18%	23%
Total grams	3	18	23
In 1 g	0.03	0.18	0.23
Calories per gram	0.12	1.62	0.92

(0.03 × 4.0 kcal) + (0.18 × 9.0 kcal) + (0.23 × 4.0 kcal)
Total calories per gram: 0.12 + 1.62 + 0.92 = 2.66 kcal
Total calories per 100 g: 2.66 × 100 = 266 kcal
Percentage of calories from lipid: (18 g × 9.0 kcal·g^{-1}) ÷ 266 kcal × 100 = 60.9%

water. Thus, each gram of ice cream contains 0.03 g protein, 0.18 g lipid, and 0.23 g carbohydrate. Using these compositional values and the Atwater factors, the following represents the kilocalorie value per gram of the chocolate chip ice cream: Net kilocalorie values show that 0.03 g of protein contains 0.12 kcal (0.03 × 4.0 kcal·g^{-1}), 0.18 g of lipid contains 1.62 kcal (0.18 × 9 kcal·g^{-1}), and 0.23 g of carbohydrate contains 0.92 kcal (0.23 × 4.0 kcal·g^{-1}). Combining the separate values for the nutrients yields a total energy value for each gram of chocolate chip ice cream of 2.66 kcal (0.12 + 1.62 + 0.92). A 100-g serving yields a caloric value 100 times as large, or 266 kcal. The percentage of total calories derived from lipid equals 60.9% (162 lipid kcal ÷ 266 total kcal). Similar computations estimate the caloric value for *any* food serving. Of course, increasing or decreasing portion sizes (or adding lipid-rich sauces or creams or using fruits or calorie-free substitutes) affects caloric content accordingly.

Computing the caloric value of foods is time-consuming and laborious. Various governmental agencies in the United States and abroad have evaluated and compiled nutritive values for thousands of foods. The most comprehensive data bank resources include the US Nutrient Data Bank (USNDB) maintained by the US Department of Agriculture's (USDA) Consumer Nutrition Center[12] and a computerized data bank maintained by the Bureau of Nutritional Sciences of Health and Welfare Canada.[8] Many commercial software programs incorporate the original USDA nutritional databases, which are available for download to the public for a nominal fee. (The USDA Nutrient Database can be viewed at **www.nal.usda.gov/fnic/foodcomp/search/**; the Nutrient Data Laboratory can be accessed at **www.ars.usda.gov/main/site_main.htm?modecode=12-35-45-00**; and the Food and Nutrition Information Center, National Agricultural Library, Agricultural Research Service of the USDA can be accessed at **fnic.nal.usda.gov/nal_display/index.php?info_center=4&tax_level=1**).

Appendix A presents energy and nutritive values for common foods, including specialty and fast-food items. Compute nutritive values for specialty dishes such as chicken or beef tacos from standard recipes; actual values vary considerably depending on the preparation method. Examination of Appendix A reveals large differences among the energy values of various foods. Consuming an equal number of calories from diverse foods often requires increasing or decreasing the quantity of a particular food. For example, to consume 100 kcal from each of six common foods—carrots, celery, green peppers, grapefruit, medium-sized eggs, and mayonnaise—one must eat 5 carrots, 20 stalks of celery, 6.5 green peppers, 1 large grapefruit, 1¼ eggs, but only 1 tbsp of mayonnaise. Consequently, an average sedentary adult woman would need to consume 420 celery stalks, 105 carrots, 136 green peppers, or 26 eggs, yet only 1½ cup of mayonnaise or 8 oz of salad oil, to meet her daily 2100-kcal energy needs. These examples dramatically illustrate that foods high in lipid content contain considerably more calories than foods low in lipid with correspondingly higher water content.

Calories Equal Calories

A calorie reflects food energy regardless of the food source. From an energy standpoint, 100 calories from mayonnaise equals the same 100 calories in 20 celery stalks, or 100 calories of Ben and Jerry's Chocolate Macadamia ice cream still equals 100 calories of asparagus spears! For example, the caloric equivalent of a Carl's Jr. Guacamole Bacon Six Dollar Burger (1040 total kcal; 650 kcal from fat [72 g or 62.5%; 24 g saturated fat]) remains the equivalent of 208 celery stalks! Or stated somewhat differently, consuming 208 celery stalks would provide the same number of total calories as this super-sized burger. A person's caloric intake equals the sum of *all* energy consumed from either small or large quantities of foods. It should be clear that even celery and asparagus spears would become "fattening" foods if consumed in excess. Chapter 7 considers variations in daily energy intake among sedentary and active persons, including diverse groups of athletes.

PERSONAL HEALTH AND EXERCISE NUTRITION 6.1

Nutrient Timing to Optimize Muscle Response to Resistance Training

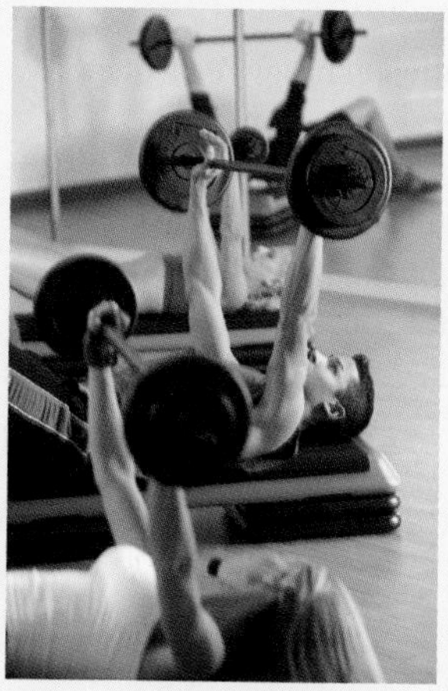

New research findings in sports and exercise nutrition emphasize not only the specific type and mixture of nutrients but also the timing of nutrient intake to enhance performance. The goal of nutrient timing is knowing when to eat and what to eat to help athletes, recreational competitors, and exercise enthusiasts achieve their most advantageous exercise performance and subsequent recovery. Knowing about nutrient timing enables one to blunt the catabolic state (release of the hormones glucagon, epinephrine, norepinephrine, cortisol) and activate the natural muscle-building hormones (testosterone, growth hormone, insulin-like growth factor-1, insulin) to facilitate recovery from exercise and maximize muscle growth. The three phases for optimizing specific nutrient intake include

1. The **energy phase** (a) enhances nutrient intake to spare muscle glycogen and protein, (b) enhances muscular endurance, (c) limits immune system suppression, (d) reduces muscle damage, and (e) facilitates recovery in the postexercise period. Consuming a carbohydrate/protein supplement in the immediate pre-exercise period and during exercise extends muscular endurance; the ingested protein promotes protein metabolism, thus reducing demand for muscle's release of amino acids. Carbohydrates consumed during exercise suppress cortisol release. This blunts the suppressive effects of exercise on immune system function and reduces branched-chain amino acids generated by protein breakdown for energy.

> *The recommended* energy phase *supplement profile contains the following nutrients: 20 to 26 g of high-glycemic carbohydrates (glucose, sucrose, maltodextrin), 5 to 6 g of whey protein (rapidly digested, high-quality protein separated from milk in the cheese-making process), 1 g of leucine, 30 to 120 mg of vitamin C, 20 to 60 IU of vitamin E, 100 to 250 mg of sodium, 60 to 100 mg of potassium, and 60 to 220 mg of magnesium.*

2. The **anabolic phase** consists of the 45-min postexercise metabolic window—a period that enhances insulin sensitivity for muscle glycogen replenishment and muscle tissue repair and synthesis. This shift from catabolic to anabolic state occurs largely by blunting the action of cortisol and increasing the anabolic, muscle-building effects of insulin by consuming a standard high-glycemic carbohydrate/protein supplement in liquid form (e.g., whey protein and high-glycemic carbohydrates). In essence, the high-glycemic carbohydrate consumed after exercise serves as a nutrient activator to stimulate insulin release, which in the presence of amino acids increases muscle tissue synthesis and decreases protein degradation.

> *The recommended* anabolic phase *supplement profile contains the following nutrients: 40 to 50 g of high-glycemic carbohydrates (glucose, sucrose, maltodextrin), 13 to 15 g of whey protein, 1 to 2 g of leucine, 1 to 2 g of glutamine, 60 to 120 mg of vitamin C, and 80 to 400 IU of vitamin E.*

3. The **growth phase** extends from the end of the anabolic phase to the beginning of the next workout. It represents the time period to maximize insulin sensitivity and maintain an anabolic state to accentuate gains in muscle mass and muscle strength. The *rapid segment*, which involves the first several hours of this phase, helps maintain increased insulin sensitivity and glucose uptake to maximize glycogen replenishment. It also aims to speed elimination of metabolic wastes via increases in blood flow and stimulation of tissue repair and muscle growth. The *sustained segment*, which involves the next 16 to 18 h, maintains a positive nitrogen balance. This occurs with a relatively high daily protein intake (between 0.91 and 1.2 g of protein per pound of body weight), which fosters sustained but slower muscle tissue synthesis. An adequate carbohydrate intake emphasizes glycogen replenishment.

> *The recommended* growth phase *supplement profile contains the following nutrients: 14 g of whey protein, 2 g of casein, 3 g of leucine, 1 g of glutamine, and 2 to 4 g of high-glycemic carbohydrates.*

Ivy J, Portman R. *Nutrient Timing: The Future of Sports Nutrition.* North Bergen, NY: Basic Health Publications Inc., 2004.
Skolnik H, Chernus A. *Nutrient Timing for Peak Performance.* Champaign, IL: Human Kinetics Press, 2010.

SUMMARY

1. A kilocalorie, or kcal, represents a measure of heat that expresses the energy value of food.
2. Burning food in the bomb calorimeter directly quantifies the food's energy content.
3. The heat of combustion represents the amount of heat liberated by the complete oxidation of a food in the bomb calorimeter. Average gross energy values equal 4.2 $kcal \cdot g^{-1}$ for carbohydrate, 9.4 $kcal \cdot g^{-1}$ for lipid, and 5.65 $kcal \cdot g^{-1}$ for protein.
4. The coefficient of digestibility indicates the proportion of food consumed that the body digests and absorbs.
5. Coefficients of digestibility average 97% for carbohydrates, 95% for lipids, and 92% for proteins. Thus, the net energy values (known as Atwater general factors) are 4 $kcal \cdot g^{-1}$ of carbohydrate, 9 $kcal \cdot g^{-1}$ of lipid, and 4 $kcal \cdot g^{-1}$ of protein.
6. The Atwater calorific values allow one to compute the caloric content of any meal from the food's carbohydrate, lipid, and protein content.
7. The calorie represents a unit of heat energy regardless of food source. From an energy standpoint, 500 kcal of chocolate ice cream topped with whipped cream and hazelnuts is no more fattening than 500 kcal of watermelon, 500 kcal of cheese and pepperoni pizza, or 500 kcal of a bagel with salmon, onions, and sour cream.

MEASUREMENT OF HUMAN ENERGY EXPENDITURE

ENERGY RELEASED BY THE BODY

All of the metabolic processes within the body ultimately result in heat production. Thus, the rate of heat production from cells, tissues, or even the whole body operationally defines the rate of energy metabolism. The calorie represents the basic unit of heat measurement, and the term *calorimetry* defines the measurement of heat transfer. **Direct calorimetry** and **indirect calorimetry**, two different measurement approaches illustrated in **FIGURE 6.2**, accurately quantify the energy generated by the body during rest and physical activity.

Direct Calorimetry

Heat represents the ultimate fate of all of the body's metabolic processes. The early experiments of French chemist Antoine Lavoisier (1743–1794; see Connections to the Past in this chapter) and his contemporaries in the 1770s provided the impetus to directly measure energy expenditure during rest and physical activity (**scienceworld.wolfram.com/biography/Lavoisier.html**). The idea, similar to that used in the bomb calorimeter depicted in Figure 6.1, provides a convenient although elaborate way to directly measure heat production in humans.

The human calorimeter illustrated in **FIGURE 6.3** consists of an airtight chamber with an oxygen supply where a person lives and works for an extended period.[1] A known water volume at a specified temperature circulates through a series of coils at the top of the chamber. This water absorbs the heat produced and radiated by the person while in the calorimeter. Insulation protects the entire chamber, so any change in water temperature relates directly to the person's energy metabolism. For adequate ventilation, the person's exhaled air continually passes from the room through chemicals that remove moisture and absorb carbon dioxide. Oxygen added to the air recirculates through the chamber. Direct measurement of heat production in humans has considerable theoretical implications, yet its application is limited. Accurate measurements of heat production in the calorimeter require considerable time and expense and formidable engineering expertise. Thus, use of the calorimeter remains inapplicable for energy determinations for most sport, occupational, and recreational activities.

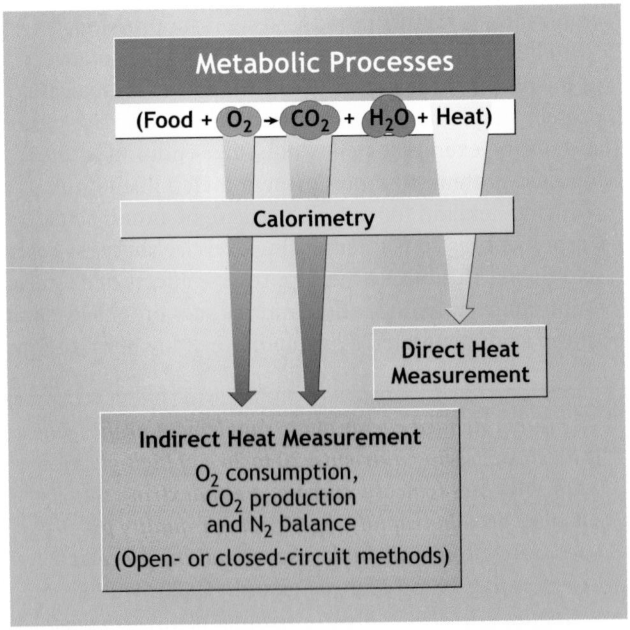

FIGURE 6.2. The measurement of the body's rate of heat production gives a direct assessment of metabolic rate. Heat production (metabolic rate) can be estimated indirectly by measuring the exchange of carbon dioxide and oxygen gases during the breakdown of food macronutrients and nitrogen excretion.

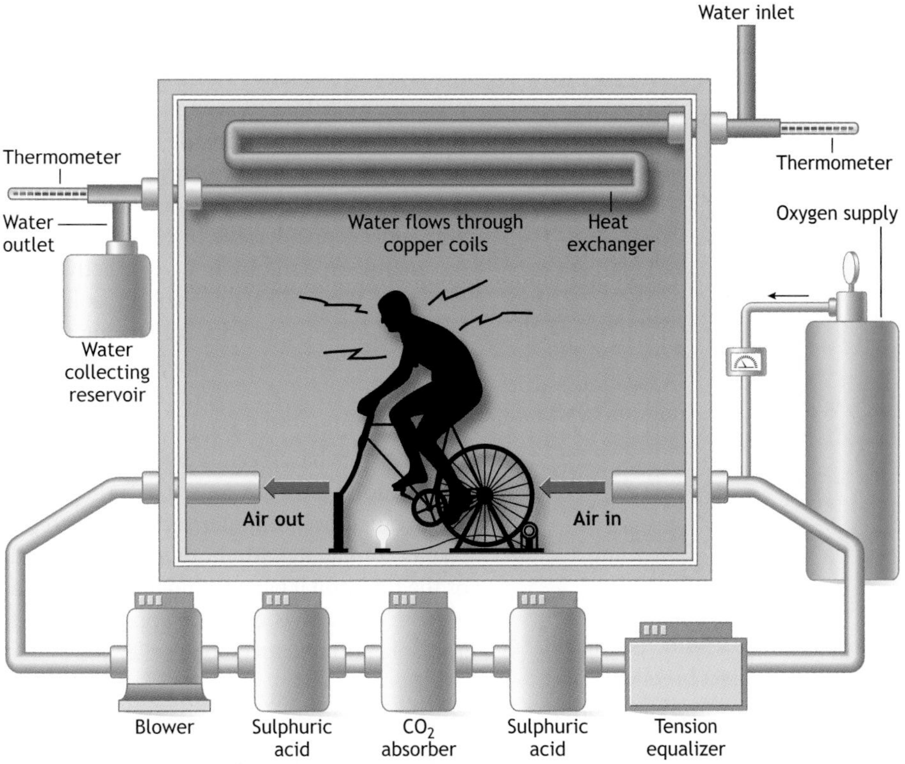

FIGURE 6.3. A human calorimeter directly measures energy metabolism (heat production). In the Atwater-Rosa calorimeter, a thin copper sheet lines the interior wall to which heat exchangers attach overhead and through which water passes. Water cooled to 2°C moves at a high flow rate, rapidly absorbing the heat radiated from the subject during exercise. As the subject rests, warmer water flows at a slower flow rate. In the original bicycle ergometer shown in the schematic, the rear wheel contacts the shaft of a generator that powers a light bulb. In a later version of the ergometer, copper made up part of the rear wheel. The wheel rotated through the field of an electromagnet, producing an electric current to accurately determine power output.

Indirect Calorimetry

All energy-releasing reactions in the body ultimately depend on oxygen use. Measuring a person's oxygen uptake therefore provides an indirect yet accurate estimate of energy expenditure. Indirect calorimetry remains relatively simple to operate and less expensive to maintain and staff than direct calorimetry.

Caloric Transformation for Oxygen

Research with the bomb calorimeter shows that approximately 4.82 kcal release when a blend of carbohydrate, lipid, and protein burns in 1 L of oxygen. Even with large variations in the metabolic mixture, this calorific value for oxygen varies only slightly within 2 to 4%. Assuming the metabolism of a mixed diet, a rounded value of 5.0 kcal · L^{-1} of oxygen consumed designates the appropriate conversion factor to estimate energy expenditure under steady-rate conditions of aerobic metabolism. An energy-oxygen equivalent of 5.0 kcal · L^{-1} provides a convenient yardstick to transpose any aerobic physical activity to a caloric (energy) frame of reference. In fact, indirect calorimetry through oxygen uptake measurement serves as the basis to quantify the energy or caloric stress of most physical activities (refer to Appendix B).

Closed-circuit spirometry and open-circuit spirometry represent the two common methods of indirect calorimetry.

Closed-Circuit Spirometry

FIGURE 6.4 illustrates the technique of closed-circuit spirometry developed in the late 1800s and still used in hospitals and some laboratories dedicated to human nutrition research to estimate resting energy expenditure. The subject breathes 100% oxygen from a prefilled container called a spirometer. The equipment consists of a "closed system" because the person rebreathes only the gas in the spirometer. A canister of soda lime (potassium hydroxide) in the breathing circuit absorbs the carbon dioxide in the exhaled air. A drum attached to the spirometer revolves at a known speed and records oxygen uptake from changes in the system's volume.

Oxygen uptake measurement with closed-circuit spirometry becomes problematic during exercise. The subject must remain close to the bulky equipment, the circuit's resistance to the large breathing volumes in exercise is considerable, and during intense exercise the speed of carbon dioxide removal becomes inadequate. For these reasons, open-circuit spirometry remains the most widely used procedure to measure exercise oxygen uptake.

Open-Circuit Spirometry

With open-circuit spirometry, a subject inhales ambient air with a constant composition of 20.93% oxygen, 0.03%

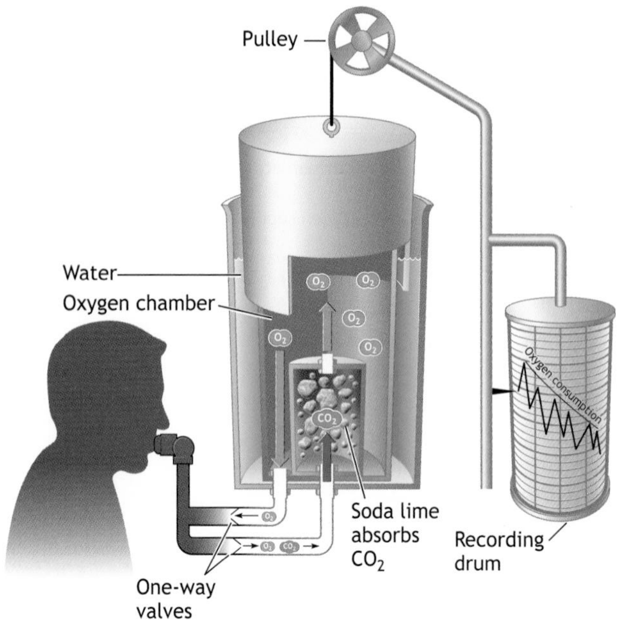

FIGURE 6.4. The closed-circuit method uses a spirometer prefilled with 100% oxygen. As the subject breathes from the spirometer, soda lime removes the expired air's carbon dioxide content. The difference between the initial and final volumes of oxygen in the calibrated spirometer indicates oxygen consumption during the measurement interval.

carbon dioxide, and 79.04% nitrogen. The nitrogen fraction also includes a small quantity of inert gases (e.g., argon 0.93%; krypton 0.00011%; xenon 0.0000087%). The changes in oxygen and carbon dioxide percentages in expired air compared with those in inspired ambient air indirectly reflect the ongoing process of energy metabolism. Thus, analysis of two factors—volume of air breathed during a specified time period and composition of exhaled air—provides a useful way to measure oxygen uptake and infer energy expenditure.

Five common indirect calorimetry procedures measure oxygen uptake under various conditions:

1. Portable spirometry
2. Bag technique
3. Ventilated hood technique
4. Computerized instrumentation
5. Doubly labeled water technique

Portable Spirometry: German scientists in the early 1940s perfected a lightweight, portable system first devised by German respiratory physiologist Nathan Zuntz (1847–1920) at the turn of the 20th century to determine indirectly the energy expended during physical activity.[13] Activities included war-related operations such as traveling over different terrain with full battle gear, operating transportation vehicles including tanks and aircraft, and physical tasks that soldiers encounter during combat operations. The subject carried a backpack-like, 3-kg, box-shaped apparatus. Ambient inspired air passed through a two-way valve, and the expired air exited through a gas meter. The meter measured total expired air volume and collected a small gas sample for later analysis of oxygen and carbon dioxide content. Subsequent determination was made of oxygen uptake and energy expenditure for the measurement period. Carrying the portable spirometer allows considerable freedom of movement for estimating energy expenditure in diverse activities such as mountain climbing, downhill skiing, sailing, golf, and common household activities (Appendix B). During vigorous activity, however, the equipment becomes cumbersome. Also, the meter under records airflow volume during intense exercise with rapid breathing.[15] Subsequently, many different, smaller portable systems have been designed, tested, and used in various applications. For the most part, these systems use the latest advances in computer technology to produce acceptable results compared with more fixed, dedicated desktop systems or the traditional bag technique described in the next section. **FIGURE 6.5** shows exercise applications of a commercially available portable metabolic collection system.

CALORIES ADD UP WITH REGULAR EXERCISE

For distance runners who train up to 100 miles weekly, or slightly less than the distance of four marathons at close to competitive speeds, the weekly caloric expenditure from training averages about 10,000 kcal. For the serious marathon runner who trains year-round, the total energy expended in training for 4 years before an Olympic competition exceeds 2 million kcal—the caloric equivalent of 555 pounds of body fat. This more than likely contributes to the low levels of body fat (3–5% of body mass for men, 12–17% for women) of these highly conditioned yet efficient "metabolic machines."

Bag Technique: **FIGURE 6.6** depicts an application of the classic bag technique to measure oxygen consumption during exercise. In this example, a subject performs front-crawl swimming exercise wearing headgear with a two-way, high-velocity, low-resistance breathing valve. He breathes ambient air through one side of the valve and expels it from the other side. The air then passes into either large canvas or plastic Douglas bags (named for distinguished British respiratory physiologist Claude G. Douglas [1882–1963]) or rubber meteorologic balloons or directly through a gas meter that continually measures expired air volume. The meter collects a small sample (aliquot) of expired air for analysis of oxygen and carbon dioxide composition. Assessment of oxygen uptake (as with all indirect calorimetric techniques) uses an appropriate calorific transformation for oxygen to compute energy expenditure.[8]

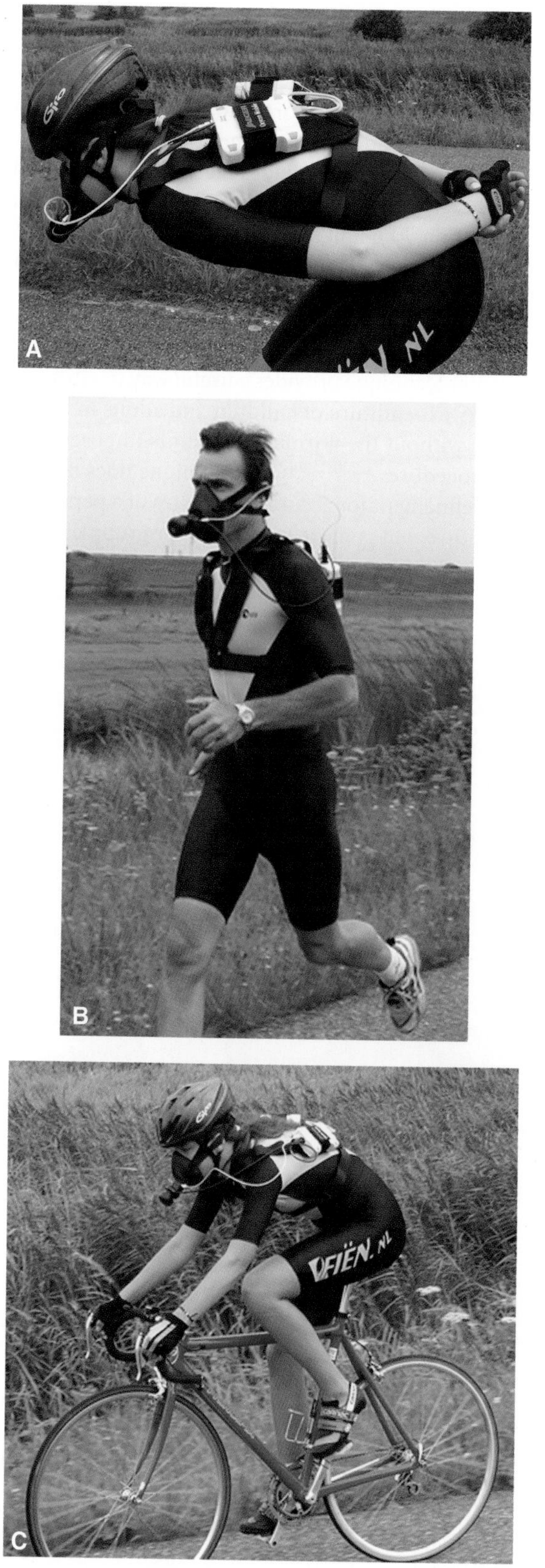

FIGURE 6.5. Portable metabolic collection systems use the latest in miniature computer technology. Built-in oxygen and carbon dioxide analyzer cells coupled with a highly sensitive micro-flow meter measure oxygen uptake by the open-circuit method during different activities such as **(A)** in-line skating, **(B)** running, and **(C)** cycling.

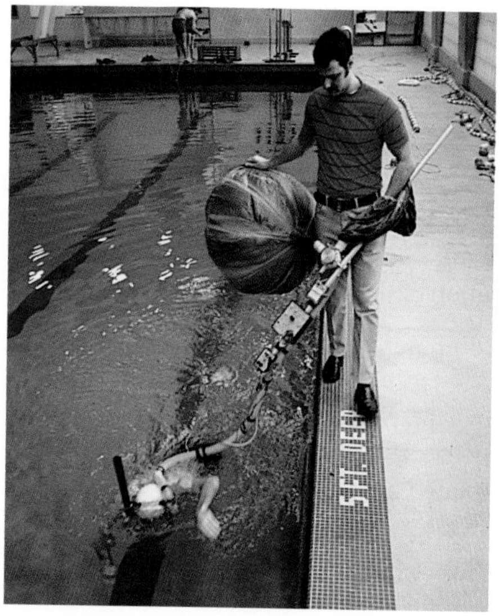

FIGURE 6.6. Measurement of oxygen uptake with open-circuit spirometry (bag technique) during front-crawl swimming.

VENTILATED HOOD TECHNIQUE: The open ventilated hood technique represents an application of open-circuit spirometry (**FIG. 6.7**). With this technique, a flexible cone or tent surrounds the patient's head and shoulders so the expired gasses are captured by the airflow pumped through the tent to oxygen and carbon dioxide gas analyzers. This method permits continuous monitoring over longer periods than tolerated with the restriction imposed by mouthpieces, nose clips, and hoses with the typical methods of open-circuit spirometry. This technique remains the method of choice to estimate basal and resting energy expenditure during longer durations of rest and sleep.

COMPUTERIZED INSTRUMENTATION: With advances in computer and microprocessor technology, the exercise scientist can rapidly measure metabolic and

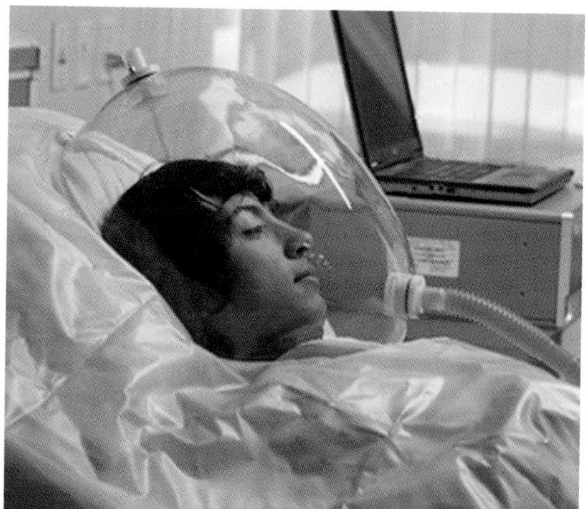

FIGURE 6.7. Ventilated hood system of open-circuit spirometry.

physiologic responses to exercise, although some have raised concern about the accuracy of a widely used computerized breath-by-breath system.[8]

A computer interfaces with at least three instruments:

1. System that continuously samples the subject's expired air
2. Flow-measuring device that records air volume breathed
3. Oxygen and carbon dioxide analyzers that measure the composition of the expired gas mixture

The computer performs metabolic calculations based on electronic signals it receives from the instruments. A printed or graphic display of the data appears throughout the measurement period. More advanced systems include continuously automated blood pressure, heart rate, and temperature monitors with preset instructions to regulate speed, duration, and workload of a treadmill, bicycle ergometer, stepper, rower, swim flume, or other exercise apparatus. **FIGURE 6.8** depicts a modular computerized systems approach for collecting, analyzing, and displaying metabolic and physiologic responses during exercise.

Newer portable systems include wireless telemetric transmission of data for metabolic measurement—pulmonary ventilation and oxygen and carbon dioxide analysis—during a broad range of exercise, sport, and occupational activities.[4] The lightweight and miniaturized components include a voice-sensitive chip that provides feedback on pacing, duration of exercise, energy expenditure, heart rate, and pulmonary ventilation. The unit's microprocessor stores "real-time" exercise or telemetry data for later downloading to a host or satellite computer or storage via "cloud" computing.

DOUBLY LABELED WATER TECHNIQUE: The doubly labeled water technique provides a useful way to estimate total daily energy expenditure of children and adults in free-living conditions without the normal constraints imposed by other indirect procedures.[18,20,21,24] The technique does not furnish sufficient refinement for accurate estimates of a person's energy expenditure, but is more applicable for group estimates.[19] Relatively few subjects participate in research studies with this technique because of the expense involved in using doubly

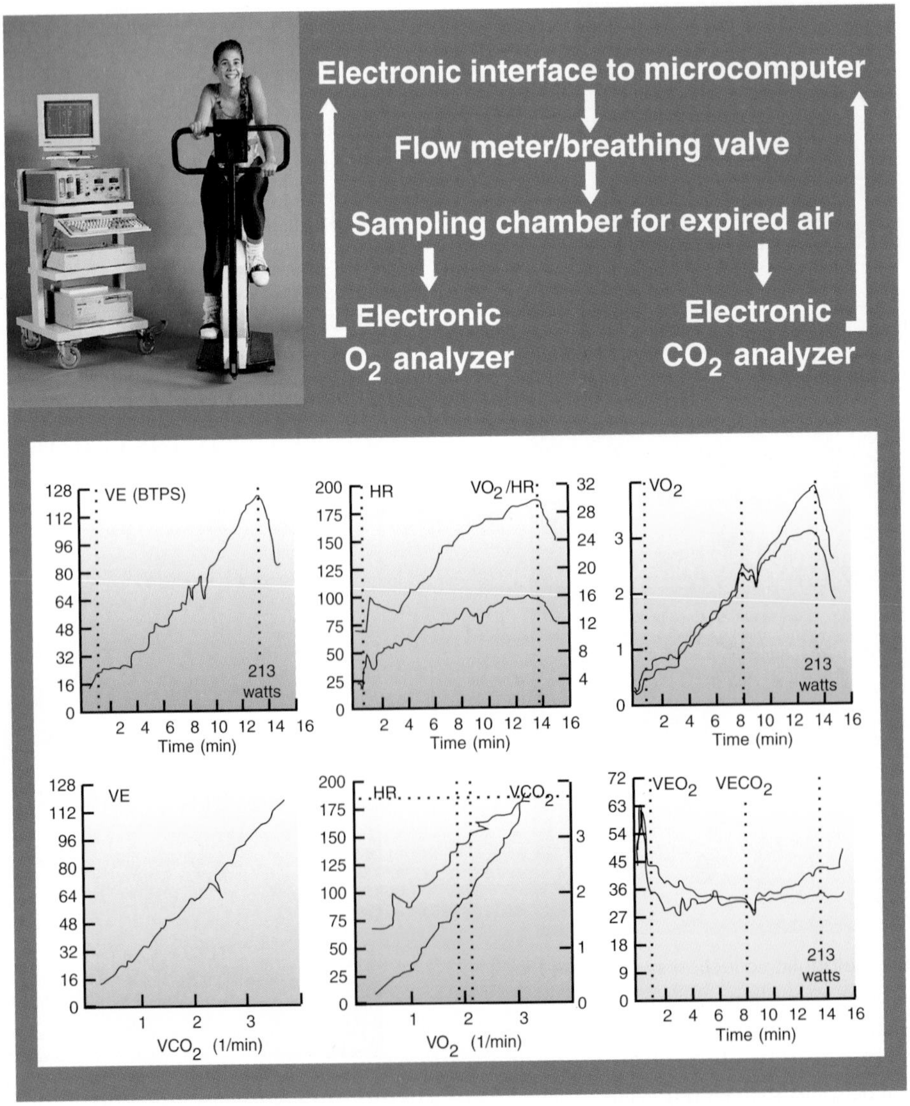

FIGURE 6.8. Computer systems approach to the collection, analysis, and output of physiologic and metabolic data.

labeled water. The high technical accuracy of the method allows doubly labeled water to serve as a criterion for validating other methods (e.g., physical activity questionnaires and physical activity records) to estimate total daily energy expenditure of groups over prolonged time periods.[3,17,21]

The subject consumes a quantity of water containing a known concentration of the stable isotopes of hydrogen (^{2}H or deuterium) and oxygen (^{18}O or oxygen-18)—hence the term *doubly labeled water*. The isotopes distribute throughout all body fluids. Labeled hydrogen leaves the body as water (^2H_2O) in sweat, urine, and pulmonary water vapor, while labeled oxygen leaves as water ($H_2{}^{18}O$) and carbon dioxide ($C^{18}O_2$) produced during macronutrient oxidation in energy metabolism. An isotope ratio mass spectrometer determines the differences between the two isotopes' elimination relative to the body's normal "background" levels. This procedure allows for precise measurement of mixtures of stable isotopes and estimates total carbon dioxide production during the measurement period. Oxygen consumption is estimated based on carbon dioxide production and an assumed or measured respiratory quotient value of 0.85.

Control baseline values for ^{18}O and ^{2}H are determined by analyzing the subject's urine or saliva before ingesting the doubly labeled water. The ingested isotopes require about 5 h to distribute throughout the body water. The initial enriched urine or saliva sample is then measured daily or weekly for the study's duration, usually up to 2 or 3 weeks. The progressive decrease in the sample concentrations of the two isotopes permits computation of carbon dioxide production rate.[19] Accuracy of the doubly labeled water technique versus energy expenditure with oxygen consumption in controlled settings averages between 3 and 5%. This magnitude of error probably increases in field studies, particularly among physically active person's.[24]

The doubly labeled water technique provides an ideal way to assess total energy expenditure of groups over prolonged time periods, including bed rest and during extreme activities such as climbing Mt. Everest, cycling the Tour de France, rowing, and endurance running and swimming.[11,16,21] Major drawbacks of the method include the cost of enriched ^{18}O and the expense of spectrometric analysis of the two isotopes.

Direct Versus Indirect Calorimetry

Energy metabolism studied simultaneously with direct and indirect calorimetry provides convincing evidence for the validity of the indirect method to estimate human energy expenditure. At the turn of the 20th century, Atwater and Rosa compared direct and indirect calorimetric methods for 40 days with three men who lived in calorimeters similar to the one in Figure 6.3. Their daily caloric outputs averaged 2723 kcal when measured directly by heat production and 2717 kcal when computed indirectly using closed-circuit measures of oxygen consumption. Other experiments with animals and humans based on moderate exercise also have demonstrated close agreement between the two methods; the difference averaged mostly less than ±1%. In the Atwater and Rosa experiments, the ±0.2% method error represents a remarkable technical achievement given that these experiments relied on handmade instruments.

THE RESPIRATORY QUOTIENT

Research in the early part of the 19th century discovered a way to evaluate the metabolic mixture in exercise from measures of gas exchange in the lungs.[12] The complete oxidation of a molecule's carbon and hydrogen atoms to carbon dioxide and water end products requires different amounts of oxygen. Thus, the substrate metabolized (whether carbohydrate, fat, or protein) determines the quantity of carbon dioxide produced relative to oxygen consumed. The **respiratory quotient (RQ)** refers to this ratio of metabolic gas exchange as follows:

$$RQ = CO_2 \text{ produced} \div O_2 \text{ consumed}$$

The RQ provides a convenient guide to approximate the nutrient mixture catabolized for energy during rest and aerobic exercise. The caloric equivalent for oxygen differs depending on the macronutrients oxidized, so precisely determining the body's heat production or energy expenditure requires knowledge of both RQ and oxygen uptake.

Respiratory Quotient for Carbohydrate

The complete oxidation of one glucose molecule requires six oxygen molecules and produces six molecules of carbon dioxide and water as follows:

$$C_6H_{12}O_6 + 6\,O_2 \rightarrow 6\,CO_2 + 6\,H_2O$$

Gas exchange during glucose oxidation produces a number of carbon dioxide molecules equal to the oxygen molecules consumed; therefore, the RQ for carbohydrate equals 1.00.

$$RQ = 6\,CO_2 \div 6O_2 = 1.00$$

Respiratory Quotient for Lipid

The chemical composition of lipid differs from carbohydrate because lipid contains considerably fewer oxygen atoms in proportion to carbon and hydrogen atoms. The 2:1 ratio of hydrogen to oxygen in carbohydrate matches the ratio in water, whereas fatty acids have a much larger ratio. Consequently, catabolizing fat for energy requires considerably more oxygen consumed relative to carbon dioxide produced. Palmitic acid, a typical fatty acid, oxidizes to carbon dioxide and water. This reaction produces 16 carbon dioxide molecules for every 23 oxygen molecules consumed. The following equation summarizes this exchange to compute RQ:

$$C_{16}H_{32}O_2 + 23\,O_2 \rightarrow 16\,CO_2 + 16\,H_2O$$
$$RQ = 16\,CO_2 \div 23\,O_2 = 0.696$$

Generally, a value of 0.70 represents the RQ for lipid, with variation ranging between 0.69 and 0.73. The value depends on the oxidized fatty acid's carbon chain length.

Respiratory Quotient for Protein

Proteins do not simply oxidize to carbon dioxide and water during energy metabolism. Rather, the liver first deaminates the amino acid molecule. The body excretes nitrogen and sulfur fragments in the urine, sweat, and feces. The remaining "keto acid" fragment then oxidizes to carbon dioxide and water to provide energy for biologic work. These short-chain keto acids, as with fat catabolism, require more oxygen consumed relative to carbon dioxide produced to achieve complete combustion. The protein albumin oxidizes as follows:

$$C_{72}H_{112}N_2O_{22}S + 77\ O_2 \rightarrow 63\ CO_2 + 38\ H_2O + SO_3 + 9\ CO(NH_2)_2$$

$$RQ = 63\ CO_2 \div 77\ O_2 = 0.818$$

The general value of 0.82 characterizes the RQ for protein.

Estimating Energy Expenditure Using the Weir Method

In 1949, J. B. Weir, a Scottish physician/physiologist from Glasgow University, presented a simple but highly accurate method to estimate caloric expenditure from measures of pulmonary ventilation and the expired oxygen percentage. The Weir method, accurate to within ±1% of the traditional RQ method, is widely used in clinical research.[23]

Basic Equation

Weir showed that the following formula calculates caloric expenditure ($kcal \cdot min^{-1}$) if energy production from protein breakdown averages about 12.5% of total energy expenditure (a reasonable percentage for most persons under typical conditions):

$$kcal \cdot min^{-1} = \dot{V}_{E(STPD)} \times (1.044 - [0.0499 \times \%O_{2E}])$$

where $\dot{V}_{E(STPD)}$ represents expired ventilation per minute (corrected to STPD conditions), and $\%O_{2E}$ represents expired oxygen percentage. The value in parentheses, $(1.044 - [0.0499 \times O_{2E}])$, represents the "Weir factor." **TABLE 6.3** displays Weir factors for different $\%O_{2E}$ values.

To use the table, find the $\%O_{2E}$ and corresponding Weir factor. Compute energy expenditure as $kcal \cdot min^{-1}$ by multiplying the Weir factor by $\dot{V}_{E(STPD)}$.

Example

During a steady-rate jog on a treadmill, $\dot{V}_{E(STPD)} = 50$ $L \cdot min^{-1}$ and $O_{2E} = 16.0\%$. Energy expenditure by the Weir method computes as follows:

$$\begin{aligned} kcal \cdot min^{-1} &= \dot{V}_{E(STPD)} \times (1.044 - [0.0499 \times \%O_{2E}]) \\ &= 50 \times (1.044 - [0.0499 \times 16.0]) \\ &= 50 \times 0.2456 \\ &= 12.3 \end{aligned}$$

Respiratory Quotient for a Mixed Diet

During activities ranging from complete bed rest to moderate aerobic exercise such as walking or slow jogging, the RQ seldom reflects the oxidation of pure carbohydrate or pure fat. Instead, metabolism of a mixture of these two nutrients occurs with an RQ intermediate between 0.70 and 1.00. *For*

TABLE 6.3 Weir Factors for Different Expired Oxygen Percentages ($\%O_{2E}$)

$\%O_{2E}$	Weir Factor	$\%O_{2E}$	Weir Factor	$\%O_{2E}$	Weir Factor	$\%O_{2E}$	Weir Factor
14.50	.3205	15.80	.2556	17.10	.1907	18.30	.1308
14.60	.3155	15.90	.2506	17.20	.1807	18.40	.1268
14.70	.3105	16.00	.2456	17.30	.1857	18.50	.1208
14.80	.3055	16.10	.2406	17.40	.1757	18.60	.1168
14.90	.3005	16.20	.2366	17.50	.1658	18.70	.1109
15.00	.2955	16.30	.2306	17.60	.1707	18.80	.1068
15.10	.2905	16.40	.2256	17.70	.1608	18.90	.1009
15.20	.2855	16.50	.2206	17.80	.1558	19.00	.0969
15.30	.2805	16.60	.2157	17.90	.1508	19.10	.0909
15.40	.2755	16.70	.2107	18.00	.1468	19.20	.0868
15.50	.2705	16.80	.2057	18.10	.1308	19.30	.0809
15.60	.2556	16.90	.2007	18.20	.1368	19.40	.0769
15.70	.2606	17.00	.1957				

Formulas used to calculate data from Weir JB. New methods for calculating metabolic rate with special reference to protein metabolism. J Physiol 1949;109:1. If $\%O_2$ expired does not appear in the table, compute individual Weir factors as $1.044 - 0.0499 \times \%O_{2E}$.

most purposes, we assume an RQ of 0.82 from the metabolism of a mixture of 40% carbohydrate and 60% fat, applying the caloric equivalent of 4.825 kcal per liter of oxygen for the energy transformation. Using 4.825, a value of 4% represents the maximum error possible to estimate energy metabolism from steady-rate oxygen uptake.

TABLE 6.4 presents the energy expenditure per liter of oxygen uptake for different nonprotein RQ values, including their corresponding percentages and grams of carbohydrate and fat used for energy. The nonprotein value assumes that the metabolic mixture comprises *only* carbohydrate and fat. Interpret the table as follows.

Suppose oxygen uptake during 30 min of aerobic exercise averages 3.22 $L \cdot min^{-1}$ with carbon dioxide production of 2.78 L·min−1. The RQ, computed as $\dot{V}CO_2 \div \dot{V}O_2$ (2.78 ÷ 3.22), equals 0.86. From Table 6.4, this RQ value (left column)

TABLE 6.4 Thermal Equivalents of Oxygen for the Nonprotein Respiratory Quotient (RQ), Including Percentage Kilocalories and Grams Derived from Carbohydrate and Lipid

Nonprotein RQ	kcal per L O_2	Percentage Kilocalories Derived from		Grams per L O_2	
		Carbohydrate	Lipid	Carbohydrate	Lipid
0.707	4.686	0.0	100.0	0.000	0.496
0.71	4.690	1.1	98.9	0.012	0.491
0.72	4.702	4.8	95.2	0.051	0.476
0.73	4.714	8.4	91.6	0.090	0.460
0.74	4.727	12.0	88.0	0.130	0.444
0.75	4.739	15.6	84.4	0.170	0.428
0.76	4.750	19.2	80.8	0.211	0.412
0.77	4.764	22.8	77.2	0.250	0.396
0.78	4.776	26.3	73.7	0.290	0.380
0.79	4.788	29.9	70.1	0.330	0.363
0.80	4.801	33.4	66.6	0.371	0.347
0.81	4.813	36.9	63.1	0.413	0.330
0.82	4.825	40.3	59.7	0.454	0.313
0.83	4.838	43.8	56.2	0.496	0.297
0.84	4.850	47.2	52.8	0.537	0.280
0.85	4.862	50.7	49.3	0.579	0.263
0.86	4.875	54.1	45.9	0.621	0.247
0.87	4.887	57.5	42.5	0.663	0.230
0.88	4.889	60.8	39.2	0.705	0.213
0.89	4.911	64.2	35.8	0.749	0.195
0.90	4.924	67.5	32.5	0.791	0.178
0.91	4.936	70.8	29.2	0.834	0.160
0.92	4.948	74.1	25.9	0.877	0.143
0.93	4.961	77.4	22.6	0.921	0.125
0.94	4.973	80.7	19.3	0.964	0.108
0.95	4.985	84.0	16.0	1.008	0.090
0.96	4.998	87.2	12.8	1.052	0.072
0.97	5.010	90.4	9.6	1.097	0.054
0.98	5.022	93.6	6.4	1.142	0.036
0.99	5.035	96.8	3.2	1.186	0.018
1.00	5.047	100.0	0.0	1.231	0.000

corresponds to an energy equivalent of 4.875 kcal · L^{-1} of oxygen uptake or an exercise energy output of 13.55 kcal · min^{-1} (2.78 L $O_2 \cdot min^{-1}$ × 4.875 kcal). Based on a nonprotein RQ, 54.1% of the calories come from the combustion of carbohydrate and 45.9% from fat. The total calories expended during the 30-min exercise equals 406 kcal (13.55 kcal · min^{-1} × 30).

> **OXYGEN UPTAKE AND BODY SIZE**
>
> To adjust for the effects of variations in body size on oxygen consumption (i.e., bigger people usually consume more oxygen), researchers frequently express oxygen consumption in terms of body mass (termed **relative oxygen consumption**), as milliliters of oxygen per kilogram of body mass per minute ($mL \cdot kg^{-1} \cdot min^{-1}$). At rest, this averages about 3.5 $mL \cdot kg^{-1} \cdot min^{-1}$ **(1 MET)**, or 245 $mL \cdot min^{-1}$ **(absolute oxygen consumption)** for a 70-kg person. Other means of relating oxygen consumption to aspects of body size and body composition include milliliters of oxygen per kilogram of fat-free body mass per minute ($mL \cdot kg\ FFM^{-1} \cdot min^{-1}$) and sometimes milliliters of oxygen per square centimeter of muscle cross-sectional area per minute ($mL \cdot cm\ MCSA^{-2} \cdot min^{-1}$).

THE RESPIRATORY EXCHANGE RATIO

Application of the RQ assumes that oxygen and carbon dioxide exchange measured at the lungs reflects the actual gas exchange from macronutrient metabolism in the cell. This assumption remains reasonably valid for rest and during steady-rate mild to moderate aerobic exercise without lactate accumulation. However, factors such as hyperventilation (overbreathing) can spuriously alter the exchange of oxygen and carbon dioxide in the lungs so the ratio of gas exchange no longer reflects only the substrate mixture in cellular energy metabolism. Respiratory physiologists term the ratio of carbon dioxide produced to oxygen consumed under such conditions the **respiratory exchange ratio** (**R** or **RER**). This ratio computes in exactly the same manner as RQ.

For example, carbon dioxide elimination increases during hyperventilation because the breathing response increases to disproportionately high levels compared with actual metabolic demand. By overbreathing, the normal carbon dioxide level in blood decreases as this gas "blows off" in expired air. A corresponding increase in oxygen uptake does not occur with this additional carbon dioxide elimination; thus, the rise in R cannot be attributed to the oxidation of foodstuff. In such cases, R usually increases above 1.00.

Exhaustive exercise presents another anomaly that causes R to rise above 1.00. In such cases, sodium bicarbonate in the blood buffers or "neutralizes" the lactate generated during anaerobic metabolism to maintain proper acid-base balance in the following reaction:

$$HLa + NaHCO_3 \rightarrow NaLa + H_2CO_3 \rightarrow H_2O + CO_2 \rightarrow Lungs$$

Buffering of lactate produces the weaker carbonic acid. In the pulmonary capillaries, carbonic acid degrades to carbon dioxide and water components, and carbon dioxide readily exits through the lungs. The R increases above 1.00 because buffering adds "extra" carbon dioxide to the expired air, in excess of the quantity normally released during energy metabolism.

Relatively low values for R occur following exhaustive exercise when carbon dioxide remains in cells and body fluids to replenish the bicarbonate that buffered the accumulating lactate. This action reduces the expired carbon dioxide without affecting oxygen uptake. This causes the R to dip below 0.70.

MEASUREMENT OF HUMAN ENERGY-GENERATING CAPACITIES

We all possess the capability for anaerobic and aerobic energy metabolism, although the capacity for each form of energy transfer varies considerably among person's. **FIGURE 6.9** shows the involvement of the anaerobic and aerobic energy transfer systems for different durations of all-out exercise. At the initiation of either high- or low-speed movements, the intramuscular phosphagens adenosine triphosphate (ATP) and phosphocreatine (PCr) provide immediate and nonaerobic energy for muscle action. Following the first few seconds of muscular movement, the glycolytic energy system (initial phase of carbohydrate breakdown) provides an increasingly greater proportion of total energy. Continuation of exercise places a progressively greater demand on aerobic metabolic pathways for ATP resynthesis.

Some physical activities require the capacity of more than one energy transfer system, whereas other activities rely predominantly on a single system. All activities activate each energy system to some degree depending on exercise intensity and duration. Greater demand for anaerobic energy transfer occurs for higher intensity and shorter duration activities.

Both direct and indirect calorimetric techniques estimate the power and capacity of the different energy systems during different physical activities. **TABLE 6.5** lists some of the direct and indirect physiologic performance tests in common use for such purposes.

ENERGY EXPENDITURE DURING REST AND PHYSICAL ACTIVITY

Three factors determine total daily energy expenditure (**FIG. 6.10**):

1. Resting metabolic rate, which includes basal and sleeping conditions plus the added energy cost of arousal
2. Thermogenic influence of food consumed
3. Energy expended during physical activity and recovery

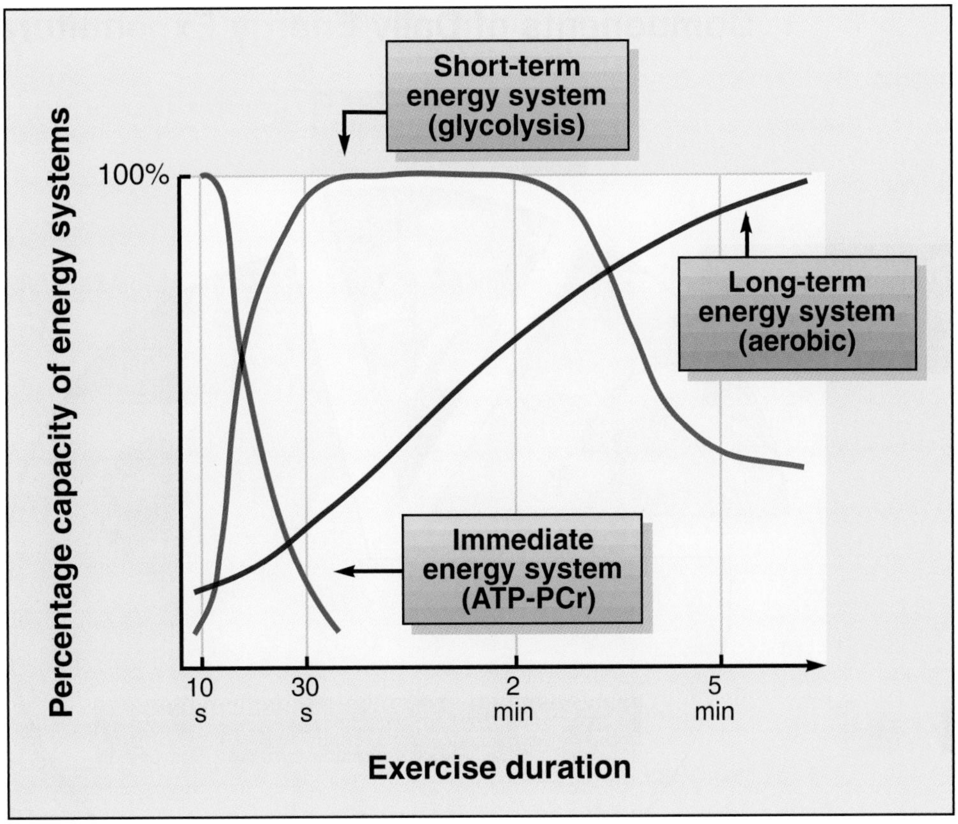

FIGURE 6.9. Three energy systems and their percent contribution to total energy output during all-out exercise of different durations.

Basal Metabolic Rate

For each person, a minimum energy requirement sustains the body's functions in the waking state. Measuring oxygen consumption under the following three standardized conditions quantifies this requirement called the **basal metabolic rate (BMR)**:

1. No food consumed for at least 12 h before measurement; the **postabsorptive state** describes this condition
2. No undue muscular exertion for at least 12 h before measurement
3. Measured after the person has been lying quietly for 30 to 60 min in a dimly lit, temperature-controlled (thermoneutral) room

Maintaining controlled conditions provides a standardized way to study the relationship between energy expenditure and body size, gender, and age.[26] The BMR also establishes an important energy baseline for implementing a prudent program of weight control using food restraint, exercise, or a combination of both. In most instances, basal values measured in the laboratory remain only marginally lower than values

TABLE 6.5 Common Direct (Physiologic) and Indirect (Performance) Tests of Human Energy-Generating Capacities

Energy System	Direct (Physiologic) Measures	Indirect (Performance Test) Measures
Immediate (anaerobic) system	Changes in ATP/PCr levels for all-out exercise, ≤ 30 s	Stair sprinting; power jumping; power lifting
Short-term (anaerobic) system	Lactate response/glycogen depletion to exercise, ≤ 3 min	Sprinting; all-out cycle ergometry (e.g., all-out Wingate Test), running and swimming tests
Long-term (aerobic) system	$\dot{V}O_{2max}$[a] assessment; 4–20 min duration of maximal incremental exercise	Walk/jog/run/step/cycle tests; submaximal and maximal tests; heart rate response to exercise

[a]*Highest oxygen uptake achieved per minute during maximal endurance exercise.*

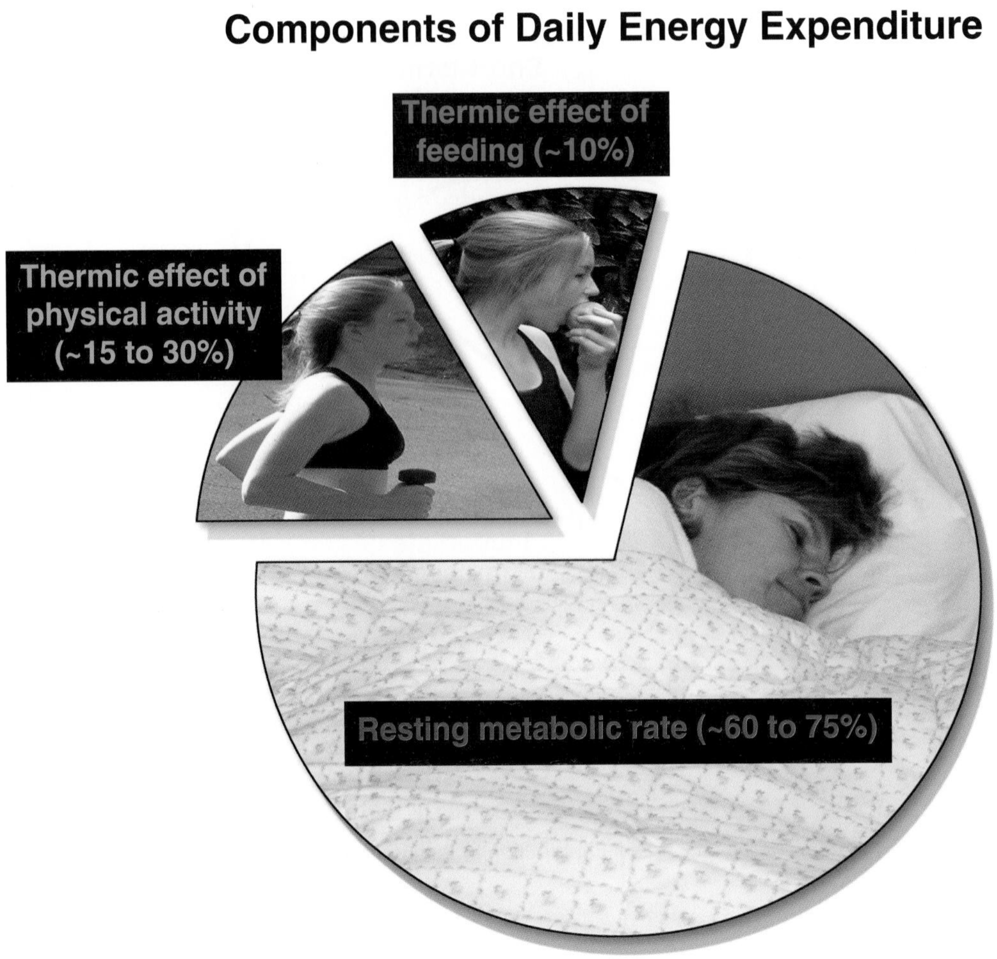

FIGURE 6.10. Components of daily energy expenditure.

> **REGULAR EXERCISE SLOWS THE DECREASE IN METABOLISM WITH AGE**
>
> Increases in body fat and decreases in fat-free body mass (FFM) largely explain the 2% decline in BMR per decade through adulthood. Regular physical activity blunts the age-related decrease in BMR. An accompanying 8% increase in resting metabolism occurred when 50- to 65-year-old men increased FFM with intense resistance training. In addition, an 8-week aerobic conditioning program for older adults increased resting metabolism by 10% without any change in FFM, indicating that endurance and resistance exercise training can offset the decrease in resting metabolism usually observed with aging.

for the resting metabolic rate measured under less stringent conditions. One example would include measurement 3 to 4 h after a light meal without physical activity. The terms basal metabolism and resting metabolism often are applied interchangeably.

Influence of Body Size on Resting Metabolism

FIGURE 6.11 shows that BMR (expressed as kilocalories per square meter of body surface area per hour; $kcal \cdot m^{-2} \cdot h^{-1}$) averages 5 to 10% lower in females compared with males at all ages. A female's larger percentage of body fat and smaller muscle mass relative to body size help explain her lower metabolic rate per unit of surface area. From ages 20 to 40 years, average values for BMR equal 38 $kcal \cdot m^{-2} \cdot h^{-1}$ for men and 35 $kcal \cdot m^{-2} \cdot h^{-1}$ for women.

Estimating Resting Daily Energy Expenditure

Use the curves in **FIGURE 6.11** to estimate a person's **resting daily energy expenditure (RDEE).** For example, between ages 20 and 40 years, the BMR of men averages about 38 $kcal \cdot m^{-2} \cdot h^{-1}$, whereas for women, the corresponding value

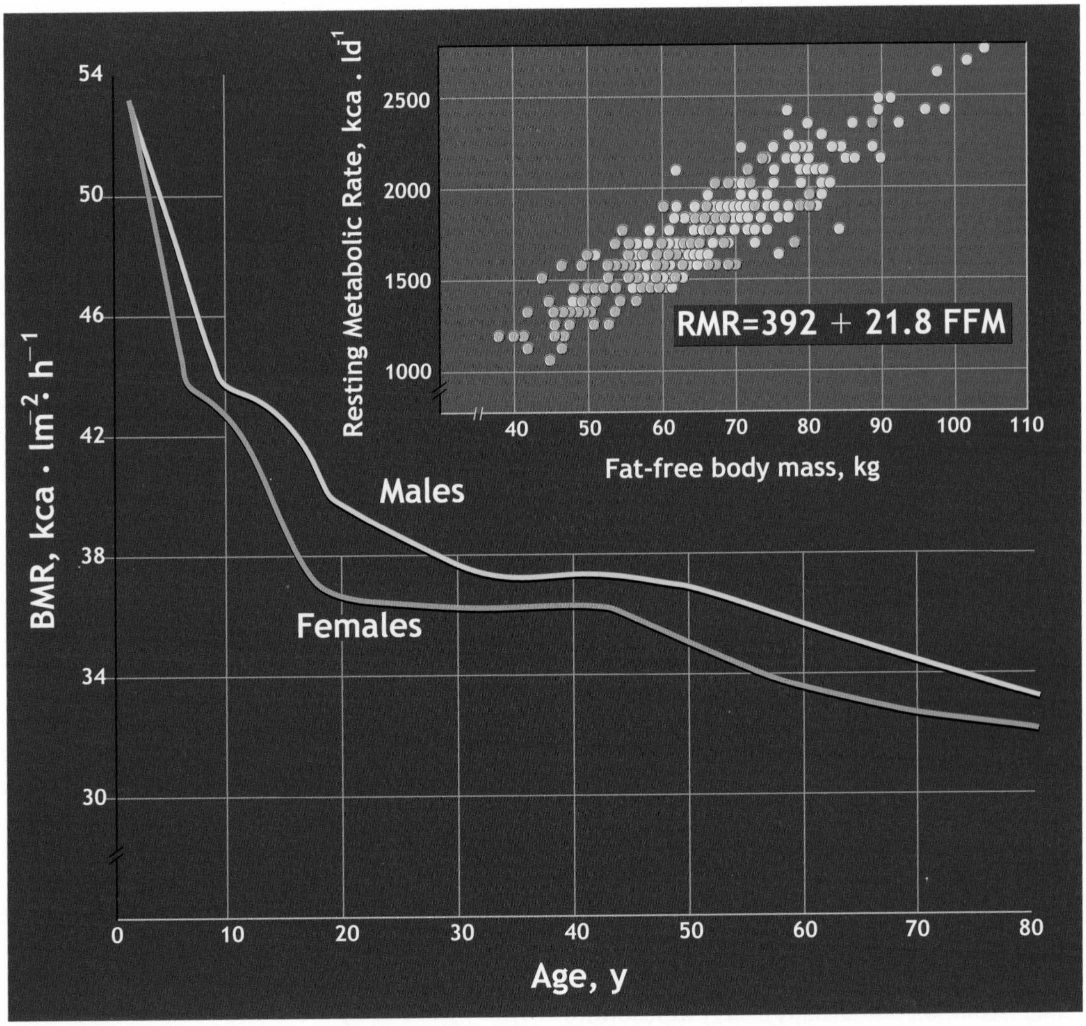

FIGURE 6.11. BMR as a function of age and gender. (Data from Altman PL, Dittmer D. *Metabolism*. Bethesda, MD: Federation of American Societies for Experimental Biology, 1968.) Inset graph shows the strong relationship between fat-free body mass and daily resting metabolic rate for men and women. (From Ravussin E, et al. Determination of 24-h energy expenditure in man: methods and results using a respiratory chamber. *J Clin Invest* 1986;78:1568.)

equals 35 $kcal \cdot m^{-2} \cdot h^{-1}$. To estimate total metabolic rate per hour ($kcal \cdot h^{-1}$), multiply the BMR value by the person's body surface area (BSA). This hourly total provides important information to estimate the daily energy baseline requirement for caloric intake.

Accurate measurement of BSA poses a considerable challenge. Experiments in the early 1900s provided the data to determine BSA. The studies clothed eight men and two women in tight whole-body underwear and applied melted paraffin and paper strips to prevent modification of their body surface. The treated cloth was then removed and cut into flat pieces to allow precise measurements of body surface area (length × width). The close relationship between height (stature in centimeters) and body weight (mass in kilograms) and BSA enabled derivation of the following empirical formula to predict BSA:

$$\text{BSA, m}^2 = 0.20247 \times \text{Stature}^{0.725} \times \text{Body mass}^{0.425}$$

where stature is height in meters (multiply inches by 0.254 to convert to meters) and body mass is weight in kilograms (divide pounds by 2.205 to convert to kilograms).

Sample BSA computation for a man who is 70 in tall (1.778 m) and weighs 165.3 lb (75 kg):

$$\text{BSA} = 0.20247 \times 1.778^{0.725} \times 75^{0.425}$$
$$= 0.20247 \times 1.51775 \times 6.2647$$
$$= 1.925 \text{ m}^2$$

For a 20-year-old man, for example, the estimated BMR equals 36.5 kcal·m^{-2}·h^{-1}. If his BSA was 1.925 m^{-2} (see related box for BSA computations), the hourly energy expenditure would equal 70.3 kcal (36.5 × 1.925 m^2). On a 24-h basis, this amounts to an RDEE of 1686 kcal (70.3 × 24).

Predicting Resting Daily Energy Expenditure

Body mass (BM, kg), stature (S; in centimeters), and age (A; in years) can estimate RDEE with sufficient accuracy using the following equations for women and men:

$$\text{Women: RDEE} = 655 + (9.6 \times \text{BM}) + (1.85 \times \text{S}) - (4.7 \times \text{A})$$
$$\text{Men: RDEE} = 66.0 + (13.7 \times \text{BM}) + (5.0 \times \text{S}) - (6.8 \times \text{A})$$

Examples

Woman

$$\text{BM} = 62.7 \text{ kg}; \text{S} = 172.5 \text{ cm}; \text{A} = 22.4 \text{ y.}$$
$$\begin{aligned}\text{RDEE} &= 655 + (9.6 \times 62.7) + (1.85 \times 172.5) - (4.7 \times 22.4)\\ &= 655 + 601.92 + 319.13 - 105.28\\ &= 1471 \text{ kcal}\end{aligned}$$

Man

$$\text{BM} = 80 \text{ kg}; \text{S} = 189.0 \text{ cm}; \text{A} = 30 \text{ y.}$$
$$\begin{aligned}\text{RDEE} &= 66.0 + (13.7 \times 80) + (5.0 \times 189.0) - (6.8 \times 30.0)\\ &= 66.0 + 1096 + 945 - 204\\ &= 1903 \text{ kcal}\end{aligned}$$

THREE MAIN FACTORS THAT AFFECT ENERGY EXPENDITURE

Three important factors affect **total daily energy expenditure (TDEE)**:

1. Physical activity
2. Dietary-induced thermogenesis
3. Climate

Pregnancy also affects TDEE mainly through its effect of increasing the energy cost of many modes of weight-bearing physical activity.

Physical Activity

Physical activity profoundly affects human energy expenditure.[2,3,5,9,11,15,22,25] Three to four hours of intense training by world-class athletes nearly doubles their daily caloric output. Most people can sustain metabolic rates that average 10 times the resting value during "big muscle" fast walking and hiking exercise and running, cycling, and swimming. *Physical activity generally accounts for between 15 and 30% of TDEE.*

Dietary-Induced Thermogenesis

Consuming food increases energy metabolism from the energy-requiring processes of digesting, absorbing, and assimilating nutrients. **Dietary-induced thermogenesis** (DIT; also termed **thermic effect of food,** or TEF) typically reaches maximum within 1 h after eating depending on food quantity and type. The magnitude of DIT ranges between 10 and 35% of the ingested food energy. A meal of pure protein, for example, elicits a thermic effect often equaling 25% of the meal's total energy content.

> **TAKE A WALK AFTER EATING**
>
> Persons with poor control over body weight often have a depressed thermic response to eating, an effect most likely related to a genetic predisposition. This can contribute to considerable body fat accumulation over a period of years. Exercising after eating augments a person's normal thermic response to food intake. This supports the wisdom of "going for a brisk walk" following a meal.

Climate

Environmental factors influence resting metabolic rate. The resting metabolism of people who live in tropical climates, for example, averages 5 to 20% higher than counterparts in more temperate regions. Exercise performed in hot weather also imposes a small additional metabolic load; it causes about a 5% elevation in oxygen uptake compared with the same work performed in a thermoneutral environment. The increase in metabolism occurs from a direct thermogenic effect of elevated core temperature plus additional energy required for sweat gland activity and altered metabolism.

Pregnancy

Maternal cardiovascular dynamics follow normal response patterns during pregnancy. Moderate exercise generally presents no greater physiologic stress to the mother other than imposed by the additional weight gain and possible encumbrance of fetal tissue. Pregnancy does not compromise the absolute value for aerobic capacity expressed in L·min^{-1}. As pregnancy progresses, increases in maternal body weight add considerably to exercise effort during weight-bearing walking, jogging, and stair climbing and may also reduce the economy of physical effort.

ENERGY EXPENDITURE DURING PHYSICAL ACTIVITY

An understanding of resting energy metabolism provides an important frame of reference to appreciate the potential of humans to increase daily energy output. According to numerous surveys, *physical inactivity* (e.g., watching television or playing computer games, lounging around the home, and other sedentary activities) accounts for about one third of a person's waking hours. This means that regular physical activity has the potential to considerably boost the TDEE of large numbers of men and women. Actualizing this potential depends on the intensity, duration, and type of physical activity performed.

Additional Insights

Can Extra Vitamins Boost Ability to Generate Energy?

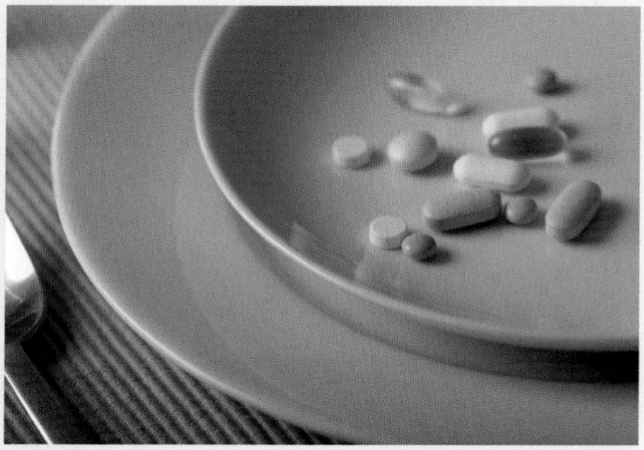

One sure way to sell vitamins and vitamin-enriched energy drinks, energy bars, water, and breakfast cereals is to claim they boost energy level, enhance sports performance, and counter any fatiguing effects of strenuous physical activity. Labels abound with slogans like "ultimate strength B-vitamin formula for all day energy" and "unlock your energy potential." Centrum vitamin company's website (**www.centrum.com/OurProducts/Energy.aspx**) claims that its Centrum Performance Specialist supplement "helps unlock your energy with higher levels of B-vitamins." It further states that "Centrum Specialist naturally helps your body produce energy, while still giving you all the benefits of a Centrum multivitamin."

Some truth and some fiction often cloud such supplement advertisements. We must emphasize that vitamins contain *no useful energy* for the body; instead, they serve as essential links and regulators in metabolic reactions that *release* energy from food. Our bodies do require small amounts of thiamin (vitamin B_1), niacin (vitamin B_3), pantothenic acid (vitamin B_5), and pyridoxine (vitamin B_6) for energy metabolism and protein synthesis. However, adequate quantities of these vitamins are readily available from a wide variety of food in a well-balanced diet. Once the vitamin requirement is met, additional quantities serve no useful purpose and do not "supercharge" the body's energy transfer systems. Also, no credible evidence exists that one's level of regular physical activity increases the recommended level for vitamin intake or that extra vitamin intake above recommended levels increases energy capacity or reduces overall or specific body fatigue. At high levels of daily physical activity, food intake generally increases to sustain the added exercise energy requirements. Additional food consumed through a variety of nutritious meals proportionately increases vitamin and mineral intakes.

Related References

Lavie CJ, Milani JN. Do antioxidant vitamins ameliorate the beneficial effects of exercise training on insulin sensitivity? *J Cardiopulm Rehabil Prev* 2011;31:211.

Sahlin K. Boosting fat burning with carnitine: an old friend comes out from the shadow. *J Physiol* 2011;589:1509.

Singh A, et al. Neuroendocrine response to running in women after zinc and vitamin E supplementation. *Med Sci Sports Exerc* 1999;31:536.

Theodorou AA, et al. No effect of antioxidant supplementation on muscle performance and blood redox status adaptations to eccentric training. *Am J Clin Nutr* 2011;93:1373.

Yfanti C, et al. Effect of antioxidant supplementation on insulin sensitivity in response to endurance exercise training. *Am J Physiol Endocrinol Metab* 2011;300:E761.

Zwart SR, et al. Vitamin K status in spaceflight and ground-based models of spaceflight. *J Bone Miner Res* 2011;26:948.

Researchers have measured the energy expended during diverse activities such as brushing teeth, house cleaning, mowing the lawn, walking the dog, driving a car, playing ping-pong, bowling, dancing, swimming, rock climbing, and physical activity during space flight within the space vehicle and outside during work tasks (extravehicular activity).[9,15] Consider an activity such as rowing continuously at 30 strokes per minute for 30 min. If the amount of oxygen consumed averaged 2.0 L · min^{-1} during each minute of rowing, then in 30 min the rower would consume 60 L of oxygen. A reasonably accurate estimate of the energy expended in rowing can be made because 1 L of oxygen generates about 5 kcal of energy. In this example, the rower expends 300 kcal (60 L × 5 kcal) during the exercise. This value represents **gross energy expenditure** for the exercise period. The **net energy expenditure** attributable solely to rowing equals gross energy expenditure (300 kcal) minus the energy requirement for rest for an equivalent time.

One can estimate TDEE by determining the time spent in daily activities (using a diary) and determining the activity's corresponding energy requirement. Listings of energy expenditure for a wide range of physical activities are available in Appendix B or on the Internet.

Energy Cost of Recreational and Sport Activities

TABLE 6.6 illustrates the energy cost among diverse recreational and sport activities.[11] Notice, for example, that volleyball requires about 3.6 $\text{kcal} \cdot \text{min}^{-1}$ (216 $\text{kcal} \cdot \text{h}^{-1}$) for a person who weighs 71 kg (157 lb). The same person expends more than twice this energy, or 546 $\text{kcal} \cdot \text{h}^{-1}$, swimming the front crawl. Viewed somewhat differently, 25 min spent swimming expends about the same number of calories as playing 1 h of recreational volleyball. Energy expenditure increases

TABLE 6.6 Gross Energy Cost (kcal) for Selected Recreational and Sport Activities in Relation to Body Mass

kg	50	53	56	59	62	65	68	71	74	77	80	83
lb	110	117	123	130	137	143	150	157	163	170	176	183
ACTIVITY												
Volleyball	12.5	2.7	2.8	3.0	3.1	3.3	3.4	3.6	3.7	3.9	4.0	4.2
Aerobic dancing	6.7	7.1	7.5	7.9	8.3	8.7	9.2	9.6	10.0	10.4	10.8	11.2
Cycling, leisure	5.0	5.3	5.6	5.9	6.2	6.5	6.8	7.1	7.4	7.7	8.0	8.3
Tennis	5.5	5.8	6.1	6.4	6.8	7.1	7.4	7.7	8.1	8.4	8.7	9.0
Swimming, slow crawl	6.4	6.8	7.2	7.6	7.9	8.3	8.7	9.1	9.5	9.9	10.2	10.6
Touch football	6.6	7.0	7.4	7.8	8.2	8.6	9.0	9.4	9.8	10.2	10.6	11.0
Running, 8-min mile	10.8	11.3	11.9	12.5	13.11	3.6	14.2	14.8	15.4	16.0	16.5	17.1
Skiing, uphill racing	13.7	14.5	15.3	16.2	17.0	17.8	18.6	19.5	20.3	21.1	21.9	22.7

Copyright © from Fitness Technologies, Inc. 5043 Via Lara lane. Santa Barbara, CA. 93111
Note: Energy expenditure computes as the number of minutes of participation multiplied by the kcal value in the appropriate body weight column. For example, the kcal cost of 1 h of tennis for a person weighing 150 lb (68 kg) equals 444 kcal (7.4 kcal × 60 min).

proportionately if the pace of the swim increases or volleyball becomes more intense.

Effect of Body Weight

Body weight plays an important contributing role in exercise energy requirements. This occurs because the energy expended during **weight-bearing exercise** increases directly with the body weight transported. *Such a strong relationship exists that one can predict energy expenditure during walking or running from body weight with almost as much accuracy as measuring oxygen consumption under controlled laboratory conditions.* In non–weight-bearing or **weight-supported exercise** (e.g., stationary cycling), little relationship exists between body weight and exercise energy cost.

From a practical standpoint, walking and other weight-bearing exercises require a substantial calorie burn for heavier people. Notice in **TABLE 6.6** that playing tennis or volleyball requires considerably greater energy expenditure for a person who weighs 83 kg than for someone 20 kg lighter. Expressing caloric cost of weight-bearing exercise in relation to body weight as kilocalories per kilogram of body weight per minute ($kcal \cdot kg^{-1} \cdot min^{-1}$) greatly reduces the difference in energy expenditure among persons of different body weights. The absolute energy cost of the exercise ($kcal \cdot min^{-1}$) still remains greater for the heavier person.

AVERAGE DAILY RATES OF ENERGY EXPENDITURE

A committee of the US Food and Nutrition Board (www.iom.edu/) proposed various norms to represent average rates of energy expenditure for men and women in the United States. These values apply to people with occupations considered between sedentary and active and who participate in some recreational activities (i.e., weekend swimming, golf, and tennis). **TABLE 6.7** shows that between 2900 and 3000 kcal for males and 2200 kcal for females between the ages of 15 and 50 years represent the average daily energy expenditures. Note in the lower part of the table that the typical person spends about 75% of the day in sedentary activities. This predominance of physical *inactivity* has prompted some sociologists to refer to the modern-day American as *homo sedentarius*. Compelling evidence supports this descriptor because at least 60% of American adults do not obtain enough physical activity to generate positive health benefits. In fact, more than 25% of adults receive no additional physical activity at all during leisure time. Physical activity decreases with age,[25] and sufficient activity becomes less common among women than men, particularly among those with lower incomes and less formal education. Unfortunately, nearly one half of youths age 12 to 21 years are not vigorously active on a regular basis.

THE METABOLIC EQUIVALENT

Values for oxygen consumption and kcal commonly express differences in exercise intensity. As an alternative, a convenient way to express exercise intensity classifies physical effort as multiples of resting energy expenditure with a unit-free measure. To this end, scientists have developed the concept of metabolic equivalents (**METs**), an acronym derived from the term *M*etabolic *E*quivalen*T*. One MET represents an adult's average seated resting oxygen consumption or energy expenditure—about 250 mL $O_2 \cdot min^{-1}$, 3.5 mL $O_2 \cdot kg^{-1} \cdot min^{-1}$, 1 $kcal \cdot kg^{-1} \cdot h^{-1}$, or 0.017 $kcal \cdot kg^{-1} \cdot min^{-1}$

TABLE 6.7 Average Rates of Energy Expenditure for Men and Women Living in the United States[a]

	Age, y	Body Mass kg	Body Mass lb	Stature cm	Stature in	Energy Expenditure, kcal
Males	15–18	66	145	176	69	3000
	19–24	72	160	177	70	2900
	25–50	79	174	176	70	2900
	51+	77	170	173	68	2300
Females	15–18	55	120	163	64	2200
	19–24	58	128	164	65	2200
	25–50	63	138	163	64	2200
	50+	65	143	160	63	1900

AVERAGE TIME SPENT DURING THE DAY

Activity	Time (h)
Sleeping and lying down	8
Sitting	6
Standing	6
Walking	2
Recreational activity	2

Data from Food and Nutrition Board, National Research Council: Recommended Dietary Allowances, revised. Washington, DC: National Academy of Sciences. 1989.

[a]The information in this table was designed for the maintenance of practically all healthy people in the United States.

ORIGIN OF THE TERM MET

In the early 1900s, researchers began to study the effectiveness of varied exercise protocols on human physiologic responses to hot and cold environmental stressors. The basic need in cold environments was efficient clothing to withstand extreme environmental stress. One concern was how to balance thermal qualities of clothing with metabolic heat production at rest and during increasing exercise intensities. One strategy defined the thermal characteristics of clothing to provide optimal protection from the cold to maintain a stable thermal equilibrium or central core body temperature. Seventy years ago, three environmental physiologists—Drs. A. Pharo Gagge from Yale University, Alan Burton from the University of Toronto, and H.C. Bazett, MD, from the University of Pennsylvania—first proposed a practical system of measurement units to describe heat exchange applicable to persons of varying body sizes and shapes. They were first to coin the term *MET* to indicate a heat unit to represent a thermal constant of metabolic heat to maintain body temperature. One MET (or metabolic equivalent) to maintain body heat was shown to vary in absolute amounts based on an a person's size. They ascribed 1 MET as an amount of heat generated by a 100-W light bulb by a resting man of average size. Their empirically derived thermal constants that related to energy metabolism provided the early impetus for future experimentation in temperature regulation and clothing design, which includes the thermally balanced modern space suits in use today.

($1\ \text{kcal} \cdot \text{kg}^{-1} \cdot \text{h}^{-1} \div 60\ \text{min} \cdot \text{h}^{-1} = 0.017$). For example, a 2-MET activity requires twice the resting metabolism, or about 500 mL of oxygen per minute; a 3-MET intensity level requires three times as much energy as expended at rest, and so on for additional MET increments.

The MET provides a convenient way to rate exercise intensity with respect to a resting baseline (i.e., multiples of resting energy expenditure). Conversion from MET to $\text{kcal} \cdot \text{min}^{-1}$ requires body weight and use of the following conversion: $1.0\ \text{kcal} \cdot \text{kg}^{-1} \cdot \text{h}^{-1} = 1$ MET. For example, if a person weighing 70 kg bicycles at 10 mph (listed as a 10-MET activity), the corresponding kcal expenditure calculates as follows:

$$\begin{aligned} 10.0\ \text{METs} &= 10.0\ \text{kcal} \cdot \text{kg}^{-1} \cdot \text{h}^{-1} \times 70\ \text{kg} \div 60\ \text{min} \\ &= 700\ \text{kcal} \div 60\ \text{min} \\ &= 11.7\ \text{kcal} \cdot \text{min}^{-1} \end{aligned}$$

Table 6.7 presents a five-level classification of physical activity based on energy expenditure and corresponding MET levels for untrained men and women.

PERSONAL HEALTH AND EXERCISE NUTRITION 6.2

Predicting Energy Expenditure During Treadmill Walking and Running

A linear relationship exists between oxygen uptake or energy expenditure and walking speeds between 3.0 and 5.0 $km \cdot h^{-1}$ (1.9 and 3.1 mph) and running at speeds faster than 8.0 $km \cdot h^{-1}$ (5–10 mph). Adding the resting oxygen uptake to the oxygen requirements of both the horizontal and vertical components of the walk or run makes it possible to estimate total (gross) exercise oxygen uptake ($\dot{V}o_2$) and energy (kcal) expenditure.

Basic Equation

$\dot{V}o_2$ ($mL \cdot kg^{-1} \cdot min^{-1}$) = Resting component (1 metabolic equivalent [MET]; 3.5 mL $O_2 \cdot kg^{-1} \cdot min^{-1}$) + horizontal component (speed, $m \cdot min^{-1}$ × oxygen cost of horizontal movement) + vertical component (percent grade × speed, $m \cdot min^{-1}$ × oxygen cost of vertical movement).

[To convert mph to $m \cdot min^{-1}$, multiply by 26.82; to convert $m \cdot min^{-1}$ to mph, multiply by 0.03728.]

1. Walking: Oxygen cost equals 0.1 $mL \cdot kg^{-1} \cdot min^{-1}$ for the horizontal component of movement and 1.8 $mL \cdot kg^{-1} \cdot min^{-1}$ for the vertical component.
2. Running: Oxygen cost equals 0.2 $mL \cdot kg^{-1} \cdot min^{-1}$ for the horizontal component of movement and 0.9 $mL \cdot kg^{-1} \cdot min^{-1}$ for the vertical component.

Predicting Energy Cost of Treadmill Walking

Problem 1

A 55-kg person walks on a treadmill at 2.8 mph (2.8 × 26.82 = 75 $m \cdot min^{-1}$) up a 4% grade. Calculate: (1) $\dot{V}o_2$ ($mL \cdot kg^{-1} \cdot min^{-1}$), (2) METs, and (3) energy expenditure ($kcal \cdot min^{-1}$). [Note: express % grade as a decimal value; i.e., 4% grade = 0.04.]

Predicting Energy Cost of Treadmill Running

Problem 2

A 55-kg person runs on a treadmill at 5.4 mph (5.6 × 26.82 = 145 $m \cdot min^{-1}$) up a 6% grade. Calculate: (1) $\dot{V}o_2$ in $mL \cdot kg^{-1} \cdot min^{-1}$, (2) METs, and (3) energy expenditure ($kcal \cdot min^{-1}$).

thePoint *Visit* **thePoint.lww.com/MKKSEN4e** *to find the answers to these questions.*

SUMMARY

1. Direct calorimetry and indirect calorimetry are two methods to determine the body's rate of energy expenditure. Direct calorimetry measures actual heat production in an appropriately insulated calorimeter. Indirect calorimetry infers energy expenditure from measurements of oxygen uptake and carbon dioxide production using closed-circuit spirometry, open-circuit spirometry, or doubly labeled water technique.
2. The doubly labeled water technique estimates energy expenditure in free-living conditions without the normal constraints of laboratory procedures. The method serves as a gold standard for other long-term energy expenditure estimates, but drawbacks include the cost of enriched ^{18}O and the expense of spectrometric analysis of the two isotopes.
3. The complete oxidation of each macronutrient requires a different quantity of oxygen uptake compared to carbon dioxide production. The ratio of carbon dioxide produced to oxygen consumed, termed the *respiratory quotient*, or *RQ*, provides key information about the nutrient mixture catabolized for energy. The RQ equals 1.00 for carbohydrate, 0.70 for fat, and 0.82 for protein.
4. For each RQ value, a corresponding caloric value exists for each liter of oxygen consumed. This RQ–kilocalorie relationship provides an accurate estimate of exercise expenditure during steady-rate exercise.
5. The RQ does not indicate specific substrate use during non–steady-rate exercise because of nonmetabolic carbon dioxide production in the buffering of lactate.
6. The R reflects pulmonary exchange of carbon dioxide and oxygen under various physiologic and metabolic conditions; R does not fully mirror the macronutrient mixture catabolized.
7. BMR reflects the minimum energy required for vital functions in the waking state. BMR relates inversely to

SUMMARY *(continued)*

age and gender, averaging 5 to 10% lower in women than men.

8. TDEE represents the sum of energy required in basal and resting metabolism, thermogenic influences (particularly the thermic effect of food), and energy generated in physical activity.
9. Body mass, stature, and age, or approximations of fat-free body mass (FFM), provide for estimates of resting daily energy expenditure.
10. Physical activity, dietary-induced thermogenesis, and environmental factors (and to a lesser extent pregnancy) significantly affect TDEE.
11. Energy expenditure can be expressed in gross or net terms. Gross (total) values include the resting energy requirement, whereas net energy expenditure reflects the energy cost of the activity that excludes resting metabolism over an equivalent time interval.
12. Daily rates of energy expenditure classify different occupations and sports professions. Heavier persons expend more energy in most physical activities than lighter counterparts simply from the energy cost of transporting the additional body mass.
13. Different classification systems rate the strenuousness of physical activities. These include rating based on energy cost expressed in $kcal \cdot min^{-1}$, oxygen requirement expressed in $L \cdot min^{-1}$, or multiples of the resting metabolic rate (METs).

thePoint *Visit* **thePoint.lww.com/MKKSEN4e** *to view the following animations related to content presented in Chapter 6:* ***Oxygen consumption*** *and* ***Oxygen transport****.*

TEST YOUR KNOWLEDGE ANSWERS

1. **True:** In nutritional terms, 1 calorie expresses the quantity of heat needed to raise the temperature of 1 kg (1 L) of water 1°C (specifically, from 14.5 to 15.5°C). Thus, kilogram-calorie or kilocalorie (kcal) more accurately defines a calorie.

2. **False:** Laboratories use the bomb calorimeter to measure the total energy value of the various food macronutrients. Bomb calorimeters operate on the principle of direct calorimetry to measure the heat liberated as the food burns completely.

3. **False:** Heat of combustion refers to the heat liberated by oxidizing a specific food; it represents the food's total energy value assessed by bomb calorimetry. The oxidation pathways of food in the intact organism and bomb calorimeter differ, yet the energy liberated in the complete breakdown of food remains identical regardless of the combustion pathways.

4. **False:** The heat of combustion for carbohydrate varies depending on the arrangement of atoms in the particular carbohydrate molecule. On average, for 1 g of carbohydrate, a value of 4.2 kcal generally represents the average heat of combustion.

5. **False:** The heat of combustion for lipid varies with the structural composition of the triacylglycerol molecule's fatty acid components. The average heat of combustion for lipid equals $9.4\ kcal \cdot g^{-1}$.

6. **False:** The coefficient of digestibility represents the percentage of an ingested macronutrient digested and absorbed by the body. The quantity of food remaining unabsorbed in the intestinal tract voids in the feces. The relative percentage digestibility coefficients average 97% for carbohydrate, 95% for lipid, and 92% for protein.

7. **False:** The doubly labeled water technique estimates total daily energy expenditure of children and adults in free-living conditions without the normal constraints imposed by other procedures of indirect calorimetry. It involves the ingestion of stable isotopes of hydrogen and oxygen, which distribute throughout all body fluids. Differences between elimination rates of the two isotopes relative to the body's normal "background" level estimate total carbon dioxide production from energy metabolism during the measurement period.

8. **False:** The average net energy values can be rounded to simple whole numbers referred to as Atwater general factors as follows: $4\ kcal \cdot g^{-1}$ for carbohydrate, $9\ kcal \cdot g^{-1}$ for lipid, and $4\ kcal \cdot g^{-1}$ for protein.

9. **True:** The more one eats of any food, the more calories one consumes. A person's caloric intake equals the sum of *all* energy consumed from either small or large food quantities. Thus, celery becomes a "fattening" food when consumed in excess. Achieving this excess involves consuming a considerable quantity of celery. For example, the typical sedentary woman needs to consume 420 celery stalks, yet only 8 oz of salad oil, to meet her daily 2100-kcal energy needs.

10. **True:** Inherent chemical differences in the composition of carbohydrates, lipids, and proteins mean that the complete oxidation of a molecule's carbon and hydrogen atoms to carbon dioxide and water end products requires different amounts of oxygen. Gas exchange during glucose oxidation produces six carbon dioxide molecules for six oxygen molecules consumed. Therefore, the RQ (CO_2 produced ÷ O_2 consumed) for carbohydrate equals 1.00 (RQ = 6 CO_2 ÷ 6 O_2 = 1.00).

Key References

ACSM's Resource Manual for Guidelines for Exercise Testing and Prescription. 6th ed. Baltimore: Lippincott Williams & Wilkins, 2009.
Ainsworth BE, et al. Compendium of physical activities: classification of energy costs of human physical activities. *Med Sci Sports Exerc* 1993;25:71.
Atwater WO, Rosa EB. Description of a new respiration calorimeter and experiments on the conservation of energy in the human body. US Department of Agriculture, Office of Experiment Stations, Bulletin No. 63. Washington, DC: Government Printing Office, 1899.
Atwater WO, Woods CD. The chemical composition of American food materials. US Department of Agriculture Bulletin No. 28. Washington, DC: US Department of Agriculture, 1896.
Bailey BW, McInnis K. Energy cost of exergaming: a comparison of the energy cost of 6 forms of exergaming. *Arch Pediatr Adolesc Med* 2011;165:597.
Conway JM, et al. Comparison of energy expenditure estimates from doubly labeled water, a physical activity questionnaire, and physical activity records. *Am J Clin Nutr* 2002;75:519.
Durnin JVGA, Passmore R. *Energy, Work and Leisure.* London: Heinemann, 1967.
Ekelund U, et al. Energy expenditure assessed by heart rate and doubly labeled water in young athletes. *Med Sci Sports Exerc* 2002;34:1360.
Gagnon D, Kenny GP. Exercise-rest cycles do not alter local and whole-body heat loss responses. *Am J Physiol Regul Integr Comp Physiol* 2011;300:R958.
Gibson RS. *Principles of Nutritional Assessment.* 2nd Ed. New York: Oxford University Press, 2006.
Gunn SM, et al. Determining energy expenditure during some household and garden tasks. *Med Sci Sports Exerc* 2002;34:895.
Health and Welfare Canada. Nutrient value of some common foods. Health Services and Promotion Branch, Health and Welfare Canada, Ottawa, Canada. Available at: www.hc-sc.gc.ca/fn-an/nutrition/fiche-nutri-data/index-eng.php. Accessed August 4, 2011.
Keys A, et al. Basal metabolism and age of adult men. *Metabolism* 1973;22:579.
Krogh A, Lindhard J. The relative value of fat and carbohydrate as sources of muscular energy. *Biochem J* 1920;14:290.
McCance A, Widdowson EM. *The Composition of Foods.* 5th ed. London: Royal Society of Chemistry, Ministry of Agriculture, Fisheries and Food, 2002.
Montoye HJ, et al. *Measuring Physical Activity and Energy Expenditure.* Boca Raton, FL: Human Kinetics, 1996.
Pennington JA, Spungen MS. *Bowes and Church's Food Values of Portions Commonly Used.* 19th ed. Philadelphia: Lippincott, 2009.
Poehlman ET, et al. Resting metabolic rate and post prandial thermogenesis in highly trained and untrained males. *Am J Clin Nutr* 1988;47:793.
Segal KR, et al. Thermic effects of food and exercise on lean and obese men of similar lean body mass. *Am J Physiol* 1987;252:E110.
Speakman JR. The history and theory of the doubly labeled water technique. *Am J Clin Nutr* 1998;68(Suppl):932S.
Thiel C, et al. Energy cost of youth obesity exercise modes. *Int J Sports Med* 2011;32:142.
Weir JB. New methods for calculating metabolic rate with special reference to protein metabolism. *J Physiol* 1949;109:1.
Withers RT, et al. Energy metabolism in sedentary and active 49- to 70-yr-old women. *J Appl Physiol* 1998;84:1333.
Wouters-Adriaens MP, Westerterp KR. Basal metabolic rate as a proxy for overnight energy expenditure: the effect of age. *Br J Nutr* 2006;95:1166.
Zamparo P, Capelli C, Pendergast D. Energetics of swimming: a historical perspective. *Eur J Appl Physiol* 2011;111:367.

thePoint *Visit* **thePoint.lww.com/MKKSEN4e** *for a list of the references cited in this chapter, including additional, relevant references.*

Optimal Nutrition for the Physically Active Person: Making Informed and Healthful Choices

PART 3

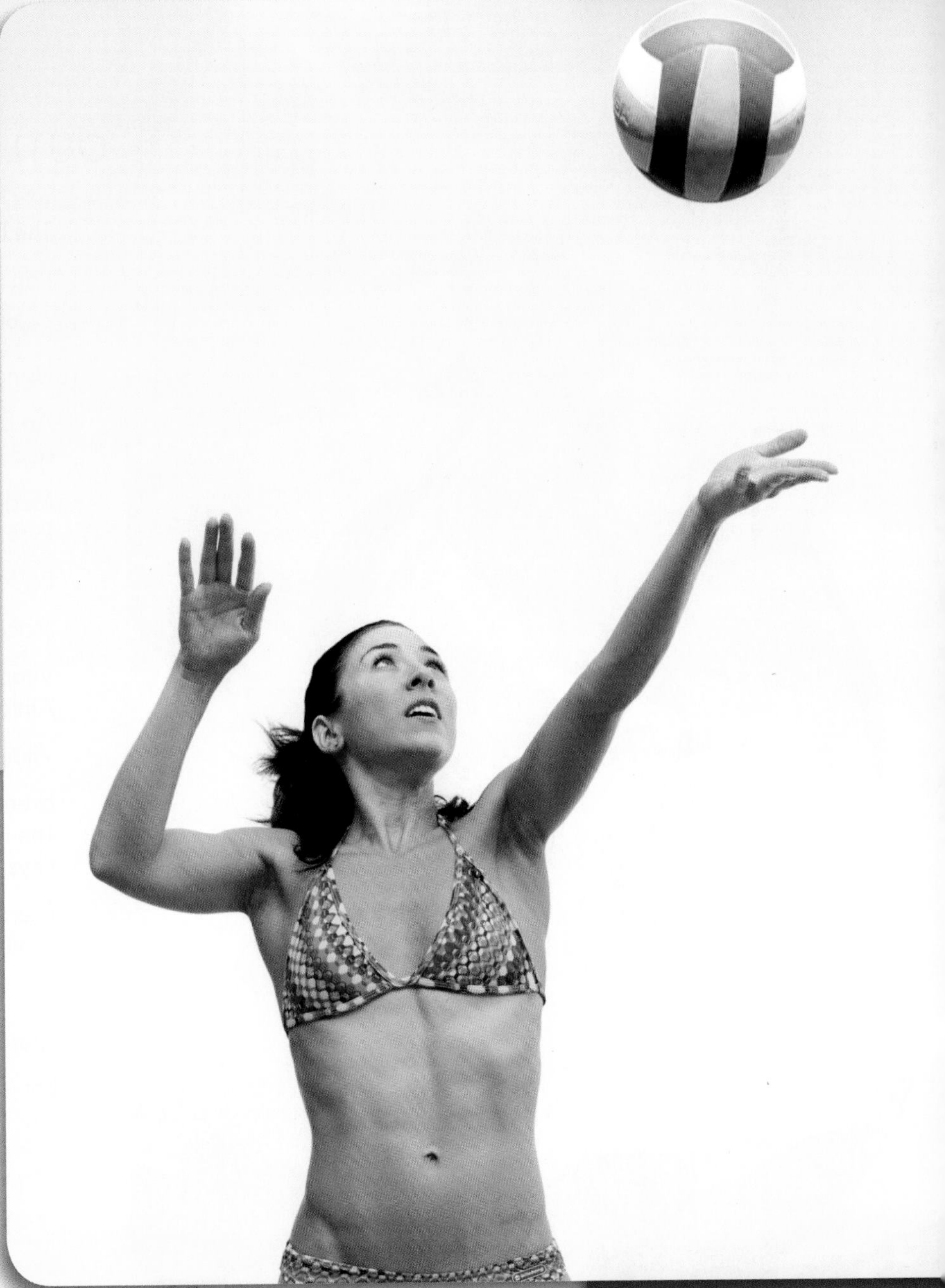

CONTENTS

CHAPTER 7

Nutritional Recommendations for the Physically Active Person

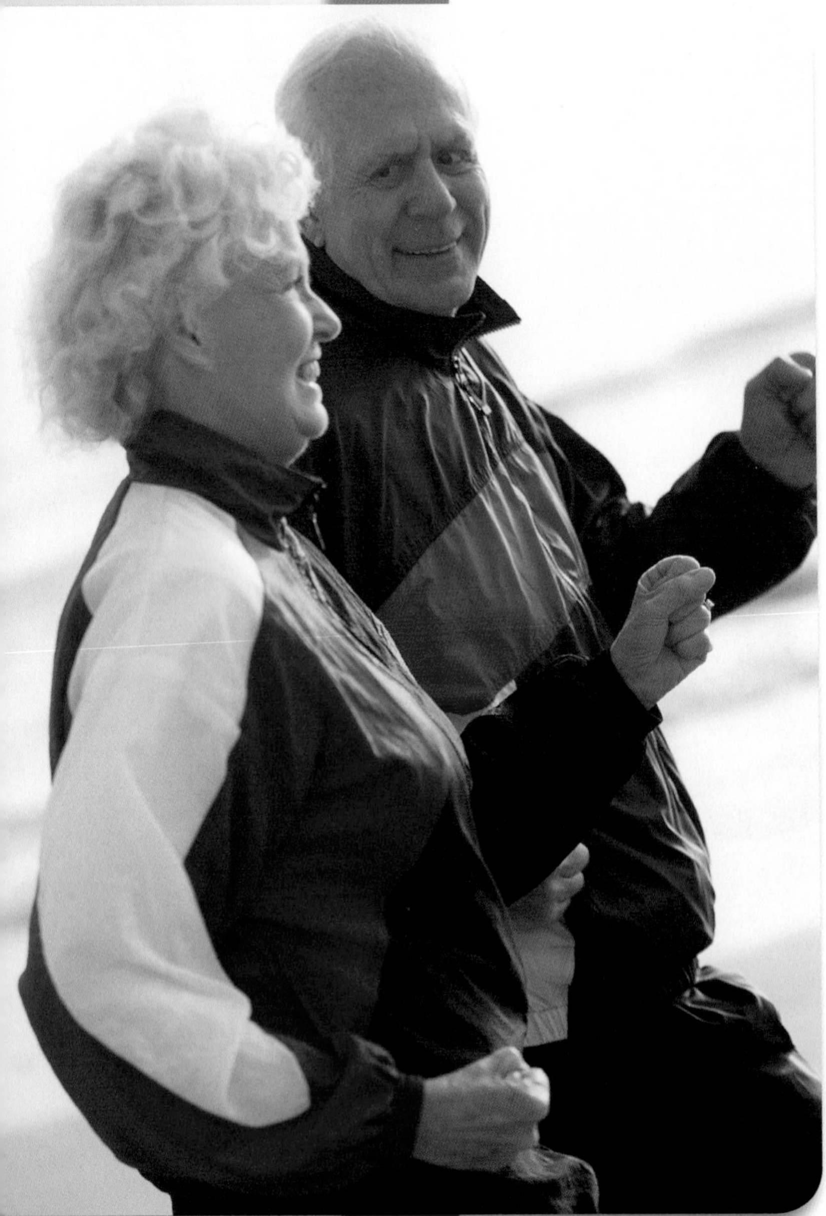

OUTLINE

TEST YOUR KNOWLEDGE

Select true or false for the 10 statements below, then check out the answers at the end of the chapter. Retake the test after you've read the chapter; you should achieve 100%!	True	False
1. Humans differ from machines in that they do not conform to the laws of thermodynamics, at least in terms of energy balance.	❍	❍
2. One pound of stored body fat contains approximately 3500 kcal of energy.	❍	❍
3. A potential problem with MyPlate is that it lumps all foods within a food category together (e.g., bread, cereal, rice, and pasta group) without distinguishing between healthful and not so healthful foods within that category.	❍	❍
4. Recent government guidelines for good nutrition emphasize specific numeric goals for different individual nutrients.	❍	❍
5. Physically active individuals require additional micronutrients above recommended values to support their increased level of energy expenditure.	❍	❍
6. Serious weight trainers benefit from taking high doses of amino acid supplements to provide the required "building blocks" to increase muscle mass.	❍	❍
7. To promote good health, lipid intake should not exceed 10% of total caloric intake.	❍	❍
8. High-carbohydrate (60–70% total caloric intake), high-fiber (30–50 $g \cdot d^{-1}$) diets do not promote good health because they deprive an individual of needed quantities of lipid.	❍	❍
9. Athletes who train intensely require vitamin and mineral intake above recommended values for optimal physical performance and training responsiveness.	❍	❍
10. Saturated fatty acids provide an excellent source of antioxidant vitamins.	❍	❍

An optimal diet supplies required nutrients in adequate amounts for tissue maintenance, repair, and growth without excess energy intake. Proper nutrition helps in four ways[6]:

1. Improves physical performance
2. Optimizes programs of physical conditioning
3. Improves recovery from fatigue
4. Avoids injury

Dietary recommendations for physically active men and women must account for the energy requirements of a particular activity or sport and its training demands, including individual dietary preferences. Although no "one" food or diet exists for optimal health and exercise performance, careful planning and evaluation of food intake should follow sound nutritional guidelines. The physically active person must obtain sufficient energy and macronutrients to replenish liver and muscle glycogen, provide amino acid building blocks for tissue growth and repair, and maintain a desirable body weight. Lipid intake must also provide essential fatty acids and fat-soluble vitamins. Supplementing with vitamins and minerals is unnecessary provided a well-balanced diet provides for the body's energy needs. Unfortunately, the nutrition knowledge of athletes and its impact on their dietary intake is probably no greater than that of the general population.[46] The box titled "Six Ways That Exercise Nutritionists Can Help Physically Active Individuals and Competitive Athletes" outlines the recommendations of a joint position statement from the American College of Sports Medicine, American Dietetic Association (ADA), and Dietitians of Canada about how qualified health, exercise, and nutrition professionals can counsel individuals who engage regularly in physical activity.

SIX WAYS THAT EXERCISE NUTRITIONISTS CAN HELP PHYSICALLY ACTIVE INDIVIDUALS AND COMPETITIVE ATHLETES

1. Educate athletes about energy requirements for their sport and the role of food in fueling the body. Discourage unrealistic weight and body composition goals and emphasize the importance of adequate energy intake for good health, prevention of injury, and exercise performance.
2. Assess the body size and composition of an athlete for the determination of an appropriate weight and composition for the sports in which he or she participates. Provide the athlete with nutritionally sound techniques for maintaining an appropriate body weight and composition without the use of fad or severe diets. Undue pressure on athletes for weight loss or the maintenance of a lean body build can increase the risk of restrictive eating behaviors and, in extreme cases, lead to a clinical eating disorder.
3. Assess the athlete's typical dietary and supplement intake during training, competition, and the off-season. Use this assessment to provide appropriate recommendations for energy and nutrient intakes for the maintenance of good health, appropriate body weight and composition, and optimal sport performance throughout the year. Give specific guidelines for making good food and fluid selections while traveling and eating away from home.
4. Assess the fluid intake and weight loss of athletes during exercise and make appropriate recommendations regarding total fluid intake and fluid intake before, during, and after exercise. Help athletes to determine appropriate types and amounts of beverages to use during exercise, especially if the athlete is exercising in extreme environments.
5. For athletes such as the vegetarian athlete with special nutrition concerns, provide appropriate nutritional guidelines to ensure adequate intakes of energy, protein, and micronutrients.
6. Carefully evaluate any vitamin/mineral or herbal supplements, ergogenic aids, or performance-enhancing drugs an athlete wants to use. These products should be used with caution and only after careful review of their legality and the current literature pertaining to the ingredients listed on the product label; these products should not be recommended until after evaluating the athlete's health, diet, nutrition needs, current supplement and drug use, and energy requirements.

From American College of Sports Medicine, American Dietetic Association, and Dietitians of Canada. Joint position statement. Nutrition and athletic performance. *Med Sci Sports Exerc* 2000;32:2130.

THE ENERGY BALANCE EQUATION

The concept of energy balance most typically applies to body weight maintenance and weight loss, as discussed in Chapter 14. Proper attainment of energy balance also becomes an important goal for physically active people, particularly during intense training or multiple daily workouts when maintaining energy balance with proper nutrient intake optimizes exercise performance and the training response.

THERE IS NO CIRCUMVENTING THE LAWS OF THERMODYNAMICS!

The human body functions in accord with the immutable, fundamental laws of thermodynamics, which originated from the fields of mathematics, thermodynamics, physics, and chemistry in the 1800s. These laws, directly applicable to metabolic systems in the biological sciences, state that if total calories from food exceed daily energy expenditure, excess calories accumulate as fat in adipose tissue.

One must consider the rationale underlying the **energy balance equation** when replenishing the body's macronutrient energy reserves in training or in planning to favorably modify body weight and body composition. *In accord with the first law of thermodynamics, the energy balance equation dictates that body mass remains constant when caloric intake equals caloric expenditure.* **FIGURE 7.1** depicts factors that contribute to daily energy balance and imbalance. The middle example shows what happens all too frequently when energy input exceeds energy output and the calories consumed in excess of daily requirements become stored as fat in adipose tissue. Weight gain occurs with a long-term positive energy imbalance that often results from subtle regulatory alterations between energy intake and energy expenditure. *Thirty-five hundred "extra" kcal through either increased energy intake or decreased energy output approximates 1 lb (0.45 kg) of stored body fat.* The lower example illustrates what happens when energy output exceeds energy input. In this case, the body obtains the required calories from its energy stores, resulting in reduced body weight and body fat. Little fluctuation occurs in body weight if an equilibrium exists in which energy input (calories in food) balances energy output (calories expended in daily activities), as shown in the top panel of the figure. This situation mostly applies to physically active individuals who must regularly replenish the energy to power exercise through nutrient-rich food sources as outlined in sections that follow.

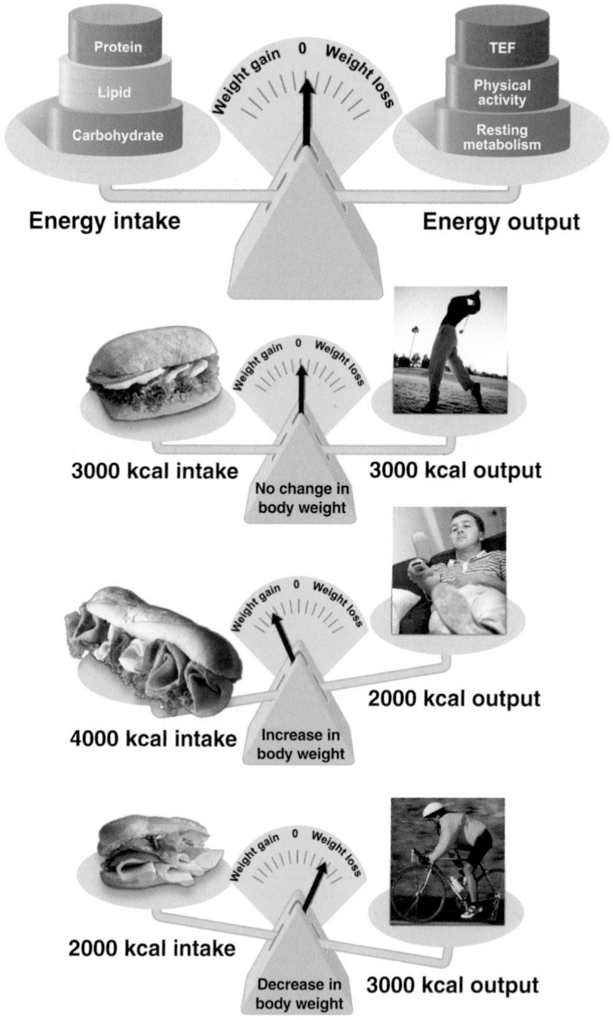

FIGURE 7.1. The energy balance equation (*TEF*, thermic effect of food).

MORE LIPID EQUALS MORE CALORIES

Lipid-rich foods contain a higher energy content than foods that are relatively fat free. One glass of whole milk, for example, contains 160 kcal, whereas the same quantity of skim milk contains only 90 kcal. If a person who normally consumes one quart of whole milk each day switches to skim milk, the total calories ingested each year would be reduced by the equivalent calories in 25 pounds of body fat. Thus, following this switch for just 3 years theoretically represents the equivalent energy in 75 pounds of body fat. Equally dramatic, consider the consumption of a popular fast-food item over the same 3-year period. Eating only 30 medium orders of essentially nonnutritious French fries from McDonald's or other fast-food restaurants yearly (total of 90 orders at 380 kcal or 171 grams of fat per order) represents the total energy equivalent of 34,200 kcal consumed (9.8 lb of body fat) and 15,390 grams of fat (542 oz or 34 lb of pure fat!). This is enough "energy" to power a round-trip walk from Los Angeles, CA, to San Diego, CA, or the outskirts of Ann Arbor, MI, to Chicago,IL.

PRINCIPLES OF GOOD EATING

Key principles of good eating include *variety*, *balance*, and *moderation*. A healthful diet requires some simple planning that does not demand a lifetime of deprivation and misery.

Variety

Choosing foods from a variety of food sources creates a diet that contains sufficient amounts of all required nutrients and reduces risk of developing lifestyle-related illness. For example, each vegetable form contains a unique set of phytochemicals (see Personal Health and Exercise Nutrition 6.1, p. 189), so consuming a variety of vegetables provides a broad array of these beneficial food constituents. A diverse diet also makes mealtimes more interesting and something to look forward to. Available data suggest that the average American consumes less than 20 different foods during any given week, whereas Australians consume nearly 30 different foods per day, the goal established by the Australian government (**www.nutritionaustralia.org/national/resource/food-variety**).

Balance

Balance in one's diet indicates the intake of nutrients from all the major food groups and thus enables the person to benefit from the variety of accessory nutrients unique to each food. Prolonged intake of a diet that inordinately focuses on one food group often creates nutritional deficiency, despite intake of sufficient energy. For example, if a person dislikes milk or milk products (yogurt, ice cream, and cheese), the likelihood of calcium deficiency increases because this food group constitutes the major source of calcium.

Moderation

Eating moderately requires appropriate planning to maintain a balanced nutrient intake throughout the day. For example, if one meal contains high-fat foods, other meals during the day must contain less fat. A good action plan moderates rather than eliminates the intake of certain foods. In this way, one can enjoy all types of foods during the day.

MYPLATE: THE NEW HEALTHY EATING GUIDE

In the typical American diet, energy-dense but nutrient-poor foods frequently substitute for more nutrient-rich foods. This pattern of food intake increases the risk for obesity, marginal

FOOD VARIETY CHECKLIST

Use the Food Variety Checklist for 1 week to test the variety of your diet. Give yourself 1 point for each food category you have eaten throughout 1 week. Count each food category only once.

Food Variety Checklist	Your Score
Fruit	
Stone fruit (e.g., apricot, avocado, cherries, nectarine, olive, peach, plum, prune)	______
Citrus (e.g., oranges, lemons, limes)	______
Apples	______
Bananas	______
Berries (e.g., raspberry, strawberry)	______
Grapes (including raisins, sultanas)	______
Melons (e.g., honeydew, rockmelon, watermelon, cantaloupe)	______
Pears	______
Tropical fruit (e.g., guava, jackfruit, mango, papaya, pineapple)	______
Dates, kiwifruit, passion fruit	______
Vegetables	
Root vegetables (e.g., carrots, sweet potatoes, potatoes, bamboo shoots, beetroot, ginger, parsnip, radish, water chestnut)	______
Leafy greens (e.g., spinach, cabbage, Brussels sprouts, chard)	______
Marrow-like vegetables (e.g., cucumber, eggplant, marrow, pumpkin, squash, turnip, zucchini)	______
Flowers (e.g., broccoli, cauliflower, endive, chicory, lettuce)	______
Stalks (e.g., celery)	______
Onions (e.g., sweet onion, garlic, leek)	______
Peppers (e.g., capsicum)	______
Tomatoes, okra	______
Legumes/Pulses	
Beans (e.g., green beans, snow peas, snap beans, dried peas)	______
Adzuki, baked beans, black beans, black eyed beans, cranberry beans, navy beans, chickpeas kidney beans, lentils, lima beans, beans sprouts, pinto beans, soy beans (sprouts), soy milk, bean curd	______
Grains and Cereals	
Wheat (including ready-to-eat cereals such as bran flakes and whole meal/white bread)	______
Rye (includes ready-to-eat products)	______
Barley (includes ready-to-eat products)	______
Oats (includes ready-to-eat products)	______
Rice (includes ready-to-eat products)	______
Corn (includes ready-to-eat products)	______

Food Variety Checklist	Your Score
All other grains and cereals (e.g., buckwheat, millet, quinoa, semolina, tapioca)	______
Meat	
Pork (including ham and bacon)	______
Lamb, beef, veal	______
Poultry (e.g., chicken, turkey, duck)	______
Game (e.g., quail, wild duck, pigeon)	______
Liver, brain, all other organ meats	______
Seafood	
Shellfish and mollusks (e.g., mussels, squid, clams, oysters, scallops)	______
Crustaceans (e.g., prawns, lobster, crabs, shrimps)	______
Fatty fish (e.g., anchovies, tuna, salmon, sardines, herring, mackerel, kipper, pilchards)	______
Fish (saltwater)	______
Fish (freshwater)	______
Roe (caviar)	______
Dairy	
Milk, yogurt (without live culture), ice cream, cheese	______
Live cultures (yogurt with live culture, e.g., acidophilus, bifid bacteria)	______
Eggs	
All varieties	______
Fats	
Oil	______
Hard/soft spreads	______
Herbs and Spices	
Use regularly	______
Nuts and Seeds	
Almond, brazil, cashew, chestnut, coconut, hazelnut, peanuts, peanut butter, pecan, pine nut, pistachio, pumpkin seed, sesame seed, sunflower seed, walnut	______
Fermented Foods	
Miso, tempeh, soy sauce	______
Sauerkraut	______
All other varieties	______
Beverages	
Nonalcoholic (e.g., tea, coffee, cocoa)	______
Alcoholic	______
Other	
Sugar, syrup, honey, confectionary, jam, marmalade, chocolate, soft drinks	______
Yeast (e.g., vegemite, marmite, brewer's yeast)	______
Water including mineral and spring water	______
TOTAL AMOUNT OF DIFFERENT FOODS	______

Score Your Food Variety

Total Food Variety Score	Dietary Adequacy
>30 per week	Very good
25–29 per week	Good
10–24 per week	Fair
<20 per week	Poor
<10 per week	Very poor

References: Savige GS, et al. Food variety as nutritional therapy. Curr Ther 1997:62. Walker J, Fisher G. Food Secrets. Brisbane: The Australian Nutrition Foundation (Qld Div) Inc., 1997.

RECOMMENDED MEAL COMPOSITION

The suggested composition of a 2500-kcal diet based on recommendations of an expert panel of the Institute of Medicine of the National Academies (www.iom.edu) is as follows:

	Carbohydrate	Lipid	Protein
Percentage	60	15	25
kcal	1500	375	625
Grams	375	94	69
Ounces	13.2	3.3	2.4

DIET–HEART LINKS

Research published in the *Archives of Internal Medicine* based on an analysis of over 200 studies involving millions of people indicates that vegetables, nuts, and the Mediterranean diet, which is rich in vegetables, nuts, whole grains, fish, and olive oil, make the list of "good" heart-healthy foods, whereas foods on the "bad" list include starchy carbohydrates like white bread and the *trans* fats in many cookies and French fries. Insufficient evidence exists to conclude that meat, eggs, and milk are either good or bad for the heart.

micronutrient intakes, low high-density lipoprotein (HDL) and high low-density lipoprotein (LDL) cholesterol levels, and elevated homocysteine levels.

On June 2, 2011, the US Department of Agriculture (USDA) unveiled **MyPlate**, a new icon with nutritional guidelines for healthy eating. MyPlate provides a stylized and colorful color-coded dinner plate to replace the 2005 MyPyramid. Supporters of the new icon claim it has greater practicality and intuitiveness than its MyPyramid predecessor, which many nutritionists and healthcare professionals claimed was confusing and difficult to understand. The MyPlate strategy, emphasizing more plant-based eating habits from a variety of vegetables from all five subgroups, attempts to help Americans become healthier in their battle against the obesity crisis. The new guide, illustrated in **FIGURE 7.2A**, has different-sized plate portions to symbolize the recommended food groups and builds on the messages of the government's revised 2010 *Dietary Guidelines for Americans*.[60,70] Fruits and vegetables occupy one half of the plate, with vegetables making up the major part of the half. Grains, particularly whole grains and proteins, make up the other half of the plate, with grains taking up a majority of that half. This eliminates the old pyramid's references to sugars, fats, or oils. A new category replaces the old "proteins" category. Meat & Beans can include meat, poultry, seafood, eggs, and vegetarian options such as beans and peas, nuts and seeds, and tofu. A blue circle adjoining the plate icon indicates dairy products such as a glass of skim or reduced-fat milk, cheese, or yogurt. Daily caloric intake, portion size, fat intake, and energy expenditure are not represented. Similar to the new *Guidelines*, MyPlate stresses balanced portions among the different food categories. The government website (www.ChooseMyPlate.gov) provides more detailed advice about the *Guidelines*.

POTENTIAL PROBLEMS WITH MYPLATE

As with the previous 2005 MyPyramid guidelines, the MyPlate guidelines are not without flaws and concerns.

- The "Fruits" section makes no distinction between fruit juice and the actual fruit—a half cup of fruit juice is listed as equivalent to a half cup of fruit. This ignores the fact that the glycemic load is far higher in fruit juice than in fruit.
- The "Grains" section makes no distinction between true whole grains and grains ground into flour. As with fruits, whole and intact grains, rather than those pulverized and processed, slow digestion and stabilize blood sugar.
- As with the MyPyramid, protein is listed as a food section and not as a macronutrient found in different foods. This listing is confusing: Is it the point to recommend nutrients or foods that contain certain nutrients? Because most people acquaint meat with protein, it seems that the recommendation is to eat more meat.
- Placement of the "Dairy" section as a circle image to the side suggests that the recommendation is to drink a glass of milk with every single meal. Is the suggestion to "drink milk" or to recommend an increase in calcium intake?

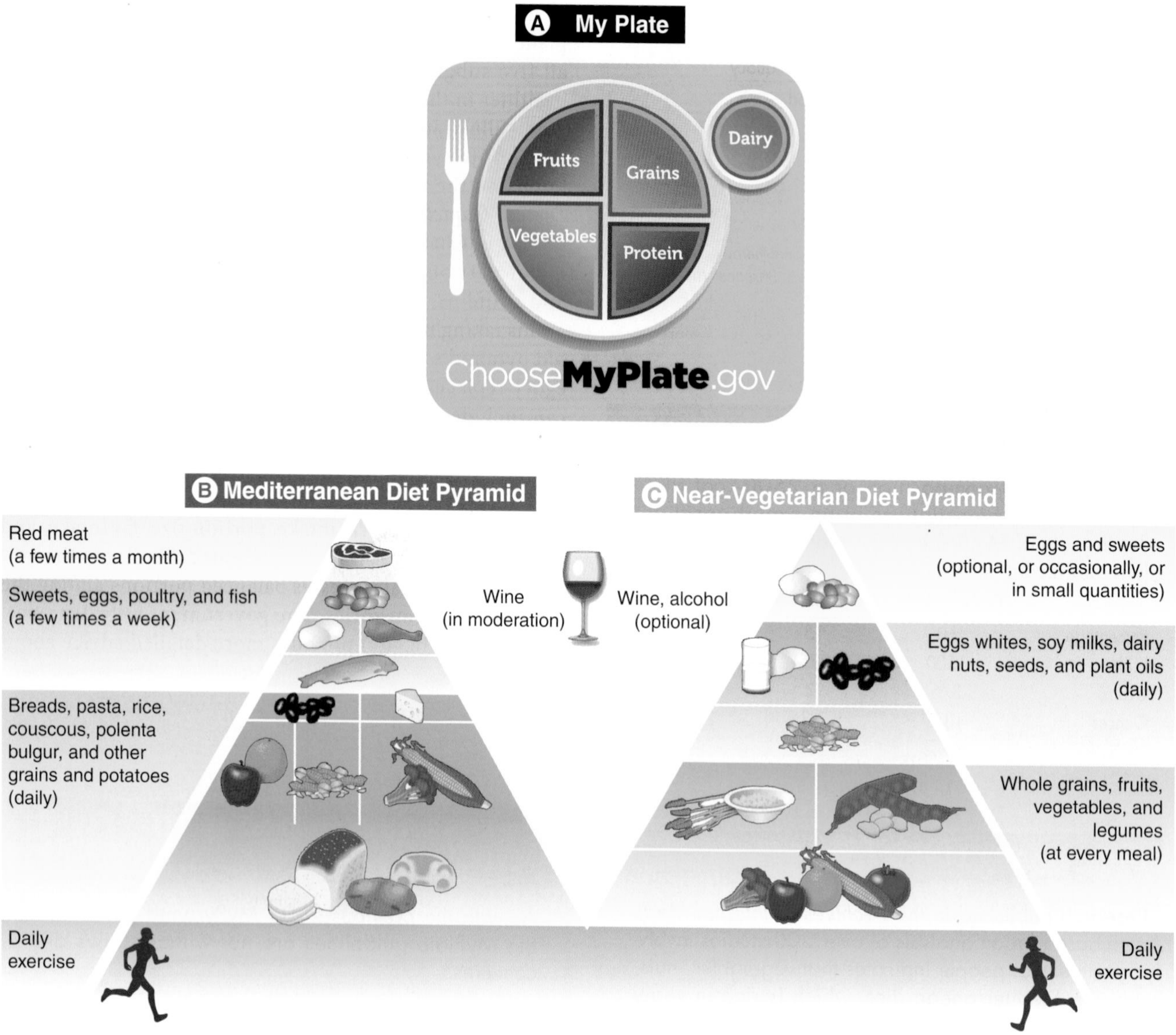

FIGURE 7.2. A. MyPlate: The new healthy eating guide. **B.** Mediterranean Diet Pyramid application to individuals whose diet consists largely of foods from the plant kingdom, or fruits, nuts, vegetables, and all manner of grains, and protein derived from fish, beans, and chicken, with dietary fat composed mostly of monounsaturated fatty acids and with mild alcohol consumption. **C.** Near-Vegetarian Pyramid without meat or dairy products consumed. The focus of the two pyramids in **B** and **C** on fruits and vegetables, particularly cruciferous and green leafy vegetables and citrus fruit and juice, also reduces risk for ischemic stroke and may potentiate the beneficial effects of cholesterol-lowering drugs.

The *Dietary Guidelines for Americans, 2010* (**www.cnpp.usda.gov/DietaryGuidelines.htm**), formulated for the general population, also provide a sound framework for meal planning for physically active individuals. The mission of the guidelines is as follows:

> "Based on the most recent scientific evidence review, this document provides information and advice for choosing a healthy eating pattern—namely, one that focuses on nutrient-dense foods and beverages, and that contributes to achieving and maintaining a healthy weight. Such a healthy eating pattern also embodies food safety principles to avoid foodborne illness."

The principle message advises consuming a varied but balanced diet. To maintain a healthful body weight, attention must focus on portion size, number of calories, and daily physical activity. A major point is to consume a reduced-sodium diet rich in fruits and vegetables, cereals and whole grains, nonfat and low-fat dairy products, legumes, nuts, fish, poultry, and lean meats with a concomitant reduction in calories from solid fats, added sugars, and refined grains.[8,15,23,56,64] **FIGURE 7.3** illustrates how the typical American diet compares to recommended intakes or limits set forth in the *Guidelines.* According to this report, Americans eat too many calories with too much solid fat, added sugars, refined grains, and sodium. They also consume too little potassium; dietary fiber; calcium; vitamin D; unsaturated fatty acids from oils, nuts, and seafood; and other important nutrients found mostly in vegetables, fruits, whole grains, and low-fat milk and milk products.

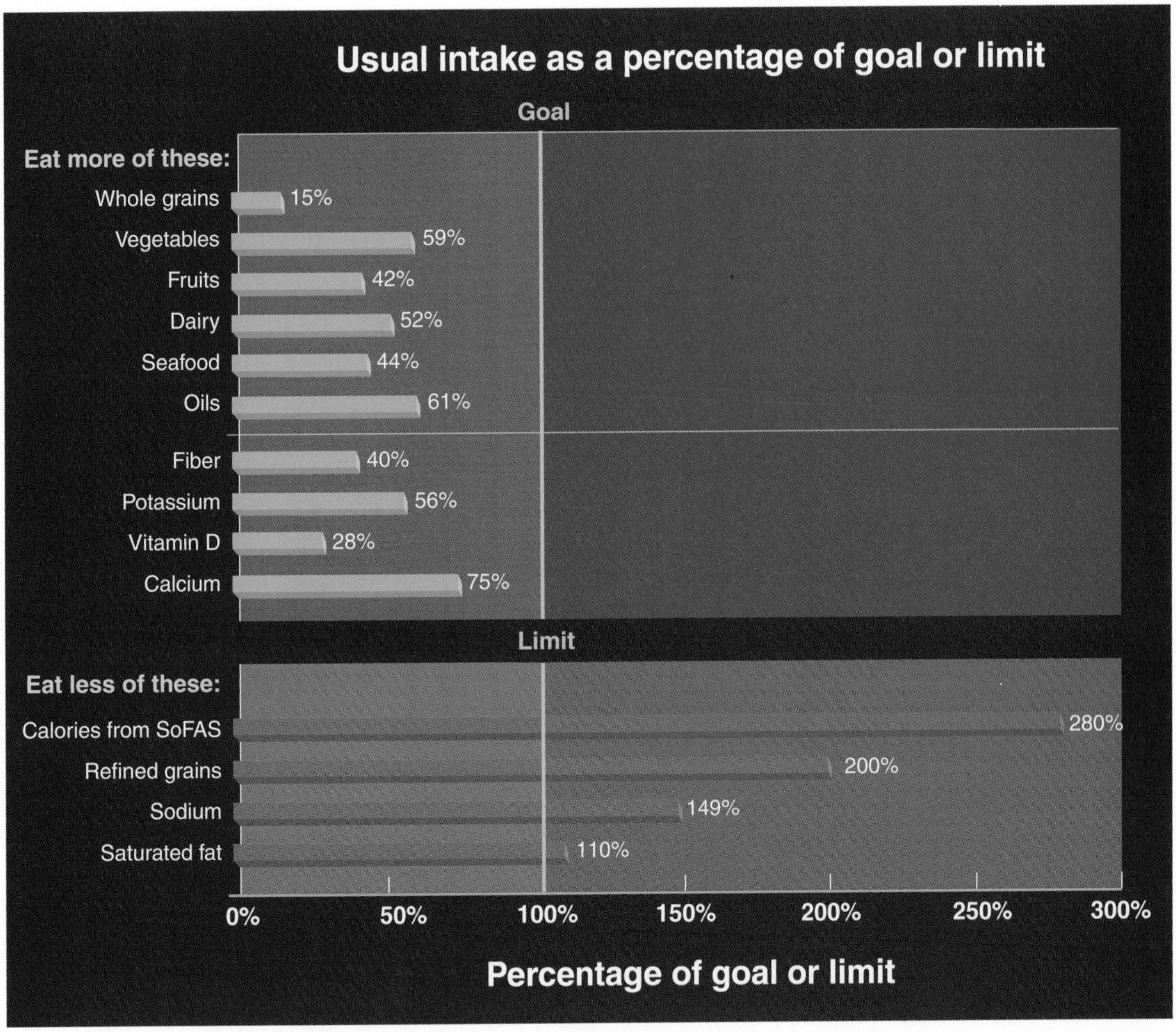

FIGURE 7.3. Comparison of typical American diets to recommended intake levels or limits.

PERSONAL HEALTH AND EXERCISE NUTRITION 7.1

A Brief History of USDA Food Guides and Guidelines

1916–1930s: "Food for Young Children" and "How to Select Food"

- Established guidance based on food groups and household measures
- Focus was on "protective foods"

1940s: A Guide to Good Eating (Basic Seven)

- Foundation diet for nutrient adequacy
- Included daily number of servings needed from each of seven food groups
- Lacked specific serving sizes
- Considered complex

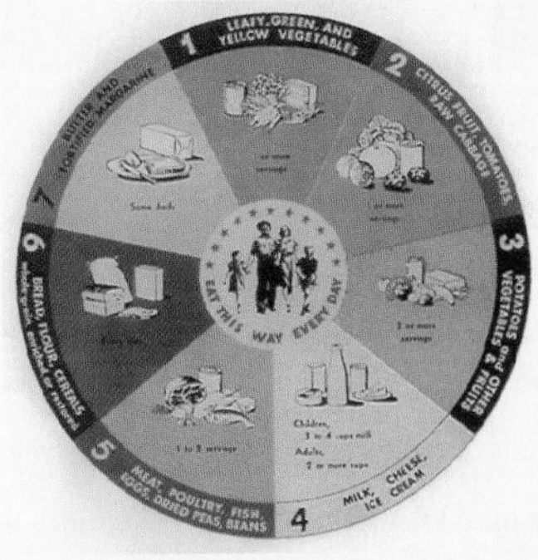

1956–1970s: Food for Fitness, A Daily Food Guide (Basic Four)

- Foundation diet approach—goals for nutrient adequacy
- Specified amounts from four food groups
- Did not include guidance on appropriate fats, sugars, and calorie intake

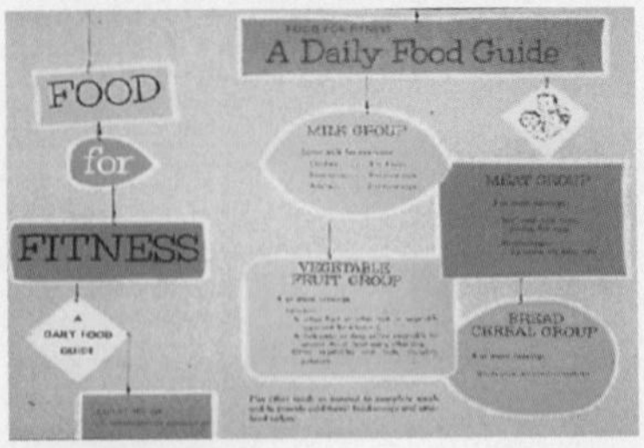

1979: Hassle-Free Daily Food Guide

- Developed after the 1977 Dietary Goals for the United States were released
- Based on the Basic Four, but also included a fifth group to highlight the need to moderate intake of fats, sweets, and alcohol

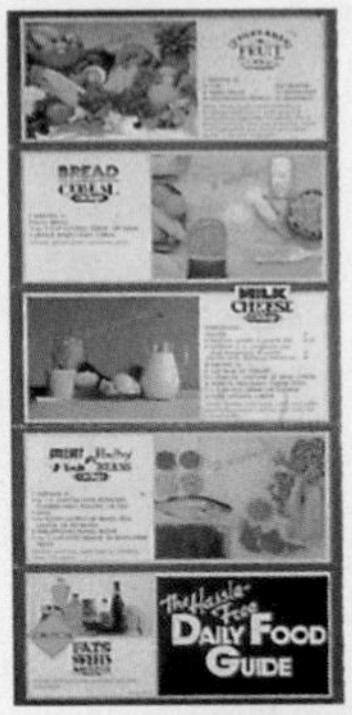

1984: Food Wheel: A Pattern for Daily Food Choices

- Total diet approach included goals for both nutrient adequacy and moderation
- Five food groups and amounts formed the basis for the Food Guide Pyramid
- Daily amounts of food provided at three calorie levels
- First illustrated for a Red Cross nutrition course as a food wheel

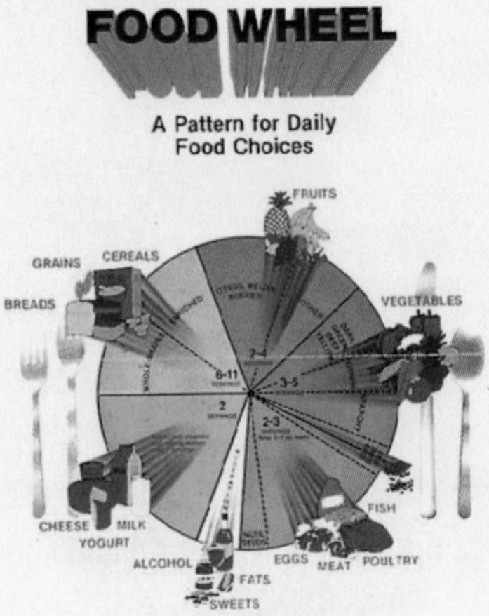

1992: Food Guide Pyramid

- Total diet approach—goals for both nutrient adequacy and moderation
- Developed using consumer research, to bring awareness to the new food patterns
- Illustration focused on concepts of variety, moderation, and proportion
- Included visualization of added fats and sugars throughout five food groups and in the tip
- Included range for daily amounts of food across three calorie levels

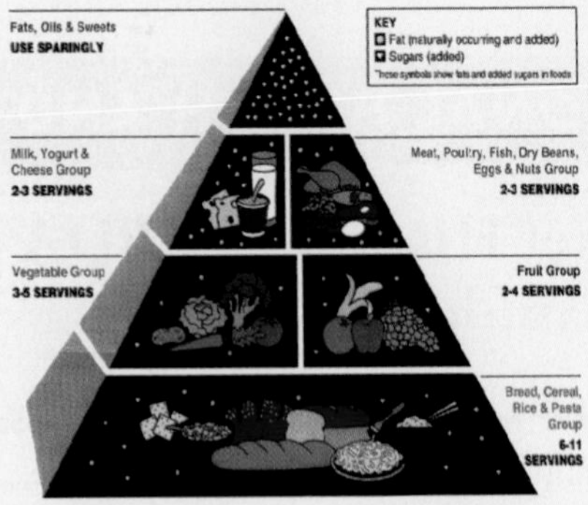

2005: MyPyramid Food Guidance System

- Introduced along with updating of Food Guide Pyramid food patterns for the *2005 Dietary Guidelines for Americans,* including daily amounts of food at 12 calorie levels
- Continued "pyramid" concept, based on consumer research, but simplified illustration. Detailed information provided on website "MyPyramid.gov"
- Added a band for oils and the concept of physical activity
- Illustration could be used to describe concepts of variety, moderation, and proportion

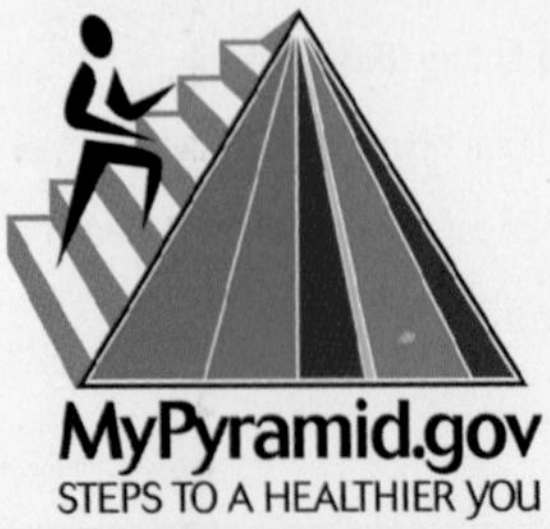

2011: MyPlate

- Introduced along with updating of USDA food patterns for the *2010 Dietary Guidelines for Americans*
- Different shape to help grab consumers' attention with a new visual cue
- Icon that serves as a reminder for healthy eating, not intended to provide specific messages
- Visual is linked to food and is a familiar mealtime symbol in consumers' minds, as identified through testing
- "My" continues the personalization approach from MyPyramid

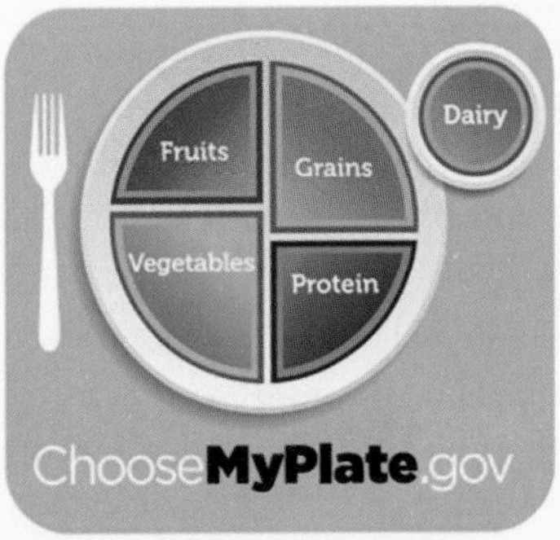

From: US Department of Agriculture. A brief history of USDA food guides. Available at: www.choosemyplate.gov/downloads/MyPlate/ABriefHistoryOfUSDAFoodGuides.pdf.

PERSONAL HEALTH AND EXERCISE NUTRITION 7.2

2010 Recommendations from the *Dietary Guidelines for Americans*

By law (Public Law 101–445, Title III, 7 U.S.C. 5301 et seq.), *Dietary Guidelines for Americans* (*Guidelines*) are reviewed, updated if necessary, and published every 5 years. The USDA and the US Department of Health and Human Services jointly create each edition. The newest version, the *Dietary Guidelines for Americans, 2010,* is based on the latest report from these agencies. The complete report can be found at www.health.gov/DietaryGuidelines. Following are excerpts from the *Dietary Guidelines for Americans, 2010* (www.health.gov/dietaryguidelines/dga2010/DietaryGuidelines2010.pdf).

The intent of the Dietary Guidelines is to summarize and synthesize knowledge about individual nutrients and food components into an interrelated set of recommendations for healthy eating that can be adopted by the public. Taken together, the recommendations encompass two over-arching concepts:

1. **Maintain calorie balance over time to achieve and sustain a healthy weight.** People who are most successful at achieving and maintaining a healthy weight do so through continued attention to consuming only enough calories from foods and beverages to meet their needs and by being physically active. To curb the obesity epidemic and improve their health, many Americans must decrease the calories they consume and increase the calories they expend through physical activity.
2. **Focus on consuming nutrient-dense foods and beverages.** Americans currently consume too much sodium and too many calories from solid fats, added sugars, and refined grains.[2] These replace nutrient-dense foods and beverages and make it difficult for people to achieve recommended nutrient intake while controlling calorie and sodium intake. A healthy eating pattern limits intake of sodium, solid fats, added sugars, and refined grains and emphasizes nutrient-dense foods and beverages—vegetables, fruits, whole grains, fat-free or low-fat milk and milk products,[3] seafood, lean meats and poultry, eggs, beans and peas, and nuts and seeds.

Key Recommendations

- Prevent and/or reduce overweight and obesity through improved eating and physical activity behaviors.
- Control total calorie intake to manage body weight. For people who are overweight or obese, this means consuming fewer calories from foods and beverages.
- Increase physical activity and reduce time spent in sedentary behaviors.
- Maintain appropriate calorie balance during each stage of life—childhood, adolescence, adulthood, pregnancy and breastfeeding, and older age.

Foods and Food Components to Reduce

- Reduce daily sodium intake to less than 2300 milligrams (mg) and further reduce intake up to 1500 mg among persons age 51 and older and those of any age who are African American or have hypertension, diabetes, or chronic kidney disease. The 1500 mg recommendation applies to about one-half of the U.S. population, including children and majority of adults. *(Interestingly, this recommendation disregards guidance from the Dietary Guidelines Advisory Committee and the American Heart Association [AHA] experts, which recommended a daily sodium reduction to 1500 mg across the board.)*

- Consume less than 10% of total calories from saturated fatty acids by replacing them with monounsaturated and polyunsaturated fatty acids.
- Consume less than 300 mg a day of dietary cholesterol.
- Keep *trans* fatty acid consumption as low as possible, especially by limiting foods that contain synthetic sources of *trans* fats such as partially hydrogenated oils, and by limiting other solid fats.

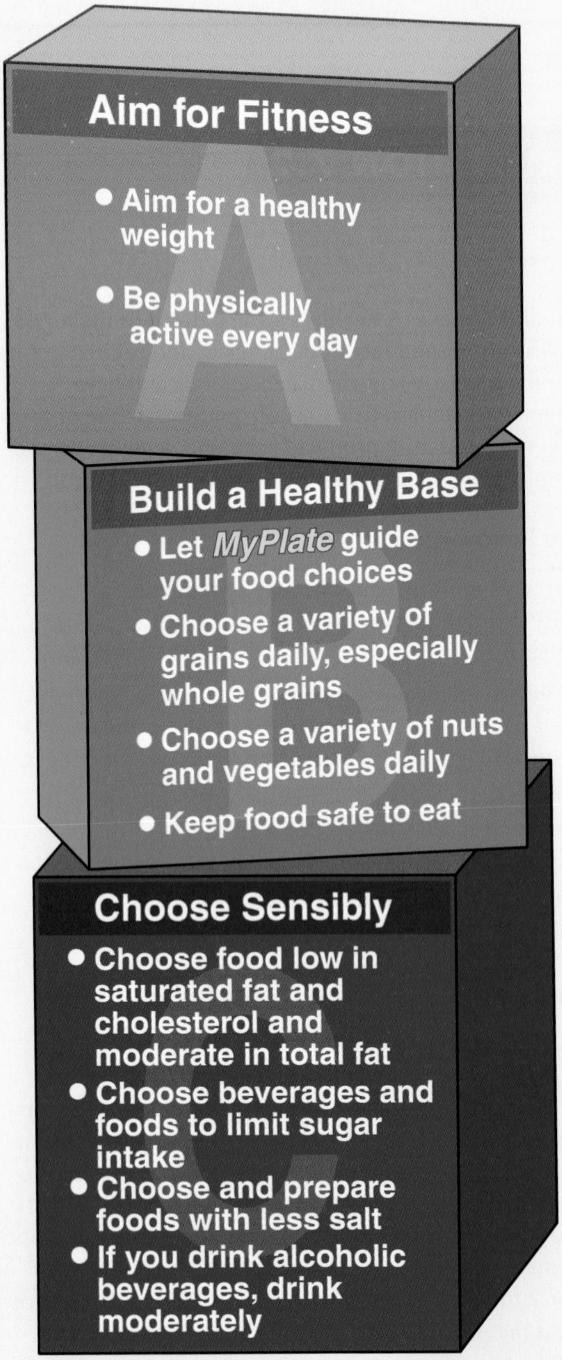

Aim for Fitness
Aim for a healthy weight
Be physically active every day
Build a Healthy Base
Let MyPlate guide your food choices
Choose a variety of grains daily, especially whole grains
Choose a variety of nuts and vegetables daily
Keep food safe to eat
Choose Sensibly
Choose food low in saturated fat and cholesterol and moderate in total fat
Choose beverages and foods to limit sugar intake
Choose and prepare foods with less salt
If you drink alcoholic beverages, drink moderately

- Reduce the intake of calories from solid fats and added sugars.
- Limit the consumption of foods that contain refined grains, especially refined grain foods that contain solid fats, added sugars, and sodium.
- If alcohol is consumed, it should be consumed in moderation—up to one drink a day for women and two drinks a day for men—and only by adults of legal drinking age.

Foods and Nutrients to Increase

- Increase vegetable and fruit intake.
- Eat a variety of vegetables, especially dark-green and red and orange vegetables and beans and peas.
- Consume at least one-half of all grains as whole grains. Increase whole-grain intake by replacing refined grains with whole grains.
- Increase intake of fat-free or low-fat milk and milk products, such as milk, yogurt, cheese, or fortified soy beverages.
- Choose a variety of protein foods, which include seafood, lean meat and poultry, eggs, beans and peas, soy products, and unsalted nuts and seeds.
- Increase the amount and variety of seafood consumed by choosing seafood in place of some meat and poultry.
- Replace protein foods that are higher in solid fats with choices that are lower in solid fats and calories and/or are sources of oils.
- Use oils to replace solid fats where possible.
- Choose foods that provide more potassium, dietary fiber, calcium, and vitamin D, which are nutrients of concern in American diets. These foods include vegetables, fruits, whole grains, and milk and milk products.

Recommendations for Women Capable of Becoming Pregnant

- Choose foods that supply heme iron (which is more readily absorbed by the body), additional iron sources, and enhancers of iron absorption such as vitamin C-rich foods.
- Consume 400 micrograms (μg) a day of synthetic folic acid from fortified foods and/or supplements) including food forms of folate from a varied diet.

Recommendations for Women Who Are Pregnant or Breastfeeding

- Consume 8–12 ounces of seafood a week from a variety of seafood types.
- Due to their methyl mercury content, limit white (albacore) tuna to 6 ounces a week and do not eat the following four types of fish: tilefish, shark, swordfish, and king mackerel.

- If pregnant, take an iron supplement as recommended by an obstetrician or other health care provider.

Recommendations for Individuals Age 50 and Older

- Consume foods fortified with vitamin B_{12}, such as fortified cereals, or dietary

Building Healthy Eating Patterns

- Select an eating pattern that meets nutrient needs over time at an appropriate calorie level (assess calorie needs to establish levels of food intake).
- Account for all foods and beverages consumed and assess how they fit within a total healthy eating pattern. Focus on nutrient-dense foods, reduce intake of calorie-dense beverages, and consider supplements and fortified foods if needed.
- Follow food safety recommendations when preparing and eating foods to reduce the risk of food-borne illnesses (**clean** hands, food contact surfaces, and vegetables and fruits; **separate** raw, cooked, and ready-to-eat foods while shopping, storing, and preparing foods; **cook** foods to a safe temperature; **chill** [refrigerate] perishable foods promptly).

Helping Americans Make Healthy Choices

1. Ensure that all Americans have access to nutritious foods and opportunities for physical activity.
2. Facilitate individual behavior change through environmental strategies.
3. Set the stage for lifelong healthy eating, physical activity, and weight management behaviors.

FIGURE 7.4 illustrates the important components of the whole-grain seed and the nutrient loss for 13 nutrients in the refining of whole-wheat flour. For example, refined flour (yellow bars) has just 13% of vitamin B_6, 20% of niacin, and 30% of the iron contained in whole-wheat form. The left side of the figure describes the whole-grain seed and its nutritional value.

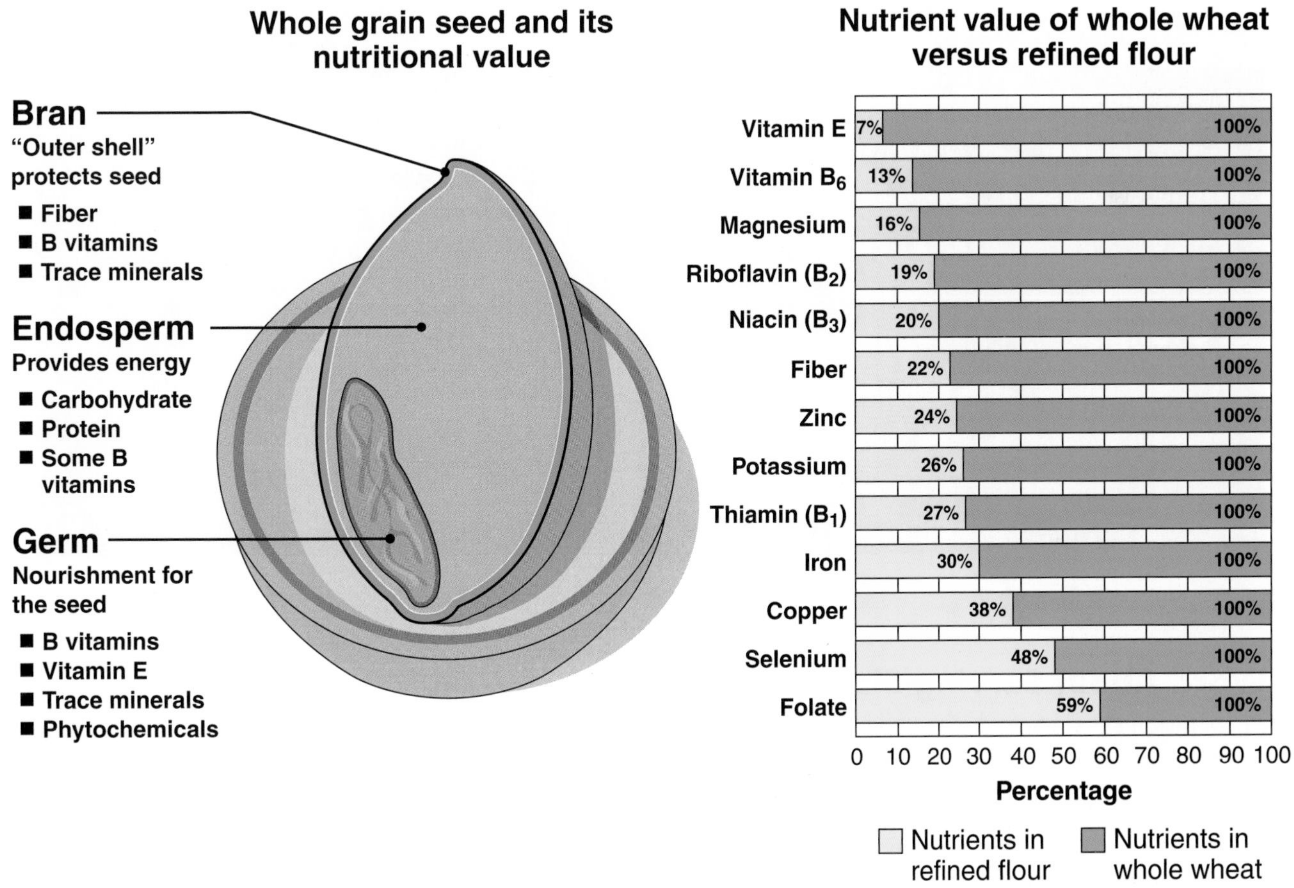

FIGURE 7.4. Whole grains provide a rich nutritional package.

TEN SUPER FOODS YOU SHOULD EAT

1. Cantaloupe
One-fourth of a melon supplies the recommended daily requirement for vitamins A and C.

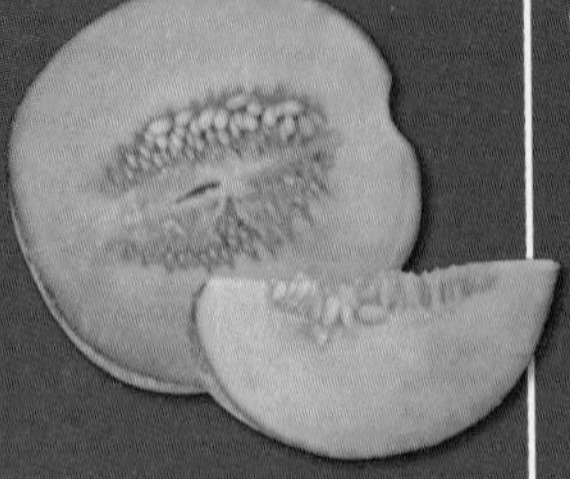

2. Sweet potatoes
Rich in carotenoids, vitamin C, potassium, and fiber.

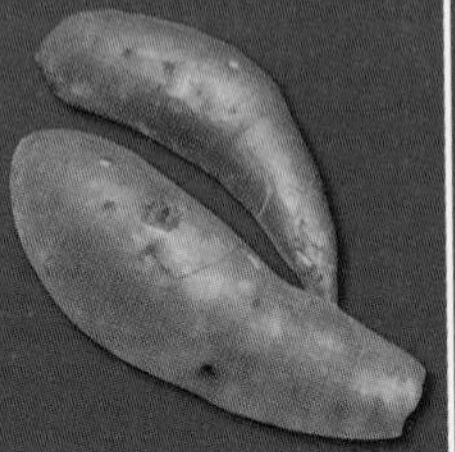

3. Fat free or low-fat 1% milk (including soy milk)
Rich in calcium and vitamins with minimal fat and cholesterol.

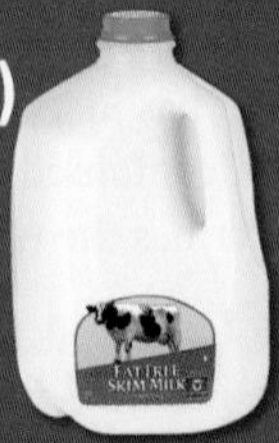

4. Salmon or other fatty fish
The omega-3 fats in fatty fish such as salmon, swordfish, and rainbow trout help to reduce the risk of sudden-death from heart attack.

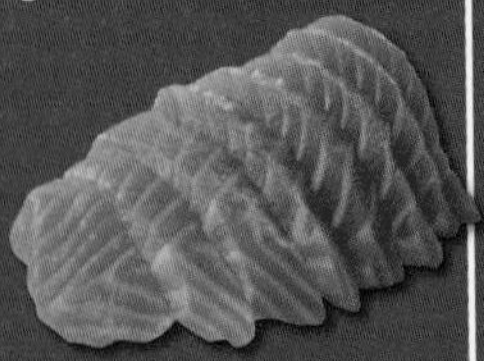

5. Oranges
Rich in vitamin C, folic acid, and fiber.

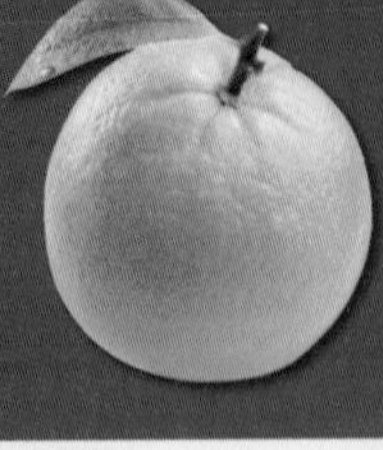

6. Broccoli
Rich in vitamin C, carotenoids, and folic acid.

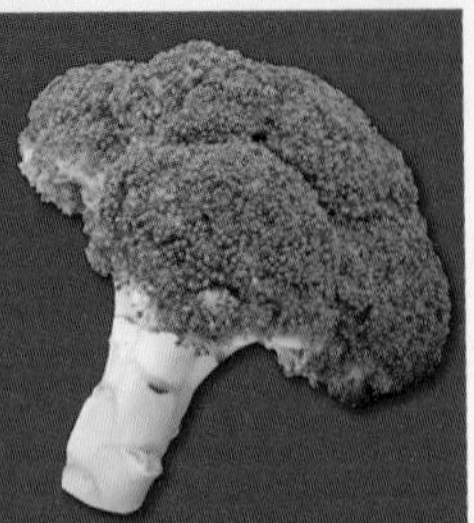

7. Whole grain bread
Richer in fiber, vitamins, and minerals than enriched white bread or "wheat" bread.

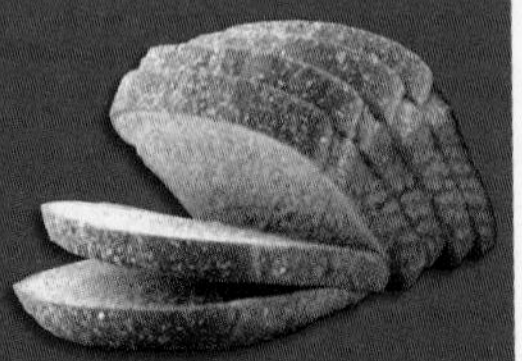

8. 100% bran cereal
One-half-cup serving provides about one-third of the daily requirement for fiber, helping to reduce the risk of constipation, diverticulosis, and heart disease.

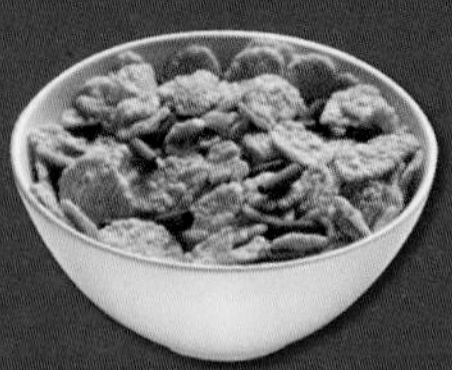

9. Beans
Rich in protein, iron, folic acid, and fiber. Examples include garbanzo, pinto, black, navy, and kidney beans, and lentils.

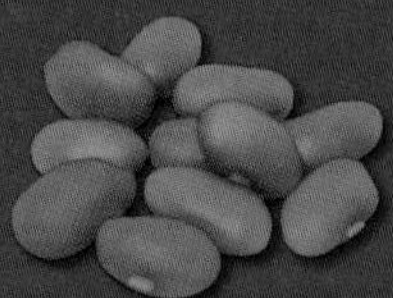

10. Spinach or kale
Rich in carotenoids, calcium, and fiber.

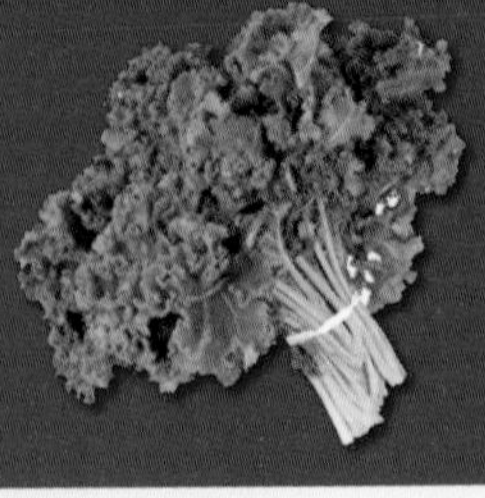

A Word About Serving Size

Much confusion exists about serving size and portion size. For example, the USDA defines a standard *serving* of pasta as 1/2 cup, whereas the Food and Drug Administration (FDA; www.fda.gov), which regulates food labels, claims a standard serving is 1 cup. Contrast these sizes with a typical restaurant pasta *portion* that averages about 3 cups—equal to six servings from MyPlate. To add further confusion, most people consider a serving to be the amount of food they typically consume (actually a portion), when, for the government's purpose, it represents a far smaller standard unit of measure. Within the perspective of "real-world" standards and government standards, the USDA recommendation to consume 6 to 11 servings of grains or breads daily seems an unattainable goal. Keep in mind that one serving by government standards represents a relatively small portion size (see box labeled picture portions on p. 224): a 6-oz glass of fruit or vegetable juice; 1 medium-sized orange, banana, or apple; 1 cup of salad greens—about the size of your fist; 1 egg; 1 cup of milk or yogurt; 1 slice of bread; 2 tablespoons of peanut butter—about the size of a ping-pong ball; 1/2 cup of chopped fruits and vegetable—3 medium asparagus spears, 8 carrot sticks, 1 ear of corn, or 1/4 cup of dried fruit like raisins; 3 oz of meat, fish, or poultry—about the size of a deck of playing cards; 1 teaspoon of butter or mayonnaise—the size of a fingertip; or 2 oz of cheese—the size equivalent of two thumbs.

A BIG PLUS FOR WHOLE GRAINS

According to the government's *Dietary Guidelines for Americans*, prudent nutrition includes eating "at least 3 ounces of whole-grain cereals, breads, crackers, rice, or pasta every day." Increasing one's intake of whole grains can lower risk of stroke, type 2 diabetes, obesity, abdominal fat accumulation, constipation, and particularly heart disease.[64,87]

The *Dietary Guidelines for Americans* recommends diet and lifestyle choices to promote health, support physically active lives, and reduce chronic disease risks. It also includes advice to exercise moderately for 30 minutes (e.g., walking, jogging, bicycling, and lawn, garden, and house work) most, but preferably all, days of the week. The *Guidelines* advise children to exercise moderately for 60 minutes daily. The *Guidelines* acknowledge that good nutrition and regular exercise provide an important approach to ensure good health and combat the obesity epidemic. The *Guidelines* separate fruits and vegetables from grains and emphasize whole-grain consumption. The *Guidelines* also recommend replacing foods in the diet with more nutrient-dense options, yet no consistent standards or criteria exist for such categorization.[29]

DIETARY GUIDELINES FOR AMERICANS, 2010: MODIFICATIONS TO RECOMMENDATIONS

1. Saturated fat intake is reduced from 10% of total daily calories to 7%; emphasis is placed on substituting more healthful monounsaturated and polyunsaturated fatty acids.
2. Cholesterol intake remains unchanged at 300 mg daily for healthy adults and less than 200 mg for those with heart disease risks.
3. *Trans* fatty acid intake is halved from 1% to 0.5% of total calories.
4. Recommended daily sodium intake is reduced from 2300 mg to 1500 mg. Increased intake of potassium is urged to help counter the elevating effects of sodium on blood pressure.
5. Recommended intake of seafood calls for two 4-oz servings per week with the goal of averaging 250 mg of the omega-3 fatty acids docosahexaenoic acid and eicosapentaenoic acid daily.
6. There is a shift to more plant-based carbohydrate and protein foods and a focus on nutrient-rich rather than energy-dense foods.

USING THE DIETARY GUIDELINES

Proper use of the *Guidelines* involves making changes in typical food choices to adhere more closely to guideline recommendations. **TABLE 7.1** lists examples of food substitutions in line with the *Guidelines*.

American Heart Association Recommendations

Dietary guidelines from the AHA (www.heart.org) for the general public over the age of 2 years address the growing rates of obesity, hypertension, and type 2 diabetes in the United States.[69,75] Because of the strong association between excess body weight and cardiovascular disease, the recommendations also emphasize achieving and maintaining a healthful body weight. Lifestyle modifications include increasing the level of regular physical activity and eliminating all tobacco. These guidelines are essentially similar to guidelines from other agencies (including the USDA). They place great emphasis on the adoption of healthy eating patterns and lifestyle behaviors instead of targeting specific numeric goals, such as the number of grams of dietary fat to consume. **TABLE 7.2** outlines four major goals and associated

TABLE 7.1 Examples of Appropriate Substitutions to Bring Existing Eating Behaviors More in Line with the *Dietary Guidelines for Americans*

If you eat this	Try this
White bread	Whole-wheat or whole-grain bread
Breakfast cereal with sugar	Low-sugar cereal; shredded wheat
Coleslaw/potato salad	Bean salad with yogurt
Chips/salty snacks	Low-salt baked pretzels
Donuts	Bran muffin; cornbread
Vegetables, boiled	Vegetables, steamed
Vegetables, canned	Vegetables, frozen
Fried foods	Broiled or barbequed foods
Whole milk	Nonfat or low-fat milk
Ice cream	Sherbet or frozen yogurt
Mayonnaise-based dressings	Oil and vinegar or diet salad dressing
Cookies	Air-popped corn
Salted foods	Flavor foods with herbs and spices or lemons

PICTURE PORTIONS

A portion is the amount of food you actually eat. It may be more or less than a standard serving, which is the amount listed on food labels and listed in food composition tables. The different food items and corresponding picture portion sizes can be used for reference

Food Item	Picture Portion
Medium potato (computer mouse)	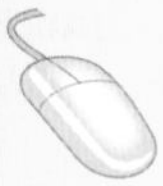
Medium-sized fruit or vegetable (tennis ball)	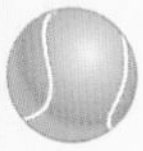
One-fourth cup dried fruit or raisins (golf ball)	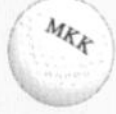
Average bagel (hockey puck)	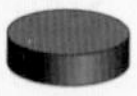
Pancake or slice of bread (DVD)	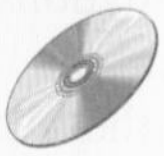
Cup of fruit (baseball)	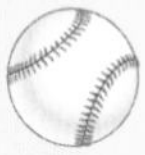
Cup of lettuce (four leaves)	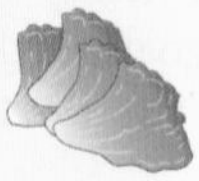
Three ounces cooked meat or poultry (cassette tape)	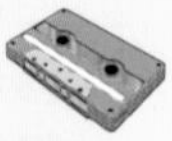
Three ounces grilled fish (your checkbook)	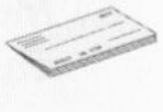
One ounce cheese (four dice)	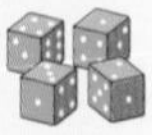
One teaspoon butter or margarine (postage stamp)	
One tablespoon salad dressing (thumb tip)	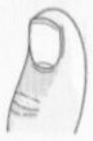
Two tablespoons peanut butter (ping pong ball)	
One cup cooked dry beans (tennis ball)	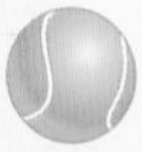
One ounce nuts or candies (one small handful)	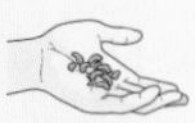
One ounce chips or pretzels (one large handful)	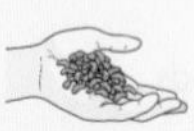

RECOMMENDATIONS FROM THE AHA

The American Heart Association (AHA) guidelines (*Guide to the Primary Prevention of Cardiovascular Diseases*) to prevent heart attacks and strokes list secondhand smoke for the first time as a risk factor. They also recommend screening for risk factors beginning at age 20 and every 5 years thereafter to assess smoking habits, family medical history, and blood pressure. Men should maintain a waistline of 40 inches or less and women a waistline of 35 inches or less. Persons 40 years of age and older should be screened for additional risk factors such as cholesterol levels. The new guidelines drop passages that recommended hormone supplements and antioxidant vitamins to reduce cardiovascular risk. Also, a daily dose of aspirin, previously recommended for individuals who have already suffered a heart attack or stroke, is now also suggested for those whose risk assessment indicates at least a 10% risk of a heart attack in the next decade.

guidelines for the general population; **TABLE 7.3** presents specific dietary recommendations for the general population and for men and women at higher disease risk (formerly known as the "Step 2" diet).

The principle message advises consuming a varied but balanced diet. To maintain a healthful body weight, attention must focus on portion size and number. Importance is placed on consuming a diet rich in fruits and vegetables, cereals and whole grains, nonfat and low-fat dairy products, legumes, nuts, fish, poultry, and lean meats.[8,52]

AN EXPANDING EMPHASIS ON HEALTHFUL EATING AND REGULAR PHYSICAL ACTIVITY

Scientists have responded to the rapidly rising number of adults and children who are overweight or obese and the increasing incidence of comorbidities associated with the overweight condition. In September 2002, the Institute of Medicine (**www.iom.edu**), the medical division of the National Academies, issued guidelines as part of their *Dietary Reference Intakes* (see Chapter 2).[11] They recommend that Americans spend at least *1 hour* (equivalent of about 400–500 kcal expended) over the course of each day in moderately intense brisk walking, swimming, or cycling to maintain health and normal body weight. This amount of regular physical activity—based on an assessment of the amount of exercise healthy persons engage in each day—represents twice that previously recommended in 1996 in a report from the US Surgeon General! The advice agrees with the 2003 recommendations by the World Health Organization (WHO; **www.who.int**), recommendations by the

TABLE 7.2 Major Nutritional Guidelines for the General Population

Population Goals	Major Guidelines
Overall healthy eating program	• Consume a varied diet that includes foods from each of the major food groups with an emphasis on fruits, vegetables, whole grains, low-fat or nonfat dairy products, fish, legumes, poultry, and lean meats. • Monitor portion size and number to ensure adequate, not excess, intake.
Appropriate body weight BMI ≤ 25	• Match energy intake to needs. • When weight loss is desirable, make appropriate changes to energy intake and expenditure (physical activity). • Limit foods with a high sugar content and those with a high caloric density.
Desirable cholesterol profile	• Limit foods high in saturated fat, *trans* fat, and cholesterol. • Substitute unsaturated fat from vegetables, fish, legumes, and nuts.
Desirable blood pressure Systolic <140 mm Hg Diastolic <90 mm Hg	• Maintain a healthy body weight. • Consume a varied diet with emphasis on vegetables, fruits, and low-fat or nonfat dairy products. • Limit sodium intake. • Limit alcohol intake.

BMI, body mass index (kg·m^{-2}).

Source: Krauss RM, et al. AHA dietary guidelines revision 2000: a statement for healthcare professionals from the Nutrition Committee of the American Heart Association. Circulation 2000;102:2284.

Food and Agriculture Organization of the United Nations (www.fao.org) and, more recently, the International Association for the Study of Obesity (www.iaso.org/iotf),[120] and research findings that point to the health and weight-loss benefits of longer duration weekly physical activity.[51,56] The advice represents a *bold increase* in exercise duration, considering that 30 minutes of similar-type exercise on most days decreases disease risk, more than 60% of the US population fails to incorporate even a moderate level of exercise into their lives, and 25% of the US population does not exercise at all.

The team of 21 experts also recommended for the first time a range for macronutrient intake plus how much dietary fiber to consume in the daily diet. These recommendations

TABLE 7.3 Specific Dietary Recommendations for the General Population and for Men and Women at Higher Disease Risk

For the General Population	For Populations at Higher Risk[a]
1. Restrict total fat to ≤30% of total calories. 2. Restrict saturated fat to ≤10% of total calories. 3. Limit the total intake of cholesterol-raising fatty acids (saturated and *trans*) to ≤10% of calories. 4. Limit cholesterol intake to ≤300 mg·d^{-1}. 5. Replace cholesterol-raising fatty acids with whole grains and unsaturated fatty acids from fish, vegetables, legumes, and nuts. 6. Limit sodium intake to ≤2400 mg·d^{-1} (≤6.0 g·d^{-1} of salt). 7. If alcohol is consumed, limit intake to 2 drinks per day for men, 1 drink per day for women. 8. Eat at least 2 servings of fish per week. 9. Eat 5 or more servings of vegetables and fruits per day. 10. Eat 6 or more servings of grain products per day. 11. Emphasize daily intake of low-fat or non-fat dairy products.	***Elevated LDL-cholesterol or preexisting cardiovascular disease*** 1. Restrict saturated fat to ≤7% of total calories. 2. Limit cholesterol intake to ≤200 mg·d^{-1}. 3. Weight loss when appropriate. 4. Include soy protein with isoflavones. ***Dyslipidemia characterized by low HDL-cholesterol, elevated triglycerides, and small, dense LDL-cholesterol*** 1. Replace saturated fat calories with unsaturated fat. 2. Limit carbohydrate intake, especially sugars and refined carbohydrates. 3. Weight loss when appropriate. 4. Increase physical activity. ***Diabetes mellitus and insulin resistance*** 1. Restrict saturated fat to ≤7% of total calories. 2. Limit cholesterol intake to ≤200 mg·d^{-1}. 3. When selecting carbohydrates, choose those with high fiber content.

Modified from Krauss RM, et al. AHA dietary guidelines revision 2000: a statement for healthcare professionals from the Nutrition Committee of the American Heart Association. Circulation 2000;102:2284.

[a] LDL, HDL.

Additional Insights

Foods That Comprise a Healthy Diet: The Evolution of Nutritional Recommendations

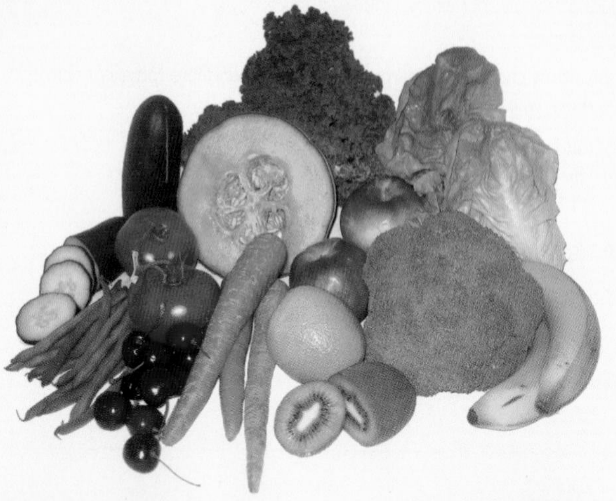

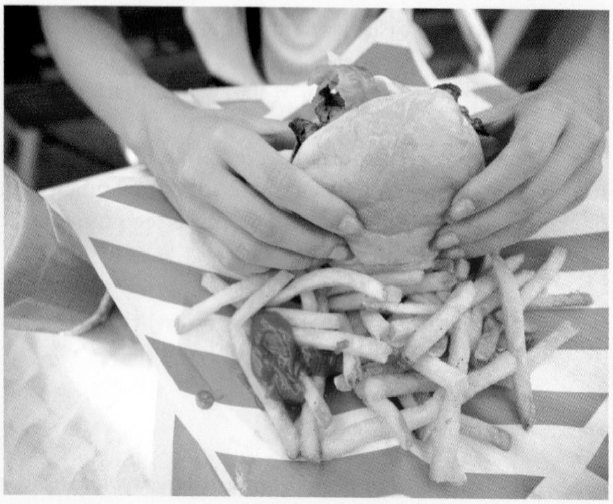

The good food–bad food controversy evolved from public health attempts during the 1950s to identify foods that promote "good health." Included were foods with optimal sources of vitamins and minerals as specified in the first Recommended Dietary Allowances (RDAs) legislation that listed specific amounts of vitamins, minerals, and protein to prevent nutrient deficiencies. This approach seemed appropriate at the time to help in the battle against malnutrition. For example, citrus fruits were recommended to avoid scurvy, thereby making such fruits "good-to-eat foods" because they contained high vitamin C concentrations. Likewise, carrots were advocated as being a good food to stave off vitamin A deficiency and potential night blindness, while milk was included as a good source of needed calcium. For the next two decades, the good-food nutrition message, which covered hundreds of foods, continued to center on the positive health benefits the recommended foods provided.

In the 1970s, nutrition research began to focus on dietary modifications related to risk for heart disease with primary emphasis on consuming foods low in cholesterol and saturated fatty acids. Because eggs and processed meats were high in both of these lipids, the public health message tilted toward restriction of bad foods relative to good foods. The 1980s saw the first *Dietary Guidelines for Americans* recommend a reduction in the intake of "bad" foods with high fat, sugar, and sodium, such as French fries, mayonnaise-rich foods, potato chips, candy, and sugar-sweetened beverages. Thus, the focus continued on what *not* to eat, instead of the more positive approach of what *to* eat.

In contrast to "good" versus "bad" foods, the ADA (www.ada.org) currently favors a *total* dietary approach to food choices. They argue that the totality of what a person eats, rather than any one particular food consumed (or omitted), determines a "healthy diet." This total dietary approach to sound nutrition is supported by the current *Dietary Guidelines* (see page 219) that stress balance, moderation, and variety in food choices. Each variant of the *Guidelines* allows consumers to choose small amounts of less nutrient-dense foods (i.e., foods high in fats, sugars, and alcohol) while still meeting daily nutrient needs within age and gender caloric limits. This message, that limited quantities of bad foods are acceptable provided that nutrient-dense foods comprise the major portion of one's choices, supports the total diet approach that no single food is either good or bad. Unfortunately, the classification of good or bad foods is not simply determined by its nutrient density or "healthfulness," but also is influenced by seemingly unrelated factors that impact nutritional policy in the United States. On many levels, politics remains first and foremost as the largest influence on nutritional recommendations, followed by financial interest among large, multinational food conglomerates, rather than the validity of scientific inquiry about nutrition and its relation to health and disease. The history of the recommendations of the USDA (www.usda.org) and *Dietary Guidelines for Americans* have been clouded by big business interests and the need to gather support of the American agricultural industry, which includes nonstop lobbying efforts by powerful organizations from the meat and dairy industry. Thus, it should occasion little surprise that despite strong scientific evidence to the contrary, foods of animal origin, such as dairy products, eggs, and meat, still serve as primary components of the US diet. The science on the matter is difficult to ignore—promotion of optimum health and disease avoidance should emphasize more nutrient-rich, plant-based foods, the bulk of which should consist of whole unprocessed foods, whole-grain breads and cereal products, legumes such as beans and peas, vegetables, and fruits, with foods of animal origin representing no more than a side dish.

Related References

Ashe M, et al. Changing places: policies to make a healthy choice the easy choice. *Public Health* 2011; 125:889.

Butler D, Pearson H. Dietary advice: flash in the pan? *Nature* 2005;433:794.

Flock MR, Kris-Etherton PM. Dietary Guidelines for Americans 2010: implications for Cardiovascular disease. *Curr Atheroscler Rep* 2011; 13:499.

Kirkhus B, et al. Effects of similar intakes of marine n-3 fatty acids from enriched food products and fish oil on cardiovascular risk markers in healthy human subjects. *Br J Nutr* 2011;15:1.

Krebs-Smith SM, et al. Healthfulness of the U.S. food supply: little improvement despite decades of dietary guidance. *Am J Prev Med* 2010;38:472.

Rehm CD, et al. The quality and monetary value of diets consumed by adults in the United States. *Am J Clin Nutr* 2011; 94:1333.

US Department of Health and Human Services. 2010 Dietary Guidelines for Americans. Available at: http://health.gov/DietaryGuidelines/.

Watts ML, et al. The art of translating nutritional science into dietary guidance; history and evolution of the Dietary Guidelines for Americans. *Nutr Rev* 2011;69:404.

are intended for professional nutritionists and the general public. To meet daily energy and nutrient needs while minimizing risk for heart disease and type 2 diabetes, adults should consume between 45 and 65% of total calories from carbohydrates. This relatively wide range provides for flexibility in recognition that both the high-carbohydrate, low-fat diet of Asian peoples and the higher fat diet of peoples from the Mediterranean region with its high monounsaturated fatty acid olive oil content contribute to good health. The maximum intake of added sugars—the caloric sweeteners added to manufactured foods and soda, candy, fruit drinks, cakes, cookies, and ice cream—is placed at 25% of total calories. This relatively high 25% level represented the threshold above which a significant decline would occur for several important micronutrients such as vitamin A and calcium. Acceptable lipid intake ranges between 20 and 35% of caloric intake, a range at the lower end of most recommendations and at the upper end of the 30% limit set by the AHA, American Cancer Society, and National Institutes of Health. The panel noted that very low fat intake combined with high intake of carbohydrate tends to lower HDL cholesterol and raise triacylglycerol levels. Conversely, high intake of dietary fat and accompanying increased caloric intake contributes to obesity and its related medical complications. Moreover, high-fat diets usually link with an increased saturated fatty acid intake, raising plasma LDL cholesterol concentrations, which further potentiates coronary heart disease risk. The panel recommended "as low as possible" saturated fat intake; they also recognized that no safe level existed for *trans* fatty acid intake.

Recommended protein intake ranges between 10 and 35% of calories, which remains consistent with prior recommendations. For the first time, age-based recommendations are provided for all of the essential amino acids contained in dietary protein. **TABLE 7.4** presents an example of the macronutrient composition for a 2500-kcal diet based on these new guidelines.

The panel's recommendations for dietary fiber intake are discussed in Chapter 1. Particularly important is the consumption of water-soluble fibers (pectin from fruits and oat and rice bran); these reduce plasma cholesterol levels and slow digestion to increase satiety and decrease the risk of overeating.

TABLE 7.4 Possible Macronutrient Composition of a 2500-kcal Diet Based on Recommendations of the Expert Panel of the Institute of Medicine, National Academies

	Composition of 2500-kcal Intake		
	Carbohydrate	Lipid	Protein
Percentage	60	15	25
kcal	1500	375	625
Grams	375	94	69
Ounces	13.2	3.3	2.4

MEDITERRANEAN AND VEGETARIAN DIET PYRAMIDS

The illustrations in **FIGURE 7.2B and 7.2C** present diet pyramids for application to individuals whose diet consists largely of the following:

1. Fruits, nuts, vegetables, legumes, and all manner of unrefined grains, and protein derived from fish and less meat, beans, and chicken, with dietary fat composed mostly of monounsaturated fatty acids with mild ethanol consumption (**Mediterranean Diet Pyramid**).
2. Foods primarily from the plant kingdom (**Near-Vegetarian Diet Pyramid**).

A Mediterranean-type diet—possibly mediated via several plant foods in the diet—substantially reduces the rate of recurrence after a first myocardial infarction, perhaps from its association with increased total antioxidant capacity and low LDL cholesterol levels.[27,35,108] Its high monounsaturated fatty acid content (generally olive oil with its associated phytochemicals) also staves off age-related memory loss, heart disease, cancer, and overall mortality rate in healthy, elderly people.[27,33,74,129,135] The dietary focus of both pyramids on fruits and vegetables, particularly cruciferous and green leafy

MEAT CONSUMPTION IN THE UNITED STATES

Meat consumption in the United States and the rest of the developed world continues to rise. Despite a shift toward higher poultry consumption, red meat still represents the largest proportion of meat consumed in the United States (58%), where meat is consumed at more than three times the global average. Twenty-two percent of the meat consumed is processed. In light of the epidemiologic evidence linking red and processed meat intake to cancer and chronic disease risk, understanding factors that determine trends in meat consumption should be helpful to public health professionals aiming to reduce chronic disease worldwide.

Dietary Modifications to Reduce Disease Risk

What scientists call *N-nitroso compounds* can cause cancer. They seem to form in the digestive tract when heme iron (the kind in red meat) and intestinal bacteria trigger meat protein to combine with nitr*ites* that are added to processed meats or with the nitrites that the body makes from the nitr*ates* in water and in some vegetables such as spinach and carrots.

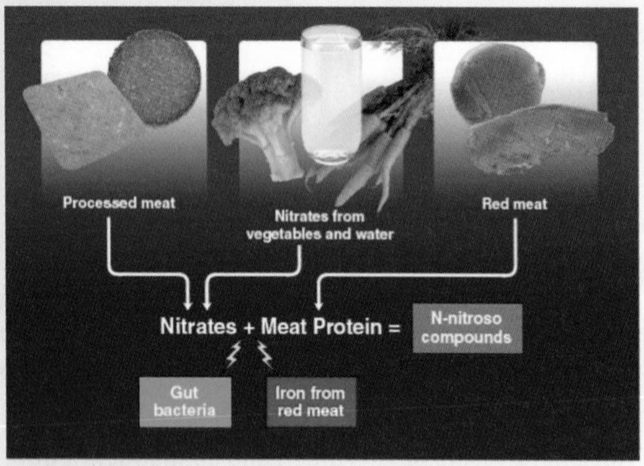

Do the following to reduce this risk:

- Cut back on red and processed meats. Aim for only about one serving a week.
- Replace red meat with poultry, fish, beans, nuts, and soy-based veggie meats. Look for nitrite-free deli meats.
- Aim for adequate calcium intake: 1000 mg daily for ages 50 or younger and 1200 mg above age 50.

Source: Daniel CR, et al. Trends in meat consumption in the USA. *Public Health Nutr* 2010;12:1.

Nutrition Action Health Letter, June 2009.

ONE SIZE DOES NOT FIT ALL

Clearly, no one food or meal provides optimal nutrition and associated health-related benefits. Perhaps the following statement best summarizes the metabolic, epidemiologic, and clinical trial evidence over the past several decades regarding diet and lifestyle behaviors and coronary heart disease.[52]

> "Substantial evidence indicates that diets using nonhydrogenated unsaturated fats as the predominant form of dietary fat, whole grains as the main form of carbohydrates, an abundance of fruits and vegetables, and adequate omega-3 fatty acids can offer significant protection against coronary heart disease. Such diets, together with regular physical activity, avoidance of smoking, and maintenance of a healthy body weight, may prevent the majority of cardiovascular disease in Western populations."

vegetables and citrus fruit and juice, also reduces risk for ischemic stroke,[62] may enhance the beneficial effects of cholesterol-lowering drugs,[63] and protects against the metabolic syndrome, a cluster of precursors of heart disease and type 2 diabetic symptoms[66] that include hypertension and unhealthy blood sugar levels.

GOOD FOR THE NERVOUS SYSTEM

People who follow a Mediterranean-style meal plan (diet) are 40% less likely to develop Alzheimer's disease compared with individuals who do not follow this diet. The diet includes eating diverse vegetables, legumes, fruits, cereals, and fish, while limiting intake of meat and dairy products, drinking moderate amounts of alcohol, and emphasizing monounsaturated fats over saturated fats, a dietary focus that also reduces heart disease risk.

This diet may also produce slower rates of mental decline in the elderly. A recent report analyzed data from a continuing study with prospective design, large sample, and use of a well-validated dietary questionnaire of 3790 Chicago residents 65 and older that began in 1993. Subjects' mental acuity was tested at 3-year intervals, and their degree of adherence to the diet was tracked on a 55-point scale. High scores for adherence to the diet associated with slower rates of cognitive decline, even after controlling for smoking, education, obesity, hypertension, and other factors. Those in the top third for adherence were cognitively the equivalent of 2 years younger than those in the bottom third.

Source: Tangney CC, et al. Adherence to a Mediterranean-type dietary pattern ad cognitive decline in a community population. *Am J Clin Nutr* 2011;305:1348.

Connections to the Past

Russel Henry Chittenden (1856–1943)

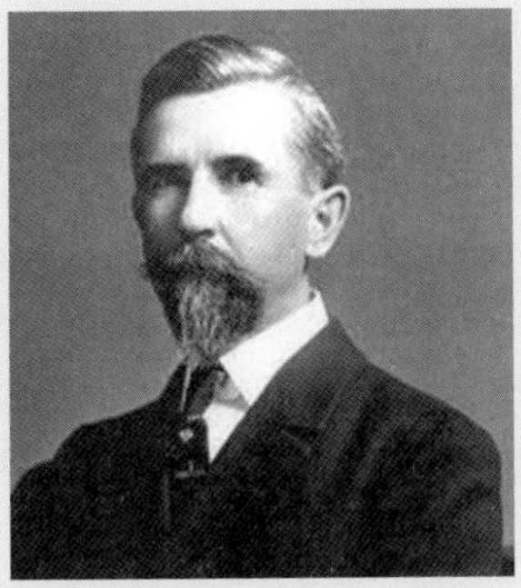

Russel H. Chittenden excelled in chemistry at Yale University's Sheffield Scientific School, where his senior project investigated why leftover scallops tasted sweeter when recooked. Chittenden discovered that muscle tissue contained large amounts of free glycogen. With encouragement from his mentor, Chittenden published his paper in the *American Journal of Science* (1875; republished in a British and German journal).Chittenden published 144 scientific papers, including "Physiological Economy in Nutrition, With Special Reference to the Minimal Proteid Requirement of the Healthy Man. An Experimental Study." It refocused attention on man's minimal protein requirement while resting or exercising and influenced future research in nutrition and exercise physiology. After studying laborers who consumed approximately 3100 kcal (12,977 kJ) daily, the Germans Rubner and Voit maintained that protein intake should be either 118 $g \cdot d^{-1}$ (Voit) or 127 $g \cdot d^{-1}$ (Rubner); the American scientist Atwater (see p. 170) recommended a protein intake similar to Rubner's.

thePoint *Visit* **thePoint.lww.com/MKKSEN4e** *for more details about how Chittenden influenced future research in nutrition and exercise physiology with experiments that evaluated low-protein diets.*

PERSONAL ASSESSMENT

An objective assessment of energy and nutrient intake provides the frame of reference for judging the adequacy of one's diet related to recommended guidelines. Such determinations from careful daily food intake records provide a reasonably close estimate compared with more direct measurements. Appendix C outlines the *Three-Day Dietary Survey* procedure to assess a diet's adequacy.

Diet Quality Index

The **Diet Quality Index** focuses on the nutritional elements of a diet considered the most important relative to good health and disease prevention. This instrument, designed for use for individuals 18 years and older, measures overall quality of one's diet that reflects a risk gradient for diet-related chronic disease. It provides a score based on a composite of the eight food- and nutrient-based recommendations (total fat, saturated fat, cholesterol, fruit and vegetables, grains and legumes, protein, sodium, and calcium) of the National Academy of Sciences. This index presented in **FIGURE 7.5** offers a simple scoring schema based on the risk gradient associated with diet and the major diet-related chronic diseases.[121] Respondents who meet or exceed a given dietary goal receive a score of 0; a score of 1 applies to an intake that falls within 30% of a dietary goal; the score becomes 2 when intake fails to fall within 30% of the goal. The scores for all eight categories are then totaled. The index ranges from 0 to 16, with the lower score representing a higher quality diet. A score of *4 or less* reflects a more healthful diet, whereas an index of *10 or higher* pinpoints a less healthful diet needing improvement.

The Healthy Eating Index

The USDA designed the **Healthy Eating Index (HEI)** presented in **TABLE 7.5** for nutrition promotion activities and to monitor changes in diet quality over time. This 100-point analytic tool evaluates how well a person's diet conforms to recommendations based on dietary balance, moderation, and variety.[45,137] Total scores can range from a "poor" diet (HEI score <65) to a "good" diet (HEI score >85), with scores of 65 to 74 and 75 to 84 being in between. HEI scores for each component of the index are defined as "poor" (score <5), "needs improvement" (score between 5 and 8), and "good" (score >8).

KEEP THEM UNREFINED, COMPLEX, AND LOW GLYCEMIC

Little health risk exists in subsisting chiefly on a variety of fiber-rich complex carbohydrates if intake also supplies essential amino acids, fatty acids, minerals, and vitamins. The most desirable complex carbohydrates exhibit slow digestion and absorption rates. Moderate- to low-glycemic foods include whole-grain breads, cereals, pastas, legumes, most fruits, and milk and milk products.

MACRONUTRIENT NEEDS FOR THE PHYSICALLY ACTIVE

Many physically active individuals receive either inadequate or incorrect information concerning prudent dietary practices. *Research in exercise nutrition, although far from complete, indicates that teenagers, adults, and competitive athletes who exercise regularly to keep fit do not require additional nutrients*

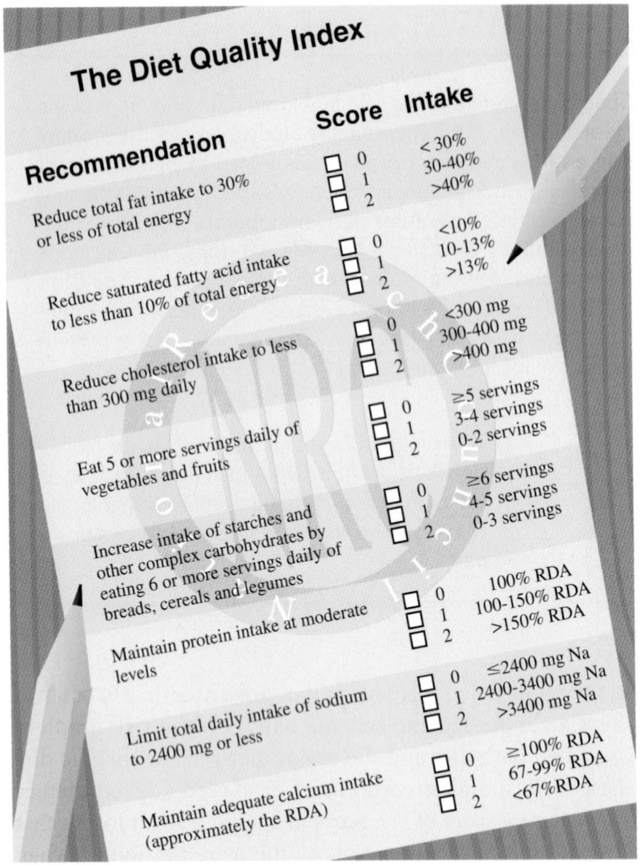
The Diet Quality Index
Recommendation
Score
Intake
Reduce total fat intake to 30% or less of total energy
0 1 2
< 30%
30-40%
>40%
Reduce saturated fatty acid intake to less than 10% of total energy
0 1 2
<10%
10-13%
>13%
Reduce cholesterol intake to less than 300 mg daily
0 1 2
<300 mg
300-400 mg
>400 mg
Eat 5 or more servings daily of vegetables and fruits
0 1 2
≥5 servings
3-4 servings
0-2 servings
Increase intake of starches and other complex carbohydrates by eating 6 or more servings daily of breads, cereals and legumes
0 1 2
≥6 servings
4-5 servings
0-3 servings
Maintain protein intake at moderate levels
0 1 2
100% RDA
100-150% RDA
>150% RDA
Limit total daily intake of sodium to 2400 mg or less
0 1 2
≤2400 mg Na
2400-3400 mg Na
>3400 mg Na
Maintain adequate calcium intake (approximately the RDA)
0 1 2
≥100% RDA
67-99% RDA
<67%RDA

FIGURE 7.5. The revised Diet Quality Index assesses risk for chronic diseases associated with overall dietary pattern. A score of 0 indicates that a respondent's diet meets the desired dietary goal for the item; a score of 1 means the intake falls within 30% of the goal; and an intake that fails to fall within 30% of the goal receives a score of 2. Scores are then added (range from 0 to 16), with the lower score indicating a better quality of diet. (Available from the National Academies Press at www.nap.edu/openbook.php?record_id=1222&page=R1. Additional sources include Haines PS, et al. The Diet Quality Index revised: a measurement instrument for populations. *J Am Diet Assoc* 1999;99:697; Newby PK, et al. Reproducibility and validity of the Diet Quality Index Revised as assessed by use of a food-frequency questionnaire. *Am J Clin Nutr* 2003;78:941; and Kim EH, et al. Diet quality indices and postmenopausal breast cancer survival. *Nutr Cancer* 2011;63:381.)

beyond those obtained by consuming a nutritionally well-balanced diet.

What the Physically Active Actually Eat

Inconsistencies exist among studies that relate diet quality to physical activity level and/or physical fitness. Some studies have shown a positive association between healthier diets and higher physical activity levels, whereas others have not. Part of the inconsistency results from use of relatively crude and imprecise self-reported measures of physical activity, small sample size, and unreliable dietary assessments.[42,82] **TABLE 7.6** contrasts the nutrient and energy intakes with national dietary recommendations of a large population-based cohort of nearly 7059 men and 2453 women classified as low, moderate, and high for cardiorespiratory fitness who participated in the Aerobics Center Longitudinal Study. The four most significant findings of this study indicate the following:

1. A progressively lower BMI was seen for men and women with increasing levels of physical fitness.
2. Remarkably small differences were observed in energy intake in relation to physical fitness classification of women (94 $kcal \cdot d^{-1}$) and men (82 $kcal \cdot d^{-1}$), with the moderate fitness group consuming the fewest calories for both sexes.
3. A progressively higher dietary fiber intake and a lower cholesterol intake across fitness categories were seen.
4. Men and women with higher fitness levels consumed diets that more closely approached dietary recommendations with respect to dietary fiber, percentage of energy from total fat, percentage of energy from saturated fat, and dietary cholesterol than peers of lower fitness.

FIGURE 7.6 lists the recommended intakes for protein, lipid, and carbohydrate and food sources for these macronutrients for active men and women. A daily energy requirement of 2000 kcal for women and 3000 kcal for men represents average values for typical young US adults. *After meeting basic nutrient requirements (as recommended in* **FIG. 7.6***)*, a variety of food sources based on individual preference supply the extra energy needs for physical activity.

Proteins

As discussed in Chapter 1, 0.8 $g \cdot kg^{-1}$ of body mass (0.35 $g \cdot lb^{-1}$) represents the RDA for protein intake. Thus, a person weighing 77 kg (170 lb) requires about 62 g or 2.2 oz of protein daily. Assuming that even during exercise relatively little protein loss occurs through energy metabolism (an assumption not entirely correct), this protein recommendation remains adequate for most active individuals. Also, the protein intake for the typical American exceeds the protein RDA; the competitive athlete's diet usually contains two to four times more protein than recommended values. One nutritional dilemma for the physically active vegetarian concerns obtaining an adequate balance of essential amino acids from a diet that obtains its protein from the plant kingdom. Chapter 1 discusses the use of complementary protein food sources to minimize this problem. It remains unclear whether physically active children and adolescents require more protein for optimal growth and development than their sedentary counterparts.

TABLE 7.5 Healthy Eating Index—2005: Components and Standards for Scoring[a]

Component	Maximum points	Standard for maximum score	Standard for minimum score of zero
Total fruit (includes 100% juice)	5	≥0.8 cup equiv. per 1000 kcal	No fruit
Whole fruit (not juice)	5	≥0.4 cup equiv. per 1000 kcal	No whole fruit
Total vegetables	5	≥1.1 cup equiv. per 1000 kcal	No vegetables
Dark green and orange vegetables and legumes[b]	5	≥0.4 cup equiv. per 1000 kcal	No dark green and orange vegetables and legumes
Total grains	5	≥3.0 oz equiv. per 1000 kcal	No grains
Whole grains	5	≥1.5 oz equiv. per 1000 kcal	No whole grains
Milk[c]	10	≥1.3 oz equiv. per 1000 kcal	No milk
Meat and beans	10	≥2.5 oz equiv. per 1000 kcal	No meat or beans
Oils[d]	10	≥12 grams per 1000 kcal	No oil
Saturated fat	10	≤7% of energy[e]	≥15% of energy
Sodium	10	≤0.7 gram per 1000 kcal	≤2.0 grams per 1000 kcal
Calories from solid fat, alcohol, and added sugar (SoFAAS)	20	≤20% of energy	≤50% of energy

[a] *Intakes between the minimum and maximum levels are scored proportionately, except for saturated fat and sodium, see note e.*
[b] *Legumes are counted as vegetables only after meat and beans standard is met.*
[c] *Includes all milk products, such as fluid milk, yogurt, and cheese.*
[d] *Includes nonhydrogenated vegetable oil and oils in fish, nuts, and seeds.*
[e] *Saturated fat and sodium get a score of 8 for the intake levels that reflect the 2005 Dietary Guidelines for Americans,[67,78] <10% of calories from saturated fat and 1.1 grams of sodium per 1000 kcal, respectively.*

TABLE 7.6 Average Values for Nutrient Intake Based on 3-Day Diet Records by Levels of Cardiorespiratory Fitness in 7059 Men and 2453 Women

Variable	Men		
	Low Fitness[a,b] (*N* = 786)	Moderate Fitness[c] (*N* = 2457)	High Fitness (*N* = 4716)
Demographic and health data			
Age (y)	47.3 ± 11.1[a,b]	47.3 ± 10.3[c]	48.1 ± 10.5
Apparently healthy (%)	51.5[a,b]	69.1[c]	77.0
Current smokers (%)	23.4[a,b]	15.8[c]	7.8
BMI ($kg \cdot m^{-2}$)	30.7 ± 5.5[a,b]	27.4 ± 3.7[c]	25.1 ± 2.7
Nutrient data			
Energy (kcal)	2378.6 ± 718.6[a]	2296.9 ± 661.9[c]	2348.1 ± 664.3
$Kcal \cdot kg^{-1} \cdot d^{-1}$	25.0 ± 8.1[a]	26.7 ± 8.4[c]	29.7 ± 9.2
Carbohydrate (% kcal)	43.2 ± 9.4[b]	44.6 ± 9.1[c]	48.1 ± 9.7
Protein (% kcal)	18.6 ± 3.8	18.5 ± 3.8	18.1 ± 3.8
Total fat (% kcal)	36.7 ± 7.2[b]	35.4 ± 7.1[c]	32.6 ± 7.5
SFA (% kcal)	11.8 ± 3.2[b]	11.3 ± 3.2[c]	10.0 ± 3.2
MUFA (% kcal)	14.5 ± 3.2[a,b]	13.8 ± 3.1[c]	12.6 ± 3.3
PUFA (% kcal)	7.4 ± 2.2[a,b]	7.5 ± 2.2	7.4 ± 2.3
Cholesterol (mg)	349.5 ± 173.2[b]	314.5 ± 147.5[c]	277.8 ± 138.5
Fiber (g)	21.0 ± 9.5[b]	22.0 ± 9.7[c]	26.2 ± 11.9

TABLE 7.6 Average Values for Nutrient Intake Based on 3-Day Diet Records by Levels of Cardiorespiratory Fitness in 7059 Men and 2453 Women *(Continued)*

	Men		
Variable	Low Fitness[a,b] (N = 786)	Moderate Fitness[c] (N = 2457)	High Fitness (N = 4716)
Calcium (mg)	849.1 ± 371.8[a,b]	860.2 ± 360.2[c]	924.4 ± 386.8
Sodium (mg)	4317.4 ± 1365.7	4143.0 ± 1202.3	4133.2 ± 1189.4
Folate (μg)	336.4 ± 165.2[b]	359.5 ± 197.0[c]	428.0 ± 272.0
Vitamin B6 (mg)	2.4 ± 0.9[b]	2.4 ± 0.9[c]	2.8 ± 1.1
Vitamin B12 (μg)	6.6 ± 5.5[a]	6.8 ± 6.0	6.6 ± 5.8
Vitamin A (RE)	1372.7 ± 1007.3[a,b]	1530.5 ± 1170.4[c]	1766.3 ± 1476.0
Vitamin C (mg)	117.3 ± 80.4[b]	129.2 ± 108.9[c]	166.0 ± 173.2
Vitamin E (AE)	11.5 ± 9.1[b]	12.1 ± 8.6[c]	13.7 ± 11.4
	Women		
Variable	Low Fitness[a,b] (N = 233)	Moderate Fitness[c] (N = 730)	High Fitness (N = 1490)
Demographic and health data			
Age (years)	47.5 ± 11.2[b]	46.7 ± 11.6	46.5 ± 11.0
Apparently healthy (%)	55.4[a,b]	71.1c	79.3
Current smokers (%)	12.0[a,b]	9.0c	4.2
BMI ($kg \cdot m^{-2}$)	27.3 ± 6.7[a,b]	24.3 ± 4.9[c]	22.1 ± 3.0
Nutrient data			
Energy (kcal)	1887.4 ± 607.5[a]	1793.0 ± 508.2[c]	1859.7 ± 514.7
$kcal \cdot kg^{-1} \cdot d^{-1}$	27.1 ± 9.4[a]	28.1 ± 8.8[c]	31.7 ± 9.8
Carbohydrate (% kcal)	47.7 ± 9.6[b]	48.2 ± 9.0[c]	51.1 ± 9.4
Protein (% kcal)	17.6 ± 3.7[a]	18.1 ± 3.9	17.7 ± 3.9
Total fat (% kcal)	34.8 ± 7.6[b]	33.7 ± 6.8[c]	31.3 ± 7.5
SFA (% kcal)	11.1 ± 3.3[b]	10.6 ± 3.2[c]	9.6 ± 3.1
MUFA (% kcal)	13.4 ± 3.4[a,b]	12.8 ± 3.0[c]	11.9 ± 3.2
PUFA (% kcal)	7.5 ± 2.2	7.5 ± 2.2	7.4 ± 2.4
Cholesterol (mg)	244.7 ± 132.8[b]	224.6 ± 115.6[c]	204.1 ± 103.6
Fiber (g)	18.9 ± 8.2[a,b]	20.0 ± 8.3[c]	23.2 ± 10.7
Calcium (mg)	765.2 ± 361.8[a,b]	774.6 ± 342.8[c]	828.3 ± 372.1
Sodium (mg)	3350.8 ± 980.8	3256.7 ± 927.7	3314.4 ± 952.7
Folate (μg)	301.8 ± 157.6[a,b]	319.7 ± 196.2	356.2 ± 232.5
Vitamin B6 (mg)	2.0 ± 0.8[b]	2.0 ± 0.8[c]	2.2 ± 0.9
Vitamin B12 (μg)	4.7 ± 4.2	4.9 ± 4.2	5.0 ± 4.2
Vitamin A (RE)	1421.9 ± 1135.3[b]	1475.1 ± 1132.9[c]	1699.0 ± 1346.9
Vitamin C (mg)	116.7 ± 7.5[b]	131.5 ± 140.0	153.5 ± 161.1
Vitamin E (AE)	10.8 ± 7.5	10.3 ± 6.5[c]	11.5 ± 8.1

From Brodney S, et al. Nutrient intake of physically fit and unfit men and women. Med Sci Sports Exerc 2001;33:459.

SFA, saturated fatty acid; PUFA, polyunsaturated fatty acid; MUFA, monounsaturated fatty acid; RE, retinol equivalents; AE, α-tocopherol units.

[a] *Significant difference between low and moderate fitness. P<.05.*

[b] *Significant difference between low and high fitness. P<.05.*

[c] *Significant difference between moderate and high fitness. P<.05.*

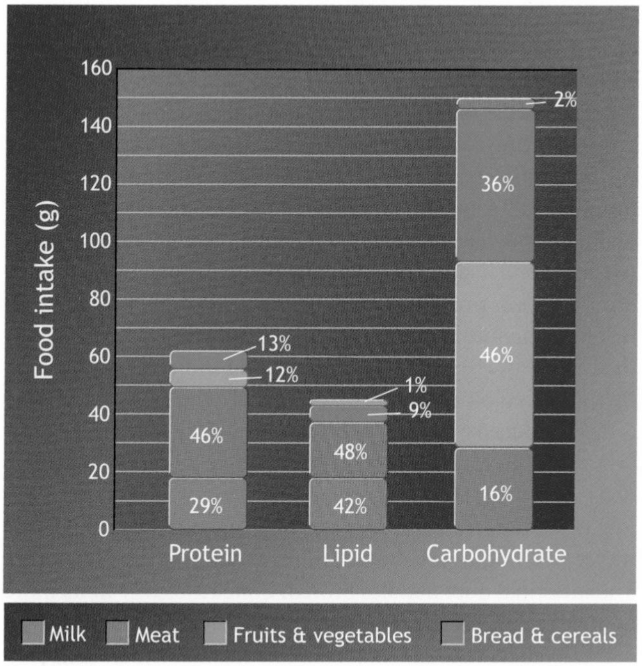

FIGURE 7.6. Basic recommendations for carbohydrate, lipid, and protein components and the general categories of food sources in a balanced diet.

Is the RDA Really Enough?

Studies of human protein needs in the mid-1800s postulated that muscular contraction destroyed a portion of the muscle's protein content to provide energy for biologic work. Based on this belief, prevailing wisdom recommended a high-protein diet for persons involved in heavy physical labor and intense exercise to provide for the structural content of skeletal muscle and its energy needs. In many ways, many modern-day athletes mimic these beliefs and practices. For men and women who devote considerable time and effort training with resistive equipment, dietary protein often represents their most important macronutrient. For one reason, many fitness enthusiasts believe that resistance training in some way damages or "tears down" a muscle's inherent protein structure. This drain of muscle protein would require additional dietary protein above the RDA for subsequent tissue resynthesis to a new, larger, and more powerful state. Many endurance athletes also believe that training increases protein catabolism to sustain the energy requirements of exercise, particularly when glycogen reserves are low. They thus believe that consuming added dietary protein offsets the protein–energy drain and provides building blocks to resynthesize depleted muscle mass. To some extent, the reasoning of both groups of athletes has merit. The relevant question concerns whether the protein RDA provides a sufficient reserve should intense training increase demands for protein synthesis or catabolism.

Is Some Modification Required For Recommended Protein Intake?: Much of the current understanding of protein dynamics in exercise derives from studies that expanded the classic method to determine protein breakdown by measuring urea excretion. For example, the output of "labeled" carbon dioxide from amino acids either injected or ingested increases during exercise in proportion to metabolic rate. As exercise progresses, the concentration of plasma urea also increases, coupled with a dramatic rise in nitrogen excretion in sweat. This often occurs without any change in urinary nitrogen excretion. These observations run counter to prior conclusions concerning minimal protein breakdown during endurance exercise, because the early studies only measured nitrogen in urine. **FIGURE 7.7** illustrates that the sweat mechanism serves an important role in excreting the nitrogen from protein breakdown during exercise. Urea production does not reflect all aspects of protein breakdown because the oxidation of both plasma and intracellular leucine (a branched-chain essential amino acid) increases during moderate exercise, independent of changes in urea production.

FIGURE 7.7 also shows that protein use for energy reaches its highest level during exercise in a glycogen-depleted state (indicated by *low CHO*). This emphasizes the important role carbohydrate plays as a protein sparer. It further indicates that carbohydrate availability inhibits protein catabolism in exercise. Protein breakdown for energy and its role in gluconeogenesis undoubtedly serve important needs in endurance exercise (or in frequent intense training) when glycogen reserves diminish.

Eating a high-carbohydrate diet with adequate energy intake conserves muscle protein in individuals who chronically engage in intense training. The potential for increased protein use for energy (and the depression of protein synthesis) during strenuous exercise helps to explain why individuals who

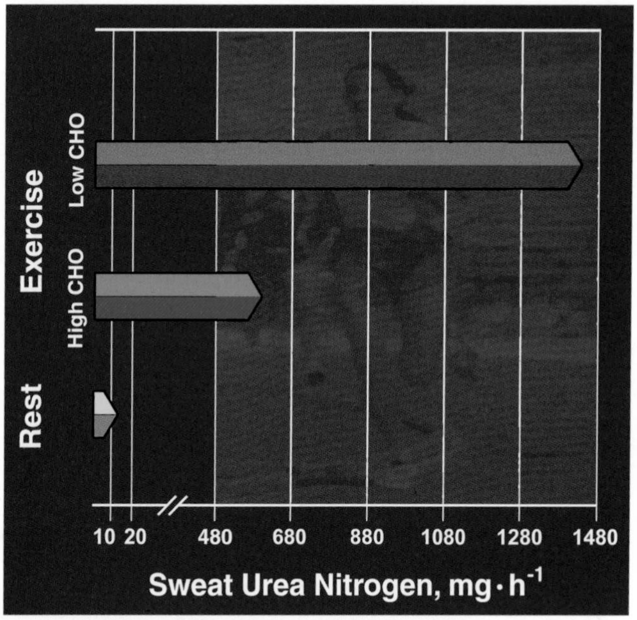

FIGURE 7.7. Excretion of urea in sweat at rest and during exercise after carbohydrate loading *(High CHO)* and carbohydrate depletion *(Low CHO)*. The largest use of protein (as reflected by sweat urea) occurs with low glycogen reserves. (From Lemon PWR, Nagel F. Effects of exercise on protein and amino acid metabolism. *Med Sci Sports Exerc* 1981;13:141.)

PROLONGED EXERCISE AND STARVATION: A SIMILAR METABOLIC MIXTURE

Increased protein catabolism during endurance exercise and intense training often mirrors the metabolic mixture during short-term starvation. With depleted glycogen reserves, gluconeogenesis from amino acid–derived carbon skeletons largely sustains the liver's glucose output. More than likely, augmented protein breakdown reflects the body's attempt to maintain blood glucose concentration for central nervous system functioning.

resistance train to augment muscle size generally refrain from glycogen-depleting, endurance-type exercise.

The beginning phase of an exercise training regimen also places a transient but increased demand on body protein, perhaps resulting from both muscle injury and associated increased energy requirements. A continuing area of controversy concerns whether initial increased protein demand contributes to a true long-term increase in protein requirement *above* the RDA. *Although a definitive answer remains elusive, protein breakdown above the resting level occurs during endurance exercise (and with resistance training) to a degree greater than previously believed.* Protein catabolism becomes most apparent when exercising with low carbohydrate reserves or low energy intake. Protein use may increase from a need to repair exercise-induced damaged tissue and from extra protein required for gains in lean tissue mass. Unfortunately, research has yet to pinpoint the protein requirements for individuals who train 4 to 6 hours daily by resistance-type exercise.

At this point in time (and without convincing evidence to the contrary), it seems prudent that those in endurance training should consume between 1.2 and 1.4 g of high-quality protein per kilogram of body mass daily; those who resistance train may benefit from 1.8 g per kilogram of body mass. This level of protein intake falls within the range typically consumed by physically active men and women, thus obviating the need to consume supplementary protein.

Preparations of Simple Amino Acids

The usual reasons for using protein and amino acid supplements include stimulation of muscle growth and strength, enhanced energy capacity, and increased growth hormone output (see Chapter 12).[143] Supplement manufacturers often advertise that *only* simple amino acids are absorbed from the gut into the blood at a rate fast enough to stimulate muscle growth during resistance training. Male and female weightlifters, bodybuilders, and other power athletes consume up to four times the RDA for protein. This level of excess takes the form of liquids, powders, or pills of "purified" protein at a cost often in excess of $50 a pound of actual protein. Such preparations often contain proteins "predigested" to simple amino acids through chemical action in the laboratory. Advocates believe the body absorbs the simple amino acid molecule more readily (increased bioavailability) to optimize the expected muscle growth induced by training or to improve strength, power, and "vigor" in the short term for a strenuous workout. This simply does not occur. The healthy intestine absorbs amino acids rapidly when they exist in more complex dipeptide and tripeptide molecules, not just in simple amino acid form (see Chapter 3). The intestinal tract handles protein quite efficiently in its more complex forms. A concentrated amino acid solution creates an osmotic effect that draws water into the intestine, often precipitating irritation, cramping, and diarrhea. In addition, carbohydrate remains the preferred energy source to power the anaerobic energy system primarily relied on in resistance training. Multiple sets of single exercises can reduce a muscle's glycogen content by 40%. *Simply stated, adequate research design and methodology has not shown that protein (amino acid) supplementation in any form above the RDA increases muscle mass or improves muscular strength, power, or endurance.* Most individuals obtain adequate protein to sustain muscle growth with resistance training by consuming ordinary foods in a well-balanced diet. Provided caloric intake balances energy output by consuming a wide variety of foods, no need exists to consume supplements of protein or simple amino acids.

VEGETARIANS MAY REQUIRE A BIT MORE PROTEIN

Vegetarians should increase recommended protein intake values by 10% to adjust for less efficient digestion of plant protein. If protein intake remains adequate, consuming animal sources of protein does not facilitate muscle strength or size gains with resistance training compared with a similar protein intake from plant sources.

Lipids

No firm standards exist for optimal lipid intake. The amount of dietary lipid varies widely according to personal taste, money spent on food, and availability of lipid-rich foods. For example, lipid furnishes only about 10% of the energy in the average diet of people living in Asia, whereas in many Western countries, lipid accounts for 40 to 45% of the energy intake. *To promote good health, lipid intake should probably not exceed 30% of the diet's energy content. Of this, at least 70% should come from unsaturated fatty acids.* For those who consume a Mediterranean-type diet rich in monounsaturated fatty acids, a somewhat higher total fat percentage (35–40%) becomes the norm.

No exercise performance benefit occurs by reducing the percentage of lipid intake below the 30% value. In fact, significant reductions in dietary lipid compromise exercise performance. A diet of 20% lipid produced poorer endurance performance scores than a diet of identical caloric value containing about 40% lipid.[103] Such findings further fuel the controversy concerning the importance of dietary lipid for individuals involved in intense training and endurance competition (see "High-Fat Versus Low-Fat Diets for Endurance

Training and Exercise Performance" in Chapter 8). Consuming a low-fat diet during strenuous training also creates difficulty in increasing carbohydrate and protein intake enough to furnish energy to maintain body weight and muscle mass. In addition, essential fatty acids and fat-soluble vitamins enter the body in dietary lipids; thus, sustaining a low-fat or "fat-free" diet could create a relative state of malnutrition. A low-fat diet (i.e., 20% total calories as lipid; see Chapter 12) also blunts the normal rise in plasma testosterone following a short-term bout of resistance exercise.[139] A low-fat intake may in fact be contraindicated for intense resistance training.

Carbohydrates

The negative end of the nutrition continuum includes low-calorie "semistarvation" diets and other potentially harmful practices such as high-fat, low-carbohydrate diets, "liquid-protein" diets (essentially carbohydrate free), and single food-centered diets. These extreme diet plans often sacrifice good health, exercise performance, and optimum body composition. *A low-carbohydrate diet rapidly compromises energy reserves for vigorous physical activity or regular training.* Excluding sufficient carbohydrate energy from the diet causes an individual to train in a state of relative glycogen depletion,[12] which eventually may produce "staleness" and unfortunately hinder exercise performance.[13,53,77]

The prominence of dietary carbohydrates varies widely throughout the world, depending on availability and relative cost of lipid-rich and protein-rich foods. Complex carbohydrate–rich unrefined grains, starchy roots, and dried peas and beans usually are cheapest compared with their energy value. In East Asia, carbohydrates (rice) contribute 80% of the total energy intake; in contrast, in the United States, carbohydrate supplies only about 40 to 50% of the energy intake. *No hazard to health exists when subsisting chiefly on a variety of fiber-rich complex unrefined carbohydrates, with adequate intake of essential amino acids, fatty acids, minerals, and vitamins.*

ABSOLUTE CARBOHYDRATE AMOUNT COUNTS

Carbohydrate intake recommendations for physically active individuals assume that daily energy intake balances energy expenditure. Unless this condition exists, even consuming a relatively large *percentage* of carbohydrate calories will not adequately replenish this important energy macronutrient.

Stored muscle glycogen and bloodborne glucose become prime energy contributors in maximal exercise with inadequate oxygen supply to active muscles. Stored glycogen also provides substantial energy during intense aerobic exercise. Consequently, dietary carbohydrate plays an important role for individuals who maintain a physically active lifestyle. *Their diet should contain at least 55 to 60% of calories as carbohydrates, predominantly starches from unprocessed grains, fruits, and vegetables.* For competitive swimmers, rowers, and speed skaters, the importance of maintaining a relatively high daily carbohydrate intake relates more to the considerable and prolonged energy demands of their training than to the short-term demands of actual competition.

More Specific Carbohydrate Recommendations

General recommendations for carbohydrate intake range between 6 and 10 $g \cdot kg^{-1}$ of body mass daily. This amount varies with an individual's daily energy expenditure and mode of exercise performed. *Individuals undergoing endurance training should consume, on a daily basis, 10 g of carbohydrate per kilogram of body mass.* Thus, the daily carbohydrate intake for a small 46-kg (100-lb) person who expends about 2800 kcal each day should be approximately 450 g or 1800 kcal. In contrast, a person weighing 68 kg (150 lb) should consume 675 g of carbohydrate (2700 kcal) daily to sustain an energy requirement of 4200 kcal. In both examples, carbohydrates represent 65% of total energy intake. Chapter 12 presents specific diet and exercise techniques to facilitate glycogen storage in the days before endurance competition.

Carbohydrate and the "Overtraining Syndrome"

Endurance runners, swimmers, cross-country skiers, and cyclists frequently experience chronic fatigue in which successive days of hard training become progressively more difficult. Normal exercise performance usually deteriorates because the individual experiences increasing difficulty recovering from exercise training. The overtrained condition, commonly termed the **overtraining syndrome**, represents more than just a short-term inability to train as usual or a slight dip in competition-level performance. Rather, it reflects chronic fatigue experienced during workouts and in subsequent recovery periods. It also relates to increased incidence of infections, injuries, persistent muscle soreness, and general malaise and loss of interest in sustaining high-level training. Specific symptoms of overtraining are highly individualized. The symptoms outlined in the box titled "The Overtraining Syndrome: Six Symptoms of Staleness" generally represent the most common consequences of overtraining; they usually persist until the person rests. Complete recovery requires weeks or even months.

THE OVERTRAINING SYNDROME: SIX SYMPTOMS OF STALENESS

1. Unexplained, persistently poor performance
2. Disturbed mood states characterized by general fatigue, depression, and irritability
3. Elevated resting pulse, painful muscles, and increased susceptibility to upper respiratory infections and gastrointestinal disturbances
4. Insomnia
5. Weight loss
6. Overuse injuries

It Takes Time to Replenish Glycogen

Even with a high-carbohydrate diet, muscle glycogen does not rapidly replenish to pre-exercise levels. It takes a minimum of 24 hours to replenish muscle glycogen levels following prolonged exhaustive exercise; liver glycogen restores at a faster rate. *One to two days of rest (or lighter exercise) combined with a high-carbohydrate intake re-establishes pre-exercise muscle glycogen levels after exhaustive training or competition.* Chapter 8 discusses in detail how to facilitate carbohydrate replenishment following exhaustive exercise.

Unmistakably, if a person performs unduly intense exercise on a regular basis, carbohydrate intake must adjust to permit glycogen resynthesis to maintain optimal training. This certainly provides a nutritional justification for the recommendation of many coaches and trainers to gradually reduce or *taper* workout intensity several days before competition while still maintaining a high-quality, carbohydrate-rich diet. The box titled "Practical Nutritional Guidelines for Prevention of Chronic Athletic Fatigue Among Athletes" outlines practical nutritional guidelines to diminish the likelihood of chronic athletic fatigue or **staleness**. These guidelines were prepared for competitive swimmers, but the recommendations apply to all individuals in intense training.

PRACTICAL NUTRITIONAL GUIDELINES FOR PREVENTION OF CHRONIC ATHLETIC FATIGUE AMONG ATHLETES[a]

1. Consume easily digested high-carbohydrate drinks or solid foods 1–4 h before training and/or competition. Roughly 1 g of carbohydrate/kg body weight is the recommended intake 1 h before exercise, and up to 5 g of carbohydrate/kg body weight/h is suggested if the feeding occurs 4 h prior to exercise. For example, a 70-kg swimmer could drink 350 mL (12 oz) of a 20% carbohydrate beverage 1 h before exercise or eat 14 "energy bars," each containing 25 g carbohydrate, 4 h before exercise.
2. Consume an easily digested, high-carbohydrate, liquid or solid food containing at least 0.35–1.5 g of carbohydrate/kg body weight/h immediately after exercise for the first 4 h after exercise. Thus, a 70-kg swimmer could drink 100–450 mL (3.6–16 oz) of a 25% carbohydrate beverage or 1–4.5 energy bars, each containing 25 g of carbohydrate, immediately after exercise and every hour thereafter for 4 h.
3. Consume a 15–25% carbohydrate drink or a solid high-carbohydrate supplement with each meal. For example, reduce consumption of normal foods by 250 kcal and consume a high-carbohydrate beverage or solid food containing 250 kcal of carbohydrate with each meal.
4. Maintain a stable body weight during all phases of training by matching energy consumption to the energy demands of training. This will also help maintain body carbohydrate reserves.

[a] In cooperation with a nutritionist or dietitian, athletes should maintain a record of foods consumed so that an accurate assessment can be made of total energy and total carbohydrate intake. Based on this assessment, dietary adjustments can be made to ensure that during intense training seasons, the athlete consumes roughly 10 g of carbohydrate/kg body weight daily.

From Sherman WJ, Maglischo EW. Minimizing chronic athletic fatigue among swimmers: special emphasis on nutrition. *Sports Sci Exchange, Gatorade Sports Sci Inst* 1991;35:4.

VITAMINS AND EXERCISE PERFORMANCE: THE ATHLETE'S DILEMMA

About 160 million Americans take dietary supplements on a daily basis believing these compounds bask in a health halo for their ability to ward off disease and enhance well-being. The *Nutrition Business Journal* (newhope360.com/nutrition-business-journal) reports that Americans expended nearly $27 billion on dietary supplements in 2009, up from $20.4 billion in 2004. Vitamin–mineral pills represent the most common form of nutritional supplement used by the general public. Estimates indicate that between 75 and 100 million Americans take a daily multivitamin supplement. This accounts for 34% of total supplement sales, which total $1.9 billion. Particularly susceptible marketing targets include the exercise enthusiast, the competitive athlete, and others who assist athletes to achieve peak performance. The following excerpts (including the letter writer's emphasis in italics) were taken from a letter to a college athletic trainer from a physician extolling his concoction of micronutrients (with dosages as high as 15–25 times recommended levels) developed for the "unique" needs of the physically active individual. Such pseudoscientific promotional pitches from so-called experts continually bombard coaches, athletic trainers, and all individuals involved in regular exercise:

> Dear ___________:
>
> I'm a physician with an interest in *biochemistry* and nutrition and the effects of both on *athletes*. Today, *good nutrition requires supplementation*.
>
> The product I developed is an "*all-natural* nutritional foundation for building strong, healthy bodies that perform at peak levels *without harmful side effects*. Using this formula, athletes notice increased energy and improved performance." This product "is an alternative to steroids and other quick fixes."
>
> This product "is the *only complete supplement* of its kind that combines *23 essential vitamins, minerals and antioxidants* in the proper amounts needed for powerful performance. (You may be startled to see how dramatically my formulation *exceeds* the RDAs.) The amounts shown on the back of this letter are based on the latest research in nutrition . . . NOT outdated government information."
>
> While developing this product, "I consulted with world famous biochemists . . . collaborated with leading nutritionists

(the same ones physicians have ignored for years) ... walked miles and miles in health food stores ... *completed a comprehensive search of current medical literature*."

This letter applies the typical psychological "tools" of advertising: *respect for authority* (I'm a physician, of course I am correct), *safety* (try it, it can't hurt you and it might help); *disdain for the conventional wisdom of science and governmental agencies* (the new scientists have the answers, but the "old club" will not publish them), *prestige by association* (I've checked with experts [unnamed biochemists and nutritionists] and gone to the library), and *if a little is good, more must be better* (you'll get a dose dramatically above recommended values). One of the few items missing is a testimonial from a renowned athlete, perhaps wearing a nostril-dilating adhesive strip!

More than 50% of athletes in certain sports regularly consume vitamin–mineral supplements. They undertake such practices either to ensure adequate micronutrient intake or to achieve excess in hopes of enhancing exercise performance and training responsiveness. If vitamin–mineral deficiencies become apparent in active people, they often occur among the following groups:

1. Vegetarians or groups with low energy intake (dancers, gymnasts, and weight-class sport athletes who continually strive to maintain or reduce body weight)
2. Individuals who eliminate one or more food groups from their diet
3. Individuals who consume large amounts of processed foods and simple sugars with low micronutrient density (endurance athletes)

Under these adverse situations, a multivitamin–mineral supplement at recommended dosages can upgrade the micronutrient density of the daily diet.

GET YOUR VITAMINS FROM FOOD, NOT FROM SUPPLEMENTS

The food sources below not only provide a rich source for the specific vitamins but supply them in a nutrient-rich package of accessory nutrients with potential health-promoting benefits.

Vitamin A (carotenoids): organ meats, carrots, cantaloupe, sweet potatoes, pumpkin, apricots, spinach, milk, collards, eggs
Vitamin C: guava, citrus fruits and juices, red, yellow, and green peppers, papaya, kiwi, broccoli, strawberries, tomatoes, sweet and white potatoes, kale, mango, cantaloupe
Vitamin D: salmon, tuna, sardines, mackerel, oysters, cod liver oil, egg yolks, fortified milk, fortified orange juice, fortified breakfast cereal
Vitamin E: vegetable oils, nuts, seeds, spinach, kiwi, wheat germ
Vitamin K: spinach, kale, collards, Swiss chard, broccoli, romaine lettuce
Vitamin B_1 (thiamin): sunflower seeds, enriched bread, cereal, pasta, whole grains, lean meats, fish, beans, green peas, corn, soybeans
Vitamin B_2 (riboflavin): lean meats, eggs, legumes, nuts, green leafy vegetables, dairy products, enriched bread
Vitamin B_3 (niacin): dairy products, calf's liver, poultry, fish, lean meat, nuts, eggs, fortified bread and cereal
Pantothenic acid: calf's liver, mushrooms, sunflower seeds, corn, eggs, fish, milk, milk products, whole-grain cereal, beans
Biotin: eggs, fish, milk, liver and kidney, milk products, soybeans, nuts, Swiss chard, whole-grain cereal, beans
Vitamin B_6: beans, bananas, nuts, eggs, meat, poultry, fish, potato, fortified bread and ready-to-eat cereals
Vitamin B_{12}: liver, meat, eggs, poultry, fish (trout and salmon), shellfish, milk, milk products, fortified breakfast cereal
Folate (folic acid): beef liver, green leafy vegetables, avocado, green peas, enriched bread, fortified breakfast cereals

VITAMIN SUPPLEMENTS: THE COMPETITIVE EDGE?

Over 50 years of research fails to support the use of vitamin supplements to improve aerobic and anaerobic exercise performance or ability to train arduously in nutritionally adequate healthy people.[34,110,132,133,141] When vitamin intakes achieve recommended levels, supplements neither improve exercise performance nor increase the blood levels of these micronutrients. They exert *no effect* on the physical responses to strenuous training and do not protect against muscle damage from intense exercise.[85,144] The facts, unfortunately, remain clouded by "testimonials" from coaches and elite athletes who attribute their success to a particular dietary modification or specific vitamin supplements.

As noted in Chapter 2, many vitamins serve as coenzyme components or precursors of coenzymes to help regulate energy metabolism. **FIGURE 7.8** illustrates that B-complex vitamins play a key role as coenzymes in important energy-yielding reactions during carbohydrate, fat, and protein catabolism. They also contribute to hemoglobin synthesis and red blood cell production. The belief that "if a little is good, more must be better" has led many coaches, athletes, fitness enthusiasts, and even some "expert" scientists to advocate supplementing with vitamins above recommended levels.

Supplementing with vitamin B_6 (pyridoxine), an essential cofactor in glycogen and amino acid metabolism, did not benefit the metabolic mixture metabolized by women during intense aerobic exercise.[81] In fact, the status of athletes for this vitamin normally equals reference standards for the general population[79]; levels of vitamin B_6 do not decrease with strenuous exercise to levels warranting supplementation.[114]

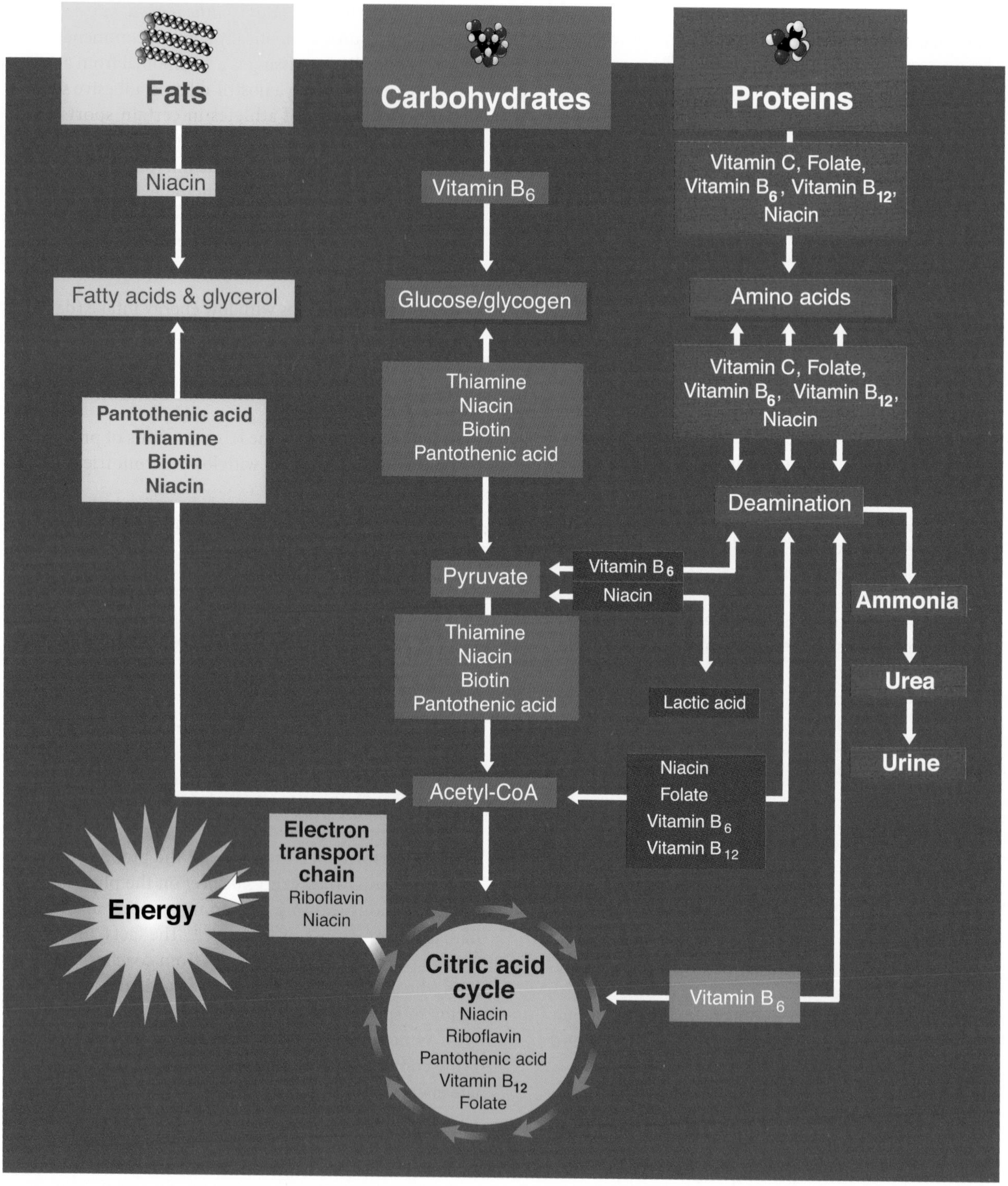

FIGURE 7.8. General schema for the role of water-soluble vitamins in the metabolism of carbohydrates, fats, and proteins.

Supplementing for 4 days with a highly absorbable derivative of thiamin—a component of the five-enzyme complex pyruvate dehydrogenase that catalyzes movement of pyruvate into the citric acid cycle—offered no advantage over a placebo on measures of oxygen uptake, lactate accumulation, and cycling performance during exhaustive exercise.[141] The loss of water-soluble vitamins in sweat, even during extreme physical activity, is probably negligible.

No exercise benefit exists for vitamins C and E with intakes above recommended values. Vitamin C, for example, serves as a factor to synthesize collagen and the adrenal hormone norepinephrine. Supplementing with vitamin C has negligible effects on endurance performance and does not alter the rate, severity, and duration of injuries compared with placebo treatment. Vitamin C status assessed by serum concentration and urinary ascorbate levels in diverse groups of highly trained athletes does not differ from untrained subjects despite large differences in daily physical activity level.[117] Other investigators report similar findings for this and other vitamins.[32,44,116] Furthermore, the energy intake of active persons usually increases to match the increased energy requirement of physical activity; thus a proportionate increase also occurs in micronutrient intake, often in amounts greatly exceeding recommended levels.

Vitamin E deficiencies may impair muscular function,[22] yet no scientific data have established that vitamin E consumed in excess of the RDA benefits stamina, circulatory function, or energy metabolism. Chronic high-potency multivitamin–mineral supplementation for well-nourished healthy individuals does not benefit aerobic fitness, muscular strength, neuromuscular performance following prolonged running, or athletic performance.[36,125]

A Unique Case for Vitamin C

Consuming vitamin C above recommended daily levels (75 mg for women and 90 mg for men) does not protect the general population against upper respiratory tract infection (URTI). Daily supplements of 500 to 1500 mg of vitamin C may confer some benefit to individuals engaged in strenuous exercise who experience frequent viral infections.[48,104,106]

Moderate exercise heightens immune function, whereas a prolonged period of intense physical activity such as marathon running or an exceedingly intense training session transiently suppresses and stresses the body's first line of defense against infectious agents. This increases risk of URTI within 1 or 2 weeks of exercise stress. For these individuals, additional vitamin C and E and perhaps carbohydrate ingestion before, during, and after a training workout may boost the normal immune mechanisms for combating infection.[57,90,95] Page 243 presents a more complete discussion of exercise, nutritional supplementation, and URTI.

AN INDUSTRY THAT CONTINUES TO EXPAND

Vitamin and other dietary supplements continue to gain in popularity. The percentage of adults in the United States who take supplements grew from 42% in 1988 to 1994, during the last National Health and Nutrition Examination Survey, to 50% in the most recent survey performed in 2003 to 2006, according to the National Center for Health Statistics, which conducted the survey. Vitamins and minerals are the most commonly used supplements, with about 40% of men and women saying they take them. Use of calcium increased from 28% to 61% among women aged 60 and older, whereas vitamin D use increased among both men and women.

In 2010, $25 billion worth of all types of supplements were sold in vitamin shops, supermarkets, drug stores, and online. According to the supplements trade group the Council for Responsible Nutrition (www.crnusa.org), nearly 53% of Americans supplement daily with a multivitamin, costing $4.5 billion annually. However, available data indicate that the most effective approach is to get your vitamins from food in a well-balanced, healthful diet rather than dietary supplements to reduce overall mortality risk, diverse cancer risks, and cardiovascular risk. Exceptions include calcium and iron; folic acid in pregnant women; and vitamin B_{12} (e.g., for those over age 50 years who may be unable to absorb it from food); and vitamin D for those with darker skin or insufficient exposure to sunlight; this is the only supplement use supported by research and not marketing hype.

Megavitamins

Most nutritionists believe little harm occurs in consuming a multivitamin capsule containing the recommended quantity of each vitamin. For some people, the psychological effects of supplementation may even confer a benefit. Of concern are those individuals who believe that "if a little is good, more must be better" and who take **megavitamins** (doses at least 10 and up to 1000 times those required to prevent deficiency), hoping that "supercharging" with vitamins improves overall health, exercise performance, and training responsiveness. Such practices can be harmful, except in the case of a serious medical illness that requires prescribed, above-normal vitamin intake.

Vitamins Behave as Chemicals

Once the enzyme systems catalyzed by specific vitamins become saturated, any excess taken in a megadose functions as a chemical or drug in the body. For example, a megadose of water-soluble vitamin C raises serum uric acid levels and precipitates gout in people predisposed to this disease. At intakes above 1000 mg daily, urinary excretion of oxalate (a breakdown product of vitamin C) increases, accelerating kidney stone formation in susceptible individuals. Also, some American Blacks, Asians, and Sephardic Jews have a genetic metabolic deficiency that becomes activated to hemolytic anemia with excessive vitamin C intake. For iron-deficient individuals, megadoses of vitamin C may destroy significant

MORE AND "NATURAL" NOT NECESSARILY BETTER

Vitamins synthesized in the laboratory are no less effective for bodily functions than vitamins from natural sources. Compared with the deficient state, vitamin supplements reverse the symptoms of vitamin deficiency and improve exercise performance. Once a person is cured of a deficiency, taking additional supplements does not further improve normal nutritional status. Of course, when adequate vitamin intake is achieved via food intake, the added benefit of the food's content of additional diverse nutrients provides a substantial added bonus.

amounts of vitamin B_{12}. In healthy persons, vitamin C supplements frequently irritate the bowel and cause diarrhea.

Excess vitamin B_6 can induce liver disease and nerve damage. Excessive riboflavin (vitamin B_2) can impair vision, whereas a megadose of nicotinic acid (niacin) acts as a potent vasodilator and inhibitor of fatty acid mobilization during exercise. A blunted fatty acid metabolism could cause a more rapid than normal depletion of muscle glycogen during exercise. Folate in concentrated supplement form can trigger an allergic response that produces hives, light-headedness, and breathing difficulties. Possible side effects of a vitamin E megadose include headache, fatigue, blurred vision, gastrointestinal disturbances, muscular weakness, and low blood sugar. It is difficult to "construct" a vitamin E-deficient diet because unsaturated fatty acids usually contain vitamin E. The toxicity to the nervous system of megadoses of vitamin A and the damaging effects to the kidneys of excess vitamin D are well known.

If vitamin supplementation does offer benefits to physically active individuals, they would only apply to those with marginal vitamin stores or those who restrict energy intake or make poor dietary choices.[80]

EXERCISE, FREE RADICALS, AND ANTIOXIDANTS: THE POTENTIALLY PROTECTIVE MICRONUTRIENTS FOR PHYSICALLY ACTIVE PEOPLE

The benefits of physical activity are well known, but the possibility for negative effects remains controversial. Potentially negative effects occur because elevated aerobic exercise metabolism increases the production of free radicals (see Chapter 2).[4,17,91,99,136] Free radical production in humans and subsequent tissue damage are not directly measured, but rather inferred from markers of free radical by-products. Increased free radicals could possibly overwhelm the body's natural defenses and pose a health risk from an elevated oxidative stress level. Free radicals also play a role in muscle injury from exercise, particularly eccentric muscle actions and unaccustomed exercise. Muscle damage of this nature releases muscle enzymes and initiates inflammatory cell infiltration into the damaged tissue.

The opposing position maintains that although free radical production increases during exercise, the body's normal antioxidant defenses remain either adequate or improve as natural enzymatic defenses become "upregulated" through exercise training adaptations.[47,54,124] Upregulation of antioxidant defenses accompanies a reduced exercise-induced lipid peroxidation in red blood cell membranes, increasing their resistance to subsequent oxidative stress.[89] *Convincing epidemiologic evidence supports the beneficial effects of regular aerobic exercise on cancer and heart disease incidence, the occurrences of which are linked to oxidative stress.*

> **GREEN TEA AND HEALTH BENEFITS**
>
> The belief that drinking green tea confers health benefits has increased in popularity in recent years. However, federal regulators have correctly, in our opinion, rejected a petition to allow green tea labels to claim that drinking at least 5 oz of green tea a day (or green tea extract) reduces heart disease risk. The FDA's review of 105 articles and other publications submitted with the petition concluded that no credible evidence exists to support claims of health benefits. A health claim characterizes a relationship between consuming a particular substance and a reduced risk of contracting a particular disease. The bottom line is that green tea is rich in plant compounds that may protect laboratory animals from diverse diseases, but the jury is still out as to whether it protects humans against heart disease, strokes, cancer, or cognitive decline.

Increased Metabolism and Free Radical Production

Exercise produces reactive oxygen (free radicals) in at least two ways. The first occurs via a mitochondrial electron leak, probably at the cytochrome level, that produces superoxide radicals. The second happens during alterations in blood flow and oxygen supply—underperfusion during intense exercise followed by reperfusion in recovery, which triggers excessive free radical generation. Some argue that the potential for free radical damage increases during trauma, stress, and contraction-induced muscle damage from exercise, and also from environmental pollutants including smog. With exercise, the risk depends on intensity and the participant's state of training because exhaustive exercise by the untrained often produces oxidative damage in active muscles. **FIGURE 7.9** illustrates how regular exercise affects oxidative response and potential for tissue damage, including protective adaptive responses.

Important Questions

Two questions arise concerning physical activity and free radical production:

1. Are physically active individuals more prone to free radical damage?
2. Are nutritional agents with antioxidant properties required in increased quantities by the physically active person?

In answer to the first question, research suggests that for well-nourished individuals, the body's natural defenses respond adequately to increased physical activity. A single bout of exercise increases oxidant formation, but the natural antioxidant defenses cope effectively in both healthy individuals and trained heart transplant recipients.[59] Even after repeating multiple exercise bouts on consecutive days, several indices of oxidative stress indicated no depletion of antioxidant defenses. The second question requires an equivocal answer. Some evidence indicates that exogenous antioxidant compounds either slow exercise-induced free radical

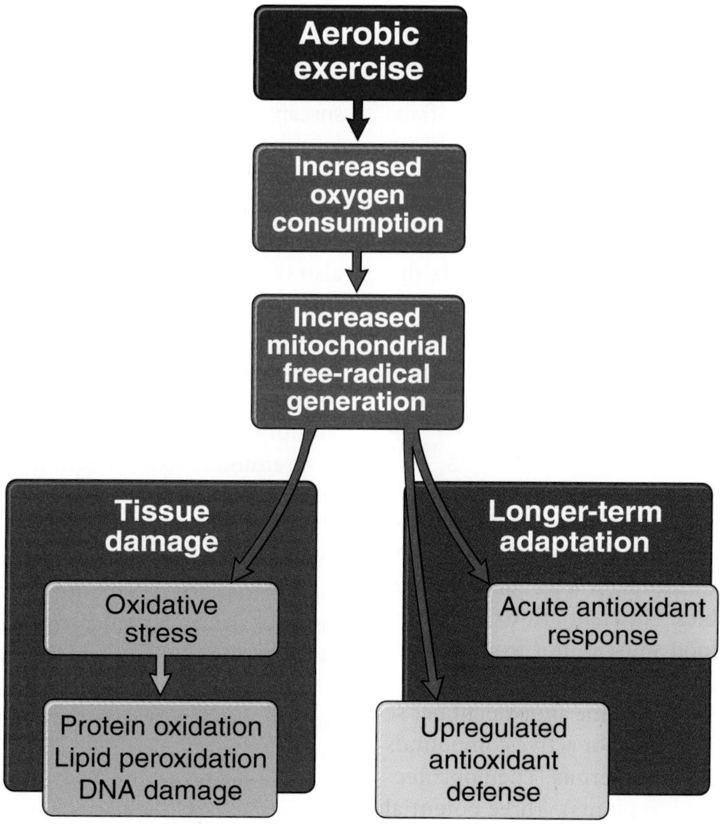

FIGURE 7.9. Cascade of events and adaptations produced by regular aerobic exercise that lessen the likelihood of tissue damage.

formation or augment the body's natural antioxidant defense system. This would limit the extent and progression of muscle damage following an acute exercise bout.

If supplementation proves beneficial, vitamin E may be the most important antioxidant related to exercise.[21,55,115] In one study, vitamin E-deficient animals began exercise with plasma membrane function compromised from oxidative damage. These animals reached exhaustion earlier than animals with normal vitamin E levels. For animals fed a normal diet, vitamin E supplements diminished exercise-induced oxidative damage to skeletal muscle fibers[39] and myocardial tissue.[40] Humans fed a daily antioxidant vitamin mixture of β-carotene, ascorbic acid, and vitamin E had lower serum and breath markers of lipid peroxidation at rest and following exercise than subjects not receiving supplements.[65] Five months of vitamin E supplementation in racing cyclists produced a protective effect on markers of oxidative stress induced by extreme endurance exercise. Two weeks of daily supplementation with 120 IU of vitamin E decreased free radical interaction with cellular membranes and slowed muscle tissue disruption from heavy resistance training.[85] In contrast, 30 days of vitamin E supplementation (1200 IU $\cdot$ d^{-1}) produced a 2.8-fold increase in serum vitamin E concentration without affecting contraction-induced indices of muscle damage including postexercise force decrement or inflammation caused by eccentric muscle actions.[9] Similarly, a 4-week daily vitamin E supplement of 1000 IU produced no positive effect on biochemical or ultrastructural indices of muscle damage in experienced runners following a half-marathon.[26] No evidence emerged that vitamin E supplements effectively reduced oxidative damage induced by resistance training exercises.[138] Differences in exercise severity and oxidative stress could account for discrepancies in research findings.

Selenium and the trace minerals copper, manganese, and zinc possess antioxidant properties due to their incorporation within the structure of glutathione peroxidase and other enzymes that protect plasma membranes from free radical damage. In a double-blind, placebo-controlled cancer prevention trial, individuals received a selenium supplement of 200 μg daily or about three to four times the recommended value.[20] Supplementation reduced incidence of and mortality from prostate (71%), esophageal (67%), colorectal (62%), and lung (46%) cancers.

Four proposed mechanisms for selenium's protection include the following:

1. Its function as an essential component of antioxidant enzymes
2. It alters carcinogen metabolism and inhibits tumor growth
3. It affects the endocrine and immune systems
4. It acts through molecular mechanisms to regulate the programmed death (*apoptosis*) of damaged precancerous cells

The recommended daily selenium intake is 70 μg for adult men and 55 μg for women; intakes in excess of 1000 μg can produce toxicity, including hair and fingernail loss and gastrointestinal dysfunction. Selenium-rich foods include bran (wheat, rice, oats) and other grains, Brazil nuts, shellfish (oysters, mussels, whelk), fish (orange roughy, canned tuna and canned anchovies, swordfish, pickled herring), liver, bacon and pork chops, lobster and crab, sunflower seeds, mushrooms, and asparagus.

Coenzyme Q_{10} probably acts as an antioxidant either singularly within the respiratory chain or as a recycler of vitamin E. Little evidence exists that coenzyme Q_{10} exerts the same direct antioxidant effect as vitamin E.

A Prudent Recommendation: In general, antioxidant supplementation with vitamins C and E in individuals with no previous deficiencies in these vitamins has no effect on physical adaptations to strenuous endurance training.[41,144] Some supplementing with various antioxidant compounds, however, slows exercise-induced free radical formation and may augment the body's natural defense system. A prudent recommendation includes consuming a well-balanced diet of fruits, grains, and vegetables. Nutrient antioxidants are best obtained from diverse food sources, not from supplements. We endorse this position because of uncertainty about whether health protection derives from the antioxidant per se or its interaction with the broad array of active compounds within the food source (e.g., the numerous "chemoprotectant" phytochemicals contained in plants). Three potential mechanisms for antioxidant health benefits include:

1. Influencing molecular mechanisms and gene expression
2. Providing enzyme-inducing substances that detoxify carcinogens
3. Blocking uncontrolled growth of cells

EXERCISE, INFECTIOUS ILLNESS, CANCER, AND THE IMMUNE RESPONSE

"Don't exercise until you're fatigued or you'll get sick" is a common perception held by many parents, athletes, and coaches that too much strenuous exercise increases susceptibility to certain illnesses. In contrast, the belief also exists that regular, more moderate exercise improves health and reduces susceptibility to infectious illnesses such as the common cold.

Studies as early as 1918 reported that most cases of pneumonia among boys in boarding school occurred among athletes. Respiratory infections seemed to progress toward pneumonia after intense sports training. Anecdotal reports also related the severity of poliomyelitis to participation in intense physical activity at a critical time of infection. Current epidemiologic and clinical findings from the flourishing field of **exercise immunology**—the study of the interactions of physical, environmental, and psychological factors on immune function—support the contention that unusually strenuous physical activity affects immune function to increase susceptibility to illness, particularly URTI.

The immune system comprises a highly complex and self-regulating grouping of cells, hormones, and interactive modulators that defend the body from invasion from outside bacterial, viral, and fungal microbes, foreign macromolecules, and abnormal cancerous cell growth. This system has two functional divisions: (1) **innate immunity** and (2) **acquired immunity**. The innate immune system includes anatomic and physiologic components (skin, mucous membranes, body temperature, and specialized defenses such as natural killer [NK] cells, diverse phagocytes, and inflammatory barriers). The acquired immune system consists of specialized B- and T-lymphocyte cells. These cells, when activated, regulate a highly effective immune response to a specific infectious agent. If infection does occur, an optimal immune system blunts the severity of illness and speeds recovery.

FIGURE 7.10 proposes a model for interactions among exercise, stress, illness, and the immune system. Within this framework, exercise, stress, and illness interact, each with its own effect on immunity. For example, exercise affects susceptibility to illness, and certain illnesses clearly affect exercise

THREE RICH DIETARY SOURCES OF VITAMIN ANTIOXIDANTS

1. β-Carotene: pigmented compounds or carotenoids that give color to yellow, orange, and green leafy vegetables and fruits; examples include carrots; dark-green leafy vegetables such as spinach, broccoli, turnip, beet, and collard greens; sweet potatoes; winter squash; apricots; cantaloupe; mangos; and papaya
2. Vitamin C: citrus fruits and juices; cabbage, broccoli, and turnip greens; cantaloupe; green and red sweet peppers; and berries
3. Vitamin E: poultry, seafood, vegetable oils, wheat germ, fish liver oils, whole-grain breads and fortified cereals, nuts and seeds, dried beans, green leafy vegetables, and eggs

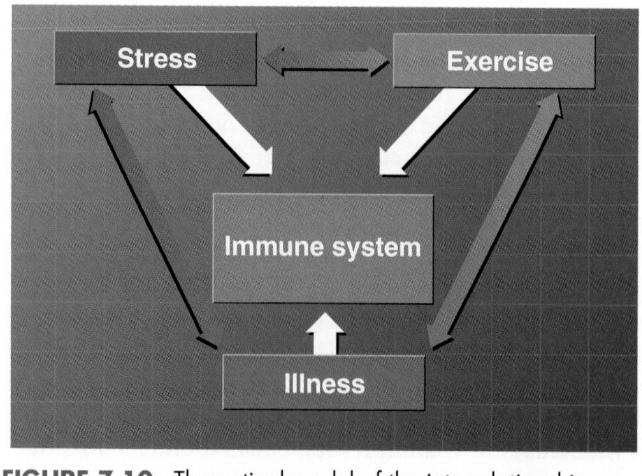

FIGURE 7.10. Theoretical model of the interrelationships among stress, exercise, illness, and the immune system. (From MacKinnon LT. Current challenges and future expectations in exercise immunology: back to the future. *Med Sci Sports Exerc* 1994;26:191.)

capacity. Likewise, psychological factors via links between the hypothalamus and immune function and other forms of stress, including nutritional deficiencies and acute alterations in normal sleep schedule, influence resistance to illness. Concurrently, exercise either positively or negatively moderates the body's response to stress. Each factor—stress, illness, and short- and long-term exercise—exerts an independent effect on immune status, immune function, and resistance to disease.

Upper Respiratory Tract Infections

FIGURE 7.11 displays the general J-shaped curve to describe the relationship between short-term exercise (and unusually intense training) and susceptibility to URTI. The figure also indicates that markers of immune function follow an inverted J-shaped curve. One may draw overly simplistic implications from these relationships, but regular light-to-moderate physical activity does appear to offer more protection against URTI; its frequency, symptoms, and severity; and possibly diverse cancers than a sedentary lifestyle.[61,78,84] For example, the frequency of colds among individuals who were physically active five or more times a week was up to 46% less than sedentary counterparts. The number of days the individuals experienced cold symptoms also was less among the physically active. Those who rated high in physical fitness experienced 34% fewer days of cold symptoms (and less severe symptoms) than those rated the least fit.[98] In addition, moderate exercise does not exacerbate the severity and duration of illness if infection does occur.[142] In contrast, strenuous physical activity (marathon run or intense training session) provides an "open window" (3–72 hours) of decreased antiviral and antibacterial resistance and increased risk of URTI (by two to six times) that manifests itself within 1 or 2 weeks.[25,118]

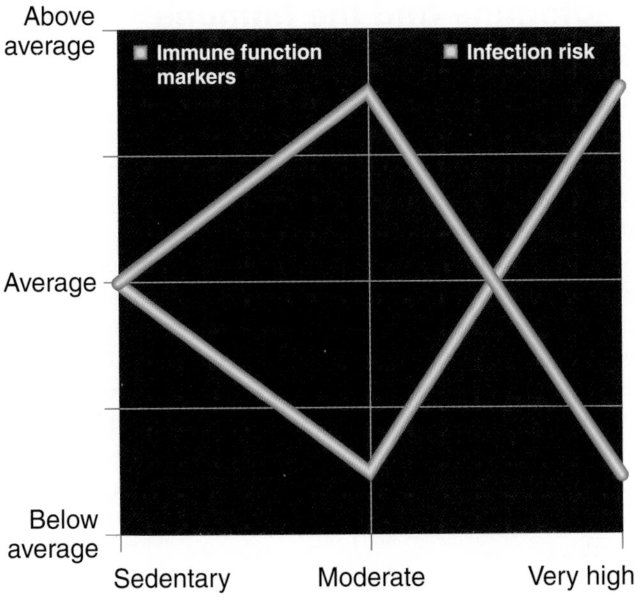

FIGURE 7.11. Exercise intensity affects immune function and risk of infection.

For example, approximately 13% of the participants in a Los Angeles marathon reported an episode of URTI during the week following the race. For runners of comparable ability who did not compete for reasons other than illness, the infection rate approximated 2%.[92]

Two Acute Exercise Effects

1. **Moderate exercise:** *A bout of moderate exercise boosts natural immune functions and host defenses for up to several hours.*[68,83] Noteworthy effects include the increase in NK cell activity. These phagocytic lymphocyte subpopulations enhance the blood's disease-fighting capacity. They also provide the body's first line of defense against diverse pathogens. The NK cell does not require prior or specific sensitization to foreign bodies or neoplastic cells. Rather, these cells demonstrate spontaneous cytolytic activity that ultimately ruptures and/or inactivates viruses and the metastatic potential of tumor cells.

A HEALTHFUL WAY TO REDUCE COLD RISK

For overweight, sedentary, postmenopausal women who participated in a program of moderate-intensity exercise 5 days a week for 12 months, the risk of colds decreased by more than threefold compared to a control group of women who attended once-weekly stretching sessions.[18]

2. **Exhaustive exercise:** *A prolonged period of exhaustive exercise (or other form of extreme stress or increased training) severely impairs the body's first line of defense against infection.*[67,72,103] Repeated cycles of unusually intense exercise further compound the risk. For example, impaired immune function from strenuous exercise "carries over" to a second bout of exercise on the same day to produce even more pronounced changes in neutrophils, lymphocytes, and select CD cells.[119] Elevated temperature, cytokines, and various stress-related hormones (epinephrine, growth hormone [GH], cortisol, β-endorphins) with exhaustive exercise may mediate depression of the body's innate (NK cell and neutrophil activity) and adaptive (T- and B-cell function) immune defenses.[7,93,131] The transient but diminished immunity after strenuous exercise remains apparent in the mucosal immune system of the upper respiratory tract.[83,89]

Chronic Exercise Effects

Aerobic training positively affects natural immune functions and resistance to stress in young and older individuals and in the obese during periods of weight loss.[30,31,121] Areas of improvement include enhanced functional capacity of natural cytotoxic immune mechanisms (e.g., antitumor actions of NK cell activity) and slowing of the age-related decrease in

T-cell function and associated cytokine production. The cytotoxic T cells defend directly against viral and fungal infections and contribute to regulating other immune mechanisms.

If exercise training enhances immune function, one might question why trained individuals show increased susceptibility to URTI after intense competition. The **open window hypothesis** maintains that an inordinate increase in training or actual competition exposes even the highly conditioned person to "nonnormal" stress that transiently but severely depresses NK cell function. This period of immunodepression ("open window") decreases natural resistance to infection.[64] The inhibitory effect of strenuous exercise on adrenocorticotropic hormone output and cortisol's maintenance of optimal blood glucose concentrations may negatively affect the immune process. For individuals who exercise regularly but only at moderate levels, the window of opportunity for infection remains "closed," thus preserving the protective benefits of regular exercise on immune function.

Resistance Training: Nine years of prior resistance exercise training did not affect resting NK cell number or activity level when compared with sedentary controls.[94] Comparisons indicated that resistance training activated monocytes more than typically observed for regular aerobic exercise. Monocyte activation releases prostaglandins that downregulate NK cells following exercise; this inhibits the long-term positive effect of exercise on NK cells. These investigators had previously shown that NK cells increase a substantial 225% following an acute bout of resistance exercise, a response similar to the immediate effect of moderate aerobic exercise.[100,101]

Perhaps a Role for Nutritional Supplements

Nutritional factors influence immune function (and possibly susceptibility to infection) in response to strenuous exercise and training.[2,37,122,123] For example, consuming a fat-rich diet containing 62% energy from lipids negatively affected the immune system compared with a carbohydrate-rich diet (65% energy from carbohydrates).[102] Supplementing with a 6% carbohydrate beverage (0.71 L before; 0.25 L every 15 minutes during; and 500 mL every hour throughout a 4.5-hour recovery) beneficially lowered cytokine levels in the inflammatory cascade after 2.5 hours of endurance running.[90] Subsequent research by the same laboratory showed that ingesting carbohydrates at 4 mL per kilogram of body mass every 15 minutes during 2.5 hours of high-intensity running or cycling maintained higher plasma glucose levels in 10 triathletes during exercise than a placebo.[96] A 6% carbohydrate solution ingested during exercise by young adult male competitive cyclists and triathletes attenuated the exercise-induced immune response and stress, particularly by phagocytizing cells by the reduced release of cortisol, as effectively as a 12% beverage.[122] Similar beneficial results with carbohydrate ingestion for cortisol and select anti-inflammatory cytokines have been observed following competition, regardless of age or gender.[97] A blunted cortisol response and diminished proinflammatory and anti-inflammatory cytokine response accompanied the higher plasma glucose levels with carbohydrate supplementation in exercise. *This suggests a carbohydrate-induced reduction in overall physiologic stress in prolonged intense exercise.*

Combined supplementation with the antioxidant vitamins C and E produces more prominent immunopotentiating effects (enhanced cytokine production) in young, healthy adults than supplementation with either vitamin alone.[57] In addition, a 200-mg daily vitamin E supplement enhanced clinically relevant indices of T-cell–mediated function for healthy elderly subjects.[88] However, long-term daily supplementation with a physiologic dose of vitamins and minerals or with 200 mg of vitamin E did not lower the incidence and severity of acute respiratory tract infections in noninstitutionalized persons age 60 and older. Among individuals experiencing an infection, those receiving vitamin E had *longer* total illness duration and restriction of activity.[43]

Daily supplementation with vitamin C does appear to benefit individuals engaged in strenuous exercise, particularly those predisposed to frequent viral URTIs.[48,107] Runners who received a 600-mg daily vitamin C supplement before and for 3 weeks after a 90-km ultramarathon competition experienced significantly fewer symptoms of URTI—running nose, sneezing, sore throat, coughing, and fever—than runners receiving a placebo.[104] Interestingly, infection risk inversely related to race performance; those with the fastest times suffered more symptoms. URTI also appeared most frequently in runners with strenuous training regimens. For these individuals, additional vitamin C and E and perhaps carbohydrate ingestion before, during, and after prolonged stressful exercise may boost normal immune mechanisms to combat infection.[93,95] More than likely, the presence of other stressors—lack of sleep, mental stress, poor nutrition, or weight loss—magnifies the stress on the immune system from a single bout (or repeated bouts) of exhaustive exercise.

Glutamine and the Immune Response

The nonessential amino acid glutamine plays an important role in normal immune function. One protective aspect of glutamine concerns its use as an energy fuel for nucleotide synthesis by disease-fighting cells, particularly the lymphocytes and macrophages that defend against infection. Sepsis (infection), injury, burns, surgery, and endurance exercise lower glutamine levels in plasma and skeletal muscle. Lowered plasma glutamine most likely occurs because glutamine demand by the liver, kidneys, gut, and immune system exceeds its supply from the diet and skeletal muscle. A lowered plasma glutamine concentration contributes to the immunosuppression that accompanies extreme physical stress.[10,49,128] Thus, glutamine supplementation might reduce susceptibility to URTI following strenuous physical exertion.

Marathoners who ingested a glutamine drink (5 g of L-glutamine in 330 mL of mineral water) at the end of a race and then 2 hours later reported fewer URTIs than unsupplemented runners.[14] Subsequent studies by the same researchers to determine a possible mechanism for glutamine's protective effect on postexercise infection risk reported no effect of supplementation on changes in blood lymphocyte distribution.[16] Appearance of URTI in athletes during intense training does not fluctuate with changes in plasma glutamine concentration. Pre-exercise glutamine supplementation does not affect the immune response following a single bout of sustained high-intensity exercise or repeated bouts of intense exercise.[71,113,149] Glutamine supplements taken 0, 30, 60, and 90 minutes following a marathon race prevented the decrease in glutamine concentrations following the race but did not influence three factors: (1) lymphokine-activated killer cell activity, (2) the proliferative responses, or (3) exercise-induced changes in leukocyte subpopulations. *Currently, insufficient data exist to recommend glutamine supplements to reliably blunt immunosuppression from exhaustive exercise.*

A General Recommendation

Optimum immune function generally occurs with a lifestyle that emphasizes the following:

1. Regular physical activity
2. Maintenance of a well-balanced diet
3. Reducing stress to a minimum
4. Adequate sleep

For prudent weight loss, use a gradual approach because more rapid weight loss with accompanying severe caloric restriction suppresses immune function. With prolonged, intense exercise, carbohydrate ingestion (about 1 $L \cdot h^{-1}$ of a typical sports drink) lessens the negative changes in immunity brought about by physiologic stress and carbohydrate depletion. In general, endurance athletes who ingest carbohydrate during a race experience much lower disruption in hormonal and immune measures than do athletes not consuming carbohydrate. These responses indicate a diminished level of physiologic stress.

MINERALS AND EXERCISE PERFORMANCE

The use of single-mineral supplements is ill advised unless prescribed by a physician or registered dietitian because of potential adverse consequences. Excess magnesium supplementation, for example, can cause gastrointestinal disturbances, including diarrhea. Magnesium intake can impair iron and zinc nutrition, whereas a 15-mg zinc excess per day inhibits copper absorption and adversely affects HDL cholesterol concentrations. Concern also exists about the long-term effects of chromium supplementation on tissue chromium accumulation and toxic side effects. *Short- and long-term mineral supplementation above recommended levels does not benefit exercise performance or enhance training responsiveness.*

Mineral Losses in Sweat

Loss of water and accompanying mineral salts, primarily sodium chloride and some potassium chloride in sweat, poses an important challenge during prolonged exercise, especially in hot weather. Excessive water and electrolyte loss impairs heat tolerance and exercise performance and can cause severe dysfunction in the form of heat cramps, heat exhaustion, or heat stroke. The yearly number of heat-related deaths during spring and summer football practice tragically illustrates the importance of fluid and electrolyte replacement. The most recent tragedies occurred in severe heat conditions during July 2011 in Florida, Georgia, and South Carolina. Five teenage high school football players and one coach died from heat-related injuries during off-season workouts in preparation for the upcoming fall season. During practice or a game, an athlete may lose up to 5 kg of water from sweating. This corresponds to about 8.0 g of salt depletion because each kilogram (1 L) of sweat contains about 1.5 g of salt (40% of NaCl represents sodium). *Replacement of water lost through sweating, however, becomes the crucial and immediate need.* As indicated in Chapter 10, some salt added to the ingested fluid facilitates this process.

Defense Against Mineral Loss

Vigorous exercise triggers a rapid and coordinated release of the hormones **vasopressin** and **aldosterone** and the enzyme **renin** to minimize sodium and water loss through the kidneys. Sodium conservation by the kidneys occurs even under extreme conditions such as running a marathon in warm, humid weather when sweat output often reaches 2 L an hour. Electrolytes lost in sweat are usually replenished by adding a slight amount of salt to fluid or food ingested. Runners in a 20-day road race in Hawaii maintained plasma minerals at normal levels by consuming an unrestricted diet without mineral supplements.[28] Ingesting "athletic drinks" offers no special benefit in replacing the minerals lost through sweating compared with consuming the same minerals in a well-balanced diet. Salt supplements may be necessary for prolonged exercise in the heat when fluid loss exceeds 4 or 5 kg. One can achieve proper supplementation by drinking a 0.1 to 0.2% salt solution (adding 0.3 tsp of table salt per liter of water). Chapter 10 presents more specific recommendations for electrolyte replacement via the rehydration beverage.

A mild potassium deficiency occurs with intense exercise during heat stress, but a diet with the recommended amount of potassium generally ensures adequate levels. Drinking an 8-oz glass of orange or tomato juice replaces the calcium, potassium, and magnesium lost in 3 L (7 lb) of sweat, a sweat loss not likely to occur with less than 60 minutes of vigorous exercise.

Trace Minerals and Exercise

Many coaches and athletes believe that supplementing with certain trace minerals enhances exercise performance and counteracts the demands of heavy training. Strenuous exercise may increase excretion of the following four trace elements:

1. *Chromium:* Necessary for carbohydrate and lipid catabolism and proper insulin function and protein synthesis

2. *Copper:* Required for red blood cell formation; influences specific gene expression and serves as a cofactor or prosthetic group for several enzymes
3. *Manganese:* Component of superoxide dismutase in the antioxidant defense system
4. *Zinc:* Component of lactate dehydrogenase, carbonic anhydrase, superoxide dismutase, and enzymes related to energy metabolism, cell growth and differentiation, and tissue repair

Urinary losses of zinc and chromium were 1.5- and 2.0-fold higher on the day of a 6-mile run than on a rest day.[5] A relatively large loss of copper and zinc occurs in sweat during exercise.[24,73] The normal plasma volume expansion with aerobic training combined with zinc redistribution from the plasma to other body tissues (e.g., liver and skeletal muscles) dilutes plasma zinc concentrations to indicate an *apparent* zinc inadequacy.

Trace mineral losses with exercise do not necessarily mean that physically active individuals should supplement with these micronutrients. No benefit occurred from short-term 25-mg daily zinc supplementation on metabolic and endocrine responses and performance during strenuous exercise in eumenorrheic women.[126] Collegiate football players who supplemented with 200 μg of chromium (as chromium picolinate) daily for 9 weeks showed no beneficial changes in body composition or muscular strength during intense weightlifting compared with a control group that received a placebo.[19] Power and endurance athletes had higher, not lower, plasma levels of copper and zinc than nontraining controls.[112] Men and women who train strenuously (with large sweat production) and show marginal nutrition and low body weight (e.g., weight-class wrestlers, endurance runners, ballet dancers, female gymnasts) should carefully monitor trace mineral intake to prevent overt deficiency.[76] For most physically active men and women, only transient, trace mineral losses occur with exercise, without impairing exercise performance, training responsiveness, and overall health.

Iron, zinc, and copper interact and compete for the same carrier during intestinal absorption. Thus, excessive intake of one mineral often causes deficiency in the other. For example, consuming excess iron reduces zinc absorption, whereas excess zinc blunts copper absorption. In addition, supplementing with zinc above recommended levels can lower HDL cholesterol, diminishing the beneficial effect of aerobic exercise on this cardioprotective plasma lipoprotein. Chapter 12 discusses the possible ergogenic effects of chromium supplements and other trace minerals such as boron and vanadium. **TABLE 7.7** outlines exercise-related functions and food sources of four minerals—zinc, copper, chromium, and selenium—associated with exercise and training.

EXERCISE AND FOOD INTAKE

Balancing energy intake with energy expenditure represents a primary goal for the physically active individual of normal body weight. Energy balance not only optimizes physical performance, but it also helps to maintain lean body mass, training responsiveness, and immune and reproductive function. Physical activity represents the most important factor affecting daily energy expenditure (see Chapter 14). A person can estimate daily energy requirements from tabled energy cost values for diverse activities (considering frequency, intensity, and duration) such as those presented in Appendix B.

FIGURE 7.12 illustrates age-related average daily energy intakes for males and females in the US population. Energy intakes peak between ages 16 and 29 years and then decline for succeeding age groups. A similar pattern occurs for males and females, although males achieve higher energy intakes than females at all ages. Between ages 20 and 29 years, women consume on average 35% fewer kcal than men on a daily basis (3025 kcal [12,657 kJ] vs 1957 kcal [8188 kJ]). Thereafter, the sex-related difference in energy intake becomes smaller; at age 70, women consume about 25% fewer kcal than male counterparts.

Physical Activity Makes a Difference

Individuals who engage regularly in moderate-to-intense physical activity eventually increase daily energy intake to match their higher level of energy expenditure. Lumber workers, who expend approximately 4500 kcal daily, unconsciously adjust energy intake to balance energy output. Consequently, body mass remains stable despite a relatively large food intake. The body requires several days to attain energy equilibrium when balancing food intake to meet a new level

TABLE 7.7 Exercise-Related Functions and Food Sources of Selected Trace Minerals

	Function	Prominent Food Sources
Zinc	Component of several enzymes involved in energy metabolism; cofactor to carbonic anhydrase	Oysters, wheat germ, beef, dark poultry meat, whole grains, liver
Copper	Required to synthesize cytochrome oxidase and for use of iron; constituent of ceruloplasmin; constituent of superoxide dismutase	Liver, kidney, shellfish, whole grains, legumes, nuts, eggs
Chromium	Enhances action of insulin	Mushrooms, prunes, nuts, whole-grain bread and cereal, brewer's yeast
Selenium	Functions as an antioxidant with glutathione peroxidase; complements vitamin E function	Seafood, kidney, liver

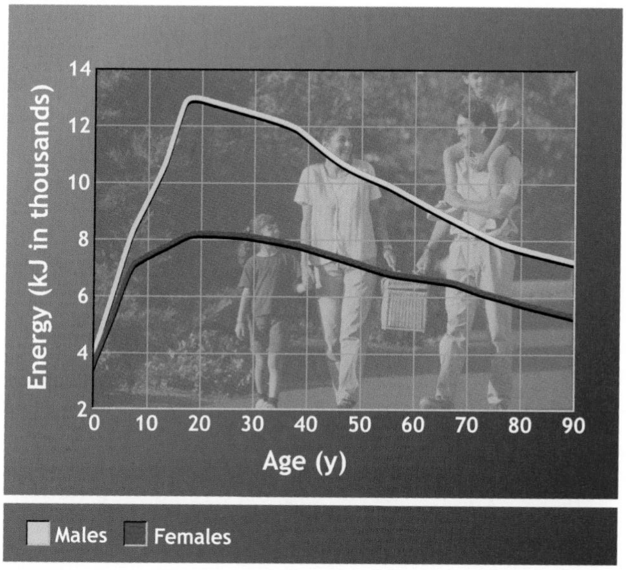

FIGURE 7.12. Average daily energy intake for males and females by age in the US population during the years 1988 to 1991. (From Briefel RR, et al. Total energy intake of the U.S. population: the Third National Health and Nutrition Examination Survey, 1988–1991. *Am J Clin Nutr* 1995;62(Suppl):10725; and Troiano RP. Energy and fat intake of children and adolescents in the United States: data from the National Health and Nutrition Survey. *Am J Clin Nutr* 2000;72:13435.)

of energy output. *Sedentary persons often do not maintain a fine energy balance, thereby allowing energy intake to exceed daily energy expenditure.* The lack of precision in regulating food intake at the low end of the physical activity spectrum undoubtedly contributes to the "creeping obesity" in highly mechanized and technically advanced sedentary societies.

Daily food intake of athletes in the 1936 Olympics reportedly averaged more than 7000 kcal, or roughly three times the average intake.[1] These often-quoted energy values justify what many believe to be an enormous food requirement of athletes in training. These figures represent estimates because objective dietary data did not appear in the original report. In all likelihood, they are inflated estimates of the energy expended (and required) by the athletes. For example, distance runners who train upward to 100 miles a week (6 minutes a mile pace at about 15 kcal per minute) do not expend more than 800 to 1300 "extra" calories daily. For these endurance athletes, about 4000 kcal from daily food intake should balance the increased exercise energy expenditure.

Potential for Negative Energy Balance with High-Volume Training

Many athletes, particularly females, do not meet energy intake recommendations. Research with elite female swimmers, using the doubly labeled water technique described in Chapter 6, noted that total daily energy expenditure increased to 5593 kcal daily during high-volume training. This value represents the highest level of sustained daily energy expenditure reported for female athletes.[134] Daily energy intake did not increase enough to match training demands and averaged only 3136 kcal, implying a negative energy imbalance. The possibility of a negative energy balance in the transition from moderate to intense training may ultimately compromise a person's full potential to train efficiently and compete.

FIGURE 7.13 presents energy intakes from a large sample of elite male and female endurance, strength, and team sport athletes in the Netherlands. For the men, daily energy intake ranged between 2900 and 5900 kcal, whereas the intakes of women competitors ranged between 1600 and 3200 kcal. With the exception of the large energy intakes of athletes at extremes of performance and training, daily energy intake generally did not exceed 4000 kcal for the men and 3000 kcal for the women.

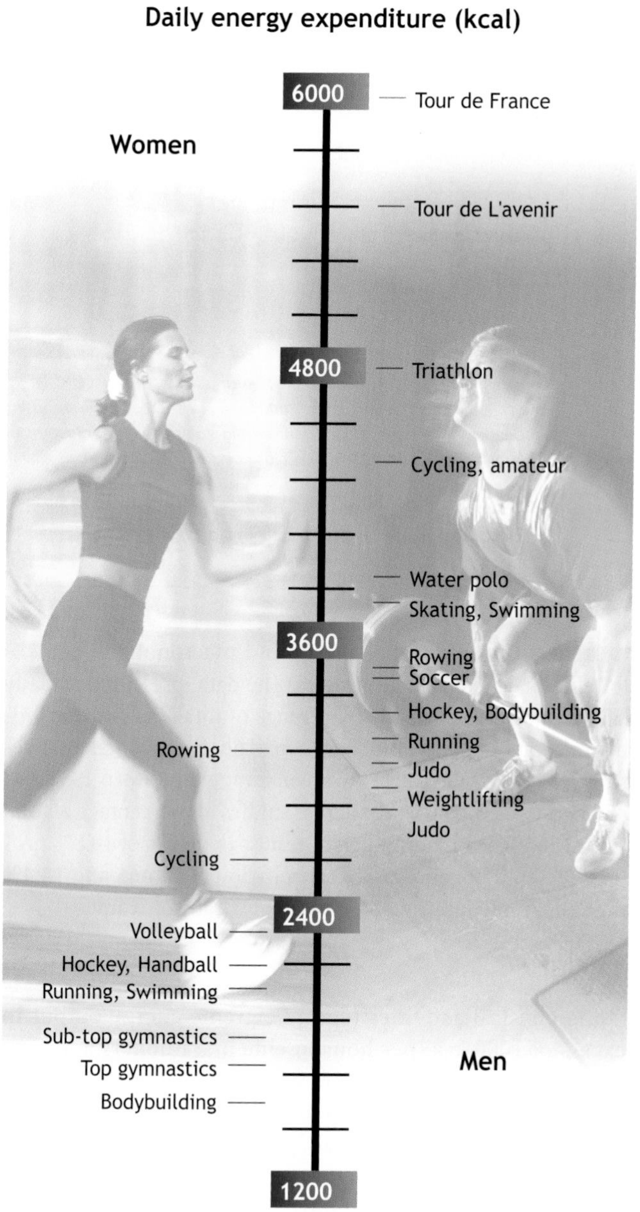

FIGURE 7.13. Daily energy intake (in kcal) of elite male and female endurance, strength, and team sport athletes. (Modified from van Erp-Baart AMJ, et al. Nationwide survey on nutritional habits in elite athletes. *Int J Sports Med* 1989;10:S11.)

TABLE 7.8 Examples of Daily Intakes of Energy, Protein, Lipid, and Carbohydrate (CHO) of Well-Trained Male and Female Athletes

Group	Energy Intake (kcal)	Protein		Lipid		CHO		Research Study
		(g)	(%)	(g)	(%)	(g)	(%)	
Well-Trained Males								
Distance runners (*n* = 50)	3170	114	14	116	33	417	52	7
Distance runners (*n* = 10)	3034	128	17	115	34	396	49	4
Triathletes (*n* = 25)	4095	134	13	127	27	627	60	2
Marathon runners (*n* = 19)	3570	128	15	128	32	487	52	2
Football players (*n* = 56)	3395	126	15	141	38	373	44	2
Weightlifters (*n* = 19)	3640	156	18	155	39	399	43	2
Soccer players (*n* = 8)	4952	170	14	217	39	596	47	6
Swimmers (*n* = 22)	5222	166	12	248	43	596	45	1
Swimmers (*n* = 9)	3072	108	15	102	30	404	55	5
Well-Trained Females								
Distance runners (*n* = 44)	1931	70	19	60	28	290	53	7
Distance runners, eumenorrheic (*n* = 33)	2489	81	12	97	35	352	53	3
Distance runners, amenorrheic (*n* = 12)	2151	74	13	67	27	344	60	3
Swimmers (*n* = 21)	3573	107	12	164	41	428	48	1
Swimmers (*n* = 11)	2130	79	16	63	28	292	55	5

From Williams C. Carbohydrate needs of elite athletes. In: Simopoulos AP, Parlou KN, eds. Nutrition and Fitness for Athletes. Basel: Karger, 1993.

1 *Berning JR, et al. The nutritional habits of adolescent swimmers. Int J Sports Nutr 1991;1:240.*

2 *Burke LM, et al. Dietary intakes and food use of groups of elite Australian male athletes. Int J Sports Nutr 1991;1:278.*

3 *Deuster PA, et al. Nutritional intakes and status of highly trained amenorrheic and eumenorrheic women runners. Fertil Steril 1986;46:636.*

4 *Grandjean AC. Macro-nutrient intake of US athletes compared with the general population and recommendations for athletes. Am J Clin Nutr 1989;49:1070.*

5 *Hawley JA, Williams MM. Dietary intakes of age-group swimmers. Br J Sports Med 1991;25:154.*

6 *Jacobs I, et al. Muscle glycogen concentration and elite soccer players. Eur J Appl Physiol 1982;48:297.*

7 *Courtesy of V. Katch (unpublished).*

TABLE 7.8 lists additional energy and macronutrient intakes for elite male and female athletes. The data, presented as daily caloric intake, include the percentage of total energy as carbohydrate, protein, and lipid. For men, daily energy intake ranges from 3034 to 5222 kcal; for women, it ranges between 1931 and 3573 kcal. Averaging values across studies for percentage of total calories for each macronutrient results in values of 14.8% protein, 35.0% lipid, and 49.8% carbohydrate for men and 14.4% protein, 31.8% lipid, and 54.0% carbohydrate for women.

Tour de France

Some physical activities require extreme energy output in excess of 1000 kcal per hour in elite marathoners and professional cyclists. This occurs with a correspondingly large energy intake during competition or periods of high-intensity training. For example, the daily energy requirements of elite cross-country skiers during 1 week of training averaged 3740 to 4860 kcal for women and 6120 to 8570 kcal for men.[127] These values for women agree with recent evaluations of daily energy expenditure of seven elite lightweight female rowers, which averaged 3957 kcal over a 14-day training period.[51] **FIGURE 7.14** outlines variation in daily energy expenditure for a male competitor during the most grueling event in sports, the Tour de France professional cycling race. Daily energy expenditure averaged 6500 kcal for nearly 3 weeks. Large variation occurred, depending on the level of activity for a particular day; energy expenditure decreased to 3000 kcal on a "rest" day and increased to 9000 kcal cycling over a mountain pass. By combining liquid nutrition with normal meals, this cyclist nearly matched daily energy expenditure with energy intake.

Ultraendurance Running Competition

Energy balance has been studied during a 1000-km (approximately 600-mile) race from Sidney to Melbourne, Australia. The Greek ultramarathon champion Yiannis Kouros completed the race in 5 days, 5 hours, and 7 minutes, finishing 24 hours and 40 minutes ahead of the next competitor. Kouros did not sleep during the first 2 days of competition. He covered 463 km (287.8 miles) at an average speed of 11.4 $km \cdot h^{-1}$ during day 1 and 8.3 $km \cdot h^{-1}$ on day 2. During the remaining days, he took frequent rest periods, including periodic breaks for short "naps." Weather ranged from spring to winter conditions (30-8°C), and terrain varied. **TABLE 7.9** lists the pertinent details of distance covered, energy expenditure, and food and water intake.

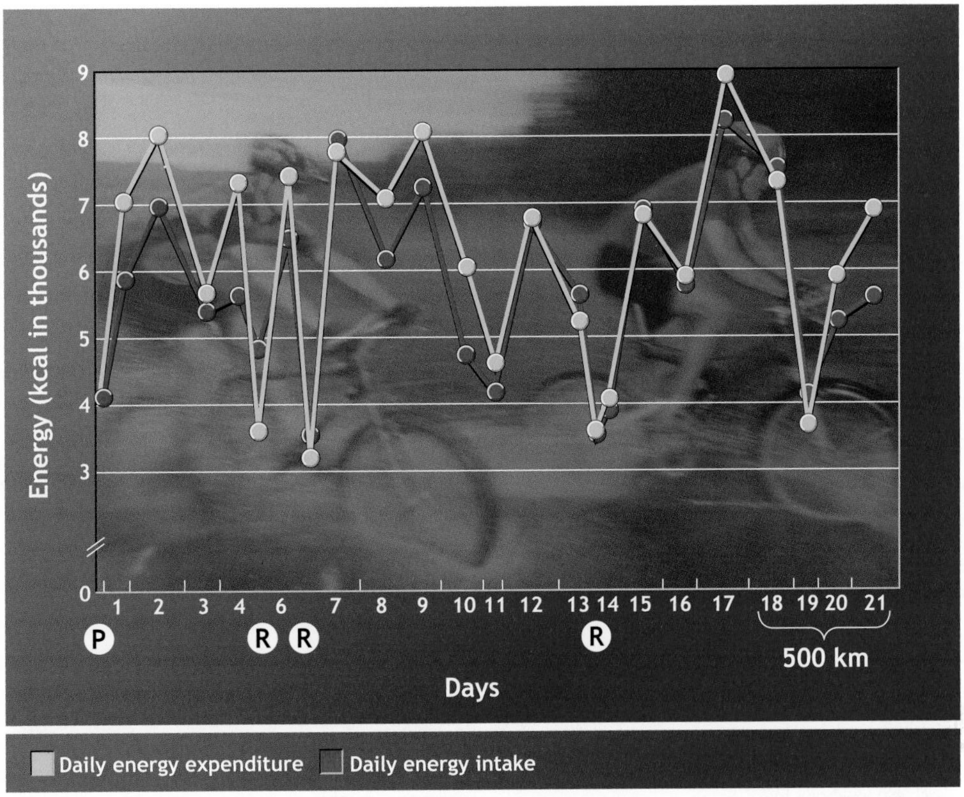

FIGURE 7.14. Daily energy expenditure *(yellow circles)* and energy intake *(red circles)* for a cyclist during the Tour de France competition. For 3 weeks in July, nearly 200 cyclists push themselves over and around the perimeter of France covering 2405 miles, more than 100 miles daily (only 1 day of rest), at an average speed of 24.4 mph. Note the extremely high energy expenditure values and ability to achieve energy balance with liquid nutrition plus normal meals. *P*, stage; *R*, rest day. (Modified from Saris WHM, et al. Adequacy of vitamin supply under maximal sustained workloads; the Tour de France. In: Walter P, et al., eds. *Elevated Dosages of Vitamins*. Toronto: Huber Publishers, 1989.)

The near equivalence between Kouros' estimated total energy intake (55,970 kcal) and energy expenditure (59,079 kcal) represents a remarkable aspect of energy homeostasis during extremes of physical exertion. Of the total energy intake from food, carbohydrates represented 95.3%, lipids 3%, with the remaining 1.7% proteins. Protein intake from food averaged considerably below the RDA level (although protein supplements were taken in tablet form). The unusually large daily energy intake (8600–13,770 kcal) came from Greek sweets (baklava, cookies, and donuts), some chocolate, dried fruit and nuts, various fruit juices, and fresh fruits. Every 30 minutes after the first 6 hours of running, Kouros replaced sweets and fruit with a small biscuit soaked in honey or jam. He consumed a small amount of roasted chicken on day 4 and drank coffee every morning. He took a 500-mg vitamin C supplement every 12 hours and a protein tablet twice daily.

The remarkable achievement by this champion exemplifies a highly conditioned athlete's exquisite regulatory control for energy balance during strenuous exercise. Kouros performed at a pace requiring a continuous energy supply averaging 49% of aerobic capacity during the first 2 days of competition and 38% for Days 3 to 5. He finished the competition without compromising overall health and without muscular injuries or thermoregulatory problems, and his body mass remained unchanged. Reported difficulties included a severe bout of constipation during the competition and frequent urination that persisted for several days after the race.

Another case study of a 37-year-old male ultramarathoner further demonstrates the tremendous capacity for prolonged, high daily energy expenditure. The doubly labeled water technique evaluated energy expenditure during a 2-week period of a 14,500-km run around Australia in 6.5 months (average 7–90 $km \cdot d^{-1}$) with no days for rest.[50] Daily energy expenditure over the measurement period averaged 6321 kcal; daily water turnover equaled 6.1 L. The subject ran about the same distance each day over the study period as in the entire race period. As such, these data likely represent energy dynamics for the entire run.

High-Risk Sports for Marginal Nutrition

Gymnasts, ballet dancers, ice dancers, and weight-class athletes in boxing, wrestling, and judo engage in arduous training. Yet due to the nature of their sport, these men and women continually strive to maintain a lean, light body mass (**TABLE 7.10**). As a result, energy intake often intentionally falls short of energy expenditure and a relative state of malnutrition develops. The daily nutrient intake (% of RDA) of 97 competitive female gymnasts 11 to 14 years of age indicates that nutritional supplementation could prove beneficial to these individuals (**FIG. 7.15**). Twenty-three percent of the girls consumed less than 1500 kcal daily, and more than 40% consumed less than two thirds of the RDA for vitamin

TABLE 7.9 Distance Covered and Daily and Total Energy Balance, Nutrient Distributions in Food, and Water Intake During an Elite Ultra Distance Running

Day of the Race	Distance Covered	Estimated Energy Expenditure	Estimated Energy Intake	Carbohydrates			Lipids			Proteins			H_2O
	(km)	(kcal)	(kcal)	(g)	(%)	(kcal)	(g)	(%)	(kcal)	(g)	(%)	(kcal)	(L)
1	270	15,367	13,770	3375	98.0	13,502	20	1.3	180	22	0.7	88	22.0
2	193	10,741	8600	1981	92.2	7923	53	5.5	477	50	2.3	200	19.2
3	152	8919	12,700	3074	96.8	12,297	27	1.9	243	40	1.3	160	22.7
4	165	9780	7800	1758	90.1	7032	56	6.5	504	66	3.4	264	14.3
5	135	7736	12,500	3014	96.4	12,058	30	2.2	270	43	1.4	172	18.3
5 h	45	2536	550	138	100.0	550	—	—	—	—	—	—	3.2
Total	960	55,079	55,970	13,340		53,364	186		1674	221		734	99.7

Modified from Rontoyannis GP, et al. Energy balance in ultramarathon running. Am J Clin Nutr 1989;49:976.
The runner weighed 65 kg, was 171 cm tall, had a percentage body fat of 8%, and a $\dot{V}O_2max$ of 62.5 mL·kg^{-1}·min^{-1}.

TABLE 7.10 High-Risk Sports for Marginal Nutrition

Criterion	Sports Discipline
Low weight—chronically low energy intakes to achieve low body fat	Gymnastics, jockeys, ballet, dancing, rhythmic gymnastics, ice dancing, aerobics
Competition weight—drastic weight loss regimens to achieve desired weight category	Weight class sports (e.g., judo, boxing, wrestling, rowing, ski jumping)
Low fat—drastic fat loss to achieve lowest possible fat	Bodybuilding
Vegetarian athletes	Endurance events

From Brouns F. *Nutritional Needs of Athletes.* New York: John Wiley & Sons, 1993.

E, folate, iron, magnesium, calcium, and zinc. Clearly, a large number of these adolescent gymnasts needed to upgrade the nutritional quality of their diets or consider supplementation. For such athletes, carbohydrate intake fails to reach the level required by intense training. Consequently, they often train and perform in a carbohydrate-depleted state. Some protein supplementation to achieve a daily intake between 1.2 and 1.6 g per kilogram of body mass also may be warranted to maintain nitrogen balance and reduce the potential for impaired training status.

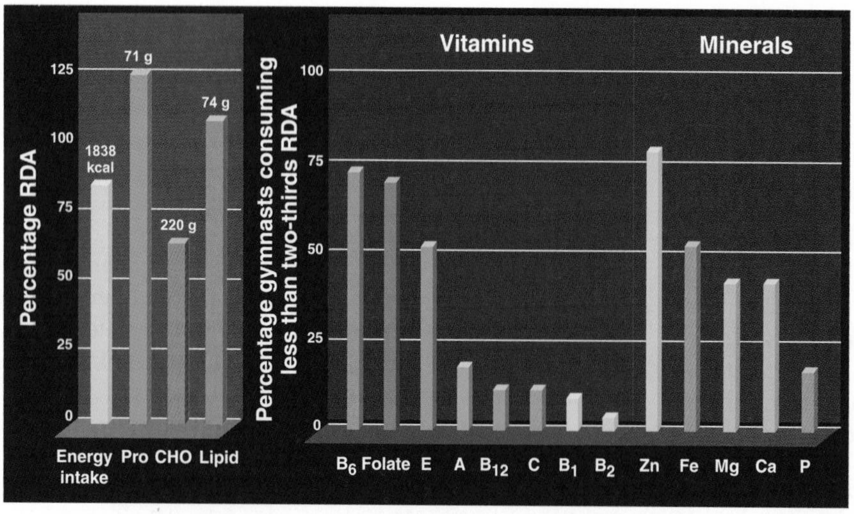

FIGURE 7.15. Average daily nutrient intake of 97 adolescent female gymnasts (11–14 years old) related to recommended values. The RDA on the *y* axis reflects only protein, whereas energy, carbohydrate (CHO), and lipid reflect "recommended" values *(left)*. Percentage of gymnasts consuming less than two thirds of the RDA *(right)*. Mean age, 13.1 years; mean stature, 152.4 cm (60 in); mean body mass, 43.1 kg (94.8 lb). (Modified from Loosli AR, Benson J. Nutritional intake in adolescent athletes. *Pediatr Clin N Am* 1990;37:1143.)

EAT MORE, WEIGH LESS

The energy intakes of 61 middle-aged men and women who ran 60 km per week ranged between 40 and 60% more calories per kilogram of body mass than intakes of sedentary controls. The extra energy required to run between 8 and 10 km daily accounted for the runners' larger caloric intake. Paradoxically, the most active runners who ate considerably more on a daily basis weighed considerably less than runners who exercised at a lower total caloric expenditure. These data agree with other studies of physically active people; they also support the argument that regular exercise provides an effective way to "eat more yet weigh less" while maintaining a lower percentage of body fat. Chapter 14 more fully explores the important role of regular exercise for weight control.

SUMMARY

1. MyPlate provides recommendations for healthful nutrition for physically active men and women. It emphasizes fruits, grains, and vegetables and de-emphasizes foods high in animal protein, lipids, and dairy products.
2. The Diet Quality Index, a composite score based on eight food and nutrient recommendations of the National Academy of Sciences, provides a general indication of the "healthfulness" of one's diet.
3. Within rather broad limits, a balanced diet provides the nutrient requirements of athletes and other individuals who engage in exercise training programs. Well-planned menus of about 1200 kcal daily offer the vitamin, mineral, and protein requirements. Consuming additional food (depending on physical activity level) then meets daily energy needs.
4. The protein RDA of 0.8 g per kilogram of body mass represents a liberal requirement believed to be adequate for all people regardless of physical activity level.
5. A protein intake between 1.2 and 1.8 g per kilogram of body mass should adequately meet the possibility for added protein needs during strenuous training and prolonged exercise.
6. Physically active individuals readily achieve optimal protein values because they consume two to five times the protein RDA with their increased energy intake.
7. Precise recommendations do not exist for daily lipid and carbohydrate intake. A prudent recommendation suggests not to exceed 30 to 35% of daily calories from lipids; of this amount, strive for 90% unsaturated fatty acids.
8. For physically active people, carbohydrates should provide 60% or more of the daily calories (400-600 g), particularly as unrefined polysaccharides.
9. The AHA recommends lifestyle modifications that include increasing regular physical activity and eliminating use of all tobacco products.
10. A proper diet emphasizes fruits and vegetables, cereals and whole grains, nonfat and low-fat dairy products, legumes, nuts, fish, poultry, and lean meats.
11. To address the nation's obesity epidemic, the AHA urges men to maintain a waistline of 40 inches or less and women to maintain a waistline of 35 inches or less.
12. Americans should devote at least 1 hour daily to moderately intense physical activity (brisk walking, swimming, or cycling) to maintain good health and a desirable body weight.
13. To meet daily energy and nutrient needs and minimize chronic disease risk, adults should consume between 45 and 65% of total calories from carbohydrates, with maximum intake of added sugars placed at 25% of total calories.
14. Acceptable lipid intake ranges between 20 and 35% of caloric intake, with protein intake between 10 and 35%.
15. Successive days of intense training gradually deplete carbohydrate reserves, even when maintaining the recommended carbohydrate intake. This could lead to "staleness," making continued training more difficult.
16. Vitamin supplementation above amounts in a well-balanced diet does not improve exercise performance or the potential for training. Serious illness can result from regularly consuming an excess of fat-soluble and, in some instances, water-soluble vitamins.
17. Elevated metabolism in physical activity increases the production of potentially harmful free radicals. To reduce the possibility for oxidative stress and cellular damage, the daily diet should contain foods rich in antioxidant vitamins and minerals.
18. A J-shaped curve generally describes the relationship between short-term exercise intensity and susceptibility to URTI.
19. Light-to-moderate physical activity offers greater protection against URTI and diverse cancers than a sedentary lifestyle. A bout of intense physical activity provides an "open window" that decreases antiviral and antibacterial resistance and increases URTI risk.
20. Glutamine supplements are not recommended to reliably blunt immunosuppression from exhaustive exercise.
21. Excessive sweating during exercise causes loss of body water and related minerals. Mineral loss should be replaced following exercise through well-balanced meals.
22. Intensity of daily physical activity largely determines energy intake requirements. The daily caloric needs of athletes in strenuous sports probably do not exceed 4000 kcal unless body mass is large or training level or competition is extreme.

thePoint *Visit* **thePoint.lww.com/MKKSEN4e** *to view the following animation related to content presented in Chapter 7:* ***Vitamin C as an antioxidant.***

TEST YOUR KNOWLEDGE ANSWERS

1. **False:** The human body functions in accord with the laws of thermodynamics. This also includes the dynamics of energy balance. In accord with the first law of thermodynamics, the energy balance equation dictates that body mass remains constant when caloric intake equals caloric expenditure. If the total food calories exceed daily energy expenditure, excess calories accumulate as fat in adipose tissue. Conversely, weight loss occurs when daily energy expenditure exceeds daily energy intake.

2. **True:** Thirty-five hundred "extra" kcal through either increased energy intake or decreased energy output approximates the energy contained in 1 pound (0.45 kg) of stored body fat.

3. **True:** As with the previous *MyPyramid* guidelines, the *MyPlate* guidelines are not without flaws and concerns. For example, the "Fruits" section makes no distinction between fruit juice and the actual fruit—a half cup of fruit juice is listed as equivalent to half cup of fruit. This ignores the fact that the glycemic load is far higher in fruit juice than in fruit. Also, the "Grains" section makes no distinction between true whole grains and grains ground into flour. As with fruits, whole and intact grains, rather than those pulverized and processed, slow digestion and stabilize blood sugar.

4. **False:** Guidelines from the US government are similar to those advocated by other agencies (including the USDA); they place great emphasis on adopting healthy eating patterns and lifestyle behaviors rather than focusing on specific numeric goals such as for dietary fat intake.

5. **False:** Research in exercise nutrition, although far from complete, indicates that the large number of teenagers and adults who exercise regularly to keep fit, including competitive athletes, do not require additional nutrients beyond those obtained through the regular intake of a nutritionally well-balanced diet. Endurance athletes and others who engage regularly in intense training must maintain adequate energy and protein intake and appropriate carbohydrate consumption to match this macronutrient's use for energy during exercise. However, attention to proper diet does not mean that a physically active person must join the ranks of the more than 40% of Americans who take supplements (spending about $6 billion yearly) to micromanage nutrient intake.

6. **False:** Adequate research design and methodology have not shown that amino acid supplementation in any form above the RDA significantly increases muscle mass or improves muscular strength, power, or endurance. Most individuals obtain adequate protein to sustain muscle growth with resistance training by consuming ordinary foods in a well-balanced diet. Provided caloric intake balances energy output (and one consumes a wide variety of foods), no need exists to consume protein supplements or simple amino acids.

7. **False:** Standards for optimal lipid intake are not firmly established, but to promote good health, lipid intake should probably not exceed 25 to 30% of the diet's energy content. Of this, at least 70% should come from unsaturated fatty acids.

8. **False:** No hazard to health exists when subsisting chiefly on a variety of fiber-rich complex unrefined carbohydrates, with adequate intake of essential amino acids, fatty acids, minerals, and vitamins.

9. **False:** Over 50 years of research fails to support the use of vitamin supplements by nutritionally adequate healthy people to improve exercise performance or the ability to train arduously. When vitamin intake achieves recommended levels via diet, supplements neither improve performance nor increase the blood levels of these micronutrients.

10. **False:** The best sources of antioxidants are β-carotene found in pigmented compounds that give color to yellow and orange vegetables and fruits, including carrots; dark-green leafy vegetables such as spinach, broccoli, turnips, and beet and collard greens; and sweet potatoes, winter squash, apricots, cantaloupe, mangos, and papaya; vitamin C found in citrus fruits and juices, cabbage, broccoli, turnip greens, cantaloupe, green and red sweet peppers, and berries; and vitamin E found in poultry, seafood, vegetable oils, wheat germ, fish liver oils, whole-grain breads and fortified cereals, nuts and seeds, dried beans, green leafy vegetables, and eggs.

Key References

Aoi W, et al. Exercise and functional foods. *Nutr J* 2006;5:15.

Brooks GA, et al. Chronicle of the Institute of Medicine physical activity recommendation: how a physical activity recommendation came to be among dietary recommendations. *Am J Clin Nutr* 2004;79:921S.

Burke LM. Fueling strategies to optimize performance: training high or training low? *Scand J Med Sci Sports* 2010;20(Suppl 2):48.

Carter P, et al. Fruit and vegetable intake and incidence of type 2 diabetes mellitus: systematic review and meta-analysis. *BMJ* 2010;341:4229.

Chubak J, et al. Moderate-intensity exercise reduces incidence of colds among postmenopausal women. *Am J Med* 2006;119:937.

Cordain L, et al. Origins and evolutions of the Western diet: health implications for the 21st century. *Am J Clin Nutr* 2005;81:341.

Drewnowski A. Concept of a nutritious food: toward a nutrient density score. *Am J Clin Nutr* 2005;82:721.

Frisardi V, et al. Nutraceutical properties of Mediterranean diet and cognitive decline: possible underlying mechanisms. *J Alzheimers Dis* 2010;22:715.

Gaskins AJ, et al. Adherence to a Mediterranean diet and plasma concentrations of lipid peroxidation in premenopausal women. *Am J Clin Nutr* 2010;92:146.

Gauche E, et al. Vitamin and mineral supplementation and neuromuscular recovery after a running race. *Med Sci Sports Exerc* 2006;38:2110.

Heaney C, et al. Nutrition knowledge in athletes: a systematic review. *IJSNEM* 2011;21:248.

Hu FB, Willett WC. Optimal diets for prevention of coronary heart disease. *JAMA* 2002;288:2569.

Jeffery RW, et al. Physical activity and weight loss: does prescribing higher physical activity goals improve outcome? *Am J Clin Nutr* 2003;78:684.

Kakanis MW, et al. The open window of susceptibility to infection after acute exercise in healthy young male elite athletes. *Exerc Immunol Rev* 2010;16:119.

Kastorini CM, et al. The effect of Mediterranean diet on metabolic syndrome and its components: a meta-analysis of 50 studies and 534,906 individuals. *J Am Coll Cardiol* 2011;57:1299.

Krauss RM, et al. AHA dietary guidelines revision 2000: a statement for health care professionals from the Nutrition Committee of the American Heart Association. *Circulation* 2000;102:2284.

Lauber RP, Sheard NF. The American Heart Association dietary guidelines for 2000: a summary report. *Nutr Rev* 2001;59:298.

Matthews CE, et al. Moderate to vigorous physical activity and risk of upper-respiratory tract infection. *Med Sci Sports Exerc* 2002;34:1242.

McGinley C, et al. Does antioxidant vitamin supplementation protect against muscle damage? *Sports Med* 2009;39:1011.

Nieman DC. Immune response to heavy exertion. *J Appl Physiol* 1997;82:1385.

Pattwell DM, Jackson MJ. Contraction-induced oxidants as mediators of adaptation and damage in skeletal muscle. *Exer Sport Sci Rev* 2004;32:14.

Pedersen BK, Hoffman-Goetz L. Exercise and the immune system: regulation, integration, and adaptation. *Physiol Rev* 2000;80:1055.

Sarris WWM, et al. How much physical activity is enough to prevent unhealthy weight gain? Outcome of the IASO 1st Stock Conference and consensus statement. *Obesity Rev* 2003;4:1201.

Wolfe RR. Protein supplements and exercise. *Am J Clin Nutr* 2000;72(Suppl):551S.

Yfanti C, et al. Antioxidant supplementation does not alter endurance training adaptation. *Med Sci Sports Exerc* 2010;42:1388.

thePoint *Visit* **thePoint.lww.com/MKKSEN4e** *for a list of the references cited in this chapter, including additional, relevant references.*

CHAPTER 8

Nutritional Considerations for Intense Training and Sports Competition

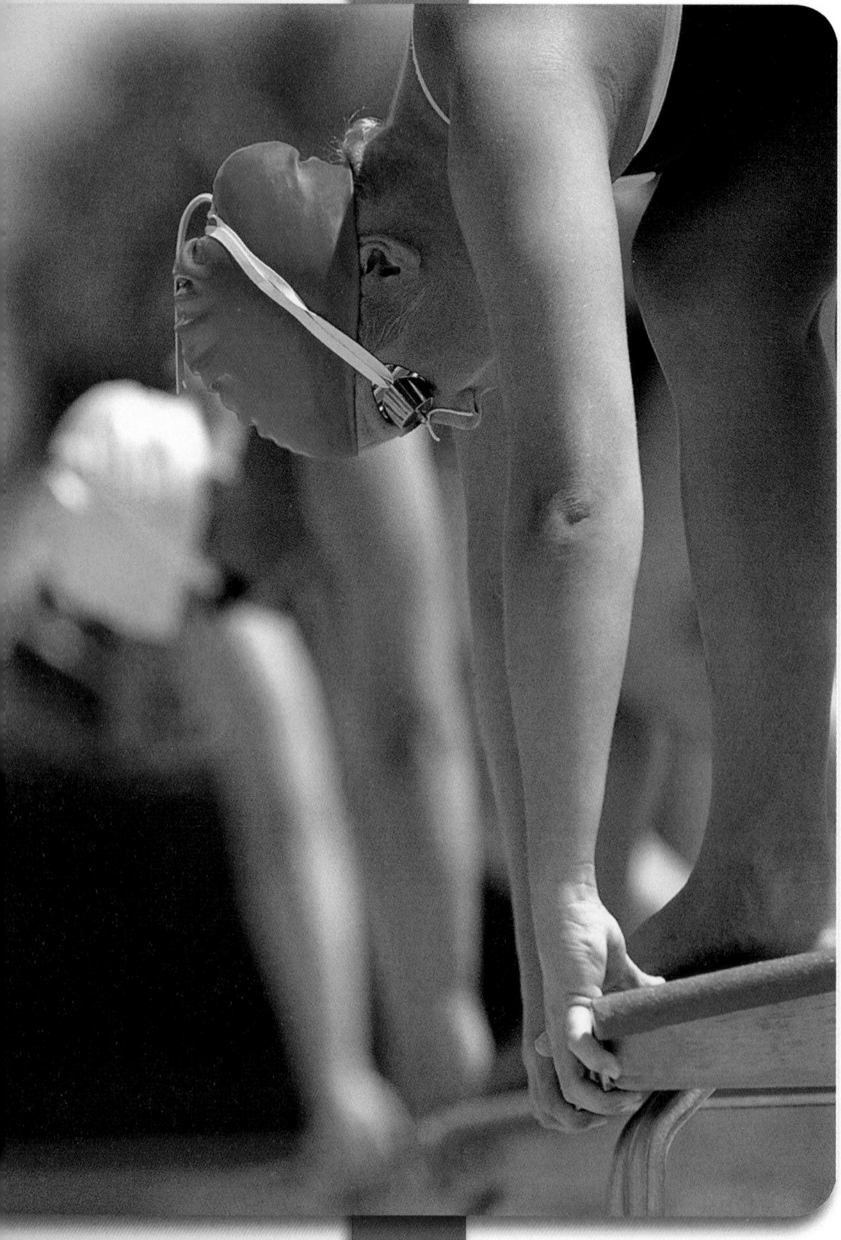

OUTLINE

TEST YOUR KNOWLEDGE

Select true or false for the 10 statements below, and then check out the answers at the end of the chapter. Retake the test after you've read the chapter; you should achieve 100%!	True	False
1. One should fast for 24 h before sports competition or intense training to avoid an upset stomach caused by undigested food	❍	❍
2. The ideal precompetition meal consists of high-protein foods to ensure elevated levels of muscle protein during competition.	❍	❍
3. It is unwise to eat during intense aerobic exercise.	❍	❍
4. The glycemic index indicates the number of calories in different forms of carbohydrate.	❍	❍
5. Consuming high-glycemic carbohydrates provides the most effective means to rapidly replenish depleted glycogen following intense endurance exercise.	❍	❍
6. Glycogen reserves in muscle and liver usually replenish within 12 h when consuming high-glycemic carbohydrates in the immediate postexercise period.	❍	❍
7. Avoid drinking liquids immediately before vigorous exercise to minimize intestinal discomfort and impaired exercise performance.	❍	❍
8. Plain cold water serves as the optimal oral rehydration beverage for consumption during exercise.	❍	❍
9. Research supports the wisdom of adding some sodium to an oral rehydration solution, particularly during prolonged exercise in the heat.	❍	❍
10. Drinking a concentrated sugar drink before and during exercise facilitates rehydration and enhances exercise performance.	❍	❍

The need to maintain optimal nutrient intake to sustain the energy and tissue-building requirements of regular physical activity also requires unique dietary modifications to facilitate intense training and enhance sports competition.

THE PRECOMPETITION MEAL

Athletes often compete in the morning following an overnight fast. As noted in Chapter 1, considerable depletion occurs in carbohydrate reserves over an 8- to 12-h period without eating, even if the person normally follows appropriate dietary recommendations. Consequently, precompetition nutrition takes on an important new role. *The precompetition meal should provide adequate carbohydrate energy and ensure optimal hydration.* Within this framework, fasting before competition or intense training makes no sense physiologically because it rapidly depletes liver and muscle glycogen and impairs subsequent exercise performance. If a person trains or competes in the afternoon, breakfast becomes the important meal to optimize glycogen reserves. For late afternoon training or competition, lunch becomes the important source for topping off glycogen stores. Consider the following three factors when individualizing the precompetition meal plan:

1. Food preferences
2. Psychological set
3. Food digestibility

As a general rule, eliminate foods high in lipid and protein content on the day of competition because these foods digest slowly and remain in the digestive tract longer than carbohydrate foods of similar energy content. Timing of the precompetition meal also deserves consideration. The increased stress and tension that usually accompany competition decrease blood flow to the digestive tract, depressing intestinal absorption. *A carbohydrate-rich, precompetition meal requires 1 to 4 h to digest, absorb, and replenish muscle and liver glycogen.*

Protein or Carbohydrate?

Many athletes become psychologically accustomed to the classic "steak and eggs" precompetition meal, but such a meal provides no benefit to exercise performance. To the contrary, this type of meal with its low carbohydrate content can negatively impact optimal exercise performance.

There are five reasons to modify or even abolish the high-protein precompetition meal in favor of a high-carbohydrate meal:

1. Dietary carbohydrates replenish liver and muscle glycogen depletion that occurs during sleep, an essentially fasting state.
2. Carbohydrates digest and absorb more rapidly than proteins or lipids. They provide energy faster and reduce the feeling of fullness following a meal.
3. A high-protein meal elevates resting metabolism considerably more than a high-carbohydrate meal because of the greater energy requirements for digestion, absorption, and assimilation. The additional metabolic heat produced during these processes can strain the body's heat-dissipating mechanisms and impair exercise performance in hot weather.
4. Protein breakdown for energy facilitates dehydration during exercise because the by-products of amino acid breakdown require water for urinary excretion. For example, approximately 50 mL of water "accompanies" the excretion of each gram of urea in urine.
5. Carbohydrate serves as the primary energy nutrient or "fuel" for short-term anaerobic activity and for prolonged, intense aerobic exercise.

Make It Carbohydrate Rich

The ideal precompetition meal maximizes muscle and liver glycogen storage and provides glucose for intestinal absorption during exercise. The meal should attain these three requirements:

1. Contain 150 to 300 g carbohydrate (3–5 $g \cdot kg^{-1}$ of body mass in either solid or liquid form)
2. Be consumed 3 to 4 h before exercising
3. Contain relatively little fat and fiber to facilitate gastric emptying and minimize gastrointestinal distress

The importance of precompetition feeding occurs only if the person maintains a nutritionally sound diet throughout training. Pre-exercise feedings cannot correct existing nutritional deficiencies or inadequate nutrient intake in the weeks before competition.

LIQUID AND PREPACKAGED BARS, POWDERS, AND MEALS

Commercially prepared nutrition bars, powders, and liquid meals offer an alternative approach to precompetition feeding or supplemental feedings during periods of competition.[41] Nutrient supplements also effectively enhance energy and nutrient intake in training, particularly if energy output exceeds energy intake from lack of interest or mismanagement of feedings.

Liquid Meals

Liquid meals provide high-carbohydrate content but contain enough lipid and protein to contribute to satiety. A liquid meal digests rapidly, leaving essentially no residue in the intestinal tract. Liquid meals prove particularly effective during day-long swimming and track meets or during tennis, soccer, softball, and basketball tournaments. In these outings, the person usually has little time for or interest in food. Liquid meals offer a practical approach to supplementing caloric intake during the high-energy output phase of training. Athletes also can use liquid nutrition to help maintain body weight and as a ready source of calories to gain weight.

Nutrition Bars

Nutrition bars (called "energy bars," "protein bars," and "diet bars") contain a relatively high protein content that ranges between 10 and 30 g per bar. The typical 60-g bar contains 25 g (100 kcal) of carbohydrate (equal amounts of starch and sugar), 15 g (60 kcal) of protein, and 5 g (45 kcal) of lipid (3 g or 27 kcal of saturated fat), with the remaining weight as water. This represents about 49% of the bar's total 205 calories from carbohydrates, 29% from protein, and 22% from lipid. The bars often include vitamins and minerals at 30 to 50% of recommended values, and some contain dietary supplements such as β-hydroxy-methylbutyrate and are labeled as dietary supplements rather than foods.

NUTRIENT COMPOSITION OF NUTRITION BARS VARIES WITH PURPOSE

So-called energy bars contain a greater proportion of carbohydrates, whereas "diet" or "weight loss" bars are lower in carbohydrate content and higher in protein. "Meal replacement bars" have the largest energy content (240–310 kcal), with proportionately more of the three macronutrients. "Protein bars" simply contain a larger amount of protein.

Nutrition bars provide a relatively easy way to obtain important nutrients. They should not, however, totally substitute for normal food intake because they lack the broad array of plant fibers and phytochemicals found in food, and they typically contain a relatively high level of saturated fatty acids. As an added insight, these bars are generally sold as dietary supplements; no independent assessment by the Food and Drug Administration (FDA) through the Dietary Supplement Health and Education Act of 1994 (www.health.gov/

dietsupp/ch1.htm) or other federal or state agency exists to validate the labeling claims for nutrient content and composition.

Nutrition Powders and Drinks

A high protein content between 10 and 50 g per serving represents a unique aspect of nutrition powders and drinks. They also contain added vitamins, minerals, and other dietary supplement ingredients. The powders come in canisters or packets that readily mix with water or other liquid forms premixed in cans. These products often serve as an alternative to nutrition bars; they are marketed as meal replacements, dieting aids, energy boosters, or concentrated protein sources.

The nutrient composition of powders and drinks varies considerably from nutrition bars. Most nutrition bars contain at least 15 g of carbohydrates to provide texture and taste, whereas powders and drinks do not. This accounts for the relatively high protein content of powders and drinks. Nutrition powders and drinks generally contain fewer calories per serving than do bars, but this can vary for a powder depending on the liquid used for mixing.

The recommended serving of a powder averages about 45 g (about 1.5 oz), the same amount as a nutrition bar minus its water content, but with wide variation in this recommendation. A typical serving of a high-protein powder mix contains about 10 g of carbohydrate (two thirds as sugar), 30 g of protein, and 2 g of lipid. This amounts to 178 kcal, or 23% of calories from carbohydrate, 67% from protein, and 10% from lipid. When mixed in water, these powdered nutrient supplements exceed the recommended protein intake percentage and fall below recommended lipid and carbohydrate percentages. A drink typically contains slightly more carbohydrate

NUTRIENT CONTENT AND SAFETY OF ENERGY BEVERAGES VERSUS SPORTS DRINKS

The United States is the world's largest consumer of energy beverages (EBs) by volume, with more than 400 million gallons consumed in 2010 (more than 1 gallon person yearly) mostly among persons 11 to 35 years of age. Sales of EBs will exceed $9 billion in 2012, up from $6.6 billion in 2007. No governmental standards exist to regulate sales of EBs, so manufacturers are free to include controversial ingredients without fear of governmental oversight or regulation. Unfortunately, EB consumption associates positively with high-risk behaviors (e.g., increased illicit drug use, sexual risk taking, fighting, failure to use seat belts, taking risks on a dare, smoking, excessive alcohol abuse). Whereas sports drinks (SD) serve as hydrating agents and as a means to replenish electrolytes and carbohydrates, elevated levels of caffeine and other substances in EBs create undesirable physiologic side effects. Researchers searched the English-language scientific literature using the MEDLINE and EMBASE databases and the Google Internet search engine during January 1976 through May 2010. **TABLE 1** compares the ingredients in four popular EBs (Red Bull, Rockstar, Monster, and Full Throttle). **TABLE 2** summarizes the recommendations based on the literature for consumption of EB and SD beverages.

Source: Higgins JP, et al. Energy beverages: content and safety. *Mayo Clin Proc* 2010;85:1022.

TABLE 1 Comparison of Ingredients in Energy Beverages[a]

	Red Bull	Rockstar	Monster	Full Throttle
Calories	220	280	200	220
Carbohydrates	54 g Sucrose, glucose	62 g Sucrose, glucose	54 g Sucrose, glucose, sucralose, maltodextrin	57 g High-fructose corn syrup, sucrose
Sodium	Only listed as sodium citrate	80 mg sodium citrate	360 mg 16% RDA Sodium citrate, sodium chloride	160 mg Sodium citrate
Caffeine	160 mg	160 mg Part of a 1.35-g "energy blend"	Only listed as part of a 5000-mg "energy blend"	141 mg Part of a 3000-mg "energy blend"
Taurine	2000 mg	2000 mg Part of a 1.35-g "energy blend"	2000 mg Part of a 5000-mg "energy blend"	Only listed as part of a 3000-mg "energy blend"
Glucuronolactone	Only listed (1200 mg)[b]	None listed	only listed as part of a 5000-mg "energy blend"	None listed
Niacin (B_3)	200% RDA Niacinamide (40 mg)[b]	40 mg 200% RDA Niacinamide	40 mg 200% RDA Niacinamide	100% RDA Niacinamide
Inositol (B_8)	Only listed	50 mg Part of a 1.35-g "energy blend"	Only listed as part of a 5000-mg "energy blend"	None listed
Pyridoxine hydrochloride (B_6)	500% RDA (10 mg)[b]	4 mg 200% RDA	4 mg 200% RDA	200% RDA

(continued)

TABLE 1 Comparison of Ingredients in Energy Beverages[a] *(Continued)*

	Red Bull	Rockstar	Monster	Full Throttle
Cyanocobalamin (B_{12})	160% RDA Listed as vitamin B_{12} (10 μg)[b]	12 μg 200% RDA	12 μg 200% RDA	200% RDA
Riboflavin (B_2)	None listed	6.8 mg 400% RDA	3.4 mg 200% RDA	None listed
Pantothenic acid (B_5)	100% RDA Calcium Pantothenate (10 mg)[b]	20 mg 200% RDA Calcium pantothenate	None listed	None listed
Ginseng extract	None listed	50 mg Part of a 1.35-g "energy blend"	400 mg	Only listed as part of a 3000-mg "energy blend"
Guarana extract	None listed	50 mg Part of a 1.35-g "energy blend"	Only listed as part of a 5000-mg "energy blend"	Only listed as part of a 3000-mg "energy blend"
Ginkgo biloba leaf extract	None listed	300 mg Part of a 1.35-g "energy blend"	None listed	None listed
Milk thistle extract	None listed	40 mg Part of a 1.35-g "energy blend"	None listed	None listed
L-carnitine	None listed	50 mg Part of a 1.35-g "energy blend"	Only listed as part of a 5000-mg "energy blend"	Only listed as part of a 3000-mg "energy blend" Carnitine fumarate
Sorbic acid	None listed	Yes	Yes	No
Sodium benzoate	None listed	Yes Benzoic acid	Yes Benzoic acid	Yes
Citric acid	None listed	Yes	Yes	Yes
Natural flavors	Yes	Yes	Yes	Yes
Artificial flavors	Yes	Yes	None listed	None listed
Coloring	"Colors"	"Caramel"	"color added"	Blue 1, Red 40

[a]*As listed on 16-oz can unless otherwise noted. RDA = recommended daily allowance.*

[b]*This amount is not listed on the can; the corporate office was called and this was all the information given.*

TABLE 2 Recommendations Regarding Energy Beverage and Sports Drink Consumption

For the nonathlete consumer	1. Limit your consumption of EBs to no more than 500 mL or 1 can per day. 2. Do not mix EBs with alcohol; this can mask intoxication and may be extremely dehydrating. 3. Rehydrate with water or an appropriately formulated SD after exercise or intense physical activity. 4. If you experience an adverse reaction to an EB, report it to your healthcare professional or organization. 5. If you are being treated for hypertension, avoid using EBs. 6. If you have a serious underlying medical condition, including coronary artery disease, heart failure, or arrhythmia, consult with your physician before using EBs.
For the athlete participating in exercise lasting *less than 1 h*	1. Do not use EBs. 2. SDs appear safe, but do not consume EBs while exercising because of the possibility of dehydration, elevation of blood pressure, and lack of equivocal benefits versus water or SDs.
For the athlete participating in exercise *lasting 1 h or longer*	1. Do not use EBs. 2. SDs containing carbohydrates and electrolytes help prevent dehydration and restore important minerals lost through perspiration, and they produce better hydration than water.

Higgins, JP et al. Energy beverages: content and safety. Mayo Clin Proc 2010;85:1033. NACS Online. Energy Drink Sales Expected to Exceed $9 Billion by 2011. Available at: www.nacsonline.com/NACS/News/Daily_News_Archives/December2007/Pages/nd1210074.aspx. Accessed July 30, 2011.

and less protein than does a powder. As with nutrition bars, the FDA and other federal or state agencies make no independent assessment of the validity of labeling claims for macronutrient content and composition.

TABLE 8.1 provides the macronutrient composition for commercially packaged liquid food supplements (rapid stomach emptying with low residue and gastrointestinal distress), high-carbohydrate drinks, and "high-energy" bars typically advocated for physically active persons. Prudent use of some of these supplements can replenish glycogen reserves before and after intense exercise and competition, especially because an athlete's appetite for "normal" food wanes.

CARBOHYDRATE FEEDING BEFORE, DURING, AND FOLLOWING INTENSE EXERCISE

The "vulnerability" of the body's glycogen stores during intense, prolonged exercise has focused considerable research on potential benefits of carbohydrate feedings immediately before and during exercise. Failure to maintain adequate muscle and liver glycogen depots can quickly bring strenuous exercise to a grinding halt as often occurs during intense endurance competitions. This need to optimize glycogen storage also includes ways to most effectively replenish carbohydrate in the postexercise recovery period.

Carbohydrate Feedings Before Exercise

Confusion exists about potential endurance benefits of pre-exercise ingestion of simple sugars. One could argue that consuming high-glycemic, rapidly absorbed carbohydrates (see **FIG. 8.3**) within 1 h before exercising would negatively affect endurance performance in one of two ways:

1. Inducing an overshoot in insulin from the rapid rise in blood sugar. Insulin excess causes a relative hypoglycemia called **rebound hypoglycemia**. Blood sugar reduction impairs central nervous system function during exercise to produce a fatiguing effect.
2. Facilitating glucose influx into muscle through large insulin release to increase carbohydrate catabolism for energy in exercise. Simultaneously, high insulin levels inhibit lipolysis, reducing free fatty acid mobilization from adipose tissue. Both augmented carbohydrate breakdown and depressed fat mobilization contribute to premature glycogen depletion and early fatigue.

Research in the late 1970s indicated that drinking a highly concentrated sugar solution 30 min before exercise precipitated early fatigue in endurance activities. For example, endurance on a bicycle ergometer declined 19% when subjects consumed a 300-mL solution containing 75 g of glucose 30 min before exercise compared with riding time preceded by the same volume of plain water or a liquid meal of protein, lipid, and carbohydrate.[31] Paradoxically, consuming the concentrated pre-event sugar drink (in contrast to drinking plain water) hastily depleted muscle glycogen reserves. This occurred because the dramatic rise in blood sugar within 5 to 10 min after ingestion produced an overshoot in insulin release from the pancreas known as **accentuated hyperinsulinemia**, followed by rebound hypoglycemia as glucose moved rapidly into muscle.[38,121] At the same time, insulin inhibited fat mobilization for energy, an effect that can last for several hours after consuming a concentrated sugar solution. During exercise, intramuscular carbohydrate catabolized to a greater degree than under normal conditions, increasing the rate of glycogen depletion.

These negative research findings seem impressive and their explanation reasonable, yet such results have *not* been replicated in subsequent investigations of healthy subjects[1,21,29,36] or patients with type 1 diabetes.[80] In fact, pre-exercise glucose ingestion *increased* muscle glucose uptake but *reduced* liver glucose output during exercise, to conserve liver glycogen.[60] The discrepancy among studies has no clear explanation. One way to eliminate any potential for negative effects of pre-exercise simple sugars is to consume them at least 60 min prior to exercise. This provides sufficient time to re-establish hormonal balance before exercise begins. In all likelihood, individual differences exist in the response to specific carbohydrate ingestion before exercise and subsequent insulin release. The person's pre-exercise glucose or glycogen status plays a role including a food's glycemic index (GI) (see page 263).

SUPPLEMENT USE AMONG ELITE ATHLETES

A recent survey of high-performance Canadian athletes indicated that 88.4% reported taking one or more dietary supplements during the previous 6 months. Of the supplements used, sport drinks (22.4%), sport bars (14.0%), multivitamins and minerals (13.5%), protein supplements (9.0%), and vitamin C (6.4%) were the most frequently reported.[27]

Pre-exercise Fructose: Not a Good Alternative

Fructose, a six-carbon isomer of glucose (same molecular formula but structurally different), was discovered in 1847 by French chemist Augustin-Pierre Dubrunfaut (1797–1881). The fructose molecule, the sweetest of all the naturally occurring carbohydrates—1.73 times as sweet as sucrose—absorbs more slowly from the gut than either glucose or sucrose. Fructose, with the lowest GI of 19 compared to all the natural sugars, causes only minimal insulin response with essentially no decline in blood glucose. Recall that carbohydrates that degrade quickly during digestion and release glucose rapidly into the bloodstream have a high GI, whereas carbohydrates that degrade more slowly release glucose more gradually into the bloodstream and have a low GI. These observations have stimulated debate about the possible benefits of fructose as an immediate pre-exercise exogenous carbohydrate fuel source for prolonged exercise. From a practical but undesirable standpoint, consuming a high-fructose beverage often produces vomiting and diarrhea, which obviously would negatively impact subsequent exercise performance. Once absorbed by the small intestine, fructose must first enter the liver for conversion to glucose. We have previously pointed out that fructose exists in foods as either a monosaccharide (free fructose) or a unit of the sucrose disaccharide molecule. The small intestine directly absorbs free fructose. But when consumed in the form of sucrose, fructose digestion

TABLE 8.1 Composition of Commercial Carbohydrate Supplements in Liquid and Solid Form

Beverage	kcal per 8-oz Serving	Carbohydrate, g	Lipid, g	Protein, g
GatorPro Sports Nutrition	360	58 (65%)	7 (17%)	16 (18%)
Nutrament	240	34 (57%)	6.5 (25%)	11 (18%)
SportShake	310	45 (58%)	10 (29%)	11 (13%)
SegoVery	180	30 (67%)	2.5 (13%)	9 (20%)
Go	190	27 (56%)	3 (13%)	15 (31%)
Sustacal	240	33 (55%)	5.5 (21%)	14.5 (24%)
Ensure	254	35 (54%)	9 (32%)	9 (14%)
Endura Optimizer	279	57 (82%)	<1 (2%)	11 (16%)
Metabolol II	258	40 (62%)	2 (7%)	20 (31%)
ProOptibol	266	44 (66%)	2 (7%)	18 (27%)
Muscle Pep	261	45 (69%)	1 (3%)	18 (28%)
Protein Repair Formula	200	26 (52%)	1.5 (8%)	20 (40%)

High Carbohydrate Beverages

Beverage	Carbohydrate, type	Serving Size, oz	Carbohydrate, g per oz	% Carbohydrate
GatorLode	Maltodextrin & glucose	12	5.9	20
Carboplex	Maltodextrin		7.1	24
Exceed	Maltodextrin & sucrose	32	7.1	24
Carbo Fire	Glucose, polymers, fructose		7.1	24
Ultra Fuel	Maltodextrin	16	6.25	23
Carbo Power	Maltodextrin, high-fructose corn syrup		7.9	18

Sports Energy Bars

Bar	Size, oz	Total kcal	Carbohydrate, g	Protein, g	Lipid, g
Power Bar	2.25	225	42 (75%)	10 (17%)	2 (8%)
Exceed Sports Bar	2.9	280	53 (76%)	12 (17%)	2 (7%)
Edgebar	2.5	234	44 (75%)	10 (17%)	2 (8%)
K-Trainer	2.25	220	40 (73%)	10 (18%)	2 (9%)
Tiger Sport	2.3	230	40 (70%)	11 (19%)	3 (11%)
Thunder Bar	2.25	220	41 (74%)	10 (18%)	2 (8%)
Ultra Fuel	4.87	290	100 (82%)	15 (12%)	3 (6%)
Clif Bar	2.4	252	52 (80%)	5 (8%)	3 (12%)
Gator Bar	2.25	220	48 (87%)	3 (5%)	2 (8%)
Forza	2.5	231	45 (78%)	10 (18%)	1 (4%)
BTU Stoker	2.6	252	46 (73%)	10 (16%)	3 (11%)
PR Bar	1.6	190	19 (40%)	14 (30%)	6 (30%)

Carbohydrate content of common foods: 4 chocolate chip cookies = 28 g; 1 cup Wheaties (1 oz) = 23 g; 1 apple = 21 g; 1 cup apple juice = 29 g; 1 banana = 27 g
Protein content of common foods: 1 cup milk = 8 g; 3 oz baked salmon = 21 g; 1 cup cooked peas = 16 g; 3 oz steak = 22 g; 1 large egg = 6 g.

occurs only in the upper portion of the small intestine. As sucrose contacts the intestinal membranes, the enzyme sucrase catalyzes the cleavage of sucrose to produce one unit each of glucose and fructose. Fructose then enters the hepatic portal vein that drains blood from the gastrointestinal tract and spleen to capillary beds in the liver, further limiting how quickly fructose becomes available as an energy source.

KEEP IT GLUCOSE

Do not substitute exogenous fructose for glucose during prolonged exercise because less fructose oxidizes when consuming equivalent amounts of both sugars.[62]

Carbohydrate Feedings During Exercise: Some Added Protein May Help

Intense aerobic exercise for 1 h decreases liver glycogen by about 55%, whereas a 2-h strenuous workout almost totally depletes the glycogen content of the liver and exercised muscle fibers. Even maximal, repetitive, 1- to 5-min bouts of exercise interspersed with periods of lower intensity exercise—as in soccer, ice hockey, field hockey, European handball, and tennis—dramatically lower liver and muscle glycogen reserves.[41,94,101] Physical and mental performance improves with carbohydrate supplementation during exercise.[2,98,112,116,119] Carbohydrate feedings during prolonged exercise also allow persons to exercise at greater intensity, although their perception of physical effort remains no different than for a placebo group.[104]

The addition of protein to the carbohydrate-containing beverage may extend time to fatigue and reduce muscle damage compared to supplementation during exercise with carbohydrate only.[4,53,70,89] Two studies shed light on the importance of adding protein to carbohydrate-rich supplements during aerobic exercise. In one study,[30] researchers determined if consuming a supplement containing a mixture of different carbohydrates (glucose, maltodextrin, and fructose) plus a moderate amount of protein during endurance exercise would increase time to exhaustion, despite containing 50% less total carbohydrate than a carbohydrate-only supplement (CHO). Fifteen trained male and female cyclists exercised on two separate occasions at intensities alternating between 45 and 70% $\dot{V}O_{2max}$ for 3 h, after which the workload increased to between 74 and 85% $\dot{V}O_{2max}$ until voluntary exhaustion. Supplements (275 mL) were consumed every 20 min during exercise; they consisted of either a 3% carbohydrate plus 1.2% protein supplement (MCP) or a 6% CHO. With exercise at or below the ventilatory threshold (VT; indirect pulmonary indicator of point of blood lactate accumulation), time to exhaustion with the MCP supplement was significantly greater than with the CHO-only supplement (45.64 vs 35.47 min, respectively). The results suggested that a carbohydrate mixture plus a moderate amount of protein improved aerobic endurance at exercise intensities near the VT, despite containing a lower total carbohydrate and caloric content.

A second study[67] investigated the effects of a low mixed carbohydrate plus moderate protein supplement compared to a traditional 6% carbohydrate supplement consumed during endurance exercise on time to exhaustion. Fourteen trained female cyclists and triathletes cycled on two separate occasions for 3 h at intensities that varied between 45 and 70% $\dot{V}O_{2max}$, followed by a ride to exhaustion at an intensity approximating each person's VT (average 75% $\dot{V}O_{2max}$). Supplements (275 mL) were provided every 20 min during exercise and were composed of a carbohydrate mixture (1% each of dextrose, fructose, and maltodextrin) plus 1.2% protein (CHO + PRO) or 6% dextrose-only (CHO). Time to exhaustion was significantly greater when exercising with the CHO + PRO supplement (49.9 min) compared to the CHO-only supplement (42.4 min). Improved performance occurred despite the fact that the CHO + PRO supplement contained a lower carbohydrate and caloric content than the CHO-only supplement. The researchers speculated that the greater performance with CHO + PRO supplement resulted from the combined effects of protein and

CHEAPER MORE HEALTHFUL ALTERNATIVE WITH SIMILAR EFFECTIVENESS

Entrepreneurs continue to expand into the sports nutrition marketplace. As the ergogenic importance of consuming a carbohydrate supplement (usually in drink form) during endurance exercise to maintain muscle, liver, and blood carbohydrate levels becomes well established, business ventures have inserted diverse products for consumers to consider. One such product, Sport Beans – Energizing Jelly Beans, provides carbohydrate in gel form for ready and regular consumption during exercise to provide, in the company's words, "quick energy for sports performance." While consumption of such a product may prove beneficial, what remains unanswered is whether a cheaper and perhaps more nutritious product may prove equally beneficial. To test this hypothesis, researchers examined the effects of a natural carbohydrate source in the form of sun-dried raisins versus Sport Beans on endurance performance of trained cyclists and triathletes.[1,2] Randomized exercise trials administered in crossover fashion consisted of a 120-min, constant-load, glycogen depletion period followed by a 10-km time trial. During each trial, subjects consumed an isocaloric quantity of either the raisins or the Sport Beans at 20-min intervals. No significant differences emerged between trials for endurance performance, power output, or ratings of perceived exertion. However, sensory acceptance scores (product pleasantness) rated higher for the raisins. The conclusion is that sun-dried raisins are a natural, pleasant-tasting, cost-effective carbohydrate alternative to commercial jelly beans as a supplement during moderate-to-intense aerobic exercise.

1. Campbell C, et al. Carbohydrate-supplement form and exercise performance. *Int J Sport Nutr Exerc Metab* 2008;18:179.
2. Rietschier HL, et al. Sun-dried raisins are a cost-effective alternative so sports jelly beans in prolonged cycling. *J Strength Cond Res* 2011;25:3150.

carbohydrate plus the mixture of diverse carbohydrate sources within the supplement.

Although no beneficial effects occurred in experienced rugby players on functional and metabolic markers of *recovery* from a rugby union-specific shuttle running protocol with carbohydrate plus protein supplementation compared to a CHO,[85] positive effects of such supplementation *during* endurance performance were confirmed in a meta-analysis of 88 randomized crossover studies involving consumption of carbohydrate or carbohydrate plus protein supplements.[107]

The results revealed the following salient findings:

1. Effects of carbohydrate supplements ranged from clear, large improvements of 6% to moderate impairments of 2%.
2. The most effective supplement consisted of a 3 to 10% carbohydrate-plus-protein drink that provided $0.7\ g \cdot kg^{-1} \cdot h^{-1}$ of glucose polymers, $0.2\ g \cdot kg^{-1} \cdot h^{-1}$ of fructose, and $0.2\ g \cdot kg^{-1} \cdot h^{-1}$ of protein.
3. Increases in the benefit of a supplement were *small* with an additional 9-h fast and $0.2\ g \cdot kg^{-1} \cdot h^{-1}$ of protein, *probably small to moderate* with ingesting the first bolus not at the start of exercise but 1 to 4 h before exercise, and *possibly small* with increasing the frequency of ingestion by three boluses an hour.
4. The effects of exercise duration depend on the concentration of the supplement's carbohydrate plus protein content.

No Abnormal Insulin Response During Exercise

Consuming high-glycemic sugars *during* exercise does *not* augment the insulin response and possible hypoglycemia that could occur with sugar consumption in the pre-exercise condition. This occurs because sympathetic nervous system hormones in exercise inhibit insulin release. Concurrently, exercise facilitates glucose uptake by muscle so the exogenous glucose moves into these cells with a lower insulin requirement.

Consuming about 60 g of liquid or solid carbohydrates each hour benefits intense, long-duration (≥1 h) aerobic exercise and repetitive short bouts of near-maximal effort.[3,16,17,50,66] As reviewed in Chapter 5, sustained exercise at or below 50% of maximum intensity relies primarily on energy from fat oxidation, with relatively little demand on carbohydrate breakdown. This level of exercise does not tax glycogen reserves to a degree that would hinder endurance. In contrast, glucose feedings provide supplementary carbohydrate during intense exercise when glycogen demand for energy increases greatly. In fact, mixtures of glucose, fructose, and sucrose ingested simultaneously at a rate between 1.8 and $2.4\ g \cdot min^{-1}$ result in a 20 to 55% higher exogenous carbohydrate oxidation rate peak as high as $1.7\ g \cdot min^{-1}$ (with reduced oxidation of endogenous carbohydrate) compared with ingestion of an isocaloric amount of glucose.[12,14,49,87,88]

Exogenous carbohydrate intake during exercise provides the following two benefits:

1. Spares muscle glycogen, particularly in the type I, slow-twitch muscle fibers, because the ingested glucose powers exercise.[102,103]
2. Maintains a more optimal level of blood glucose. This elevates plasma insulin levels and lowers cortisol and growth hormone levels and prevents headache, lightheadedness, nausea, and other symptoms of central nervous system distress.[11,73,111,122] Blood glucose maintenance also supplies muscles with glucose when glycogen reserves deplete in the later stages of prolonged exercise.[20,38]

FIGURE 8.1 shows that training status does not alter the ability to oxidize glucose during exercise when trained and untrained persons exercise at the same relative intensity. Seven trained cyclists and seven untrained subjects exercised for 2 h at 60% of aerobic capacity. At the onset of exercise, each subject consumed $8\ mL \cdot kg^{-1}$ body mass of an 8% naturally labeled [^{13}C]-glucose solution with $2\ mL \cdot kg^{-1}$ body mass of the fluid ingested every 20 min thereafter. Total exogenous [^{13}C]-glucose use ($3.2\ kcal \cdot min^{-1}$) was similar in both groups despite a 24% higher absolute oxygen uptake in the trained subjects (36 vs $29\ mL\ O_2 \cdot kg^{-1} \cdot min^{-1}$; **FIG. 8.1A**) and higher total fat oxidation. *About 1.5 to 1.7 g (6.0–6.8 kcal) per minute represents the upper limit for oxidizing exogenous carbohydrate.*[49,51,113,114] Equivalence in exogenous glucose use between trained and untrained

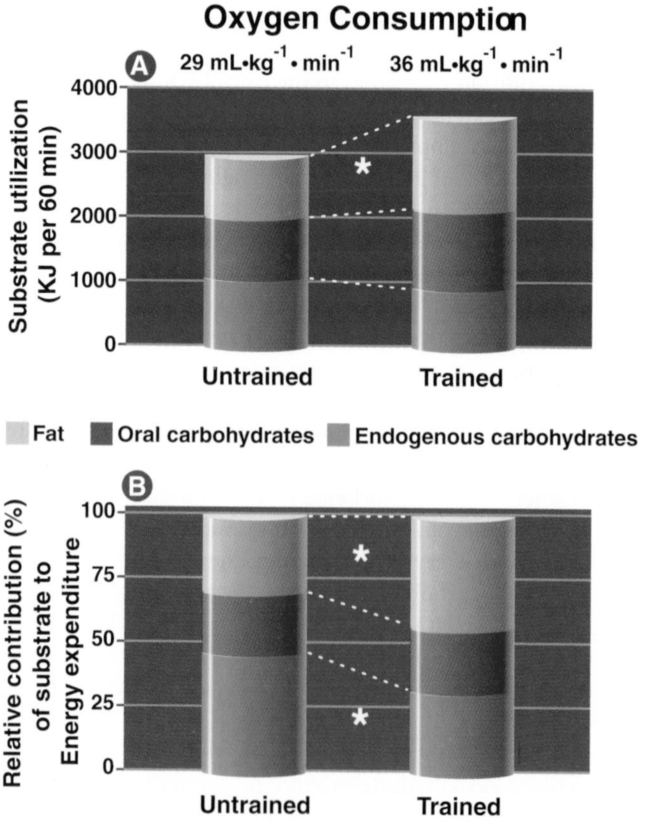

FIGURE 8.1. **(A)** Absolute (kJ per 60 min of exercise) and **(B)** relative (%) contributions of substrates to energy expenditure in endurance-trained and untrained men. (*) Statistically significant difference between trained and untrained men. Multiply by 0.239 to convert kilojoules to kilocalories. (From Jeukendrup AE, et al. Exogenous glucose oxidation during exercise in endurance-trained and untrained subjects. *J Appl Physiol* 1997;83:835.)

subjects occurred even with a relatively smaller contribution of exogenous and endogenous carbohydrate to the higher total energy expenditure of the trained subjects (**FIG. 8.1B**). This suggests that carbohydrate absorption from the gastrointestinal tract into the circulation limits ingested carbohydrate's catabolism rate during exercise independent of training state.

A Distinct Ergogenic Advantage in Intense Aerobic Exercise

Carbohydrate feeding during exercise at 60 to 80% of aerobic capacity postpones fatigue by 15 to 30 min, with performance improvement generally ranging between 15 and 35%. This effect, potentially important in long-distance running, occurs because fatigue in well-nourished persons usually becomes noticeable after 2 h of intense exercise. A person can deflect fatigue and extend endurance with a single concentrated carbohydrate feeding consumed approximately 30 min before anticipated fatigue. **FIGURE 8.2** shows that this feeding restores the level of blood glucose, which then sustains the energy needs of active muscles.

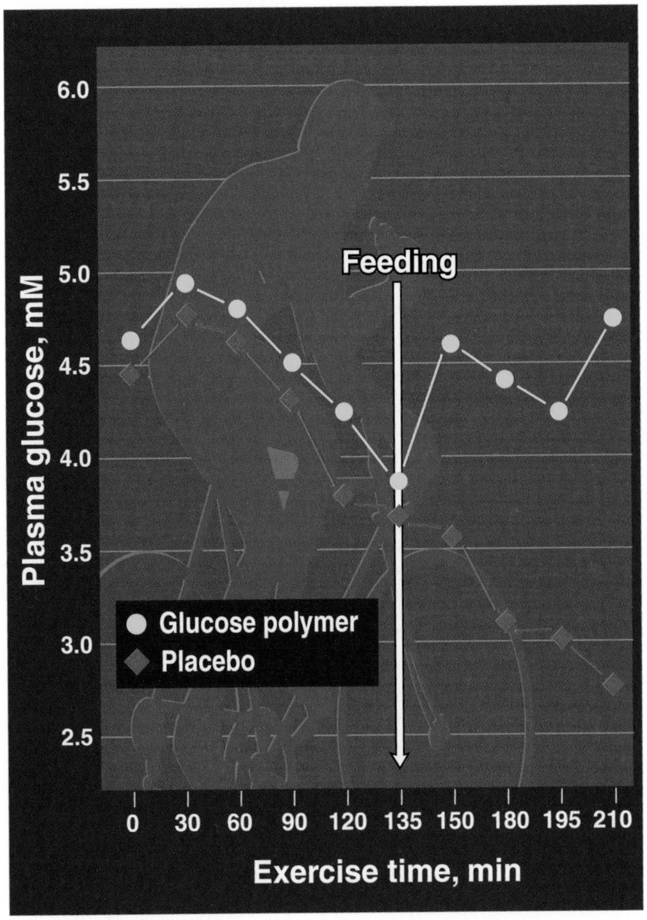

FIGURE 8.2. Average plasma glucose concentration during prolonged high-intensity aerobic exercise when subjects consumed either a placebo or glucose polymer (3 g · kg^{-1} body mass in a 50% solution). (Modified from Coggan AR, Coyle EF. Metabolism and performance following carbohydrate ingestion late in exercise. *Med Sci Sports Exerc* 1989;21:59.)

Endurance benefits from carbohydrate feedings become apparent at about 75% of aerobic capacity. When exercise initially exceeds this intensity, a person must reduce intensity to the 75% level during the final stages to maintain the benefits from carbohydrate intake.[20] Repeated feedings of solid carbohydrate (43 g sucrose with 400 mL water) at the beginning and at 1, 2, and 3 h during exercise maintain blood glucose and slow glycogen depletion during 4 h of cycling. Maintaining blood glucose and glycogen reserves also enhances intense exercise performance to exhaustion at the end of the activity.[3,6,59,83,96] The winner of a marathon run is usually the athlete who sustains intense aerobic effort and sprints to the finish.

REPLENISHING GLYCOGEN RESERVES: REFUELING FOR THE NEXT BOUT OF INTENSE TRAINING OR COMPETITION

All carbohydrates do not digest and absorb at the same rate. Plant starch composed primarily of amylose represents a more resistant carbohydrate because of its relatively slow hydrolysis rate. Conversely, starch with relatively high amylopectin content digests and absorbs more rapidly.

The Glycemic Index

The ***GI*** *serves as a relative (qualitative) indicator of how carbohydrate-containing food affects blood glucose levels.* The rise in blood sugar—termed the *glycemic response*—is determined after ingesting a food containing 50 g of a digestible carbohydrate (total carbohydrate minus fiber) and comparing it over a 2-h period with a "standard" for carbohydrate (usually white bread or glucose) with an assigned value of 100.[8,120] The GI, formulated in 1980 to 1981 by University of Toronto researchers,[46,47] expresses the percentage of total area under the blood glucose response curve for a specific food compared with glucose (**FIG. 8.3**). Thus, a food with a GI of 45 indicates that ingesting 50 g of the food raises blood glucose concentrations to levels that reach 45% of that reached with 50 g of glucose. The GI provides a more useful physiologic concept than simply classifying a carbohydrate on the basis of its chemical configuration as simple or complex, sugar or starch, or available or unavailable. One international listing of GI values contains nearly 1300 entries that represent values of more than 750 different food types.[32] Differences in values exist within the literature, depending on the laboratory and exact food type evaluated (e.g., slight variations in type of white bread, rice, and potatoes used as the standard of comparison). Do not view the GI as an unwavering standard because considerable variability exists among persons consuming a specific carbohydrate-containing food. A high GI rating does not necessarily indicate poor nutritional quality.[78] For example, carrots, brown rice, and corn, with their rich quantities of health-protective micronutrients, phytochemicals, and dietary fiber, have relatively high GIs.

The GI reflects individual differences in response to how food is digested, its preparation, and its ripeness. For example,

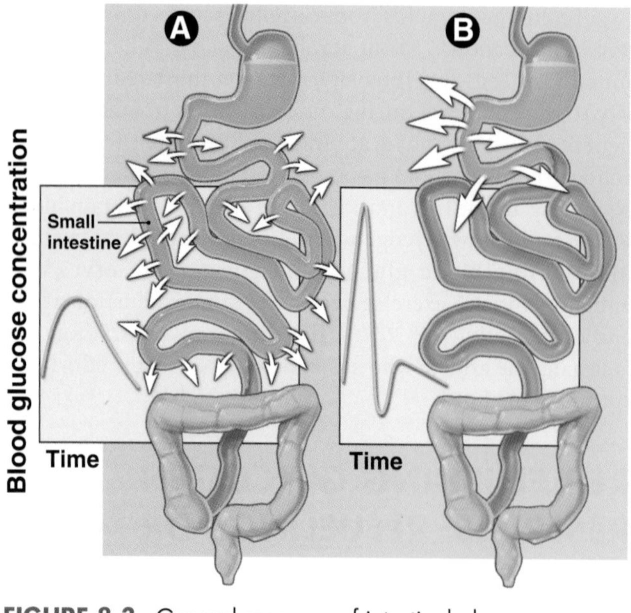

FIGURE 8.3. General response of intestinal glucose absorption following feeding of foods with either **(A)** low GI or **(B)** high GI such as glucose. The low-glycemic food absorbs at a slower rate throughout the full length of the small intestine to produce a more gradual rise in blood glucose.

NOT SIMPLY THE CARBOHYDRATE FORM

The GI is a function of glucose appearance in the systemic circulation and its uptake by peripheral tissues, which is influenced by the properties of the carbohydrate-containing food. For example, a food's high amylose-to-amylopectin ratio or high fiber and fat content slow intestinal glucose absorption, whereas the protein content of the food may augment insulin release to facilitate glucose uptake by the cells.[90]

a ripe banana has a higher GI than a "greener" banana. Once foods are combined (i.e., a ripe banana eaten with three flavors of ice cream topped with nuts and chocolate fudge), the meal's GI for that combination of foods differs from the GI for the separate items.

The revised GI listing also includes the **glycemic load** associated with the specified serving sizes of different foods. Whereas the GI compares equal quantities of a carbohydrate-containing food, the glycemic load quantifies the overall glycemic effect of a typical food *portion*. This represents the

Connections to the Past

August Krogh (1874–1949)

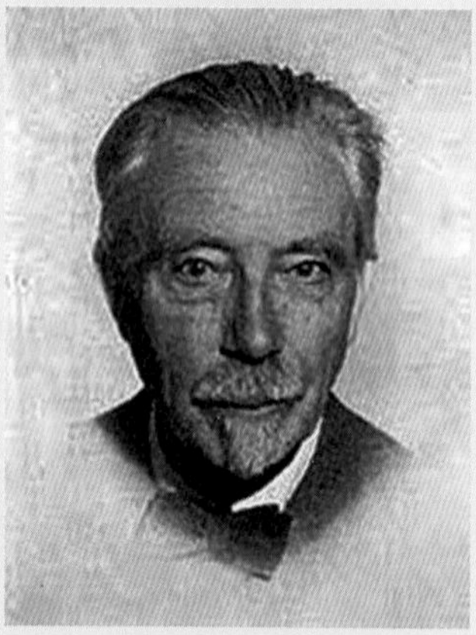

August Krogh began his career in the laboratory of the noted Danish physician-physiologist Christian Harald Bohr (1855–1911; father of physicist and 1922 Physics Nobel laureate Niels Henrik Bohr (1885-1962) and mathematician Harald Bohr; (1887–1951), who himself had been trained by physiologist Carl Ludwig (1816–1895) in Leipzig. Bohr had already clarified the dynamics of muscle contraction and solubility of oxygen in different fluids including blood. His studies of oxygen influenced Krogh's early experiments of tissue respiration in animals. Krogh devised equipment to measure respiratory gas exchange in snails, frogs, and fishes. Krogh's *An Account of the Structure and Function of the Lungs and Air Sacks of Birds*, the equivalent of a Master's thesis (1899), proved oxygen diffused rapidly through the thin pulmonary membranes, while the skin eliminated carbon dioxide. Subsequent experiments in gas transport corrected the prevailing view that lungs were gland-type structure that *secreted* oxygen and carbon dioxide. Krogh's highly accurate equipment analyzed respiratory gases, and established that pulmonary gas was exchanged by the mechanism of diffusion, not secretion. The problem solved by Krogh was whether nitrogen or nitrogenous gases were released from the body as a normal by-product of metabolism. In 1906, he proved that gaseous nitrogen remained constant, solving a vexing question in physiology. Krogh's fresh approach to this and other problems using respiratory methods to quantify nitrogen dynamics also won fame. The methods succeeded without using the traditional German method that measured nitrogen in ingested food and fluid and excreted nitrogen in feces and urine. Krogh published nearly 300 research papers, many of which are considered "classics" in exercise physiology. He also devised a bicycle ergometer with magnets and weights to quantify power output and exercise intensity. He was awarded the 1920 Nobel Prize in Physiology or Medicine for the discovery of the mechanism of regulation of the capillaries in skeletal muscle.

thePoint

Visit **thePoint.lww.com/MKKSEN4e** *for more details about how Nobel Prize winner August Krogh's insightful experiments influenced basic and applied research in the biological sciences, including the emerging field of exercise physiology.*

product of the amount of available carbohydrate in that serving and the food's GI. A high glycemic load reflects a greater expected elevation in blood glucose and a greater insulin release. An increased risk for type 2 diabetes and coronary heart disease coincides with the chronic consumption of a diet with a high glycemic load.[45,58]

Not All Carbohydrates Are Equal

FIGURE 8.4 *(top)* lists the GI for common items in various food groupings. **FIGURE 8.4** *(bottom)* gives examples of high- and low-GI meals of similar calorie and macronutrient composition. For easy identification, we have placed foods into high, moderate, and low GI categories. Interestingly, a

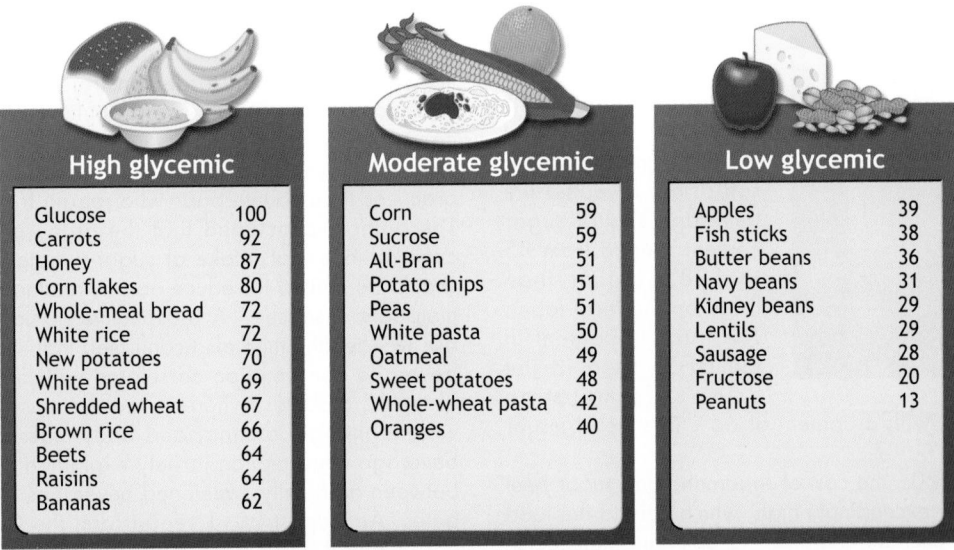

High glycemic	
Glucose	100
Carrots	92
Honey	87
Corn flakes	80
Whole-meal bread	72
White rice	72
New potatoes	70
White bread	69
Shredded wheat	67
Brown rice	66
Beets	64
Raisins	64
Bananas	62

Moderate glycemic	
Corn	59
Sucrose	59
All-Bran	51
Potato chips	51
Peas	51
White pasta	50
Oatmeal	49
Sweet potatoes	48
Whole-wheat pasta	42
Oranges	40

Low glycemic	
Apples	39
Fish sticks	38
Butter beans	36
Navy beans	31
Kidney beans	29
Lentils	29
Sausage	28
Fructose	20
Peanuts	13

High GI Diet	CHO (g)	Contribution to Total GI	Low GI Diet	CHO (g)	Contribution to Total GI
Breakfast			**Breakfast**		
30 g Corn Flakes	25	9.9	30 g All-Bran	24	4.7
1 banana	30	7.8	1 diced peach	8	1.1
1 slice whole meal bread	12	3.8	1 slice grain bread	14	2.2
1 tsp margarine			1 tsp margarine		
			1 tsp jelly		
Snack			**Snack**		
1 crumpet	20	6.4	1 slice grain fruit loaf	20	4.1
1 tsp margarine			1 tsp margarine		
Lunch			**Lunch**		
2 slices whole-meal bread	23.5	7.6	2 slices grain bread	28	4.5
2 tsp margarine			2 tsp margarine		
25 g cheese			25 g cheese		
1 cup diced cantaloupe	8	10.4	1 apple	20	3.6
Snack			**Snack**		
4 plain sweet biscuits	28	10.4	200 g low-fat fruit yogurt	26	4.1
Dinner			**Dinner**		
120 g lean steak			120 g lean minced beef		
1 cup of mashed potatoes	32	12.1	1 cup boiled pasta	34	6.4
1/2 cup of carrots	4	1.7	1 cup of tomato and onion sauce	8	2.5
1/2 cup of green beans	2	0.6	Green salad with vinaigrette	1	0.6
50 g broccoli					
Snack			**Snack**		
290 g watermelon	15	5.1	1 orange	10	2.1
1 cup of reduced-fat milk throughout day	14	1.9	1 cup of reduced-fat milk throughout day	14	1.9
Total	**212**	**69.8**	**Total**	**212**	**39.0**

For each diet, the carbohydrate choices are maximized for differences between the two diets.

FIGURE 8.4. *Top.* GI categorization of common food sources of carbohydrates. *Bottom.* Examples of high– and low–GI diets that contain the same amounts of energy and macronutrients and derive 50% of energy from carbohydrate (CHO) and 30% of energy from lipid. (Diets from Brand-Miller J, Foster-Powell K. *Nutr Today* 1999;34:64.)

Additional Insights

Does Consumption of Sugar-Sweetened Beverages Increase Disease Risk—A Devil in Disguise?

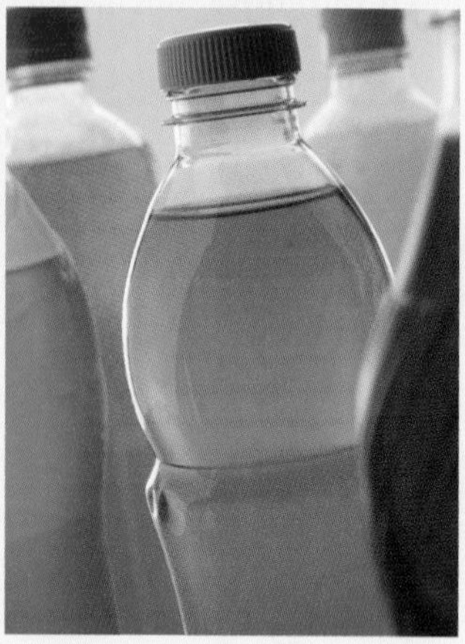

Background

High-fructose corn syrup (HFCS), originally developed in 1921, derives from glucose. Analysis of the fructose content of 20 of the most popular soft drinks revealed the beverage's *total* sugar content ranged from 85 to 128% higher than listed on the food label: The fructose content in the HFCS used in the drink's formulation *averaged* 59% with a content of 65% in several major brands.

In the mid-1970s, the cost of sugarcane and sugar beet imports became exceedingly high, which caused the food industry to seek alternative sweeteners. Soft drink manufacturers quickly began to replace sugar with the cheaper HFCS, and by the mid-1980s, all nondiet soft drinks contained HFCS. The average American currently consumes between 50 and 70 g (1.7–2.5 oz) of HFCS in sugar-sweetened beverages daily, which translates to an extra daily consumption of 200 to 250 kcal.

Health Impact

The association of sugar-sweetened beverage consumption with weight gain and risks of overweight and obesity has led some researchers to suggest that consumption of refined carbohydrates (of which HFCS represents the most prevalent) is likely to cause even greater metabolic damage than saturated fat. A recent meta-analysis of 11 studies with approximately 300,000 participants warns that the consumption of beverages sweetened with sugar and HFCS, including fruit juice concentrate, boosts type 2 diabetes risk—with the risk persisting even if the calories do not contribute to added body weight. Examples of such sugar-sweetened drinks include soft drinks, fruit drinks, iced tea, and energy and vitamin water beverages. The study showed that persons who drink one or two nondiet drinks daily increased their type 2 diabetes risk by 26% compared to those drinking less than one drink monthly. A 20% greater risk was also noted for the drinkers of sweetened beverages for central obesity, hypertension, abnormal cholesterol, insulin resistance, and lack of exercise, a cluster of factors that increase the risk of cardiovascular disease, stroke, and type 2 diabetes. Adjusting for body mass index reduced the risk, but it did not eliminate it, which indicates a separate effect of the sweetened drinks on disease risk.

The authors cautioned that this observational analysis was not designed to demonstrate a cause-and-effect relationship. The relationship could simply reflect that consumers of nondiet drinks lead an overall less healthy lifestyle that includes a lack of exercise and poor dietary practices than counterparts who refrain from such drinks. The authors concluded that the data "provide empirical evidence that intake of sugar-sweetened beverages should be limited to reduce obesity-related risk of chronic metabolic diseases." A prospective 20-year follow-up of 40,389 healthy men also confirmed that sugar-sweetened beverage consumption correlated with an elevated risk of type 2 diabetes, whereas health status, pre-enrollment weight change, dieting, and body mass index and *not* beverage consumption largely explained the association between artificially sweetened beverages and type 2 diabetes. An August 2011 report form the Centers for Disease Control and Prevention (CDC; www.cdc.gov/nchs/data/databriefs/db71.htm) revealed that 50% of Americans drink a soda or other sugary beverage each day with 1 in 20 people drinking the equivalent of more than four cans of soda daily.

Sources:

deKoning L, et al. Sugar-sweetened and artificially sweetened beverage consumption and risk of type diabetes in men. *Am J Clin Nutr* 2011;93:1321.

Ho CT. Soda warning? High-fructose corn syrup linked to diabetes, new study suggests. *Science Daily*, August 23, 2007.

Malik VS, et al. Sugar-sweetened beverages and risk of metabolic syndrome and type 2 diabetes: a meta-analysis. *Diabetes Care* 2010;33:2477.

Related References

Andreyeva T, et al. Exposure to food advertising on television: associations with children's fast food and soft drink consumption and obesity. *Econ Hum Biol* 2011:221.

Fung TT, et al. Sweetened beverage consumption and risk of coronary heart disease in women. *Am J Clin Nutr* 2009;89:1037.

Ogden CL, et al. Consumption of sugar drinks in the United States, 2005–2008. NCHS data brief, no 71. Hyattsville, MD: National Center for Health Statistics, 2011.

Ventura EE, et al. Sugar content of popular sweetened beverages based on objective laboratory analysis: focus on fructose content. *Obesity* 2011;19:868.

food's index rating does not depend simply on its classification as a "simple" (monosaccharides and disaccharides) or "complex" (starch and fiber) carbohydrate. This is because the plant starch in white rice and potatoes has a higher GI than the simple sugars (particularly fructose) in apples and peaches. A food's fiber content slows digestion rate; thus, peas, beans, and other legumes have a low GI. Ingesting lipids and proteins tends to slow the passage of food into the small intestine, thus reducing the GI of the meal's accompanying carbohydrate content. *Clearly, the most rapid method to replenish glycogen following exercise is to consume foods with moderate to high GIs rather than foods rated low,*[15,21,22,95,115] *even if the replenishment meal contains a small amount of lipid and protein.*[14] In fact, the addition of liquid protein to the carbohydrate supplement may even enhance the magnitude of glycogen resynthesis.[7] During the first 2 h of recovery, with muscle glycogen content at its lowest level, consuming a glucose polymer solution with low osmolality restores glycogen more rapidly than an energy-equivalent solution of monomers with high osmolality.[77] This beneficial effect of low-osmolality solutions on glycogen replenishment probably results from two factors:

1. More rapid gastric emptying and glucose delivery to the small intestine
2. Augmented postexercise-stimulated, non–insulin-dependent glucose uptake by the muscles. The addition of L-arginine to a carbohydrate-containing beverage offers no additional benefit to carbohydrate replenishment.[84]

The need for glycogen in previously active muscle augments glycogen resynthesis in the postexercise period.[75] When food becomes available following exercise, four factors facilitate cellular glucose uptake:

1. Hormonal milieu reflected by elevated insulin
2. Increased tissue sensitivity to insulin and other transporter proteins; examples include GLUT1 and GLUT4, members of a family of facilitative monosaccharide transporters that mediate glucose transport activity
3. Low catecholamine levels
4. Increased activity of glycogen synthase, a specific form of the glycogen-storing enzyme

To speed glycogen replenishment following intense training or competition, one should consume high-glycemic, carbohydrate-rich foods as quickly as possible. Follow this practical advice to rapidly restore depleted glycogen reserves:

1. Within 15 min after stopping exercise, consume 50 to 75 g (2–3 oz, or 1.0–1.5 g·kg^{-1} body mass) of high- to moderate-glycemic carbohydrates.
2. Continue eating 50 to 75 g of carbohydrate every 2 h until achieving 500 to 700 g (7–10 g·kg^{-1} body mass) or until eating a large high-carbohydrate meal.
3. If immediately ingesting carbohydrate following exercise proves impractical, an alternative strategy involves eating meals that contain 2.5 g of high-glycemic carbohydrate per kilogram of body mass at 2, 4, 6, 8, and 22 h after exercise. This regimen replenishes glycogen to levels similar to those achieved with the same protocol begun immediately after exercise.[54,74]

COMPARISON OF THE SUGAR CONTENT IN 12-OZ COKE AND PEPSI SOFT DRINKS

According to the Centers for Disease Control and Prevention, approximately one half of the US population consumes sugar drinks on any given day, with males consuming more sugar drinks than females, and teenagers and young adults consuming more sugar drinks than other age groups.

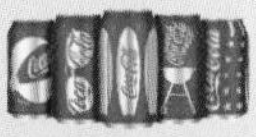

	Fluid, oz	Sugar, g	g·oz^{-1}
Cherry Coke	12	42	3.50
Coca-Cola Vanilla	12	42	3.50
Coca-Cola caffeine free	12	39	3.25
Coca-Cola Classic	12	40.5	3.38
Coca-Cola Regular	12	39	3.25
Mello Yello	12	48	4.00
Fanta Orange	12	44	3.67
Minute Maid Fruit Punch	12	43	3.58

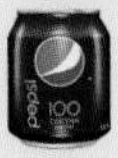

Pepsi Caffeine Free	12	41	3.42
Pepsi Wild Cherry	12	42	3.50
Pepsi-Cola	12	41	3.33
Pepsi Throwback	12	40	3.33
Sierra Mist Cranberry Splash	12	40	3.33
Mountain Dew	12	46	3.92
Citrus Blast	12	38	3.17
Mug Cream Soda	12	47	3.92

Sources: *Nutrition Connection. Available at:* http://productnutrition.thecoca-colacompany.com/welcome. *Accessed September 24, 2011; Pepsico. Available at:* www.pepsicobeveragefacts.com. *Accessed September 24, 2011.*

Ogden CL, et al. Consumption of sugar drinks in the United States, 2005–2008. NCHS Data Brief, No 71. Hyattsville, MD: National Center for Health Statistics, 2011. Available at: www.cdc.gov/nchs/data/databriefs/db71.htm/. Accessed January 20, 2012.

REPLACE FLUID AND ENERGY DURING EXERCISE

To optimize water and carbohydrate absorption, consume a 6% carbohydrate–electrolyte solution that combines fructose and sucrose, each transported by separate noncompetitive pathways.

Insulin-Stimulating Effect of Protein Ingestion in Recovery: Does It Augment Glycogen Replenishment?

Consuming an amino acid–protein mixture of whey protein hydrolysate with free leucine and phenylalanine ($0.4\ g \cdot kg^{-1} \cdot h^{-1}$) in a carbohydrate-containing beverage ($0.8\ g \cdot kg^{-1} \cdot h^{-1}$) facilitates more muscle glycogen storage without gastrointestinal discomfort than ingesting a carbohydrate-only beverage of the same concentration.[106] This advantage appears to relate to the insulinotropic effect of a higher level of plasma amino acids.[105,123] The benefit of added protein and/or amino acids and associated increased insulin release on glycogen replenishment is no greater than simply adding additional carbohydrate to the recovery supplement.[86] Trained athletes attained glycogen synthesis rates equivalent to those with a glucose plus protein supplement with a carbohydrate-only intake of $1.2\ g \cdot kg^{-1} \cdot h^{-1}$.[106] Supplements taken at 30-min intervals over a 5-h recovery period produced maximal glycogen resynthesis. Additional intake of protein or amino acids does not increase glycogen synthesis rate.

Defining the Optimal Nutritional Approach

Research has addressed the following question: Is it better to consume large meals or more frequent snacks of high-glycemic carbohydrates to optimize glycogen replenishment? One study compared 24-h carbohydrate replenishment with the following two patterns of consuming an energy-equivalent meal of high-glycemic carbohydrates[15]:

1. "Gorging" on a single large meal, with its greater incremental glucose and insulin response
2. "Nibbling" on frequent smaller snacks, which produces a more stable glucose and insulin response

The two styles of eating produced *no difference* in final glycogen levels. Thus, persons should eat high-glycemic carbohydrates following intense exercise; the frequency of the meals and snacks should dovetail with a person's appetite and availability of food following exercise.

Glycogen Replenishment Takes Time

Avoid legumes, fructose, and milk products when rapidly replenishing glycogen reserves because of their slow rates of intestinal absorption. More rapid glycogen resynthesis takes place if the person remains inactive during recovery.[19] *With optimal carbohydrate intake, glycogen stores replenish at about 5 to 7% an hour. Even under the best of circumstances, it takes at least 20 h to re-establish glycogen stores following a glycogen-depleting exercise bout.*

Optimal glycogen replenishment benefits persons involved in these three types of activities:

1. Regular intense training
2. Tournament competition with qualifying rounds
3. Competitive events scheduled with only 1 or 2 days for recuperation

Before current methods for establishing a wrestler's minimal wrestling weight (see Chapter 14), wrestlers who lost considerable glycogen (and water) using food and fluid restriction before the weigh-in to "make weight" also benefited from a proper glycogen replenishment strategy.[44] For collegiate wrestlers, short-term weight loss through energy restriction without dehydration also impaired anaerobic exercise capacity.[81] Anaerobic performance recovered to near-baseline values when these athletes then consumed meals containing 75% carbohydrate over the next 5 h (equivalent to $21\ kcal \cdot kg^{-1}$ body mass). No improvement occurred if the refeeding diet contained only 45% carbohydrate. Even without full glycogen replenishment, some replenishment in recovery benefits endurance in the next exercise bout. For example, replenishing carbohydrate after only a 4-h recovery period from glycogen-depleting exercise yields better endurance in subsequent exercise than a similar scenario without carbohydrate consumed in recovery.

THE IDEAL ORAL REHYDRATION BEVERAGE

1. Tastes good
2. Absorbs rapidly
3. Causes little or no gastrointestinal distress
4. Maintains extracellular fluid volume and osmolality
5. Offers the potential to enhance exercise performance

Choose the Right Form of Carbohydrate

To evaluate the influence of a carbohydrate's structure on glycogen replenishment, eight male cyclists decreased the glycogen content of the vastus lateralis muscle with 60 min of cycling at 75% $\dot{V}O_{2max}$ followed by six 1-min sprints at 125% $\dot{V}O_{2max}$.[52] Twelve hours after the glycogen-depleting exercise, they consumed a 3000-kcal meal (ratio of 65%:20%:15% carbohydrate to lipid to protein). A solution of glucose, maltodextrin (glucose polymer), waxy starch (100% amylopectin), or resistant starch (100% amylose) provided all of the recovery meal's carbohydrate. Muscle biopsies taken 24 h into recovery (**FIG. 8.5**) revealed a lower glycogen repletion level from the resistant starch meal (high amylose content, low GI) than from meals with the other, more rapidly hydrolyzed carbohydrates. Keeping to the prescribed carbohydrate intake in the immediate recovery period produces more desirable glycogen replenishment than letting athletes eat the amount they wish.

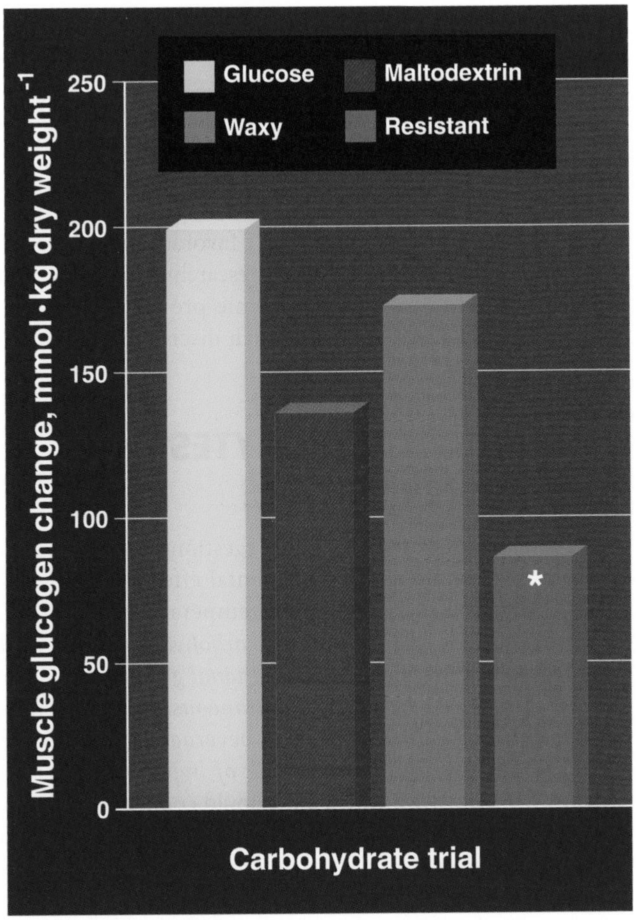

FIGURE 8.5. Changes in muscle glycogen with various carbohydrate feedings of similar energy content in the 24-h period following glycogen-depleting exercise. (*) Denotes significantly lower value than glucose, maltodextrin, and waxy starch. (From Jozsi AC, et al. The influence of starch structure on glycogen resynthesis and subsequent cycling performance. *Int J Sports Med* 1996;17:373.)

INGESTED PROTEIN DURING ENDURANCE EXERCISE MAY DELAY FATIGUE

Leucine, valine, and isoleucine, the branched chain amino acids (BCAAs) from muscle, can oxidize in energy metabolism during exercise, which suggests they may play important roles during endurance activities.[1] It remains unclear, however, whether consuming a protein supplement *during* exercise provides an ergogenic boost. Two lines of research suggest that protein consumption during exercise could benefit endurance performance:

1. Increased insulin stimulation: A combination carbohydrate plus protein supplement consumed during exercise stimulates insulin secretion, which in turn conserves muscle and liver glycogen as exercise progresses.[2]
2. Suppression of central fatigue: The level of circulating BCAAs decrease as endurance exercise progresses. Concurrently, the essential amino acid tryptophan unloads from albumin at a high rate into plasma. Thus, BCAAs and tryptophan compete for the same transporters that facilitate their transfer across the blood-brain barrier. When BCAA levels decrease, a higher percentage of tryptophan attaches to the transporters to increase the brain's tryptophan uptake. Tryptophan then converts to serotonin to produce a relaxation effect that ultimately causes a fatigued sensation and resulting decrease in exercise performance.[3,4] This suggests that ingesting BCAAs during exercise to maintain their plasma concentration should delay serotonin-induced fatigue and subsequently enhance endurance performance. Mixed support for this hypothesis continues to generate new research.[5–11]

1. Grahm TE, et al. Training and muscle ammonia amino acid metabolism in humans during prolonged exercise. *J Appl Physiol* 1995;69:287.
2. Ivy JL, et al. Effect of a carbohydrate-protein supplement on endurance performance during exercise of varying intensity. *Int J Sport Nutr Exerc Metabol* 2003;13:382.
3. Davis JM, Bailey SP. Possible mechanisms of central nervous system fatigue during exercise. *Med Sci Sports Exerc* 1997;29:45.
4. Davis JM. Carbohydrates, branched-chain amino acids, and endurance: the central fatigue hypothesis. *Int J Sport Nutr* 1995;5:S29.
5. Bailey SJ, et al. Acute L-arginine supplementation reduces the O_2 cost of moderate-intensity exercise and enhances high-intensity exercise tolerance. *J Appl Physiol* 2010;109:1394.
6. Blomstrand E, et al. Administration of branched-chain amino acids during sustained exercise: effects on performance and on plasma concentration of some amino acids. *Eur J Appl Physiol* 1991;63:83.
7. Blomstrand E, et al. Effect of branched-chained amino acid and carbohydrate supplementation on the exercise-induced change in plasma and muscle concentration of amino acids in human subjects. *Acta Physiol Scand* 1996;153:87.
8. Hsu MC, et al. Effects of BCAA, arginine and carbohydrate combined drink on post-exercise biochemical response and psychological condition. *Chin J Physiol* 2011;54:71.
9. Javierre C, et al. L-tryptophan supplementation can decrease fatigue perception during an aerobic exercise with supramaximal intercalated anaerobic bouts in young healthy men. *Int J Neurosci* 2010;120:319.
10. Mittleman KD, et al. Branched-chain amino acids prolong exercise during heat stress in men and women. *Med Sci Sports Exerc* 1998;30:83.
11. Van Hall G, et al. Ingestion of branched-chain amino acids and tryptophan during sustained exercise in man; failure to affect performance. *J Physiol* 1995;486:789.

THE GLYCEMIC INDEX AND PRE-EXERCISE FEEDINGS

Use the GI to formulate the immediate pre-exercise feeding. The ideal meal immediately before exercising should provide a source of glucose to maintain blood sugar and sustain muscle metabolism; it also should not trigger a spike in insulin release. A relatively normal plasma insulin level theoretically preserves blood glucose availability and optimizes fat mobilization and catabolism while sparing glycogen reserves. As mentioned previously, consuming simple sugars (i.e., concentrated high-glycemic carbohydrates) immediately before exercising causes blood sugar to rise rapidly (called the **glycemic response**), often triggering excessive insulin release (called the **insulinemic response**). The following resulting cascade of three factors negatively affects endurance exercise performance:

1. Rebound hypoglycemia
2. Depressed fat catabolism
3. Early depletion of glycogen reserves

Consuming low-GI foods (e.g., starch with high amylose content) immediately before exercise provides a relatively slow rate of glucose absorption into the blood. This eliminates any possible insulin surge, while a steady supply of "slow-release" glucose becomes available from the digestive tract as exercise progresses. This effect theoretically proves beneficial during long-term, intense exercise, particularly in unusual long-distance events such as ocean swimming or 100-mile, nonstop hikes where the practicality of consuming carbohydrate during such extreme physical activities remains a challenge.[118]

Several studies support the wisdom of consuming low-glycemic carbohydrates (starch with high amylose content or moderate-glycemic carbohydrate with high dietary fiber content) in the immediate 45- to 60-min period before exercise. The response to such a regimen allows for a slower rate of glucose absorption, thus reducing the potential rebound glycemic response. For trained cyclists who performed intense aerobic exercise, a pre-exercise low-glycemic meal of lentils extended endurance compared with feedings of either glucose or a high-glycemic meal of potatoes of equivalent carbohydrate content.[13] Higher blood glucose levels near the end stages of exercise accompanied the low-glycemic, pre-exercise feeding.[25,37] Despite inducing potentially favorable alterations in blood glucose and fat catabolism, all research has not observed ergogenic benefits from low-glycemic pre-exercise carbohydrates.[29,36,100] The reasons for such discrepancies remain unknown.

GLUCOSE, ELECTROLYTES, AND WATER UPTAKE

As we discuss in Chapter 10, fluid ingestion before and during exercise minimizes the detrimental effects of dehydration on cardiovascular dynamics, temperature regulation, and exercise performance. *Adding carbohydrate to the* ***oral rehydration beverage*** *provides additional glucose energy for exercise as glycogen reserves simultaneously deplete. Adding electrolytes to the rehydration beverage maintains the thirst mechanism and reduces risk of hyponatremia* (see Chapter 10). Coaches and athletes should cooperate to determine the optimal fluid/carbohydrate mixture and volume to minimize fatigue and prevent dehydration. Concern focuses on the dual observations that a large fluid volume intake impairs carbohydrate uptake, while a concentrated sugar/electrolyte solution impairs fluid replacement.

Important Considerations

Stomach emptying rate greatly affects fluid and nutrient absorption by the small intestine. **FIGURE 8.6** illustrates major factors

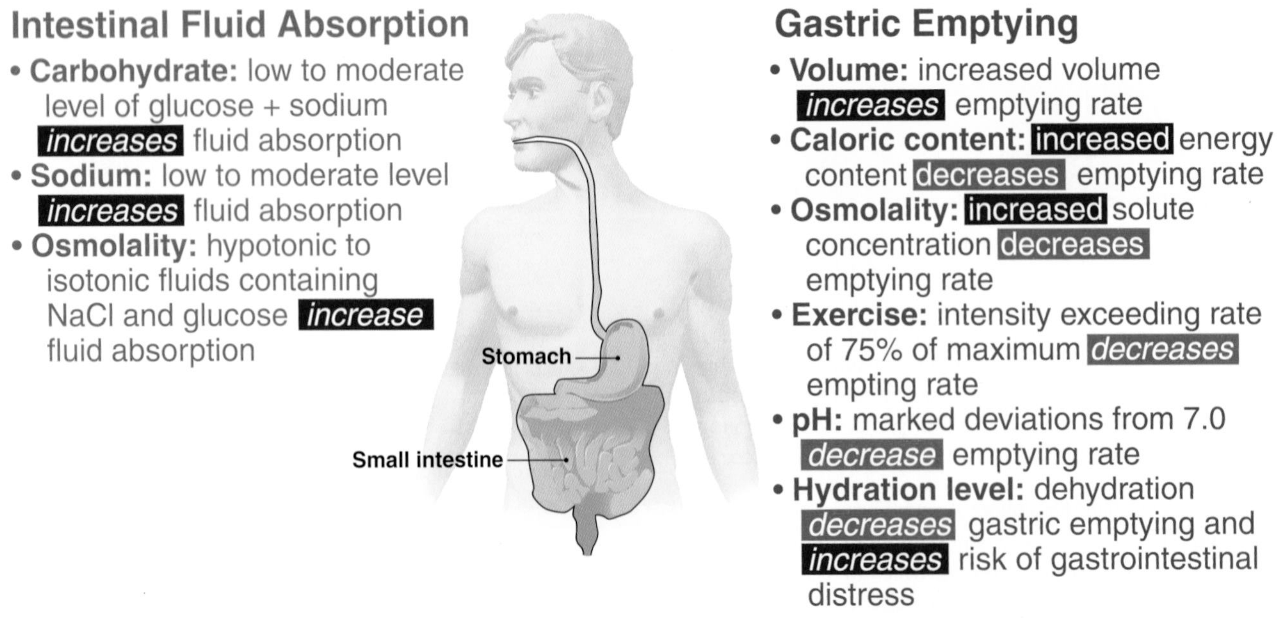
Intestinal Fluid Absorption
• Carbohydrate: low to moderate level of glucose + sodium increases fluid absorption
• Sodium: low to moderate level increases fluid absorption
• Osmolality: hypotonic to isotonic fluids containing NaCl and glucose increase fluid absorption
Stomach
Small intestine
Gastric Emptying
• Volume: increased volume increases emptying rate
• Caloric content: increased energy content decreases emptying rate
• Osmolality: increased solute concentration decreases emptying rate
• Exercise: intensity exceeding rate of 75% of maximum decreases empting rate
• pH: marked deviations from 7.0 decrease emptying rate
• Hydration level: dehydration decreases gastric emptying and increases risk of gastrointestinal distress

FIGURE 8.6. Major factors that affect gastric emptying (stomach) and fluid absorption (small intestine).

that influence gastric emptying in the stomach and fluid absorption in the small intestine. Little negative effect of exercise on gastric emptying occurs until an intensity of about 75% of maximum, after which emptying rate slows.[57] Gastric volume, however, greatly impacts gastric emptying because emptying rate declines exponentially as the stomach's fluid volume decreases. *Maintaining a relatively large stomach fluid volume represents a major factor that speeds gastric emptying to compensate for any inhibitory effects of the beverage's carbohydrate content.*

Practical Recommendations

Consuming 400 to 600 mL of fluid 20 min before exercise optimizes the beneficial effect of increased stomach volume on fluid and nutrient passage into the small intestine. Regularly ingesting 150 to 250 mL of fluid at 15-min intervals throughout exercise continually replenishes fluid passed into the intestine; this maintains a relatively large and constant gastric volume.[5,26,55,72] This protocol delivers about 1 L of fluid each hour to the small intestine, a volume that meets the needs of most endurance athletes. Prior research indicated that colder fluid empties from the stomach more rapidly than fluid at room temperature, yet fluid temperature does *not* exert a major influence during exercise. Beverages containing alcohol or caffeine induce a diuretic effect (with alcohol the most pronounced), which facilitates water loss. Both beverages are contraindicated as a means for fluid replacement.

Consider Fluid Concentration

Concern exists about the potential negative effect of consuming sugary drinks on water absorption from the digestive tract. Gastric emptying slows when ingested fluids either contain increased concentrations of particles in solution (osmolality) or possess high caloric content.[9,82] Rehydration beverages hypertonic to plasma (>280 $mOsm \cdot kg^{-1}$) retard the intestine's net fluid uptake. This negatively affects prolonged exercise in hot weather, when adequate fluid intake *and* absorption play prime roles in the participant's health and safety. The negative effect of concentrated sugar molecules on gastric emptying is diminished (and plasma volume maintained) if the drink contains a short-chain glucose polymer or **maltodextrin** rather than simple sugars. Short-chain polymers of 3 to 20 glucose units derived from cornstarch breakdown reduce the number of particles in solution. Fewer particles facilitate water movement from the stomach for intestinal absorption.

Adding a small amount of glucose and sodium (glucose being the more important factor) to the oral rehydration solution does not negatively affect gastric emptying. It also facilitates fluid uptake by the intestinal lumen because rapid cotransport of glucose–sodium across the intestinal mucosa stimulates water's passive uptake by osmotic action.[33,34,92]

Water replenishes effectively, and the additional glucose uptake contributes to blood glucose maintenance. This glucose serves two purposes:

1. Spares muscle and liver glycogen
2. Provides blood glucose should glycogen reserves decline during the later stage of exercise

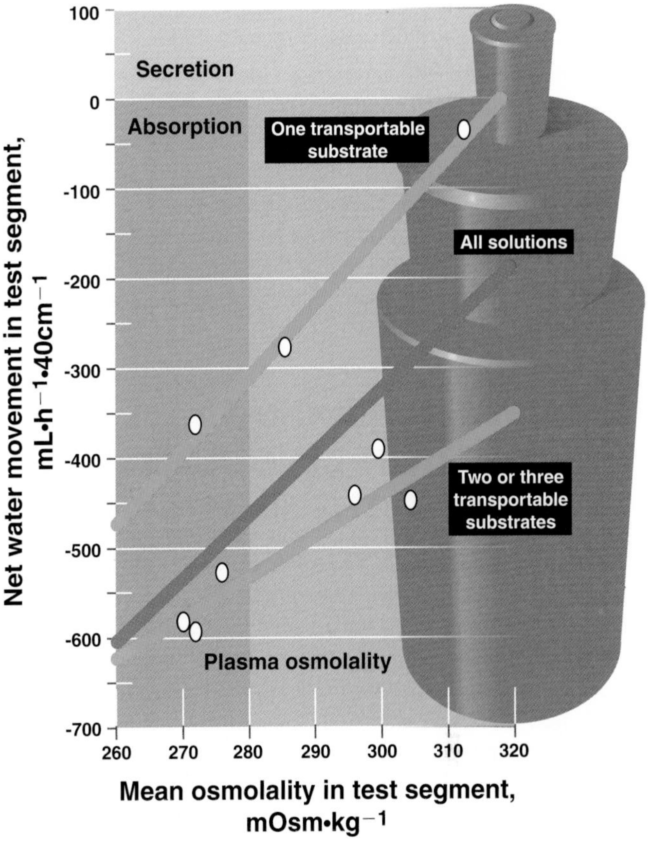

FIGURE 8.7. Net water movement related to mean osmolality in the intestinal test segment. Water absorption from the intestine shows as a negative value (high negative values indicate greater absorption), whereas secretion into the intestinal lumen shows as a positive value. The *pink line* shows the relationship among the three test solutions containing one transportable substrate, whereas the *orange line* refers to six solutions containing two or three transportable substrates. The middle line *(red)* represents the relationship among all test solutions. For each test solution, net water absorption increases as osmolality decreases. For any osmolality value, greater net water absorption occurs from the gut into the body with solutions containing more than one transportable substrate. (From Shi X, et al. Effects of carbohydrate type and concentration and solution osmolality on water absorption. *Med Sci Sports Exerc* 1995;27:1607.)

Rehydration solutions that combine two different transportable carbohydrate substrates (glucose, fructose, sucrose, or maltodextrins) produce greater water uptake at a particular intestinal lumen osmolality than solutions containing only one substrate from enhanced solute flux and thus water flux from the intestine[24] (**FIG. 8.7**).

The second substrate stimulates more intestinal transport mechanisms, thus facilitating net water absorption by osmosis.

Potential Benefit of Sodium: Adding moderate amounts of sodium to ingested fluid minimally affects glucose absorption and does not alter the contribution of ingested glucose to the total energy yield in prolonged exercise.[35,40,61] The extra sodium, the most abundant ion in the extracellular space (0.5–0.7 $g \cdot L^{-1}$) does, however, help to maintain plasma sodium concentrations. This effect benefits ultraendurance athletes at risk for hyponatremia, a potentially fatal condition that occurs from a large sweat–sodium loss coupled with drinking copious amounts of plain water. Maintaining plasma osmolality with added sodium in the rehydration beverage also reduces urine output and sustains the sodium-dependent osmotic drive to drink. These factors promote continued fluid intake *and* fluid retention during recovery.[63,64,117] Chapter 10 discusses the optimal characteristics of a rehydration beverage following exercise-induced dehydration.

RECOMMENDED ORAL REHYDRATION BEVERAGE: EVALUATING THE SPORTS DRINKS

A 5 to 8% carbohydrate–electrolyte beverage consumed while exercising in the heat helps to regulate temperature and fluid balance as effectively as plain water. As an added bonus, this drink maintains glucose metabolism by providing an intestinal delivery rate of 5.0 kcal · min^{-1} *and preserves glycogen during prolonged exercise.*[64,65,68,69,93] Consuming such a solution in recovery from prolonged exercise in a warm environment also improves endurance capacity for subsequent exercise.

To determine the percentage carbohydrate in a drink, divide carbohydrate content (in grams) by fluid volume (in milliliters) and multiply by 100. For example, 80 g of carbohydrate in 1 L (1000 mL) of water provides an 8% solution ($80 \div 1000 \times 100$). A typical Gatorade drink contains about 14 g of sugar in a 240-mL bottle, equivalent to about 6 g per 100 mL or 6%. The competitor drink Powerade contains 8% sugar. Both rehydration beverages fall within the generally recommended range of 4 to 8% sugar content.

Environmental and exercise conditions interact to influence the rehydration solution's optimal composition. Fluid replenishment becomes significant to health and safety when intense aerobic effort in hot, humid weather lasts between 30 and 60 min. In this type of environment, we recommend a more dilute carbohydrate–electrolyte solution containing less than 5% carbohydrate. In cooler weather, when dehydration is not a major factor, a more concentrated beverage of 15% carbohydrate suffices. Little difference exists among liquid glucose, sucrose, or starch as the preferred ingested carbohydrate fuel source during exercise.

Optimal carbohydrate replenishment ranges between 30 and 60 g (about 1–2 oz) an hour. **TABLE 8.2** compares the carbohydrate and mineral content and osmolality of popular fluid replacement beverages. **FIGURE 8.8** presents a general guideline for fluid intake each hour during exercise for a given amount of carbohydrate replenishment. Although a trade-off exists between carbohydrate ingestion and gastric emptying, the stomach empties up to 1700 mL of water per hour, even when drinking an 8% carbohydrate solution. Approximately 1000 mL (about 1 quart) of fluid consumed per hour probably represents the optimal volume to offset dehydration, because larger fluid intakes can cause gastrointestinal discomfort.

PRACTICAL RECOMMENDATIONS FOR FLUID AND CARBOHYDRATE REPLACEMENT DURING EXERCISE

1. Monitor dehydration rate from changes in body weight. Require urination before postexercise body weight determination. Each pound of weight loss corresponds to 450 mL (15 fl oz) of dehydration.
2. Drink fluids at the same or somewhat greater rate as their estimated depletion (or at least at a rate close to 80% of the sweating rate) during prolonged exercise with accompanying cardiovascular stress, high metabolic heat, and dehydration.
3. Endurance athletes can meet both carbohydrate (30–60 $g \cdot h^{-1}$) and fluid requirements by drinking during each hour 625 to 1250 mL (average about 250 mL every 15 min) of a beverage that contains 4 to 8% carbohydrate.

HIGH-FAT VERSUS LOW-FAT DIETS FOR ENDURANCE TRAINING AND EXERCISE PERFORMANCE

Debate concerns the wisdom of maintaining a high-fat diet (or even fasting) during training or before endurance competition.[23,28,71,109,110] Adaptations to high-fat diets consistently show a shift in substrate use toward higher fat oxidation during exercise.[16,42,43,99,124] Proponents of high-fat diets argue that a long-term increase in dietary fat stimulates fat burning by augmenting the capacity to mobilize and catabolize fat. Any fat-burning enhancement should conserve glycogen reserves and/or contribute to improved endurance capacity under low-glycogen conditions. To investigate possible benefits, research compared endurance capacity in two groups of 10 young men matched for aerobic capacity who consumed either a high-carbohydrate diet (65% kcal from carbohydrate) or high-fat diet (62% kcal from lipid) for 7 weeks. Each group trained for 60 to 70 min at 50 to 85% of aerobic capacity, 3 days a week during weeks 1 to 3 and 4 days a week during weeks 4 to 7. After 7 weeks of training, the group consuming the high-fat diet switched to the high-carbohydrate diet. **FIGURE 8.9** displays the exercise performance for both groups. Endurance results were clear: The group consuming the high-carbohydrate diet performed significantly better after 7 weeks of training (102.4 min) than the group consuming the high-fat diet (65.2 min). When the high-fat diet group switched to the high-carbohydrate diet during week 8, only a small additional improvement in endurance of 11.5 min occurred. Consequently, total overall endurance improvement over the 8-week period reached 115% for the high-fat diet group, whereas endurance for the group on the high-carbohydrate diet improved by 194%. The inset table shows daily energy and nutrient intakes before the experimental treatment (habitual diet) and during the 7-week experimental diet. The high-fat diet produced suboptimal adaptations in endurance performance, which were not fully remedied by switching to a high-carbohydrate diet.

TABLE 8.2 Comparison of Various Beverages Used by Athletes to Replace Fluid Lost in Exercise

Beverages	Flavors	CHO Source	CHO conc (%)	Sodium (mg)	Potassium (mg)	Other Minerals and Vitamins	Osmolality ($mOsm \cdot L^{-1}$)
GATORADE[a] Thirst Quencher Stokely-Van Camp, Inc., a subsidiary of the Quaker Oats Company	Lemon-lime, lemonade, fruit punch, orange, citrus cooler	S/G (powder) S/G syrup solids (liquid)	6	110	25	Chloride, phosphorus	280–360
Exceed[a] Ross Laboratories	Lemon-lime, orange	G polymers/F	7.2	50	45		
Quickick[a] Cramer Products, Inc.	Lemon-lime, fruit punch, orange, grape, lemonade,	F/S	4.7	116	23	Chloride, calcium, magnesium, phosphorus	250
Sqwincher, the Activity Drink Universal Products, Inc	Lemon-lime, fruit punch, lemonade, orange, grape, strawberry, grapefruit	G/F	6.8	60	36	Calcium, chloride, phosphorus	305
10-K Beverage Products, Inc.	Lemon-lime, orange, fruit punch, lemonade, iced tea	S/G/F	6.3	52	26	Chloride, phosphorus, calcium, magnesium, vitamin C	470
USA Wet Texas Wet, Inc	Lemon-lime, orange, fruit punch	S	6.8	62	44	Vitamin C, chloride, phosphorus	350
Coca-Cola Coca-Cola, USA	Regular, Classic, Cherry	HFCS/S	10.7–11.3	9.2	trace		
Sprite Coca-Cola, USA	Lemon-lime	HFCS/S	10.2	28	trace	Chloride, phosphorus	450
Cranberry juice cocktail		HFCS/S	15	10	61		
Orange juice		F/S/G	11.8	2.7	510	Phosphorus	600–715
Water				low[b]	low[b]		
PowerAde		HFCS/M	8	73	33		695
All-Sport		HFCS	8–9	55	55	Phosphorus, vitamin C	890
10 K		S/G/F	6.3	54	25	Phosphorus, calcium, iron, vitamins C and A, niacin, riboflavin, thiamine	690
Cytomax		FCS/S	7–11	10	150		
Breakthrough		M/F	8.5	60	45		
Everlast		S/F	6	100	20		
Hydra Charge		M/F	8	–	trace		
SportaLYTE		M/F/G	7.5	100	60		

[a]*Serving size, 8 fluid oz.*
[b]*Depends on water source.*
S = sucrose; F = fructose; G = glucose; HFCS= high fructose corn syrup; M = maltodextrin

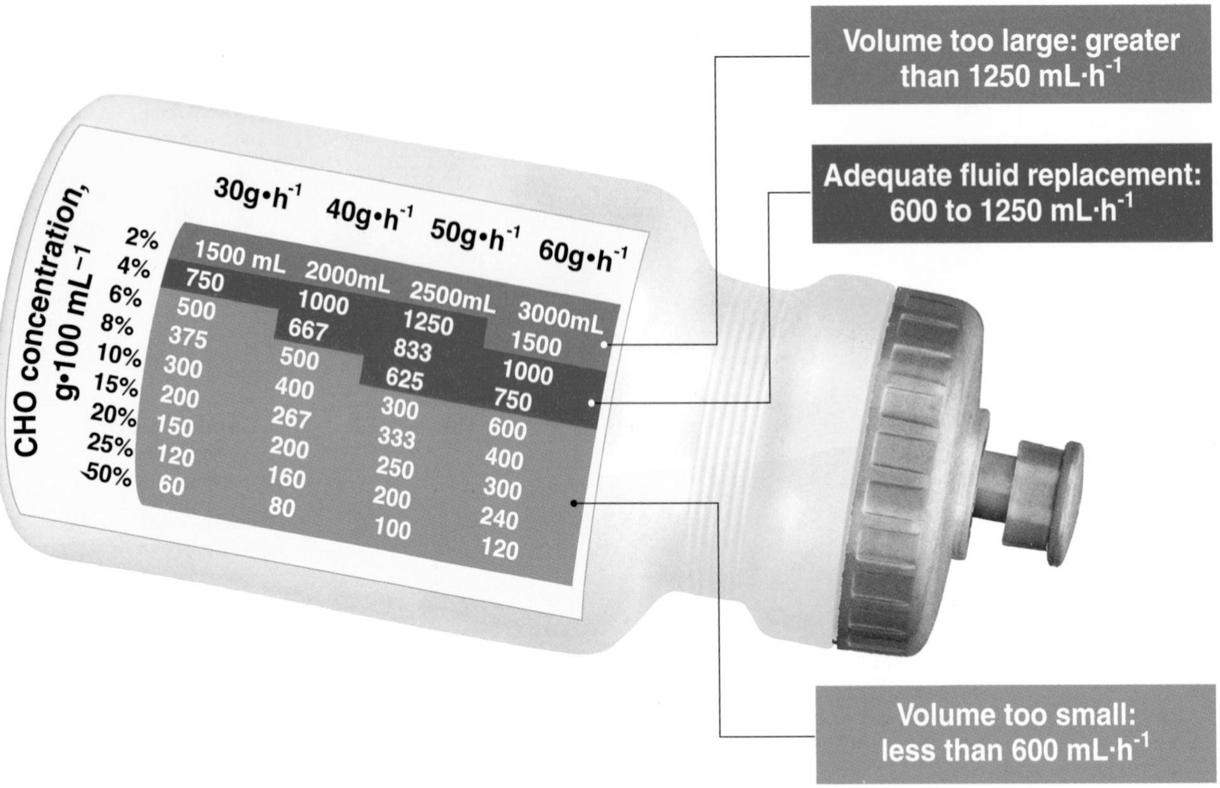

FIGURE 8.8. Fluid volume to ingest each hour to obtain the noted amount of carbohydrate (CHO). (Modified from Coyle EF, Montain SJ. Benefits of fluid replacement. *Med Sci Sports Exerc* 1992;24:S324.)

HIGH-FAT VERSUS LOW-FAT EFFECTS ON EXERCISE ECONOMY: TRAINING MAY MAKE A DIFFERENCE

Seven days of consuming a high-fat diet containing 74% of calories from fat reduces whole-body exercise economy (i.e., increases the oxygen cost of a set exercise task) by more than 10% in sedentary men. This diet also significantly increased simple reaction times and decreased cognitive function as measured by the power of attention. Just about any increase in the oxygen cost of exercise would profoundly affect performance in intense endurance activities. To test whether a similar diet would negatively affect whole-body exercise efficiency in endurance-trained men and thus hinder aerobic exercise performance, 16 endurance-trained men received in random order a short-term, high-fat (70% kcal from fat) or moderate-carbohydrate (50% kcal from carbohydrate) diet. Exercise efficiency was assessed on a bicycle ergometer, and aerobic exercise performance was measured with a 1-h time trial. Muscle biopsies assessed mitochondrial protein content. Despite the 60% higher level of plasma free fatty acids with the high-fat compared to the moderate-carbohydrate diet, no change occurred in whole-body efficiency or in mitochondrial function. However, endurance exercise performance decreased on the high-fat diet, which probably resulted from early glycogen depletion. The researchers concluded that prior exercise training blunts the deleterious effect of short-term, high-fat feeding on whole body efficiency.[1,2]

1. Edwards LM, et al. Short-term consumption of a high-fat diet impairs whole body efficiency and cognitive function in sedentary men. *FASEB J* 2011;25:1088.
2. Edwards LM, et al. Endurance exercise training blunts the deleterious effect of high-fat feeding on whole body efficiency. *Am J Physiol Regul Integr Comp Physiol* 2011;301:R320.

Subsequent research from the same laboratory failed to demonstrate any endurance-enhancing effect of a high-fat diet containing only moderate carbohydrate (15% total kcal) in rats, regardless of their training status. For sedentary humans, maintaining either a low or high dietary fat intake for 4 weeks did not affect maximal or submaximal aerobic exercise performance.[79] A 6-day exposure to a high-fat, low-carbohydrate diet, followed by 1 day of carbohydrate restoration with a high-carbohydrate diet, increased fat oxidation during prolonged submaximal exercise. This carbohydrate-sparing effect did not enhance 1-h time trial performance after 4 h of continuous cycling.[18]

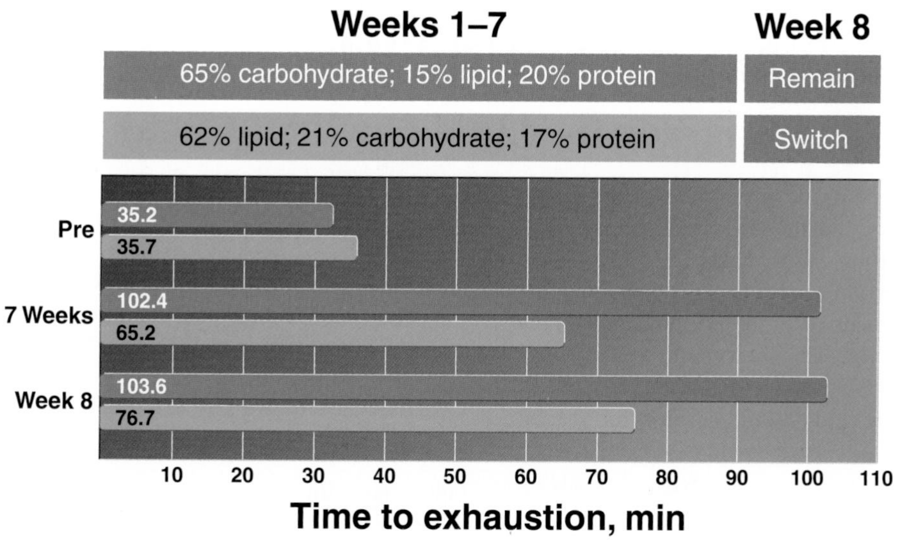

Daily intake of energy and nutrients in the subjects' habitual dient and during 7 weeks on an experimental diet

	Units	Habitual diet CHO	Habitual diet Lipid	Experimental diet CHO	Experimental diet Lipid
Energy, E	MJ	13.6	11.9	14.3	13.7*†
Protein	E%	13.2	14.3	14.6	16.5*†
	g	105.0	101.0	123.0	133.0*†
Carbohydrate	E%	48.2	53.4	65.0	22.0*†
	g	386.0	373.0	546.0	177.0*†
	g • kg body wt^{-1}	4.7	5.0	6.8	2.4*†
Simple sugars	E%	11.0	10.0	7.0	2.2*†
Dietary fiber	g • MJ^{-1}	2.3	2.6	4.3	2.2*†
Lipid	E%	34.3	39.0	20.4	62.0*†
	g	118.0	94.0	75.0	217.0*†
Cholesterol	mg • MJ^{-1}	31.0	29.0	26.0	44.0*†
Essential FA	E%	4.4	4.3	4.0	11.2*†
P/S ratio		0.39	0.43	0.53	0.62*†

Values are means; *significantly different between the habitual and the experimental diet; †significantly different between the two experimental diets; MJ, megajoule; E%, percent of total energy

FIGURE 8.9. Effects of a high-carbohydrate (CHO) versus a high-fat diet on endurance performance. The group consuming the high-fat diet for 7 weeks switched to the high-CHO diet during week 8. The endurance test consisted of pedaling a bicycle ergometer at the desired rate. The inset table compares the average daily energy and nutrient intakes during the habitual and experimental diets. P/S ratio, polyunsaturated-to-saturated fatty acid ratio. (From Helge JW, et al. Interaction of training and diet on metabolism and endurance during exercise in man. *J Physiol* 1996;492:293.)

PERSONAL HEALTH AND EXERCISE NUTRITION 8.1

How to Assess and Upgrade the Lipid Quality of Your Diet

The typical Western diet contains too much total lipid, too much saturated fat, and too much cholesterol. Dietary lipids represent about 36% of total caloric intake, with the average person consuming 15% of total calories as saturated fatty acids. Health professionals recommend that lipid intake should not exceed 30% of the diet's total energy content, and consuming less (about 20%) may confer even greater health benefits. Unsaturated fatty acids should account for at least 70% of the total lipid intake, equally distributed between polyunsaturates and monounsaturates, with cholesterol intake below 300 $mg \cdot day^{-1}$.

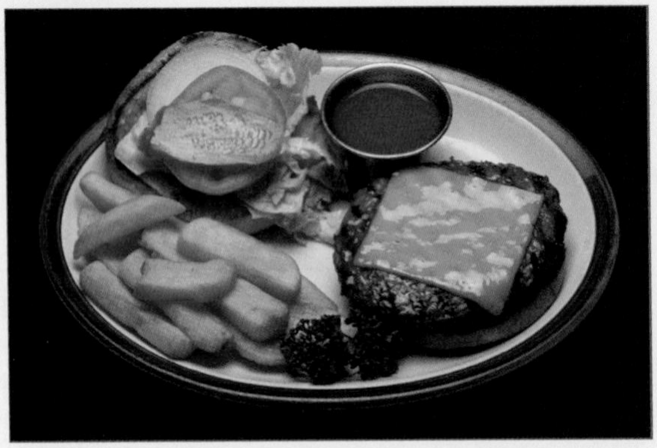

Estimating the Percentage of Total Calories Consumed from Fat

Based on research correlating food intake from a diary with data from a simple questionnaire, it is possible to estimate the percentage of total calories from fat.

Choosing Among the Different Fats in Your Diet

Lipids (fats) not only provide fuel for energy but also aid in the absorption of fat-soluble vitamins, are an integral part of the plasma membrane, provide for hormone synthesis (steroids), and aid in insulation and protection of vital organs. Most lipids store in adipose tissue for subsequent release into the bloodstream as free fatty acids, which broadly classify as monounsaturated, polyunsaturated, and saturated. Each exerts different effects on cholesterol and lipoprotein deposition in arteries and subsequent coronary heart disease risk.

Choosing the Proper Dietary Fat

TABLE 1 shows the available food choices for different types of lipids based on how they affect total cholesterol and the different lipoprotein fractions.

TABLE 1 Choose the Right Fat for Your Diet

Best Choice Monounsaturated Fatty Acids	Good Choice Polyunsaturated Fatty Acids	Occasional Choice Saturated/Hydrogenated Fatty Acids
Effects on Cholesterol and Lipoproteins		
• Decreases total cholesterol	• Decreases total cholesterol	• Increases total cholesterol
• Decreases LDL-cholesterol	• Decreases LDL-cholesterol	• Increases LDL-cholesterol
• No effect on HDL-cholesterol	• Decreases HDL-cholesterol	• Decreases HDL-cholesterol
	Food Examples	
Vegetable oils: avocado, canola, olive, peanut	**Vegetable oils:** corn, safflower, sesame, soybean, sunflower, transfat-free margarine, mayonnaise, Miracle Whip	**Tropical vegetable oils:** coconut, palm, palm kernel, cocoa butter
		Hydrogenated oils: margarine, shortening
Nuts: acorns, almonds, beechnuts, cashews, chestnuts, hazelnuts, hickory, macadamia, natural peanut butter, peanuts, pecans, pistachios	**Nuts:** Brazil, butternuts, pine, walnuts	**Animal fats:** bacon, beef fat, chicken fat, egg yolk, fatty meats, lamb fat, lard, pepperoni, pork fat, salt pork, sausage, kielbasa
Other: fish fat (omega-3 fatty acids)	**Seeds:** sesame, pumpkin, sunflower	**Dairy products:** butter, cheese (regular, light, low fat), cream cheese, half & half, ice cream, sour cream, whole milk, 2% milk

Information collated from the American Heart Association (www.aha.org), Centers for Disease Control (www.CDC.gov), and American College of Sports Medicine (www.acsm.org).

Questionnaire

HOW MUCH FAT DO YOU CONSUME? THINK OF YOUR DIET OVER THE PAST 3 MONTHS AND ANSWER THE FOLLOWING QUESTIONS.

Choices: Place the number in the space below 1 = Usually/always; 2 = Often; 3 = Sometimes; 4 = Rarely/never

1. When I eat bread, rolls, muffins, or crackers, I eat them without butter or margarine.
2. When I eat cooked vegetables, I eat them without butter, margarine, salt pork, or bacon fat.
3. When I eat cooked vegetables, they are cooked by a method other than frying.
4. When I eat potatoes, they are cooked by a method other than frying.
5. When I eat boiled or baked potatoes I eat them without butter, margarine, or sour cream.
6. When I eat green salads, I eat them without dressing.
7. When I eat dessert, I eat it without cream or whipped-cream topping.
8. When I eat spaghetti or noodles, I eat it plain or use a meatless sauce.
9. My main meal for the day is usually meatless.
10. When I eat fish, it is broiled, baked, or poached.
11. When I eat chicken, it is broiled or baked.
12. When I eat chicken, I remove the skin.
13. When I eat red meat, I trim off all visible fat.
14. When I eat ground beef, I choose extra lean.
15. When I drink milk I choose skim or 1% fat milk instead of 2% fat or whole milk.
16. When I eat cheese, it is the reduced-fat variety.
17. When I eat a frozen dessert, it is sherbet, ice milk, or nonfat versions of ice cream or yogurt.
18. When I eat green salads with dressing, I use a low-fat or nonfat dressing.
19. When I sauté or pan fry food, I use a nonstick spray instead of oil, margarine, or butter.
20. When I use mayonnaise or a mayonnaise-type dressing, I usually use a low-fat or nonfat variety.
21. When I eat dessert, I usually eat fruit.
22. When I eat snacks, I usually eat raw vegetables.
23. When I eat snacks, I usually eat fresh fruit.

Scoring

Total your score and divide by 23.

Your average	Percentage kcal from fat
1.0 to 1.5	Less than 25%
1.5 to 2.0	25 to 29%
2.0 to 2.5	30 to 34%
2.5 to 3.0	35 to 39%
3.0 to 3.5	40 to 44%
3.5 to 4.0	45%+

A high-fat diet stimulates adaptive responses that assist fat catabolism, yet reliable research has not demonstrated consistent exercise or training benefits from this dietary modification. Compromised training capacity and symptoms of lethargy, increased fatigue, and higher ratings of perceived exertion usually accompany exercise when subsisting on a high-fat diet.[16,42,97] One must carefully consider the potential detrimental health risks when recommending a diet with 60% of total calories from lipid. This concern may prove unwarranted for athletes with high levels of daily energy expenditure. Increasing the diet's percentage of lipid calories to 50% for physically active persons who maintain a stable body weight does not adversely affect heart disease risk factors, including plasma lipoprotein profiles.[10,56] Overall, available research does not support the popular notion that reducing carbohydrate while increasing fat intake above a 30% level optimizes the metabolic "zone" for endurance performance.[91,108] Conversely, restriction of dietary fat intake considerably below recommended levels also impairs endurance exercise performance.[42,106,108]

SUMMARY

1. The precompetition meal should include readily digestible foods and contribute to the energy and fluid requirements of exercise. Meals high in carbohydrates and relatively low in lipids and proteins serve this purpose. Three hours should provide sufficient time to digest and absorb the precompetition meal.
2. Commercially prepared liquid meals offer a practical approach to precompetition nutrition and energy supplementation. These "meals" (1) provide balance in nutritive value, (2) contribute to fluid needs, and (3) absorb rapidly, leaving practically no residue in the digestive tract.
3. Intense aerobic exercise for 1 h decreases liver glycogen by about 55%, whereas a 2-h strenuous workout nearly depletes the glycogen content of the liver and specifically exercised muscles.
4. Carbohydrate-containing beverages consumed during exercise enhance endurance performance by maintaining blood sugar concentration. Glucose supplied in the blood can (1) spare existing glycogen in active muscles or (2) serve as "reserve" blood glucose for later use should muscle glycogen become depleted. Adding some protein to the beverage enhances the effectiveness of these drinks.
5. All carbohydrates do not digest and absorb at the same rate. The GI provides a relative measure of blood glucose increase after consuming a food containing 50 g of a digestible carbohydrate (total carbohydrate minus fiber) and compares it over a 2-h period to a "standard" for carbohydrate (usually white bread or glucose) with an assigned value of 100. The glycemic load quantifies the overall glycemic effect of a typical portion of food.
6. For rapid carbohydrate replenishment after exercise, begin immediately to consume moderate- to high-glycemic index carbohydrate-containing foods (50–75 g of carbohydrate each hour). With optimal carbohydrate intake, glycogen stores replenish at a rate of about 5 to 7% an hour.
7. Use the GI to formulate the immediate pre-exercise feeding. Foods with a low GI digest and absorb at a relatively slow rate. Ingesting these carbohydrates in the immediate pre-exercise period provides a steady supply of "slow-release" glucose from the intestinal tract during exercise.
8. Maintaining a relatively large stomach fluid volume throughout exercise enhances gastric emptying. Optimal gastric volume occurs by consuming 400 to 600 mL of fluid immediately before exercise, followed by regular fluid ingestion of 250 mL every 15 min thereafter.
9. Drinking concentrated sugar-containing beverages slows the gastric emptying rate. This could negatively upset fluid balance during exercise and heat stress.
10. The ideal oral rehydration beverage contains between 5 and 8% carbohydrates. This formulation permits carbohydrate replenishment without adversely affecting fluid balance and thermoregulation.
11. Adding moderate amounts of sodium to the ingested fluid helps to maintain plasma sodium concentration. This benefits the ultraendurance athlete at risk for hyponatremia.
12. Maintaining plasma osmolality with added sodium in the rehydration beverage reduces urine output and sustains the sodium-dependent osmotic drive to drink.
13. A high-fat diet stimulates adaptive responses that augment fat use, but reliable research has yet to demonstrate consistent exercise or training benefits from this dietary modification approach.

thePoint *Visit* **thePoint.lww.com/MKKSEN4e** *to view the following animations related to content presented in Chapter 8:* ***Insulin functions*** *and* ***Glycogen synthesis.***

TEST YOUR KNOWLEDGE ANSWERS

1. **False:** Significant depletion occurs in carbohydrate reserves over an 8- to 12-h period without eating, even if the person normally follows appropriate dietary recommendations. Thus, fasting before competition or intense training makes no sense physiologically because it rapidly depletes liver and muscle glycogen, which subsequently impairs exercise performance. In individualizing the precompetition meal plan, consider the following factors: (1) food preference, (2) "psychological set" of the competitor, and (3) digestibility of the foods.

2. **False:** The ideal precompetition meal maximizes muscle and liver glycogen storage and provides glucose for intestinal absorption during exercise. The meal should contain 150 to 300 g of carbohydrate (3–5 $g \cdot kg^{-1}$ body mass in either solid or liquid form), be consumed 3 to 4 h before exercising, and contain relatively little fat and fiber to facilitate gastric emptying and minimize gastrointestinal distress.

3. **False:** Intense aerobic exercise for 1 h decreases liver glycogen by about 55%, whereas a 2-h strenuous workout almost totally depletes the glycogen content of the liver and the exercised muscle fibers. Also, maximal, repetitive, 1- to 5-min bouts of exercise interspersed with periods of lower intensity exercise—as occurs in soccer, ice hockey, field hockey, European handball, and tennis—dramatically lower liver and muscle glycogen reserves. Research shows that physical and mental performance under such conditions improves with carbohydrate supplementation during exercise. Carbohydrate feedings during intense, prolonged exercise also enable persons to exercise at greater intensity of effort.

4. **False:** The GI serves as an indicator of a carbohydrate's ability to raise blood glucose levels. This index expresses the percentage of total area under the blood glucose response curve for a specific food, compared with glucose. Blood sugar increase—termed the *glycemic response*—is determined after ingesting a food containing 50 g of a carbohydrate and comparing it over a 2-h period with a "standard" for carbohydrate (usually white bread or glucose) with an assigned value of 100.

5. **True:** The most rapid method of replenishing carbohydrate after exercise requires consuming foods with moderate to high glycemic indices rather than foods rated low, even if the replenishment meal contains a small amount of lipid and protein. Furthermore, ingesting lipids and proteins slows the passage of food into the small intestine, reducing the GI of the meal's accompanying carbohydrate content.

6. **False:** More-rapid glycogen resynthesis takes place if the person remains inactive during recovery. With optimal carbohydrate intake (high-glycemic foods), glycogen stores replenish at a rate of about 5 to 7% per hour. Thus, even under the best of circumstances, it takes at least 20 h to re-establish glycogen stores following a glycogen-depleting exercise bout.

7. **False:** Consuming 400 to 600 mL of fluid 20 min before exercise optimizes the beneficial effect of an increased stomach volume on fluid and nutrient passage into the small intestine. Then, regularly ingesting 150 to 250 mL of fluid (at 15-min intervals) throughout exercise continually replenishes fluid in the stomach; this maintains a relatively large and constant gastric volume. Such a protocol delivers about 1 L of fluid per hour to the small intestine, a volume that meets the needs of most endurance athletes.

8. **False:** A 5 to 8% carbohydrate–electrolyte beverage consumed during exercise in the heat contributes to temperature regulation and fluid balance as effectively as plain water. As an added bonus, this drink aids in maintaining glucose metabolism (providing an intestinal delivery rate of 5.0 $kcal \cdot min^{-1}$) and glycogen reserves in prolonged exercise.

9. **True:** Adding moderate amounts of sodium to ingested fluids exerts a minimal effect on glucose absorption or the contribution of ingested glucose to the total energy yield in prolonged exercise. The extra sodium (0.5–0.7 $g \cdot L^{-1}$) contributes to maintaining plasma sodium concentrations and benefits the ultraendurance athlete at risk for hyponatremia. Hyponatremia occurs from large sweat–sodium loss coupled with drinking large amounts of plain water. Maintaining plasma osmolality with added sodium in the rehydration beverage also reduces urine output and sustains the sodium-dependent osmotic drive to drink.

10. **False:** Drinking concentrated sugar-containing beverages slows gastric emptying rate, which could ultimately upset fluid balance during exercise and heat stress. The ideal oral rehydration solution contains between 5 and 8% carbohydrates. This beverage formulation permits carbohydrate replenishment without adversely affecting fluid balance and thermoregulation.

Key References

Baty JJ, et al. The effect of a carbohydrate and protein supplement on resistance exercise performance, hormonal response, and muscle damage. *J Strength Cond Res* 2007;21:321.

Berardi JM, et al. Postexercise muscle glycogen recovery enhanced with a carbohydrate-protein supplement. *Med Sci Sports Exerc* 2006;38:1106.

Brouns F, Beckers E. Is the gut an athletic organ? *Sports Med* 1993;15:242.

Burelle Y, et al. Oxidation of an oral [^{13}C] glucose load at rest and prolonged exercise in trained and sedentary subjects. *J Appl Physiol* 1999;86:52.

Burke LM. Nutrition for distance events. *J Sports Sci* 2007;25(Suppl 1):S29.

Burke LM, et al. Muscle glycogen storage after prolonged exercise: effect of the frequency of carbohydrate feeding. *Am J Clin Nutr* 1996;64:115.

Burke LM, et al. Energy and carbohydrate for training and recovery. J *Sports Sci* 2006;24:675.

Coyle EF. Timing and method of increased carbohydrate intake to cope with heavy training, competition and recovery. *J Sports Sci* 1991;9:29.

Coyle EF. Substrate utilization during exercise in active people. *Am J Clin Nutr* 1995;61(Suppl):968S.

Currell K, Jeukendrup AE. Superior endurance performance with ingestion of multiple transportable carbohydrates. *Med Sci Sports Exerc* 2008;40:275:2008.

DeMarco HD, et al. Pre-exercise carbohydrate meals: application of the glycemic index. *Med Sci Sports Exerc* 1999;31:164.

Erlenbusch M, et al. Effect of high-fat or high-carbohydrate diets on endurance exercise: a meta-analysis. *Int J Sport Nutr Exerc Metabol* 2005;15:1.

Foster-Powell K, et al. International table of glycemic index and glycemic load values: 2002. *Am J Clin Nutr* 2002;76:5.

Jentjens RL, et al. High oxidation rates from combined carbohydrates ingested during exercise. *Med Sci Sports Exerc* 2004;36:1551.

Maugham RJ, et al. Dietary supplements. *J Sports Sci* 2004;22:2004.

McCleave EL, et al. A low carbohydrate-protein supplement improves endurance performance in female athletes. *J Strength Cond Res* 2011;25:879.

Morrison PJ, et al. Adding protein to a carbohydrate supplement provided after endurance exercise enhances 4E-BP1 and RPS6 signaling in skeletal muscle. *J Appl Physiol* 2008;104:1029.

Noakes TD, et al. The importance of volume in regulating gastric emptying. *Med Sci Sports Exerc* 1991;23:307.

Pabkin JAM, et al. Muscle glycogen storage following prolonged exercise: effect of timing of ingestion of high glycemic index food. *Med Sci Sports Exerc* 1997;29:220.

Roy LP, et al. High oxidation rates from combined carbohydrates ingested during exercise. *Med Sci Sports Exerc* 2004;36:1551.

Shirreffs SM, et al. Fluid and electrolyte needs for preparation and recovery from training and competition. *J Sports Sci* 2004;22:57.

Vandenbogaerde TJ, Hopkins WG. Effects of acute carbohydrate supplementation on endurance performance: a meta-analysis. *Sports Med* 2011;41:773.

van Loon KJC, et al. Maximizing postexercise muscle glycogen synthesis: carbohydrate supplementation and the application of amino acid or protein hydrolysate mixtures. *Am J Clin Nutr* 2000;72:106.

Wagenmakers AJ. Carbohydrate feedings improve 1 h time trial cycling performance. *Med Sci Sports Exerc* 1996;28:S37.

Williams C, Serratose L. Nutrition on match day. *J Sports Sci* 2006;24:687.

thePoint

Visit **thePoint.lww.com/MKKSEN4e** *for a list of the references cited in this chapter, including additional, relevant references.*

CHAPTER 9

Making Wise Choices in the Nutrition Marketplace

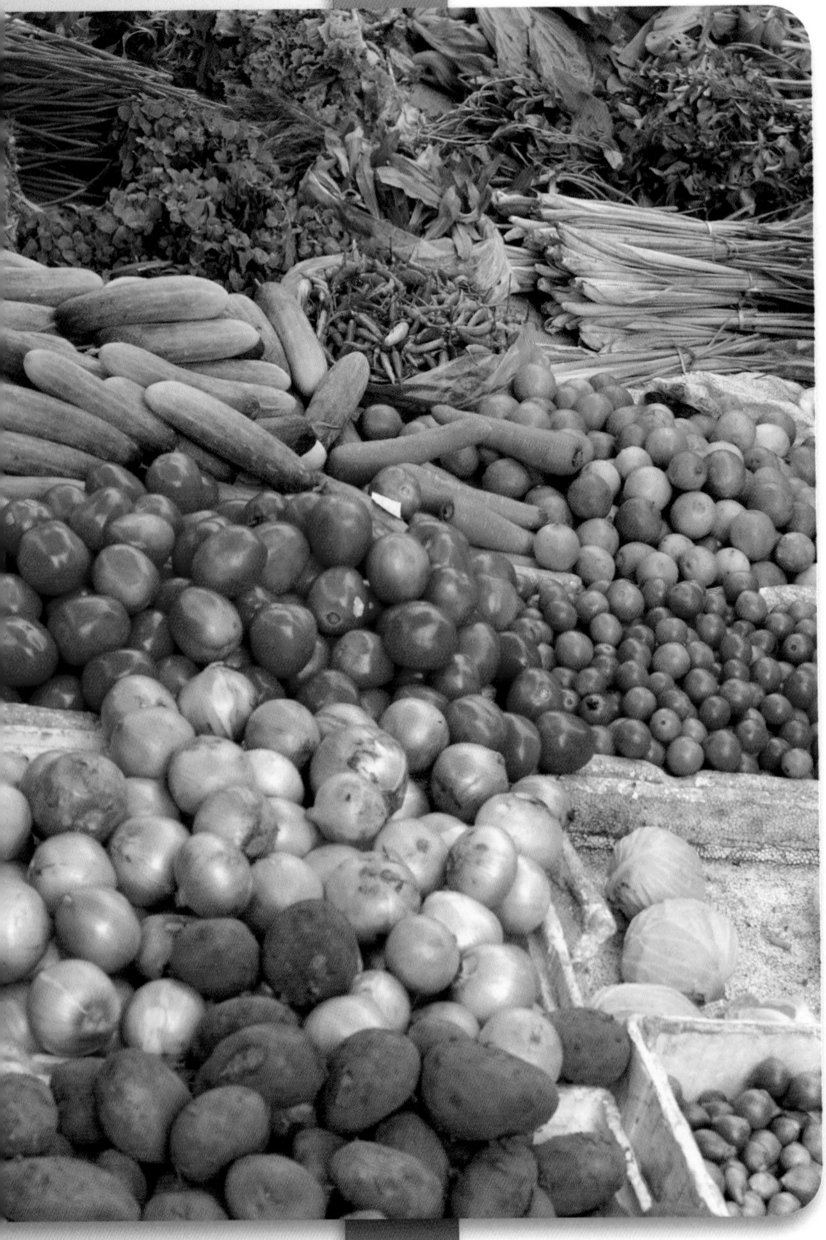

OUTLINE

- What Does Food Mean to You?
- Regulating What We Eat: Food and Nutrition Policy
- Food Advertising and Packaging
- Government "Watchdog" Agencies
- The Food Label (Nutrition Panel)
- Daily Values
- Nutrient Content Descriptors
- Nutrition Facts Panels for Meat and Poultry Products
- Food Additives
- Baby Foods
- Health Claims
- Labeling of Ingredients
- New Menu and Vending Machine Labeling Requirements
- Determining the Nutrient Percentage in a Food
- What People Eat
- Supersizing: An American Trend
- Active People on the Go: Eating at Fast-Food Restaurants
- The Hunger–Obesity Paradox
- The Organics Movement

TEST YOUR KNOWLEDGE

Select true or false for the 10 statements below, then check out the answers at the end of the chapter. Retake the test after you have read the chapter; you should achieve 100%!	True	False
1. Most people choose food based on two major variables—taste and nutritional value.	❍	❍
2. FTC stands for Federal Trade Commission; it regulates food-product advertising in different media.	❍	❍
3. A food's nutritional quality is based solely on its protein-to-fat ratio.	❍	❍
4. Federal law dictates that sellers of dietary supplements must guarantee their products as safe and effective.	❍	❍
5. Dietary supplements must provide precise information about their contents clearly listed on the package.	❍	❍
6. The ATF stands for the Bureau of Alcohol, Tobacco, Firearms, and Explosives; it enforces federal laws related to alcohol, tobacco, firearms, and explosives.	❍	❍
7. The Daily Reference Values on food labels assume a 3000-kcal daily intake as representative of the average caloric intake for most adults.	❍	❍
8. The term "healthy" can be used on a food label without meeting any established criteria for making a claim for health benefits.	❍	❍
9. The *Hunger–Obesity Paradox* refers to the theory that overfat persons are always hungry.	❍	❍
10. Obesity continues to grow at an epidemic rate in the United States despite any significant change in eating patterns and behaviors.	❍	❍

WHAT DOES FOOD MEAN TO YOU?

Our bodies have changed little from our ancient ancestors, but over the last century the world we live in has changed dramatically. The technologic era has allowed industrialized countries to create an abundant low-cost, high-calorie food supply, massive transportation and communication networks to distribute it, and the luxuries of convenience foods and high-speed cooking equipment to support it. Individuals now have the freedom to choose foods from a far greater variety in local markets than ever before. Consequently, many factors interact to influence a person's food selections and eating behaviors.

Factors Affecting Food Choices

About one fourth of the US population consumes inordinately large quantities of calorically dense food that often exceeds daily energy requirements. Besides hunger, food satisfies deep personal and social needs. Understanding the factors that compel us to eat certain foods helps to make wise decisions regarding food choices.

Age-Old Tradition

Seeking food and the pleasures of eating often intertwine with other human drives deeply embedded in our culture. Food, for example, has become a central part of sharing. We offer food and drink to visitors in our homes; most of us also accept food and drink when we visit another's home, even if we are not hungry or do not particularly care for the food. Athletes learn what foods to eat from coaches who may advocate steak and eggs or special drinks, yet have never taken a formal course in sport and exercise nutrition or read reputable resource materials in the area. Such food experiences gleaned from coaches, trainers, and even parents often persist well into adulthood and pass on as part of one's "eating tradition."

Early Experiences: Emotion and Family

Early food experiences become entangled with strong emotional forces, particularly from our caregivers or parents. For many, food equates with security and love and can associate with feelings of comfort and "good" times (e.g., family gatherings, holidays, desserts, special occasions) or of "bad" times (e.g., punishment, lack of money, lack of food availability). As adults, we may reject some of these earlier food choices, but we still crave them because they connect us with positive childhood experiences.

Positive and Negative Associations

Specific memories of past events often influence food choices. In early childhood, sweets and snacks are often used as rewards for good behavior or denied as punishment. Thus, these foods become a personal reward for achieving something good or are used to make us feel good, or they are rejected because they associate with negative experiences. This learned response plays a significant role in our food choices and may help to explain why many adults overeat in an attempt to make themselves feel good.

A noxious experience paired with the eating of a particular food can imprint an aversion to that food. The food aversion persists, although the specific experience may be forgotten. Many athletes who experience a change in performance often associate this change with a particular food or meal. This sets the stage for some bizarre practices before athletic events such as eating precisely the same foods (at the same time) prior to every competition or performance.

Fear of Foods

Children often resist eating new or different foods and only eat familiar foods provided by their caregiver. Unfortunately, as we age, we often classify foods we consume as "normal" and different foods consumed by others as "odd" or "weird." This dictates certain food preferences that create a fear of some foods that carries over from one generation to the next. Athletes who travel to other "far away" countries often cringe at foods they never considered eating (e.g., boiled dragonflies, blubber, cooked rat, grilled dog or cat meat, squirrel and monkey brains, fried ants and beetles, bull penis, raw snails) and perform poorly because they avoid the available but nutritious unaccustomed foods. Developing a varied palate at an early age expands an individual's eating pleasures later in life.

Convenience/Availability

Although food habits develop slowly as we age, food availability plays a considerable role in developing these habits. For example, fast-food chains exist within easy reach of most individuals in North America and Europe; they offer relatively inexpensive, calorie-laden alternatives to home-cooked meals. Busy parents often rely on such foods to feed their children, totally neglecting fresh fruits and vegetables usually absent from the food menus. Many fast-food establishments cater to young children by offering indoor or outdoor "playlands" and providing "free" toys and a place where children can readily interact with other children. It is not surprising that, over the years, children grow accustomed to eating with distractions or that they "cry on demand" for certain foods they do not like just to get the toy. Vending machines in schools and the workplace substitute for homemade meals. Indeed, the rush to find and eat cheap, high-fat, high-sugar meals has replaced the traditional family dinner that typically consisted of whole grains, lean meats, fruits, and vegetables. Most Western nations now have become "fast-food nations," fixated on convenience and availability with little consideration for the food's nutritional value.

Pleasure

Many factors determine the pleasure of food, including biological, psychological, and cultural factors. The biological needs for satiety and nourishment play a primal role in the pleasure derived from feeding ourselves. Other factors such as taste, texture, color, and aroma of food, individually or in combination, also influence this biological drive via chemical factors known to trigger the brain's pleasure-sensing areas.

Taste

Taste (or gustation; adjectival form, *gustatory*) represents one of the traditional five senses and refers to the ability to detect food flavor, certain minerals, and poisons through the sensory taste bud organs concentrated on the tongue's upper surface. Taste can be categorized into five basic tastes:

1. Sweetness
2. Bitterness
3. Sourness
4. Saltiness
5. Umami

UMAMI: THE FIFTH BASIC TASTE

Umami, a Japanese word used universally in all major languages, means "pleasant savory taste." In 1985, umami was officially recognized as the scientific term to describe the taste of glutamates and nucleotides. Umami, often described as a pleasant "brothy" or "meaty" taste, has a long-lasting, mouth-watering, and coating sensation over the tongue. Sensation of umami represents detection of the carboxylate anion of glutamate in specialized receptor cells present on the tongues of human and other primates.

Umami has a mild but lasting aftertaste difficult to describe in words. It induces salivation and a furriness sensation on the tongue, stimulating the throat, roof, and back of the mouth. By itself, umami is not palatable, but it makes foods have a pleasant taste in the presence of a matching aroma. However, like other basic tastes (with the exception of sucrose), umami is pleasant only within a relatively narrow concentration range. Many foods are rich in umami, mainly those that contain high levels of L-glutamate, IMP (inosinic acid or inosine monophosphate), and GMP (guanosine monophosphate, also known as 5′-guanidylic acid or guanylic acid). Examples include fish; shellfish; cured meats; varied vegetables such as mushrooms, ripe tomatoes, Chinese cabbage, spinach, or green tea; and fermented and aged cheeses, shrimp pastes, and soy sauce. Humans' first encounter with umami is often breast milk, as it contains roughly the same amount of umami as different broths.

All basic tastes classify as either appetitive or aversive, depending on the food's effect on our bodies. The basic tastes contribute only partially to food's sensation and flavor in the mouth; other contributing factors include smell detected by the olfactory epithelium of the nose, texture detected through a variety of mechanoreceptors and muscle sensors, and temperature detected by thermoreceptors.

Pleasure associated with taste, texture, and aroma is learned within a perceptual and cultural context. For example, food preferences, tastes, and pleasures in East Asia differ vastly compared with those in Western Europe or North America. Moreover, taste intimately links to olfactory sensations; those who lose the ability to smell exhibit remarkable changes in taste and food pleasure preferences. Many food manufacturers capitalize on the link between smell, taste, and food pleasure by adding chemicals that mimic specific smells and tastes. It now is possible to purchase almost any "food" chemically altered to taste like something else. Manufacturers have even found a way to chemically reproduce the taste of beef, chicken, or lamb and add this "flavor" to nonmeat products and advertise them as, for example, "meat-flavored vegetables."

A search on the Internet of different flavored potato chips worldwide reveals a staggering variety of chemically flavored chips (**TABLE 9.1**).

TABLE 9.1 Different Flavored Potato Chips Around the World

Country	Chip Flavor
Argentina 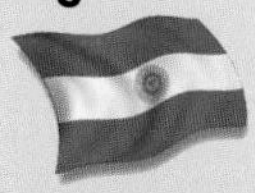	Steak with Onions and Sweet Peppers
	Patagonia Lamb
	Grilled Provolone Cheese
	Tomato and Herbs
Canada 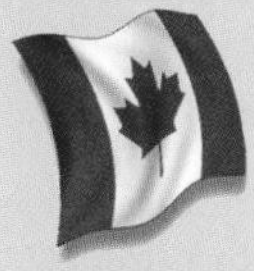	Buffalo Wings
	Cheddar & Sour Cream
	Crispy Bacon
	Dill Pickle
	Ketchup
	Onion and Garlic
USA 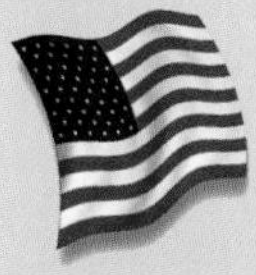	New York Cheddar with Herbs
	Honey Dijon
	Yogurt & Green Onion
	Roasted Red Pepper with Goat Cheese
	Spicy Thai
	Cheddar Beer
New Zealand 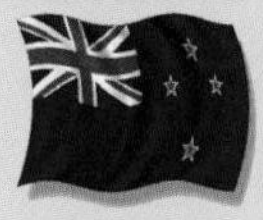	Chili & Sour Cream
	Feta & Italian Herbs
	Honey Soy Chicken
	Caramelized Onion
	Roast Chicken, Sage, & Onion
	Roast Lamb & Mint
	Smoked Salmon & Capers
	Sundried Tomato & Balsamic Vinegar
United Kingdom 	Black Olive & Garlic
	Black Pepper & Ginger
	Horseradish & Sour Cream
	Mature Cheddar & Red Onion
	Sundried Tomato & Basil
	Heinz Tomato Ketchup
	Lamb & Mint
	Marmite Yeast Extract
	Pickled Onion
	Prawn Cocktail
	Steak & Onion
Japan 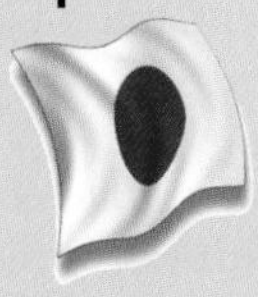	American Burger
	Caesar Salad
	Caramel Butter
	Cheese Cake
	Cheese Curry
	Consommé
	Cream Croquette
	Cream of Corn
	Deep Fried Battered Pork
	Gorgonzola
	Ham and Cream
	Indian Curry
	Mushroom & Bacon
	Spicy Pork
	Tandoori Chicken
	Tofu in a Spicy Pork Sauce

Cost

Food cost plays an important role in determining food choice. Beginning in the 1950s, the industrialization of food production; the initiation of food subsidies for mostly wheat, corn, and soy; and the commercialization of the beef, chicken, and pork industries dramatically changed food choices. This trend resulted in the production of cheap, plentiful food as evidenced by the dramatic increase in fast-food outlets on six continents. Americans now spend more money on fast food ($110 billion) than on movies, music, books, magazines, and newspapers combined. McDonalds, the largest of the fast-food restaurants, has 32,000 restaurants in 117 countries worldwide with 1.7 million employees that feed 46 million people daily (more than Spain's population)! Compared with people 30 years ago, individuals in industrialized nations share the following four characteristics regarding "food":

1. They consume more total food
2. They consume more snacks
3. They consume larger food portions
4. They consume more calories

Also playing a role are new product introductions, particularly more convenient ones, less costly imports, growth in the away-from-home food sector, expanded advertising programs, and changes in food enrichment standards.

Beverages provide an example of how government subsidies, marketing, and related forces have changed food consumption patterns and trends. In 1945, Americans drank more than four times more milk as carbonated soft drinks; in 2010, they downed nearly four times more soda than milk! Milk consumption has decreased, alcohol consumption has leveled off and decreased slightly, and soft drink and bottled water consumption have dramatically increased in the last 10 years.[9,10]

HIGH-GLYCEMIC CARBOHYDRATES ON THE RISE SINCE 1970

Americans now consume about 45% more calories from grains than in 1970, with about 90% in refined form. In 1970, daily consumption averaged 430 kcal; by 2008, the typical daily caloric intake from grains averaged 625 kcal, and in 2011, it increased to about 700 kcal. This excess has paralleled the nation's increase in excess body fat and type 2 diabetes. Consumption of these "empty calories" also displaces the nutrient-rich vegetables, fruits, beans, nuts, and whole grains that could help to lower blood pressure and positively improve the overall health profile. The statistics are staggering: Since 1970, on a yearly basis, Americans now consume about 25% more refined grains; three times more cheese; almost double the amount of meat, poultry, and seafood (120 pounds yearly); and about 20 pounds more per person of sugars (100 pounds of sugars per person; roughly one half from cane or beet sugar and one half from high-fructose corn syrup).

Choosing Food Based on Nutritional Value

Choosing foods based on nutritional value, unlike the other reasons for choosing foods, is a consciously learned behavior. Choosing nutritious foods can coexist with other gratifications including physical pleasure, emotional satisfaction, cost economy, and convenience. Learning to eat nutritiously requires motivation, knowledge, and commitment, but once learned, it can become a lifelong "habit."

Choosing Foods Based on Nutrient Density: Determining a food's **nutrient density** or "healthfulness" provides useful information about its nutritional quality.[4,5] This should be of particular interest to athletes and others who train on a regular basis for reasons related to achieving optimal nutrition and sports performance. One concept of nutrient density considers the quantity of a specific nutrient (protein, vitamins, minerals) per 100 g or per 1000 kcal of the food. In essence, comparing foods for nutrient density conveniently determines the better food source for a particular nutrient. Computing a food's **Index of Nutritional Quality (INQ)** makes this practical. Usually, the numerator of the INQ refers to the nutrient amount per 100 g of food divided by the Recommended Dietary Allowance (RDA) for that nutrient. The denominator represents the number of kcal per 100 g divided by the population average for daily energy intake (3000 kcal for men and 2000 kcal for women). An INQ greater than 1.0 means the food provides an adequate source of that nutrient; an INQ below 1.0 indicates an inadequate nutritional source. For convenience in classification, a food considered "good" has an INQ between 2 and 6, whereas an INQ above 6 denotes an "excellent" source of the nutrient.

INQ = (Amount of nutrient per 100 g ÷ RDA for that nutrient) ÷ (kcal in 100 g ÷ Population average for daily energy intake)

The following calculations determine which food provides the best source of protein: whole milk, 2% milk, 1% low-fat milk, a raw egg, chocolate chip cookies, or a McDonald's Big Mac hamburger. The calculations apply to an adult male (age 25–50 years) with an average daily energy intake of 3000 kcal.

First, refer to Appendix A for the protein content for 100 g (3.52 oz) of each of the six foods. The following example illustrates how to compute the INQ for protein in one raw egg:

Step 1. Compute the amount of protein in 100 g of egg. Appendix A presents the values in 1 oz, or 28.4 g. Because there is 3.52 g of protein per 28.4 g of egg (0.124 g of protein per 1 g of egg), 100 g of egg yields 12.4 g of protein.

Step 2. Divide the **Step 1** result by 63 g (protein RDA for adult males, age 25–50 years); 12.4 g ÷ 63 g = 0.17.

Step 3. Compute the number of kcal in 100 g of egg. Because 1 oz (28.34 g) yields 40 kcal (1.41 kcal per 1 g of egg), then 100 g of egg yields 141 kcal.

Step 4. Divide the **Step 3** result by 3000 kcal (daily energy expenditure for average adult male): 141 kcal ÷ 3000 kcal ÷ 0.047.

Step 5. Divide the **Step 2** result by the **Step 4** result to obtain the INQ for the protein in egg: 0.17 ÷ 0.047 = 4.2.

The other food items have the following protein INQ values: whole milk, 2.67; 2% milk, 3.24; 1% low-fat milk, 3.75; chocolate chip cookies, 0.61; and Big Mac, 0.525. The inescapable conclusion is that egg ranks first and 1% low-fat milk second as the best protein sources per quantity of food compared with the other food items.

A food's excellent INQ rating for a single nutrient does not reflect an equivalent rating for other nutrients. No single food ranks excellent for all of its nutrients. *In essence, no perfect food exists; some foods are just more nutritious for a particular nutrient per amount of food consumed.*

The Aggregate Nutrient Density Index Gains in Popularity: The **Aggregate Nutrient Density Index** (ANDI; **www.eatrightamerica.com/andi-superfoods**) provides an alternative way to calculate a food's nutritional quality. The index was developed to include the influence of many known healthful nutrients, not just protein, vitamins, and minerals as with the INQ. The following 20 nutrients are included in the ANDI:

1. Calcium
2. Beta-carotene
3. Alpha-carotene
4. Lutein
5. Zeaxanthin
6. Lycopene
7. Fiber
8. Folate
9. Glucosinolates
10. Iron
11. Magnesium
12. Niacin
13. Selenium
14. Vitamin B_1 (thiamin)
15. Vitamin B_2 (riboflavin)
16. Vitamin B_6
17. Vitamin B_{12}
18. Vitamin C
19. Vitamin E
20. Zinc

A nonnutrient, the Oxygen Radical Absorbance Capacity (ORAC) score, is also included (see the box titled "ORAC: A New Measure of Antioxidant Phytochemical Influence").

The Whole Foods Market chain (**www.wholefoodsmarket.com/healthstartshere/andi.php**) uses the ANDI score as part of an initiative to help consumers choose more "healthful foods" without having to count calories or obsess over any one nutrient like lipid. ANDI nutrient quantities, which normally are expressed using different measurements (e.g., milligrams, micrograms, International Units), are converted to a percentage of their reference daily intake (RDI) so that a common value is considered for each nutrient. Because no RDI currently exists for carotenoids, glucosinolates, or the ORAC score, creating goal values is based on available research and current understanding of the benefits of these factors. All nutrients are weighted equally except for the food's ORAC score. The ORAC score has a weighting factor of 2 (as if it were two nutrients) due to the supposed importance of antioxidant nutrients to good health. The sum of the food's total nutrient value is then multiplied by a fraction to make the highest number (i.e., most nutritious) equal 1000, so that all foods could be considered on a numerical scale of 1 to 1000.

The following are the ANDI scores for 20 common foods:

Food	ANDI	Food	ANDI
Kale	1000	White potato	31
Collards	1000	Skim milk	36
Spinach	73	Chicken breast	27
Bok choy	824	Tofu	37
Brussels sprouts	672	Ground beef	20
Carrots	240	White (regular) pasta	18
Strawberries	212	Potato chips	11
Oranges	10	Vanilla ice cream	9
Sweet potatoes	83	French fries	7
Pistachio nuts	48	Cola	0.6

ORAC: A NEW MEASURE OF ANTIOXIDANT PHYTOCHEMICAL INFLUENCE

The Oxygen Radical Absorbance Capacity unit (ORAC value or ORAC score) represents a method to quantify antioxidant capacity in biological samples. The precise relationship between the food's ORAC value and its health benefit has not been firmly established, yet many nutritionists believe that foods higher on the ORAC scale will more effectively neutralize damaging free radicals than foods lower on the scale. According to the free radical theory of aging, consuming foods with a high ORAC score slows oxidative processes and subsequent free radical damage that can contribute to age-related tissue degeneration and disease.

Kohri S, et al. An oxygen radical absorbance capacity-like assay that directly quantifies the antioxidant's scavenging capacity against AAPH-derived free radicals. *Anal Biochem* 2009;386:167.

Guidance for Industry, Food Labeling; Nutrient Content Claims; Definition for "High Potency" and Definition for "Antioxidant" for Use in Nutrient Content Claims for Dietary Supplements and Conventional Foods. US Department of Health and Human Services, Food and Drug Administration, Center for Food Safety and Applied Nutrition, June 2008.

Litescu SC, et al. Methods for the determination of antioxidant capacity in food and raw materials. *Adv Exp Med Biol* 2011;68:241.

Appetite Versus Hunger: Appetite and hunger do not have the same meanings. Appetite represents the desire to eat and is affected by external and psychological factors; it addresses the question, "What do I want to eat?" The answer is influenced by smell, sight, temperature, humidity, learned preferences, and the situational context of the meal (who you are with, location, time of day, and medication and metabolic influences). Hunger represents an internal drive to eat largely based on central (hypothalamus, vagus nerve) and peripheral physiologic modulations (blood glucose levels, increases in the hormones glucagon, ghrelin [hormone produced in the stomach and pancreas that stimulates appetite], and leptin [hormone produced by adipose tissue than counters the actions of ghrelin and insulin]) and addresses the question, "When can or will I eat?"

CONTRARIAN VIEW OF THE US DIETARY GUIDELINES FOR AMERICANS: TIME TO CHANGE STRATEGIES TO IMPROVE OVERALL HEALTH?

The *US Dietary Guidelines for Americans* have a major impact on Americans' diets because federal food policies, including standards for schools and many federal food-assistance programs, must comply with their recommendations. Agroindustrial interests stand to gain or lose from their implementation of carefully monitored *Guidelines* development. Drs. Willett and Ludwig of the Harvard School of Public Health argue that, although important progress has been made, Americans should rely on multiple sources for information about diet and health until the process of formulating the *Guidelines* fundamentally improves. They make a case for real reform that focuses on foods rather than individual nutrients because (1) the relationship between diet and chronic disease cannot be adequately predicted from the effects of individual nutrients, and (2) people choose foods, not nutrients, when deciding what to consume. The researchers also posit that the *Guidelines* represent the assessments of a relatively small group of experts with limited time who must summarize and interpret a vast, complex, often inconsistent, and rapidly growing body of data. Within this context, prior beliefs and/or biases may weigh heavily on opinions given. The following recommendations warrant consideration in formulating future *Guidelines*:

1. Move primary responsibility for *Guideline* development to the Centers for Disease Control and Prevention or Institute of Medicine to avoid conflicts of interest at the US Department of Agriculture arising from its institutional mission to promote commodities.
2. Provide the advisory committee with adequate funds to ensure a comprehensive scientific review.
3. Regularly update nutrient DRIs (used to inform the *Guidelines*).
4. Conduct all stages of *Guideline* development in open meetings.
5. Prepare public recommendations with direct input from advisory committee members.
6. Base recommendations primarily on foods, not nutrients.
7. Write *Guidelines* that explicitly state which foods should be consumed less by Americans to reduce risk for chronic disease.

Source: Willett WC, Ludwig DS. The 2010 Dietary Guidelines—The Best Recipe for Health? *N Engl J Med* 2011; 365:1563.

REGULATING WHAT WE EAT: FOOD AND NUTRITION POLICY

For the past 60 years, both positive and negative dramatic changes have impacted the food and nutrition scene. The most blatant example of negativism concerns how multinational companies laser focus on profit rather than consumer well-being. Collectively, companies allocate billions of dollars annually to espouse supposed "health benefits" of vitamins and minerals, specialty foods, and diverse dietary supplements. Similarly, manufacturers of home exercise equipment often succumb to false and deceptive advertising to entice customers to purchase their products. Undoubtedly, big-budget advertising pays off. Almost 200 million Americans purchase billions of dollars of dietary supplements, including over $3 billion worth of exercise equipment that includes abdominal and thigh burner "slimming" boards and gadgets, stationary bicycles, rowers, beltless treadmills, "gliders," face and neck "shapers," and countless exercise DVDs that tout exercise routines for getting fit and reducing body weight and excess body fat.

The US Food and Drug Administration (FDA; www.fda.gov/) is the government agency tasked to regulate the following eight categories of products:

1. Food
2. Drugs (prescription, over-the-counter, generics)
3. Medical devices (e.g., pacemakers, contact lenses, hearing aids)
4. Biologics (e.g., vaccines)
5. Animal feed and drugs
6. Cosmetics
7. Radiation-emitting products (e.g., cell phones, lasers, microwaves)
8. Combination products

The FDA also regulates dietary supplements but under a different set of regulations than "conventional" food and drug products.[13] The **Dietary Supplement Health and Education Act of 1994** (**DSHEA**; www.fda.gov/food/dietarysupplements/default.htm) requires that the dietary supplement manufacturer assume responsibility for ensuring that a supplement meets all safety requirements before marketing it. The FDA can take legal action against any unsafe dietary supplement product after it reaches the market. Generally, manufacturers do not need to register their dietary supplement products with the FDA or receive FDA approval before producing or selling them. Manufacturers must ensure that product label information remains truthful and not deceptive or misleading.

The FDA's postmarketing responsibilities include monitoring safety, such as voluntary dietary supplement adverse event reporting, and product information, including labeling, claims, package inserts, and accompanying literature. Another important agency, the Federal Trade Commission (FTC; www.ftc.gov/) regulates dietary supplement advertising.

The Nutrition Labeling and Education Act of 1990 (**NLEA**; www.fda.gov/ICECI/Inspections/InspectionGuides/ucm074948.htm) defines commonly consumed dietary supplements in the marketplace in the form of capsules, tablets, liquids, or powders. This also includes vitamins, essential minerals, protein, amino acids, botanicals such as ginseng and yohimbe, extracts from animal glands, garlic extract, fish oils, fibers such as acacia guar gum, compounds not generally recognized as foods or nutrients such as bioflavonoids, enzymes, germanium, nucleic acids, para-aminobenzoic acid, and rutin, and mixtures of these ingredients.

FOOD ADVERTISING AND PACKAGING

In the late 1970s, renewed interest in nutrition and healthful eating occurred when the medical community linked cholesterol-rich diets to high blood cholesterol, a primary risk factor for heart disease. In addition, large-scale epidemiologic studies linked many forms of cancer to dietary practices. Coincidentally, the emerging physical fitness movement that swept North America beginning in the 1960s superimposed on the diet–heart disease and diet–cancer connections. Health clubs flourished, and articles in the lay press championed the latest tips on how to improve physical fitness and overall health by eating well and exercising regularly.

Advertising's Goal: To Shape Behavior

Advertising purposely attempts to create, shape, and alter perceptions about what we eat and how we exercise. The food industry spends more than $45 billion a year on advertising and promotion to sell its products and hundreds of millions more for lobbying. In 2006, 44 major US food and beverage marketers spent $1.6 billion to promote their products to children under age 12 and adolescents age 12 to 17. The companies integrate television, packaging, in-store advertising, sweepstakes, and the Internet to market their products. Not surprisingly, television advertising plays the greatest role—children and adolescents view up to 6100 televised food advertisements yearly or nearly 17 ads every day. Approximately one third of the ads are for candy and snacks, one fourth are for cereal, and one tenth tout fast food. Only 5% are devoted to healthy foods and beverages. No ads specifically target fruits and vegetables. This represents a real disconnect between federal guidelines that emphasize eating a healthy diet versus the large food manufacturers that effectively short circuit the efforts to get people to alter their eating habits by making healthy food choices.

Food companies also provide funds to academic departments and research institutes; they support conventions, meetings, and conferences and contribute to the production of "fact sheets." Companies such as *Coca-Cola*, *Monsanto*, *Procter & Gamble*, and *Slim-Fast* often sponsor nutrition journals and help to sponsor scientific conferences. Food and drug companies underwrite the cost of publishing journal supplements of papers presented at conferences they frequently support. In some instances, corporate funding underwrites entire departments at universities.

McDonald's Corporation, the largest purchaser in the United States of pork, beef, and potatoes and the second largest purchaser of chicken, spends more than any other company in the world to advertise its products. In 2008, McDonald's spent $823 million on advertising, which skyrocketed in 2011 to over $1.7 billion on direct media advertising (radio, television, print). Contrast this sum with the less than $1 million the National Cancer Institute spends to promote good nutrition! Soft drink manufacturers commit over $1 billion or more each year to advertise products. According to the National Soft Drink Association (NSDA; **www.everyday-wisdom.com/soft-drink-consumption.html**), soft drink consumption now exceeds 600 12-oz (340.19 g) servings per person per year. Compared to 40 years ago, soft drink consumption in the United States has doubled for females and tripled for males. The highest consumers are young males age 12 to 29 years whose average consumption is 0.5 gallons daily, or 160 gallons per year, double that of annual milk consumption!

A CONTRIBUTING FACTOR TO THE OBESITY EPIDEMIC

For every $1 spent on ads that urge us to eat multiple servings of fruits and vegetables daily, the food and beverage industries spend $1100 enticing us to buy fast-food meals, soft drinks, sugary breakfast cereals, and other foods that contribute to the country's massive waist sprawl.

Governmental agencies try to police the food industry by legislating how manufacturers can advertise their products. Unfortunately, no state or federal guidelines require that a company disclose all the facts about a product to support a particular claim. Manufacturers of many dietary supplements, for example, retain the luxury of interpreting the "facts" about their product's effectiveness. Consequently, the consumer must decipher what the advertising actually means and interpret the information on food labels.

GOVERNMENT "WATCHDOG" AGENCIES

TABLE 9.2 presents an overview of the different agencies that ensure food safety in the United States. The agencies listed in the table also work with other governmental agencies such as the Consumer Product Safety Commission (www.cpsc.gov) to enforce the Poison Prevention Packaging Act (www.cpsc.gov/businfo/pppa.pdf); the Federal Bureau of Investigation (FBI; www.fbi.gov) to enforce the Federal Anti-Tampering Act (www.fda.gov/opacom/laws/fedatact.htm); and the US

TABLE 9.2 Us Food Safety Team. The United States Maintains a Monitoring System to Monitor Food Production and Distribution at Every Level (Local, State, and National). Monitoring Proceeds by Food Inspectors, Microbiologists, Epidemiologists, and Other Food Scientists Working for City and County Health Departments, State Public Health Agencies, and Different Federal Departments and Agencies

Agency	Functions
US Department of Health and Human Services	
Food and Drug Administration www.cfsan.fda.gov/list.html;	Oversees all domestic and imported food sold in interstate commerce, including shell eggs, but not meat and poultry **http://www.fda.gov/cvm/**
Centers for Disease Control and Prevention www.cdc.gov	Oversees all foods; investigates with local, state, and other federal officials sources of food-borne disease outbreaks; develops and advocates public health policies to prevent food-borne diseases; conducts research to help prevent food-borne illness
US Department of Agriculture	
Food Safety and Inspection Service www.fsis.usda.gov	Oversees domestic and imported meat and poultry and related products, such as meat- or poultry-containing stews, pizzas and frozen foods, processed egg products (generally liquid, frozen, and dried pasteurized egg products)
Cooperative State Research, Education, and Extension Service www.reeusda.gov	Oversees all domestic foods, some imported (with US colleges and universities, develops research and education programs on food safety for farmers and consumers)
National Agricultural Library Usda/Fda Foodborne Illness Education Information Center www.nal.usda.gov/fnic/	Oversees all foods (maintains a database of computer software, audiovisuals, posters, games, teachers' guides, and other educational materials on preventing food-borne illness)
US Environmental Protection Agency www.epa.gov	Oversees drinking water (regulates toxic substances and wastes to prevent their entry into the environment and food chain, assists states in monitoring quality of drinking water and finding ways to prevent contamination of drinking water, determines safety of new pesticides, sets tolerance levels for pesticide residues in foods, and publishes directions on safe use of pesticides)
US Department of Commerce	
National Oceanic And Atmospheric Administration http://seafood.nmfs.noaa.gov/	Oversees fish and seafood products (through its fee-for-service seafood inspection program; inspects and certifies fishing vessels, seafood processing plants, and retail facilities for federal sanitation standards)
US Department of the Treasury	
Bureau of Alcohol, Tobacco and Firearms www.atf.treas.gov/alcohol/index.htm	Oversees alcoholic beverages except wine beverages containing less than 7% alcohol (enforces food safety laws governing production and distribution of alcoholic beverages; investigates cases of adulterated alcoholic products, sometimes with help from FDA)
US Customs Service www.customs.ustreas.gov	Oversees imported foods (works with federal regulatory agencies to ensure that all goods entering and exiting the United States do so according to US laws and regulations)
US Department of Justice www.usdoj.gov.	Oversees all foods (prosecutes companies and individuals suspected of violating food safety laws; through US marshals service, seizes unsafe food products not yet in the marketplace, as ordered by courts)
Federal Trade Commission/www.ftc.gov	Oversees all foods (enforces a variety of laws that protect consumers from unfair, deceptive, or fraudulent practices, including deceptive and unsubstantiated advertising)
State and Local Governments	Oversee all foods within their jurisdictions (work with FDA and other federal agencies to implement food safety standards for fish, seafood, milk, and other foods produced within state borders; inspect restaurants, grocery stores, and other retail food establishments, as well as dairy farms and milk processing plants, grain mills, and food manufacturing plants within local jurisdictions; embargo [stop the sale of] unsafe food products made or distributed within state borders)

Postal Service (**www.usps.com**) to enforce laws prohibiting mail fraud.

Federal Trade Commission

The FTC regulates food product advertising in various media (television, radio, newsprint) and pursues legal action against manufacturers who advertise unsubstantiated claims or deceptive ads. For example, if a television ad states, "Consuming this supplement reduces your chances of colon cancer," the FTC can require the manufacturer to substantiate the claim. The FTC has authority to remove a product from the marketplace if the product's claims lack verification.

The FTC describes its mission as follows: *"To enforce a variety of federal antitrust and consumer protection laws. The commission seeks to ensure that the nation's markets function competitively, and are vigorous, efficient, and free of undue restrictions."* The FTC also works to enhance the smooth operation of the marketplace by eliminating unfair or deceptive acts or practices. With regard to exercise and fitness, the FTC maintains vigilance concerning false and misleading claims for workout gear and all types of exercise equipment. As the nation's consumer protection agency, the FTC offers tips to separate fitness facts from physical fiction. The FTC warns that some advertisers promote—without evidence—that their shoes, clothing, equipment, or other exercise add-ons offer a quick, easy way to shape up and get fit. The FTC provides useful tips for buying exercise equipment (**www.ftc.gov/bcp/consumer/products/pro10.shtm**) as part of *Project Workout*, the FTC consumer education campaign (**www.ftc.gov/opa/1997/06/workout.shtm**). In general, the FTC's efforts are directed toward stopping actions that threaten consumers' opportunities to exercise informed choice. The FTC also undertakes economic analysis to support its law enforcement efforts and to contribute to the policy deliberations of Congress, the executive branch, other independent agencies, and state and local governments when requested.

FTC FINES REEBOK $25 MILLION FOR DECEPTIVE SHOE ADVERTISING

The FTC continues to prosecute equipment manufacturers of exercise-related equipment for fraudulent and misleading advertisements concerning their products. The most recent high-profile settlement ordered the shoe and clothing manufacturer Reebok to pay $25 million in customer refunds to settle charges it deceptively advertised its *EasyTone* walking shoes and *RunTone* running shoes that Reebok claimed would measurably strengthen the leg, thigh, and buttocks muscles. The FTC's complaint against Reebok included that they falsely claimed their "toning" footwear had made a 28% gain in strength and tone in the buttock muscles, 11% more strength and tone in the hamstring muscles, and 11% more strength and tone in the calf muscles than regular walking shoes. Beginning in early 2009, Reebok advertised its claims through print, television, and the Internet. The claims also appeared on shoe boxes and counter displays in retail stores. As part of the settlement, Reebok was barred from making such claims without proper scientific evidence, and further misrepresenting any tests, studies, or research results regarding toning shoes and other toning apparel.

Source: www. ftc.gov/opa/2011/09/reebok.shtm

Connections to the Past

Edward Smith (1819–1874)

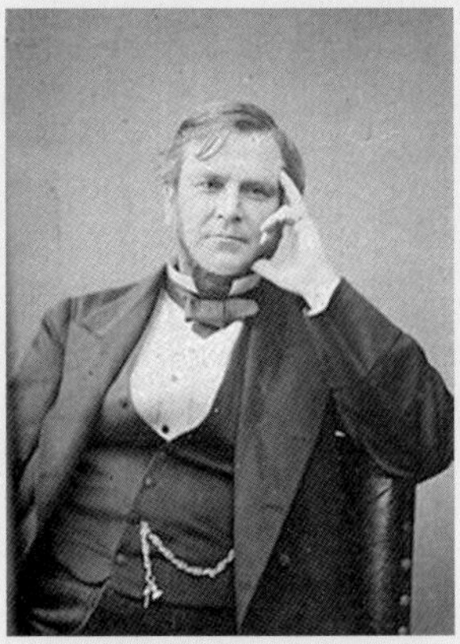

Edward Smith, a physician, public health advocate, and social reformer, advocated better living conditions for Britain's lower classes, including prisoners. He believed they were maltreated because they received no additional food while toiling on the exhausting "punitive treadmill." In 1863, the first government-sponsored survey of food consumption in low-income families, supervised by Smith, proved the inadequacy of their diet. Bread was the staple (19.1 lb [8.7 kg] per adult per week), followed by potatoes (2.4 lb; 10.9 kg), milk (16 oz; 453.6 g), meats (0.8 lb; 362.9 g), sugar (0.5 lb; 0.23 kg), and fats (0.3 lb; 0.14 kg). A daily food intake of 2190 kcal (9167 kJ) consisted of 370 g of carbohydrate, 53 g of fat, and 55 g of protein. Smith argued that prisoners consuming a diet consisting of 93% carbohydrate would become ill. Thus, diet had social consequences. Disabled by weakness, prisoners would be unable to perform hard labor after release and would be more likely to resort to crime.

Smith had observed prisoners climbing up a treadwheel, whose steps resembled the side paddle wheels of a Victorian steamship. Prisoners climbed for 15 minutes, followed by a 15-minute rest, for a total of 4 hours of work three times a week. To overcome resistance from a sail on the prison roof attached to the treadwheel, each man traveled the equivalent of 1.43 miles up a steep hill.

thePoint *Visit* **thePoint.lww.com/MKKSEN4e** *for more details about how Smith used closed-circuit spirometry to demonstrate that protein was not the main fuel for exercise.*

Food and Drug Administration

The FDA represents one of 13 agencies within the Department of Health and Human Services (DHHS; www.hhs.gov). With the exception of poultry and meat products, the FDA regulates what manufacturers can state on food labels; the safety of cosmetics, medicines, and medical devices; and feed and drugs for pets and farm animals. The FDA also decides what additives manufacturers can add to foods, including potential hazards with food additives (contaminants), foodborne infections, toxicants, artificially constituted foods, biologics, medical devices, radiological products, and pesticide residues.

One of six major FDA agencies (see TABLE 9.2), the **Center for Food Safety and Applied Nutrition** (CFSAN; **www.fda.gov/food/default.htm**) regulates billions of dollars of imported food and cosmetic products sold across state lines. The CFSAN employs about 800 people to carry out its mission that (1) the food supply remains safe, nutritious, and wholesome and (2) labels on foods and cosmetics maintain a high degree of accuracy. These two goals make sense when one considers that about one fifth of every consumer dollar in the United States goes for food and cosmetic products. Consumers spend 25 cents of every consumer dollar on products regulated by the FDA. Of this amount, approximately 75% is spent on food.

The CFSAN specialized support staff includes chemists, microbiologists, toxicologists, food technologists, pathologists, pharmacologists, nutritionists, physicians, epidemiologists, mathematicians, and sanitarians. Their five main areas of responsibility include the following:

1. Cosmetics and colors
2. Food labeling
3. Plant and dairy foods and beverages
4. Premarket approval
5. Special nutritionals such as dietary supplements and infant formulas

The law defines a "**dietary supplement**" (typically sold in the form of tablets, capsules, soft gels, liquids, powders, or bars) as a product taken by mouth that contains a "dietary ingredient" intended to supplement the diet. "Dietary ingredients" may include vitamins, minerals, herbs or other botanicals, amino acids, and substances (e.g., enzymes, organ tissues, glandular material, and metabolites). Dietary supplements may also be extracts or concentrates from plants or foods. Products sold as dietary supplements must be clearly labeled as dietary supplements.

The DSHEA of 1994 reduced the FDA's control over vitamin, mineral, enzyme, hormone, botanical, amino acid, and herb supplements, which were reclassified as "foods" not drugs. Under the DSHEA, FDA approval stringently requires proof of purity, safety, and effectiveness (via clinical trials) for public consumption of over-the-counter and prescription pharmaceuticals. Marketing of dietary supplements does *not* require such approval because they are considered "foods." In contrast to medicines, which must meet safety and efficacy requirements before they come to market, legislation places the burden on the FDA to prove that a supplement is harmful before it can remove it from the market. Extolling the benefits of a supplement can progress with *only* the manufacturer's assurance of safety provided the supplement does not claim disease-fighting benefits. Since DSHEA passage, dietary supplements in the United States have skyrocketed, jumping from $5 billion in 1994 to nearly $10 billion in 1997 to over $29 billion in 2011. Estimates indicate the global supplement industry as a $200 billion per year business that is growing steadily at approximately 35% annually. Sixty-five percent of adult Americans, or approximately 150 million people, consider themselves supplement users according to a 2009 survey conducted for the Council for Responsible Nutrition (CRN; founded in 1973; **www.crnusa.org**). In the sports nutrition and weight-loss category of sales, sales growth achieved 9% in 2010 to reach $23 billion.

A manufacturer of an iron-containing supplement cannot make a specific unsubstantiated health claim about a product such as "This product cures anemia." However, more generalized "structure and function" claims are permissible, such as "Iron is important in the synthesis of hemoglobin in red blood cells." The frightening aspect of lessened control over the supplement industry means that many supplements consumed in excess mimic the harmful effects of illegally obtained chemicals and drugs.

Rules for Dietary Supplements

To add strength to the 1994 DSHEA, the FDA approved a dietary supplement bill in September 1997. The FDA published final rules that provided consumers with somewhat more complete information in the labeling of dietary supplement products. These rules implement some of the major provisions of the 1994 DSHEA designed to facilitate public access to "natural" medicines. The act requires the FDA to develop labeling requirements specifically designed for products containing ingredients such as vitamins, minerals, herbs, or amino acids intended to supplement the diet.

The new rules require these products to be labeled as dietary supplements (e.g., "Vitamin C Dietary Supplement") and to carry a "Supplement Facts" panel (see page 291) with information similar to the "Nutrition Facts" panel that appears on most processed foods (see page 294). The rules also set parameters for use of the terms *high potency* and *antioxidant* when used in the labeling of dietary supplements. *Despite this attempt by the government to upgrade industry standards, consumers must recognize that quality control does not fully exist for dietary supplements.*

The rules also require that the labels of products containing botanical ingredients identify the part of the plant used. In addition, the source of the dietary ingredient may either follow the name or be listed in the ingredient statement below the "Supplement Parts" panel.

The following two guidelines apply for use of the terms *high potency* and *antioxidant* on food labels:

SUMMARY OF NUTRITIONAL LABELING RULES FOR DIETARY SUPPLEMENTS, UPDATED 2003

The FDA has mandated that all supplements contain consistent information on a "Supplement Facts" panel. The label must contain a title, a clear identity statement, and a complete list of all ingredients. The "Supplement Facts" panel must contain the following eight requirements:

1. Title: "Supplement Facts" to allow for easy identification.
2. Information must be listed "per serving." Serving sizes are determined by manufacturers' recommendations for consumption at one occasion.
3. Nutrients required in nutrition labeling of conventional foods must be listed when present and omitted when not present.
4. "Other dietary ingredients" (e.g., botanicals, phytochemicals) that do not have recommendations for daily consumption are listed as part of the label shown in the insert. The quantity present must be stated and identified as having no recommendations for consumption.
5. The list of dietary ingredients in the nutrition label (nutrients and nonnutrients) may include the source ingredient. If so, the source need not be listed again in the ingredient list.
6. Botanicals must state the part of the plant present and be identified by their common usual name. In addition, the Latin binomial name is needed if the common or usual name is not listed in *Herbs of Commerce,* published by the American Herbal Products Association.
7. Proprietary blends may be listed with the weight given for the total blend only. When this is done, components of the blend must be listed in descending order of predominance by weight.
8. When present at 0.5 g or more, *trans* fat must be listed in the Supplement Facts panel of a dietary supplement on a separate line under the listing of saturated fat.

SUPPLEMENT FACTS
Serving Size Four (4) Capsules

Amount per Serving		%DV
Natural beta carotene Plus mixed carotenoids	5000 iu	100%
Alpha carotene	1000 iu	*
Vit. C (ascorbic acid)	1000 mg	1167%
Bioflavonoids	50 mg	*
Ascorbyl palmitate	50 mg	*
Vit. D3 (cholecalciferol)	1000 iu	250%
Vit. E (natural) (succinate)	200 iu	667%
Vit. B1 (Thiamine)	100 mg	6667%
Vit. B2 (Riboflavin)	25 mg	1470%
Vit. B3 (Niacinamide Niacin)	125 mg	625%
Vit. B5 (panthothenic acid)	250 mg	2500%
Vit. B6 (pyridoxine HCL)	50 mg	2500%
Folic acid	800 mcg	200%
Vit. B12 (cyanocobalamin)	500 mcg	833%
Biotin	600 mcg	200%
Magnesium (citrate)	100 mg	25%
Calcium (citrate)	100 mg	10%
Iodine (kelp)	150 mcg	100%

Zinc (L-Monomethionine)	25 mg	167%
Selenium (GarliSelect®)	200 mcg	285%
Copper	1 mg	50%
Manganese	3 mg	150%
Chromium (ChromeMate®)	300 mcg	375%
Molydenum	125 mcg	169%
Boron	3 mg	*
Silica (horsetail)	5 mg	*
PABA	50 mg	*
Trimethylglycine (TMG)	50 mg	*
Alpha lipoic acid	50 mg	*
Lutein (OptiLut®)	6 mg	*
Lycopene	3 mg	*
Resveratrol (50% extract)	25 mg	*
Grape seed extract (Std. 95% polyphenols)	25 mg	*
Green tea extract (Std. 98% polyphenols)	25 mg	*
Milk thistle extract (Std. 70% silymarin)	25 mg	*
Bilberry extract (Std. 25% anthocyanidins)	25 mg	*

Other ingrediunts: Cellulose, Magnesium stearate

* Daily value (DV) not established.

1. **High potency** may be used to describe a nutrient in a food product, including dietary supplements, at 100% or more of the RDI established for that vitamin or mineral. High potency can be used with multi-ingredient products if two thirds of the product's nutrients occur at levels more than 100% of the RDI.
2. **Antioxidant** may be used in conjunction with currently defined claims for "good source" and "high" to describe a nutrient for which scientific evidence shows that following absorption of a sufficient quantity, the nutrient (e.g., vitamin C) inactivates free radicals or prevents free radical–initiated chemical reactions.

User Beware: Dietary supplements need not meet the same quality control for purity and potency as pharmaceuticals, allowing for considerable variation in the concentration of marker compounds.[12] So-called all-natural pills and powders sold as dietary supplements have caused lead poisoning, impotence, lethargy and "unarousable" sleep, nausea, vomiting, diarrhea, abnormal heart rhythms (from the presence of powerful pesticides, herbs, toxic contaminants, or potent prohibited drugs and hormones), and failed tests for illicit drug use in athletes trying to self-treat diverse ailments or improve physical function.[1]

Advertisements for "health food" preparations containing natural herbs often promise weight loss, muscle growth, increased endurance capacity, and a drug-free "herbal high." Some nutritionists believe these products are street drugs masquerading as diet supplements. To compound matters, the preparations appear as dietary supplements and thus escape the FDA's rigid control over foods and pharmaceuticals. Many compounds fail to conform to labeling requirements of the DSHEA for proper and correct identification of the strength of the product's ingredients. Simply stated, supplement manufacturers need not guarantee that all ingredients are on its label. In this regard, independent organizations such as ConsumerLab (**www.consumerlab.com**) provide their "seal of approval" about purity and quality control and the safety, effectiveness, and potential for adverse effects for numerous dietary and sport nutrition supplements. These include herbal, vitamin, and mineral supplements that affect health, wellness, and nutrition.

Bureau of Alcohol, Tobacco, Firearms and Explosives

The Bureau of Alcohol, Tobacco, Firearms and Explosives (ATF; **www.atf.gov**) regulates the qualification and operation of distilleries, breweries, wineries, and importers and wholesalers of alcohol-related products. The ATF National Laboratory, founded in 1886, tests new products coming onto the market and whether any products currently on the market pose a health risk to consumers. The ATF also ensures that alcohol beverage labels do not contain misleading information and examines all label applications for approval. The ATF maintains statistics about domestic alcohol and tobacco production.

US Department of Agriculture

The US Department of Agriculture (USDA; **www.usda.gov**) deals with farm and foreign agricultural services, food, nutrition, and consumer services, food safety, marketing and regulatory programs, natural resources and environment, research, education, economics, and rural development. The Center for Nutrition Policy and Promotion (**www.cnpp.usda.gov**) coordinates nutrition policy in the USDA and provides overall leadership in nutrition education for consumers. The goals of the program include providing needy individuals with access to a more nutritious diet, improving the eating habits of American children, and helping America's farmers find an outlet for distributing food purchased under farmer assistance authorities. The Center serves as the link between basic science and the consumer. The Center also coordinates with the DHHS the review, revision, and dissemination of the *Dietary Guidelines for Americans*, which represents the federal government's statement of nutrition policy, formed by a consensus of professionals in science and medicine. The USDA regulates food labels for poultry and meat products.

The USDA's Food and Nutrition Information Center (FNIC) maintains an Internet presence (**www.nal.usda.gov/fnic/**) where users may read, download, or print information. Individuals can access full texts of the FNIC's bibliographies, resource lists, and fact sheets covering nutrition education, human nutrition, and food service management. The FNIC also maintains a 2011 updated database to look up calories or nutrients in food. The output for a single food is extensive, as shown in the accompanying table for 100 grams (about 3 oz) of raw pistachio nuts.

FNIC Facts For Pistachio Nuts

Common Name: Pistachios
Scientific Name: *Pistacia veralist*
Nutrient Values and Weights for the Edible Portion

Nutrient	Unit	Value per 100 Grams
Water	g	3.91
Energy	kcal	562
Energy	kJ	2352
Protein	g	20.27
Total lipid (fat)	g	45.39
Ash	g	2.91
Carbohydrate, by difference	g	27.51
Fiber, total dietary	g	10.3
Sugars, total	g	7.66
Sucrose	g	6.87
Glucose (dextrose)	g	0.32
Fructose	g	0 .24
Lactose	g	0.00
Maltose	g	0.17
Starch	g	1.67
Minerals		
Calcium, Ca	mg	105
Iron, Fe	mg	3.92
Magnesium, Mg	mg	121
Phosphorus, P	mg	490
Potassium, K	mg	1025
Sodium, Na	mg	1
Zinc, Zn	mg	2.20
Copper, Cu	mg	1.300
Manganese, Mn	mg	1.200
Fluoride, F	µg	3.4
Selenium, Se	µg	7.0
Vitamins		
Vitamin C, total ascorbic acid	mg	5.6
Thiamin	mg	0.870
Riboflavin	mg	0.160
Niacin	mg	1.300
Pantothenic acid	mg	0.520
Vitamin B-6	mg	1.700
Folate, total	µg	51
Folic acid	µg	0
Folate, food	µg	51
Folate, DFE	µg_DFE	51
Vitamin B-12	µg	0.00

Vitamin A, RAE	µg_RAE	21
Retinol	µg	0
Carotene, beta	µg	249
Carotene, alpha	µg	0
Cryptoxanthin, beta	µg	0
Vitamin A, IU	IU	415
Lutein + zeaxanthin	µg	1405
Vitamin E (alpha-tocopherol)	mg	2.30
Tocopherol, beta	mg	0.00
Tocopherol, gamma	mg	22.60
Tocopherol, delta	mg	0.80
Vitamin D (D2 + D3)	µg	0.0
Vitamin D	IU	0
Lipids		
Fatty acids, total saturated	g	5.556
4:0	g	0.000
6:0	g	0.000
8:0	g	0.000
10:0	g	0.000
12:0	g	0.000
13:0	g	0.000
14:0	g	0.000
15:0	g	0.000
16:0	g	4.994
17:0	g	0.000
18:0	g	0.476
20:0	g	0.043
22:0	g	0.044
24:0	g	0.000
Fatty acids, total monounsaturated	g	23.820
14:1	g	0.000
16:1 undifferentiated	g	0.473
18:1 undifferentiated	g	23.174
20:1	g	0.174
22:1 undifferentiated	g	0.000
24:1 c	g	0.000
20:2 n-6 c,c	g	0.000
Fatty acids, total polyunsaturated	g	13.744
18:2 undifferentiated	g	13.485
18:3 undifferentiated	g	0.259
18:4	g	0.000
20:3 undifferentiated	g	0.000
20:4 undifferentiated	g	0.000
20:5 n-3 (EPA)	g	0.000
22:5 n-3 (DPA)	g	0.000
22:6 n-3 (DHA)	g	0.000
Fatty acids, total trans	g	0.000
Cholesterol	mg	0
Phytosterols	mg	214
Stigmasterol	mg	5
Campesterol	mg	10
Beta-sitosterol	mg	198
Amino acids		
Tryptophan	g	0.271
Threonine	g	0.667
Isoleucine	g	0.893
Leucine	g	1.542
Lysine	g	1.142
Methionine	g	0.335
Cystine	g	0.355
Phenylalanine	g	1.054
Tyrosine	g	0.412
Valine	g	1.230
Arginine	g	2.012
Histidine	g	0.503
Alanine	g	0.914
Aspartic acid	g	1.803
Glutamic acid	g	3.790
Glycine	g	0.946
Proline	g	0.805
Serine	g	1.216
Other		
Alcohol, ethyl	g	0.0
Caffeine	mg	0
Theobromine	mg	0

DIFFERENCES BETWEEN THE "NUTRITION FACTS" PANEL AND THE "SUPPLEMENT FACTS" PANEL

Nutrition Facts Panel	Supplement Facts Panel
Must list ingredients with RDIs or DRVs.	Must list dietary ingredients without RDIs or DRVs.
Cannot list the source of a dietary ingredient.	May list the source of a dietary ingredient.
Cannot list the part of a plant from which the food derives.	Must include the part of the plant from which a dietary ingredient is derived.
Must list "zero" amounts of nutrients.	Cannot list "zero" amounts of nutrients.
	Not required to list the source of a dietary ingredient in the ingredient statement if it is listed in the "Supplement Facts" panel.

THE FOOD LABEL (NUTRITION FACTS PANEL)

The FDA and the Food Safety and Inspection Service (FSIS; **www.fsis.usda.gov/**) of the USDA issue regulations concerning nutritional information contained in food labels to (1) help consumers choose more healthful diets and (2) offer an incentive to food companies to improve the nutritional qualities of their products. In addition, the Nutritional Labeling and Education Act (with 1998 updates to the regulations) now requires food manufacturers to strictly adhere to regulations about what can and cannot be printed on food labels. Nine key provisions of food label reform include the following:

1. Nutrition labeling for almost all foods to assist consumers in making more healthful food choices
2. Information on labels on the amount per serving of saturated fat, cholesterol, dietary fiber, and other

nutrients considered of major health concern to consumers

3. The amount of *trans* fatty acids on nutrition labels in light of mounting evidence that *trans* fatty acids increase heart disease risk
4. Nutrient reference values on labels, expressed as % daily values, to help consumers determine how a food fits into an overall daily diet
5. Uniform definitions for terms that describe a food's nutrient content, such as "light," "low-fat," and "high-fiber," to ensure that such terms have the same meaning for any product on which they appear
6. Substantiating claims about the relationship between a nutrient or food and a disease or health-related condition, such as calcium and osteoporosis, and fat and cancer
7. Standardized serving sizes to make nutritional comparisons among similar products easier
8. Declaration of total percentage of juice in juice drinks so consumers can determine a product's juice content
9. Voluntary nutrition information for many raw foods

The food label also must list ingredients according to how much of the ingredient the food contains. In 2006, food makers were required to clearly state on food labels whether the product contained allergens such as milk, eggs, peanuts, wheat, soy, fish, shellfish, and tree nuts. In July 2011, the American Academy of Allergy Asthma & Immunology (www.aaaai.org) estimated that food allergies affect up to 2 million or 8% of children in the United States.

Nutrition Panel Title

The food label displayed in **FIGURE 9.1**, entitled "Nutrition Facts," differs from the previous title (Nutrition Information per Serving) and represents a more distinctive and easy to read label.

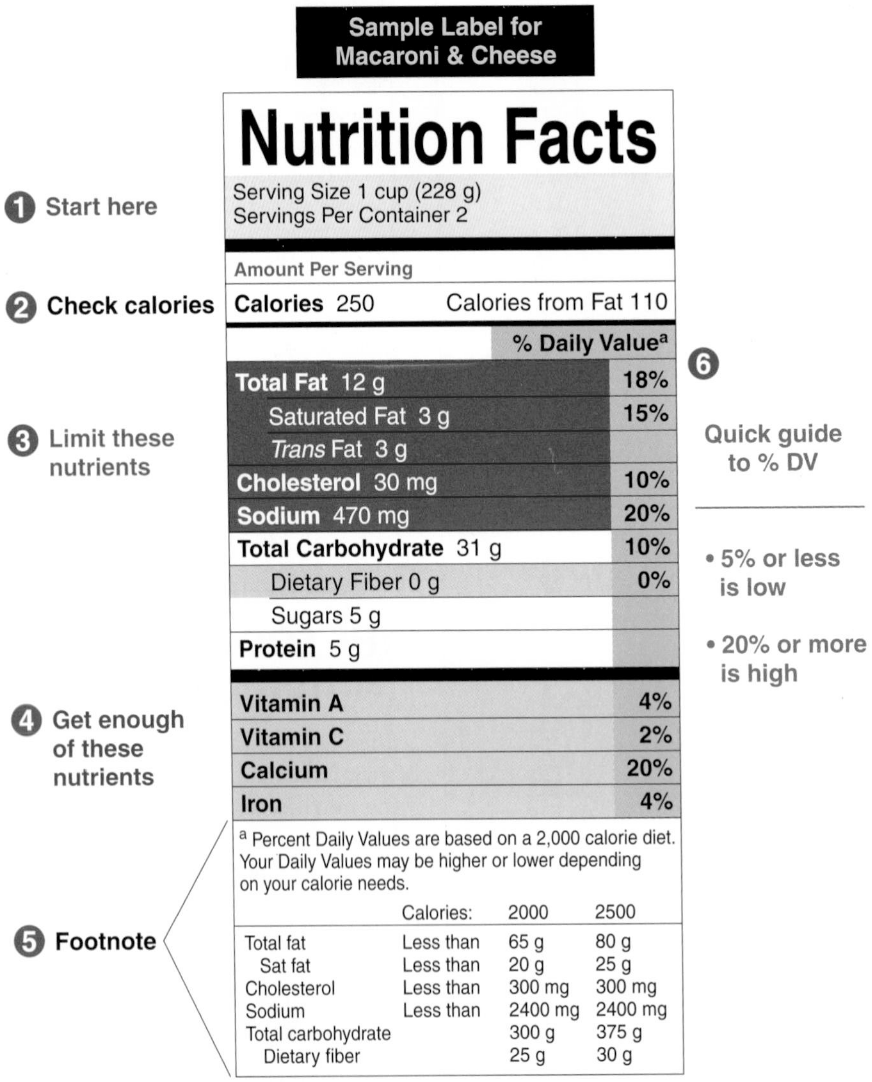

FIGURE 9.1 Reading the Nutrition Facts panel. Food labels help one make informed choices. Foods that contain only a few of the nutrients required on the standard label have a shorter label format. What is on the label depends on what is in the food. Small- and medium-sized packages with limited label space also can use the short form.

Nutrients Listed on Label

The following information must be listed on all food labels:

1. Calories from fat/calories from saturated fat
2. Total fat
3. Saturated fat, stearic acid, polyunsaturated fat, monounsaturated fat, *trans* fat
4. Cholesterol
5. Sodium
6. Potassium
7. Total carbohydrate
8. Dietary fiber (soluble and insoluble fiber)
9. Sugars (sugar alcohols)
10. Other carbohydrates
11. Protein
12. Vitamins and minerals (for which RDIs have been established)

Definitions

The definitions for each of the seven nutrients listed on the label are as follows:

1. **Total fat:** Total lipid fatty acids expressed as triglycerides
2. **Saturated fat:** The sum of all fatty acids containing no double bonds
3. **Polyunsaturated fat:** *cis,cis*-methylene interrupted polyunsaturated fatty acids
4. **Monounsaturated fat:** *cis*-monounsaturated fatty acids
5. **Total carbohydrate:** Amount calculated by subtraction of the sum of crude protein, total fat, moisture, and ash from the total weight of food
6. **Sugars:** The sum of all free monosaccharides and disaccharides
7. **Other carbohydrate:** The difference between total carbohydrate and the sum of dietary fiber, sugars, and, when declared, sugar alcohol

DAILY VALUES

The Nutrition Facts panel must contain two sets of label reference values collectively termed Daily Values. These include Daily Reference Values (DRVs) and RDIs.

Daily Reference Value

Only the DRV term appears on the label to make label reading less confusing. DRVs established for macronutrients include sources of energy (fat, carbohydrate [including fiber], and protein) and non–calorie-contributing cholesterol, sodium, and potassium. A daily intake of 2000 kcal serves as the reference number of calories for determining the DRVs for the energy-producing nutrients. The 2000-kcal level was chosen in part because it approximates the caloric requirements for postmenopausal women, the group with the highest risk for excessive calorie and fat intake.

DRVs for the seven nutrients listed below are based on a 2000-kcal diet:

1. Total fat: 65 g
2. Saturated fat: 20 g
3. Cholesterol: 300 mg
4. Total carbohydrate: 300 g
5. Dietary fiber: 25 g
6. Sodium: 2400 mg
7. Protein: 50 g

Reference Daily Intake

The RDI replaces the term "US RDA" introduced in 1973 as a label reference value for vitamins, minerals, and protein in voluntary nutrition labeling. The name change was sought because of confusion over "US RDA" values determined by the FDA and used on food labels versus "RDA" values determined by the National Academy of Sciences for various population groups and used by the FDA to determine the US RDAs. The values for the new RDIs remain the same as the old US RDAs.

RDIs have been established for the following 25 nutrients:

1. Vitamin A
2. Vitamin C
3. Calcium
4. Iron
5. Vitamin D
6. Vitamin E
7. Vitamin K
8. Thiamin
9. Riboflavin
10. Niacin
11. Vitamin B_6
12. Folate
13. Vitamin B_{12}
14. Biotin
15. Pantothenic acid
16. Phosphorus
17. Iodine
18. Magnesium
19. Zinc
20. Selenium
21. Copper
22. Manganese
23. Chromium
24. Molybdenum
25. Chloride

Nutrition Panel Format

The format for showing nutrient content per serving must be declared as percentages of the Daily Values—the new label reference values. The amount of nutrients expressed in grams or milligrams, such as fat, cholesterol, sodium, carbohydrates, and protein, must be listed to the immediate right of each named nutrient. A column headed "% Daily Value" also must appear on the label.

Declaring nutrients as a percentage of the Daily Values should prevent misinterpretations that arise with quantitative values. For example, one could mistake a food with 140 mg of sodium as a high-sodium food because the number 140 seems relatively large. In actuality, this amount represents less than 6% of the 2400-mg Daily Value for sodium. In contrast, a food with 5 g of saturated fat could be construed as low in that nutrient, yet that food provides one fourth of the total 20-g Daily Value for saturated fat based on a 2000-kcal diet. The % Daily Value listing carries a footnote declaring that percentages are based on a 2000-kcal diet.

NUTRIENT CONTENT DESCRIPTORS

TABLE 9.3 presents the guidelines for the claims and descriptions that manufacturers can use in food labeling to promote their products.

Additional Definitions

The labeling regulations also provide guidelines for additional definitions:

Percent fat free: A product bearing this claim must be a low-fat or a fat-free product. In addition, the claim must accurately reflect the amount of fat present in 100 g of the food. Thus, if a food contains 2.5 g fat per 50 g, the claim must be "95% fat free."

Implied: These types of claims are prohibited when they wrongfully imply that a food contains or does not contain a meaningful nutrient level. For example, a product claiming to include an ingredient known as a source of fiber (i.e., "made with oat bran") is prohibited unless the product contains enough oat bran to meet the definition for "good source" of fiber. As another example, a claim that a product contains "no tropical oils" is allowed, but only for foods "low" in saturated fat because consumers have come to equate tropical oils with high saturated fat.

Meals and main dishes: Claims that a meal or main dish is "free" of a nutrient such as sodium or cholesterol must meet the same requirements as those for individual foods. Other claims can be used under special circumstances. For example, "low-calorie" means the meal or main dish contains 120 kcal or less per 100 g. "Low-sodium" means the food has 140 mg or less per 100 g. "Low-cholesterol" means the food contains 20 mg of cholesterol or less per 100 g and no more than 2 g of saturated fat. "Light" means the meal or main dish is low fat or low calorie.

Standardized foods: Any nutrient content claim such as "reduced-fat," "low-calorie," and "light" may be used in conjunction with a standardized term if the new product meets these three guidelines:

1. The product has been specifically formulated to meet the FDA's criteria for that claim.
2. The product is not nutritionally inferior to the traditional standardized food.
3. The product complies with compositional requirements established by the FDA.

A new product bearing a claim also must have performance characteristics similar to those of the referenced, traditional standardized food. If the product does not and the differences materially limit the product's use, its label must state the differences to inform consumers (e.g., not recommended for baking).

What Does "Fresh" Mean?

The FDA has issued informal, nonmandatory guidelines for use of the term "fresh." The agency took this step because of concern over possible misuse of this term on some food labels. The regulation defines "fresh" to suggest that a food

TABLE 9.3 Requirements for Manufacturers' Claims on Food Labels

Claim	Requirements That Must Be Met Before Using the Claim in Food Labeling
Fat-free	Less than 0.5 g of fat per serving, with no added fat or oil
Low fat	3 g or less of fat per serving
Less fat	25% or less of fat than the comparison food
Saturated fat free	Less than 0.5 g of saturated fat and 0.5 g of *trans* fatty acids per serving
Cholesterol-free	Less than 2 mg of cholesterol per serving, and 2 g or less of saturated fat per serving
Low cholesterol	20 mg or less of cholesterol per serving and 2 g or less of saturated fat per serving
Reduced calorie	At least 25% fewer calories per serving than the comparison food
Low calorie	40 calories or less per serving
Extra lean	Less than 5 g of fat, 2 g of saturated fat, and 95 mg of cholesterol per (100 g) serving of meat, poultry, or seafood
Lean	Less than 10 g of fat, 4.5 g of saturated fat, and 95 mg of cholesterol per (100 g) serving of meat, poultry, or seafood
Light (fat)	50% or less of the fat than in the comparison food (e.g., 50% less fat than a company's regular cheese)
Light (calories)	1/3 fewer calories than the comparison food
High-fiber	5 g or more fiber per serving
Sugar-free	Less than 0.5 g of sugar per serving
Sodium-free or salt-free	Less than 5 mg of sodium per serving
Low sodium	140 mg or less per serving
Low sodium	35 mg or less per serving
Healthy	A food low in fat, saturated fat, cholesterol, and sodium, and contains at least 10% of the Daily Values for vitamin A, vitamin C, iron, calcium, protein, or fiber
"High," "Rich in," or "Excellent Source"	20% or more of the Daily Value for a given nutrient per serving
"Less," "Fewer" or "Reduced"	At least 25% less of a given nutrient or calories than the comparison food
"Low," "Little," "Few," or "Low Source of"	An amount that would allow frequent consumption of the food without exceeding the Daily Value for the nutrient; can only make the claim as it applies to all similar foods
"Good Source of," "More," or "Added"	The food provides 10% more of the Daily Value for a given nutrient than the comparison food

is raw or unprocessed. In this context, "fresh" can describe a raw food, a food that has never been frozen or heated, and one that contains no preservatives (irradiation at low levels is allowed). "Fresh frozen," "frozen fresh," and "freshly frozen" can describe foods quickly frozen while still fresh. Blanching is allowed (brief scalding before freezing to prevent nutrient breakdown). Other uses of the term "fresh," as in "fresh milk" or "freshly baked bread," remain unaffected.

HOW SWEETNESS IS MEASURED

Splenda (sucralose) is 600 times sweeter than sugar and three times sweeter than Equal (aspartame or NutraSweet). How does one compare sweetness? Scientists measure the relative degree of sweetness with panels of trained participants who compare samples of plain water to those with progressively higher concentrations of sweetener until they notice a difference. The "threshold value" for a compound occurs when 50% of the testers detect a change from the taste of the nonsweetened water. Scientists measure relative sweetness by comparing the threshold values for various types of sugars and sugar substitutes. The average person can detect a solution of approximately 0.5% sucrose (1 tsp of table sugar dissolved in a glass of water). The artificial nonnutritive sweetener and flavor enhancer neotame made by NutraSweet (**www.nutrasweet.com**; FDA approved in 2002) is 7000 to 13,000 times sweeter than sucrose. The benefits of such a product to food manufacturers include its lower cost of production compared to sugar or high-fructose corn syrup (due to lower amounts to achieve the same sweetening). The benefits to consumers include fewer "empty" sugar calories and lower impact on blood sugar. Neotame also is approved for use by the European Union (EU), Australia, and New Zealand.

NUTRITION FACTS PANELS FOR MEAT AND POULTRY PRODUCTS

Beginning January 1, 2012, the familiar nutrition label required on all packaged food items will be required on 40 of the most commonly purchased cuts of beef, poultry, pork, and lamb. This Nutrition Facts panel will include the number of calories and the grams of total fat and saturated fat a product contains. Additionally, any product that lists a lean percentage statement such as "76% lean" on its label also must list its fat percentage, making it easier for the consumer to understand the product's amounts of lean protein and fat.

The panel's intent is to provide consumers with sufficient information at the store to assess the nutrient content of the major cuts, enabling them to select meat and poultry products that fit into a healthful diet that meets family or individual needs. Examples of the major cuts of raw, single-ingredient meat and poultry products include, but are not limited to, whole or boneless chicken breasts and other pieces, and beef whole cuts such as brisket or tenderloin steak. Examples of ground or chopped meat and poultry products include, but are not limited to, hamburger and ground turkey.

Information provided on the meat label may shock some people because it shows that, for example, a 4-oz (113.39 g) serving of 73% lean ground beef contains 350 kcal, 270 kcal of which come from fat. This makes up 60% of the suggested daily intake of saturated fat in a 2000-kcal diet. **FIGURE 9.2** shows a sample of a product food label for meat.

FOOD ADDITIVES

A manufacturer wishing to include an additive in a food must follow specific FDA guidelines. The manufacturer must test to ensure the additive meets its claims. The FDA also requires that the additive be detected and measured in the product and that it produces no undesirable health effects

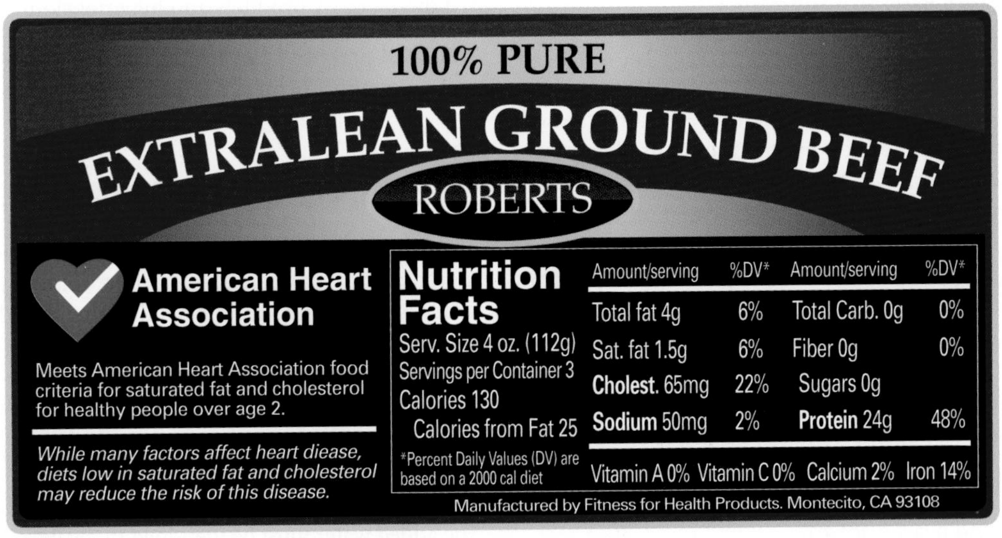
100% PURE
EXTRALEAN GROUND BEEF
ROBERTS
American Heart Association
Meets American Heart Association food criteria for saturated fat and cholesterol for healthy people over age 2.
While many factors affect heart diease, diets low in saturated fat and cholesterol may reduce the risk of this disease.
Nutrition Facts
Serv. Size 4 oz. (112g)
Servings per Container 3
Calories 130
Calories from Fat 25
*Percent Daily Values (DV) are based on a 2000 cal diet
Amount/serving %DV* Amount/serving %DV*
Total fat 4g 6% Total Carb. 0g 0%
Sat. fat 1.5g 6% Fiber 0g 0%
Cholest. 65mg 22% Sugars 0g
Sodium 50mg 2% Protein 24g 48%
Vitamin A 0% Vitamin C 0% Calcium 2% Iron 14%
Manufactured by Fitness for Health Products. Montecito, CA 93108

FIGURE 9.2 A sample of the new meat product food label.

(e.g., cancer or birth defects) when given in large doses to animals. Strict guidelines exist once the FDA approves an additive.

Approximately 700 additives were initially included on a list of additives **generally recognized as safe** (referred to as GRAS). An expanded **GRAS** list currently includes about 2000 flavoring agents and 200 coloring agents. These substances do not receive permanent approval but face periodic review. Additives include emulsifiers, stabilizers, and thickeners (to provide texture, smoothness, and consistency); nutrients such as vitamin C added to fruit juice or potassium iodide added to salt (to improve nutritive value); flavoring agents (to enhance taste); leavening agents (to make baked goods rise or to control acidity or alkalinity); preservatives, antioxidants, sequestrants, and antimycotic agents (to prevent spoilage, rancidity of fats, and microbial growth); coloring agents (to increase attractiveness); bleaches (to whiten foods and speed up the maturing of cheese); and humectants and anticaking agents (to retain moisture and keep products such as salts and powders free flowing).

BABY FOODS

The FDA does not allow the broad use of nutrient claims on infant and toddler foods. The agency may propose later claims specifically for these foods. The terms "unsweetened" and "unsalted" can be used on these foods because they relate to taste and not nutrient content.

HEALTH CLAIMS

Current regulations now permit claims for relationships between the intake of a nutrient or food and the risk of disease or health-related condition. Claims can be made in four ways:

1. Through third-party references such as the National Cancer Institute or the American Heart Association
2. Statements
3. Symbols such as a heart
4. Vignettes or descriptions

Whatever the choice, the claim must meet requirements for authorized health claims. For example, a claim cannot state the degree of risk reduction; it can only use "may" or "might" in discussing the nutrient–disease or food–disease relationship. In addition, claims must state that other factors play a role in that disease. Health claims also must be phrased so consumers understand the relationship between the nutrient and the disease and the nutrient's importance to a daily diet. The following exemplifies an appropriate health claim: "While many factors affect heart disease, diets low in saturated fat and cholesterol may reduce the risk of this disease." Nutrient–disease relationship claims are as follows:

Approved health claims

- Soluble fiber and heart disease
- Dietary fat and cancer
- Saturated fat/cholesterol and heart disease
- Calcium and osteoporosis
- Fiber-containing grain products, fruits, and vegetables and cancer
- Folate and neural tube defects
- Dietary sugar alcohols and dental caries
- Whole oats and psyllium and heart disease
- Soy protein and heart disease
- Calcium and hypertension
- Plant sterol and plant sterol esters (collectively, *phytosterols*) and heart disease

Approved authoritative health claim statements

- Whole grains and heart disease and cancer (first health claim approved under the FDA Modernization Act of 1997; **www.fda.gov/RegulatoryInformation/Legislation/FederalFoodDrugandCosmeticActFDCAct/SignificantAmendmentstotheFDCAct/FDAMA/FullTextofFDAMAlaw/default.htm**)
- Potassium and high blood pressure

Qualified health claims (supportive but not conclusive research)

- Heart-healthy benefits of omega-3 fatty acids
- Eating 1.5 oz (42.52 g) of walnuts a day may reduce coronary heart disease risk
- Eating 2 tbsp (23 g) of olive oil daily may reduce the risk of coronary heart disease due to the monounsaturated fat in olive oil

Health claims denied approval

- Dietary fiber and cancer (wheat bran and colon cancer)
- Dietary fiber and cardiovascular disease
- Antioxidant vitamins and cancer
- Zinc and immune function in the elderly

Possible future health claims (1–5 years)

- Folic acid/vitamin B_6/vitamin B_{12} and heart disease
- Low-fat dairy products and hypertension

TABLE 9.4 presents rules for the use of allowable health claims and an example of an accompanying label statement.

LABELING OF INGREDIENTS

The ingredient list on a food label represents the listing of each ingredient in descending order of predominance. Descending order of predominance means that the ingredients are listed in order of predominance by weight (i.e., the ingredient that weighs the most is listed first, followed by the ingredient that weighs least listed last).

Example: INGREDIENTS: Pinto beans, water, and salt

Water added in making a food is considered an ingredient. The added water must be identified in the list of ingredients and listed in its descending order of predominance by weight.

Additional Insights

Is *Trans* Fat–Free Really Heart Healthy?

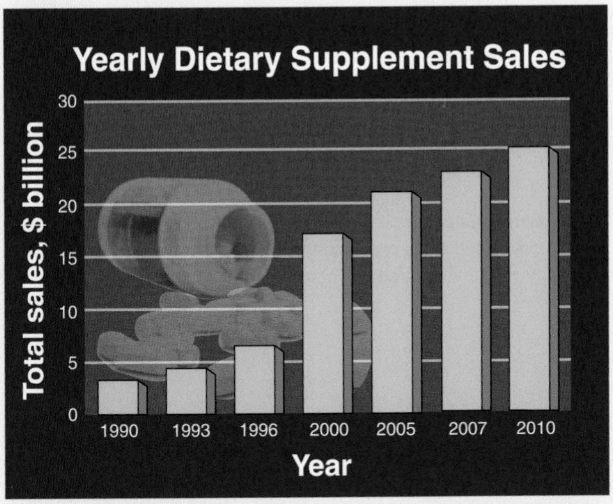

Most health professionals agree that limiting dietary saturated and *trans* fat consumption reduces risk for heart disease, yet little attention has focused on replacement fats that could be just as unhealthy to cardiovascular health. During the period from 1920 to 1945 when butter and other solid animal fats were scarce, people began using margarine and other shortenings containing *trans* fatty acids as a primary replacement, so consumption of these substances in hundreds of foods became widespread.

In the late 1990s, following a report describing how *trans* fats generated more damage to heart health than saturated fats and were "likely responsible for at least 30,000 premature US deaths yearly," health advocacy and governmental groups began to recommend reductions in *trans* fat consumption. In 2005, the US Department of Agriculture *Dietary Guidelines for Americans* recommended a limit on fats and oils high in saturated and/or *trans* fatty acids, and in 2006, the FDA (**www.fda.org**) required food manufacturers to include grams of *trans* fat on food labels. Some cities including California have banned foods containing *trans* fats sold in restaurants. Fearing lost sales, the processed food industry created alternative ways to produce products lacking *trans* fat. One fat substitution technique produced "interesterified fats" (IF), achieved by blending highly saturated hard fats like palm oil (functional characteristics similar to *trans* fats), palm stearin (used to formulate *trans*-free fats such as margarine and shortening), and fully dehydrogenated vegetable oils (largely saturated fats) with liquid edible oils to produce fats with intermediate characteristics. The term "interesterified" refers to the "ester" bonds that attach fatty acids to the molecule's glycerol backbone. Unlike partial hydrogenation, which produces *trans* fatty acids, interesterification produces a unique oil where the fatty acids are moved from one triglyceride molecule to another without altering the fatty acid's structure. These repurposed fats have the stability and solidity of solid fats like partially hydrogenated vegetable oils, but technically classify as "*trans* fat free."

The FDA permits the listing IF on food labels as *high-stearate, stearic-rich fats*, or as *interesterified fats*, and thus avoids the politically negative buzz words *hydrogenated* or *partially hydrogenated* associated with *trans* fat. If a processed food label includes *vegetable oil* as an ingredient, most likely the item contains IF or *trans* fat.

What's Wrong with Interesterified Fats?

Research shows that IF raises blood glucose and depresses insulin production about twice that of *trans* fat. These effects commonly serve as precursors to type 2 diabetes and become particularly troublesome to those already afflicted with diabetes. Also, IF may reduce the beneficial high-density lipoprotein cholesterol by almost the same levels as *trans* fat.

A dose–response relationship may exist with IF intake and health risk. Detection of adverse affects appears to arise at a critical level of consumption depending on numerous factors including dilution by other dietary fats. One can assume that effects are initiated, even if undetected, at a lower intake similar to the effects with *trans* fat consumption. Accordingly, more research is warranted to determine the appropriateness of IF consumption, particularly before this fat form insidiously embeds in the food supply and intake levels compromise long-term health.

Related References

Ascherio A, et al. Trans-fatty acids intake and risk of myocar dial infarction. *Circulation* 1994;89:94.

Hayes KC, Pronczuk A. Replacing trans fat: the argument for palm oil with a cautionary note on interesterification. *J Am Coll Nutr* 2010;29(Suppl):253S.

Katan MB, et al. Trans fatty acids and their effects on lipoproteins in humans. *Ann Rev Nutr* 1995;15:473.

Mensink RP, Katan MB. Effect of dietary trans fatty acids on high-density and low-density lipoprotein cholesterol levels in healthy subjects. *N Engl J Med* 1990;323:439.

Willett WC, et al. Intake of trans fatty acids and risk of coronary heart disease among women. *Lancet* 1993;341:581.

Zhang L, et al. Crystallization of fully hydrogenated and interesterified fat and vegetable oil. *J Oleo Sci.* 2011;60:287.

Example: INGREDIENTS: Water, navy beans, and salt

Always listed is the common or usual name for ingredients unless a regulation exists that provides for a different term. For instance, the term "sugar" is used instead of the scientific name "sucrose."

Example: INGREDIENTS: Apples, sugar, water, and spices

Listing trace ingredients depends on whether the trace ingredient is present in a significant amount and has a function in the finished food. If a substance is an incidental additive and has no function or technical effect in the finished

TABLE 9.4 Requirements for Approved Health Claims with an Example of Label Statement

Nutritional Requirements for Claims	Example of Label Statement
Dietary Fat and Cancer	
The food must meet the criteria for "low-fat."	Development of cancer depends on many factors. A diet low in total fat may reduce the risk of some cancers.
Saturated Fat/Cholesterol and Heart Disease	
The food must meet the criteria for "low-fat," "low saturated fat," and "low cholesterol."	Although many factors affect heart disease, diets low in saturated fat and cholesterol may reduce the risk of this disease.
Calcium and Osteoporosis	
The food must meet the criteria for "high in calcium." The calcium in the product must be bioavailable. The food shall not contain more phosphorus than calcium on a weight basis. *(For foods containing >40% recommended dietary intake of calcium, special requirements exist.)*	Regular exercise and a healthy diet with enough calcium helps teens and young adults and white and Asian women maintain good bone health and may reduce their high risk of osteoporosis later in life.
Fiber-Containing Grain Products, Fruits, Vegetables, and Cancer	
The claim is limited to foods that are or that contain a fruit, vegetable, or grain product. The food must meet the criteria for "low-fat" and "good source of fiber."	Low-fat diets rich in fiber-containing grain products, fruits, and vegetables may reduce the risk of some types of cancer, which is associated with many factors.
Fruit and Vegetables and Cancer	
The claim is limited to foods that are or that contain a fruit or vegetable. The food must meet the criteria for "low-fat." The food must meet the criteria for "good source" of vitamins A or C or dietary fiber (prior to fortification).	Low-fat diets rich in fruits and vegetables (foods that are low in fat and may contain dietary fiber, vitamins A and C) may reduce the risk of some types of cancer, which is associated with many factors.
Folate and Neural Tube Defects	
The food must meet the criteria for a "good source of folic acid."	Healthful diets with adequate folate may reduce a woman's risk of having a child with a brain or spinal cord birth defect.
Dietary Sugar and Dental Caries	
The food must meet the criteria for "sugar-free." Sugar alcohol in the food must be a xylitol, sorbitol, mannitol, maltitol, isomalt, lactitol, hydrogenated starch hydrolysates, hydrogenated glucose syrups, or a combination of these.	Frequent between-meal consumption of foods high in sugars and starches promotes tooth decay. The sugar alcohols in [name of food] do not promote tooth decay.
Oats and Psyllium and Heart Disease	
The food must meet the criteria for "low-fat," "saturated fat," and "low-cholesterol." The food must contain at least 0.75 g of soluble fiber from beta glucan or 7 g of soluble fiber from psyllium (prior to fortification)	[Number of] grams soluble fiber daily from [source of soluble fiber] such as [name of product] as part of a diet low in saturated fat and cholesterol, may reduce the risk of heart disease. [Name of product] provides [Number of] grams per [number of] cup.
Soy Protein and Heart Disease	
The food must meet the criteria for "low fat," "saturated fat," and "low-cholesterol." The food must contain at least 6.25 g of soy protein.	Diets low in saturated fat and cholesterol that include 25 g of soy protein may reduce the risk of heart disease. A serving of [name of food] provides [number of] grams soy protein.
Whole Grains and Heart Disease and Cancer	
Whole grain must contain all portions of the kernel: bran, germ, and endosperm. The food must contain at least 51% whole-grain ingredients by weight. The food must meet the criteria for "low-fat".	Low-fat diets rich in whole-grain foods and other plant foods may reduce the risk of heart disease and certain cancers.
Potassium and High Blood Pressure	
The food must meet criteria for "good source of potassium" and "low in sodium."	Diets containing foods that are good sources of potassium and low in sodium may reduce the risk of high blood pressure and stroke.
Plant Sterols and Plant Stanol Esters	
Among the foods that may qualify for claims based on plant sterol ester contents are spreads, salad dressings, snack bars, and dietary supplements in softgel form.	Foods containing at least 0.65 g per serving of plant sterol esters, eaten twice per day with meals for a total daily intake of at least 1.3 g, as part of a diet low in saturated fat and cholesterol, may reduce the risk of heart disease.

product, then it need not be declared on the label. An incidental additive is usually present because it is an ingredient of another ingredient. Sulfites are considered to be incidental only if present at less than 10 ppm.

Listing alternative fat and oil ingredients ("and/or" labeling) is permitted only in the case of foods that contain relatively small quantities of added fat or oil ingredients (foods in which added fats or oils are not the predominant ingredient) and only if the manufacturer is unable to predict which fat or oil ingredient will be used.

Example: INGREDIENTS: Vegetable oil (contains one or more of the following: Corn oil, soybean oil, or safflower oil)

When an approved chemical preservative is added to a food, the ingredient list must include both the common or usual name of the preservative and the function of the preservative by including terms or phrases such as "preservative," "to retard spoilage," "a mold inhibitor," "to help protect flavor," or "to promote color retention."

Example: INGREDIENTS: Dried bananas, sugar, salt, and ascorbic acid to promote color retention

Spices, natural flavors, or artificial flavors may be declared in ingredient lists by using either specific common or usual names or by using the declarations "spices," "flavor" or "natural flavor," or "artificial flavor."

Example: INGREDIENTS: Apple slices, water, cane syrup, corn syrup, modified corn starch, spices, salt, natural flavor, and artificial flavor

Spices, such as paprika, turmeric, saffron, and others, that are also colorings must be declared either by the term "spice and coloring" or by the actual (common or usual) names, such as "paprika."

Vegetable powders must be declared by the common or usual name such as "celery powder."

Artificial coloring agents must be listed if they are certified as coloring agents by the Federal Food, Drug, and Cosmetic Act (abbreviated FD&C). They are listed by specific or abbreviated names such as "FD&C Red No. 40" or "Red 40."

Noncertified colors are listed as "artificial color," "artificial coloring," or by their specific common or usual names such as "caramel coloring" and "beet juice."

NEW MENU AND VENDING MACHINE LABELING REQUIREMENTS

In 2010, President Obama signed the Health Care Reform Legislation into law. Section 4205 of the Patient Protection and Affordable Care Act of 2010 requires restaurants and similar retail food establishments with 20 or more locations to list calorie content information for standard menu items on restaurant menus and menu boards, including menu boards at drive-throughs. The proposed rules also apply to vending machines, coffee shops, and convenience and grocery stores, but not to movie theater concession stands.

The declaration of nutrition information on the label and food labeling must include the following 13 items:

1. Total calories
2. Calories from fat (unless the product contains <0.5 g of fat)
3. Total fat
4. Saturated fat
5. *Trans* fat
6. Cholesterol
7. Sodium
8. Total carbohydrate
9. Dietary fiber
10. Sugars
11. Protein
12. Vitamins
13. Minerals

This labeling requirement represents a major victory for consumers. Research conducted by the FDA and other organizations shows that consumers use these Nutrition Facts in making food choices. In 2011, the newly formulated umbrella healthcare law received legal challenges regarding its constitutionality. Three cases in federal courts upheld the constitutionality of the bill, while two deemed it unconstitutional. The Supreme Court could review this law as early as the end of 2011 or beginning of 2012. Full compliance with the new labeling law is not required until the FDA completes implementation of the regulations and upholding the umbrella healthcare law.

DETERMINING THE NUTRIENT PERCENTAGE IN A FOOD

TABLE 9.5 presents nutritional information for 24 of the country's most popular franchise chains that focus on selling hamburgers. Several of the food corporations fail to provide adequate information for customers to readily determine total calories as fat. The listings are from high to low for total calories. In many cases, such lack of information proves revealing and often embarrassing to manufactures who extol their "commitment to consumers to provide healthful meals." Not surprisingly, manufacturers downplay such information and leave it up to the customer to determine how much fat contributes to the food's total caloric value.

The bottom of the table lists the Daily Values for a 2000 and 2500 kcal per day caloric intake. It is astounding to realize that one hamburger, even without accompanying French fries and a sugar-laden soda drink, supplies about a full day's requirement for calories, fat, carbohydrate, protein, saturated fat, cholesterol, and sodium. Consistently consuming an excess of calories certainly helps to fuel the obesity epidemic.[17]

TABLE 9.5 Battle of the Big Burgers: In the Battle Among Fast-Food and Casual-Dining Chains to Create the Most Colossal Burger, the Clear Loser is the Consumer Concerned About the Nutritional Quality of the Food Consumed. What the Advertising Blitz Fails to Mention is the Calorie Content of Its Burgers (As High As 1971 kcal, or Just About the Daily Energy Allotment for a Sedentary Woman—and Before Adding French Fries and a Soft Drink), the Levels of Artery-Clogging Saturated Fat (As High As 44 g), or the Astonishingly High Sodium Content (up to 3378 mg)

Name	Item	Serving Size (g)	Total (kcal)	Fat (g)	Fat (kcal)	Fat (%) Total (kcal)	Saturated Fat (g)	Cholesterol (mg)	Sodium (mg)	Carbohydrate (g)	Protein (g)
Fuddruckers	The Works Burger, 1 lb w/Bun		1971	135	1222	62%	44	280	3378	119	70
Sonic	Super Sonic Bacon double cheeseburger (w/mayo)	422	1370	96	864	63%	36	260	1610	55	3378 mg
Hardee's	2/3 lb Monster Thickburger	366	1320	95	855	65%	36	210	3020	46	70
Applebee's	A1 Steakhous Burger		1250	84	756	60%	26	255	2230	68	55
Smashburger	Barbeque, Bacon & Cheese Burger		1178	74	666	57%	28	210	2057	70	52
Denny's	Western Burger		1160	65	585	50%	21	190	1820	79	63
Burger King	Triple Whopper		1140	75	675	59%	27	205	1110	51	67
Chili's	Classic Bacon Burger		1140	72	648	57%	22	205	2150	61	59
Whataburger	Whataburger, Triple Meat	492	1120	68	612	55%	26	192	1759	58	61
Wendy's	3/4 lb Triple	423	1020	62	558	55%	28	240	1820	43	71
Dairy Queen	1/2 lb Flame Thrower GrillBurger	323	1010	71	639	63%	25	190	1540	44	36
Culvers	Bacon Deluxe Triple	376	991	67	603	61%	30	250	1831	36	61
Hardee's	$6 Thick Burger		950	59	531	56%	21	130	2020	58	45
Jack in the Box	Bacon Ultimate Cheeseburger	301	940	66	594	63%	27	125	1840	45	41
Five Guys	Bacon Cheeseburger	317	920	62	558	61%	29.5	180	1310	40	51
Checker's/Rally's	Triple Buford	350	910	61	549	60%	27	165	1870	37	40
Carl's Jr	$6 Burger		890	54	486	55%	20	130	2040	58	45
Krystal	BA Double Bacon Cheese		850	59	531	62%	22	120	1580	48	32
Fatburger	Kingburger		850	41	369	43%	13	150	1490	69	50
McDonald's	Angus Bacon and Cheese	291	790	39	351	44%	17	145	2070	63	45
A&W	Papa Burger	282	690	39	351	51%	14	145	1350	44	40
In-N-Out	Double-Double w/onion	330	670	41	369	55%	18	120	1440	39	37
Big Boys	Triple Decker		600	26	234	39%	13	95	790	35	40

(continued)

TABLE 9.5 ***(continued)*** **Battle of the Big Burgers: In the Battle Among Fast-Food and Casual-Dining Chains to Create the Most Colossal Burger, the Clear Loser is the Consumer Concerned About the Nutritional Quality of the Food Consumed. What the Advertising Blitz Fails to Mention is the Calorie Content of Its Burgers (As High As 1971 kcal, or Just About the Daily Energy Allotment for a Sedentary Woman—and Before Adding French Fries and a Soft Drink), the Levels of Artery-Clogging Saturated Fat (As High As 44 g), or the Astonishingly High Sodium Content (up to 3378 mg)**

Name	Item	Serving Size (g)	Total (kcal)	Fat (g)	Fat (kcal)	Fat (%) Total (kcal)	Saturated Fat (g)	Cholesterol (mg)	Sodium (mg)	Carbohydrate (g)	Protein (g)
White Castle	Double Smokey Bacon Ranch		420	29	261	62%	8	40	1100	22	13
		Average =	**1006**	**64**	**578**	**57%**	**24**	**176**	**1801**	**54**	**51**
	Daily Value (@2000 kcal.d^{-1})		**2000**	**65**			**20**	**300**	**2400**	**375**	**53**
	Daily Value (@2500 kcal.d^{-1})		**2500**	**80**			**25**	**300**	**2400**	**375**	**70**

Location number obtained from corporate web pages as of July 2011; fat kcal = fat grams × 9.

Learn to Read Food Labels

To illustrate the importance of understanding the components of a food label, **TABLE 9.6** compares four popular products from the Hershey Foods company for protein, carbohydrate, and lipid content (www.hersheys.com). The comparison includes the caloric value (kcal) and amount (g) of the nutrient. Reading the table's footnote easily uncovers the percentage of a nutrient in relation to the product's total caloric content (not provided by the manufacturer). In Hershey's nutrition brochure widely distributed to consumers, a common question concerning their chocolate products states: "How many calories does a Hershey's Miniature Bar contain?" The manufacturer's answer: "There are 40 calories in a Hershey's Miniature Bar. This same calorie count applies for all the Hershey's Miniature Bars—Milk Chocolate, Special Dark, Mr. Goodbar, and Krackel." The brochure fails to reveal that the chocolate bars contain approximately 50% fat for small or large-size bars! A consumer does not need the skills of a detective to make such discoveries. This applies to any food; just perform the same computations as done for the chocolate products listed in TABLE 9.6.

WHAT PEOPLE EAT

Comparisons of foods consumed around the world reveal startling facts and trends that give insight to the worldwide epidemics of obesity and type 2 diabetes. **FIGURE 9.3** displays food consumption data for 10 industrialized nations for processed factory foods versus fresh food for the year 2009. No country has embraced the movement toward dried prepackaged food as readily as the United States. Americans eat 31% more packaged food than fresh food; they consume more packaged food per person than counterparts in nearly all

TABLE 9.6 Consumer Beware: Learn to Interpret the Nutritional Label to Determine the Percentage of a Particular Nutrient in Relation to a Food's Total Energy Content

Item	Amount	Total kcal	Protein		Carbohydrate		Lipid	
			g	% kcal[a]	G	% kcal[a]	g	% kcal[a]
Hershey's chocolate milk (2% low fat)	1 cup (8 oz)	190	8	16.8	29	61.0	5	23.7
Hershey's chocolate kisses	9 pieces (1.5 oz)	220	3	5.5	23	41.8	13	53.0
Hershey's Reese's Peanut Butter Cup	2 cups (1.8 oz)	280	6	8.6	26	37.1	17	54.6
Hershey's New Trail Granola Snack Bars, chocolate-covered cocoa crème	1.3 oz	190	2	4.2	24	50.5	9	42.6

[a]*This column, which represents the percentage of total calories for each of the macronutrients, was not provided by the manufacturer. To compute the percentage contribution of a particular nutrient, multiply the caloric value for the nutrient (protein and carbohydrate =; 4 kcal·g^{-1}; lipid =; 9 kcal·g^{-1}) times the number of grams. Express the value in relation to the total number of calories. For example, to compute the percentage of lipid in Hershey's chocolate kisses (last column), multiply 9 (kcal·g^{-1}) × 13 (number of grams) to obtain 117 kcal. Then, (117 ÷ 220) × 100 =; 53%, which is the percentage of total calories supplied by lipid!*

Data from Nutrition Information for Consumers. Hershey Foods, Consumer Relations Department, P.O. Box 815, Hershey, PA 17033-0815. The percentage values were computed from the nutrient information listed in the table provided by Hershey's; data on percentages were not included as part of their table.

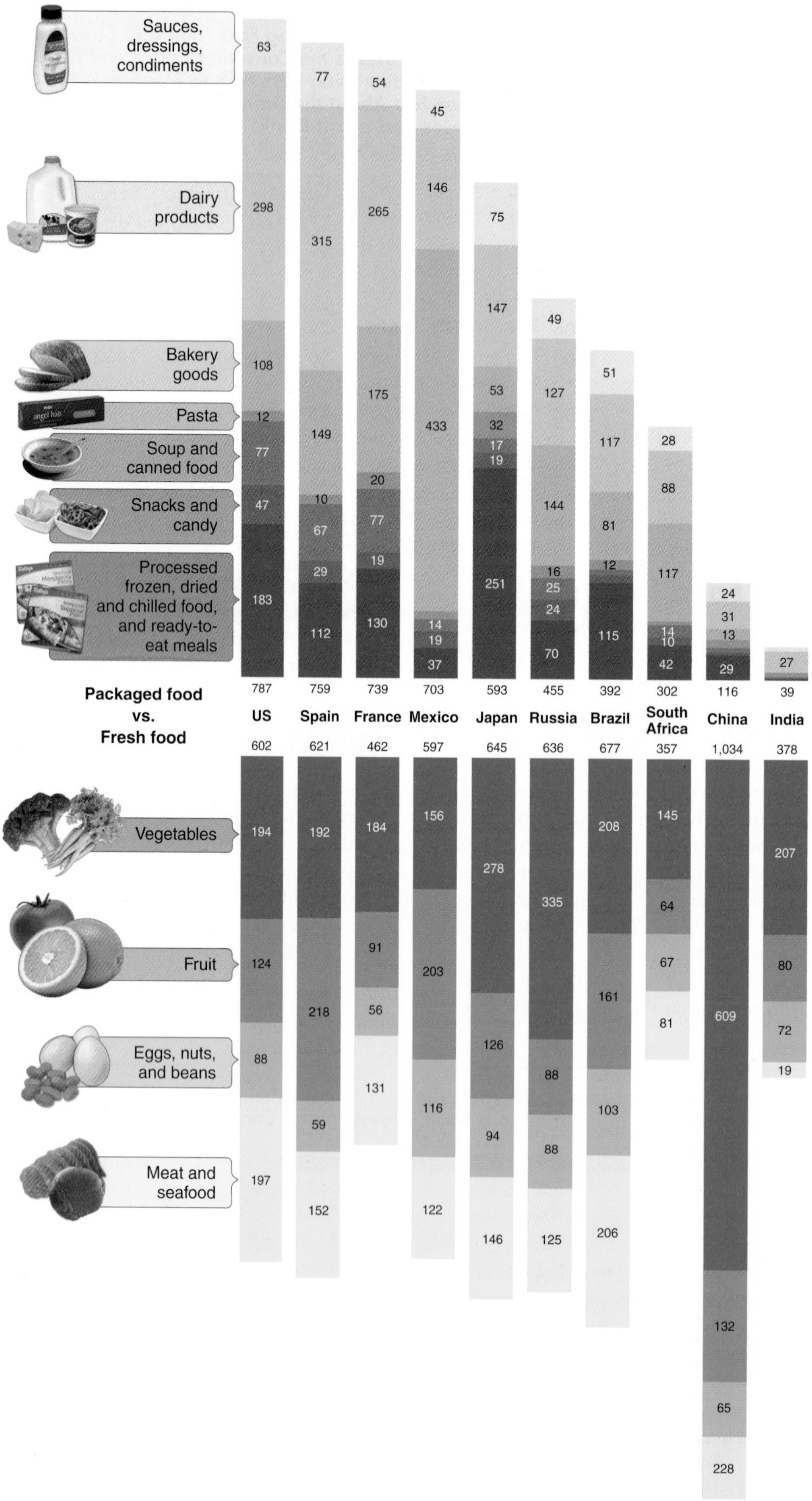

FIGURE 9.3 Consumption for 10 industrialized nations for processed factory foods versus fresh food for the year 2009.

other countries. Ready-to-eat frozen pizzas, microwave dinners, and sweet or salty snack foods comprise a sizable part of the typical American diet.

Americans consume more salt, sugar, and fat than any other nation. Epidemiologic studies have shown that diets with higher levels of these nutrients are associated with higher rates of heart disease, type 2 diabetes, and obesity. The Japanese eat large amounts of packaged frozen seafood, but the food is seldom processed and contains few chemical additives. Some Europeans eat a similar amount of packaged food per capita as Americans, but much of it is bakery bread and dairy products, not frozen toaster pastries, artificial nondairy creamers, and processed products that may contain 50 different added ingredients.

FIGURE 9.4 presents the specifics of American food consumption for the year 2010. Average consumption on a yearly basis includes 86 pounds of fats and oils, 110 pounds of red meat including 62 pounds of beef, 47 pounds of pork, 74 pounds of poultry, 60 pounds of chicken, 16 pounds of fish and shellfish, and 33 pounds of eggs. Americans also consume 31 pounds of cheese and 601 pounds of noncheese dairy products; they drink 181 pounds of beverage milks, 12 pounds of flour and cereal products, 134 pounds of wheat flour, 142

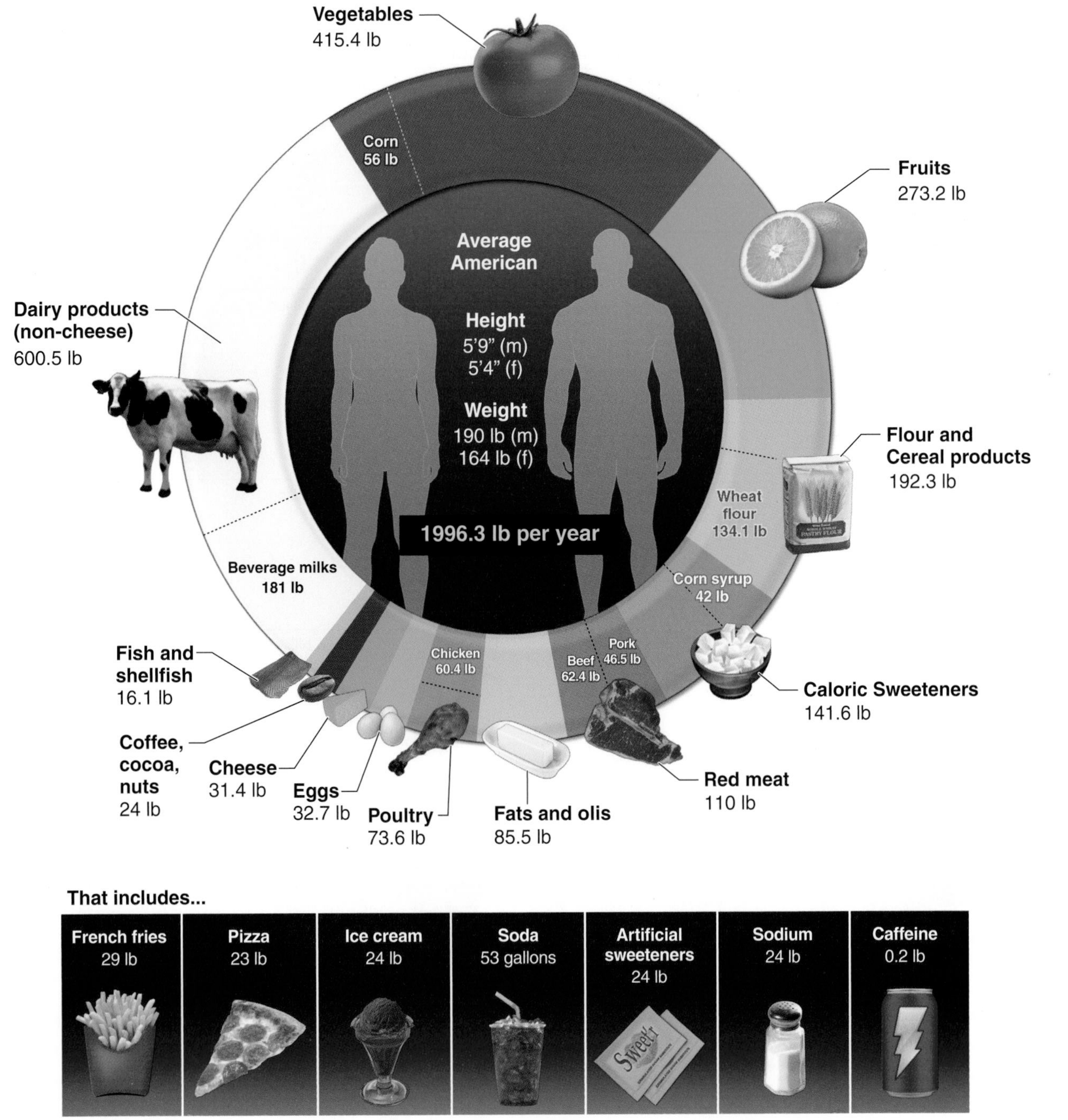

FIGURE 9.4 What the average American consumes in a year. (From The Credit Blog. Food consumption in America. Available at: www.creditloan.com/blog/2010/07/12/food-consumption-in-america/. Accessed April 11, 2012.)

ANIMALS USED FOR FOOD

Worldwide estimates for 2009 to 2010 of the number of individuals who eat no meat range between 18 and 20% (**www.esri.ie/UserFiles/publications/WP340.pdf**). Tajikistan has the highest proportion of nonmeat consumers (48% of the population); India is second with about 34.5%. Estimates of nonmeat eaters in the United States range between 3 and 8% of the population. Clearly, the majority of humans on the planet are omnivores, and estimates of the number and variety of animals needed to feed the world are staggering. The table below lists some of the latest figures for the numbers of land animals worldwide and in the United States required to feed the world's meat eaters.

Number of Land Animals Used for Food (2009)

Animal	Number of Animals Worldwide	Number of Animals in the United States
Camels 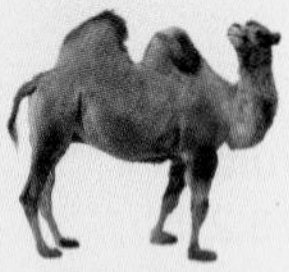	1.7 million	
Water buffalo 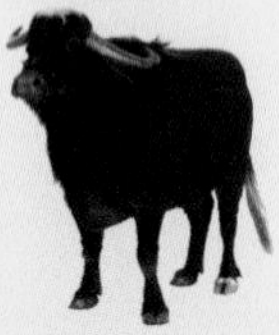	24 million	
Cows 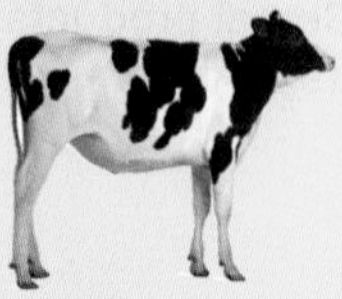	23 million	3.7 million
Goats 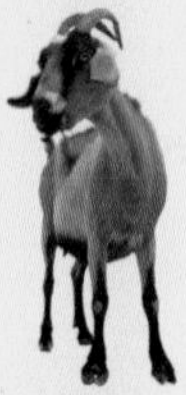	38 million	
Sheep (lamb) 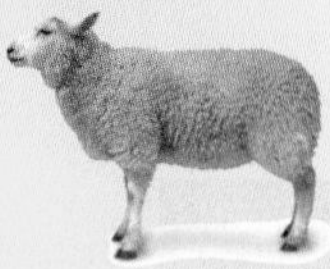	518 million	
Turkeys 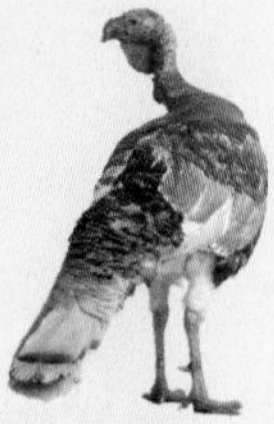	633 million	27.5 million
Rabbits 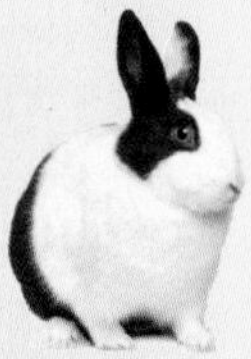	1.1 billion	
Pigs 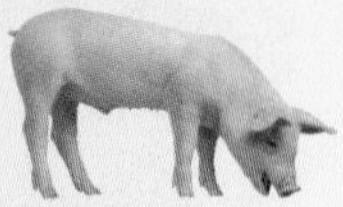	1.3 billion	118 million
Ducks 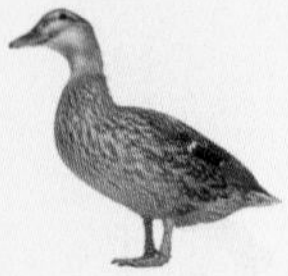	2.6 billion	22 million
Chickens 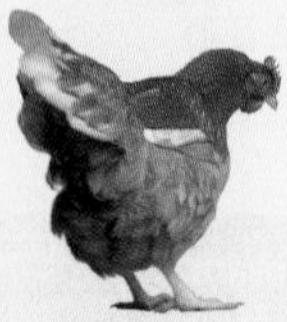	52 billion	9 billion

Source: National Geographic, May, 2011, Available at: www.blog.farmusa.org/number-of-farmed-animals-killed-in-usa-drops/; http://freefromharm.org/farm-animal-welfare/59-billion-land-and-sea-animals-killed-for-food-in-the-us-in-2009/.

pounds of caloric sweeteners including 42 pounds of corn syrup, 56 pounds of corn, and 415 pounds of vegetables. Every year, Americans consume 24 pounds of coffee, cocoa, and nuts and 273 pounds of fruit. Food intake also includes 2 pounds of French fries, 23 pounds of pizza, and 24 pounds of ice cream. Americans drink 53 gallons of soda annually, averaging about 1 gallon a week.[11] They consume 24 pounds of artificial sweeteners, 2.74 pounds of sodium (47% more than recommended), and 0.2 pounds (about 90,700 mg) of caffeine yearly.

Portion Size Distortion

Changing trends in eating behaviors coincide with the current classification by the Centers for Disease Control and Prevention of about two thirds of US adults age 20 to 70 years as either overweight or obese.[15] Part of this upswing in body weight relates to the nearly 350% increase between 1965 and 2005 in the proportion of foods that children consume from restaurants and fast-food outlets. Supersized servings of French fries and sodas are often two to five times larger than when first introduced.[9] For example, in 1955 McDonald's French fries weighed 2.4 oz (only a small size was available) and contained 210 kcal; in 2011, McDonald's offers three sizes: small, 2.5 oz and 230 kcal; medium, 4.1 oz and 380 kcal; and large, 5.4 oz and 500 kcal!

Ordering a medium popcorn and soda combo from a movie theater equates with eating three McDonald's Quarter Pounders with 12 pats of butter in terms of caloric content! According to laboratory analysis conducted by the Center for Science in the Public Interest (CSPI; www.cspinet.org), a large popcorn purchased from one of the country's large movie chains contains 1160 kcal and a whopping 60 g of fat. A small popcorn contains 670 kcal—the same as a Pizza Hut Personal Pepperoni Pan Pizza (www.cspinet.org/nah/12_09/cover.pdf).

Average portion sizes have grown to such an extent over the past 20 years that the plate arrives with enough food for two or even three people[6,10] (**TABLE 9.7**). These growing portion sizes also are changing what Americans think of and expect as a "normal" portion at home.

TABLE 9.7 Comparison of Portion Size and Caloric Content from 20 Years Ago and Today

	20 Years Ago		Today	
Item	**Portion**	**Calories**	**Portion**	**Calories**
Bagel	3-in diameter	140	6-in diameter	350
Cheeseburger	1	333	1	590
Spaghetti with meatballs	1 cup sauce, 3 small, meatballs	500	2 cups sauce, 3 large meatballs	1,020
Soda	6.5 oz	82	20 oz	250
Blueberry muffin	1.5 oz	210	5 oz	500

From: National Heart Lung and Blood Institute. Portion distortion and serving size. Available at: http://www.nhlbi.nih.gov/health/public/heart/obesity/wecan/eat-right/distortion.htm. Accessed August 25, 2011. For more eye-opening examples, check out the National Heart Lung and Blood Institute's Portion Distortion website at http://hp2010.nhlbihin.net/portion/index.htm.

SUPERSIZING: AN AMERICAN TREND

The increasing size of American food portions links to the US food industry's growing reliance on *value marketing*, a technique used to increase profits. This process encourages customers to spend a little extra money to purchase larger portion sizes, which supposedly leaves the customer with the feeling that they have "gotten a deal."

DOESN'T SEEM SO "BIG" NOW

McDonald's Big Mac with 540 kcal was marketed in 1967 to compete with the two-patty hamburger sold by rival Burger King. It certainly doesn't seem so "big" now when compared with Burger King's Whopper (670 kcal), McDonald's Angus burgers (750–790 kcal), and Wendy's Bacon Deluxe Triple hamburger (1150 kcal).

The negative nutritional and caloric costs of getting "deals" at fast-food restaurants, convenience stores, and other retail food establishments are enormous. Upgrading to larger serving sizes often increases price only modestly but substantially increases calorie and fat content, which invariably contributes to overeating and obesity.[16]

For food companies, the actual monetary costs of larger portions are relatively small because the cost of food itself is low (on average about 20% of retail costs) relative to labor, packaging, transportation, marketing, and other related costs. Thus, even the relatively small amounts of extra money consumers spend when "upgrading" to larger portion sizes translate to larger corporate profits.

In addition to using price to encourage the purchase of larger portion sizes, fast-food restaurants in particular actively encourage consumers to "upgrade" to larger sizes with point-of-purchase displays and verbal sales prompts from employees. They also encourage consumers to combine their entrée with high-profit-margin, high-calorie soft drinks and side dishes such as French fries ("Value Meal," "Combo Meal")—a food industry technique known as "bundling." This practice profoundly influences customer food choices and eventual health.[9]

A Small Cost Increase Yields a Supersize Calorie Increase

For a small price increase, customers can purchase larger portions and end up consuming substantially more calories and saturated fat. Consider the following example that one of the

PERSONAL HEALTH AND EXERCISE NUTRITION 9.1

Take the Portion Distortion Quiz

You have probably noticed that food portions in restaurants and other eating places have grown in size and often provide enough food for at least two people per serving. Undoubtedly, these larger portion sizes can lead to bigger waistlines and accompanying weight gain.

Take the Portion Distortion Quiz below to see if you know how today's portions compare to the portions available 20 years ago and the amount of physical activity required to burn off the extra calories provided by today's larger portions.

1. A bagel 20 years ago was 3 inches in diameter and had 140 calories. How many calories do you think are in today's bagel?
   a. 150 calories
   b. 250 calories
   c. 350 calories
2. A cheeseburger 20 years ago had 333 calories. How many calories do you think are in today's cheeseburger?
   a. 590 calories
   b. 620 calories
   c. 700 calories
3. A 6.5-oz portion of soda had 85 calories 20 years ago. How many calories do you think are in today's portion?
   a. 200 calories
   b. 250 calories
   c. 300 calories
4. Twenty years ago, 2.4 oz of French fries had 210 calories. How many calories do you think are in today's portion?
   a. 590 calories
   b. 610 calories
   c. 650 calories
5. A portion of spaghetti and meatballs 20 years ago had 500 calories. How many calories do you think are in today's portion of spaghetti and meatballs?
   a. 600 calories
   b. 800 calories
   c. 1025 calories
6. A cup of coffee with milk and sugar 20 years ago was 8 oz and had 45 calories. How many calories do you think are in today's mocha coffee?
   a. 100 calories
   b. 350 calories
   c. 450 calories
7. A muffin 20 years ago was 1.5 oz and had 210 calories. How many calories do you think are in a muffin today?
   a. 320 calories
   b. 400 calories
   c. 500 calories
8. Two slices of pepperoni pizza 20 years ago had 500 calories. How many calories do you think are in today's large pizza slices?
   a. 850 calories
   b. 1000 calories
   c. 1200 calories
9. A chicken Caesar salad had 390 calories 20 years ago. How many calories do you think are in today's chicken Caesar salad?
   a. 520 calories
   b. 650 calories
   c. 790 calories
10. A box of popcorn had 270 calories 20 years ago. How many calories do you think are in today's tub of popcorn?
    a. 520 calories
    b. 630 calories
    c. 820 calories

The next time you eat out, think twice about the size of food portions.

Source: *National Heart and Lung Institute. Available at:* www.nhlbi.nih.gov/health/public/heart/obesity/wecan/downloads/portion-quiz.pdf.

thePoint *Visit* **thePoint.lww.com/MKKSEN4e** *website to find the answers to the Portion Distortion Quiz!*

authors recently observed regarding the popcorn available at a local movie theater:

Popcorn Item	Calories	Total Fat (g)	Saturated Fat (g)	Price ($)
Small (85 oz, no butter)	300	20	14	5.00
Small (85 oz with butter)	470	37	22	5.00
Medium (130 oz, no butter)	650	43	31	6.00
Medium large (130 oz, no butter)	900	60	43	6.50
Medium large (150 oz, with butter)	1200	7	56	6.50
Large (175 oz, no butter)	1160	77	55	7.00
Large (175 oz, with butter)	1640	126	73	7.00

Upgrading from a small to medium-size bag of popcorn costs 20% more money, but it adds 350 more calories, a 116% increase. An upgrade to a large popcorn increases the cost by only 40% yet increases the caloric load by 286%! In this example, while adding butter minimally increases the cost, the increase in calories and fat skyrockets.

Tips to Avoid Portion Size Distortion

The trend for portion size increase has spilled over into grocery stores and vending machines, where a bagel has become a "BAGEL" and an "individual" bag of chips can easily feed more than one. The following are some tips to help avoid common portion size pitfalls:

Practice Portion Control When Eating Out

- Eat a portion of low-calorie raw vegetables before going out; it's okay to try and "spoil" your dinner with this approach.
- Split an entrée with a friend.
- Ask the wait-person for a "to-go" box, and wrap up one half of your meal when your meal arrives.
- Ask if the appetizer of choice can be "upgraded" in size to substitute for a full meal (it still would be smaller than a full-size entrée portion).

Practice Portion Control When Eating at Home

- Replace the candy dish with a fruit bowl.
- To minimize temptations of second and third helpings, serve food on individual plates instead of using serving dishes on the table.
- Keep excess food out of reach to discourage overeating.
- Eat a portion of low-calorie raw vegetables; it's okay to try and "spoil" your dinner.
- Drink a glass of water before eating.

Practice Portion Control in Front of the TV and When Snacking

- If possible, try to never eat in front of the TV.
- Put the amount that you plan to eat into a bowl or container instead of eating straight from the package.
- Prepare low-calorie snacks like raw vegetables if you know you are going to watch TV during dinner.
- Be aware of large packages; larger packages mean more food consumed.
- Divide up the contents of one large package into a smaller container and put away the extra "to go."
- Replace the candy dish with a bowl of fruit.
- Store tempting foods like cookies, chips, or ice cream out of immediate eyesight, such as on a high shelf or at the back of the freezer. Move the healthier food to the front at eye level.
- Add plain popcorn without butter to your diet.
- Snack on whole-grain cereals or plain popcorn instead of chips and candy.

ACTIVE PEOPLE ON THE GO: EATING AT FAST-FOOD RESTAURANTS

Athletes and physically active men and women who follow prudent guidelines for food consumption still must select from a plethora of foods. Like the typical person, these individuals endure a continual stream of advertising to lure them to consume a particular brand of food or to "take a break" and eat at a favorite restaurant. Many athletes eat their meals at sport-specific "training tables" during the competitive season. The off season and summer months provide a unique challenge to maintain optimum nutrition that minimizes total fat intake and emphasizes unrefined complex carbohydrates, while ensuring adequate vitamins and minerals from the main food groups.

An *occasional* trip to a fast-food eatery may temporarily disrupt the recommended intake of higher complex-carbohydrate, high-fiber, and lower-fat foods. However, *regular* visits to franchise fast-food establishments can wreak havoc on nutritional recommendations. For example, having lunch at McDonald's and eating two Big Macs, one 4-oz order of French fries, and a 16-oz chocolate triple shake "costs" 2040 total calories with 28 g of fat (40% of the 2040 kcal)! And that doesn't include breakfast and dinner calories, not to mention "snacks" at other times to make up the total daily calories consumed. The dinner meal would easily exceed 1500 kcal, and even eating a "healthy" breakfast would add another 400 kcal. The bottom line is that this typical daily eating plan containing 4300 kcal puts the athlete on a collision course for weight gain, despite expending a generous 1000 kcal from workouts or competition. Many physically active individuals stray from planned nutritional regimens. Attending parties, going out to dinner with friends, and "hanging out" often include eating foods that provide energy-dense, nonnutritious, or "empty calorie" foods.

Ethnic Sources for Poor Nutrition

The nongovernmental CSPI publishes information about a variety of food and health-related topics, including analyses of menu items from different ethnic eateries. Consider the nutritional consequences of eating at Chinese and Mexican restaurants. For the analysis of typical foods from Chinese restaurants, CSPI bought dinner-size takeout portions of 15 popular dishes from 20 midpriced Chinese restaurants in Washington, DC, Chicago, and San Francisco. For the Mexican dishes, they purchased takeout portions of 15 popular appetizers and main dishes at 19 midpriced Mexican restaurants (including large and medium-sized chains, for example Chi-Chi's, El Torito, Chevys, El Chico) in Chicago, Dallas, San Francisco, and Washington, DC. The CSPI constructed a "composite" from nine samples of each dish (e.g., equal portions of nine restaurants' chicken tacos were mixed together). An independent laboratory analyzed the food for total calories, lipid, saturated fat, cholesterol, and sodium. **TABLE 9.8** provides examples of the lipid content of typical Chinese and Italian food, including appetizers, entrees, and side dishes from noted theme restaurants (Chili's, T.G.I. Friday's, Bennigan's, Hard Rock Cafe, and Planet Hollywood). The high fat content of such popular food items should serve as a beacon that the nutritional quality of many foods at popular ethnic and chain restaurants remains a nutritional quagmire. Consult Appendix A to compare the lipid content of foods in TABLE 9.8 with the lipid content of foods at 11 popular fast-food restaurants.

The following eight conclusions from the CSPI food analyses illustrate that "eating out" regularly at ethnic restaurants does not qualify as more healthful eating than eating at popular fast-food restaurants such as Arby's, Burger King, Kentucky Fried Chicken, McDonald's, Taco Bell, or Wendy's.

1. The average Chinese dinner contains more sodium than the daily requirement. It also has 70% of a day's lipid, 80% of a day's cholesterol, and almost one half of a day's saturated fatty acid recommendation.
2. An order of lo mein contains as much salt as a whole Pizza Hut cheese pizza.
3. An order of kung pao chicken (52% lipid) contains as much lipid as four McDonald's Quarter Pounders.
4. An order of beef and cheese nachos contains the lipid in 10 glazed doughnuts from Dunkin' Donuts.
5. A chicken burrito dinner yields 1 day's worth of sodium.
6. A chile relleno dinner contains as much saturated fatty acid as 27 slices of bacon.
7. An oriental chicken salad contains more fat than a foot-long Subway cold-cut sub washed down with a Dunkin' Donuts Bavarian Kreme donut.
8. Nine fried mozzarella sticks contain as much lipid as one-half stick of butter (1/4 cup or 4 tbsp).

THE HUNGER–OBESITY PARADOX

That hunger and obesity exist side-by-side throughout the industrialized world remains counterintuitive, but research shows that both coexist within the same person and within the same household. This phenomenon, called the **hunger–obesity paradox**, was first proposed in 1995 in the case study, "Does Hunger Cause Obesity?"[2]

Because obesity connotes excessive energy intake and hunger reflects an inadequate food supply, the increased prevalence of obesity and hunger in the same population seemed paradoxical. It was hypothesized that the association of hunger and obesity in the same person (or group) might be explained by increased fat content of food eaten when the person lacked money. An alternative explanation was that obesity might represent an adaptive response to episodic food insufficiency. If obesity associates with food insufficiency as the hypothesis suggested, then obesity prevention in impoverished populations might require increased food supplementation rather than food restriction to achieve a more uniform pattern of food consumption.

Since the introduction of this hypothesis, a number of studies have shown a link between obesity and hunger.[14] For example, a 1999 study demonstrated in a population-based, randomly selected sample of 193 women age 20 to 30 years, that the mean body mass index (BMI) in the household food-insecure group was 28.2 compared with a BMI of 25.6 in food-secure households.[12] In addition, 37% of the women in the food-insecure households had a BMI greater than 29 compared with only 26% of women in food-secure households.

A 2001 study showed that the prevalence of overweight among women progressively increased as food insecurity increased, moving from 34% for those who were food secure to 41% for those mildly food insecure, to 52% for those moderately food insecure.[16] The researchers concluded that food insecurity remained a significant predictor of overweight status in women, with mildly food-insecure women 30% more likely to be overweight than food-secure women. Furthermore, subsequent research has shown, paradoxically, that providing extra food to food-insecure girls caused them to gain less weight.[7] For these girls, a food-assistance program reduced the odds of being at risk for overweight by 68% compared to nonparticipating counterparts in the program.

Poverty and Obesity Connect to Hunger and Food Insecurity

The Life Sciences Research Office (www.lsro.org) describes food insecurity as "existing whenever the availability of nutritionally adequate and safe foods or the ability to acquire acceptable food in socially acceptable ways is limited or uncertain."[8] Hunger, in the broadest interpretation, represents the uneasy or painful sensation caused by a lack of food, a consequence of food insecurity with its obvious relation to

TABLE 9.8 Lipid Content of Foods from Chinese and Italian Eateries and Appetizers, Main Dishes, and Side Dishes at Popular "Theme" (Chain) Restaurants

Food	Total Calories	Lipid (g)	Lipid (kcal)	Lipid (%)
Chinese[a]				
Kung pao chicken	1275	75	675	53
Egg roll	190	75	99	52
Moo shu pork	1220	64	576	47
Sweet & sour pork	1635	71	639	39
Beef with broccoli	1180	46	414	35
General Tso's chicken	1607	59	531	33
Orange (crispy) beef	1798	66	594	33
Hot and sour soup	109	4	36	32
House lo mein	1048	36	324	31
House fried rice	1498	50	450	30
Chicken chow mein	1067	32	288	28
Hunan tofu	931	28	252	27
Shrimp with garlic sauce	972	27	243	25
Stir fried vegetables	778	19	171	22
Szechwan shrimp	949	19	171	18
Italian				
Fettucini Alfredo	1505	97	873	58
Lasagna	954	53	477	50
Cheese manicotti	697	38	342	49
Eggplant parmigiana	1212	62	558	46
Cheese ravioli	615	26	234	38
Veal parmigiana	1070	44	396	37
Spaghetti with sausage	1025	39	351	34
Chicken marsala with side of spaghetti	1155	39	351	30
Spaghetti with meatballs	1170	39	351	30
Spaghetti with meat sauce	900	25	225	25
Linguini with red clam sauce	899	23	207	23
Spaghetti with tomato sauce	850	17	153	18
Olive Garden (Italian chain restaurant) Garlic bread, 8 oz	818	40	360	44
Fried calamari	1032	70	630	61
Antipasto (assorted meats, cheeses, marinated vegetables, dressings, tomato, lettuce)	631	47	423	67
Hot artichoke spinach dip with garlic crisps	266	15	135	51
Bread sticks & dipping sauce, 1 stick	116	2.6	23	20
Chicken giardino	484	11	99	20
Capellini primavera	281	4.7	42	15
Appetizers				
Chili, 1 cup	350	16	144	41
Buffalo wings, 12 pieces (13 oz)	700	48	432	62
Fried mozzarella sticks, 9 pieces (8 oz)	830	51	459	55
Stuffed potato skins, 8 pieces (12 oz)	1120	79	711	64

(continued)

TABLE 9.8 (*continued*) Lipid Content of Foods from Chinese and Italian Eateries and Appetizers, Main Dishes, and Side Dishes at Popular "Theme" (Chain) Restaurants

Food	Total Calories	Lipid (g)	Lipid (kcal)	Lipid (%)
Entrée & side dishes				
Grilled chicken, 6 oz	270	8	72	27
with baked potato + 1 Tbsp sour cream + 1 cup vegetable	640	14	126	20
with loaded potato + 1 cup vegetable	950	42	378	40
Sirloin steak, 7 oz	410	20	180	44
with baked potato + 1 Tbsp sour cream + 1 cup vegetable	780	26	234	30
with 2 cups french fries + 1 cup vegetable	1060	54	486	46
with loaded baked potato + 1 cup vegetable	1090	54	486	45
Chicken Caesar salad with dressing	660	46	414	63
Bacon & cheese grilled chicken sandwich	650	30	270	42
with 2 cups French fries	1230	61	549	45
with 11 onion rings	1550	94	846	55
Steak fajitas with 4 tortillas	860	31	279	32
with guacamole, sour cream, pico de gallo, diced cheese	1190	63	567	48
Chicken fajitas with 4 tortillas	840	24	216	26
Oriental chicken salad with dressing	750	49	441	59
Chicken fingers, 5 pieces (9 oz)	620	34	306	49
with 2 cups French fries + 1 cup cole slaw + 4 Tbsp dressing	1640	106	954	58
Hamburger with trimmings	660	36	324	49
with 2 cups French fries	1240	67	603	49
with 11 onion rings	1550	101	909	59
BBQ baby back ribs, 14 ribs (16 oz)	770	54	486	63
Fudge brownie sundae (10 oz)	1130	57	513	45
Philly cheese steak sandwich (6 inch)	680	35	315	46
with 2 cups French fries	1270	66	594	47
Chicken pot pie	680	37	333	49
Turkey club sandwich (13 oz)	740	34	306	41
Subway steak & cheese sub (6 inch)	370	13	117	32
Lobster, shrimp, scallop pasta	536	23	207	39

[a] *Food portions without rice.*

poverty. Clearly, obesity follows a distinct socioeconomic gradient; among women, higher obesity rates associate with low incomes and low education levels, with the highest obesity rates linked to the lowest income levels.[5]

The higher cost of more healthful foods and the lower cost of energy-dense foods that offer empty calories may mediate the association between poverty and obesity. Cheaper and less nutritious energy-dense foods may in turn promote overconsumption. Potato chips, chocolate, doughnuts, pizza, many ethnic foods, and salty snacks offer the most dietary energy at the lowest costs, with the highest levels of palatability, pleasure, and satisfaction.

It is well established that hunger and food insecurity, which usually accompany undernutrition and poverty, commonly associate with malnutrition. Surprisingly, a state of overnutrition also can associate with malnutrition. This paradoxical condition exists because many of the diets of people living in poverty consist of adequate amounts of energy to meet or exceed daily requirements but lack the nutritional quality to optimize health and prevent chronic disease. Thus, both aspects of malnutrition—undernutrition and overnutrition—emerge from living in poverty or having an inadequate food supply, as **FIGURE 9.5** demonstrates.[3]

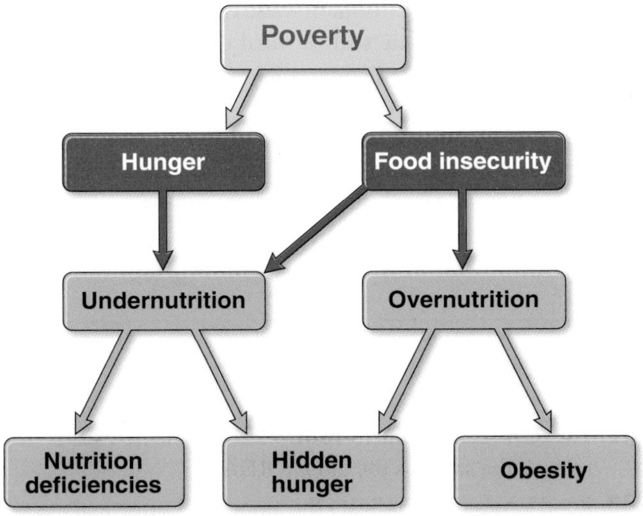

FIGURE 9.5 The hunger–obesity paradox. Definitions: *Food insecurity*: when people do not have adequate physical, social, or economic access to sufficient, safe, and nutritious food that meets their dietary needs and food preferences for an active and healthy life; *food security*: access by all people at all times to enough food for an active, healthy life, including, at a minimum, the ready availability to nutritionally adequate and safe foods and an assured ability to acquire acceptable foods in socially acceptable ways; *hidden hunger*: when an individual suffers from subclinical nutrient deficiencies (e.g., iron, folic acid, vitamin A) but does not show overt clinical signs of undernutrition. (From Dinour LM, et al. The food insecurity–obesity paradox: a review of the literature and the role food stamps may play. *J Am Diet Assoc* 2007;107:152.)

THE ORGANICS MOVEMENT

The organics movement has shown steady global growth. The first introduction in the United States occurred in 1990 with the Organic Foods Production Act of 1990 (www.farmlandinfo.org/documents/38361/Federal_Organic_Food_Production_Act.pdf), which "requires the Secretary of Agriculture to establish a National List of Allowed and Prohibited Substances which identifies synthetic substances that may be used, and the nonsynthetic substances that cannot be used, in organic production and handling operations."

Although a small part of the overall food market, "organic" purchases have grown approximately 20% a year since 1999 in the United States, while overall food sales have risen only about 3%. This trend is likely to continue as big grocers, most recently Wal-Mart, Costco, and other "big-box" retailers, expand their organic offerings.

Most industrialized countries throughout the world have established their own organic certification processes. The certification process for producers of organic food and other organic agricultural products varies from country to country and generally involves a set of production standards for growing, storing, processing, packaging, and shipping that includes the following four requirements:

1. Avoidance of synthetic chemical inputs not on the National List of Allowed and Prohibited Substances (e.g., fertilizers, pesticides, antibiotics, food additives), genetically modified organisms, irradiation, and the use of biosolids
2. Use of farmland that has been free from prohibited synthetic chemicals for a number of years (often, 3 years or more); keeping detailed written production and sales records as an audit trail
3. Maintaining strict physical separation of organic products from noncertified products
4. Undergoing periodic on-site inspections

In some countries, the government oversees certification, and commercial use of the term organic is legally restricted. Certified organic producers also are subject to the same agricultural, food safety, and other government regulations that apply to noncertified producers, although proper verification of standards among the smaller "organic" farms remains limited and controversial. The United States, the European Union, Canada, and Japan have comprehensive organic legislation, with the term "organic" used only by certified producers. Being able to include the word "organic" on a food product becomes a valuable

ABOUT ORGANIC STANDARDS

Sales of organic foods now comprise nearly 4% of total US food sales, and sales of organic fruits and vegetables are projected to grow 13% for the foreseeable future. A prime reason for the increased interest in organically grown food appears to be their supposedly higher nutrient quality and reduced levels of pesticide residues and other harmful compounds compared to conventionally grown produce.

To be classified as organic, growers need to ensure their crops adhere to the following four guidelines:

1. No synthetic fertilizers used
2. No synthetic pesticides or insecticides applied
3. No genetically engineered plants grown or animal products applied
4. Use of environmentally sound and sustainable growing practices

For organic animal products, the standard requires:

1. Use of 100% organic animal feed
2. Animals have mandatory outdoor access when weather is suitable
3. No antibiotics, growth hormones, or animal by-products in feed
4. Manure must be managed to prevent water or crop contamination

marketing advantage in today's consumer market but does not guarantee the product is legitimately organic. The purpose of organic certification is to protect consumers from misuse of the term and to make buying organics easier.

In the United States, federal organic legislation defines three levels of organics. Products made entirely with certified organic ingredients and methods can be labeled "100% organic." Products with at least 95% organic ingredients can use the word "organic." Both of these categories also may display the USDA organic seal. A third category, containing a minimum of 70% organic ingredients, can be labeled "made with organic ingredients."

Organic foods are supposed to be free of most chemical pesticides, fertilizers, antibiotics, hormones, and genetic engineering. Organic farmers and ranchers must enrich the soil and demonstrate humane animal treatment.

SUMMARY

1. Many factors affect food choices including traditions, early food experiences, emotions, food fears, food availability, and nutritional quality.
2. Pleasure associated with taste, texture, and aroma of food is learned within a perceptual and cultural context.
3. Many manufactures capitalize on the link between smell and taste and food pleasure by adding chemicals that mimic certain smells and tastes so one can purchase almost any "food" chemically altered to taste like something else.
4. Determining a food's nutrient density or "healthfulness" provides useful information about its nutritional quality referred to as the INQ.
5. Appetite and hunger refer to different entities. Appetite represents the desire to eat and is affected by external and psychological factors. Hunger represents an internal drive to eat largely based on central and peripheral physiologic systems.
6. New regulations from the FDA, under the aegis of the US Department of Agriculture's (USDA) Food Safety and Inspection Service, require manufacturers to adhere to guidelines when linking a nutrient(s) to medical or health benefits.
7. Four governmental agencies (FTC, FDA, USDA, and ATF) create the rules, regulations, and legal requirements concerning advertising, packaging, and labeling of foods and alcoholic beverages.
8. The Nutrition Labeling and Education Act of 1990 (NLEA) requires food manufacturers to strictly comply to regulations about what can and cannot be printed on food labels.
9. The format for the nutrition panel on foods must declare the nutrient content per serving as percentages of the Daily Values (the new label reference values).
10. The new "% Daily Value" comprises two sets of dietary standards: DRVs and RDIs.
11. DRVs established for macronutrients include sources of energy (lipid, carbohydrate [including fiber], and protein) and noncalorie contributors (cholesterol, sodium, and potassium).
12. The RDI replaces the term "US RDA." The new RDIs remain the same as the old US RDAs.
13. Food labels must indicate the amount of a particular nutrient, but no requirement exists to list its relative percentage in a food.
14. As of January 1, 2012, the familiar nutrition label required on all packaged food items must appear on 40 of the most commonly purchased cuts of beef, poultry, pork, and lamb.
15. The Nutrition Facts panels must include the number of calories, the grams of total fat, and saturated fat content.
16. A manufacturer wishing to include an additive in a food must follow specific FDA guidelines to ensure the additive's effectiveness (i.e., meet its claims).
17. A list of additives that are GRAS currently includes about 2000 flavoring agents and 200 coloring agents.
18. The healthcare reform legislation law of 2010 (enacted in 2012) requires restaurants and similar retail food establishments with 20 or more locations to list calorie content information for standard menu items on restaurant menus and menu boards.
19. Level of income and education, racial and ethnic background, and geographic locale and personal interests influence the amount, type, and quality of food consumed by a particular group or individual in the group.
20. People who often eat at fast-food restaurants usually double their caloric intake compared with eating at home.
21. The nongovernmental watchdog organization Center for Science in the Public Interest raises public awareness about the nutritional content of favorite foods and meals, often with alarming results about high fat content (particularly saturated fat) and excessive calorie content.
22. Hunger and obesity coexist within the same person and within the same household and link closely to "malnutrition."
23. Malnutrition from undernutrition and overnutrition emerges from living in poverty with an inadequate access to nutrient dense foods.

thePoint *Visit* **thePoint.lww.com/MKKSEN4e** *to view the following animation related to content presented in Chapter 9:* ***Diabetes.***

TEST YOUR KNOWLEDGE ANSWERS

1. **False:** Many factors determine food choice in addition to taste and nutritional value, including tradition and family preferences, emotions, fears, positive and negative associations, convenience and availability, and cost.

2. **True:** The FTC regulates food product advertising in various media (television, radio, newsprint, Internet) and pursues legal action against manufacturers who advertise unsubstantiated claims or deceptive ads. The FTC has authority to remove a product from the marketplace if the product's claims cannot be verified.

3. **False:** A food's nutritional quality or healthfulness (sometimes referred to nutrient density) is based on many factors including the number of nutrients known to promote health (protein, vitamins, minerals, fiber, phytochemical composition) in relation to the total calorie value of the food. No perfect food exits; some foods are just more nutritious than others per amount of a particular nutrient consumed.

4. **False:** The marketing of dietary supplements requires no government approval because supplements are considered foods and not drugs. In contrast to drugs, which must meet many safety and efficacy requirements before coming to market, legislation places the burden on the FDA to prove that a supplement is harmful before it can be removed from the market. Supplement marketing can progress with only the manufacturer's assurance of safety as long as the supplement does not claim disease-fighting benefits.

5. **True:** New rules in 1997 require supplements to be labeled as dietary supplements (e.g., "Vitamin C Dietary Supplement") and to carry a "Supplement Facts" panel with information similar to the "Nutrition Facts" panel that appears on most processed foods. Included on the facts panel must be an appropriate serving size; information on 14 nutrients, including sodium, vitamin A, vitamin C, calcium, and iron, when present at significant levels; other vitamins and minerals if added or part of a nutritional claim on the label; dietary ingredients with no established RDI; and if the product contains a proprietary blend of ingredients, the total amount of the blend and the identity of each dietary ingredient in the blend (although amounts of individual ingredients in the blend are not required). The rules also require that the labels of products containing botanical ingredients identify the part of the plant used.

6. **True:** The Bureau of Alcohol, Tobacco, Firearms and Explosives (ATF) is a law enforcement organization within the US Department of Treasury. It came into existence in 1972 after separating from the Internal Revenue Service (Alcohol, Tobacco, and Firearms Division). The ATF has responsibilities dedicated to reducing violent crime, collecting revenue, and protecting the public. It enforces the federal laws and regulations relating to alcohol, tobacco, firearms, explosives, and arson.

7. **False:** A daily intake of 2000 kcal serves as the reference number of calories for determining DRVs for the energy-producing nutrients. The 2000-kcal level was chosen, in part, because it approximates the caloric requirements for postmenopausal women, the group with the highest risk for excessive intake of calories and fat.

8. **False:** A "healthy" food must be low in fat and saturated fat and contain limited amounts of cholesterol and sodium. In addition, a single-item food must provide at least 10% of one or more of vitamins A or C, iron, calcium, protein, or fiber. A meal-type product, such as frozen entrees and multicourse frozen dinners, must provide 10% of two or three of these vitamins or minerals or of protein or fiber in addition to meeting the other criteria. Sodium content must be less than 360 mg per serving for individual foods and 480 mg per serving for meal-type products that carry the "healthy" claim.

9. **False:** The Hunger–Obesity Paradox refers to the counterintuitive observation that hunger and obesity coexist within the same person and within the same household. This paradox is mediated through poverty and food insecurity when people lack adequate physical, social, or economic access to sufficient, safe, and nutritious foods that meet dietary needs and food preferences for an active and healthy life. The paradox centers on the association between poverty and obesity mediated through the higher cost of more healthful foods and the lower cost of energy-dense foods that offer empty calories. Cheaper and less nutritious energy-dense foods may in turn promote overconsumption and lead to obesity.

10. **False:** Significant trends have taken place in eating behaviors. For example, Americans are supersizing their portions not just in fast-food restaurants but also in their own kitchens. A progressive increase occurred in portion size of hamburgers, burritos, tacos, French fries, sodas, ice cream, pie, cookies, and salty snacks between the 1970s and the 1990s, regardless of whether people ate out or at home. The size of hamburgers made at home increased from 5.7 oz in 1977 to 8.4 oz in 1996. Over the same time, fast-food hamburgers increased from 6.1 oz to 7.2 oz. Entrée size increase also has affected the eating behaviors of preschool children. The large, fixed size of these portions may constitute an "obesigenic" environmental influence that contributes to excessive caloric intake at meals.

Key References

Angell M, Kassirer JP. Alternative medicine: the risks of untested and unregulated remedies. *N Engl J Med* 1998;339:831.

Dietz WH. Does hunger cause obesity? *Pediatrics* 1995;95:766.

Dinour LM, et al. The food insecurity–obesity paradox: a review of the literature and the role food stamps may play. *J Am Diet Assoc* 2007;107:1952.

Drewnowski A. Concept of a nutritious food: toward a nutrient density score. *Am J Clin Nutr* 2005;82:721.

Drewnowski A, Specter SE. Poverty and obesity: the role of energy density and energy costs, *Am J Clin Nutr* 2004;79:6.

Fisher JO, et al. Children's bite size and intake of an entrée are greater with large portions than with age-appropriate or self-selected portions. *Am J Clin Nutr* 2003;77:1164.

Jones SJ, et al. Lower risk of overweight in school-aged food insecure girls who participate in food assistance. *Arch Pediatr Adolesc Med* 2003;157:780.

Life Sciences Research Office, Federation of American Societies of Experimental Biology. Core indicators of nutritional state for difficult-to-sample populations. *J Nutr* 1990;120(Suppl 11):S1559.

Nestle M. *Food Politics: How the Food Industry Influences Nutrition and Health.* Berkeley, CA: University of California Press, 2002.

Nielsen SJ, Popkin BM. Patterns and trends in food portion sizes, 1977-1998. *JAMA* 2003;289:450.

Nielsen SJ, Popkin BM. Changes in beverage intake between 1977 and 2001. *Am J Prev Med* 2004;27:205.

Olson CM. Nutrition and health outcomes associated with food insecurity and hunger. *J Nutr* 1999;129(Suppl 2):S521.

Sarubin A. Government regulation of dietary supplements. In: *The Health Professional's Guide to Dietary Supplements.* Chicago: The American Dietetic Association, 1999.

Scheier LM. What is the hunger-obesity paradox? *J Am Diet Assoc* 2005;105:883.

Sitzman K. Expanding food portions contribute to overweight and obesity. *AAOHN J* 2004;52:356.

Townsend MS, et al. Food insecurity is positively related to overweight in women. *J Nutr* 2001;131:1738.

Young LR, Nestle M. The contribution of expanding portion sizes to the U.S. obesity epidemic. *Am J Public Health* 2002;92:246.

thePoint *Visit* **thePoint.lww.com/MKKSEN4e** *for a list of the references cited in this chapter, including additional, relevant references.*

Thermoregulation and Fluid Balance During Heat Stress

PART 4

CONTENTS

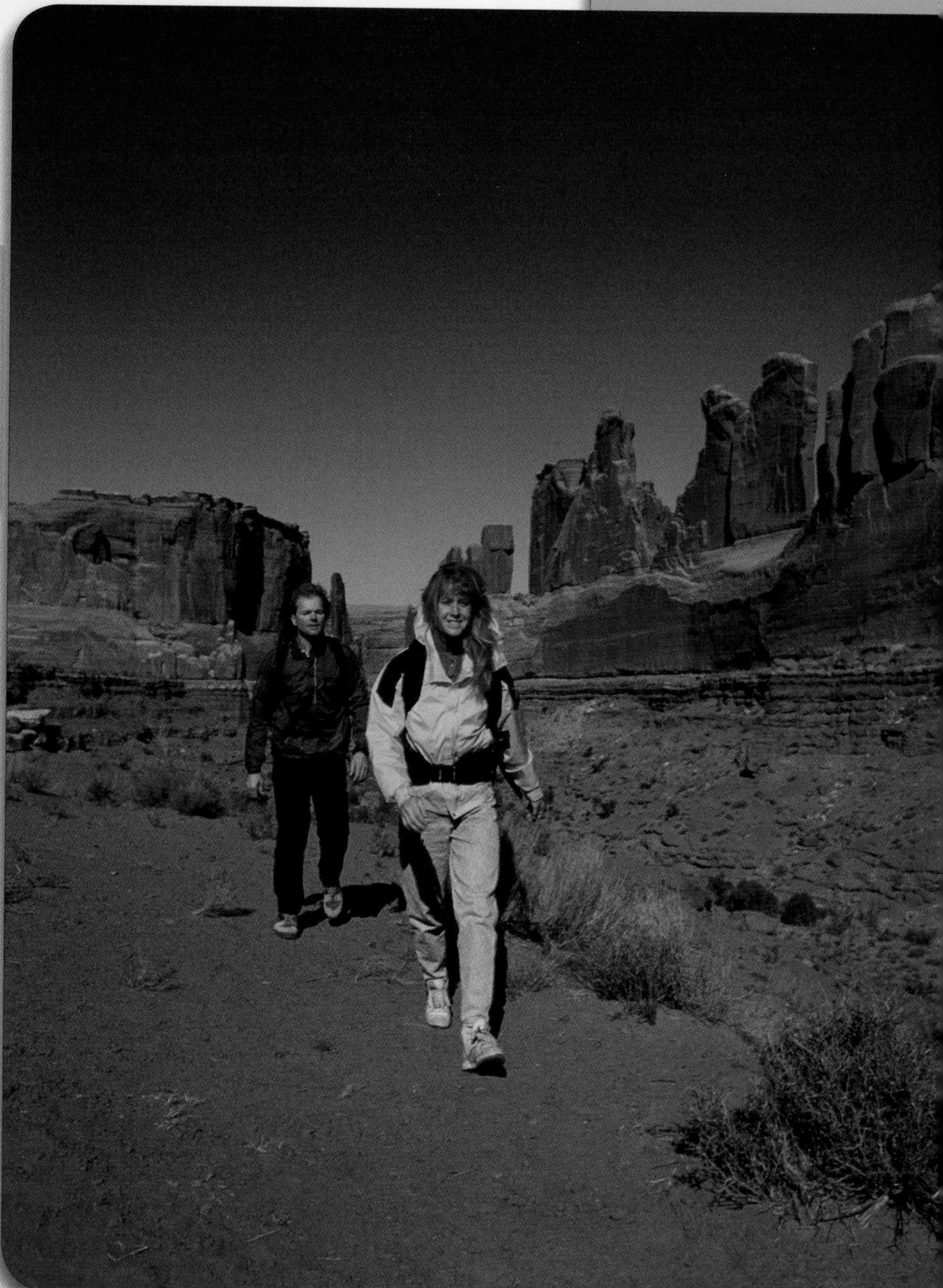

CHAPTER 10

Exercise, Thermoregulation, Fluid Balance, and Rehydration

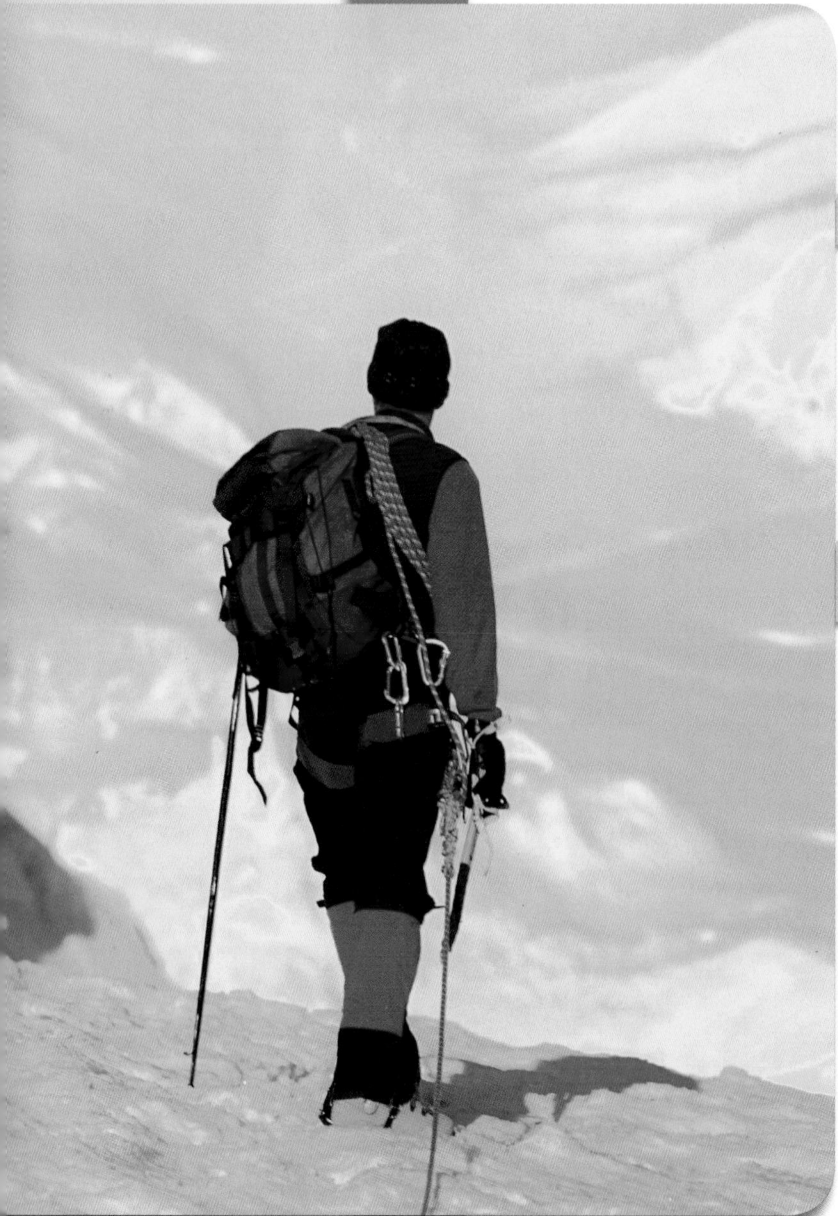

OUTLINE

- The Challenge of Environmental Stress

Mechanisms of Thermoregulation

- Thermal Balance
- Hypothalamic Regulation of Core Temperature
- Thermoregulation During Heat Stress: Heat Loss
- Evaluating Environmental Heat Stress

Thermoregulation During Exercise in the Heat

- Core Temperature During Exercise
- Water Loss in the Heat: Dehydration
- Water Replacement: Rehydration
- Hyponatremia: Reduced Sodium Concentration in Body Fluids
- Factors That Improve Heat Tolerance
- Effects of Clothing on Thermoregulation in the Heat
- Nutrition in Hot Environments
- Heat Illness: Complications from Excessive Heat Stress

TEST YOUR KNOWLEDGE

Select true or false for the 10 statements below, then check out the answers at the end of the chapter. Retake the test after you've read the chapter; you should achieve 100%!

	True	False
1. Core body temperature remains stable despite significant changes in environmental temperature.	❍	❍
2. The hypothalamus contains the central coordinating center for temperature regulation.	❍	❍
3. The body loses heat primarily via the physical mechanism of radiation.	❍	❍
4. Relative humidity refers to how dry the environment becomes in warm weather.	❍	❍
5. ADH is a major water-conserving hormone.	❍	❍
6. Exercising while dehydrated greatly increases the risk for heat injury.	❍	❍
7. The thirst mechanism provides a precise gauge to replenish water lost during exercise.	❍	❍
8. You can never consume too much water.	❍	❍
9. Air temperature primarily determines the potential physiologic strain produced by environmental heat.	❍	❍
10. Exercise in the heat requires an increase in energy intake.	❍	❍

The requirements for thermoregulation are considerable—the price of failure is death. In this chapter, we focus on the environmental challenge of high ambient temperatures. A person can tolerate a drop in deep body temperature of 10°C but an increase of only 5°C. The latter condition of **hyperthermia** occurred more than 100 times over the past 30 years among football players who died from excessive heat stress during practice or competition. Hyperthermia and dehydration were linked to the deaths of three collegiate wrestlers in the latter part of 1997. Heat injury also commonly occurs during military operations and longer duration athletic events. Athletes who illegally use erythropoietin, a hormone that boosts production of red blood cells, experience an even greater risk of heat injury. Their increased blood viscosity from increased hematocrit magnifies as dehydration progresses while exercising in the heat.

YOUTH ARE NOT IMMUNE

Government data released in August, 2011, showed that between 2001 and 2009, more than 3000 US children and teens received emergency-room treatment for nonfatal heat illness from exercise or sports participation. Data from the American Football Coaches Association (www.afca.com) and others showed that, over a 13-year period, 29 high school football players died from exertional heat stroke.

New guidelines from the American Academy of Pediatrics (www.aap.org/) entitled "Climatic Heat Stress and Exercising Children and Adolescents" published in the September 2011 issue of *Pediatrics*—released online 1 week after two Georgia high school football players died after practices in 90-plus-degree heat—replace a more restrictive policy based on past medical advice that incorrectly claimed that children were more vulnerale to heat stress than adults of equivalent training status. The current guidelines now mintain that sports participation during hot weather remains safe for healthy children and teen athletes if precautions are taken and the competitive drive does not outweigh commen sense. These athletes can reasonably play in high heat and humidity with adequate risk-reduction training of coaches and other supervisory personnel; a reasonable time to allow children to gradually acclimatize to physical activity in the heat; fluid intake before, during, and after exercise; timeouts; and emergency treatment available on the sidelines.

Council on Sports Medicine and Fitness, Council on School Health. Policy Statement–Climactic Heat Stress and Exercising Children and Adolescents. *Pediatrics*. 2012. In Press.

Knowledge of thermoregulation and the most effective ways to support its mechanisms significantly reduces heat-related tragedies. Coaches, athletes, race and event organizers, and those who provide overall nutritional advice must use strategies based on factors that contribute to heat gain and dehydration during exercise in a hot environment.[54] Concern also must focus on the most effective behavioral approaches (e.g., prudent scheduling of events, acclimatization, proper clothing, and fluid and electrolyte replacement before, during, and after exercise) to blunt the potential for negative effects on performance and safety.

THE CHALLENGE OF ENVIRONMENTAL STRESS

The human body constantly and automatically adjusts to maintain essential body nutrients and chemistry at normal levels to maintain health and support optimal performance. A change in the external environment, whether through an increase or decrease in ambient temperature or a reduction in barometric pressure at altitude, can significantly challenge the body to maintain normal stability and function. The French scientist Claude Bernard (1813–1878; see Connections to the Past in Chapter 14, p. 479) was perhaps first to recognize that the body was, for the most part, able to protect against environmental stressors and maintain stability of the internal environment through diverse mechanisms. This process of maintaining internal stability, termed by Bernard *milieu intérieur* (the environment within), represents the underlying principle of *homeostasis* first used by renowned Harvard physiologist Walter Cannon (1871–1945) who also coined the term *fight-or-flight response*.

Environmental stressors (e.g., heat, cold, hypoxia, noise, food, darkness, trauma, pathogens) challenge the milieu intérieur. The body's adaptations to counteract environmental stress may be short term (termed *accommodation*), intermediate in duration (termed *acclimation* or *acclimatization*), or long term (termed *genetic adaptation*). Accommodation and acclimation involve a complex array of adaptive responses, whereas genetic adaptation refers to semipermanent morphologic, physiologic, or other adaptations that occur over many generations within a species to successfully combat the challenge of environmental extremes.

Accommodation and acclimatization require a unique set of adaptive responses subject to substantial variability within and among individuals. Overall, most individuals adequately acclimatize to virtually all of the earth's stressful environments in about 8 to 14 days of exposure, whereas the loss of acclimatization occurs in about 14 to 28 days. Individual differences in accommodation and acclimatization depend on the following six factors:

1. Genetic characteristics
2. Available resources
3. Age (particularly in preadolescence and old age)
4. Nature and duration of previous exposures
5. Number of similar previous experiences
6. Emotional and psychological response (worry, fear, panic, self-assurance) to the environmental stress

AN ERGOGENIC AID IN ITS OWN RIGHT

Water becomes the most important performance-enhancing nutrient when exercise and heat stressors combine. The exercise nutritionist must apply knowledge of the basic physics and physiology of thermoregulation to defend effectively against the potentially lethal challenge of heat stress.

MECHANISMS OF THERMOREGULATION

THERMAL BALANCE

FIGURE 10.1 shows body temperature of the deeper tissues or **core** in dynamic equilibrium between factors that add and subtract body heat. This balance results from three integrating mechanisms that accomplish the following:

1. Alter heat transfer to the periphery or **shell**
2. Regulate evaporative cooling
3. Vary the rate of heat production

Core temperature rises quickly when heat gain exceeds heat loss as occurs during vigorous exercise in a warm environment.

TABLE 10.1 presents thermal data for heat production (oxygen consumption) and heat loss from sweating at rest and during maximal exercise. The body gains considerable heat from the reactions of energy metabolism, particularly from active muscle. Just from shivering, the total metabolic rate increases threefold to fivefold. During sustained exercise by aerobically fit men and women, metabolic rate often increases 20 to 25 times above the resting level to 20 $kcal \cdot min^{-1}$; heat production of this magnitude could theoretically increase core temperature by 1°C (1.8°F) every 5 to 7 minutes! The body also absorbs heat from the environment by solar radiation and from objects warmer than the body. Heat loss occurs by the physical mechanisms of radiation, conduction, and convection. However, water

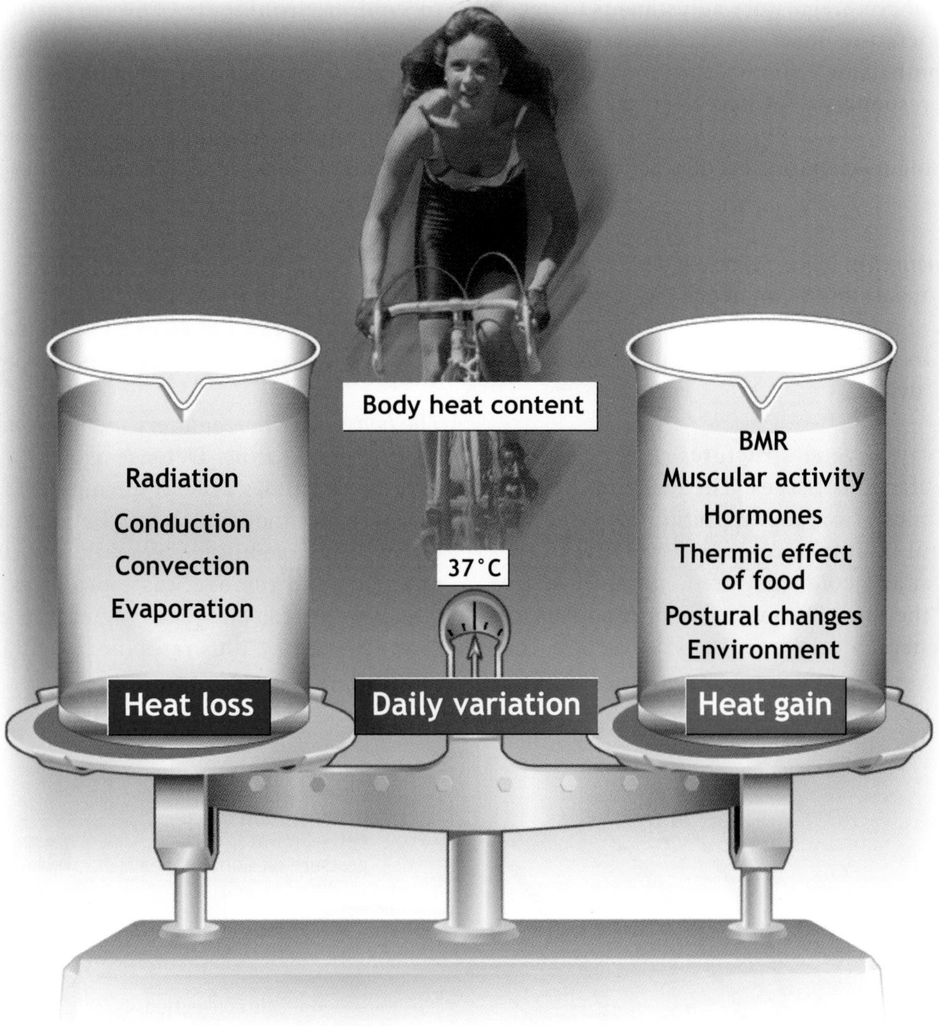

FIGURE 10.1. Factors that contribute to heat gain and heat loss to regulate core temperature at about 37°C.

vaporization or evaporation from the skin and respiratory passages provides the most important avenue for heat loss.

TABLE 10.1 Thermodynamics at Rest and During Exercise

Body's Heat Production	Rest	Maximal Exercise
(1 L O_2 uptake = ~4.82 kcal); mixed diet	~0.25 L $O_2 \cdot min^{-1}$	~4.0 L $O_2 \cdot min^{-1}$
	~1.2 $kcal \cdot min^{-1}$	~20.0 $kcal \cdot min^{-1}$
Body's Capacity for Evaporative Cooling		Maximal Sweating
(Each 1 mL sweat evaporation = ~0.6 kcal body heat loss)		30 $mL \cdot min^{-1}$ = ~18 $kcal \cdot min^{-1}$
Core temperature increase	No increase	~1°C every 5–7 min

Evaporative cooling under optimal conditions accounts for a heat loss of about 18 $kcal \cdot min^{-1}$.

Circulatory adjustments provide "fine tuning" for temperature regulation. Heat conservation occurs by rapidly shunting blood deep to the cranial, thoracic, and abdominal cavities including portions of the muscle mass. This optimizes insulation from subcutaneous fat and other areas of the body's shell. Conversely, excessive internal heat buildup dilates peripheral vessels that channel warm blood to the cooler periphery. During exercise in the heat, the strong drive for thermal balance can increase sweat rate to as high as 3.5 $L \cdot h^{-1}$.

HYPOTHALAMIC REGULATION OF CORE TEMPERATURE

*The **hypothalamus** contains the central neural coordinating center for temperature regulation.* This group of specialized neurons at the floor of the brain serves as a "thermostat" (usually set and carefully regulated at 37°C ±1°C) that makes thermoregulatory adjustments to deviations from a temperature norm. Unlike a thermostat in a building, the hypothalamus cannot "turn off" the heat; it only can initiate responses to protect the body from heat gain or heat loss.

Heat-regulating mechanisms become activated in two ways:

1. Temperature changes in blood perfusing the hypothalamus directly stimulate this thermoregulatory control center.
2. Thermal receptors in the skin provide input to modulate hypothalamic activity.

FIGURE 10.2 displays diverse structures embedded within skin and subcutaneous tissues. The inset on the right depicts the dynamics of sweat evaporation from the skin surface. Peripheral thermal receptors responsive to rapid changes in heat and cold exist predominantly as free nerve endings in the skin. The more numerous cutaneous cold receptors generally exist near the skin surface; they play an important role in initiating regulatory responses to cold environments. The cutaneous thermal receptors act as an "early warning system" that relays sensory information to the hypothalamus and cerebral cortex. This direct communication link evokes appropriate heat-conserving or heat-dissipating physiologic adjustments as the individual consciously seeks relief from the thermal challenge.

THERMOREGULATION DURING HEAT STRESS: HEAT LOSS

The body's thermoregulatory mechanisms primarily protect against overheating. Defense against a rise in core temperature becomes crucial during exercise in hot weather. Here, competition exists between mechanisms that maintain a large muscle blood flow to deliver oxygen and nutrients and remove waste products and mechanisms that provide for adequate regulation of body temperature. **FIGURE 10.3** illustrates the potential avenues for heat

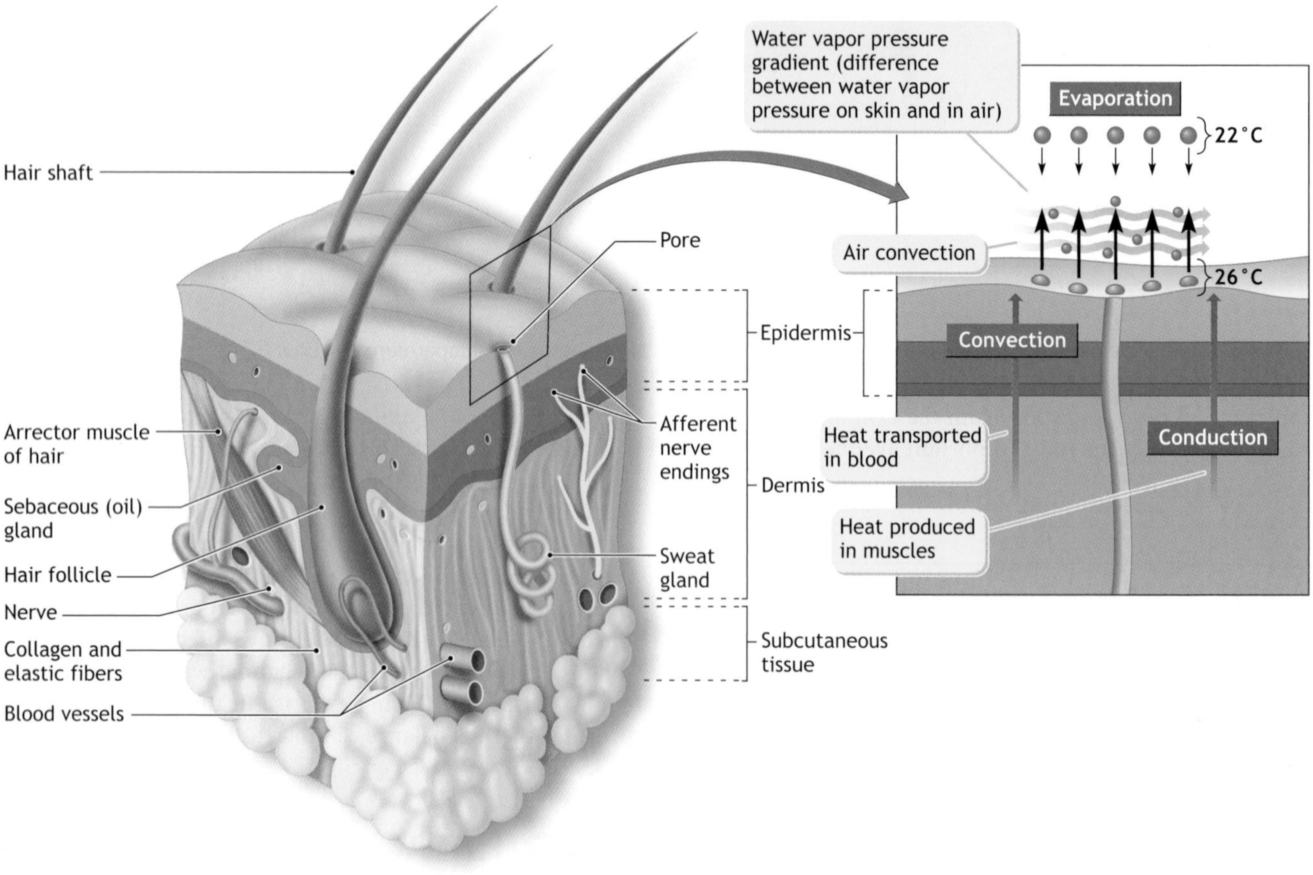

FIGURE 10.2. *Left.* Schematic illustration of the skin and underlying structures. The enlargement of the skin surface at *right* shows the dynamics of conduction, convection, and sweat evaporation for heat dissipation from the body. Each 1 L of water evaporated from the skin transfers 580 kcal of heat energy to the environment.

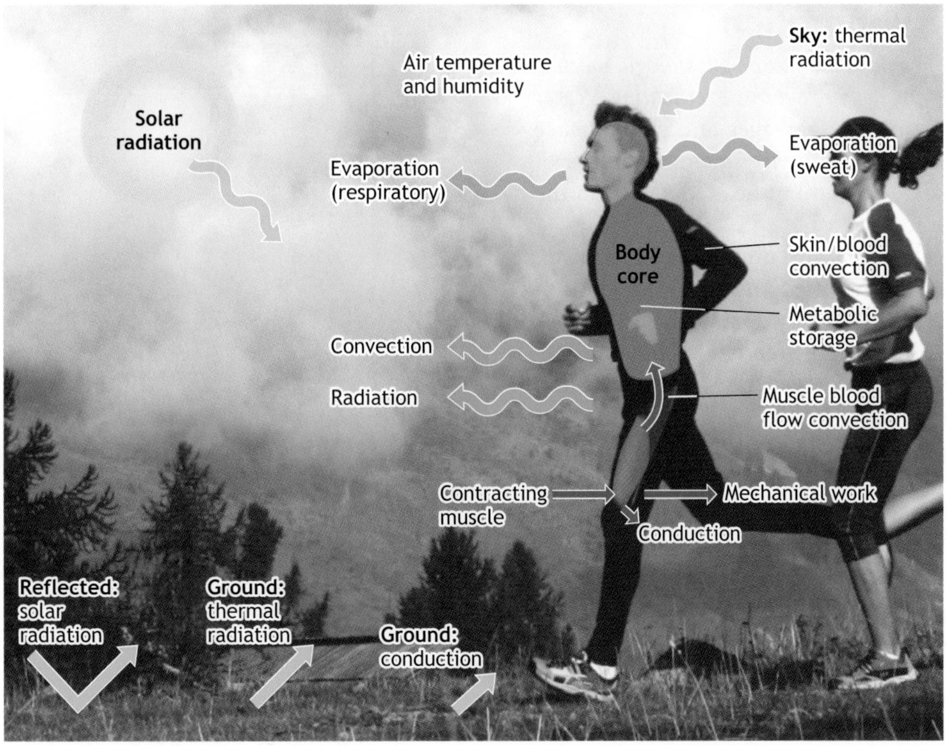

FIGURE 10.3. Heat production within active muscle and its subsequent transfer from the core to the skin. Under appropriate environmental conditions, excess body heat dissipates to the environment and core temperature stabilizes within a narrow range. (From Gisolfi CV, Wenger CB. Temperature regulation during exercise: old concepts, new ideas. *Exerc Sport Sci Rev* 1984;12:399.)

exchange in an exercising human. Body heat loss occurs in four ways:

1. Radiation
2. Conduction
3. Convection
4. Evaporation

Heat Loss by Radiation

Objects continually emit electromagnetic heat waves. Because our bodies are usually warmer than the environment, the net exchange of radiant heat energy occurs from the body through the air to nearby solid, cooler objects. This form of heat transfer, similar to how the sun's rays warm the earth, does not require molecular contact between objects. Despite subfreezing temperatures, a person can remain warm by absorbing sufficient radiant heat energy from direct sunlight (or reflected from snow, sand, or water). The body absorbs radiant heat energy when an object's temperature in the environment exceeds skin temperature.

Heat Loss by Conduction

Heat loss by conduction transfers heat directly through a liquid, solid, or gas from one molecule to another. The circulation transports most body heat to the periphery, but a small amount continually moves by conduction directly through deep tissues to the cooler surface. Conductive heat loss involves warming of air molecules and cooler surfaces in contact with skin.

The rate of conductive heat loss depends on the existence of a temperature gradient between the skin and surrounding surfaces and their thermal qualities. Warm-weather hikers gain considerable heat from their physical activity and environment. Some relief comes by lying on a cool rock shielded from the sun. Conductance between the rock's cold surface and the hiker's warmer surface facilitates loss of body heat.

Heat Loss by Convection

The effectiveness of heat loss by conduction via air depends on how rapidly air near the body exchanges once it warms. With little or no air movement or convection, warmed air next to the skin acts as a zone of insulation, thereby minimizing further conductive heat loss. Conversely, if cooler air continuously replaces warmer air that surrounds the body (as occurs on a breezy day, in a room with a fan, or during running), heat loss increases because convective currents carry heat away. For example, air currents moving at 4 mph cool twice as effectively as air moving at 1 mph.

Heat Loss by Evaporation

Evaporation of sweat provides the major physiologic mechanism for heat loss and thus defense against overheating. Water vaporization from respiratory passages and skin surface continually transfers heat to the environment. Each liter of vaporized water transfers 580 kcal of heat energy from the body to the environment.

In response to heat stress, 2 to 4 million sweat (eccrine) glands secrete large quantities of hypotonic saline solution (0.2–0.4% NaCl). Cooling occurs when sweat evaporates from skin surfaces. Cooled skin then cools blood shunted from the interior to the surface. Along with heat loss through sweating, approximately 350 mL of water seeps through the skin each day (called *insensible perspiration*) and evaporates to the environment. Also, approximately 300 mL of water vaporizes daily from the respiratory passages' moist mucous membranes.

Evaporative Heat Loss at High Ambient Temperatures

Increased ambient temperature reduces the effectiveness of heat loss by conduction, convection, and radiation. When ambient temperature exceeds body temperature, these three thermal transfer mechanisms actually contribute to heat gain. When this occurs (or when conduction, convection, and radiation *cannot* adequately dissipate a large metabolic heat load), sweat evaporation from the skin and water vaporization from the respiratory tract provide the only avenues to dissipate heat. Sweating rate increases directly with ambient temperature. For someone relaxing in a hot, humid environment, the normal 2-L daily fluid requirement often doubles or triples from evaporative fluid loss.

Heat Loss in High Humidity

FIGURE 10.4 illustrates the influence of exercise intensity and environmental conditions on sweating rate. Three factors determine sweat evaporation from the skin:

1. Surface area exposed to the environment
2. Temperature and relative humidity of ambient air
3. Convective air currents around the body

By far, relative humidity exerts the greatest impact on the effectiveness of evaporative heat loss.

Relative humidity refers to the percentage of water in ambient air at a particular temperature compared with the total quantity of moisture the air could carry. For example, 40% relative humidity means that ambient air contains only 40% of the air's moisture-carrying capacity at that specific temperature. With increasing humidity, ambient air's vapor pressure approaches that of moist skin (approximately 40 mm Hg). Consequently, evaporative heat loss becomes thwarted, even though a large quantity of sweat beads on the skin and eventually rolls off. This represents a useless water loss that can lead to dehydration and overheating. Continually drying the skin with a towel before sweat evaporates also thwarts evaporative cooling.

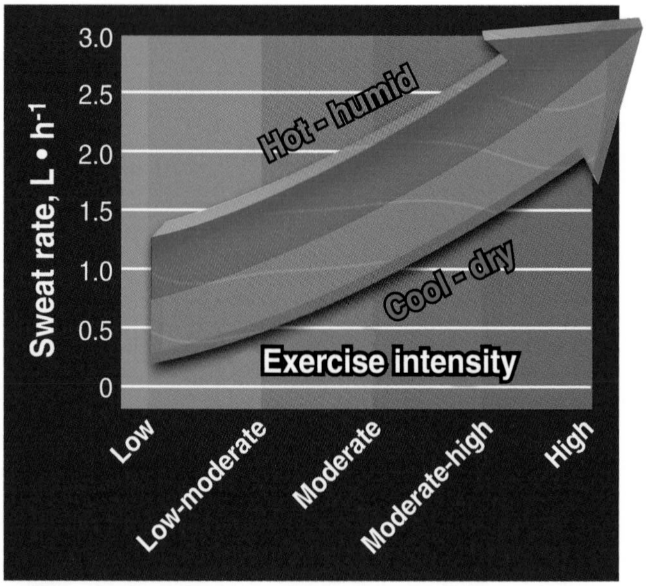

FIGURE 10.4. Approximate hourly sweating rates related to environmental conditions and exercise intensity.

> *Sweat does not cool the skin; rather, skin cooling occurs only when sweat evaporates.*

One can tolerate relatively higher environmental temperatures provided that humidity remains lower. For this reason, most people prefer the relative comfort of hot, dry desert climates to "cooler" but more humid tropical climates.

Integration of Heat-Dissipating Mechanisms

Circulation

The circulatory system serves as the main "workhorse" to control thermal balance. At rest in hot weather, heart rate and blood flow from the heart (cardiac output) increase while superficial arterial and venous blood vessels dilate to divert warm blood to the body's shell. This effect manifests as a flushed or reddened face on a hot day or during vigorous exercise. With extreme heat stress, 15 to 25% of the cardiac output passes through the skin, greatly increasing the thermal conductance of peripheral tissues. Increased peripheral blood flow favors radiative heat loss, particularly from the hands, forehead, forearms, ears, and tibial area of the lower legs.

Evaporation

Sweating begins within several seconds of the start of vigorous exercise. After about 30 minutes, sweating reaches equilibrium directly related to exercise load. A large cutaneous blood flow coupled with evaporative cooling generally produces an effective thermal defense. The cooled peripheral blood then returns to the deeper tissues to pick up additional heat on its return to the heart.

Hormonal Adjustments

Heat stress initiates hormonal adjustments to conserve the loss of salts and fluid in sweat. During heat exposure, the pituitary gland releases **antidiuretic hormone** (**ADH**; also known as vasopressin), the hormone that increases water reabsorption from the kidney tubules that causes urine to become more concentrated. Concurrently, during a single bout of exercise or with repeated days of exercise in hot weather, the adrenal cortex releases the sodium-conserving hormone **aldosterone**, which increases the renal tubules' reabsorption of sodium. Aldosterone also decreases sodium concentration in sweat (i.e., reduces sweat osmolality), which aids in additional electrolyte conservation.

AMERICAN COLLEGE OF SPORTS MEDICINE WET BULB-GLOBE TEMPERATURE RECOMMENDATIONS FOR CONTINUOUS ACTIVITIES SUCH AS ENDURANCE RUNNING AND CYCLING

- Very high risk: Above 28°C (82°F)—postpone race
- High risk: 23 to 28°C (73–82°F)—heat-sensitive individuals (e.g., obese, low physical fitness, unacclimatized, dehydrated, previous history of heat injury) should not compete
- Moderate risk: 18 to 23°C (65–73°F)
- Low risk: Below 18°C (65°F)

EVALUATING ENVIRONMENTAL HEAT STRESS

Five factors other than air temperature determine the physiologic strain imposed by heat:

1. Body size and fatness
2. Level of training
3. Acclimatization
4. Adequacy of hydration
5. External factors (convective air currents; radiant heat gain; intensity of exercise; amount, type, and color of clothing; and most importantly, relative humidity). The death of some football players from hyperthermia occurred when air temperature dipped below 75°F (23.9°C) but relative humidity exceeded 95%.

Prevention represents the most effective way to minimize or eliminate heat stress injuries. Acclimatization greatly reduces the chance for heat injury. Another defense involves use of the **wet bulb-globe temperature (WB-GT)** to evaluate the

Connections to the Past

William Harvey (1578–1657)

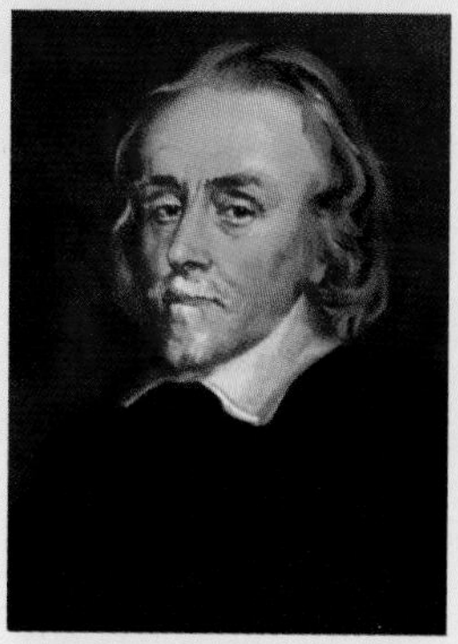

William Harvey discovered that blood circulates continuously in one direction. This monumental discovery overthrew 2000 years of ancient medical dogma that taught that blood moved from the right to left side of the heart through pores in the septum. Harvey announced his discovery during a 3-day dissection lecture at the Royal College of Physicians in London on April 16, 1616. Twelve years later, he published the details in a 72-page Latin monograph exhibited at the Frankfurt, Germany book fair, *Exercitatio Anatomica de Motu Cordis et Sanguinis in Animalibus* (*An Anatomical Treatise on the Movement of the Heart and Blood in Animals*). This monograph represents one of the most important (and famous) contributions in the distinguished history of human physiologic analysis.

By combining the new technique of experimentation on living creatures with mathematical logic and quantitative assessment, Harvey deduced that, contrary to received standard opinion, blood flowed in only one direction—from the heart to the arteries and from the veins back to the heart.

thePoint *Visit* **thePoint.lww.com/MKKSEN4e** *to find more details about Harvey's experiments on how blood circulates continuously in one direction.*

environment for its potential thermal challenge. This index of environmental heat stress, developed by the US military, incorporates ambient temperature, relative humidity, and radiant heat as follows:

$$\text{WB-GT} = 0.1 \times \text{DBT} + 0.7 \times \text{WBT} + 0.2 \times \text{GT}$$

where:

DBT = dry-bulb (air) temperature in the shade recorded by an ordinary mercury thermometer that measures air temperature.

WBT (accounts for 70% of the index) = temperature recorded by an ordinary mercury thermometer and a thermometer with a wet wick that surrounds the mercury bulb (wet bulb) exposed to rapid air movement in direct sunlight. With high relative humidity, little evaporative cooling occurs from the wetted bulb, so the temperature of this thermometer remains similar to that of the dry bulb. On a dry day, evaporation occurs from the wetted bulb. This maximizes the difference between the two thermometer readings. A small difference between readings indicates high relative humidity, whereas a large difference indicates little air moisture and a high rate of evaporation.

GT = globe temperature in direct sunlight recorded by a thermometer with a black metal sphere surrounding the bulb. The black globe absorbs radiant energy from the surroundings to provide a measure of radiant heat gain.

FIGURE 10.5 illustrates the apparatus to measure WB-GT. The top portion of the inset table presents WB-GT guidelines for athletic activities to reduce the chance of heat injury. These standards apply to lightly clothed humans; they do not consider the specific heat load imposed by football uniforms or other types of equipment. For football, the lower end of each temperature range serves as a more prudent guide.

An indication of ambient heat load also comes from the wet-bulb thermometer because this reading reflects both air temperature and relative humidity. An inexpensive wet-bulb thermometer can be purchased at most industrial supply companies. The bottom portion of the inset table of **FIGURE 10.5** presents heat stress recommendations based on wet-bulb temperature. Without the wet-bulb temperature, but knowing relative humidity via local meteorologic stations' media reports and the Internet (www.weather.com), the **heat index** (**FIG. 10.6**) devised by the US National Weather Service also evaluates relative heat stress. Sometimes referred to as the "apparent temperature," the index provides an accurate measure of how hot it feels when the relative humidity combines with the air temperature. The heat index values were determined for shady, light wind conditions, so exposure to full sunshine increases values by up to 15°F. In addition, strong winds (particularly with hot, dry air) present an extreme hazard in competitive outdoor sports. One should determine the

WB-GT Range °F	°C	Recommendations
80 – 84	26.5 – 28.8	• Use discretion,especially if unconditioned or unacclimated
85 – 87	29.5 – 30.5	• Avoid strenuous activity in the sun
> 88	> 31.2	• Avoid exercise training

WBT Range °F	°C	Recommendations
60	15.5	• No prevention necessary
61 – 65	16.2 – 18.4	• Alert all participants to problems of heat stress and importance of adequate hydration
66 – 70	18.8 – 21.1	• Insist that appropriate quantity of fluid be ingested
71 – 75	21.6 – 23.8	• Rest periods and water breaks every 20 to 30 minutes; limits placed on intense activity
76 – 79	24.5 – 26.1	• Practice curtailed and modified considerably
> 80	> 26.5	• Practice cancelled

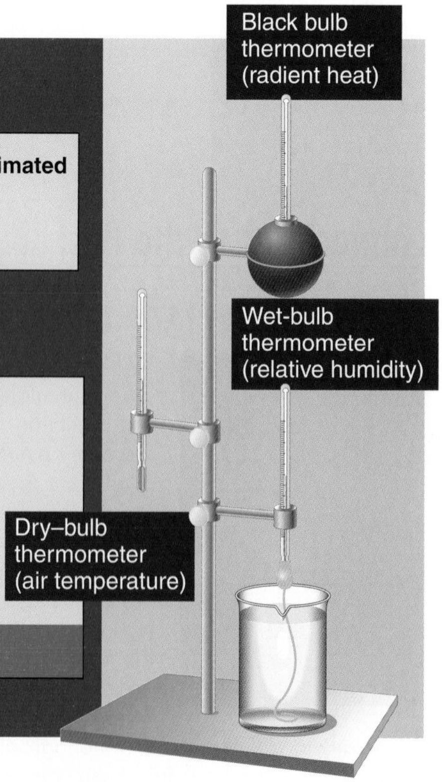

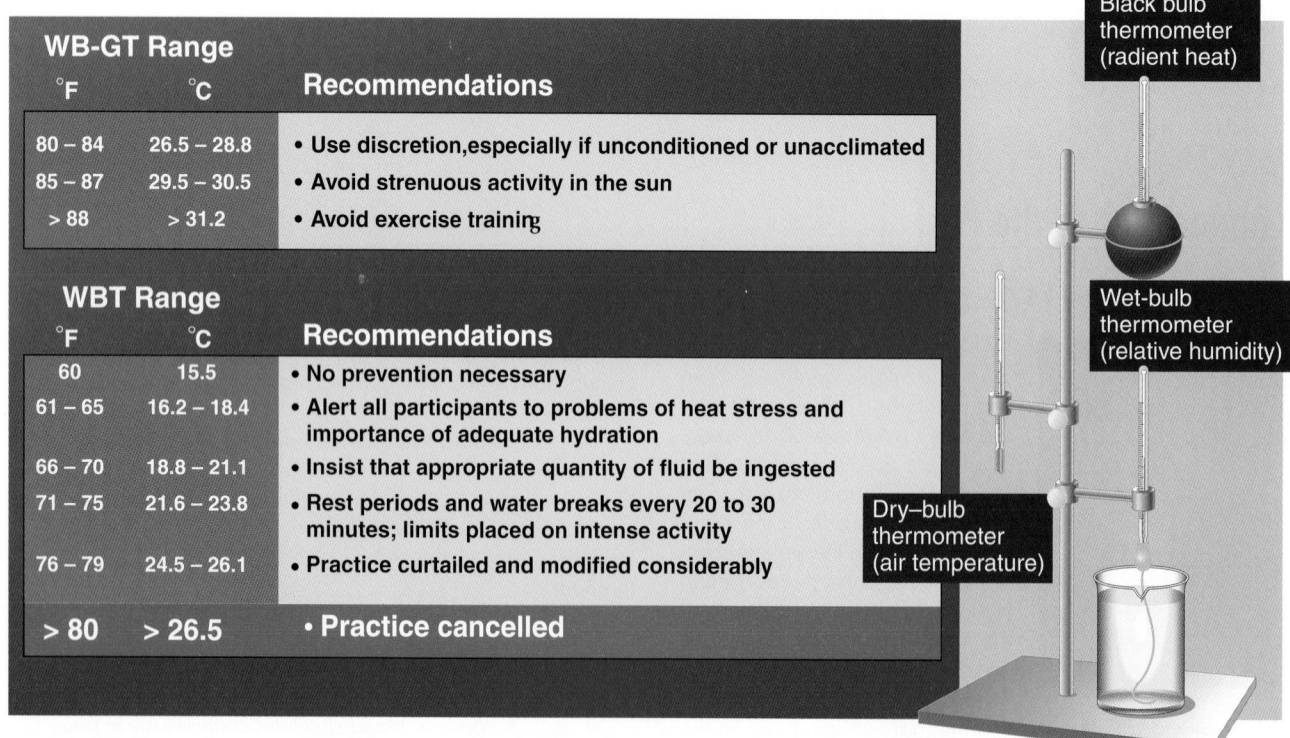

FIGURE 10.5. Wet bulb-globe temperature (WB-GT) for outdoor activities and wet-bulb temperature (WBT) guide. (Modified from Murphy RJ, Ashe WF. Prevention of heat illness in football players. *JAMA* 1965;194:650.)

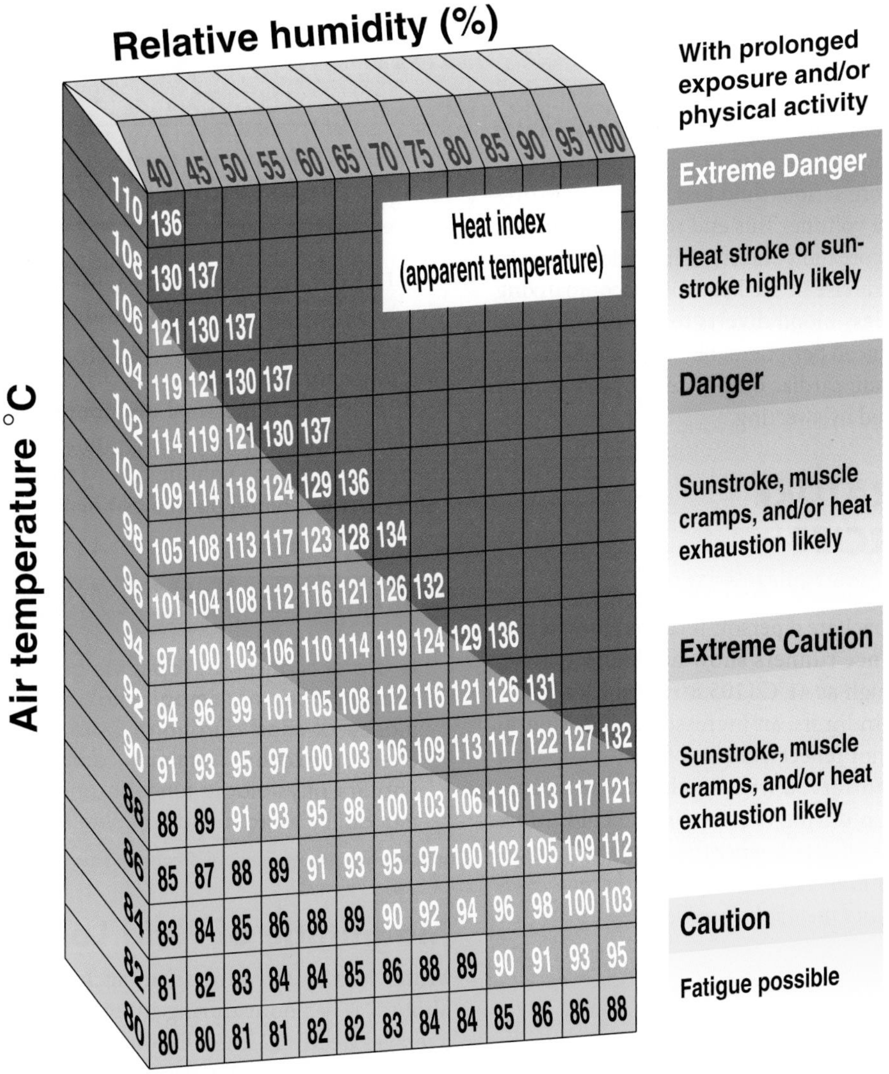

FIGURE 10.6. How hot is too hot? The heat index.

index close to the competition site to eliminate potential error from using meteorologic data some distance from the event. Data collected for the 24-hour trend of ambient temperature and relative humidity justified changing the race time for the 1996 Olympic Marathon run in Atlanta from 6:30 PM to 7:00 AM to reduce heat injury risk.

SUMMARY

1. Humans tolerate relatively small variations in internal or core temperature. Consequently, exposure to heat or cold initiates thermoregulatory mechanisms that generate and conserve heat at low ambient temperatures and dissipate heat at high temperatures.
2. The hypothalamus serves as the "thermostat" for temperature regulation. This coordination center initiates adjustments from thermal receptors in the skin and changes in hypothalamic blood temperature.
3. Warm blood diverts from the body's core to the shell in response to heat stress. Heat loss occurs by radiation, conduction, convection, and evaporation. Evaporation provides the major physiologic defense against overheating at high ambient temperatures and during exercise.
4. Warm, humid environments dramatically decrease the effectiveness of evaporative heat loss. This increases one's vulnerability to a dangerous state of dehydration and spiraling core temperature.

THERMOREGULATION DURING EXERCISE IN THE HEAT

Cardiovascular adjustments and evaporative cooling dissipate metabolic heat mainly during exercise in hot weather. Excessive sweating leads to more serious fluid loss with accompanying reductions in plasma volume. This end result can produce circulatory failure, with core temperature rising to lethal levels. During near-maximal exercise in the heat with accompanying dehydration, relatively less blood diverts to peripheral areas for heat dissipation. Reduced peripheral blood flow reflects the body's attempt to maintain cardiac output despite a diminishing plasma volume caused by sweating.

CORE TEMPERATURE DURING EXERCISE

Heat generated by active muscles can raise core temperature to fever levels that incapacitate a person if caused by external heat stress alone. Distance runners show no ill effects from rectal temperatures as high as 41°C (105.8°F) recorded at the end of a race.[13,42] Within limits, an increased core temperature with exercise does not reflect a failure of heat-dissipating mechanisms. To the contrary, a well-regulated rise in core temperature occurs even during exercise in the cold. *More than likely, a modest rise in core temperature reflects a favorable internal adjustment that creates an optimal thermal environment for physiologic and metabolic functions.*

WATER LOSS IN THE HEAT: DEHYDRATION

Dehydration refers to an imbalance in fluid dynamics when fluid intake does not replenish water loss from either hyperhydrated or normally hydrated states. A moderate exercise workout generally produces a 0.5- to 1.5-L sweat loss over a 1-hour period. Considerable water loss occurs during several hours of intense exercise in a hot environment. Even with exercise performed in less challenging thermal environments (e.g., swimming and cross-country skiing), sweating still occurs.[47] For the swimmer, immersion in water per se also stimulates body water loss through cold-induced increased urine production. Non–exercise-induced water loss occurs when boxers, weightlifters, and rowers (examples of power athletes) aggressively attempt to "make weight" through rapid weight loss induced by common dehydration techniques (e.g., heat exposure via sauna, steam room, hot whirlpool, or shower; fluid and food restriction; diuretic and laxative drugs; or vomiting). The athlete often combines techniques in hopes of achieving even faster weight loss.

Intracellular and extracellular compartments contribute to the fluid deficit (dehydration) that can rapidly reach levels that impede heat dissipation, reduce heat tolerance, and severely compromise cardiovascular function and exercise capacity.

The risk of heat illness greatly increases when a person begins exercising in a dehydrated state.

Dehydration associated with a 3% decrease in body weight slows gastric emptying rate, thus triggering epigastric cramps and feelings of nausea.[92] Avoiding dehydration not only optimizes exercise performance but also reduces the feelings of gastrointestinal discomfort associated with body fluid loss. Because sweat is hypotonic with other body fluids, the reduced plasma volume caused by sweating correspondingly increases blood plasma osmolality.

EXERCISE DURATION IS IMPORTANT

In a practical sense, rapid weight loss through dehydration does not impair maximal exercise performance of short durations up to 60 seconds. When exercise exceeds 1 minute, dehydration profoundly impairs physiologic function and compromises optimal ability to train and compete.

Magnitude of Fluid Loss

Water loss by sweating in an acclimatized person peaks at about 3 L per hour during intense exercise in the heat and averages nearly 12 L (26 lb) on a daily basis. Several hours of intense sweating can cause sweat gland fatigue, which ultimately impairs core temperature regulation. Elite marathon runners frequently experience fluid losses in excess of 5 L during competition; this represents between 6 and 10% of body mass. For slower paced marathons or ultramarathons, average fluid loss rarely exceeds 500 mL per hour. Even in a temperate climate, an average fluid loss of 2 L takes place in soccer players during a 90-minute game played at about 10°C (50°F).[49] A large sweat output and subsequent fluid loss occur in sports other than distance running; football, basketball, and hockey players also lose large quantities of fluid during a contest.

Physiologic and Performance Consequences

Any degree of dehydration impairs the capacity of circulatory and temperature-regulating mechanisms to adjust to exercise demands.

As dehydration progresses and plasma volume decreases, peripheral blood flow and sweating rate diminish and thermoregulation becomes progressively more difficult.

Cumulatively, this contributes to larger increases in heart rate, perception of effort, and core temperature than under normal hydration and premature fatigue. A fluid loss of only 1% of body mass increases rectal temperature above that with the same exercise performed when fully hydrated.

Reduced peripheral blood flow and increased core temperature during exercise relate closely to dehydration level. Dehydration of only 2% body mass impairs physical work capacity and physiologic function and predisposes to heat injury when exercising in a hot environment.[12,18,24,31,51,82,93] For each liter of sweat loss dehydration, exercise heart rate increases 8 beats·min^{-1} with a corresponding 1.0 L·min^{-1} decrease in cardiac output.[25] A large portion of water lost through sweating comes from blood plasma, so circulatory capacity progressively decreases as sweat loss progresses. Body fluid loss coincides with the following five changes in bodily functions:

1. Decreased plasma volume
2. Reduced skin blood flow for a given core temperature
3. Reduced stroke volume of the heart
4. Increased heart rate
5. General deterioration in circulatory and thermoregulatory efficiency in exercise

For exercise performance, dehydration equal to 4.3% of body mass reduced walking endurance by 18%; concurrently, $\dot{V}O_{2max}$ decreased by 22%. These same experiments showed decreased endurance performance (−22%) and $\dot{V}O_{2max}$ (−10%) when dehydration averaged only 1.9% of body mass. Clearly, even modest dehydration imposes adverse thermoregulatory and exercise performance effects during exercise. A moderate degree of hypohydration or hyperthermia exerts no effect on anaerobic exercise performance.[17]

Considerable Fluid Loss During Exercise in Winter Environments: The risk for dehydration increases during vigorous cold-weather exercise because colder air contains less moisture than air at warmer temperature, particularly at higher altitudes. Consequently, greater fluid volumes leave respiratory passages as the incoming cold, dry air fully humidifies and warms to body temperature. This air-conditioning process can create a 1-L daily fluid loss. Cold stress also increases urine production, which adds to total body fluid loss. Furthermore, many people overdress for outdoor winter activities. As exercise progresses and heat production increases, heat gain exceeds heat loss, thereby initiating a sweating response. All of these factors become magnified because many individuals consider it unimportant to consume fluids before, during, and in recovery from prolonged exercise in cold weather. **FIGURE 10.7** illustrates a back-mounted hydration system to provide ready access to water *during* prolonged winter activities as in Nordic or alpine skiing, serious outdoor winter trekking including ice and mountain climbing at high altitudes, or distance cycling or running. In the military, back-mounted hydration systems are often attached to load-bearing equipment. Many different styles and configurations of hydration systems are available at sporting goods or cycling shops and through sports equipment mail-order catalogues.

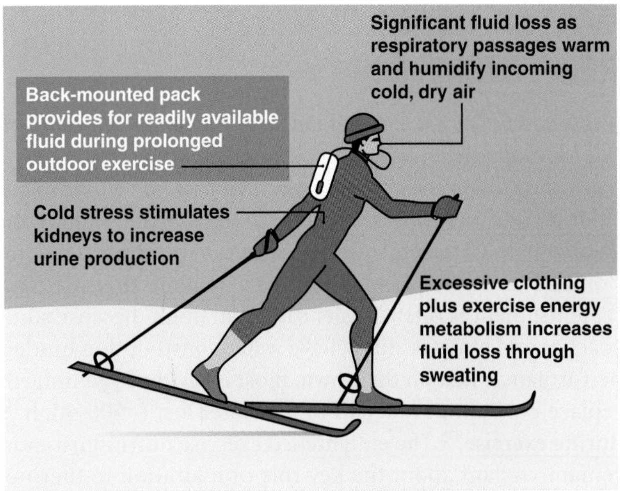

FIGURE 10.7. Factors that increase the potential for dehydration during cold-weather exercise. The illustration depicts a back-mounted hydration system to provide ready access to fluid during continuous exercise in the outdoor environment.

Diuretic Use

Athletes who use diuretics to lose body water to rapidly "make weight" place themselves at a distinct performance disadvantage. This water loss triggers a disproportionate reduction in plasma volume, which negatively impacts thermoregulation and cardiovascular function. Diuretic drugs also markedly impair neuromuscular function not noted when comparable fluid loss occurs by exercise. Athletes who induce vomiting and diarrhea to lose weight not only produce dehydration but also cause excessive mineral loss with accompanying muscle weakness and impaired neuromuscular function. This clearly gives a competitive "edge" to the opponent—a result entirely opposite than anticipated.

DON'T RELY ON ORAL TEMPERATURE

Oral temperature taken following strenuous exercise does not accurately measure deep body or core temperature. Large and consistent differences exist between oral and rectal temperatures; rectal temperature following a 14-mile race in a tropical climate averaged 103.5°F, while oral temperature remained normal at 98°F.[77] Part of this discrepancy lies in the lowering effect on oral temperature of evaporative cooling in the mouth and airways during high levels of exercise and recovery pulmonary ventilation.

WATER REPLACEMENT: REHYDRATION

Adequate fluid replacement sustains the exceptional potential for evaporative cooling of acclimatized humans. Properly scheduling fluid replacement maintains plasma volume so circulation and sweating progress optimally. Strictly following an adequate water replacement schedule prevents dehydration and its consequences, particularly hyperthermia. This replenishment is often "easier said than done" because some coaches and athletes still believe water consumption hinders performance. Left on their own, most individuals voluntarily replace only about one half of the water lost (<500 $mL \cdot h^{-1}$) during exercise.[66] The enlightened exercise nutritionist must remain vigilant about the key role of hydration in thermoregulation and its impact on exercise performance and safety.

THERE ARE RISKS AND THEN THERE ARE SERIOUS RISKS

Glycogen depletion during exercise impairs high-intensity endurance performance, yet failure to replenish this energy reserve does not impose a risk to health and safety. In contrast, inadequate water replenishment not only impairs exercise capacity but also creates life-threatening disturbances in fluid balance and core temperature.

"Cold treatments"—periodic application of cold towels to the forehead and abdomen during exercise, or taking a cold shower before exercising in a hot environment—do not facilitate heat transfer at the body's surface compared with the same exercise without skin wetting. Adequate hydration provides the most effective defense against heat stress by balancing water loss with water intake, not by pouring water over the head or body. Ingesting fluid at 4°C during exercise enhances fluid consumption and improves endurance by attenuating the rise in body temperature and thus reducing the effects of heat stress.[63] No evidence exists that restricting fluid intake during training prepares a person to perform better in the heat. *A well-hydrated individual always functions at a higher physiologic and performance level than a dehydrated one.*

Pre-exercise Hydration

Ingesting "extra" water **(hyperhydration)** before exercising in a hot environment protects to some extent against heat stress because it fosters these three effects:

1. Delays dehydration
2. Increases sweating during exercise
3. Diminishes the rise in core temperature

These outcomes contribute to enhanced exercise performance and overall safety. In addition to increasing fluid intake 24 hours before strenuous exercise in the heat, we recommend consuming 400 to 600 mL (13–20 oz) of cool water about 20 minutes before exercise. Pre-exercise fluid intake increases stomach volume, a major factor to optimize gastric emptying (see Chapter 8). A systematic regimen of hyperhydration by consuming 4.5 L of fluid daily 1 week before soccer competition by acclimated elite young players in Puerto Rico increased body water reserves (despite greater urine output) and improved temperature regulation during a soccer match in warm weather.[74] This structured sequence of pre-exercise

FLUID REPLACEMENT WITH AND WITHOUT THE CALORIES: THE ADDED COST OF REPLACING FLUID WITH SOME PRODUCTS

Beverage	Calories
Diet Pepsi (20 oz)	0
Water or club soda	0
Tea, with 2 sugar packets (8 oz)	20
Coffee, with 1 liquid creamer and 1 sugar packet (8 oz)	30
V-8 or tomato juice (8 oz)	70
Milk, fat-free (8 oz)	80
Beer, light (12 oz)	110
Orange juice (8 oz)	110
Starbucks Coffee Frappuccino Light, tall (12 oz)	110
with whipped cream	210
Gatorade (20 oz)	130
Wine, red (5 oz)	130
Cranberry juice cocktail (8 oz)	140
Grape juice (8 oz)	150
Milk, whole (8 oz)	150
Beer, regular (12 oz)	160
Dunkin' Donuts Coffee Coolatta (16 oz)	170
Gin and tonic, on the rocks (7 oz)	190
Yoplait Strawberry Smoothie (8 oz)	190
Snapple Lemonade (16 oz)	220
Coca-Cola or 7-Up (20 oz)	250
Dannon Strawberry Blend Frusion (10 oz)	260
Starbucks Caffe Latte, venti (prepared with whole milk) (20 oz)	340
Dunkin' Donuts Coffee Coolatta with cream (16 oz)	350
Nestle Nesquik Chocolate Milk (16 oz)	400
7-Eleven Super Big Gulp, Coca-Cola (44 oz)	410
Burger King Vanilla Shake, large (32 oz)	820
McDonald's Chocolate Triple Thick Shake, large (32 oz)	1160

Sources: *Company websites and US Department of Agriculture.*

hyperhydration produced a body fluid volume 1.1 L greater than produced when the players consumed their normal daily fluid volume of 2.5 L. In Chapter 12, we discuss the role of glycerol supplementation to augment pre-exercise hyperhydration.

Pre-exercise hyperhydration does not replace the need to continually replace fluid during exercise. In intense endurance activities in the heat, matching fluid loss with fluid intake often becomes impossible, because only about 1000 mL of fluid each hour empties from the stomach. This volume does not match a sweat loss that averages nearly 2000 mL per hour. Even individuals with ample access to water should be carefully monitored during exercise in the heat.

Adequacy of Rehydration

Body weight changes indicate the extent of water loss from exercise and adequacy of rehydration during and after exercise or athletic competition. Voiding small volumes of dark yellow urine with a strong odor provides a qualitative indication of inadequate hydration. Well-hydrated individuals typically produce urine in large volumes, light in color, and without a strong smell. For team athletes, assign each player a squeeze bottle for fluids to emphasize the importance of fluid replacement and monitor fluid consumed. **TABLE 10.2** recommends fluid intake with weight loss during exercise. Although these standards were developed for a 90-minute football practice, they easily adapt to most exercise situations. Menstrual cycle variations do not adversely affect rehydration.[52]

TABLE 10.2 Recommended Fluid Availability and Intake for a Strenuous 90-Minute Athletic Practice[a]

Weight Loss		Minutes Between Water Breaks	Fluid per Break		Fluid Availability for an 11-Member Squad	
lb	kg		oz	mL	gal	L
8	3.6	No practice	-	-		
7.5	3.4	Recommended	-	-		
7	3.2	10	8–10	266	6.5–8	27.4
6.5	3.0	10	8–9	251	6.5–7	25.5
6	2.7	10	8–9	251	6.5–7	25.5
5.5	2.5	15	10–12	325	5.5–6.5	22.7
5	2.3	15	10–11	311	5.5–6	21.8
4.5	2.1	15	9–10	281	5–5.5	19.9
4	1.8	15	8–9	251	4.5–5	18.0
3.5	1.6	20	10–11	311	4–4.5	16.1
3	1.4	20	9–10	281	3.5–4	14.2
2.5	1.1	20	7–8	222	3	11.4
2	0.9	30	8	237	2.5	9.5
1.5	0.7	30	6	177	1.5	5.7
1	0.5	45	6	177	1	3.8
0.5	0.2	60	6	177	0.5	1.9

[a] *Based on 80% replacement of weight loss.*

Coaches often require athletes to weigh-in before and after practice (following urination) to monitor fluid balance; each 1-lb weight loss represents 450 mL (15 fl oz) of dehydration. **FIGURE 10.8** gives a practical illustration to determine quantity and rate of exercise-induced fluid loss. To properly match fluid loss with intake, partition the estimated hourly fluid loss from a workout or competition into 10- or 15-minute periods and ingest that amount of fluid at those intervals. For example, we recommend fluid intake every 15 minutes for hourly losses up to 1000 mL, whereas fluid ingestion at 10-minute intervals optimizes replenishing fluid loss in excess of 1000 mL per hour. Make water available (and ensure it is consumed) during practice and competition. Urge individuals to rehydrate themselves because the thirst mechanism imprecisely indicates water needs, particularly in children and the elderly. The elderly generally require longer time to achieve rehydration after dehydration.[45] If rehydration were left entirely to a person's thirst, it could take several days after severe dehydration to re-establish fluid balance. *Drink at least 125 to 150% of the existing fluid loss (body weight loss) as quickly as possible after exercising. The 25 to 50% "extra" water accounts for that portion of ingested water lost in urine.*[83,84]

Flavored Drinks Help

Consuming highly palatable flavored beverages with added salt facilitates voluntary rehydration in children and young and older adults.[6,45,50,69] After exercise, dehydration, and

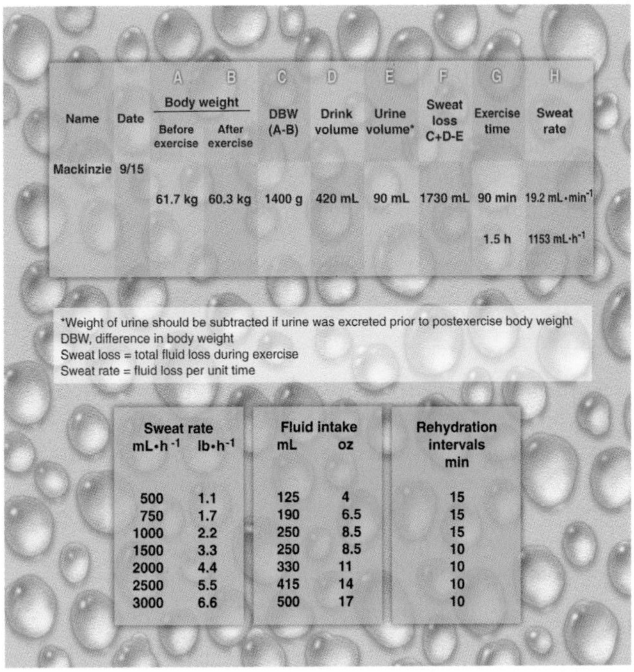

FIGURE 10.8. Computing the magnitude of sweat loss and rate of sweating in exercise. In this example, Mackinzie should drink about 1000 mL (32 oz) of fluid during each hour of activity (250 mL every 15 minutes) to remain well hydrated. (Based on a review of position stand recommendations on exercise and fluid replacement from the American College of Sports Medicine [www.acsm.org; *Med Sci Exerc Sport 1996*;20:i-vii. Review] and Gatorade Sports Science Libray regarding hydration [www.gssiweb.com/Article_Detail.aspx?articleid=667&level=2&topic=1]).

heat exposure, boys voluntarily consumed one of three beverages: (1) plain water, (2) grape-flavored water, or (3) grape-flavored water containing 6% carbohydrate (14 g/8 oz) and 18 mmol·L^{-1} NaCl (110 mg/8 oz).[95] The flavored carbohydrate–electrolyte drink elicited the largest total voluntary fluid intake (1157 mL), followed by the flavored drink (1112 mL), with the smallest volume recorded for plain water (610 mL).

Aging Affects Rehydration

Older men and women require particular attention when evaluating rehydration following exercise in the heat. Both groups do not recover from dehydration as effectively as younger adults, probably because of a depressed thirst drive. This increases susceptibility to chronic hypohydration, which creates a suboptimal plasma volume and diminished thermoregulatory capacity. When palatable fluid is readily available (e.g., carbohydrate–electrolyte solution), older adults drink enough to maintain fluid balance following exercise; the carbohydrate–electrolyte solution promotes greater voluntary fluid intake and restores plasma volume losses faster than water.[6]

Sodium Facilitates Rehydration

In Chapter 8, we pointed out that a moderate amount of sodium added to a rehydration beverage provides more complete rehydration after exercise and thermal-induced dehydration than plain water.[72,79,81] Restoring water and electrolyte balance in recovery occurs most effectively by either adding moderate to high amounts of sodium to the rehydration drink (100 mmol·L^{-1}, an amount exceeding that in commercial beverages) or combining solid food with appropriate sodium content and plain water.[48,50,53] A small amount of potassium (2–5 mmol·L^{-1}) enhances water retention in the intracellular space and may diminish extra potassium loss that results from sodium retention by the kidneys.[26]

ADDING SALT FACILITATES REHYDRATION

Pure water absorbed from the gut rapidly dilutes plasma sodium concentration. A decrease in plasma osmolality, in turn, stimulates urine production and blunts the normal sodium-dependent stimulation of the thirst mechanism. Maintaining a relatively high plasma concentration of sodium (by adding some salt sodium to ingested fluid) achieves three objectives:

1. Sustains the thirst drive
2. Promotes retention of ingested fluids (less urine output)
3. More rapidly restores lost plasma volume during rehydration

The kidneys continually form urine, so the volume of ingested fluid following exercise should exceed exercise sweat loss by 25% to 50% to restore fluid balance. Unless the beverage has a sufficiently high sodium content, excess fluid intake merely increases urine output with *no benefit* to rehydration.[85,86]

FIGURE 10.9 illustrates the effect of adding sodium to a rehydration beverage on retention of ingested fluid during exercise recovery. Six healthy men exercised in a warm, humid environment until sweating produced a 1.9% loss of body mass. They then ingested 2045 mL of one of four test drinks containing sodium in a concentration of either 2, 26, 52, or 100 mmol·L^{-1} over a 30-minute period beginning 30 minutes after exercise stopped. (Typical "sports drinks" contain between 10 and 25 mmol of sodium·L^{-1}; normal plasma sodium concentration ranges between 138 and 142 mmol·L^{-1}.) From the 1.5-hour urine sample onward, urine volume was inversely related to the rehydration beverage's sodium content. At the end of the study period, a difference in total body water content of 787 mL existed between trials using drinks with the lowest and highest sodium content. The drink containing sodium at a concentration of 100 mmol·L^{-1} contributed to the greatest fluid retention.

With prolonged exercise in the heat, sweat loss depletes the body of 13 to 17 g of salt (2.3–3.4 g·L^{-1} of sweat), about 8 g more than typically consumed daily in the diet. It seems prudent, therefore, to replace lost sodium by adding about one-third teaspoon of table salt to 1 L of water.

The American College of Sports Medicine (ACSM) recommends that sports drinks contain 0.5 to 0.7 g of sodium per liter of fluid consumed during exercise lasting more than 1 hour.[2] Moderate exercise produces negligible losses of potassium in sweat. Even at intense physical activity levels, potassium lost in sweat ranges between 5 and 18 mEq, which poses no immediate danger. One can replace potassium lost with heavy sweating by increasing intake of potassium-rich foods (citrus fruits and bananas). A glass of orange juice or tomato

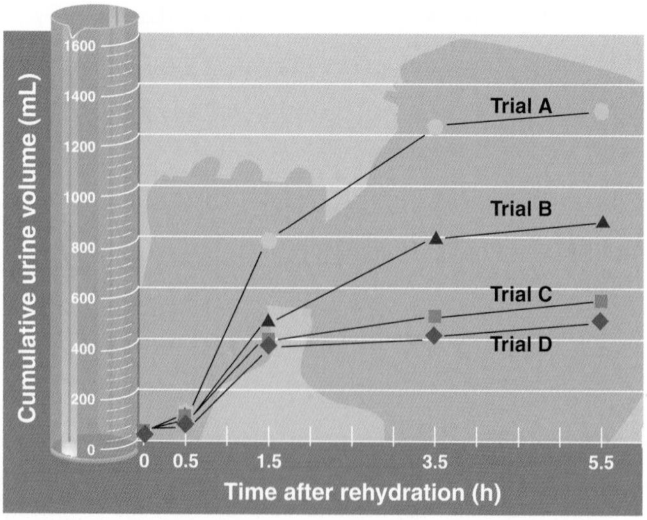

FIGURE 10.9. Cumulative urine output during recovery from exercise-induced dehydration. The oral rehydration beverages consisted of four test drinks (equivalent to 1.5 times the body weight loss, or approximately 2045 mL) containing sodium (and matching anion) in a concentration of either 2 (trial A), 26 (trial B), 52 (trial C), or 100 (trial D) mmol · L^{-1}. (From Maughan J, Leiper JB. Sodium intake and post-exercise rehydration in man. *Eur J Appl Physiol* 1995;71:311.)

TABLE 10.3 How the Drinks Stack Up: Five Major Sports Drink Categories Including Their Calorie and Carbohydrate Content plus Nutritional "Extras" per 8-oz Serving

	Calories	Carbohydrate (g)	Extras
Waters			
Tap water	0	0	Minerals—vary by source
Dasani	0	0	Spring source
Fiji	0	0	Artesian source
Penta	0	0	Purified
Fitness waters			
ChampionLyte	0	0	Electrolytes
Life O_2	0	0	10 times O_2 of tap water
Propel	10	3	Electrolytes, vitamins
Reebok	12	3	Electrolytes, vitamins, trace minerals
Sports drinks			
All Sport	70	20	No longer carbonated, vitamins B and C
G-Push (G^2)	70	18	Electrolytes, vitamins
Gatorade	50	14	Electrolytes
GU_2O	50	14	Electrolytes
Powerade	72	19	Electrolytes, vitamins
Simple sports drink	80	21	Electrolytes, vitamin C
Recovery drinks			
Endurox R^4	180	35	Electrolytes, vitamins
G-Push (G^4)	110	27	Electrolytes, vitamins, trace minerals
Gatorade energy drink	207	41	Vitamins
Energy drinks			
Red Bull	109	27	Taurine, caffeine, vitamins
SoBe adrenaline rush	135	35	Taurine, ribose, caffeine

juice replaces almost all the potassium, calcium, and magnesium excreted in 3 L of sweat. Except in unusual cases, minor adjustments in food intake and electrolyte conservation by the kidneys compensate adequately for mineral loss through sweating. **TABLE 10.3** gives examples of drinks from five major sports-beverage categories, along with their carbohydrate and calorie content per 8-oz serving. The high-carbohydrate content of beverages in the recovery drink and energy drink categories most effectively facilitates glycogen replenishment.

HYPONATREMIA: REDUCED SODIUM CONCENTRATION IN BODY FLUIDS

Four major factors are of concern in hot-weather exercise:

1. Dehydration
2. Decreased plasma volume and resulting hemoconcentration
3. Impaired physical performance and thermoregulatory capacity
4. Increased risk of heat injury (especially heat stroke)

> *The exercise physiology literature contains more than ample information about the need to consume fluid before, during, and after exercise.*

The most recommended beverage remains plain, hypotonic water. However, we now know that excessive water intake under certain exercise conditions can produce potentially serious medical complications from the syndrome termed **hyponatremia** or "water intoxication." Hyponatremia exists when serum sodium concentration falls below 135 $mEq \cdot L^{-1}$; a serum sodium concentration below 125 $mEq \cdot L^{-1}$ triggers severe symptoms. A sustained low plasma sodium concentration creates an osmotic imbalance across the blood–brain barrier that causes rapid water influx into the brain. The resulting swelling of brain tissue produces a cascade of symptoms that range from mild (headache, confusion, malaise, nausea, and cramping) to severe (seizures, coma, pulmonary edema, cardiac arrest, and death).[4,33,34,39]

SOME IMPORTANT INFLUENCING FACTORS

Data obtained from the finishers of the 2002 Boston Marathon indicate that 13% had hyponatremia.[1] The most prevalent factors associated with this disorder, which occurs in many nonelite marathoners, include:

1. Substantial pre-post race weight gain
2. Consumption of more than 3 L of fluid during race
3. Race time greater than 4 hours
4. Low body mass index

Hyponatremia More Prevalent Than Previously Thought

The exercise scenario conducive to the development of hyponatremia involves water overload during continuous high-intensity, ultramarathon-type exercise of 6 to 8 hours in duration, particularly in hot weather.[5,37,38,59,60,67,89] It can also occur in events lasting less than 4 hours such as standard marathons.[90] In a large study of more than 18,000 ultraendurance runners including triathletes, approximately 9% of collapsed individuals presented with symptoms of hyponatremia.[68] The athletes, on average, drank fluids with low a sodium chloride content less than 6.8 mmol·L^{-1}. The runner with the most severe hyponatremia with a serum sodium level of 112 mmol·L^{-1} excreted more than 7.5 L of dilute urine during the first 17 hours of hospitalization.

Researchers monitored changes in body mass and blood sodium concentration in 95 competitors receiving medical care and 169 competitors not requiring care in the 1996 New Zealand Ironman Triathlon (swim 3.8 km, cycle 180 km, run 42 km).[90] For individuals with clinical evidence of fluid or electrolyte disturbance, body mass declined 2.5 kg (–2.9 kg in competitors without medical care). Hyponatremia accounted for 9% of medical abnormalities (identical to that reported earlier).[68] One person with hyponatremia (Na = 130 mEq·L^{-1}) drank 16 L of fluid over the course of the race, with a weight gain of 2.5 kg (consistent with the hypothesis that fluid overload causes hyponatremia). An inverse relationship existed between postrace sodium concentration and percentage change in body mass; individuals who lost less weight tended to have a higher serum sodium concentration.

Level of acclimatization affects sodium loss. For example, sodium concentration in sweat ranges from 5 to 30 mmol·L^{-1} (115–690 mg·L^{-1}) in individuals fully acclimatized to the heat to 40 to 100 mmol·L^{-1} (920–2300 mg·L^{-1}) in unacclimatized individuals. In addition, some individuals produce relatively highly concentrated sweat regardless of their degree of acclimatization. *Development of hyponatremia requires extreme sodium loss through prolonged sweating coupled with dilution of existing extracellular sodium (and accompanying reduced osmolality) from consuming large fluid volumes containing low or no sodium* (**FIG. 10.10A**). A reduced extracellular solute concentration promotes movement of water into the cells (**FIG. 10.10B**). Water movement of sufficient magnitude congests the lungs, swells brain tissue, and adversely affects central nervous system function. Hyponatremia has not been reported from participation in a marathon under only mild environmental stress and where aggressive hydration practices were not promoted.[73]

Several hours of exercise in the heat can cause considerable sodium loss. Exercise in hot, humid weather produces a sweat rate of more than 1 L an hour, with a sweat sodium concentration ranging between 20 and 100 mEq·L^{-1}. Also, frequently ingesting large volumes of plain water draws sodium from the extracellular fluid compartment into the unabsorbed intestinal water, further diluting serum sodium concentration. Exercise compounds the problem because urine production decreases during exercise due to a significantly reduced renal blood flow. This reduces the body's ability to excrete excess water.

Competitive athletes, recreational participants, and occupational workers should be aware of the dangers of excessive hydration, and should ensure that fluid intake does not exceed fluid loss. We recommend the following five steps to reduce risk of overhydration and hyponatremia in prolonged exercise:

Step 1. Two to three hours before exercise, drink 400 to 600 mL (14–22 oz) of fluid.

PREDISPOSING FACTORS TO EXERCISE-ASSOCIATED HYPONATREMIA

The first reported cases of hyponatremia in Asia occurred in 2011. Three of the eight symptomatic runners admitted to the medical tent were diagnosed with hyponatremia, with blood sodium concentrations of 134 mmol·L^{-1} in a 42-km runner and 131 and 117 mmol·L^{-1} in two 84-km runners.*

Five predisposing factors include

1. Prolonged intense exercise in hot weather
2. Large sodium loss associated with sweat containing high sodium concentration; particularly prevalent in relatively unfit individuals
3. Beginning physical activity in a sodium-depleted state due to "salt-free" or "low-sodium" diet
4. Use of diuretic medication for hypertension
5. Frequent intake of large quantities of sodium-free fluid before, during, and after prolonged exercise

Source: Lee JK, et al. First reported cases of exercise-associated hyponatremia in Asia. *Int J Sports Med* 2011;32:297.

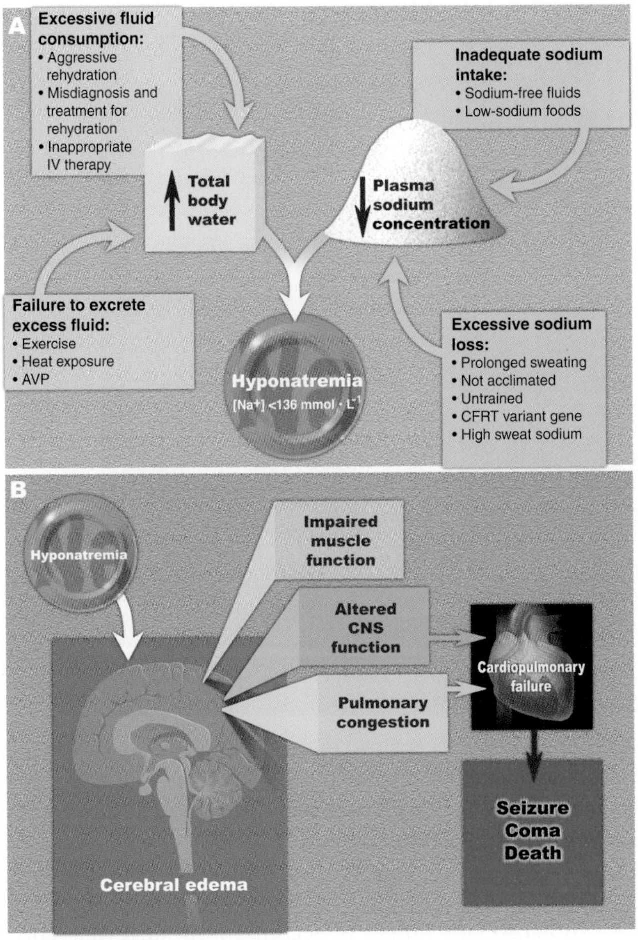

FIGURE 10.10. **A.** Factors that contribute to the development of hyponatremia. *AVP*, arginine vasopressin; *CFTR*, cystic fibrosis transmembrane regulatory gene. **B.** Physiologic consequences of hyponatremia. *CNS*, central nervous system. (Modified from Montain SJ, et al. Hyponatremia associated with exercise: risk factors and pathogenesis. *Exerc Sport Sci Rev* 2001;29:113.)

Step 2. Drink 150 to 300 mL (5–10 oz) of fluid about 30 minutes before exercise.

Step 3. Drink no more than 1000 mL·h^{-1} (32 oz) of plain water spread over 15-minute intervals during or after exercise.

Step 4. Add a small amount of sodium (approximately 1/4 to 1/2 tsp of salt per 32 oz) to ingested fluid. Commercial sports drinks are also effective in providing water, carbohydrate fuel, and electrolytes.

Step 5. Do not restrict dietary salt.

Including some glucose in the rehydration drink facilitates intestinal water uptake via the glucose–sodium transport mechanism (see Chapters 3 and 8). In addition, maintaining a high-carbohydrate status via the rehydration beverage may provide some protection against exercise-associated hyponatremia.[39]

FACTORS THAT IMPROVE HEAT TOLERANCE

Moderate exercise performed in cool weather becomes taxing if attempted on the first hot day of spring. The early stages of spring training can present a hazard for heat injury because thermoregulatory mechanisms have not yet adjusted to the dual challenge of exercise with environmental heat. *Repeated exposure to hot environments, particularly when combined with physical activity, improves capacity for exercise with less discomfort upon heat exposure.*

Acclimatization

Heat acclimatization refers to the physiologic adaptations that improve heat tolerance. **FIGURE 10.11** shows that major acclimatization to heat stress occurs during the first week of heat exposure (2–4 h daily) with essentially complete acclimatization after 10 days. In practical terms, use 15 to 20 minutes of light-intensity exercise during the first several exercise sessions in a hot environment. Thereafter, exercise sessions can increase systematically to reach the normal duration and intensity for training.

Increased Production of a More Dilute Sweat

TABLE 10.4 summarizes eight physiologic adjustments during heat acclimatization. As acclimatization progresses, larger quantities of blood shunt to cutaneous vessels to facilitate heat transfer from the core to the periphery during exercise. More effective cardiac output distribution maintains blood pressure during exercise; a lowered threshold (earlier onset) for sweating complements this cardiovascular acclimatization. An earlier onset of sweating initiates cooling before internal temperature increases too markedly. After 10 days of heat exposure, sweating capacity nearly doubles and sweat becomes dilute (less salt lost) and more evenly distributed on the skin surface. Increased sweat loss in an acclimatized individual creates a greater need to rehydrate during and following exercise. Adjustments in circulatory function and evaporative cooling enable a heat-acclimatized person to exercise with lower skin and core temperatures and heart rate than an unacclimatized individual. Optimal acclimatization necessitates adequate hydration. Also, one loses the major benefits of heat acclimatization within 2 to 3 weeks upon return to a more temperate climate.

Full Acclimatization Requires Hot-Weather Training

As one might expect, exercise "heat conditioning" in cool weather produces less effective results than acclimatization from similar exercise training in the heat. *Full heat acclimatization cannot take place without exposure to environmental heat stress.* Individuals who train and compete in hot weather show a distinct thermoregulatory advantage over those who train in cooler climates and only periodically compete in hot weather.[40]

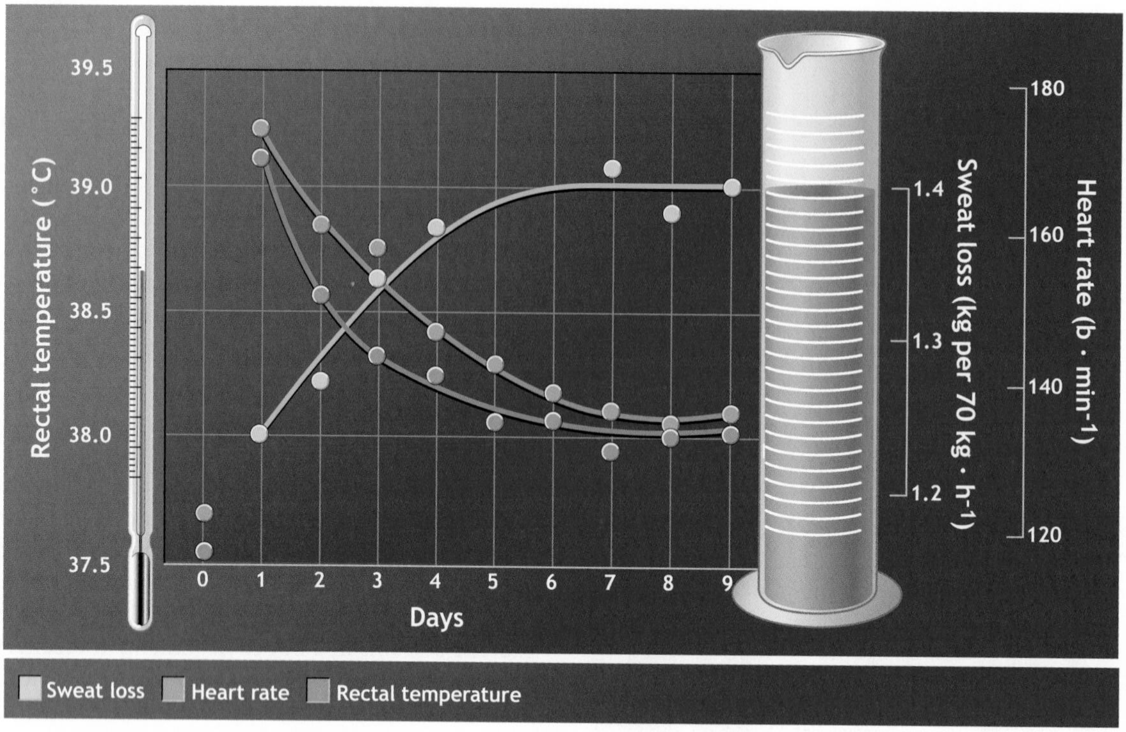

FIGURE 10.11. Average rectal temperature (blue), heart rate (orange), and sweat loss (yellow) during 100 minutes of daily heat-exercise exposure for 9 consecutive days. On day 0, the men walked on a treadmill at an exercise intensity of 300 kcal·h^{-1} in a cool climate. Thereafter, the same daily exercise took place in the heat at 48.9°C (26.7°F wet bulb). (From Lind R, Bass DE. Optimal exposure time for development of acclimatization to heat. *Fed Proc* 1963;22:704.)

Children

Prepubescent children have a greater number of heat-activated sweat glands per unit skin area than adolescents and adults, yet they sweat less and achieve higher core temperatures during heat stress.[7] These thermoregulatory differences probably last through puberty but only limit exercise capacity during extreme environmental heat stress.[30] Sweat composition differs between children and adults; adults have higher concentrations of sodium and chloride, but lower lactate, H^+, and potassium concentrations.[31,56]

Children also take longer to acclimatize to heat than adolescents and young adults. *From a practical standpoint, children exposed to environmental heat stress should exercise at reduced intensity and receive more time to acclimatize than more mature competitors.*

Male/Female Differences

Early comparisons between men and women showed that men had greater tolerance to environmental heat stress during exercise. Unfortunately, the research was flawed because women consistently exercised at higher intensities relative to

TABLE 10.4 Physiologic Adjustments During Heat Acclimatization

Acclimatization Response	Effect
Improved cutaneous blood flow	Transports metabolic heat from deep tissues to the body's shell
Effective distribution of cardiac output	Appropriate circulation to skin and muscles to meet demands of metabolism and thermoregulation; greater stability of blood pressure during exercise
Lowered threshold for start of sweating	Evaporative cooling begins early during exercise
More effective distribution of sweat over skin surface	Optimum use of effective surface for evaporative cooling
Increased sweat output	Maximizes evaporative cooling
Lowered salt concentration in sweat	Dilute sweat preserves electrolytes in extracellular fluid
Lower skin and core temperature and heart rate for standard exercise	Frees greater portion of cardiac output for distribution to active muscles
Less reliance on carbohydrate catabolism during exercise	Carbohydrate-sparing effect

AN AGE-RELATED DIFFERENCE

Age-related factors affect thermoregulatory dynamics despite equivalence between young and older adults in capacity to regulate core temperature during heat stress. Aging delays the onset of sweating and blunts the magnitude of the sweating response in possibly three ways: (1) modified sensitivity of thermoreceptors, (2) limited sweat gland output per se, and (3) dehydration-limited sweat output with insufficient fluid replacement. Aging also alters the intrinsic structure and function of the skin itself and its vasculature. Vascular changes include depressed peripheral vascular sensitivity that impairs local cutaneous vasodilation from two factors: (1) smaller release of vasomotor tone and (2) less active vasodilation once sweating begins.[46] Older adults recover less well from dehydration compared to younger counterparts because of reduced thirst drive. This places elderly individuals in a chronic state of hypohydration (with less than optimal plasma volume), which could impair thermoregulatory dynamics.[27,28]

their aerobic capacity. When comparing men and women of equal fitness, the sex differences in thermoregulation became much less pronounced.[35] *Generally, women tolerate the physiologic and thermal stress of exercise as well as men of comparable fitness and level of acclimatization; both sexes acclimatize to a similar degree.*[2,75,91]

Sweating

A distinct sex difference in thermoregulation exists for sweating. Women possess more heat-activated sweat glands per unit skin area than men, yet they sweat *less* prolifically. Women begin sweating at higher skin and core temperatures; they also produce less sweat for a similar heat-exercise load, even with acclimatization comparable to that of men.

Evaporative Versus Circulatory Cooling

Despite a lower sweat output, women show heat tolerance similar to men of equal aerobic fitness when they perform at the same exercise level. *Women rely more on circulatory mechanisms for heat dissipation, whereas greater evaporative cooling occurs in men.* Clearly, less sweat production to maintain thermal balance protects women from dehydration during exercise at high ambient temperatures.

Ratio of Body Surface Area to Body Mass

Women possess a relatively large body surface area-to-body mass ratio, a favorable dimensional characteristic for heat dissipation. Stated differently, the smaller woman has a larger external surface per unit of body mass exposed to the environment. Consequently, under identical conditions of heat exposure, women cool at a faster rate than men through a smaller body mass across a relatively large surface area. In this regard, children also possess a "geometric" advantage during heat stress, because boys and girls have larger surface areas per unit body mass than adults.

Level of Body Fat

Excess body fat negatively affects exercise performance in hot environments. Because body fat's specific heat exceeds that of muscle tissue, fat increases the insulatory quality of the shell to retard heat conduction to the periphery. The relatively large, overfat person also possesses a relatively small body surface area-to-body mass ratio for sweat evaporation compared to a leaner, smaller person.

Excess body fat directly adds to the metabolic cost of weight-bearing activities in addition to retarding effective heat exchange. The additional demands of equipment weight (such as football gear), intense competition, and a hot, humid environment compound these effects. Thus, an overfat person experiences considerable difficulty in temperature regulation and exercise performance.[32] Fatal heat stroke occurs 3.5 times more frequently in obese young adults than in individuals whose body mass falls within reasonable limits.

EFFECTS OF CLOTHING ON THERMOREGULATION IN THE HEAT

Different materials absorb water at different rates. Cottons and linens readily absorb moisture. In contrast, heavy "sweatshirts" and rubber or plastic garments produce high relative humidity close to the skin and retard the vaporization of moisture. This inhibits or even prevents evaporative cooling. Color also plays an important role; dark colors absorb light rays and add to radiant heat gain, whereas clothing of lighter color reflects heat rays away from the body.

SOME FABRICS ARE BETTER THAN OTHERS

Moisture-wicking fabrics (e.g., polypropylene, Coolmax, Drylite, *DRI-FIT*) that adhere close to the skin's surface provide optimal heat transfer and moisture from skin to the environment, particularly during high-intensity exercise in hot weather. These fabrics wick moisture *away* from the skin. They also offer benefits during exercise in cold environments because dry clothing, in contrast to sweat-drenched clothing, greatly reduces the risk for hypothermia.

Football Uniforms

Football uniforms and equipment present a considerable barrier to heat dissipation during environmental heat

Additional Insights

Beware of the American Football Uniform—Unintended Consequences

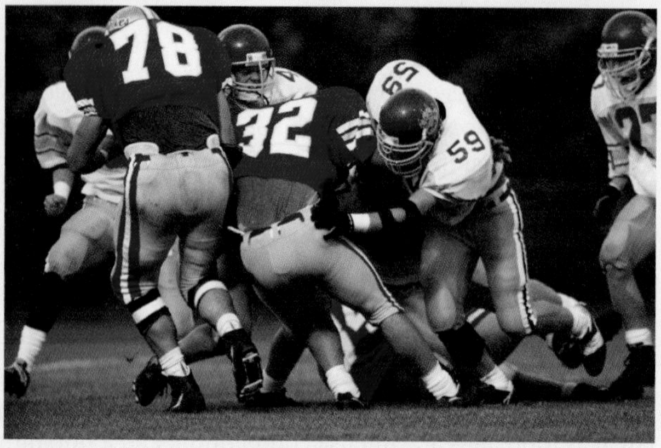

American football teams at all levels of competition often schedule practices and games that coincide with extremes in temperature, particularly the early summer months where outdoor temperatures often exceed 100°F (37.7°C). Thus, wearing the American football uniform can predispose athletes to exertional heat exhaustion or even severe exercise-induced hyperthermia at the threshold for heat stroke where rectal temperature exceeds 39°C. Kinesiology researchers have conducted randomized controlled experiments to assess how two American football uniform configurations impact exercise tolerance, including thermal, cardiovascular, hematologic, and perceptual responses in a hot, humid environment. The ultimate aim of the research was to evaluate how the physiologic and psychological responses can better monitor athlete safety.

Ten men with more than 3 years of competitive experience as football linemen (age = 23.8 years, height = 183.9 cm, body mass = 117.4 kg, percentage body fat = 30.1%) completed three controlled exercise protocols consisting of repetitive box lifting (lifting, carrying, and depositing a 20.4-kg box at a rate of 10 lifts per minute for 10 minutes), seated recovery (10 minutes), and up to 60 minutes of treadmill walking. The experiments were conducted in hot, humid environmental conditions. All men were tested wearing each of the following clothing configurations: (1) a partial uniform (PART) that included the National Football League (NFL) uniform without a helmet and shoulder pads; (2) a full uniform (FULL) that included the full NFL uniform; or (3) control clothing (CON) comprised socks, sneakers, and shorts. Exercise, meals, and hydration status were controlled. The researchers assessed sweat rate, rectal temperature, heart rate, blood pressure, treadmill exercise time, skin temperature, rating of perceived exertion, thermal perception, perception of thirst, perception of muscle pain for specific time points matched across trials, plasma volume, plasma lactate, plasma glucose, plasma osmolality, body mass, and fat mass.

During 19 of 30 experiments, participants halted exercise as a result of volitional exhaustion. Mean sweat rate, rectal temperature, heart rate, and treadmill exercise time during the CON condition differed from those measures during the PART and FULL conditions; no significant differences occurred for perceptual measurements, plasma volume, plasma lactate, plasma glucose, or plasma osmolality. Exhaustion occurred during the FULL and PART conditions at the same rectal temperature of 39.2°C. Systolic and diastolic blood pressures indicated that hypotension developed throughout exercise in all treatments. Compared with the PART condition, the FULL condition resulted in a faster rate of rectal temperature increase, decreased treadmill exercise time, and fewer completed exercise bouts. Interestingly, the increase in rectal temperature correlated highly with lean body mass during the FULL condition, and treadmill exercise positively related with total fat mass during the CON and PART conditions. No differences were found for the different perceptual scales between PART and FULL conditions.

The authors concluded the following:

1. The addition of a uniform with or without pads increased the rate of rectal temperature rise, skin temperature, and rating of perceived exertion at a given workload and decreased the amount of exercise an individual could safely perform.
2. Exercise time declined in the partial and full uniform conditions compared with the control condition, but perceptual ratings did not reflect increased thermal strain, with few perceptual differences between the control condition and partial or full uniform conditions.
3. Exercise in a full or partial uniform produced greater physiologic strain than without the uniform. These findings indicated that critical internal temperature and hypotension were concurrent with exhaustion during uncompensable (FULL) or nearly uncompensable (PART) heat stress.
4. Anthropomorphic characteristics influenced heat storage and exercise time to exhaustion.

The bottom line is that the uniform, padding, and protective armor worn by the American football player thwarts the dissipation of body heat generated during exercise to a greater extent than the clothing ensemble worn by the typical recreational exerciser. This pertains particularly to individuals of large body size. The implications for football participants are clear. The protective equipment that seals approximately 50% of the skin surface from the free flow of air in a hot, humid environment reduces heat dissipation (with a resulting increase in physiologic strain) regardless of whether the uniform is full or partial. Coaches and athletes must remain vigilant during football games and practices played in hot and humid environments to protect athletes from uncompromising physiologic and perceptual issues related to excessive heat stress.

Sources:

Armstrong LE, et al. The American football uniform: uncompensable heat stress and hyperthermic exhaustion. *J Athl Train* 2010;45:117.

Johnson EC, et al. Perceptual responses while wearing an American football uniform in the heat. *J Athl Train* 2010;45:107.

Related References

Hitchcock KM, et al. Metabolic and thermoregulatory responses to a simulated American football practice in the heat. *J Strength Cond Res* 2007;21:710.

Mora-Rodriguez R, et al. Thermoregulatory responses to constant versus variable-intensity exercise in the heat. *Med Sci Sports Exerc* 2008;40:1945.

exposure.[55] Even with loose-fitting porous jerseys, wrappings, padding (with plastic covering), helmet, and other objects of "armor" effectively seal off 50% of the body's surface from the benefits of evaporative cooling. Just wearing the 6 to 7 kg of football equipment increases metabolic load, not to mention the thermal challenge from a hot artificial playing surface and the body heat–retaining qualities of the equipment. The large body size of these athletes further magnifies heat load, particularly for offensive and defensive linemen who possess a relatively small body surface area-to-body mass ratio and a higher percentage of body fat than other players.

The Modern Cycling Helmet Does Not Thwart Heat Dissipation

Wearing a commercial cycling helmet provides considerable protection against possible head injury, but does the helmet impede thermoregulatory processes in a hot–dry or hot–humid environment? The head provides an important avenue for heat loss during exercise,[71] and many competitive cyclists believe that not wearing a helmet reduces thermal strain and physical discomfort. This belief persists even though the design of current commercial helmets remains aerodynamic and lightweight, with ventilation ports for convective and evaporative cooling. To evaluate the physiologic and perceptual responses to wearing a helmet, male and female competitive cyclists pedaled for 90 minutes at 60% peak oxygen uptake in both hot–dry (35°C, 20% relative humidity) and hot–humid (35°C, 70% relative humidity) environments with and without a protective helmet.[80] Measurements included oxygen uptake; heart rate; core, skin, and head skin temperatures; rating of perceived exertion; and perceived thermal sensations of the head and body. Results showed that exercising in a hot–humid environment produced significantly greater thermal stress, yet wearing the helmet during exercise did *not* increase the riders' level of heat strain or perceived heat sensation of the head or body.

NUTRITION IN HOT ENVIRONMENTS

Much of what researchers know about the effects of hot environments on human exercise performance and related nutritional concerns stems from research performed on military personnel from the 1930s to 1960s.[14,15,20,21,23,65]

Food Intake During Heat Exposure

Careful studies between 1941 and 1946 regarding food intake from rations provided for physically fit, active ground troops stationed in hot, humid climates (mean daily temperature from 73 to 85°F, with afternoon temperatures often ≥90°F) compared to troops stationed in a cool environment (mean daily temperature of 65°F with afternoon temperatures ≤72°F) suggest an inverse relationship between caloric intake and mean environmental temperature (**TABLE 10.5**). The researchers repor ted a consistent reduction in voluntary caloric intake per °F over the range

TABLE 10.5 Environmental Temperature and Calculated Average Nutrient Intake: US Troops in Pacific (Hawaii, Guadalcanal, Guam, Iwo Jima, Luzon: Hot Environment) Compared to Troops in North America (United States: Cool Environment)

Variable	Hawaii	Guadalcanal	Guam	Iwo Jima	Luzon	United States
Mean Temp (°F)	+73	+85	+81	+78	+83	+65
$kcal \cdot day^{-1}$	3400	3400	3500	3500	3200	3900
Carbohydrate (g)	460	450	480	470	430	520
Fat (g)	124	129	123	129	120	147
Protein total (g)	110	110	115	115	100	125

From: Institute of Medicine. Nutritional Needs in Hot Environments: Applications for Military Personnel in Field Operations. Washington, DC: National Academies Press, 1993.

of 20 to 100°F. The reduction in energy intake could not be explained by differences in basal metabolic rate (a difference of 10–20% at most), body weight, or mode of physical activity.[22]

Total protein consumed remained essentially the same in each environment, even though percentage fat and carbohydrate intake in the warm environment was less than in the cooler environment. The small differences suggested that individuals probably eat about the same regardless of environment, but with fewer calories consumed in the heat. This calorie reduction can probably be explained by two factors. First, reduced energy expenditure (and hence reduced energy intake) occurred because ofthe heat's blunting effect on physical activity level. Second, the reduced food consumption caused a corresponding reduction in the thermic effect of food (see Chapter 6) and hence reduced heat load and appetite.[8,10]

Effects of Heat and Exercise on Mineral Requirements

A significant number of athletes, coaches, and professionals believe in the positive effects of mineral supplements, yet remarkably few data exist to support a positive effect of mineral supplementation above recommended levels on exercise performance.

Prolonged strenuous exercise in the heat changes chromium, copper, iron, magnesium, and zinc metabolism, which often persists for several days into recovery.[43,44] However, the extent that these changes alter exercise performance remains untested. Some changes in plasma mineral concentrations may be attributed to an acute phase that occurs with exercise-induced tissue stress or actual tissue trauma. Also, reductions in plasma mineral concentrations may reflect increased mineral excretion in urine and sweat-induced exposure to hot temperatures.

Research must confirm if there is compromised endurance capacity, immune-antioxidant defense, or recovery from muscle injury from any changes in mineral concentrations from exercising in the heat. Also, little is known about whether dietary manipulations can attenuate any negative consequences of mineral changes from warm-weather exercise. Chapter 7, sections entitled Mineral Losses in Sweat and Trace Minerals and Exercise, provides additional discussion about this topic.

Effects of Heat and Exercise on Vitamin Requirements

Early research suggested that exercise produced significant vitamin loss in sweat during exercise. This has led some to conclude that exercise in hot environments exaggerates vitamin deficiencies and hence increases vitamin requirements. However, current consensus maintains the negligible effect of vitamin loss in sweat in the heat.[11,57,58,76]

Research is revealing whether extreme exercise in a hot environment increases requirements for certain vitamins and/or whether vitamin supplements reduce heat stress.[19,36,58] For example, the requirement for B vitamins may increase when living and working in hot environments. There is minimal loss of these vitamins in sweat, so a deficiency could occur over time from profuse sweating coupled with insufficient dietary intake. Thus, if calorie intake remains inadequate to match the energy demands of exercise in the heat, then vitamin intake could be compromised. We are unaware of any research that indicates that exposure to a hot environment with or without exercise increases the need for folic acid and vitamin B_{12} above recommended levels.

Since World War I, vitamin C has received popular attention as a nutrient to reduce the effects of heat stress. Increased vitamin C intake of 250 mg above recommended daily levels may reduce heat stress during acclimatization in individuals with adequate but low vitamin C levels.[36] Some data also have shown that long-term exposure to a hot environment may compromise vitamin C status. Thus, vitamin C supplements may support individuals who live and work in a hot environment. High-dose intakes are not recommended because excessive vitamin C adversely affects vitamin B_{12} absorption.

No compelling reason exists to recommend vitamin D supplements for people who work in the heat. Exposure to sunlight probably provides sufficient stimulus for adequate vitamin D status.[19] The antioxidant vitamins A, C, and E may reduce exercise-induced lipid peroxidation.

Gastric Emptying, Gastrointestinal Stress, and Environmental Heat Exposure

Gastric emptying rate probably decreases during heat stress. The mechanisms for this effect remain unclear, although they may associate with overall dehydration. A dehydrated state frequently occurs when individuals work in the heat, including reduced splanchnic blood flow during exercise. Elevations in core body temperature reduce stomach and intestinal motility.[41]

HEAT ILLNESS: COMPLICATIONS FROM EXCESSIVE HEAT STRESS

From the perspective of health and safety, it is far easier to prevent heat injury than remedy it. However, if one fails to heed the normal signs of heat stress—thirst, tiredness, grogginess, and visual disturbances—cardiovascular decompensation triggers a series of disabling complications termed **heat illness**. Heat-related disabilities become more apparent among overweight and poorly conditioned individuals, those with prior heat intolerance, and those who exercise when dehydrated.[3,27,32,70,88] Heat illness, in order of increasing severity, includes heat cramps, heat exhaustion, and exertional heat stroke. No clear-cut demarcation exists between these maladies because symptoms usually overlap: The cumulative effects of multiple adverse interacting stimuli can produce exercise-induced heat injury.[87] When serious heat illness occurs, only immediate corrective action using rehydration can reduce heat stress until medical help arrives.[28]

Heat Cramps

Heat cramps (involuntary muscle spasms) occur during or after intense physical activity, usually in the specific muscles exercised. Cramping most likely occurs from an imbalance in both hydration level and electrolyte concentrations. During heat exposure, sweating augments salt loss. Without electrolyte replenishment, the chances increase for muscle pain and spasm (most commonly in the muscles of the abdomen and extremities). Crampers tend to have high sweat rates and/or high sweat sodium concentrations. With heat cramps, body temperature does not necessarily increase. Prevention involves two factors: (1) providing copious amounts of water that contains salt (e.g., Gatorade or GatorLytes), and (2) increasing daily salt intake (e.g., adding a "pinch" of salt to foods at mealtime) several days before heat stress.

Heat Exhaustion

***Heat exhaustion,** the most common heat illness among the physically active, usually develops in dehydrated, untrained, and unacclimatized people; it mainly occurs during the first summer heat wave or first hard training session on a hot day.* Exercise-induced heat exhaustion occurs because of ineffective circulatory adjustments compounded by depletion of extracellular fluid (plasma volume) from excessive sweating. Blood pools in the dilated peripheral vessels. This drastically reduces the central blood volume required to maintain cardiac output. Characteristics of heat exhaustion include weak, rapid pulse; low blood pressure in the upright position; headache; nausea; dizziness; "goose bumps"; and general weakness. Sweating may decrease somewhat, but body temperature does not rise to dangerous levels (i.e., above 104°F or 40°C). A person experiencing heat exhaustion symptoms should stop exercising and move to a cooler environment; fluids should be administered orally or via intravenous therapy with 5% dextrose sugar in either 0.45% NaCl or 0.9% NaCl.[2]

Exertional Heat Stroke

***Exertional heat stroke,** the most serious and complex heat stress malady, requires immediate medical attention.* Heat stroke syndrome reflects a failure of the heat-regulating mechanisms induced by excessively high body temperature. With thermoregulatory failure, sweating usually ceases, the skin becomes dry and hot, body temperature rises to 41.5°C or higher, and the circulatory system becomes excessively strained.

Subtle symptoms often confound the complexity of exertional hyperthermia. Sweating can occur during intense exercise (e.g., 10-km running race) in young, hydrated, and highly motivated individuals. In this case, the body's heat gain greatly exceeds avenues for heat loss because of the high metabolic heat production. If left untreated, the disability becomes fatal from circulatory collapse, oxidative damage, systemic inflammatory response, and damage to the central nervous system and other organs.[16,78,96]

> ***Heat stroke represents a medical emergency!*** *While awaiting medical care, only aggressive treatment to rapidly lower elevated core temperature can avert death; the magnitude and duration of hyperthermia determine organ damage and mortality risk.*

Immediate treatment includes alcohol rubs and ice packs. Whole-body cold or ice water immersion remains the most effective treatment for a collapsed hyperthermic individual.[62,64,70] Individuals most susceptible to heat stroke include larger individuals, especially those who are unfit, poorly acclimatized to the heat, and excessively fat. This potentially fatal heat disorder also affects physically fit young individuals.[78,94]

PERSONAL HEALTH AND EXERCISE NUTRITION 10.1

Think Before You Drink

As part of a course on exercise, nutrition, and weight control, Leslie recorded all the food and beverages she consumed for 5 days. At the end of the 5 days, she analyzed her diet and was surprised to learn that more than 25% of her total caloric intake was from various beverages. This was troubling and might be an explanation for her recent weight gain—she had gained about 10 pound toward the end of her freshman year.

Leslie went to her nutrition instructor to ask for advice. During their discussion, Leslie was surprised to find that she was not alone. Beverage and snack overconsumption is a big problem for many college students. Leslie's professor pointed out the following facts regarding beverage (including snack) consumption among college-age individuals:

- ✓ The portion sizes of actual meals consumed have increased over the last 5 years.
- ✓ There is an increasing trend toward greater consumption of calorically sweetened beverages (in 2006, 23% of total kcal intake came from beverages; in 2010, the estimated kcal intake from sugar beverages was >25% of total kcal).

✓ Snacks are consistently more energy dense and less nutrient dense (calcium, fiber, folate) than meals.

✓ Beverage intake does not affect food intake (drinking more fluid does not reduce total food intake).

✓ The amount of calorically sweetened beverages sold is currently higher than at any time in history.

After reviewing her food and beverage intake history, Leslie's professor outlined the pros and cons of the different available beverages.

1. Water
   - ✓ Essential for life
   - ✓ People need to consume a minimum amount for adequate hydration
2. Tea and Coffee
   - ✓ No adverse health effects in terms of obesity and chronic diseases; the only issue is added cream and sugar
   - ✓ Animal research suggests a protective role against selected cancers (data are unclear for humans; the potential health benefits of flavonoids in tea are unclear)
   - ✓ Coffee acts as a mild antidepressant and may lower risk of type 2 diabetes
3. Low-Fat and Skim Milk and Soy Beverages
   - ✓ Skim milk: unclear benefits on weight and bone density
   - ✓ Major provider of calcium and vitamin D
   - ✓ Adult milk intake may adversely affect several chronic diseases (e.g., prostate cancer, ovarian cancer)
4. Noncalorically Sweetened Beverages
   - ✓ May condition a preference for sweetness, leading to overfatness and type 2 diabetes
5. Caloric Beverages with Some Nutrients
   - ✓ Fruit juices are high in energy content yet contribute limited nutrients
   - ✓ Vegetable juices have fewer calories but contain significant amounts of sodium

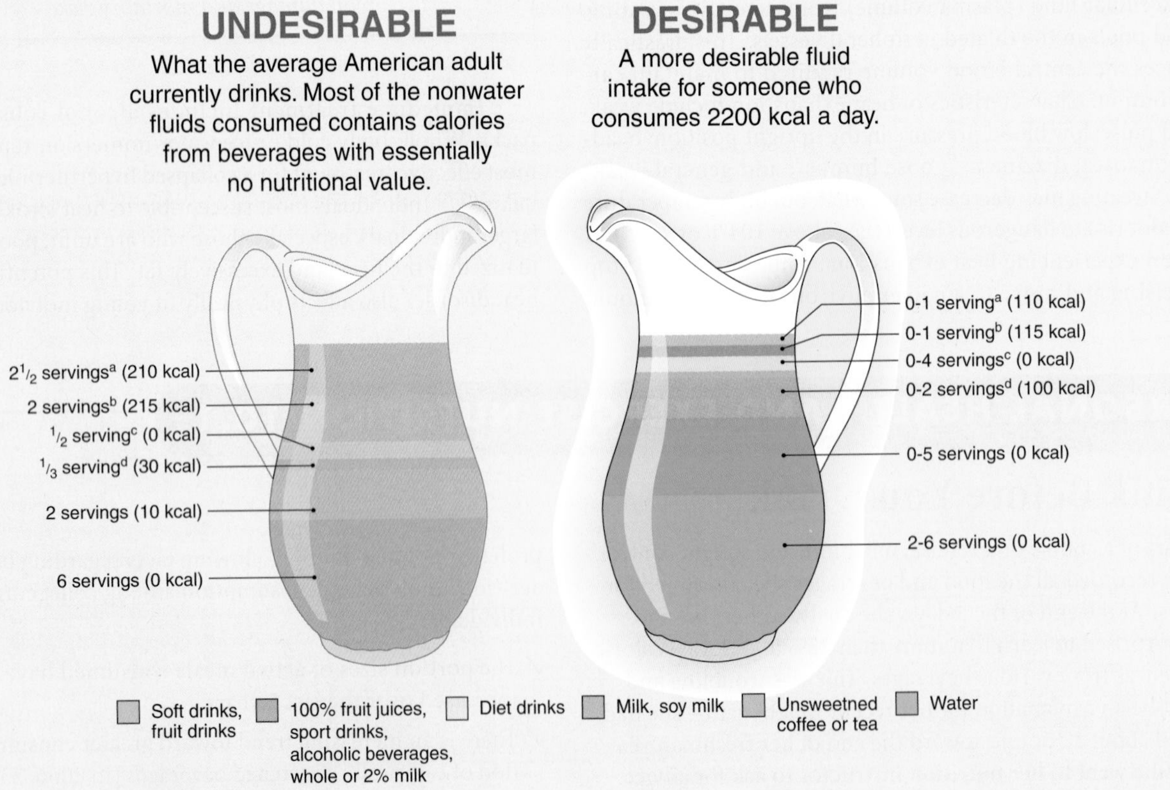

[a] 1 serving = 8 fluid oz.
[b] 0-2 servings of alcohol are okay for men
[c] Includes diet soft drinks and tea or coffee with sugar substitutes
[d] Includes fat-free or 1% milk and unsweetened fortified soy milk

✓ Whole milk contains saturated fat, which is not needed beyond infancy

✓ Sport drinks have reduced energy density compared to soft drinks and are helpful for rehydration

✓ Alcohol: Only the ethanol benefits are known (one drink daily for women, two drinks for men) and linked with reduced mortality, coronary heart disease, and type 2 diabetes

6. Calorically Sweetened Beverages

✓ Associated with increased dental caries, type 2 diabetes, and weight gain

Leslie was now ready to make an informed decision regarding her beverage consumption. She planned to try and adhere to the following guidelines, assuming she maintained her 2200-kcal diet.

✓ Water: 20 to 50 fl oz.d^{-1}

✓ Tea and Coffee (unsweetened): 0 to 40 fl oz/d (can replace water; caffeine a limiting factor—up to 400 mg/d or about 32 fl oz.d^{-1} of coffee)

✓ Low-Fat and Skim Milk and Soy Beverages: 0 to 16 fl oz.d^{-1}

✓ Noncalorically Sweetened Beverages: 0 to 32 fl oz.d^{-1} (could substitute for tea and coffee with the same limitations regarding caffeine)

✓ Caloric Beverages with Some Nutrients: 100% fruit juices 0 to 8 fl oz.d^{-1}, alcoholic beverages zero to one drink per day for women (one drink = 12 fl oz of beer, 5 fl oz of wine, or 1.5 fl oz of distilled spirits), whole milk 0 fl oz.d^{-1}

✓ Calorically Sweetened Beverages: 0 to 8 fl oz.d^{-1}

Nielsen SJ. Popkin BM. Changes in beverage intake between 1977 and 2001. *Am J Prev Med* 2004;27:205; Mucci L, et al. Cardiovascular risk and dietary sugar intake: is the link so sweet? *Intern Emerg Med* 2011 May 5; Edwards RD. Commentary: soda taxes, obesity, and the shifty behavior of consumers. *Prev Med* 2011;52:417.

SUMMARY

1. Cutaneous and muscle blood flow increase during exercise in the heat, whereas the blood supply of other tissues is temporarily compromised.

2. Core temperature normally increases in exercise; the relative stress of exercise determines the magnitude of the increase. A well-regulated temperature increase creates a more favorable environment for physiologic and metabolic functions.

3. Increased sweating strains fluid reserves, creating a relative state of dehydration. Excessive sweating without fluid replacement decreases plasma volume, and core temperature rises precipitously.

4. Exercise in a hot, humid environment poses a thermoregulatory challenge because a large sweat loss in high humidity contributes little to evaporative cooling.

5. Fluid loss in excess of 2% of body mass impedes heat dissipation, compromises cardiovascular function, and diminishes exercise capacity in a hot environment.

6. Adequate fluid replacement maintains plasma volume so circulation and sweating progress at optimal levels. The ideal replacement schedule during exercise matches fluid intake with fluid loss. This is effectively monitored by changes in body weight.

7. Each hour, the small intestine can absorb about 1000 mL of water. Prime factors that affect absorption rate include stomach volume and the osmolality of the oral rehydration beverage.

8. Excessive sweating and ingesting large volumes of plain water during prolonged exercise set the stage for hyponatremia (water intoxication). A decrease in extracellular sodium concentration causes this potentially dangerous malady.

9. A small amount of electrolytes in the rehydration beverage facilitates fluid replenishment more than drinking plain water.

10. Repeated heat stress initiates thermoregulatory adjustments that improve exercise capacity and reduce discomfort on subsequent heat exposure. Heat acclimatization triggers favorable redistribution of cardiac output and increases sweating capacity. Full acclimatization generally occurs in about 10 days of heat exposure.

11. Aging affects thermoregulatory function, yet acclimatization to moderate heat stress does not appreciably deteriorate with age.

12. When controlling for fitness and acclimatization levels, women and men show equal thermoregulatory efficiency during exercise. Women produce less sweat than men do at the same core temperature.

13. The ideal warm-weather clothing consists of lightweight, loose-fitting, and light-color clothes. Moisture-wicking fabrics against the skin optimize heat and moisture transfer from the skin to the environment.

14. Football uniforms impose a significant barrier to heat dissipation because they effectively seal off about 50% of the body's surface from the benefits of evaporative cooling. They also add to the metabolic load imposed by exercise.

15. During exercise in hot and humid environments, the modern cycling helmet does not increase the level of heat strain or perceived heat sensation of the head or body above that with the no-helmet condition.

16. In hot environments, there is a consistent reduction in voluntary energy intake per °F over the range of 20 to 100°F. The difference in intake cannot be explained by differences in basal metabolic rate, body weight, or type of physical activity.

17. Various practical heat stress indices (e.g., heat index) use ambient temperature and relative humidity to evaluate the environment's potential thermal challenge to an exercising person.

18. Heat cramps, heat exhaustion, and heat stroke are the major forms of heat illness. Heat stroke represents the most serious and complex of these maladies.

19. Oral temperature underestimates core temperature following strenuous exercise. This discrepancy results from evaporative cooling of the mouth and airways during high levels of pulmonary ventilation.

thePoint *Visit* **thePoint.lww.com/MKKSEN4e** *to view the following animation related to content presented in Chapter 10:* ***Water balance in the blood.***

TEST YOUR KNOWLEDGE ANSWERS

1. **False:** Core temperature (the temperature of deep tissues) remains in dynamic equilibrium between factors that add and subtract body heat. This balance results from integrating mechanisms that alter heat transfer to the periphery (shell), regulate evaporative cooling, and vary the rate of heat production

2. **True:** The hypothalamus contains the central coordinating center for temperature regulation. This group of specialized neurons at the floor of the brain serves as a "thermostat" (usually set and carefully regulated at 37°C ± 1°C) for making thermoregulatory adjustments to deviations from a temperature norm. Unlike a thermostat in a building, the hypothalamus cannot "turn off" the heat; it only initiates responses to protect the body from heat gain or heat loss.

3. **False:** Body heat loss occurs in four ways: radiation, conduction, convection, and evaporation. Evaporation of sweat provides the major physiologic defense against overheating. Water vaporization from the respiratory passages and skin surface continually transfers heat to the environment. For each liter of water that vaporizes, 580 kcal of heat energy transfers from the body to the environment.

4. **False:** Sweat evaporation from the skin depends on three factors: (1) surface exposed to the environment, (2) temperature and relative humidity of ambient air, and (3) convective air currents around the body. By far, relative humidity exerts the greatest impact on the effectiveness of evaporative heat loss. Relative humidity refers to the percentage of water in ambient air at a particular temperature compared with the total quantity of moisture that the air could carry. For example, 40% relative humidity means that ambient air contains only 40% of the air's moisture-carrying capacity at that specific temperature.

5. **True:** During heat stress, the pituitary gland releases ADH. ADH increases water reabsorption from the kidney tubules, causing urine to become more concentrated during heat stress. This action of ADH helps to protect against dehydration during heat stress.

6. **True:** Dehydration refers to an imbalance in fluid dynamics when fluid intake does not replenish water loss from either hyperhydrated or normally hydrated states. A moderate exercise workout generally produces a moderate 0.5- to 1.5-L sweat loss over a 1-hour period. Significant water loss occurs during several hours of intense exercise in a hot environment. The risk of heat illness greatly increases when a person begins exercising in a dehydrated state. Dehydration associated with a 3% decrease in body weight also slows the rate of gastric emptying, thus increasing epigastric cramps and feelings of nausea.

7. **False:** Urge individuals to rehydrate themselves, because the thirst mechanism imprecisely indicates water needs, particularly in children and the elderly. If left to depend on thirst, most individuals voluntarily replace only about half of the water lost during exercise. It could take several days after severe dehydration to re-establish fluid balance. Drink at least 125 to 150% of the existing fluid loss (body weight loss) as soon as possible after exercising. The 25 to 50% "extra" water accounts for that portion of ingested water lost in urine.

8. **False:** Excessive water intake under certain exercise conditions produces potentially serious medical

complications from the syndrome termed *hyponatremia* (water intoxication). Hyponatremia exists when serum sodium concentration falls below 135 $mEq \cdot L^{-1}$; a serum sodium concentration below 125 $mEq \cdot L^{-1}$ triggers severe symptoms. A sustained low plasma sodium concentration creates an osmotic imbalance across the blood-brain barrier, which causes rapid water influx into the brain. The resulting swelling of brain tissue produces a cascade of symptoms that range from mild (headache, confusion malaise, nausea, and cramping) to severe (seizures, coma, pulmonary edema, cardiac arrest, and death).

9. **False:** Factors other than air temperature determine the physiologic strain imposed by heat. These include (1) body size and fatness, (2) level of training, (3) acclimatization, (4) adequacy of hydration, and (5) external factors (convective air currents; radiant heat gain; intensity of exercise; amount, type, and color of clothing; and, most importantly, the relative humidity of ambient air).

10. **False:** Early studies of military personal stationed in the tropics suggest an inverse relationship between caloric intake and mean local ambient temperature. A consistent reduction in voluntary energy intake per °F occurs over the range of 20 to 100°F. The difference in caloric intake could not be explained by differences in basal metabolic rate, body weight, or type of physical activity.

Key References

American College of Sports Medicine, et al. American College of Sports Medicine position stand. Exertional heat illness during training and competition. *Med Sci Sports Exerc* 2007;39:556.

Armstrong LE, et al. American College of Sports Medicine position stand. Heat and cold illnesses during distance running. *Med Sci Sports Exerc* 1996;28:1.

Bar-Or O. Temperature regulation during exercise in children and adolescents. In: Gisolfi CV, Lamb DR, eds. *Perspectives in Exercise Science and Sports Medicine.* Vol. 2. Indianapolis, IN: Benchmark Press, 1989.

Brobeck JR. Food intake as a mechanism of temperature regulation. *Yale J Biol Med* 1948;20:545.

Buskirk ER, et al. Variations in resting metabolism with changes in food, exercise and climate. *Metabolism* 1957;6:144.

Consolazio CF. Energy requirements of men in extreme heat. *J Nutr* 1961;73:126.

Coyle EF, Montain SJ. Benefits of fluid replacement with carbohydrate during exercise. *Med Sci Sports Exerc* 1992;24:S324.

Donaldson GC, et al. Cardiovascular responses to heat stress and their adverse consequences in healthy and vulnerable human populations. *Int J Hyperthermia* 2003;19:225.

Gardner JW. Death by water intoxication. *Milit Med* 2002;5:432.

Haymes EM. Physiological responses of female athletes to heat stress: a review. *Phys Sportsmed* 1984;12:45.

Hubing KA, et al. Exercise-associated hyponatremia: the influence of pre-exercise carbohydrate status combined with high volume fluid intake on sodium concentrations and fluid balance. *Eur J Appl Physiol* 2011;111:797.

Institute of Medicine (IOM). *Nutritional Needs in Hot Environments: Applications for Military Personnel in Field Operations.* Washington, DC: National Academies Press, 1993.

Kenney WL, Chiu P. Influence of age on thirst and fluid intake. *Med Sci Sports Exerc* 2001;332:1524.

Kenney WL, Ho C-W. Age alters regional distribution of blood flow during moderate-intensity exercise. *J Appl Physiol* 1995;79:1112.

Maughan RJ, Sherriffs S. Exercise in the heat; challenges and opportunities. *J Sports Sci* 2004;22:917.

Maughan RJ, et al. Living, training and playing in the heat: challenges to the football player and strategies for coping with environmental extremes. *Scand J Med Sci Sports* 2010;3:117.

McCullough EA, Kenney WL. Thermal insulation and evaporative resistance of football uniforms. *Med Sci Sports Exerc* 2003;35:832.

Montain SJ, et al. Exercise associated hyponatraemia: quantative analysis to understanding etiology. *Br J Sports Med* 2006;40:98.

Noakes D. Fluid replacement during exercise. *Exerc Sports Sci Rev* 1993;21:297.

Passe DH, et al. Palatability and voluntary intake of sports beverages, diluted orange juice, and water during exercise. *Int J Sport Nutr Exerc Metab* 2004;14:272.

Rehrer NJ. The maintenance of fluid balance during exercise. *Int J Sports Nutr* 1996;15:122.

Rivera-Brown AM, et al. Exercise tolerance in a hot and humid climate in heat-acclimatized girls and women. *Int J Sports Med* 2006;27:943.

Shirreffs SM, et al. Fluid and electrolyte needs for preparation and recovery from training and competition. *J Sports Sci* 2004;22:57.

Stephenson LA, Kolka MA. Thermoregulation in women. *Exerc Sport Sci Rev* 1993;21:231.

Von Duvillard SP, et al. Fluids and hydration in prolonged endurance performance. *Nutrition* 2004;20:651.

thePoint *Visit* **thePoint.lww.com/MKKSEN4e** *for a list of the references cited in this chapter, including additional, relevant references.*

Purported Ergogenic Aids

PART 5

CONTENTS

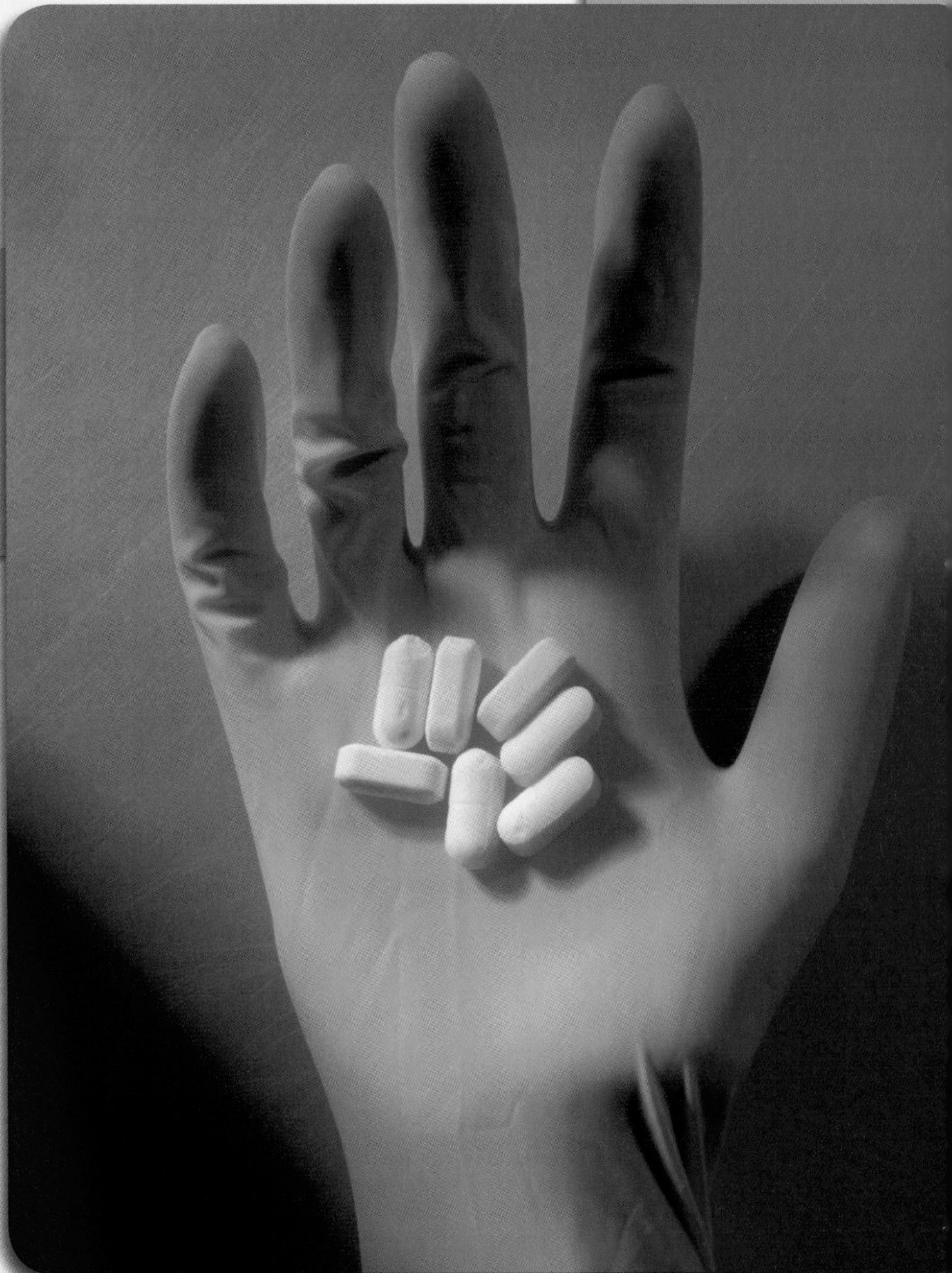

CHAPTER 11

Pharmacologic and Chemical Ergogenic Aids Evaluated

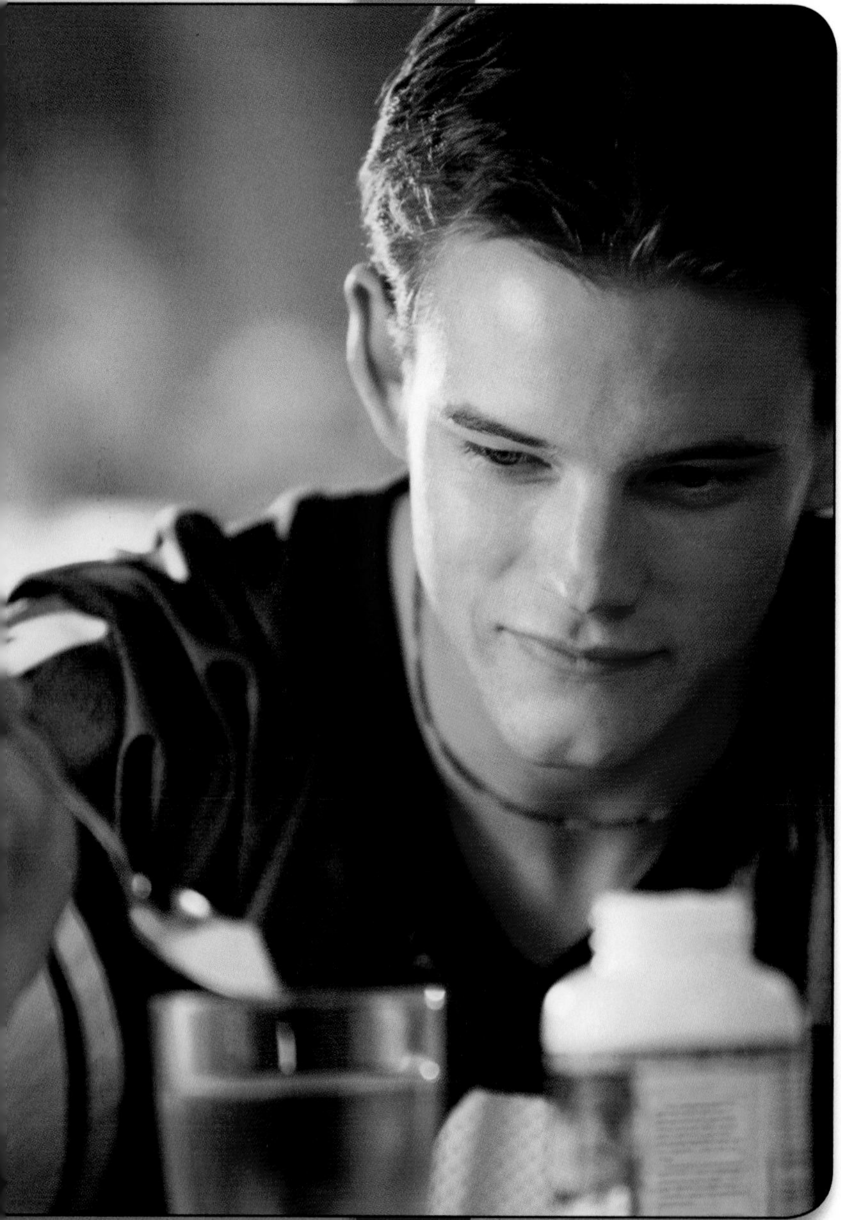

OUTLINE

TEST YOUR KNOWLEDGE

Select true or false for the 10 statements below, and then check out the answers at the end of the chapter. Retake the test after you've read the chapter; you should achieve 100%!	True	False
1. Ergogenic drug use by athletes reportedly began with the modern era (after 1900) and coincides with the ability to create "new" laboratory chemicals.	❍	❍
2. The term "placebo effect" in exercise research refers to the ability of a treatment or a compound to affect a person psychologically in a manner that improves physical performance independent of any real physiologic effect.	❍	❍
3. Anabolic steroids mimic the function of the natural human male hormone testosterone, so little chance exists for harmful side effects.	❍	❍
4. Androstenedione, an intermediate or precursor hormone between DHEA and testosterone, significantly increases endurance performance.	❍	❍
5. Amphetamines (pep pills) are dangerous and should not be taken by athletes.	❍	❍
6. Caffeine exerts no ergogenic effect other than to increase alertness in some persons.	❍	❍
7. The term *functional food* relates to the effects specific foods exert on muscular function and responsiveness to resistance training.	❍	❍
8. The herbal remedy ephedrine provides safe and positive effects for sports participants, particularly as a substance to facilitate fat loss.	❍	❍
9. Consuming a light-to-moderate amount of alcohol (e.g., a beer or two) after exercise speeds rehydration and replenishes depleted carbohydrate stores.	❍	❍
10. β-Hydroxy-β-methylbutyrate (HMB), a bioactive metabolite generated from the breakdown of the essential branched-chain amino acid leucine, decreases protein loss during stress by inhibiting protein catabolism.	❍	❍

Individuals at all levels of physical prowess use pharmacologic and chemical agents, believing that a specific drug positively influences skill, strength, power, endurance, or responsiveness to training.[135] In a drug-oriented, competitive culture, drug use for ergogenic* purposes continues to be on the upswing among high school and preadolescent-age school athletes. Among older, more highly competitive athletes (including competition surfers), illegal drug use is a cancer infecting the foundation of sports competition. When winning becomes all-important, cheating to win becomes pervasive at the highest levels of competition.[146] Often, little can be done to prevent the use *and* abuse of drugs by athletes to gain a competitive edge, despite scant "hard" scientific evidence indicating a performance-enhancing effect of many of these compounds. Ironically, athletes go to great lengths to promote all aspects of their health. They train exceptionally hard for many hours daily, generally eat well-balanced meals, and receive top-flight medical attention even for seemingly minor injuries, yet they purposely ingest synthetic agents, many of which trigger negative health effects ranging from nausea, hair loss, itching, and nervous irritability to an array of potential life-threatening conditions.

Considerable information exists concerning possible ergogenic effects of nutritional and pharmacologic aids on exercise performance and training. These include testimonials and endorsements for untested products from sports professionals and organizations, media publicity, television infomercials, and Internet home pages. This also includes research studies that extol potential performance benefits

* Ergogenic (work producing) refers to the application of a nutritional, physical, mechanical, psychological, physiologic, or pharmacologic procedure or aid to improve exercise capacity, athletic performance, and responsiveness to training. Included are aids that prepare a person to exercise, improve exercise efficiency, or facilitate the recovery process.

from alcohol, amphetamines, hormones, carbohydrates, amino acids (either consumed singularly or in combination), fatty acids, caffeine, buffering compounds, wheat-germ oil, vitamins, minerals, catecholamine agonists, steroid hormone precursors and stimulants, and even marijuana and cocaine.** **TABLE 11.1** gives examples of ingredients and the frequently *unsubstantiated* (and largely incorrect) claims advertised by makers of nutritional supplements in the physical fitness marketplace. Most persons believe these compounds enhance the response to exercise. The general population considers supplementation a way to improve physical appearance; in this regard, products aggressively marketed in the mass media to reduce fat and increase muscle mass often become instant "best sellers."

** Well-documented evidence exists about the addictive nature of cocaine and potential for significant health risks. Research has never shown that cocaine provides an ergogenic effect. Studies have been limited to animals (for obvious reasons), and results show that cocaine triggers an exaggerated catecholamine response during submaximal exercise, augments glycogen depletion in skeletal muscle, and causes lactate to rapidly accumulate in the blood.[8,21,22,41,100] These effects all impair exercise performance.

TABLE 11.1 Ingredients Commonly Advertised by Nutritional Supplement Manufacturers

The definition/alleged attributes are verbatim from literature supplied by manufacturers, product labels, promotional material about the product on the Internet, and advertisements in muscle and body building magazines.

Supplement	Alleged Attribute
American ginsengt	Restores energy after great fatigue. Reported to have invigorating and stimulating power. Acts as a general tonic. A booster.
Barley Green	Used by athletes for energy. Extremely nutritious and loaded with vitamins, proteins, minerals, chlorophyll, and enzymes.
BCAAs	Branched-chain amino acids that assist the muscles in synthesizing other amino acids to aid muscle growth. Helps muscles absorb blood sugar for energy.
Chromium (picolinate)	Activates enzymes involved in glucose and protein for burning and increasing lean body mass. Builds stamina.
Colostrum	Increases strength and lean body mass.
CoQ_{10}	Plays a role in energy production. Powerful antioxidant. Enhances the body's total systems.
Cordyceps	Renown as a supertonic. Builds physical power and mental energy.
Creatine monohydrate	Enhances energy and athletic performance and significantly increases muscle mass and strength.
DHEA	Regulates metabolism and increases muscle mass while burning fat. Strengthens and maintains the immune system and enhances energy. Increases physical well-being. A wonder supplement.
Digestive enzymes	Breaks down food particles for storage in the liver and muscles for energy. Helps to construct new muscle tissue.
Epemedium	A powerful tonic and stimulant. Helps strengthen bones and joints.
Eucommia	Superb energy tonic. Often used by athletes to strengthen the joints and the body.
Guarana extract	Increases energy and alertness. Increases fat-burning process.
Kola nut	Increases energy and alertness. Increases fat-burning process.
L-Carnitine	Controls increases in body-fat stores by converting nutrients into energy. Burns body fat and improves athletic performance.
L-Glutamine	Promotes protein and glycogen synthesis in muscles and liver. Prevents muscle catabolism. Helps buffer lactic acid buildup while training. Alleviates fatigue. Promotes recovery.
Licorice root	Strengthens muscles. Regulates blood sugar levels. Strongest detoxifier known to man without side effects.
Lipoic acid	Key compound for producing energy in muscles and normalizing blood sugar levels. Combats free radical formation.
L-Lysine	Essential building block for all proteins. Uses fatty acids required in energy production. Important for recovery from sports injuries.
Magnesium carbonate	Essential for vital enzymes. Aids in transmitting nerve and muscle impulses. Prevents muscle weakness.
Mexican wild yam	Increases physical well-being, enhances energy, and decreases body fat. Improves ability to deal with stressful situations. Clears the mind.
Muirapuama	Stimulant to enhance sports performance because of the rush it produces. Increases energy.

TABLE 11.1 Ingredients Commonly Advertised by Nutritional Supplement Manufacturers (*Continued*)

Supplement	Alleged Attribute
NAC	Reduces fatigue in muscles and improves liver metabolism. Aids the main antioxidant enzyme, glutathione peroxidase.
Nettle root	Rich in vitamins, lipids, and chlorophyll. Increases aerobic power and muscle strength. Mild anti-inflammatory and diuretic.
Orchic	Main source of natural testosterone production. Helps the body retain more protein and nitrogen to increase muscle mass and strength.
PAK	Significantly improves aerobic and anaerobic performance by increasing energy production. Reduces lactic acid.
Phosphatidyl serine	Stops exercise-induced increase in cortisol, which has an anticatabolic effect in muscles and tissues.
Plant sterols	Improves physical performance. Has general anabolic activity within muscle cells. Allows athletes to adapt to harder training loads.
Potassium chloride	Essential in maintaining fluid balance within the muscles. Aids in muscle contraction and transmission of glucose into glycogen for energy.
Quebracho bark	Highly effective stimulant. Known to elevate mood and increase energy. Builds overall strength and power. Great for endurance.
Radix angelicae	Used as a muscle building tonic. Nourishes the blood and activates blood circulation.
Radix astragali	Strengthens muscle and improves metabolic function. Potent immune system tonic. Fabulous for fighting injuries.
RNA–DNA	Increases cell energy and protein synthesis. Helps rebuild cells to ensure postworkout repair and growth. A good protein.
Royal jelly	High concentration of nutrients, especially B-complex vitamins. High concentration of vitamins, minerals, enzymes, and amino acids.
Saw palmetto	Contains plant sterols that improve physical performance and has profound effects on testosterone metabolism.
Schizandra	Increases endurance and strengthens the whole body. A powerful tonic that improves memory.
Selenium	Boosts immunity and neutralizes many free radicals and carcinogens. Vital antioxidant.
Siberian ginseng	Helps one adapt to all kinds of stresses. Improves the blood oxygen-carrying capacity. Promotes mental and physical vigor, metabolism, stamina, and endurance under stressful conditions. "Gets the body going."
Smilax	Increases muscle strength and size. Augments the body's natural production of its own testosterone.
Sumac	High in nutrients. Contains 19 different amino acids and electrolytes. Helps oxygenate the system and build and maintain lean muscle mass.
Vanadyl sulfate	Helps increase muscle growth and development and reduces body fat stores.
Vitamin C	Powerful antioxidant required for tissue growth and repair. Protects against infection and enhances immunity.
Vitamin E	A powerful antioxidant. Improves oxygen use. Enhances immune response and improves athletic performance.
Wild oats	Aids digestion and increases testosterone levels. Increases aerobic power and muscle strength. A great muscle builder.
Yerba mate	Helps to relieve fatigue and stress. Cleanses the blood and stimulates the mind. A fat-burner in vital body areas.
Yohimbe bark	Male athletes use this herb because of its reputed muscle-building effects. Improves sports performance and increases energy.
Zinc aspartate	Helps protein synthesis and collagen formation. Essential to athletes for growth and development, and to increase performance.

AN AREA OF INCREASING COMPLEXITY AND CONTROVERSY

Several explanations account for heightened interest in ergogenic factors other than innate physical ability and commitment to training that might enhance exercise capacity and training. First, more persons participate in high-level competitive amateur and professional athletics. Second, competitive success brings personal recognition and approval, but also more tangible rewards that range from college scholarships to lucrative professional contracts and commercial endorsements. Concurrently, many exercise science and applied physiology laboratories produce research about how pharmacologic agents and nutritional modification and supplementation affect energy supply, muscle metabolism, physiologic function, and growth and development.

In Use Since Antiquity

Athletes of ancient Greece from about 700 to 300 BC reportedly used hallucinogenic mushrooms, plant seeds, and ground dog testicles for ergogenic purposes, while Roman gladiator athletes ingested the equivalent of "speed" to enhance performance in the Circus Maximus (about 200–300 AD). Athletes of the Victorian era during the 15th century routinely used caffeine, alcohol, nitroglycerine, heroin, cocaine, and the rat poison strychnine for a competitive edge. In the mid-19th century in Europe, a tonic mixture of Bordeaux wine and natural cocaine extracted from cocoa leaves (marketed as *Vin tonique Marini*; **http://en.wikipedia.org/wiki/Vin_Mariani**) was sold as a curative and for medicinal and recreational purposes to "rev up" the body. Athletes would consume the drink to ward off fatigue, sometimes during the actual sport performance! Today, dietary supplements consist of nonprescription and unregulated plant extracts, vitamins, minerals, enzymes, and hormonal products. To positively influence overall health and exercise performance, these supplements must provide a nutrient undersupplied in the diet (highly unlikely for most persons) or exert a druglike influence on cellular function.

Not Without Risk

The indiscriminate use of alleged ergogenic substances increases the likelihood of adverse side effects that range from relatively benign physical discomfort to life-threatening episodes. Many of these compounds fail to conform to labeling requirements to correctly identify the strength of the product's ingredients.[70,92] Up to 20% of the nutritional supplements sampled contained substances that produce a positive result for doping, including nandrolone, testosterone, and other steroids not declared on the label. The supplements analyzed included vitamins and minerals, protein, and creatine. Such findings raise the real possibility that cross-contamination occurs in laboratories that produce both prohormone products and nutrient supplements.[9]

METHOD OF DETECTION

Testing of urine samples is the primary method for drug detection. The standard testing procedure adds chemicals to the dried urine, vaporizes it with heat, and then blows the vapor through an absorbent column and an electric or magnetic field (gas chromatography–mass spectrometry). The pattern made by the molecules deflected by the field is compared with patterns of known chemicals. Drug testing by use of gas chromatography coupled with high-resolution mass spectrometry, introduced in the 1996 Atlanta Olympic Games, detects most anabolic steroid use during the prior 18 months.

ON THE HORIZON

The day may not be far off when persons born lacking certain "lucky" genes that augment growth and development and exercise performance will simply add them, doping undetectably with DNA, not drugs. In these instances, "gene doping" misappropriates the medical applications of gene therapy that treats atherosclerosis, cystic fibrosis, and other diseases and uses them to increase the size, speed, and strength of healthy humans. For example, genes that cause muscles to enlarge would be ideal for sprinters, weightlifters, and other power athletes. In contrast, endurance athletes would benefit from genes that boost red blood cells (e.g., gene for erythropoietin) or stimulate blood vessel development (e.g., gene for vascular endothelial growth factor).

An increasing belief in the potential for selected foods to promote health has led to coining of the term **functional food**. Beyond meeting three basic nutrition needs for survival, hunger satisfaction, and preventing adverse effects, functional foods comprise those foods and their bioactive components (e.g., olive oil, soy products, omega-3 fatty acids, phytochemicals) that promote well-being, health, and optimal body function or reduce disease risk (**FIG. 11.1**).[108,129,164] Examples include many polyphenolic substances (simple phenols and flavonoids in fruits, vegetables, and nuts), carotinoids, soy isoflavones, fish oils, and components of nuts with antioxidant and other properties that decrease vascular disease and cancer risk. Primary targets for this expanding branch of food science include gastrointestinal functions, antioxidant

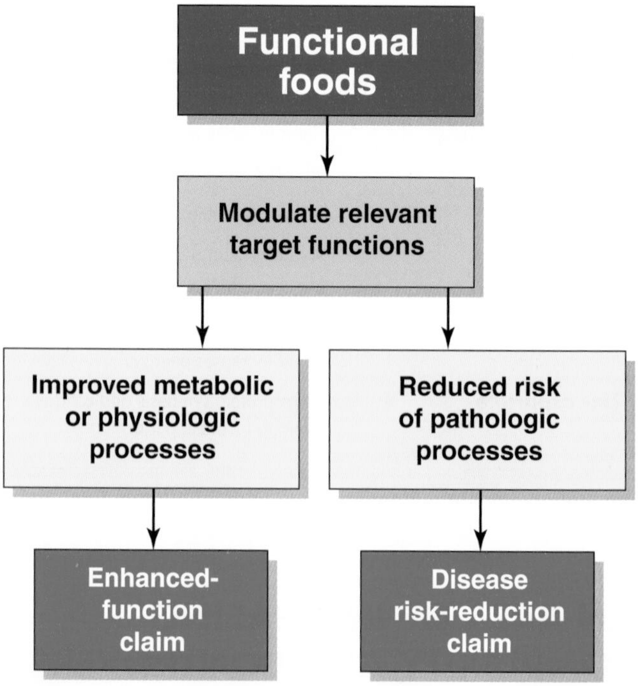

FIGURE 11.1. Strategy of functional food science. Basis for enhanced structure–function or disease risk-reduction claims. (From Roberfroid MB. Concepts and strategy of functional food science: the European perspective. *Am J Clin Nutr* 2000;71[Suppl]:1660S.)

systems, and macronutrient metabolism. Clearly, enormous implications exist to better understand nutrition's role in optimizing individual genetic potential, resistance to disease, and overall quality of exercise performance. Unfortunately, the science base generated by research in this valid field of human nutrition often falls prey to nutritional hucksterism and scam artists.

Biotechnology also has created the emerging field of **transgenic nutraceuticals**—the use of genes introduced into a host plant or animal to modify a biochemical pathway. This produces a new class of "natural" bioactive components of food in a nonfood matrix with physiologic and therapeutic functions (e.g., pharmaceutical protein vaccines and monoclonal antibodies) to promote disease prevention and treatment. Nutraceuticals differ from functional foods that deliver their active ingredients within the food matrix. By definition, nutraceutical compounds fall along the continuum from food to food supplements to drugs. Examples of such genetic engineering of nutrients include remodeling of cow mammary gland milk by adding or deleting specific milk proteins or adding oligosaccharides and development of novel food oils that do not require chemical hydrogenation without undesirable *trans* fatty acids. Through genetic tinkering, scientists can dramatically augment vitamin C levels in leaves and seeds of crop plants by increasing expression of a gene that recycles the plant's vitamin C. Undoubtedly, some of these biotechnology products will make their way into the exercise enthusiast's nutritional armamentarium to form the next wave of alleged performance enhancers.

A NEED TO CRITICALLY EVALUATE

Companies expend considerable money and effort to show a beneficial effect of a nutritional "aid." Often, a **"placebo effect,"** not the "aid," improves performance—the person performs at a higher level from the suggestive power of believing that a substance or procedure works. Sports nutritionists must evaluate the scientific merit of articles and advertisements about nutrition products.

To separate marketing "hype" from scientific fact, we pose five areas for questioning the validity of research claims concerning the efficacy of chemical, pharmacologic, and nutritional ergogenic aids:

1. **Justification**
   Scientific rationale: Does the study represent a "fishing expedition," or is a sound rationale given that the specific treatment should produce an effect? For example, a theoretical basis exists to believe that ingesting creatine elevates intramuscular creatine and phosphocreatine to possibly improve short-term power output capacity. In contrast, no rationale exists to hypothesize that hyperhydration, breathing hyperoxic gas, or ingesting medium-chain triglycerides should enhance 100-m dash performance.
2. **Subjects**
   Animals or humans: Many diverse mammals exhibit similar physiologic and metabolic dynamics, yet significant species differences exist, which limit generalizations to humans. For example, the models for disease processes, nutrient requirements, hormone dynamics, and growth and development often differ markedly between humans and other mammals.
   Sex: Sex-specific responses to the interactions between exercise, training, and nutrient requirements and supplementation limit generalizability of findings to the sex studied.
   Age: Age often interacts to influence the outcome of an experimental treatment. Effective interventions for the elderly may not apply to growing children or young and middle-aged adults.
   Training status: Fitness status and training level influence the effectiveness (or ineffectiveness) of a particular diet or supplement intervention. Treatments that benefit the untrained (e.g., chemicals or procedures that enhance neurologic disinhibition) often have little effect on elite athletes who practice and compete routinely at maximal arousal levels.
   Baseline level of nutrition: The research should establish the subjects' nutritional status before experimental treatment. Clearly, a nutrient supplement administered to a malnourished group typically improves exercise performance and training responsiveness. Such nutritional interventions fail to demonstrate whether the same effects occur if subjects received the supplement with their baseline nutrient intake at recommended levels. It should occasion little surprise, for example, that supplemental iron enhances aerobic fitness in a group with iron deficiency anemia. One cannot infer that iron supplements provide such benefits to *all* persons.
   Health status: Nutritional, hormonal, and pharmacologic interventions profoundly affect the diseased and infirmed, yet offer little or no benefit to those in good health. Research findings from diseased groups should not be generalized to healthy populations.
3. **Research sample, subjects, and design**
   Random assignment or self-selection: Apply research findings only to groups similar to the sample studied. If subject volunteers "self-select" into an experimental group, does the experimental treatment produce the results, or did a change occur from the person's motivation to enroll in the study? For example, desire to enter a weight loss study may elicit behaviors that produce weight loss independent of the experimental treatment per se. Great difficulty exists in assigning truly random samples of subjects into experimental and control groups. When subjects volunteer for an experiment, they must be randomly assigned to either a control or experimental condition, a process termed **randomization**. When all subjects receive the experimental supplement and the placebo treatment (see below), supplement administration is counterbalanced, and one half of the subjects receive the supplement first, whereas the other half take the placebo first.
   Double-blind, placebo-controlled: The ideal experiment to evaluate performance-enhancing effects of

an exogenous supplement requires that experimental and control subjects remain unaware or "blinded" to the substance administered. To achieve this goal, subjects should receive a similar quantity and/or form of the proposed aid. In contrast, control group subjects receive an inert compound or placebo. The placebo treatment evaluates the possibility of subjects performing well or responding better simply because they receive a substance they believe should benefit them (called a psychological or placebo effect). To further reduce experimental bias from influencing the outcome, those administering the treatment and recording the response must not know which subjects receive the treatment or placebo. In such a **double-blinded** experiment, it is crucial that both investigator and subjects remain unaware of the treatment condition.

Control of extraneous factors: Under ideal conditions, experiences should be as similar as possible for the experimental and control groups, except for the treatment variable. Random assignment of subjects to control or experimental groups helps to equalize factors that could unfairly influence the study's outcome.

Appropriateness of measurements: Reproducible, objective, and valid measurement tools must evaluate research outcomes. A step test to predict aerobic capacity and infrared interactance to assess body fat content represent imprecise tools to answer important questions about the efficacy of a proposed ergogenic aid.

4. **Conclusions**

Findings should dictate conclusions: The conclusions of a research study must logically follow from research findings. Frequently, investigators who study ergogenic aids extrapolate conclusions beyond the scope of their data. The implications and generalizations of research findings must remain within the context of the measurements made, subjects tested, and magnitude of subject responses. For example, increases in anabolic hormone levels in response to a dietary supplement reflect just that; they do not necessarily indicate an augmented training responsiveness or improved level of muscular function. Similarly, improvement in brief anaerobic power output capacity with creatine supplementation does not justify the conclusion that exogenous creatine improves overall "physical fitness."

Appropriate statistical analysis: Appropriate inferential statistical analysis must be applied to quantify the potential that chance caused the research outcome. Other statistics must objectify averages, variability, and degree of association or correlation among disparate variables.

Statistical versus practical significance: The finding of statistical significance of a particular experimental treatment only means a high probability exists that the results did not occur by change. One also must evaluate the magnitude of an effect for its real impact on physiology and/or performance. A reduced heart rate of three beats a minute during submaximal exercise may reach statistical significance (greater than chance occurrence), yet confer little practical effect on altering aerobic fitness or cardiovascular function.

5. **Dissemination of findings**

Published in peer-reviewed journal: High-quality research withstands the rigors of critical review and evaluation by colleagues with expertise in the specific area of investigation. **Peer review** provides a measure of quality control over scholarship and interpretation of research findings. Publications in popular magazines (e.g., *People, Glamour, Self, Men's Fitness, Muscle and Fitness, Flex*) or quasi-professional journals (e.g., *Physician and Sports Medicine, ACSM's Health & Fitness Journal*) do not undergo the same degree of review rigor as a peer-reviewed article published in a mainstream research journal. Often, no external review takes place as editors assign articles to writers for a predetermined fee for service! Even worse, self-appointed "experts" in sports nutrition and physical fitness often pay eager publishers for magazine space (or agree to write an article in exchange for ad space) to promote their particular viewpoint. In some cases, the expert owns the magazine!

Findings reproduced by other investigators: Findings from one study do not necessarily establish scientific generalizability. Conclusions become stronger and more generalizable when support emerges from the credible laboratories supervised by independent investigators without monetary connection to the sponsoring organization. Consensus reduces the influence of chance, flaws in experimental design, and investigator bias.

Table 11.2 summarizes recommendations for future research on performance-enhancing products put forth at the Conference on the Science and Policy of Performance-Enhancing Products held in January 2002.

SUPPLEMENT USE AND ABUSE AMONG ELITE ATHLETES

A survey of college student athletes by the National Collegiate Athletic Association (NCAA; www.ncaa.org) indicated that 29% of respondents used nutritional supplements during the previous year.[71] The most popular supplement, creatine (26%), was followed by amino acids (10%), with androstenedione, chromium, and ephedra each used by about 4% of athletes. Prevalence for doping occurs among athletes in sports that emphasize speed and power.[2] The International Olympic Committee (IOC; www.olympic.org/) initiated drug testing for stimulants in Olympic competition in the 1968 Mexico City games following the death of a famed Tour de France British cyclist from amphetamine overdose a year earlier. Testing has consistently expanded, with the initiation of random, unannounced drug testing in track and field in 1989 to the administration of 3500 tests before the opening ceremonies of the 2002 Winter Games in Salt Lake City, 4500 tests during the Beijing Games, and 6250 blood and urine samples planned at the 2012 London

TABLE 11.2 Research-Based Recommendations for Investigating the Optimal Dosing, Health Risks, and Efficacy of Alleged Performance-Enhancing Products

• Evaluate the risks and benefits of performance-enhancing supplements among subpopulations with diverse dietary patterns and nutrient intakes, such as adolescents, body builders, military personnel, and the elderly
• Monitoring and surveillance of the effects of chronic, prolonged use of performance-enhancing supplements, particularly androstenedione, ephedrine, and creatine
• Identification and characterization of mechanism(s) of action of performance-enhancing ingredients
• Characterization of the patterns of use (e.g., type of product, frequency) and psychosocial behavioral aspects of use among various subpopulations in the United States
• Characterization of dose–response curves for performance-enhancing supplements, particularly those containing ephedrine, alkaloids, and steroid hormone precursors such as androstenedione
• Characterization of the endocrine effects of performance-enhancing supplements, especially those containing hormonal ingredients such as androstenedione and dehydroepiandrosterone (DHEA), according to age, gender, and physiologic life stage (e.g., female athletes with amenorrhea or disordered eating or at high risk for osteoporosis)
• Comparative studies of analytical grade dietary supplement ingredients (particularly caffeine and ephedrine) with formulations currently in the marketplace
• Evaluation of the effects of combining performance-enhancing ingredients as in "stacking formulas" or the simultaneous use of multiple sports supplements
• Comparative studies that examine the effect of frequency and timing of supplementation on physical performance
• Determining targeted approaches to communicate the risks and benefits of performance-enhancing products to various segments of the US population (professional and lay audiences)
• Determining whether other stimulant and thermogenic ingredients might serve as substitutes for ephedrine alkaloids

From Fomous CM, et al. Symposium: conference on the science and policy of performance-enhancing products. *Med Sci Sports Exerc 2002;34:1685.*

Olympics. The 2011 Prohibited List from the World Anti-Doping Agency (www.wada-ama.org/) includes three categories of substances and methods:

Prohibited Substances Methods Prohibited at All Times

1. Anabolic agents
2. Peptide hormones, growth factors, and related substances
3. β_2 agonists
4. Hormone antagonists and modulators
5. Diuretics and other masking agents

Prohibited Methods

1. Enhancement of oxygen transfer
2. Chemical and physical manipulation
3. Gene doping

Substances and Methods Prohibited in Competition

1. Stimulants
2. Narcotics
3. Cannabinoids
4. Glucocorticosteroids

Substances Prohibited in Particular Sports

1. Alcohol
2. β-Blockers

The World Anti-Doping Agency (WADA) has crafted an important "core" document regarding doping in sports. The Code became effective on January 1, 2004, and has become a powerful and effective tool in antidoping efforts worldwide. The purpose, scope, and organization of the World Anti-Doping Program and the Code can be downloaded as a PDF from this site: <www.wada-ama.org/Documents/World_Anti-Doping_Program/WADP-The-Code/WADA_Anti-Doping_CODE_2009_EN.pdf>.

The purposes of the World Anti-Doping Code and the World Anti-Doping Program that supports it are

1. To protect the athletes' fundamental right to participate in doping-free sport and thus promote health, fairness, and equality for athletes worldwide
2. To ensure harmonized, coordinated, and effective antidoping programs at the international and national level with regard to detection, deterrence, and prevention of doping

In the next sections, we discuss common pharmacologic and chemical agents purported to enhance exercise performance, increase the quality and quantity of training, and augment the body's adaptation to regular exercise. Chapter 12 discusses the role of nutritional supplementation for ergogenic purposes. The following presents five mechanisms by which such foods, food components, and pharmacologic agents might enhance exercise performance:

1. Function as a central or peripheral nervous system stimulant (e.g., caffeine, choline, amphetamines, alcohol)
2. Increase storage or availability of a limiting substrate (e.g., carbohydrate, creatine, carnitine, chromium)

3. Serve as a supplemental fuel source (e.g., glucose, medium-chain triacylglycerols)
4. Reduce or neutralize performance-inhibiting metabolic by-products (e.g., sodium bicarbonate or sodium citrate, pangamic acid, phosphate)
5. Facilitate recovery (e.g., high-glycemic carbohydrates, water)

USER BEWARE

The US Anti-Doping Agency (USADA; www.usantidoping.org) sends a clear message to athletes on its website:

> The use of dietary/nutritional supplements is completely at the athlete's own risk, even if the supplements are "approved" or "verified." If you take dietary/nutritional supplements you may test positive for a prohibited substance not disclosed on the product label. This would result in a doping violation.[33,122]

ANABOLIC STEROIDS

Anabolic steroids for medical use became prominent in the early 1950s to treat patients deficient in natural androgens or with muscle-wasting (muscular dystrophy) diseases. Other legitimate steroid uses include treatment for the following:

1. Osteoporosis
2. Severe female breast cancer
3. Counter the excessive decline in lean body mass and increase in body fat often observed among elderly men
4. HIV
5. Kidney dialysis

Anabolic steroids have become an integral part of the high-technology scene of competitive American sports that began with the 1955 US weightlifting team who used Dianabol, a modified, synthetic testosterone molecule called methandrostenolone. From the 1950s until the fall of the Berlin Wall in 1989, a new era ushered in the systematic and carefully planned "drugging" of East German competitive athletes with formulations of other anabolic steroids.[59,190]

Up to 4 million athletes (90% of male and 80% of female professional bodybuilders) currently use androgens, often combined with stimulants, hormones, and diuretics, believing their use augments training effectiveness. Even in the sport of baseball, interviews with strength trainers and current players estimate that up to 30% of professionals use anabolic steroids in their quest to enhance performance.

Interestingly, a survey of 500 steroid users reported that nearly 80% are nonathletes who take these drugs for cosmetic purposes. The majority self-administer with intramuscular injections, with nearly 1 in 10 reporting hazardous injection techniques.[154]

Structure and Action

Anabolic steroids function in a manner similar to the chief male hormone testosterone. By binding with specific receptor sites on muscle and other tissues, testosterone contributes to male secondary sex characteristics. These include sex differences in muscle mass and strength that develop at puberty onset. Ninety-five percent of testosterone production takes place in the testes, with the remainder produced by the adrenal glands. One can minimize the hormone's androgenic or masculinizing effects by synthetically manipulating the steroid's chemical structure to increase muscle growth from nitrogen retention and anabolic tissue building. Nevertheless, the masculinizing effect of synthetically derived steroids still occurs despite chemical alteration, particularly in females.

Athletes who take these drugs typically combine supraphysiologic dosages of multiple steroid preparations in oral and injectable form in the belief the various androgens differ in physiologic action—a practice called "**stacking**." The term "**pyramiding**" refers to progressively increasing drug dosage usually during 4- to 18-week cycles. The athlete abstains from taking drugs between cycle stages. The drug quantities far exceed the recommended medical dose, often by 200 times or more. The athlete then progressively reduces the dosage in the months before competition to reduce risk of detection during drug testing. The difference between dosages in research studies and the excess typically abused by athletes has largely contributed to a credibility gap between scientific findings (often, no effect of steroids) and what most in the athletic community "know" to be true by taking their "normal" but still exceedingly high doses.

Designer Drug Unmasked

The Department of Molecular and Medical Pharmacology at the University of California at Los Angeles (UCLA) supports the world's largest WADA-accredited sports drug-testing facility involved with athletic doping. Founded in 1982 by a grant from the Los Angeles Olympic Organizing Committee, the UCLA facility was the first US laboratory accredited by the IOC (**www.pathnet.medsch.ucla.edu/OlympicLab/index.html**). Among its many accomplishments, the laboratory unmasked a potentially illegal "designer" compound that mimics the chemical structure similar to the prohibited steroids gestrinome and trenbolone. The researchers called the discovery a new stand-alone steroid chemical entity, not a "pro-steroid" or "precursor steroid" like many performance-boosting substances on the market—a drug with no prior record of manufacture or existence. The US Anti-Doping Agency (USADA; **www.usantidoping.org**) oversees drug testing for all sports federations under the US Olympic umbrella. The USADA said an anonymous tipster provided a syringe sample of a steroid identified as tetrahydrogestrinone (THG). Athletes who test positive face 2-year suspensions that prohibit participation in international meets.

As of October 17, 2003, the National Football League (NFL) began testing players for THG to avoid the scandal that has embarrassed track and field. For at least the past

10 years, antidoping experts have continued to criticize the NFL and Major League Baseball for not testing for human growth hormone (hGH). In early August 2011, the NFL and the players' collective bargaining union agreed on procedures to administer random drug tests at any time and place, even on game day, particularly for hGH. To their credit, baseball tests minor league players, and on August 18, 2011, a Colorado Rockies Triple-A player with considerable prior experience in the major leagues received a 50-game suspension after testing positive for hGH. He became the first North American professional athlete and eighth athlete worldwide since 2004 punished for taking the drug.

In 1987, the **American College of Sports Medicine** (**ACSM**; www.acsm.org), the largest sports medicine and exercise science organization in the world, issued a position statement that called for increased vigilance in identifying and eradicating steroid use.[5] A follow-up Position Stand in 1996 concerning blood doping concluded that such procedure used in an attempt to improve athletic performance is unethical and unfair and exposes the athlete to unwarranted and potentially serious health risks.[6] The ACSM considers such chemicals "serious threats to the health and safety of athletes, as well as detriments to the principle of fair play in sports. Any effort to veil or disguise steroid use in sports through stealth, designer, or precursor means, puts elite, amateur and even recreational athletes at risk." Both position stands are available as free PDF downloads from the following website: **http://journals.lww.com/acsm-msse/pages/collectiondetails.aspx?TopicalCollectionId=1**.

A Drug with a Considerable Following

Anabolic steroid use usually combines with resistance training and augmented protein intake to improve strength, speed, and power. The image of the steroid abuser often pictures massively developed body builders; however, abuse also occurs frequently among amateur and professional athletes in road cycling, skateboarding, surfing, tennis, track and field, baseball, hockey, football, soccer, and swimming. Federal authorities conservatively estimate that illegal trafficking in steroids exceeds $150 million yearly.

Increasingly Prevalent Among Young Athletes and Nonathletes

Steroids often are obtained on the "black market" or the legal equivalent, and androstenedione is often bought from mall nutrition stores. According to the US Drug Enforcement Agency (DEA; **www.policyalmanac.org/crime/archive/drug_trafficking.shtml**), anabolic steroids are illegally smuggled from Mexico and European countries into the United States. Recent DEA reporting indicates that Russian, Romanian, and Greek nationals are significant traffickers of steroids responsible for substantial shipments of steroids entering the United States. Unfortunately, the lack of international control over foreign supply sources makes it impossible to attack the trafficking at its source. Misinformed persons typically take massive and prolonged dosages without medical monitoring for possible harmful alterations in physiologic function. Particularly worrisome is steroid abuse among boys and girls as young as 10 and high school students who do not play team sports.[4,65] Accompanying risks including extreme virilization and irreversible premature cessation of bone growth in children who would otherwise continue to develop. Those teenagers who use steroids cite improved athletic performance as the most common reason for taking them, although 25% acknowledged enhanced appearance—simply wanting to look good—as the main reason. In this struggle for self-image, a disturbance in body image (dissatisfaction/unhappiness with upper and lower body parts and facial features), with marked symptoms of muscle dysmorphia (see Chapter 15),[28,93] contributes to anabolic steroid abuse among teenagers and young men. A unique Blue Cross/Blue Shield national survey from 1999 to 2000 noted a 25% increase in steroid and similar drug use among boys age 12 to 17. Twenty percent of these teenagers took steroids to improve their looks, not to enhance sports performance (**FIG. 11.2**).

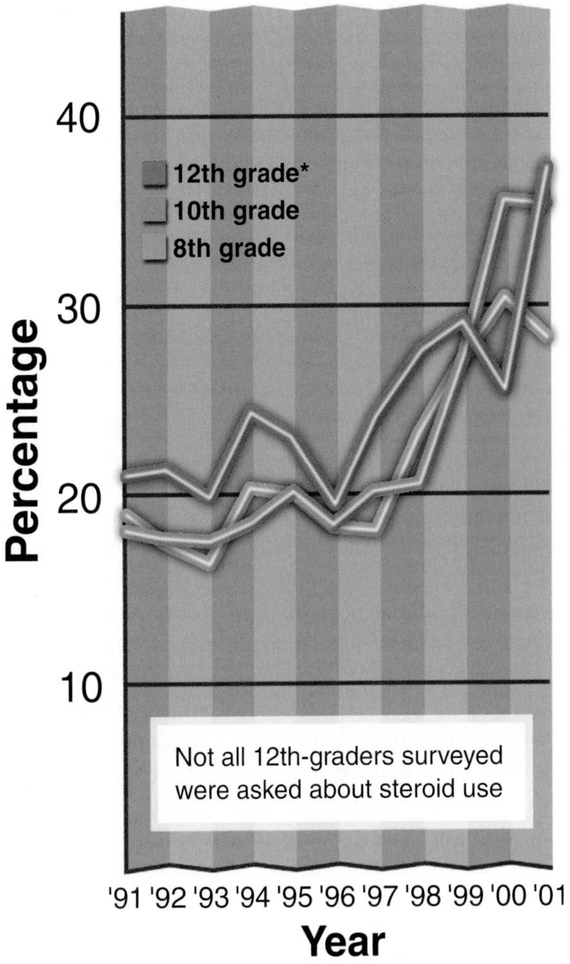

FIGURE 11.2. On the upswing: percentage of adolescent students claiming to have used anabolic steroids at least once. (Source: Blue Cross/Blue Shield; University of Michigan.)

Effectiveness Questioned

For more than six decades, researchers and athletes have debated the true effect of anabolic steroids on human body composition and exercise performance. Much of the confusion about anabolic steroids' ergogenic effectiveness stems from variations in the following nine variables[75]:

1. Experimental design
2. Poor selection of controls
3. Differences in specific drugs
4. Dosages
5. Treatment duration
6. Accompanying nutritional supplementation
7. Training intensity
8. Evaluation techniques
9. Individual differences in response

The relatively small residual androgenic effect of the steroid also may augment central nervous system function to make the athlete more aggressive (so-called roid rage), competitive, and fatigue resistant. Such facilitatory effects allow the athlete to train harder for a longer time or to believe that training improvement actually occurred. Abnormal alterations in mood and psychiatric dysfunction also are associated with androgen use.[37,163]

Early research with animals suggests that anabolic steroid treatment, when combined with exercise and adequate protein intake, stimulates protein synthesis and increases muscle protein content (myosin, myofibrillar, and sarcoplasmic factors). In contrast, other data show no benefit from steroid treatment on leg muscle weight of rats subjected to functional overload by surgically removing the synergistic muscle.[123] Anabolic steroid treatment did not complement functional overload to stimulate muscle development.

The response of humans to steroid ingestion is often difficult to interpret. Some studies show augmented body weight gains and reduced body fat with steroid use in men who train, whereas other studies show no effects on strength and power or body composition, even with sufficient energy and protein intake to support an anabolic effect.[56,74] When steroid use produced body weight gains, the compositional nature of these gains for water, muscle, and fat remained unclear.

Patients receiving dialysis and those infected with human immunodeficiency virus (HIV) commonly experience malnutrition, reduced muscle mass, and chronic fatigue. For dialysis patients, a 6-month supplement with the anabolic steroid nandrolone decanoate increased lean body mass and level of daily function.[88] Similarly, a moderate supraphysiologic androgen regimen that included the anabolic steroid oxandrolone substantially facilitated lean tissue accrual and muscle strength gains from resistance training in men with HIV compared with testosterone replacement alone.[181]

Dosage Becomes an Important Factor

Variations in drug quantity may account for confusion and create a credibility gap between scientist and steroid user about the true ergogenic effectiveness of anabolic steroids.[56] **FIGURE 11.3** illustrates changes from average baseline values for fat-free body mass (FFM), triceps and quadriceps cross-sectional muscle areas, and muscle strength (one-repetition maximum [1-RM]) after 10 weeks of treatment of 43 healthy men with some resistance training experience. The men who received the hormone while continuing to train gained about 0.5 kg (1 lb) of lean tissue weekly, with no increase in body fat over the 10-week treatment period. Even the group receiving the drug and not training increased muscle mass and strength compared with men receiving the placebo, but their increases were less than those of men who trained while taking testosterone. The researchers emphasized they did not design their study to justify or endorse steroid use for athletic purposes because of the health risks (see next section). Their data indicated the potential for medically supervised anabolic steroid treatment to restore muscle mass resulting from tissue-wasting diseases.

POPULAR WEB SITE SALES FOR ANABOLIC STEROIDS

Researchers in Italy reviewed Internet websites offering androgenic anabolic steroids (AAS) using the keywords "anabolic steroids," "anabolic steroids buy," and "anabolic steroid purchase." The analysis included the first 10 Web sites offering AAS in the first 10 pages of results. Thirty AAS-selling websites were identified, with 47% of locations in the United States and 30% in Europe. Most websites sold other anabolic/ergogenic products that included clenbuterol (77%), GH/insulin-like growth factor (IGF) (60%), thyroid hormones (47%), erythropoietin (30%), insulin (20%), or products for AAS-related adverse effects (mainly estrogen antagonists, 63%; products for erectile dysfunction, 56%; 5β-reductase inhibitors, 33%; and antiacne products, 33%). AAS were sold as medicines (70%) or as dietary supplements (30%). AAS in medicines included nandrolone (20%), methandrostenolone (18%), and testosterone (12%). Dietary supplements contained mainly DHEA and included several fake compounds. Manufacturers were declared for 98% of medicines and 67% of dietary supplements, with several manufacturers not located on the Internet. The descriptions included few adverse effects and no estrogenicity. Toxicity was seldom reported and presented as mild. Recommended doses were two- to fourfold higher than current medical recommendations. Misleading information and deceiving practices were common findings on AAS-selling Web sites, indicating their deleterious potential for public health.[42]

Do Risks Exist?

Debate exists about the health risks of anabolic steroids used by the athletic population because much of the research on steroid risk comes from medical observations. Prolonged

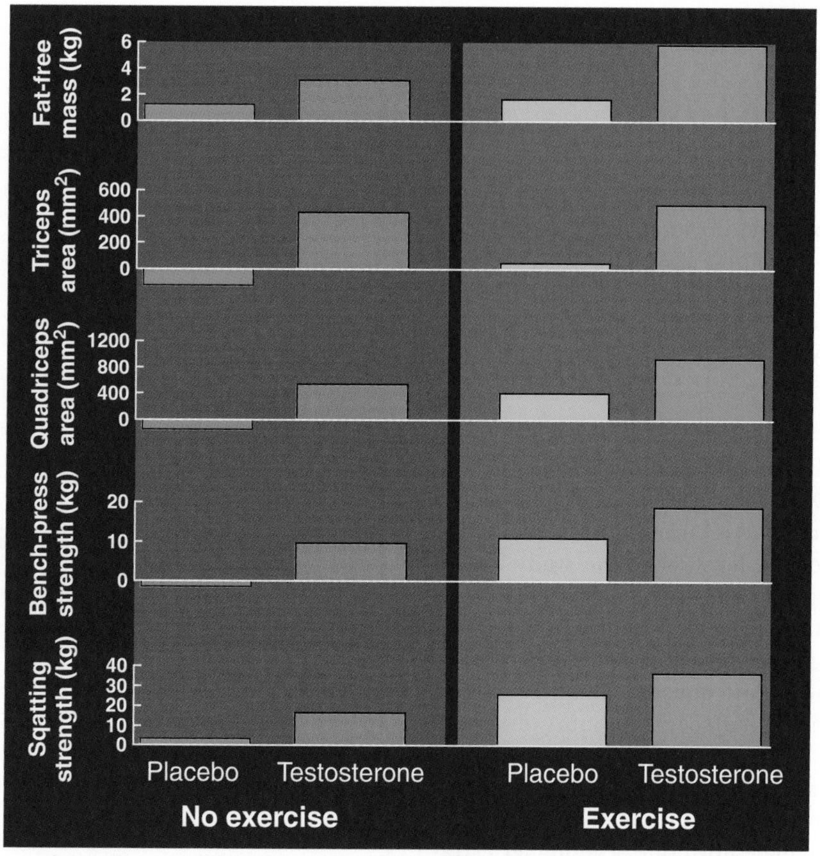

FIGURE 11.3. Changes from baseline in mean fat-free body mass, triceps and quadriceps cross-sectional areas, and muscle strength in bench press and squatting exercises over 10 weeks of testosterone treatment. (From Bhasin S, et al. The effects of supraphysiological doses of testosterone on muscle size and strength in normal men. *N Engl J Med* 1996;335:1.)

Connections to the Past

Francis Gano Benedict (1870–1957)

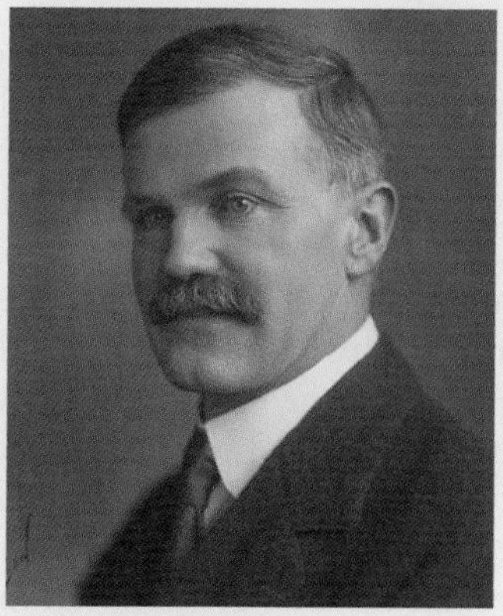

Francis G. Benedict earned his bachelor's degree at Harvard University in 1893, then his master's degree in 1894, and Ph.D. (*magna cum laude*) at Heidelberg University in 1895. A chemist, Benedict assisted Atwater in the Department of Chemistry at Connecticut's Wesleyan University. Over a 12-year period, they conducted more than 500 experiments concerning rest, exercise, and diet using the Atwater-Rosa respiration calorimeter (see chapter 6). Their results appeared in six bulletins of the Office of Experiment Stations of the U.S. Department of Agriculture under the general title *Experiments on the Metabolism of Matter and Energy in the Human Body*. In addition, Benedict published studies on the physiological action of alcohol (which proved to be controversial and opposed by the temperance organizations) and the effects of muscular exercise and mental effort on energy metabolism. When Atwater died in 1907, Benedict became Director of the Nutrition Laboratory (Boston), a post he held for 30 years until retirement. Relocating from Wesleyan to Boston provided Benedict with ready access to outstanding medical facilities. His work in respiratory metabolism complemented that of scientists in allied health fields such as renowned endocrinologist Elliot P. Joslin. Benedict studied metabolism in newborn infants, growing children and adolescents, starving people, athletes, and vegetarians; he also investigated the effects of diet, temperature regulation, and exercise on metabolism.

thePoint

Visit **thePoint.lww.com/MKKSEN4e** *for more details on Benedict's numerous research studies about calorimetry and measurement of energy expenditure using highly sophisticated, hand-made respiratory-metabolic instrumentation.*

THYROID DYSFUNCTION, STROKE RISK, AND ACUTE MYOCARDIAL INFARCTION

Increased blood platelet aggregation and impaired myocardial blood supply from steroid use could increase risk of stroke and acute myocardial infarction. For rats, anabolic steroids exerted a direct action on the thyroid gland and peripheral metabolism of thyroid hormones in a manner that also could precipitate thyroid gland dysfunction.[58]

high dosages of steroids often impair normal testosterone–endocrine function. Twenty-six weeks of steroid administration to male power athletes reduced serum testosterone to less than one half of the level when the study began; this effect lasted throughout a 12- to 16-week steroid-free follow-up.[56] Infertility, reduced sperm concentrations (azoospermia), and decreased testicular volume pose additional problems for the steroid abuser. Gonadal function usually returns to normal after several months of steroid cessation.

Other hormonal alterations that accompany steroid use in men include a sevenfold increase in estradiol concentration, the major female hormone. The higher estradiol level represents the average value for normal women and possibly explains the **gynecomastia** (excessive development of the male mammary glands, sometimes secreting milk) noted in steroid-using men. Steroid use with exercise training also causes connective tissue damage that decreases the tensile strength and elastic compliance of tendons.[110,116,140] Steroids use causes the following five worrisome responses[67,75,83,95,130,186]:

1. Chronic stimulation of the prostate gland (may increase prostate size)
2. Possible kidney malfunction
3. Injury and alterations in cardiovascular function and myocardial cell cultures
4. Possible pathologic ventricular growth and dysfunction when combined with resistance training
5. Impaired cardiac microvascular adaptation to exercise training and increased blood platelet aggregation

Steroid Use and Life-Threatening Disease

Dramatic life-shortening effects of steroids occurred in adult rats exposed to the type and relative levels of steroids taken by physically active humans. One year after terminating the 6-month steroid exposure, 52% of the mice given the high dosage had died compared with only 35% of the mice given the low dosage and 12% of the control animals not given the exogenous hormone (**FIG. 11.4**). Autopsy of steroid-treated mice revealed a broad array of pathologic effects that did not appear until long after cessation of steroid use. Most prevalent pathologies included liver and kidney tumors, lymphosarcomas, and heart damage, frequently in combinations. A 6-month exposure period represents about one fifth of a male mouse's life expectancy, a relative duration considerably longer than exposures of most humans to steroid use. Several of the pathologies, particularly liver damage, are typically seen in humans on steroids. These findings, if applicable to humans, indicate that it may require several decades before the true negative effects of chronic anabolic steroid use emerge.

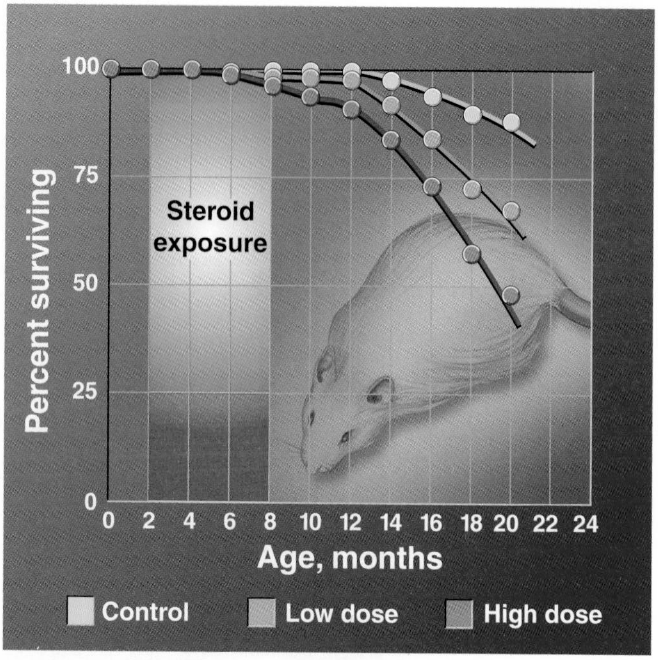

FIGURE 11.4. Life-shortening effects of exogenous anabolic steroid use in mice. (Modified from Bronson FH, Matherne CM. Exposure to anabolic-androgenic steroids shortens life span of male mice. *Med Sci Sports Exerc* 1997;29:615.)

TABLE 11.3 lists side effects and medical risks of anabolic steroid use. Concern centers on evidence about possible links between androgen abuse and abnormal liver function. The liver almost exclusively metabolizes androgens, making it particularly susceptible to damage from long-term steroid use and toxic excess. One of the serious effects of androgens on the liver occurs when it develops localized blood-filled lesions called **peliosis hepatis**. In the extreme, the liver eventually fails and the patient dies. We present these data to emphasize the potentially serious side effects, even when a physician prescribes the drug in the recommended dosage. Patients often take steroids for a longer duration than athletes, with some athletes taking steroids on and off for decades, with daily doses exceeding typical therapeutic levels (5–20 mg versus 50–200 mg used by some athletes).

Steroid Use and Plasma Lipoproteins

Anabolic steroid use, particularly orally active 17-alkylated androgens, in healthy men and women rapidly reduces high-density lipoprotein cholesterol (HDL-C), elevates both

TABLE 11.3 Side Effects and Medical Risks of Anabolic Steroids

Men		Women	
Increase	Decrease	Increase	Decrease
Testicular atrophy	Sperm count	Voice change	Breast tissue
Gynecomastia	Testosterone levels	Facial hair Menstrual irregularities Clitoral enlargement	

Men and Women		
Increase	**Decrease**	**Possible Effect**
LDL-C	HDL-C	Hypertension
LDL-C/HDL-C		Connective tissue damage
Potential for neoplastic disease of the liver		Myocardial damage
Aggressiveness, hyperactivity, irritability		Myocardial infarction
Withdrawal and depression upon stopping use		Impaired thyroid function
Acne		Altered myocardial structure
Peliosis hepatitis		

LDL-C, low-density lipoprotein cholesterol; HDL-C, high-density lipoprotein cholesterol.

low-density lipoprotein cholesterol (LDL-C) and total cholesterol, and reduces the HDL-C to LDL-C ratio. The HDL-C of weightlifters who used anabolic steroids averaged 26 $mg \cdot dL^{-1}$ compared with 50 $mg \cdot dL^{-1}$ for weightlifters not taking steroids.[94] Reduced HDL-C at this level increases a steroid user's coronary artery disease risk. HDL-C remained low among weightlifters, even after abstaining from steroid use for at least 8 weeks between consecutive steroid cycles.[169] The long-term effects of steroid use on cardiovascular morbidity and mortality remain unquantified.

Position Statement on Anabolic Steroids

As part of their long-range educational program, the ACSM has taken a stand on the use and abuse of anabolic–androgenic steroids.[6] We endorse their position, which follows.

American College of Sports Medicine Position Stand on Use of Anabolic Steroids

Based on a comprehensive survey of the world literature and a careful analysis of the claims made for and against the efficacy of anabolic–androgenic steroids in improving human physical performance, it is the position of the American College of Sports Medicine that

1. Anabolic–androgenic steroids with an adequate diet and training can contribute to increases in body weight, often in the lean mass compartment.
2. The gains in muscular strength achieved through intense exercise and proper diet can occur by the increased use of anabolic–androgenic steroids in some persons.
3. Anabolic–androgenic steroids do not increase aerobic power or capacity for muscular exercise.
4. Anabolic–androgenic steroids have been associated with adverse effects on the liver, cardiovascular system, reproductive system, and psychological status in therapeutic trials and in limited research on athletes. Until further research is completed, the potential hazards of the use of the anabolic–androgenic steroids in athletes must include those found in therapeutic trials.
5. The use of anabolic–androgenic steroids by athletes is contrary to the rules and ethical principles of athletic competition as set forth by many of the sports governing bodies. The American College of Sports Medicine supports these ethical principles and deplores the use of anabolic–androgenic steroids by athletes.

Steroid Side Effects in Females

In addition to the broad range of side effects from anabolic steroid use, females have additional concerns about their dangers. These include virilization (more apparent than in men), disruption of normal growth pattern by premature closure of the plates for bone growth (also for boys), deepened voice, altered menstrual function, dramatic increase in sebaceous gland size, acne, hirsutism (excessive body and facial hair), decreased breast size, and enlarged clitoris.

CLENBUTEROL AND OTHER β_2-ADRENERGIC AGONISTS: ANABOLIC STEROID SUBSTITUTES?

Extensive, random testing of competitive athletes for anabolic steroid use worldwide has ushered in a number of steroid "substitutes." These have appeared on the illicit health food, mail order, and "black market" drug networks as competitors try to circumvent detection. One such drug, the sympathomimetic amine **clenbuterol** (brand name examples include Broncodil, Cesbron, Clenasma, Monores, Novegan, Prontovent, Promeco, and Spiropent), has become popular among athletes because of its purported tissue-building, fat-reducing benefits. When a bodybuilder discontinues steroid use before competition to avoid detection and possible disqualification, the athlete substitutes clenbuterol to retard loss of muscle mass and facilitate fat burning to achieve the required "cut" look. Clenbuterol has particular appeal to female athletes because it does not produce similar androgenic side effects of anabolic steroids.

Clenbuterol, one of a group of chemical compounds (albuterol, clenbuterol, salbutamol, salmeterol, terbutaline) classified as a β_2-adrenergic agonist, facilitates responsiveness of adrenergic receptors to circulating epinephrine, norepinephrine, and other adrenergic amines. A review of the available studies of animals indicates that when fed to sedentary, growing livestock in dosages in excess of those prescribed in Europe for human use for bronchial asthma, clenbuterol repartitions body composition by increasing skeletal and cardiac muscle protein deposition and slows fat gain (enhanced lipolysis). Clenbuterol, in combination with angiotensin-converting enzymes, β-blockers, angiotensin II inhibitors, and aldosterone antagonists, has been used with some success in human studies of severe heart failure.[18]

CLENBUTEROL EFFECTS IN ANIMALS

1. Increases FFM and decreases fat mass when administered long term at therapeutic levels to thoroughbred racehorses partly due to changes in plasma concentrations of adiponectin and leptin.[96,97]
2. Countered the effects on muscle of aging, immobilization, malnutrition, and pathologic tissue-wasting conditions. With clenbuterol, the β_2-agonists have specific growth-promoting actions on skeletal muscle.[51,208]
3. Altered muscle fiber type distribution, inducing enlargement and increased proportion of type II muscle fibers.[44] The decreased protein breakdown and increased protein synthesis accounted for the animals' increased muscle size from clenbuterol treatment.[1,17]

Potential Negative Effects on Muscle, Bone, and Cardiovascular Function

Female rats treated with clenbuterol injected subcutaneously or sham injected with the same volume of fluid carrier each day for 14 days increased (1) muscle mass, (2) absolute maximal force-generating capacity, and (3) hypertrophy of fast- and slow-twitch muscle fibers.[47] A negative finding showed hastened fatigue during short-term, intense muscle actions. In other studies, regular exercise and regular exercise combined with clenbuterol decreased the progression of muscular dystrophy in *mdx* mice as reflected by increases in muscle force-generating capacity.[208] The group receiving clenbuterol also experienced increased muscle fatigability and cellular deformities not noted in the exercise-only group. Other research with mice indicates a decrease in force production in isolated intact skeletal muscle fiber bundles with clenbuterol administration.[124]

This negative effect on muscle structure and function may explain findings that clenbuterol treatment negated the beneficial effects of exercise training on endurance performance of animals, despite increases in muscle protein content.[84,178] Clenbuterol treatment induced muscular hypertrophy in young male rats, but it concomitantly inhibited the longitudinal growth of bones.[105] This effect may relate to clenbuterol's acceleration of epiphyseal closure in the bones of growing animals and certainly would contraindicate its use for prepubescent and adolescent humans.

Reported short-term side effects in humans accidentally "overdosing" from eating clenbuterol-tainted meat include the following eight negative effects:

1. Skeletal muscle tremor
2. Agitation
3. Palpitations
4. Dizziness
5. Nausea
6. Muscle cramps
7. Rapid heart rate (tachycardia)
8. Headache

Clenbuterol cannot be justified or recommended for use as an ergogenic aid. This drug should not be used for nonmedical applications.

Other β_2-Adrenergic Agonists

Research has focused on possible strength-enhancing effects of sympathomimetic β_2-adrenergic agonists other than clenbuterol. Men with cervical spinal cord injuries took 80 mg of **metaproterenol** daily for 4 weeks in conjunction with physical therapy. Increases occurred in estimated muscle cross-sectional area and strength of the elbow flexors and wrist extensors compared with the placebo condition.[176] **Albuterol** administration (16 mg·day^{-1} for 3 weeks) without exercise training improved muscular strength by 10 to 15%.[120] Therapeutic doses of albuterol also facilitated isokinetic strength gains from slow-speed concentric/eccentric isokinetic training.[30] **Salbutamol** ingestion over the short term and with a single dose increased maximal anaerobic power output on the Wingate anaerobic exercise test.[114]

A BLUNTED RESPONSE WITH TRAINING

Albuterol's ergogenic benefit supposedly comes from its stimulating effects on skeletal muscle β_2-receptors to increase muscle force and power. With exercise training, the muscle β_2-receptors undergo downregulation (become less sensitive to a given stimulus) from long-term exposure to training-induced elevations in blood catecholamine levels. This makes the trained athlete less responsive to a sympathomimetic drug than an untrained counterpart.

Training State Makes a Difference

Animal Research

Untrained skeletal muscle responds to the effects of β_2-adrenergic agonists. The increase in muscle mass with clenbuterol treatment plus exercise training becomes more pronounced in animals without prior training experience than in trained animals that continue training and then receive this β_2-adrenergic agonist.[139]

Human Research

Some research shows augmented muscle power output with albuterol administration.[175] No ergogenic effect on short-term performance emerged from salbutamol administration in two 10-minute cycling trials.[40] Similarly, no effect on power output during a 30-second Wingate test occurred in nonasthmatic trained cyclists who received 360 μg (twice the normal dose administered by inhaler in four measured doses of 90 μg each) 20 minutes before testing.[113] Twice the recommended dose of salbutamol (albuterol; 400 μg administered in four inhalations 20 min before exercising) did not enhance anaerobic power output, endurance performance, ventilatory threshold, or dynamic lung function of trained endurance cyclists.[147] No beneficial effect occurred in the pulmonary function and oxygen loading characteristics of the blood of trained male athletes who inhaled bronchodilators that contained β_2-adrenergic agonists before exercising.[79] Such findings support the argument that competitive athletes should not be prohibited from using these compounds because they provide no ergogenic benefit, yet they "normalize" physiologic function in persons with obstructive pulmonary disorders. Differences in the groups' training status may explain discrepancies among studies concerning albuterol's effect on short-term power output.

GROWTH HORMONE: GENETIC ENGINEERING COMES TO SPORTS

Human growth hormone (**GH** or **hGH**), also known as *somatotropin,* now competes with anabolic steroids in the illicit market of alleged tissue-building, performance-enhancing drugs. The pituitary gland's adenohypophysis produces GH. This potent anabolic and lipolytic agent plays important roles for tissue building and growth and increasing fat catabolism. Specifically, GH stimulates bone and cartilage growth, enhances fatty acid oxidation, and slows glucose and amino acid breakdown. Reduced GH secretion, which turns out to be 50% less at age 60 than age 30, accounts for some of the decreases in FFM and increases in fat mass that accompany aging. Exogenous recombinant GH supplements produced by genetically engineered bacteria can reverse these negative changes in body composition. Such results have led to a dramatic rise in the number of antiaging clinics throughout the country that provide GH to thousands of older persons looking to "turn back the clock" at a cost of $1000 or more a month. A Google Web search for the term *human growth hormone* yielded 8,810,000 results; adding the terms *antiaging* to narrow the search produced 1,750,000 Web sites! The same search on Yahoo! produced 29 million Web sites for *human growth hormone* and 37,100,000 sites when *antiaging* was added to the search.

ARE THE BENEFITS WORTH THE RISKS?

Young athletes who take GH believing they gain a competitive edge suffer increased incidence of gigantism, and adults develop acromegalic syndrome. In addition, less visual side effects include insulin resistance that leads to type 2 diabetes, water retention, and carpal tunnel compression.

Research has produced equivocal results concerning the true benefits of GH supplementation to counter the accumulated effects of aging—loss of muscle mass, thinning bones, increase in body fat (particularly abdominal fat), and a depressed energy level. For example, healthy men 70 to 85 years old who received GH supplements increased FFM by 4.3% and decreased fat mass by 13.1%.[153] Supplementation did not reverse the negative effects of aging on functional measures of muscular strength and aerobic capacity. Men receiving the supplement experienced hand stiffness, malaise (general discomfort or uneasiness), arthralgias (joint pain, a symptom of injury, infection, arthritis, or allergic reaction to medication), and lower extremity edema or swelling. One of the largest studies to date determined the effects of GH on changes in body composition and functional capacity of healthy men and women who ranged in age from mid-60s to late 80s.[19] Men who took GH gained 7 lb of lean body mass and lost a similar amount of fat mass. Women gained about 3 lb of lean body mass and lost 5 lb of body fat compared with counterparts who received

TABLE 11.4 Maximal Force Production of Knee Extensor and Flexor Muscle Groups Before and After Training With or Without Growth Hormone (GH) Supplements

	Exercise Plus Placebo			Exercise Plus GH		
Force	Initial[a]	Final[a]	% Change	Initial[a]	Final[a]	% Change
Concentric						
Knee extensors	212 ± 13	248 ± 10	+17	191 ± 11	214 ± 9	+12
Knee flexors	137 ± 11	158 ± 7	+15	122 ± 12	143 ± 6	+17
Isometric						
Knee extensors	220 ± 13	252 ± 13	+14	198 ± 15	207 ± 7	+5
Knee flexors	131 ± 8	158 ± 8	+20	127 ± 13	140 ± 16	+10

From Yarasheski KF, et al. Effect of growth hormone and resistance exercise on muscle growth in young men. Am J Physiol 1992;262:E261.

[a] Values are mean ± standard error. Maximum force (N) determined using a Cybex dynamometer. Concentric force measured at 60°·s^{-1} angular velocity. Isometric force measured at 135° of knee extension. The maximum concentric force production of the knee flexor and extensor muscles increased significantly in both groups ($P < .05$), but these increments and the increments in maximum isometric force production were not greater in the exercise plus GH group.

a placebo. The subjects remained sedentary and did not change their diet over the 6-month study period. Unfortunately, serious side effects afflicted between 24 and 46% of the subjects. These included swollen feet and ankles, joint pain, carpal tunnel syndrome (swelling of tendon sheath over a nerve in the wrist), and development of diabetes or a prediabetic condition. As in previous research, no effects were noted for GH treatment on measures of muscular strength or endurance capacity despite increased lean body mass.

Excessive GH production during the growth period produces **gigantism**, an endocrine and metabolic disorder that triggers abnormal size or overgrowth of the entire body or any of its parts. Excessive GH production following cessation of growth produces the irreversible disorder **acromegaly**. Enlarged hands, feet, and facial features characterize this malady. Medically, children who suffer from kidney failure or GH deficiency receive thrice-weekly injections of this hormone until adolescence to help achieve near-normal size. In young adults with hypopituitarism, GH replacement therapy improves muscle volume, isometric strength, and exercise capacity. It also increases endurance capacity in GH-deficient patients.[38]

Disagreement Concerning Ergogenic Effects

At first glance, GH use seems appealing to the strength and power athlete because at physiologic levels this hormone stimulates amino acid uptake and muscle protein synthesis while enhancing lipid breakdown and conserving glycogen reserves. It also seems to enhance connective tissue protein synthesis. However, few well-controlled studies have examined how GH supplements affect healthy subjects who undertake exercise training. In one study, well-trained men maintained a high-protein diet while taking either biosynthetic GH or a placebo.[43] During 6 weeks of standard resistance training with GH, percentage body fat decreased and FFM increased. No changes in body composition occurred for the group training with the placebo. Subsequent investigations have not supported these findings. Previously sedentary young men who participated in a 12-week resistance training program received daily recombinant human GH supplements (40 μg·kg^{-1}) or a placebo.[205] FFM, total body water, and whole-body protein synthesis increased more in the GH recipients. No differences emerged between groups in fractional rate of protein synthesis in skeletal muscle and torso and limb circumferences. **TABLE 11.4** shows equivalent effects of control and experimental treatments on muscle function in dynamic and static strength measures. The authors attributed the greater increase in whole-body protein synthesis in the group receiving GH to a possible increase in nitrogen retention in lean tissue other than skeletal muscle (e.g., connective tissue, fluid, and noncontractile proteins).

Until fairly recently, healthy persons could obtain GH only on the black market and often in an adulterated form. Human cadaver-derived GH (used until 1985 by US physicians to treat children of short stature) greatly increases the risk for contracting Creutzfeldt-Jakob disease, an infectious, incurable brain-deteriorating disorder that leads to rapid decreases in mental function and movement. The disease probably results from a protein called a *prion* that causes normal proteins to fold abnormally and negatively affects other proteins' functions. Currently, a synthetic form of GH (Protoropin and Humantrope) produced by genetic engineering is approved for treating GH-deficient children. But once a drug reaches market, doctors can prescribe it at their discretion.

DHEA: A WORRISOME TREND

Increased use of synthetic **dehydroepiandrosterone (DHEA)** has raised concerns about its safety and effectiveness. DHEA and its sulfated ester, DHEA sulfate or DHEAS, a relatively weak steroid hormone, are synthesized from cholesterol primarily by the adrenal cortex. A small amount of DHEA commonly referred to as the "mother hormone" and other related **prohormone compounds** are naturally derived precursors to testosterone or other anabolic steroids. **FIGURE 11.5** outlines the major pathways for synthesizing DHEA, androstenedione, and related compounds.

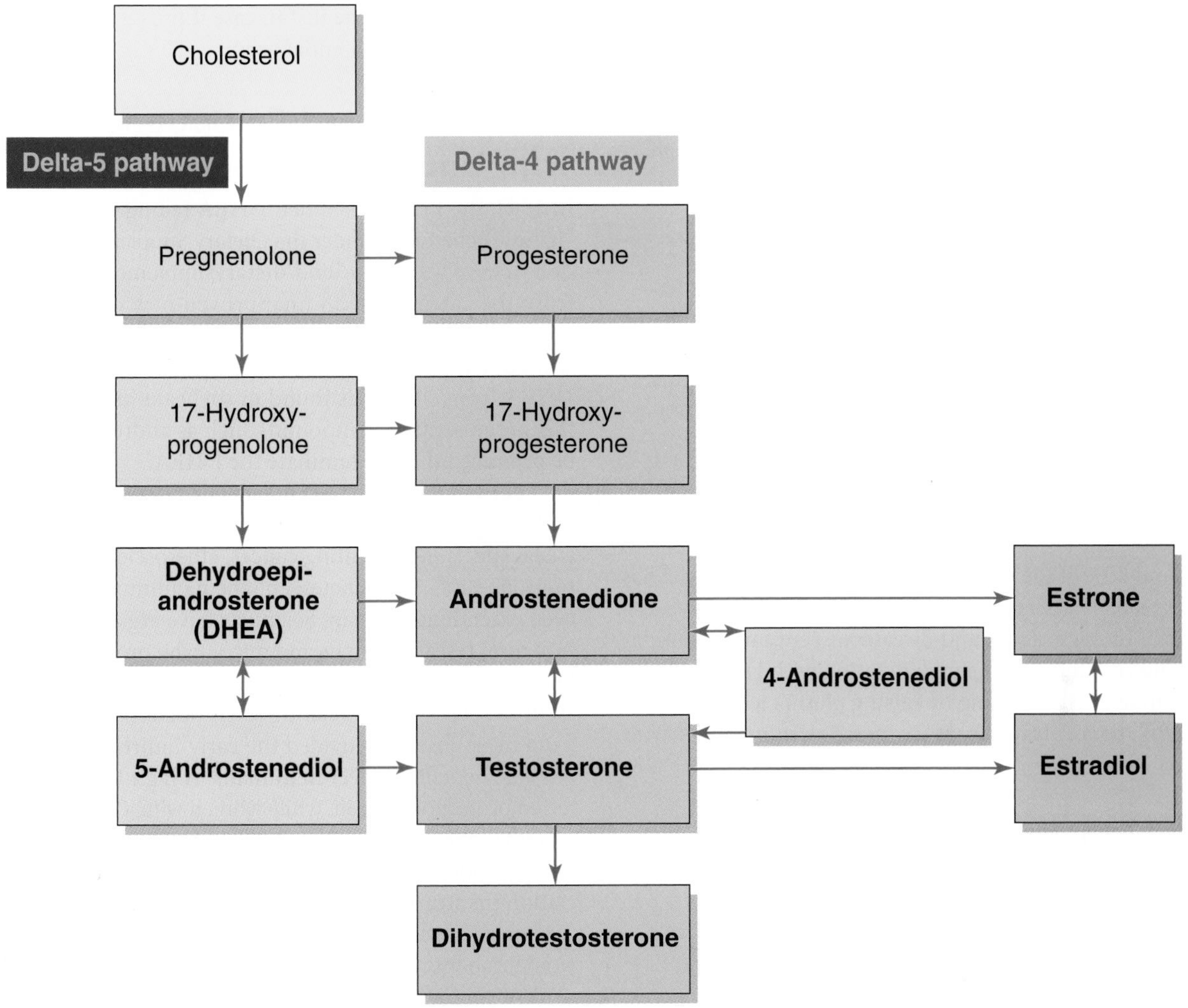

FIGURE 11.5. Proposed metabolic pathways for DHEA, androstenedione, and related compounds. *Directional arrows* signify one-way and two-way conversions. Compounds in *bold print* are products currently available on the market.

Advocates of DHEA claim that it extends life; protects against cancer, heart disease, diabetes, and osteoporosis; enhances sexual drive; facilitates lean tissue gain and body fat loss; enhances mood and memory; improves muscular capacity; and boosts immunity against various infectious diseases including AIDS. The hormone's detractors consider it "snake oil." The WADA, IOC, and US Olympic Committee (USOC)[3]* have placed DHEA on their banned substance lists at zero tolerance levels.

FIGURE 11.6 illustrates the generalized trend for plasma DHEA levels during a lifetime. For boys and girls, DHEA levels are substantial at birth and then decline sharply. A steady increase in DHEA production occurs from age 6 to 10 years, an occurrence that some researchers feel contributes to the beginning of puberty and secondary sex characteristics. Peak production occurs between ages 18 and 25 (higher in males than females). In contrast to the glucocorticoid and mineralocorticoid adrenal steroids whose plasma levels remain relatively high with aging, a long, slow decline in DHEA

BUYER BEWARE

The quantity of DHEA the body produces surpasses all other known steroids, with its largest concentrations in the brain. Its chemical structure closely resembles that of the sex hormones testosterone and estrogen. News reports and advertisements tout DHEA as a "super-hormone," a "Holy Grail" that increases testosterone production, preserves youth, invigorates sex life, and counters the debilitating effects of aging. Because DHEA occurs naturally, the Food and Drug Administration (FDA; www.fda.gov) has no control over its distribution or claims for its action and effectiveness. The lay press, mail order companies, and health food industry describe DHEA as a pill (even available as a chewing gum, each piece containing 25 mg) to cure just about any bodily ill.

*The US Olympic Committee (USOC) provides background information about prohibited substances and methods on their website (www.teamusa.org/legal/anti-doping-rules) with links to different sport organization websites (national governing bodies) and international federations. The USADA website (www.usada.org/prohibited-list/athlete-guide/) allows for a free PDF download of the "Athlete Guide to the 2011 Prohibited List."

MUCH REMAINS UNKNOWN

Despite its quantitative significance as a hormone, researchers know little about DHEA, particularly with respect to the following four areas:

1. Health and aging
2. Cellular or molecular mechanism(s) of action
3. Possible receptor sites (although its sulfate interacts with brain receptors for the neurotransmitter γ-aminobutyric acid [GABA])
4. Potential for adverse effects from exogenous dosage, particularly among young adults with normal DHEA levels

begins after age 30. By age 75, the plasma level decreases to only about 20% of the value in young adulthood. This fact has fueled speculation that plasma DHEA levels might serve as a marker of biologic aging and disease susceptibility. Popular reasoning concludes that supplementing with DHEA blunts the negative effects of aging by raising plasma levels to more "youthful" concentrations. Many persons supplement with this "natural" hormone just in case it proves beneficial, without considering its potential harm.

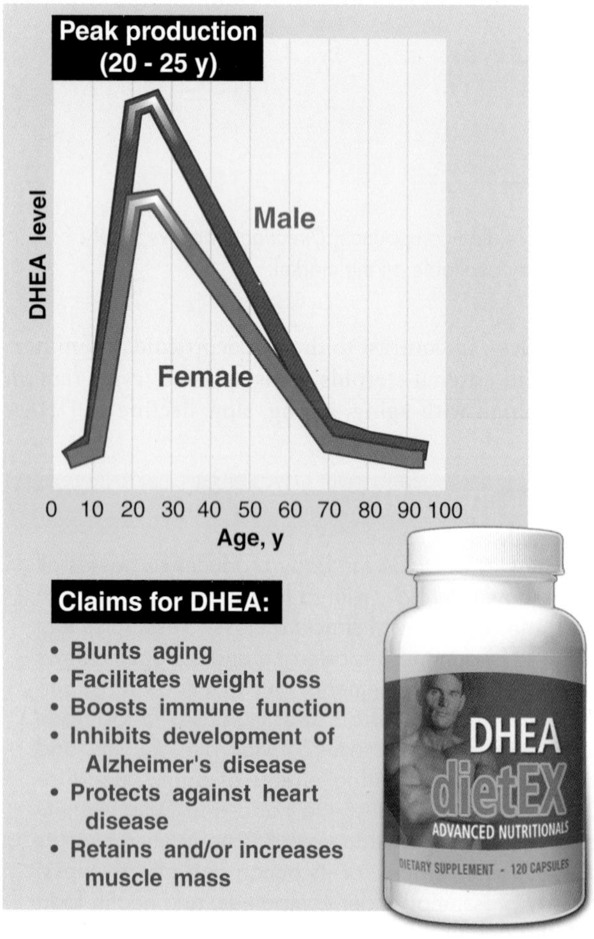

FIGURE 11.6. Generalized trend for plasma levels of DHEA for men and women during a lifetime.

An Unregulated Compound with Uncertain Safety

In 1994, the FDA reclassified DHEA (along with many other "natural" chemicals under the Dietary Supplement and Education Act; **www.fda.gov/food/dietarysupplements/default.htm**) from the category of an unapproved new drug requiring a prescription to a dietary supplement for sale over the counter without a prescription. Pharmaceutical companies synthesize DHEA from chemicals found in soybeans and wild yams. In this process, other compounds such as androstenedione may be produced that contaminate the DHEA.

Early support for DHEA came from studies of rodents fed daily supplements of this hormone. Treatment indicated beneficial effects in preventing cancer, atherosclerosis, viral infections, obesity, and diabetes; enhancing immune function; and even extending life span. Scientists have argued that the findings from research on rats and mice—who produce little, if any, DHEA—do not necessarily apply to healthy humans. Cross-sectional observations relating levels of DHEA to risk of death from heart disease provided the early indirect evidence for a possible beneficial effect in humans. A high DHEA level conferred protection in men, while women with a high DHEA level increased their heart disease risk. Subsequent research showed only a moderate protective association for men and no association for women. DHEA supplements might also provide a cardioprotective effect with aging (more beneficial in men than women), boost immune function in disease, and provide antioxidant protection during aging.

In other research on humans, middle-aged men and women received either 100 mg of DHEA or a placebo daily for 3 months and the other treatment for the next 3 months.[136] Both groups exhibited a slight increase of 1.2% in lean body mass during DHEA supplementation. Fat mass decreased in the men, but a small increase occurred for the women. Chemical markers also indicated improved immune function. An increase in muscle mass and strength induced by intense

VALID CONCERNS ABOUT DHEA

The appropriate DHEA dosage for humans has not been determined. Concern exists about possible harmful effects on blood lipids, glucose tolerance, and prostate gland health. The major reason is because medical problems associated with hormone supplementation often do not appear until years after initiation of use. A number of over-the-counter supplements contain DHEA (and other prohormones). One can readily purchase DHEA through mainstream grocery chains, drug and nutrition stores, health clubs, mail order catalogs, and the Internet. Interestingly, no data exist concerning ergogenic effects of DHEA supplements on young adult men and women.

resistance training occurred with DHEA supplementation in elderly men and women.[198] These findings suggested several possible positive effects of exogenous DHEA on muscle mass and immune system function and responsiveness to resistance training in middle-aged and elderly adults.

Research in young men evaluated short-term ingestion of 50 mg of DHEA daily on serum steroid hormones and the effect of 8 weeks of supplementation (150 mg daily) on resistance training adaptations.[25] Short-term DHEA supplementation rapidly increased serum androstenedione concentrations, although it exerted *no effect* on serum testosterone and estrogen concentrations. Furthermore, longer term DHEA supplementation raised serum androstenedione levels but had *no effect* on anabolic hormones, serum lipids, liver enzymes, muscular strength, and lean body mass compared with a placebo given to men undergoing similar training. These and similar results of other investigators indicate that relatively low dosages of DHEA do not increase serum testosterone levels, enhance muscular strength, change muscle and fat cross-sectional areas, or facilitate adaptations to resistance training.

Concern exists about the effect of unregulated long-term DHEA supplementation (particularly in doses >50 mg daily) on body function and overall health. Converting DHEA into potent androgens like testosterone in the body promotes facial hair growth in females and alters normal menstrual function. As with exogenous anabolic steroids, DHEA lowers HDL-C, which increases heart disease risk. Limited, conflicting data exist concerning its effects on breast cancer risk. Clinicians have expressed fear that elevated plasma DHEA through supplementation might stimulate growth of otherwise dormant prostate gland tumors or cause benign hypertrophy of the prostate gland itself. If cancer is present, DHEA may accelerate its growth.

On a positive note, data show that supplements of DHEA for elderly men and women decreased abdominal (visceral) fat and improved the body's use of insulin.[199] Such findings indicate a potential for DHEA in treating components of the metabolic syndrome.

DHEA supplementation also may reduce the required dose of corticosteroid medication required by patients with the autoimmune disease lupus—a systemic autoimmune disease that can affect any part of the body resulting in inflammation and tissue damage.[196] This effect would certainly reduce side effects such as accelerated osteoporosis that accompany steroid therapy.

ANDROSTENEDIONE: BENIGN PROHORMONE NUTRITIONAL SUPPLEMENT OR POTENTIALLY HARMFUL DRUG?

Many physically active persons use the legal over-the-counter "nutritional" supplement **androstenedione** (and androstenediol and norandrostenediol), believing that these steroid products accomplish the following:

1. Directly stimulate endogenous testosterone production or form androgen-like derivatives (as shown in **FIG. 11.5**)
2. Enable them to train harder, build muscle mass, and repair injury more rapidly

Androstenedione occurs naturally in meat and extracts of some plants; many of the more than 700,000 Internet sites tout androstenedione as "a prohormone, a metabolite only one step away from the biosynthesis of testosterone." Originally developed by East Germany in the 1970s to enhance performance of their elite athletes, androstenedione was first commercially manufactured and sold in the United States in 1996. By calling the substance a supplement and avoiding any claims of medical benefits, the 1994 FDA rules enable androstenedione to be marketed as a food. Many countries consider androstenedione a controlled substance, so persons travel to the United States to purchase it, further contributing to the supplement industry's increasing yearly sales. Delivery systems for androstenedione include capsules, percutaneous gels, transdermal patches, chewing gums, and steroid lozenges that dissolve under the tongue.

EIGHT RESEARCH FINDINGS CONCERNING ANDROSTENEDIONE

1. Little or no elevation of plasma testosterone concentrations
2. No favorable effect on muscle mass
3. No favorable effect on muscular performance
4. No favorable alterations in body composition
5. Elevates various estrogen subfractions
6. No favorable effects on muscle protein synthesis or tissue anabolism
7. Impairs the blood lipid profile in apparently healthy men
8. Increases likelihood of testing positive for steroid use

Androstenedione, an intermediate or precursor hormone between DHEA and testosterone, aids the liver in synthesizing other biologically active steroid hormones. Normally produced by the adrenal glands and gonads, it converts to testosterone enzymatically by 17β-hydroxysteroid dehydrogenase found in diverse body tissues. Androstenedione also serves as an estrogen precursor.

Little scientific evidence supports claims about the cryogenic effectiveness or anabolic qualities of andro-type compounds. One study showed that oral treatment with 200 mg of 4-androstene-3,17-dione or 200 mg of 4-androstene-3β,17β-diol increased peripheral plasma total and free testosterone concentrations compared with a placebo.[52] Androstenedione dosages as high as 300 mg daily have elevated testosterone levels by 34%.[110] Chronic androstenedione administration also elevates serum estradiol and estrone in men and women. This response could offset any potential anabolic effect.

COMPETITIVE ATHLETES BEWARE

Consuming trace amounts as low as 10 μg of 19-norandrostenedione daily (levels common in over-the-counter androstenedione supplements) often causes many users to test positive for 19-norandrosterone, the standard marker for the banned anabolic steroid nandrolone. Many nutritional supplements may be tainted with 19-norandrostenedione (and undisclosed by product labeling), so the caveat "buyer beware" is all too apropos. Ironically, although androgen prohormone supplements taken in large dosages may transiently increase serum testosterone, they exert no ergogenic effects on muscular strength, no favorable alterations in body composition, and no enhancement of overall health profile.

A two-phase investigation systematically evaluated whether short- or long-term androstenedione supplementation elevates blood testosterone concentrations or enhances muscle size and strength gains during resistance training.[102] In one phase, young adult men received either a single 100-mg dose of androstenedione or a placebo containing 250 mg of rice flour. **FIGURE 11.7A** shows that serum androstenedione increased 175% during the first 60 minutes following ingestion and then increased further to 350% above baseline values between minutes 90 and 270. On the other hand, short-term supplementation did not affect serum concentrations of either free or total testosterone.

In the experiment's second phase, young men received either 300 mg of androstenedione or 250 mg of a rice flour placebo daily during weeks 1, 2, 4, 5, 7, and 8 of an 8-week whole-body resistance training program. Serum androstenedione levels increased 100% in the androstenedione-supplemented

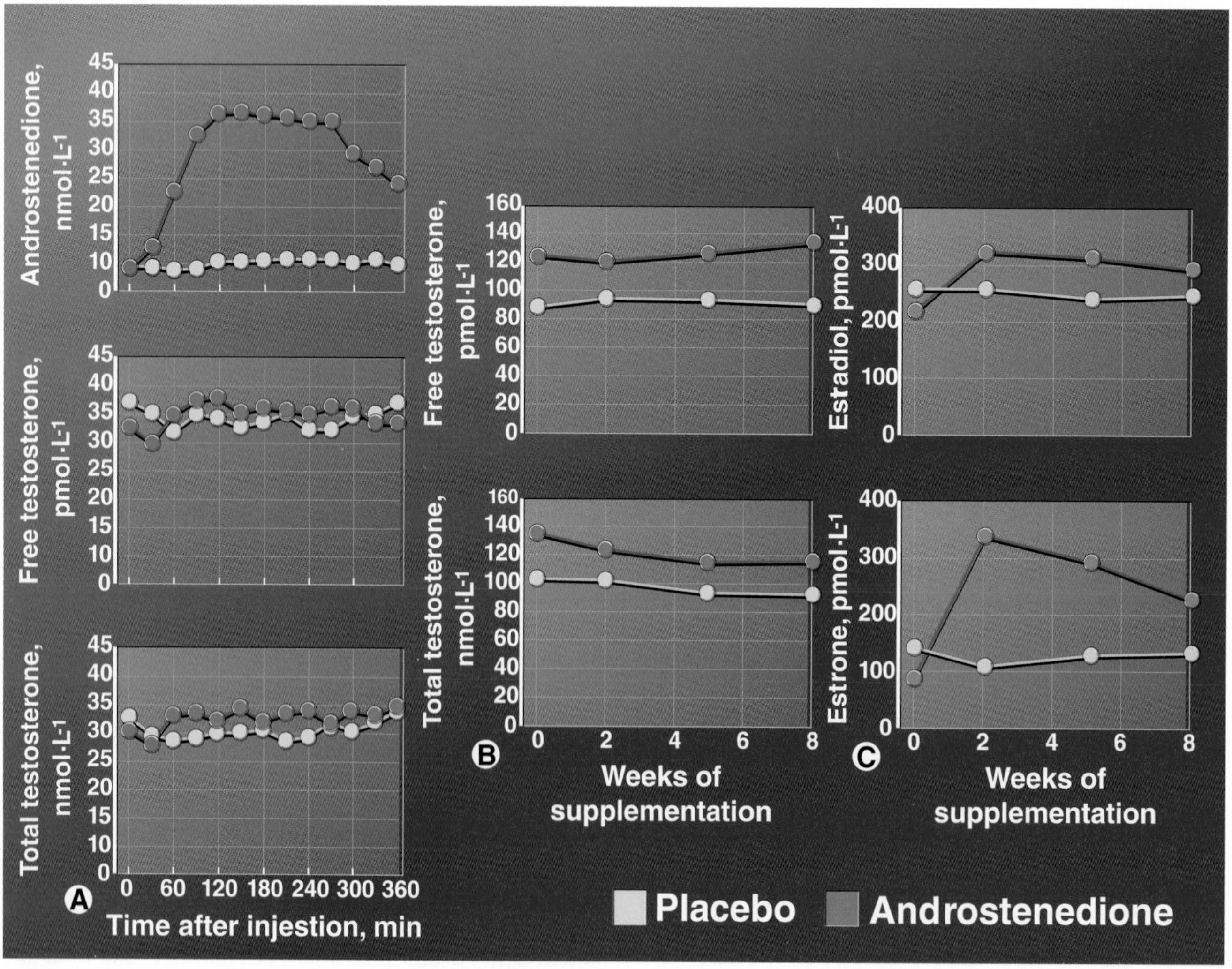

FIGURE 11.7. **(A)** Effect of short-term (single-dose) exogenous supplementation with 100 mg of androstenedione or placebo on serum concentrations of androstenedione and free and total testosterone. Serum free and total testosterone **(B)** and serum estradiol and estrone **(C)** with 300-mg daily supplementation and androstenedione (n = 9) during 8 weeks of resistance training. (From King DS, et al. Effect of oral androstenedione on serum testosterone and adaptations to resistance training in young men. *JAMA* 1999;281:2020.)

group and remained elevated throughout training. Although serum testosterone levels (**FIG. 11.7B**) remained higher in the androstenedione-supplemented group than in the placebo group before and after supplementation, they remained unaltered for both groups during the supplementation–training period. Serum estradiol and estrone concentrations increased during training in the group receiving the supplement. This suggested increased aromatization of the ingested androstenedione to estrogens (**FIG. 11.7C**). Resistance training increased muscle strength and lean body mass and reduced body fat for both groups, but no synergistic effect emerged with androstenedione supplementation. Instead, the supplement caused a 12% HDL-C *reduction* after only 2 weeks, which remained lower for the 8-week training period.[24,102] Serum liver enzyme concentrations remained within normal limits for both groups throughout the experimental period.

These findings indicate *no effect* of androstenedione supplementation on the following two factors:

1. Basal serum concentrations of testosterone
2. Training response for muscle size and strength and body composition

Worrisome are the potentially negative effects of a lowered HDL-C on overall heart disease risk and elevated serum estrogen level on gynecomastia risk and possibly pancreatic and other cancers. *The findings must be viewed within the context of this specific study because test subjects took far smaller dosages of androstenedione (≤300 mg · d^{-1}) than those routinely taken in substantial doses by bodybuilders and other athletes.*

A Modified Version

Norandrostenedione and norandrostenediol are norsteroid compounds available over the counter in the United States. They are chemically similar to androstenedione and androstenediol, respectively, with slight chemical modification that supposedly enhances anabolic properties without converting to testosterone but to the steroid nandrolone. These modifications should theoretically confer anabolic effects via the compounds' direct activation of skeletal muscle's androgen receptors. To test this hypothesis, research evaluated 8 weeks of low-dose norsteroid supplementation on body composition, girth measures, muscular strength, and mood states of young adult, resistance-trained men.[191] The men received either 100 mg of 19-nor-4-androstene-3,17-dione plus 56 mg of 19-nor-4-androstene-3,17-diol (156 mg total norsteroid per day) or a multivitamin placebo. Each subject also resistance-trained 4 days a week for the duration of the study. Norsteroid supplementation provided *no additional effect* on any of the body composition or exercise performance variables measured.

AMPHETAMINES

Amphetamines *or "pep pills" consist of pharmacologic compounds that exert a powerful stimulating effect on central nervous system function.* Athletes most frequently use amphetamine (Benzedrine) and dextroamphetamine sulfate (Dexedrine). Amphetamines are sympathomimetic because their effects mimic actions of the sympathetic hormones epinephrine and norepinephrine. These hormones increase blood pressure, pulse rate, cardiac output, breathing rate, metabolism, and blood sugar. Taking 5 to 20 mg of amphetamine usually produces an effect for 30 to 90 minutes after ingestion, although the drug's influence can persists much longer. Besides arousing sympathetic function, amphetamines supposedly increase alertness and wakefulness and augment work capacity by depressing sensations of muscle fatigue. The deaths of two famed cyclists in the 1960s during competitive road racing were attributed to amphetamine use for just such purposes. In one of these deaths in 1967, British Tour de France rider Tom Simpson overheated and suffered a fatal heart attack during the ascent of Mont Ventoux. Soldiers in World War II commonly used amphetamines to increase alertness and reduce feelings of fatigue. Consequently, it should come as little surprise that athletes use amphetamines believing they gain an ergogenic edge; ironically, little or no performance advantage exists.

Dangers of Amphetamines

The following five facts argue against amphetamine use:

1. Chronic use leads to physiologic or emotional drug dependency. This often causes cyclical use of "uppers" (amphetamines) and "downers" (barbiturates)—the barbiturates reduce or tranquilize the "hyper" state brought on by amphetamines.
2. General side effects include headache, tremulousness, agitation, insomnia, nausea, dizziness, and confusion, all of which negatively affect sports performance requiring rapid reaction and judgment and a high level of steadiness and mental concentration.
3. Taking larger doses eventually requires more drug to achieve the same effect because drug tolerance increases with prolonged use; this may aggravate or even precipitate cardiovascular and mental disorders.
4. The drugs suppress normal mechanisms for perceiving and responding to pain, fatigue, or heat stress; this effect severely jeopardizes health and safety.
5. Prolonged intake of high doses produces weight loss, paranoia, psychosis, repetitive compulsive behavior, and nerve damage.

Amphetamine Use and Athletic Performance

TABLE 11.5 summarizes the results of seven experiments on amphetamine use and physical performance. In almost all instances, amphetamines produced little or no positive effect on exercise capacity or the performance of simple psychomotor skills.

Athletes take amphetamines to get "up" psychologically for competition. On the day or evening before a contest, competitors often seem nervous and irritable and have

TABLE 11.5 Summary of Results on the Effects of Amphetamines on Athletic Performance

Study	Dose (mg)	Type of Experiment	Effect of Amphetamines
1.	10–20	Two all-out treadmill runs with 10-min rest between runs Consecutive 100-yd swims with 10-min rest intervals 220- to 440-yd swims for time 220-yd track runs for time 100-yd to 2-mile track runs for time	None None None None None
2.	10	Bench stepping to fatigue carrying weights equal to 1/3 body mass, 3 times with 3-min rest intervals	None
3.	5	100-yd swim for speed	None
4.	10	All-out treadmill runs	None
5.	10	Stationary cycling at work rates of 275–2215 $kg \cdot m \cdot min^{-1}$ for 25–35 min followed by treadmill run to exhaustion	None on submaximal or maximal oxygen uptake, heart rate, ventilation volume, or blood lactate; work time on the bicycle and treadmill increased
6.	20	Reaction and movement time to a visual stimulus	None; subjective feelings of alertness or lethargy unrelated to reaction or movement time
7.	5	Psychomotor performance during a simulated airplane flight	Enhanced performance and lessened fatigue, but if preceded by secobarbital (barbiturate), decreased performance

1. Karpovich PV. *Effect of amphetamine sulfate on athletic performance.* JAMA 1959;170:558.
2. Foltz EE, et al. *The influence of amphetamine (Benzedrine) sulfate and caffeine on the performance of rapidly exhausting work by untrained subjects.* J Lab Clin Med 1943;28:601.
3. Haldi J, Wynn W. *Action of drugs on efficiency of swimmers.* Res Q 1959;17:96.
4. Golding LA, Barnard RJ. *The effects of d-amphetamine sulfate on physical performance.* J Sports Phys Med Fitness 1963;3:221.
5. Wyndham CH, et al. *Physiological effects of the amphetamines during exercise.* S Afr Med J 1971;45:247.
6. Pierson WR, et al. *Some psychological effects of the administration of amphetamine sulfate and meprobamate on speed of movement and reaction time.* Med Sci Sports 1961;12:61.
7. McKenzie RE, Elliot LL. *Effects of secobarbital and d-amphetamine on performance during a simulated air mission.* Aerospace Med 1965;36:774.

difficulty relaxing. Under these circumstances, they take a barbiturate to induce sleep. They then regain the "hyper" condition by popping an "upper." This cycle of depressant-to-stimulant becomes potentially dangerous because the stimulant acts abnormally following barbiturate intake. The IOC, American Medical Association, and most sport-governing groups have banned amphetamine use. Ironically, most research indicates that amphetamines do *not* enhance exercise performance. Perhaps their greatest influence pertains to the psychological realm, where naive athletes believe that taking any supplement contributes to a superior performance. A placebo containing an inert substance often produces identical results.

CAFFEINE

Caffeine represents a compound whose classification and prior regulatory status depend on its use as a drug (over-the-counter migraine products), food (in coffee and soft drinks), or dietary supplement (alertness products). Caffeine is a possible exception to the general rule against taking stimulants.[98,99,107,206] In moderate doses, caffeine is well tolerated. The average American consumes 250 mg of caffeine daily, making it the most widely consumed behaviorally active substance worldwide. About 70% of caffeine is consumed in coffee, while soft drinks make up 15% and chocolate about 2%.

Caffeine belongs to a group of lipid-soluble compounds called *purines* (chemical name, 1,3,7-trimethylxanthine) found naturally in coffee beans, tea leaves, chocolate, cocoa beans, and cola nuts and often added to carbonated beverages and nonprescription medicines. Sixty-three plant species contain caffeine in their leaves, seeds, or fruits. In the United States, 75% or 14 million kg of caffeine intake comes from coffee, which amounts to 3.5 kg per person a year, 15% comes from tea, and the remainder comes from the items listed in **TABLE 11.6**. Depending on preparation, one cup of brewed coffee contains 60 to 150 mg of caffeine, instant coffee about 100 mg, brewed tea between 20 and 50 mg, and caffeinated soft drinks about 50 mg. For comparison, 2.5 cups of percolated coffee contain 250 to 400 mg of caffeine or between 3 and 6 $mg \cdot kg^{-1}$ body mass. This produces urinary caffeine concentrations within the previously established IOC acceptable limit of 12 $\mu g \cdot mL^{-1}$ and NCAA limit of 15 $\mu g \cdot mL^{-1}$. In January 2004, the IOC removed caffeine from its list of restricted substances.

TABLE 11.6 Caffeine Content (mg) of Some Common Foods, Beverages, and Over-the-Counter and Prescription Medications

Substance	Caffeine content (mg)
Beverages and Foods	
Coffee[a]	
Coffee, Starbucks, decaf, 12 oz	10
Coffee, Starbucks, grande, 16 oz	550
Coffee, Starbucks, tall, 12 oz	375
Coffee, Starbucks, short, 8 oz	250
Caffe, Starbucks, Americano, grande, 16 oz	105
Caffe, Starbucks, Americano, tall, 12 oz	70
Caffe, Starbucks, Americano, short, 8 oz	35
Caffe, Starbucks, latte or cappucinno, grande, 16 oz	70
Caffe Mocha, Starbucks, short (8 oz) or tall (12 oz)	35
Espresso, Starbucks, 8 oz	280
Brewed, drip method	110–150
Brewed, percolator	64–124
Instant	40–108
Expresso	100
Decaffeinated, brewed or instant; Sanka	2–5
Coffe Frappuccino, Starbucks, grande, 16 oz	170
Tea, 5 oz cup[a]	
Brewed, 1 min	9–33
Brewed, 3 min	20–46
Brewed, 5 min	20–50
Nestea Sweetened Lemon Ice Tea	20
Iced tea, 12 oz; instant tea	12–36
Green tea, 8oz	30
Chocolate	
Baker's semi-sweet, 1 oz; Baker's chocolate chips, 1/4 cup	13
Cocoa, 5 oz cup, made from mix	6–10
Milk chocolate candy, 1 oz	6
Sweet/dark chocolate, 1 oz	20
Baking chocolate, 1 oz	35
Chocolate bar, 3.5 oz	12–15
Jello chocolate fudge mousse	12
Ovaltine	0
Soft Drinks	
7-Eleven Big Gulp Cola, 64 oz	190
Jolt	100
Sugar Free Mr. Pibb	59
Mellow Yellow, Mountain Dew	53–54
Tab	47
Coca Cola, Diet Coke, 7-Up Gold	46
Shasta-Cola, Cherry Cola, Diet Cola	44
Dr. Pepper, Mr. Pibb	40–41
Dr. Pepper, sugar free	40
Pepsi Cola	38
Diet Pepsi, Pepsi Light, Diet RC, RC Cola, Diet Rite	36
Red Bull, 8 oz	80
Frozen Desserts	
Ben and Jerry's no fat coffee fudge frozen yogurt, 1 cup	85
Starbucks coffee ice cream, assorted flavors, 1 cup	40–60
Haagen-Dazs coffee ice cream, 1 cup	58
Haagen-Dazs coffee frozen yogurt, fat-free, 1 cup	42
Haagen-Dazs coffee fudge ice cream, low-fat, 1 cup	30
Starbucks frappuccino bar, 1 bar (2.5 oz)	15
Healthy Choice cappuccino, chocolate chunk, or cappuccino mocha fudge ice cream, 1 cup	8
Over-the-Counter Products	
Cold remedies	
Dristan, Coryban-D, Triaminicin, Sinarest	30–31
Excedrin	65
Actifed, Contac, Comtrex, Sudafed	0
Diuretics	
Aqua-ban	200
Pre-Mens Forte	100
Pain remedies	
Vanquish	33
Anacin; Midol	32
Aspirin, any brand; Bufferin, Tylenol, Excedrin P.M.	0
Stimulants	
Vivarin tablet, NoDoz maximum strength caplet, Caffedrine	200
NoDoz tablet	100
Enerjets lozenges	75
Weight control aids	
Dexatrim, Dietac	200
Prolamine	140
Pain drugs[b]	
Cafergot	100
Migrol	50
Fiorinal	40
Darvon	32

Data from product labels and manufacturers, and National Soft Drink Association, 1997.
[a]Brewing tea or coffee for longer periods slightly increases the caffeine content.
[b]Prescription, 1 oz; 30 mL.

Additional Insights
Coffee Consumption and Aggressive Forms of Cancer

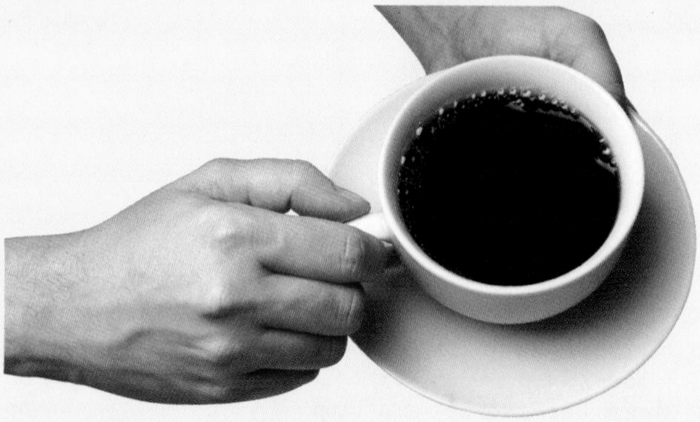

Keep coffee drinking to no more than two cups a day because more may be harmful to health. That is the warning many of us have heard over the years. Here is some news that might calm the fears of heavy coffee drinkers. Recent research from Sweden indicates that coffee consumption associates with reduced risk for the most aggressive subtype of breast cancer, the non–hormone-responsive subtype called estrogen receptor (ER) negative. Women who drank five or more cups of coffee a day had a 57% lower risk of contracting the ER-negative cancer form compared to those who drank less than one cup daily. A new study from the Harvard School of Public Health reports that men who consumed six or more cups of coffee daily experienced about a 20% lower risk of developing prostate cancer, with an even stronger 60% lower risk of developing the lethal form of this cancer. Even drinking one to three cups daily associated with a 30% lower lethal cancer risk. The risk reduction occurred whether the men drank decaffeinated or regular coffee, indicating that compounds other than caffeine provide the protective effect.

A prudent recommendation is to not necessarily boost coffee intake until the biologic mechanism for any protection is more clearly understood. However, if these findings are supported by subsequent research, coffee could provide one modifiable factor to lower risk of the most harmful forms of certain cancers. While coffee does boost blood pressure, the 1- to 3-hour spike is temporary, with no longer term effects.

Sources:

Li J, et al. Coffee consumption modifies risk of estrogen-receptor negative breast cancer. *Breast Cancer Res* 2011;13:R49.

Wilson KM, et al. Coffee consumption and prostate cancer risk and progression in the Health Professionals Follow-up Study. *J Natl Cancer Inst* 2011;103:879.

Zhang Z, et al. Habitual coffee consumption and risk of hypertension: a systematic review and meta-analysis of prospective observational studies. *Am J Clin Nutr* 2011;93:1212.

Related References

Lee AH, Binns CW. Coffee consumption and prostate cancer risk and progression in the Health Professionals Follow-up Study. *J Natl Cancer Inst* 2011;103:1481.

Turati F, et al. A meta-analysis of coffee consumption and pancreatic cancer. *Ann Oncol* 2012; 23:311.

Tverdal A, et al. Coffee intake and oral-oesophageal cancer: follow-up of 389,624 Norwegian men and women 40-45 years. *Br J Cancer* 2011;11:157.

The intestinal tract absorbs caffeine rapidly, with peak plasma concentration reached within 1 hour. Caffeine clears from the body fairly rapidly, taking about 3 to 6 hours for blood caffeine concentrations to decrease by one half. As a frame of reference, it requires about 10 hours for clearance of other stimulants like methamphetamine.

Ergogenic Effects

Drinking 2.5 cups of regularly percolated coffee 1 hour before exercising extends endurance in strenuous aerobic exercise under laboratory and field conditions, as it also does in shorter duration maximal effort and repeated exercise bouts typical of high-intensity team sports.[23,49,183] An ergogenic effect even occurs with caffeine ingestion in the minutes just before exercising.[60] Ergogenic effects during exhaustive exercise at 80% $\dot{V}O_{2max}$ that follows a 5 $mg \cdot kg^{-1}$ caffeine dose are maintained 5 hours later during a subsequent exercise challenge.[16] Thus, there is no need to ingest a smaller additional caffeine dose to preserve high blood caffeine levels to sustain the ergogenic effect during subsequent exercise within 5 hours.

CAFFEINE AND HEART ATTACKS: PERHAPS RISK RELATES TO AGE AND HOW FAST YOU METABOLIZE IT

Research published in the *Journal of the American Medical Association* indicates that coffee intake may raise heart attack risk, but only if you are younger than age 50 and possess genes that produce the enzyme that metabolizes caffeine slowly (cytochrome P450 1A2). Those who metabolize caffeine rapidly have no increased risk, even if they drink four or more cups of regular coffee daily. The same holds true for slow metabolizers age 60 and older. In contrast, younger slow metabolizers had a 64% higher risk if they drank four cups a day compared to only one cup. If additional research confirms these findings, an easy, effective method must be devised to determine if persons metabolize caffeine slowly or rapidly.

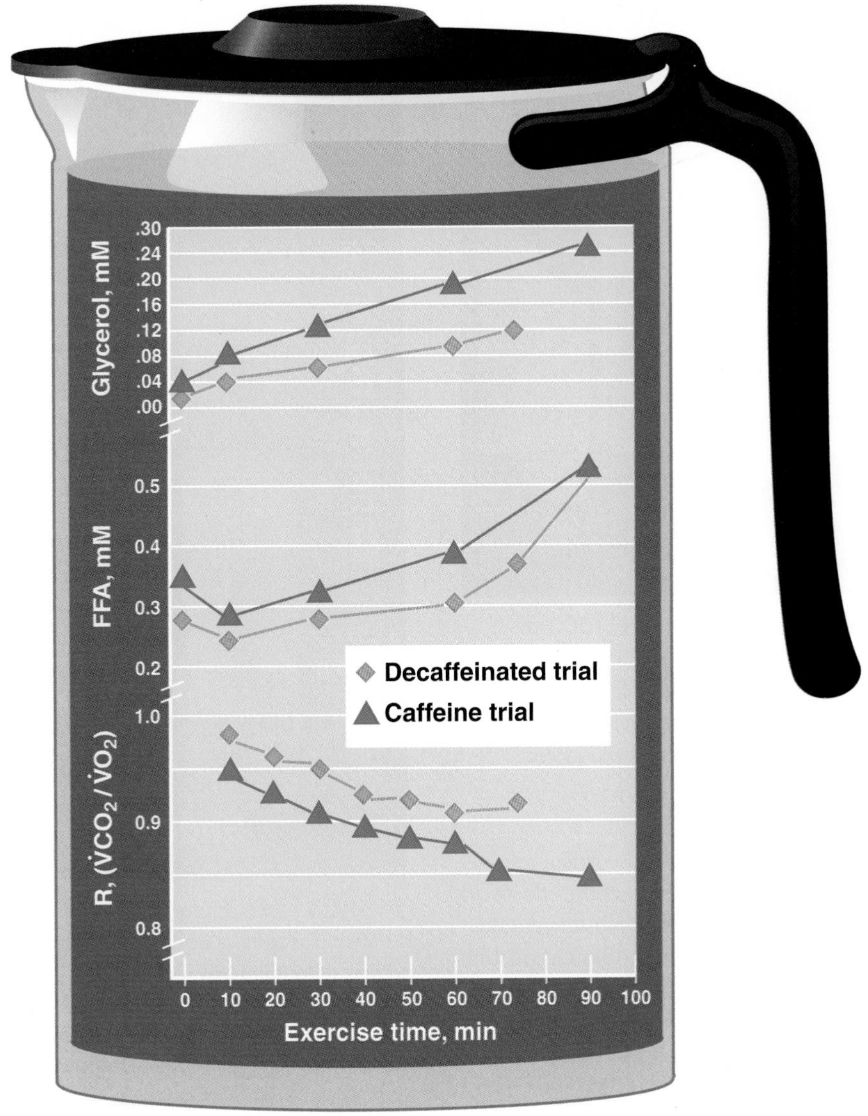

FIGURE 11.8. Average values for plasma glycerol, free fatty acids *(FFA)*, and the respiratory exchange ratio *(R)* during endurance exercise trials after ingesting caffeine and decaffeinated liquids. (From Costill DL, et al. Effects of caffeine ingestion on metabolism and exercise performance. *Med Sci Sports* 1978;10:155.)

FIGURE 11.8 reveals that subjects exercised for 90.2 minutes with 330 mg of pre-exercise caffeine compared with 75.5 minutes without it. Despite similar heart rate and oxygen uptake values during the two trials, the caffeine made the work "feel easier." Consuming caffeine 60 minutes before exercise increased exercise fat catabolism and reduced carbohydrate oxidation as assessed by plasma glycerol and free fatty acid levels and the respiratory quotient. The ergogenic effect of caffeine on endurance performance also applies to similar exercise performed at high ambient temperatures.[39]

Caffeine provides an ergogenic benefit during maximal swimming for durations less than 25 minutes. In a double-blind, cross-over research design, competent male and female distance swimmers (<25 min for 1500-m swims) consumed caffeine (6 $mg \cdot kg^{-1}$ body mass) 2.5 hours before swimming 1500 m. **FIGURE 11.9** illustrates that split times improved with caffeine for each 500 m of the swim. Total swim time averaged 1.9% faster with caffeine (20:58.6) than without it (21:21.8). Enhanced performance associated with lower plasma potassium concentration before exercise and higher blood glucose levels at the end of the trial. These responses suggest a possible caffeine effect on electrolyte balance and glucose availability.

Acute stress can impact changes in cognitive performance and mood, two factors that can play a major role in muscular

CAFFEINISM

Caffeinism refers to caffeine intoxication characterized by restlessness, tremulousness, nervousness, excitement, insomnia, flushed face, diuresis, gastrointestinal complaints, rambling flow of thought and speech, tachycardia or cardiac arrhythmia, periods of inexhaustibility, and/or psychomotor agitation.

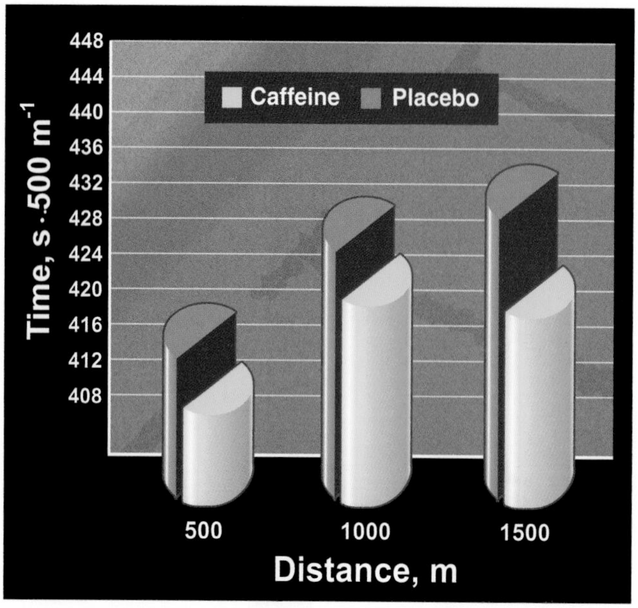

FIGURE 11.9. Split times for each 500-m of a 1500-m swim for caffeine *(yello)* and placebo *(purple)* time trials. Caffeine produced significantly faster split times. (From MacIntosh BR, Wright BM. Caffeine ingestion and performance of a 1,500-metre swim. *Can J Appl Physiol* 1995;20:168.)

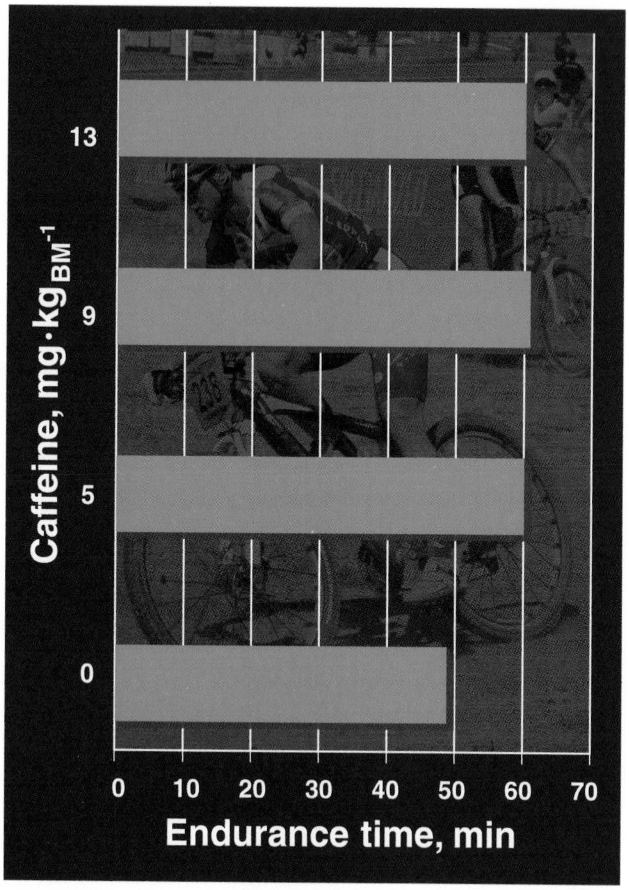

FIGURE 11.10. Endurance performances following pre-exercise dosages of caffeine in different concentrations. The cycling time (minutes) represents the average for the nine male cyclists. All of the caffeine trials were significantly better than the placebo condition (zero-dosage). No dose-response relationship occurred between caffeine concentration and endurance performance. (From Pasman WJ, et al. The effect of different dosages of caffeine on endurance performance time. *Int J Sports Med* 1995;16:25.)

performance due to a stress-related increased cortisol release. Adding glucose to a caffeine drink could impact the effects on cognition, mood, and cortisol release of both substances combined under stressful and physically demanding conditions (fire-fighting training). Using a double-blind, mixed-measures design, 81 participants were administered a 330-mL drink containing 50 g of glucose and 40 mg of caffeine or 10.25 g of fructose/glucose and 80 mg of caffeine, or a placebo drink. Grip strength and memory performance improved after consuming the 50-g glucose and 40-mg caffeine drink, and both active drinks improved performance on an intense information-processing task compared to the placebo. The drink containing 50 g of glucose and 40 mg of caffeine reduced anxiety and significantly reduced self-reported levels of stress following the fire-fighter training. Thus, in situations of stress combined with physical performance, a glucose and caffeine energy drink might be a cost-effective way to maintain mental performance levels and ameliorate negative effects of stress on mood.[184]

No Dose-Response Relationship

FIGURE 11.10 illustrates the effects of pre-exercise caffeine on endurance time of well-trained male cyclists. Subjects received a placebo or a capsule containing 5, 9, or 13 mg of caffeine per kg of body mass 1 hour before cycling at 80% of maximal power output on a $\dot{V}O_{2max}$ test. All caffeine trials improved exercise performance by 24%. No greater benefit occurred for quantities above 5 $mg \cdot kg^{-1}$ body mass. From a practical standpoint, persons should omit caffeine-containing foods and beverages 4 to 6 days before competition to optimize caffeine's potential for ergogenic effects.

Proposed Mechanism for Ergogenic Action

The ergogenic effect of caffeine (or related methylxanthine compounds) in intense, endurance exercise results from the facilitated use of fat as an exercise fuel, thus sparing the liver and muscles' limited glycogen reserves. Caffeine probably acts in either of two ways:

1. Directly on adipose and peripheral vascular tissues
2. Indirectly from stimulating epinephrine release by the adrenal medulla; epinephrine then acts to inhibit adipocyte cell adenosine receptors that normally repress lipolysis

Caffeine's inhibition of adenosine receptors on adipocyte cells increases cellular levels of cyclic-3′,5′-adenosine monophosphate (cAMP). cAMP, in turn, activates hormone-sensitive lipases to promote lipolysis, which releases free fatty acids into the plasma. Increased levels of free fatty acids contribute to increased fat oxidation, thus conserving liver and muscle glycogen. Sparing glycogen reserves benefits prolonged intense exercise; diminished glycogen in active muscles coincides with reduced capacity to sustain a high rate of power output.

Some investigators have reported the ergogenic effect to be unrelated to general hormonal or metabolic changes with caffeine.[189] This suggests possible caffeine action on specific tissues, including those of the central nervous system. Caffeine and its metabolites readily cross the blood-brain barrier to produce analgesic effects on the central nervous system. This effect would reduce the perception of effort and muscle pain during exercise.[137] Caffeine also enhances motoneuronal excitability, thus facilitating motor unit recruitment. The stimulating effects of caffeine do not result from its direct action on the central nervous system. Rather, caffeine indirectly stimulates the nervous system by blocking another chemical neuromodulator, adenosine, which calms brain and spinal cord neurons. Four factors likely interact to produce caffeine's facilitating effect on neuromuscular activity:

1. Lowered threshold for motor unit recruitment
2. Altered excitation/contraction coupling
3. Facilitated nerve transmission
4. Increased ion transport within the muscle itself

Conflicting evidence concerns the effect of pre-exercise caffeine on $\dot{V}O_{2max}$. Little effect has been noted for caffeine on repeated 20-m sprint running performance for team-sport female athletes[155] and on reactive agility time, sleep, and next-day exercise performance.[157]

CAFFEINE EFFECTS OFTEN INCONSISTENT

Prior nutrition partly accounts for the variation frequently observed among persons in their exercise response after consuming caffeine. Persons who normally consume a high-carbohydrate diet show little effect of caffeine on free fatty acid mobilization.[203] Individual differences in caffeine sensitivity, tolerance, and hormonal response from short- and long-term patterns of caffeine consumption also affect this drug's ergogenic qualities.[31,48,194,195] Interestingly, the ergogenic effects on endurance occur less for caffeine in coffee than for an equivalent dose from a caffeine capsule in water.[68] Components in coffee apparently antagonize caffeine's actions.

Effects on Muscle

Caffeine acts directly on muscle to enhance exercise capacity.[131,167,179] A double-blind research design study evaluated voluntary and electrically stimulated muscle actions under "caffeine-free" conditions and following oral administration of 500 mg of caffeine.[117] Electrically stimulating the motor nerve removed central nervous system control and quantified caffeine's direct effects on skeletal muscle. Caffeine produced no effect on maximal muscle force during voluntary or electrically stimulated muscle actions. For submaximal effort, caffeine increased force output for low-frequency electrical stimulation before and after muscle fatigue. Caffeine extended the time to exhaustion on short-term anaerobic power tests.[14] Pre-exercise caffeine administration also increased by 17% repeated submaximum isometric muscular endurance.[156] Caffeine probably exerts a direct and specific effect on skeletal muscle and its sensory processes during repetitive stimulation. In Chapter 12, we discuss how caffeine diminishes the ergogenic effect of creatine supplementation on short-term muscular power.

Warning About Caffeine

Persons who normally avoid caffeine can experience undesirable side effects when they consume it. Caffeine intoxication can increase the risk of seizures, acid-base disorders, acute hepatitis,[200] and cardiovascular events.[188]

Caffeine stimulates the central nervous system, and in quantities greater than 1.5 g daily, it can produce the following nine symptoms of caffeinism:

1. Restlessness
2. Headaches
3. Insomnia
4. Nervous irritability
5. Muscle twitching
6. Muscle tremor
7. Psychomotor agitation
8. Elevated heart rate and blood pressure (temporary spikes that usually resolve within 4 h)
9. Premature left ventricular contractions

From the standpoint of temperature regulation, caffeine's effect as a potent diuretic could cause unnecessary pre-exercise fluid loss that negatively impacts thermal balance and exercise performance in a hot environment. This dehydrating effect is probably minimal when consumed in fluids during exercise for the following reasons:

1. An exercise-induced catecholamine release greatly reduces renal blood flow (and thus urine production).
2. Enhanced renal solute reabsorption in exercise facilitates water conservation (osmotic effect).

Normal caffeine intake generally poses no significant health risk, yet death from caffeine overdose has occurred. The LD_{50} (lethal oral dose required to kill 50% of the population) for caffeine is estimated at 10 g (150 $mg \cdot kg^{-1}$ body mass). Thus, for a 50-kg woman, acute health risk occurs at a caffeine intake of 7.5 g. Moderate caffeine toxicity has been reported in small children consuming 35 $mg \cdot kg^{-1}$ body mass. This is a clear indication of the *inverted U-shaped relationship* between certain exogenous chemicals and exercise performance (and health and safety). For caffeine, if ingesting small-to-moderate quantities produces desirable effects, consuming significant excess can wreak havoc and, in the extreme, cause death.

GINSENG AND EPHEDRINE

Ginseng and ephedrine are botanical remedies commonly marketed as nutritional supplements to "reduce tension," "revitalize," "burn calories," and "optimize mental and physical performance," particularly during times of fatigue and stress. The herb ginseng also plays a role as an alternative therapy to treat diabetes, stimulate immune function, and counter male impotence. Clinically, 1 to 3 g of ginseng administered 40 minutes before an oral glucose challenge reduces postprandial glycemia in nondiabetic subjects. As with caffeine, ephedrine and ginseng occur naturally and for years have been used in folk medicine to enhance "energy."

Ginseng

Currently used in Asian medicine to prolong life, strengthen and restore sexual functions, and invigorate the body, the **ginseng** root (*Panax ginseng*, often sold as Panax or Chinese or Korean ginseng) currently serves no recognized medical use in the United States except as a soothing agent in skin ointments. Commercial ginseng root preparations generally take the form of powder, liquid, tablets, or capsules; widely marketed foods and beverages also contain various types and amounts of ginsenosides.

A common claim for ginseng in the Western world is its ability to boost energy and diminish the negative effects of overall stress on the body. Reports of an ergogenic effect often appear in nontraditional journals. Some peer-reviewed research has demonstrated a facilitating effect of ginseng on endurance performance and recovery from exercise.[101,115] A review of most research on the topic provides little objective evidence to support the effectiveness of ginseng as an ergogenic aid.[3,11,66] For example, volunteers who consumed either 200 or 400 mg of the standardized ginseng concentrate each day for 8 weeks in a double-blind research protocol showed that neither treatment affected submaximal or maximal exercise performance, ratings of perceived exertion, or physiologic parameters of heart rate, oxygen consumption, or blood lactate concentrations.[54] Similarly, no ergogenic effects emerged on diverse physiologic and performance variables following a 1-week treatment with a ginseng saponin extract administered in two doses of either 8 or 16 $mg \cdot kg^{-1}$ body mass.[134] When effectiveness has been demonstrated, the research has failed to use adequate controls, placebos, or double-blind testing protocols. *No compelling scientific evidence exists that ginseng supplementation offers any ergogenic benefit for physiologic function or exercise performance.*

Ephedrine

Based on an analysis of existing data, including commissioning a safety study by an independent research group (the Rand Corporation), the FDA announced in April 2004 a ban on ephedra, the first time this federal agency has moved to ban a dietary supplement. Unlike with ginseng, Western medicine recognizes the potent amphetamine-like alkaloid compound ephedrine (with sympathomimetic physiologic effects) found in several species of the plant ephedra (dried plant stem called ma huang [ma wong; *Ephedra sinica*]). The ephedra plant contains two major active components first isolated in 1928, ephedrine and pseudoephedrine, which exert weaker effects than ephedrine. The medicinal role of this herb has included use to treat asthma, symptoms of the common cold, hypotension, and urinary incontinence and as a central stimulant to treat depression. Physicians in the United States discontinued using ephedrine as a decongestant and asthma treatment in the 1930s in favor of safer medications. The milder pseudoephedrine remains common in nonprescription cold and flu medications and has been clinically used to treat mucosal congestion that accompanies hay fever, allergic rhinitis, sinusitis, and other respiratory conditions. In January 2004, it was removed from the banned substances list by the IOC and placed on its monitoring program because of lack of evidence showing ergogenic effect. It is now banned.

Ephedrine exerts both central and peripheral effects, with the latter reflected in increased heart rate, cardiac output, and blood pressure. Owing to its β-adrenergic effect, ephedrine produces bronchodilation in the lungs. High ephedrine dosages can produce hypertension, insomnia, hyperthermia, and cardiac arrhythmias. Other possible side effects include dizziness, restlessness, anxiety, irritability, personality changes, gastrointestinal symptoms, and difficulty concentrating. No credible evidence exists that commercial weight loss products containing a blend of ephedrine and caffeine are effective for long-term weight loss.[172]

The potent physiologic effects of ephedrine have led researchers to investigate its potential as an ergogenic aid—sold commercially before its ban by the FDA as *Ripped Fuel, Metabolift, Xenadrine RFA-1, Hyrocut,* and *ThermoSpeed.* No effect of a 40-mg dose of ephedrine occurred on indirect indicators of

NO GUARANTEE OF PURITY: WHAT YOU SEE MAY NOT BE WHAT YOU GET

Dietary supplements need not meet the same quality control for purity and potency as pharmaceuticals. The United States Pharmacopeial Convention (USP; www.usp.org/aboutUSP/) serves as a scientific nonprofit organization that sets standards for the quality, purity, identity, and strength of medicines, food ingredients, and dietary supplements manufactured, distributed and consumed worldwide. USP's drug standards are enforceable in the United States by the Food and Drug Administration. The standards are developed and relied upon in more than 130 countries worldwide. Unfortunately, many manufactures of supplement products do not adhere to standards they are asked to enforce. This allows for considerable variation in the concentrations of marker compounds in many products, for example ginseng, including levels of potentially harmful impurities and toxins such as pesticide and heavy metal contamination.[73] Neither the FDA nor other state or federal agencies routinely test ginseng-containing products or other nutritional supplements for quality or purity.

exercise performance or ratings of perceived exertion (RPE).[46] The less concentrated pseudoephedrine also produced no effect on $\dot{V}O_{2max}$, RPE, aerobic cycling efficiency, anaerobic power output (Wingate test), time to exhaustion on a bicycle ergometer[80,185] and a 40-km cycling trial,[64] or physiologic and performance measures during 20 minutes of running at 70% of $\dot{V}O_{2max}$ followed by a 5000-m time trial.[35] Conversely, a series of double-blind, placebo-controlled studies using a relatively high pre-exercise ephedrine dosage of 0.8 to 1.0 $mg \cdot kg^{-1}$ body mass, either alone or combined with caffeine, produced small but statistically significant effects on endurance performance[14,15] and anaerobic power output during the early phase of the Wingate test.[13] Also, ephedrine supplementation increased muscular endurance during the first set of traditional resistance training exercise.[87] Subsequent research has demonstrated improved 1500-m running performance with no reported side effects by male athletes who receive ephedrine 2.5 $mg \cdot kg^{-1}$ body mass compared to a maltodextrin placebo 90 minutes before the all-out run trial.[81] Ergogenic effects were attributed to central nervous system effects rather than to altered metabolism.

Numerous anecdotal reports exist of adverse effects from ephedra-containing compounds, but a cause-and-effect relationship between use and untoward responses, including death, remains hotly debated.

ALCOHOL

Alcohol, more specifically ethyl alcohol or ethanol (a form of carbohydrate), classifies as a depressant drug. Alcohol provides 7 kcal of energy per gram (mL) of pure (100% or 200 proof) substance. Adolescents and adults, athletes and nonathletes, abuse alcohol more than any other drug in the United States.

Alcohol Use Among Athletes

Statistics remain equivocal about alcohol use among athletes compared with the general population. In a study of athletes in Italy, 330 male high school nonathletes consumed more beer, wine, and hard liquor and had greater episodes of heavy drinking (including greater cigarette smoking rates) than 336 athletes.[50] Interestingly, the strongest predictor of the participants' alcohol consumption was their best friend and girlfriend's drinking habits. In other research, physically active men drank less alcohol than sedentary counterparts.[72] Some athletes possess a more negative attitude about drinking than the general population,[151] but collegiate athletes generally drink more heavily and are more likely to drive while intoxicated than their nonathletic peers.[141] In a sample of former world-class Finnish athletes who competed between 1920 and 1965, the current alcohol consumption of the endurance athletes (average age, 57.5 years) was less than that of an age-matched control group.[55] A study of the relationship between athletic participation and depression, suicidal ideation, and substance use among high school students in Kentucky reported no greater alcohol consumption for 823 athletes than for the school's general student body.[149] Athletes also reported less depression, thoughts about suicide, and cigarette smoking and marijuana use than nonathletes. Teenage male athletes also drank 25.5% less beer and 39.9% less wine and whiskey than nonathletes.[57]

Several studies indicate that athletes are more likely to engage in binge drinking.[106,112,140] A self-reported questionnaire assessed alcohol intake of randomly selected students in a representative national sample of 4-year colleges in the United States.[142] Compared with nonathletic students, athletes were at higher risk for binge drinking (five or more alcoholic drinks on at least one occasion in the past 2 weeks for men and four or more drinks for women), heavier alcohol use, and drinking-related harm. Athletes were also more likely than nonathletes to surround themselves with (1) others who binge drink and (2) a social environment conducive to excessive alcohol consumption. These findings support the position that future alcohol prevention programs targeted to athletes should address the unique social and environmental influences that affect the current athletes' heavier alcohol use.

TABLE 11.7 compares serious male and female recreational runners and matched controls on responses to the Michigan Alcoholism Screening Test (MAST). Male runners drank more (14.2 vs 5.4 drinks per week) and felt guiltier about their drinking behavior (26.6%) than nonexercising controls (3.8%). Male and female runners drank more frequently than controls (2.8 vs 2.3 times per week), whereas runners with MAST scores suggesting a history of problems with alcohol drank less than nonathletic controls with a similar score. Men also consumed more alcohol and drank more frequently (including binge drinking) than women. This study illustrates that problems associated with alcohol consumption do not exclude adult runners. Running may serve as a healthy substitute for runners prone to alcoholic behavior.

Alcohol's Action and Psychological and Physiologic Effect on Athletic Performance

Levels of Alcohol in Beverages and in the Body

One alcoholic drink contains 1.0 oz (28 g or 28 mL) of 100-proof (50%) alcohol. This translates into 12 oz of regular beer (about 4% alcohol by volume) or 5 oz of wine (11–14% alcohol by volume). The stomach absorbs between 15 and 25% of the alcohol ingested. The small intestine rapidly takes up the remainder for distribution throughout the body's water compartments, particularly the water-rich tissues of the central nervous system. The absence of food in the digestive tract facilitates alcohol absorption. Interestingly, substitution of artificially sweetened alcohol mixers for sucrose-based mixers has a marked effect on the rate of gastric emptying of alcohol, resulting in elevated blood alcohol concentrations.[166] The liver, the major organ for alcohol metabolism, removes alcohol at a rate of about 10 g per hour, equivalent to the alcohol content of one drink. Consequently, consuming more than one drink per hour increases blood alcohol concentration, expressed in grams per deciliter ($g \cdot dL^{-1}$).

TABLE 11.7 Responses from Male and Female Recreational Runners and Matched Controls to the Shortened[a] and Brief[b] Versions of the Michigan Alcoholism Screening Test (MAST)

MAST Item	Men (*N* = 536)		Women (*N* = 262)	
	Runners, % (*N*)	Controls, % (*N*)	Runners, % (*N*)	Controls, % (*N*)
1. I am not a normal drinker.[a, b]	19.1 (75)	22.8 (31)	12.1 (17)	13.9 (16)
2. My friends and relatives think I'm not a normal drinker.[a, b]	14.5 (56)	22.8 (31)	10.1 (14)	13.0 (15)
3. Attended Alcoholics Anonymous for drinking.[a, b]	4.5 (18)	8.9 (12)	2.1 (3)	4.3 (5)
4. Lost friends because of drinking.[a]	6.1 (24)	7.9 (11)	1.4 (2)	4.3 (5)
5. Trouble at work because of drinking.[a, b]	3.8 (15)	5.0 (7)	0.7 (1)	3.4 (4)
6. Feel guilty about drinking.[b]	26.6 105)	13.8 (19)	16.7 (24)	15.5 (18)
7. Neglected obligations, family, work for 2 or more days in a row due to drinking.[a, b]	4.8 (19)	5.0 (7)	1.4 (2)	0.9 (1)
8. Experienced delirium tremens.[a]	4.3 (17)	2.9 (4)	0.7 (1)	3.4 (4)
9. Unable to stop drinking when desired.[b]	5.4 (21)	7.2 (10)	4.3 (6)	3.4 (4)
10. Sought help for drinking.[a, b]	5.3 (21)	7.2 (10)	2.1 (3)	6.0 (7)
11. Hospitalized for drinking.[a, b]	1.5 (6)	4.3 (6)	0.7 (1)	3.4 (4)
12. Drinking caused problems with spouse, parent, or other relative.[b]	20.6 (81)	21.0 (29)	2.8 (4)	8.5 (10)
13. Arrested for drunk driving.[a, b]	9.4 (37)	11.5 (16)	2.8 (4)	2.6 (3)
14. Arrested for drunken behavior.[b]	5.5 (22)	5.8 (8)	0.7 (1)	1.7 (2)

Adapted from Gutgesell M, et al. Reported alcohol use and behavior in long-distance runners. Med Sci Sports Exerc 1996;28:1063.
[a]*Shortened MAST; from Binokur A, VanRooijen I. A self-administered Short Michigan Alcoholism Screening Test (SMAST). J Stud Alcohol 1975;36:117.*
[b]*Brief MAST; from Pokorny AD, et al. The brief MAST: a shortened version of the Michigan Alcoholism Screening Test. Am J Psychiatry 1972;129:342.*

Consuming two alcoholic drinks in 1 hour produces a blood alcohol concentration between 0.04 and 0.05 g·dL^{-1}. However, factors such as age, body mass, body fat content, and gender influence blood alcohol level. Depending on the state, the legal limit for alcohol intoxication generally ranges between a blood alcohol concentration of 0.11 and 0.16

Additional Insights

Caffeine plus Alcohol: An Unnecessary and Potentially Harmful Jolt

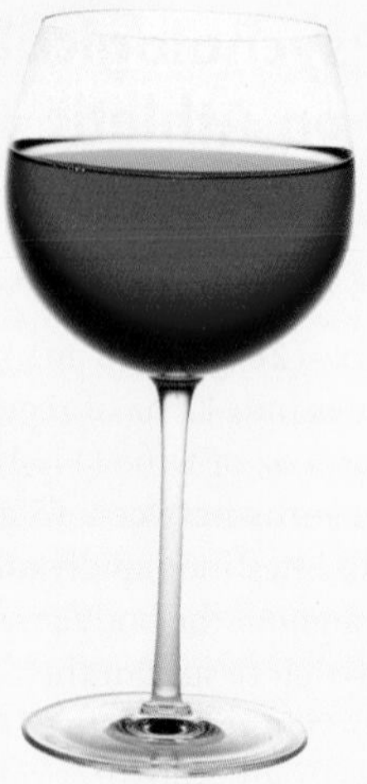

With the popularity of caffeine beverages mixed with alcohol, a new product appeared on grocery shelves in 2008—ready-made caffeine beverages mixed with alcohol. These cocktail mixers gained widespread popularity but also the scrutiny of the FDA (www.fda.gov/NewsEvents/Newsroom/PressAnnouncements/ucm234109.htm; http://www.cdc.gov/alcohol/fact-sheets/cab.htm). This watchdog agency examined the published peer-reviewed literature on the coconsumption of caffeine and alcohol[12,78,85,180]; consulted with experts in the fields of toxicology, neuropharmacology, emergency medicine, and epidemiology; and reviewed information provided by product manufacturers. The FDA also performed its own independent laboratory analysis of products sold by four companies that were warned in 2010 that their products presented a public health concern. The FDA ruled that the addition of caffeine to their malt alcoholic beverages was an "unsafe food additive."

1. Charge Beverages Corp.: *Core High Gravity HG, Core High Gravity HG Orange, and Lemon Lime Core Spiked*
2. New Century Brewing Co., LLC: *Moonshot*
3. Phusion Projects, LLC (doing business as Drink Four Brewing Co.): *Four Loko*
4. United Brands Company Inc.: *Joose and Max*

The drinks, popular among youth, are regularly consumed by 31% of 12- to 17-year-olds and 34% of 18- to 24-year-olds. Current alcohol energy drinks on the market contain anywhere from 6 to 12% alcohol by volume. The Centers for Disease Control and Prevention point out that when alcoholic beverages are mixed with energy drinks, the caffeine can mask the depressive effects of alcohol. Concomitantly, caffeine has no effect on the liver's metabolism of alcohol and thus does not reduce breath alcohol concentrations or reduce the risk of alcohol-attributable harms. Drinkers who consume alcohol mixed with energy drinks are three times more likely to binge drink based on breath alcohol levels than drinkers who do not report mixing alcohol with energy drinks.[128,187] The chart below contains the ingredients, alcohol content, container size, estimated kcal, and estimated number of standard drinks in one can. These products were sold prior to the ban.

Product	Supplier	Ingredients	Alcohol Content	Container Size	Estimated Calories[a]	Estimated number of standard drinks[b]
808	Liquid Arts Beverage Group	Cognac, vodka, liquor, caffeine and guarana	10%	12 oz.	350	2
Axis	Associated Brewing Company	Artificial flavors, wormwood oil, and certified color	1.2%	16 oz.	400	3.2
BE	Anheauser-Busch Inc.	Beer, caffeine, ginseng & guarana extract	6.60%	10 oz.	250	1.1
California Organic Brewery, Mateveza	Rave Associates, Inc.	Beer with yerba mate (caffeinated tea)	5%	22 oz.	500	1.8
Carpe Noctum A.M.	Atomic Brands, Inc.	Vodka, caffeine, taurine, natural and artificial flavors	9%	12.68 oz.	350	1.9
Core	Associated Brewing Company	Artificial flavors, wormwood oil, color	12%	23.5 oz.	700	4.8
Core	Associated Brewing Company	Malt beverage with natural and artificial flavors, taurine, guarana, ginseng, caffeine	12%	23.5 oz.	700	4.8
Four Loko beverages	Phusion Projects, LLC	Malt beverage with artificial flavors, taurine, guarana, caffeine, and FD&C	12%	23.5 oz.	700	4.8
Jack Daniel's Country Cocktail, Black Jack Cola	Brown-Forman Corportation	Malt breverage with natural flavors, artificial color, and caffeine	5%	10 oz.	200	.08
Joose, Max	United Brands Company, Inc.	Malt beverage with natural flavors, ginseng, taurine, caffeine	12%	23.5 oz.	700	4.8
Joose Mamba, Joose Orange, Panther Joose	United Brands Company, Inc.	Malt beverage with natural flavors, caffeine, ginseng, taurine, and certified colors	9.90%	23.5-24 oz.	700	5

[a]*Calories reported on Daily Burn (*http://dailyburn.com*).*
[b]*Drink estimates are calculated on the NIAAA "What's in Your Cocktail Calculator," at* http://.niaaa.nih.gov/ToolsResources/CocktailCalculator.asp.

From www2.myacpa.org/docs/publications/ACPA_Alcohol_Caffeine.pdf.
Under the Federal Food, Drug, and Cosmetic Act (see Chapter 9), a substance added intentionally to food such as the addition of caffeine to alcoholic beverages is deemed "unsafe" and unlawful unless its particular use has been FDA approved. Thus, the drinks cannot be legally marketed because the FDA has not approved the use of caffeine in alcoholic drinks.

g·dL^{-1}. Blood alcohol concentration above 0.40 ($\geq$19 drinks in 2 h) leads to coma, respiratory depression, and eventual death.

Psychological and Physiologic Effects

Athletes use alcohol to enhance performance because of its psychological and physiologic effects. In the psychological realm, some have argued that alcohol before competition reduces tension and anxiety (**anxiolytic effect**), enhances self-confidence, and promotes aggressiveness. Alcohol also facilitates neurologic "disinhibition" because of its initial, though transitory, stimulatory effect. Thus, the athlete believes that alcohol facilitates physical performance at or close to physiologic capacity, particularly for activities requiring maximal strength and power. *Research does not substantiate any ergogenic effect of alcohol on muscular strength, short-term anaerobic power, or longer term aerobic activities.*

Initially acting as a stimulant, alcohol's ultimate effect produces generalized central neurologic depression (memory, visual perception, speech, motor coordination). These effects relate directly to blood alcohol concentration. Damping of psychomotor function causes the antitremor effect of alcohol ingestion. Consequently, alcohol use has been particularly prevalent in rifle and pistol shooting and archery, which require steadiness and accuracy. Achieving an antitremor effect also provides the primary rationale for using drugs called β-blockers, such as propranolol, which diminish the arousal effect of sympathetic stimulation. Most research indicates that alcohol at best provides no ergogenic benefit; at

PERSONAL HEALTH AND EXERCISE NUTRITION 11.1

Alcohol Metabolism and Use: The Correct Approach

Background

Abraham Lincoln, who enjoyed whiskey every now and then, once said, "It is true that many were injured by intoxicating drink, but none seemed to think the injury arose from the use of a bad thing, but from the abuse of a very good thing." President Lincoln most likely knew little about the medicinal benefits of "lighter drinking"; he simply enjoyed an occasional drink, like many persons in present-day society.

Alcohol abuse among college students, however, remains a persistent problem, representing the leading cause of death among persons between ages 15 and 24. In America, more than 100,000 people die each year from alcohol-related deaths (mostly related to driving). Advertisers have touted the health benefits of "light" drinking. Many persons have used this as justification to increase alcohol consumption.

Much confusion exists regarding (1) alcohol's metabolic effects, (2) defining levels of intake, (3) determining safe intake limits, and (4) the role of alcohol as a nutrient.

Alcohol Chemistry and Metabolism

Some alcohol metabolizes in the cells lining the stomach, while most breaks down in the liver. About 10% is directly eliminated by diffusion through the kidneys or the lungs. From a structural standpoint, ethanol contains a hydroxyl group (OH^-) and therefore resembles a carbohydrate. Because it converts directly to acetyl-coenzyme A (CoA) during catabolism, it does not proceed through glycolysis, in contrast to glucose and glycogen breakdown. Consequently, ethanol cannot provide substrate for glucose synthesis (gluconeogenesis). In metabolic terms, alcohol metabolizes more like a lipid than a sugar.

Alcohol concentration varies with the type of beverage. "Proof" value indicates its concentration, which equals two times the percentage concentration. For example, an 80-proof beverage contains 40% alcohol. When discussing alcohol consumption, "one drink" refers to a 12-oz bottle of beer, a 5-oz glass of table wine, or a cocktail with 1.5 oz of 80-proof liquor. Each of these drinks contains about 0.6 oz of alcohol by weight.

Alcohol Metabolism with Low Blood Alcohol Levels

At low consumption and correspondingly low blood levels, alcohol reacts with nicotinamide adenine dinucleotide (NAD) in the cell's cytosol to form acetaldehyde and NADH under the influence of the zinc-requiring enzyme alcohol dehydrogenase. Acetaldehyde then converts to acetyl-CoA (see Chapter 4) to yield more NADH. Acetyl-CoA enters the citric acid cycle; the NADH, $FADH_2$, and guanosine triphosphate molecules produced in acetaldehyde and acetyl-CoA formation and in the citric acid cycle provide energy to synthesize adenosine triphosphate (ATP; see figure).

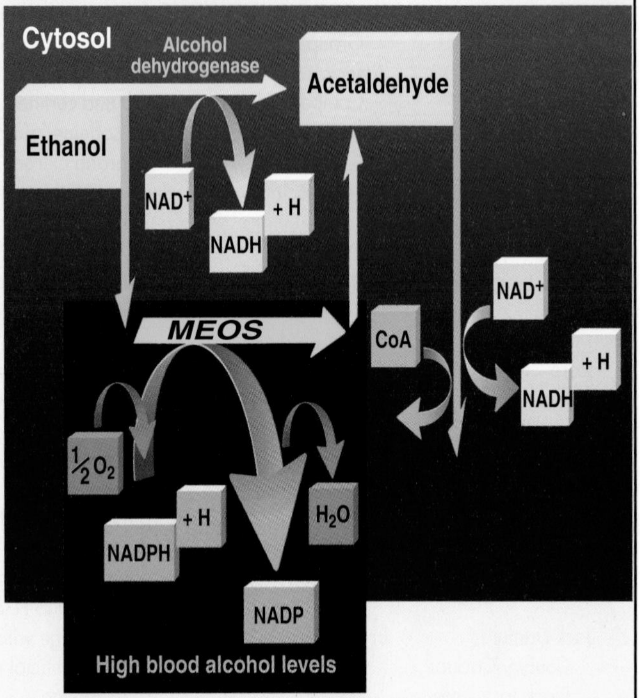

Alcohol Metabolism with High Blood Alcohol Levels

When blood alcohol levels increase with high alcohol intake, alcohol dehydrogenase cannot sustain the metabolism of all alcohol into acetaldehyde. In this situation, an alternative metabolic pathway, the microsomal ethanol-oxidizing system (MEOS), becomes activated. MEOS uses considerable energy to break down alcohol, in contrast to the simpler alcohol dehydrogenase pathway that readily produces useful energy as ATP. Normally, the MEOS metabolizes drugs and other "foreign" substances in the liver. Under the stress of excessive alcohol intake, the liver "registers" alcohol as a foreign substance for breakdown by MEOS. Chronic MEOS activation increases alcohol tolerance because high alcohol intake proportionally increases its rate of breakdown.

Rather than forming NADH by use of alcohol dehydrogenase (as occurs with moderate alcohol intake), the MEOS uses nicotinamide adenine dinucleotide phosphate (NADPH), a compound similar to NADH. However, instead of yielding potential ATP molecules via formation of NADH from the first step in alcohol breakdown, MEOS uses potential ATP energy (in the form of NADPH) as NADPH converts to NADP. The use of different pathways to catabolize alcohol, depending on intake level, helps to explain why alcoholics do not gain the weight expected based on the alcohol-derived energy consumed. High alcohol use damages liver function in a manner that hampers other metabolic pathways. This cascading effect also contributes to the reduced energy yield associated with high alcohol use. In addition, alcohol increases metabolic rate to further contribute to an alcoholic's increased weight loss.

Determining a Safe Limit of Alcohol Intake

Arbitrary limits define a "safe" alcohol intake, but "light," "moderate," and "heavy" represent the most common classifications. Historically, Anstie's rule (attributed to the British neurologist Sir Francis Edmund Anstie [1833–1874]) provided a frequently used operational definition, based on a person's ability to safely "handle" alcohol. At the time, the safe level for a typical male amounted to about three standard drinks daily (over 8 h).

We now know that three factors—age, sex, and body weight (size)—determine a person's ability to "handle" alcohol. For a standard alcohol intake, blood alcohol levels inversely relate to body weight; the lower the weight, the greater is the effect. Blood alcohol levels below 0.01% almost never impair function; levels from 0.01 to 0.04% sometimes impair function; levels from 0.05 to 0.07% usually impair function; and levels of 0.08% and above always impair function. For most persons who weigh less than 170 lb, blood alcohol levels achieve the usually impaired level with only two drinks over 2 hours. For those who exceed 170 lb, three drinks in 2 hours impair function. Consequently, consuming no more than two drinks daily classifies as light-to-moderate drinking.

Benefits and Risks of Light-to-Moderate Drinking

For adults older than 18 years, light-to-moderate drinking associates with a lower risk of coronary heart disease, decreased incidence of ischemic stroke, and reduced occurrence of gallstones compared with alcohol abstinence. Moderate drinking is not risk free, however. Obviously, any level of drinking increases addiction risk, particularly for persons with a family history of alcoholism. Links exist between light-to-moderate drinking and female breast cancer risk, harm to the fetus, and increased colon cancer risk in men and women.

Risks of Heavy Drinking

Heavy drinkers experience the highest overall risk of morbidity (contracting illness) and mortality, compared with nondrinkers or to those who drink moderately. Heavy drinking associates with diverse health problems including cirrhosis of the liver, inflammation of the pancreas and stomach, certain cancers, high blood pressure, diseases of the heart muscle, heart arrhythmias, hemorrhagic stroke, and increased accidents and suicide.

General Guidelines for Alcohol Use

Neither the Surgeon General's Office, the National Academy of Science, nor the US Department of Agriculture/Department of Health and Human Services recommends drinking alcohol. All groups caution that if adults consume alcohol, it should be in moderation and with meals (no more than two drinks a day for men and one for women). Avoid drinking any alcohol before or while driving, operating machinery, taking medications, or engaging in other activity requiring sound judgment; no alcohol should be consumed while pregnant.

Do You Have a Problem?

Asking a person about the quantity and frequency of alcohol consumption provides an important means to detect abuse and dependence. The following CAGE questionnaire is popular for use in routine health care.

CAGE Questionnaire to Screen for Alcohol Abuse

C: Have you ever felt you ought to CUT down on drinking?
A: Have people ANNOYED you by criticizing your drinking?
G: Have you ever felt bad or GUILTY about your drinking?
E: Have you ever had a drink first thing in the morning to steady your nerves or get rid of a hangover (EYE-OPENER)?

More than one positive response to the CAGE questionnaire suggests an alcohol problem.

Marks DB, et al. *Basic Medical Biochemistry.* Baltimore: Williams & Wilkins, 1996.

Mayfield D, et al. The CAGE questionnaire: validation of a new alcoholism instrument. *Am J Psychiatry* 1974;131:1121.

Suter PM. Effects of alcohol on energy metabolism and body weight regulation: is alcohol a risk factor for obesity. *Nutr Rev* 1997;55:157.

worst, it precipitates undesirable side effects that impair performance (**ergolytic effect**). For example, alcohol's depression of nervous system function profoundly impairs all sports performances requiring balance, hand–eye coordination, reaction time, and overall need to process information rapidly. These effects vary considerably among persons and become apparent in a dose-response relationship at blood alcohol levels above 0.05 $g \cdot dL^{-1}$. In the extreme, it seems unlikely that a legally intoxicated person or team could perform optimally in *any* competitive sports activity.

Alcohol impairs cardiac function. Ingesting 1 g of alcohol per kilogram of body mass during 1 hour raises blood alcohol level to just over 0.10 $g \cdot dL^{-1}$. This level, often observed among "social drinkers," acutely depresses myocardial contractility. In terms of metabolism, alcohol blunts the liver's capacity to synthesize glucose from noncarbohydrate sources via gluconeogenesis. Each of these effects impairs performance in high-intensity aerobic activities that rely heavily on cardiovascular capacity and energy from carbohydrate catabolism. Alcohol provides no benefit as an energy substrate and does not favorably alter the metabolic mixture in endurance exercise. In addition, substituting alcohol for high glycemic carbohydrates in the postexercise replenishment period decreases optimal glycogen storage in recovery.[27]

Alcohol and Fluid Replacement

Alcohol exaggerates the dehydrating effect of exercise in a warm environment; it acts as a potent diuretic by depressing antidiuretic hormone release from the posterior pituitary and blunting the arginine–vasopressin response. Both effects impair thermoregulation during heat stress, thus placing the athlete at greater risk for heat injury during exercise.

Many athletes consume alcohol-containing beverages after exercising or sports competition, so a legitimate question concerns the degree to which alcohol impairs rehydration in recovery. Alcohol's effect on rehydration has been studied following exercise-induced dehydration of about 2% of body mass.[173,174] Subjects consumed rehydration fluid volumes equivalent to 150% of fluid lost and containing 0, 1, 2, 3, or 4% alcohol. Urine volume produced during the 6-hour study period directly related to the beverage's alcohol concentration—greater alcohol consumption produced more urine. Increases in plasma volume in recovery compared with the dehydrated state averaged 8.1% when the rehydration fluid contained no alcohol, but only 5.3% for the beverage with 4% alcohol content. The bottom line: *Alcohol-containing beverages impede rehydration.* Alcohol acts as a peripheral vasodilator and should *not* be consumed during cold exposure or to facilitate recovery from hypothermia.[89] A good "stiff drink" does not warm you up!

Perhaps Some Benefit

A moderate daily alcohol intake—2 oz or 30 mL of 90-proof alcohol, three 6-oz glasses of wine, or slightly less than three 12-oz beers—reduces a healthy person's risk of heart attack and stroke, independent of physical activity level[10,53,168] and improves the likelihood of surviving a myocardial infarction.[138] The heart-protective benefit of moderate alcohol consumption also applies to persons with type 2 diabetes.[202] The mechanism for benefit remains elusive, yet moderate alcohol intake increases HDL-C, particularly its subfractions HDL_2 and HDL_3. In addition, certain components of red wine (e.g., polyphenols) may inhibit LDL-C oxidation, thus blunting a critical step in arterial plaque formation.[144] Moderate wine intake also associates with more "heart-healthy" dietary choices that positively affect plasma lipids. For nondiabetic postmenopausal women, consuming 30 g (two drinks) of alcohol each day benefited insulin and triacylglycerol concentrations and insulin sensitivity.[45] In contrast, excessive alcohol consumption offers no lipoprotein benefit and increases liver disease and cancer risk.

ALCOHOL NO ERGOGENIC BENEFIT WHATSOEVER

The major conclusions of a position statement of the American College of Sports Medicine on Alcohol use in Sports remain as germain ane today as when first published in 1982.[6] Two main conclusions emerged:

1. Acute alcohol ingestion impairs psychomotor skill, including reaction time, balance, accuracy, hand–eye coordination, and complex coordination.
2. Alcohol does not improve and may even decrease strength, power, speed, local muscular endurance, and cardiovascular endurance.

BUFFERING SOLUTIONS

Dramatic alterations occur in the acid–base balance of the intracellular and extracellular fluids during maximal exercise of between 30 and 120 seconds in duration because the muscle fibers rely predominantly on anaerobic energy transfer. In such conditions, significant lactate accumulates, with a concurrent fall in intracellular pH. Increased acidity inhibits the energy transfer and contractile capabilities of active muscle fibers, thereby causing a decline in exercise performance.

The **bicarbonate** aspect of the body's buffering system provides a major line of defense against increased intracellular H^+ concentration (see Chapter 3). Maintaining high levels of extracellular bicarbonate rapidly releases H^+ from cells and delays the onset of intracellular acidosis. Increasing bicarbonate (alkaline) reserves might enhance anaerobic exercise performance because increased H^+ concentration in intense exercise reduces the calcium sensitivity of the contractile proteins, which impairs muscle function.[36,182] Research in this area has produced conflicting results, perhaps from variations in the pre-exercise sodium bicarbonate dose and the type of exercise to evaluate the effects of pre-exercise alkalosis.[69,125,192]

To improve experimental design, one early study evaluated the effects of acute induced alkalosis on short-term fatiguing exercise that greatly increased anaerobic metabolites. Trained middle-distance runners ran an 800-m race under normal (control) conditions or after ingesting either a sodium bicarbonate solution (300 $mg \cdot kg^{-1}$ body mass) or a similar quantity of calcium carbonate placebo. **TABLE 11.8** shows that the alkaline drink raised pH and standard bicarbonate levels before exercise. Subjects ran an average of 2.9 seconds faster under alkalosis and achieved higher postexercise values for blood lactate, pH, and extracellular H^+ concentration than those under placebo or control conditions.

The ergogenic benefit of pre-exercise alkalosis also occurs in women (**FIG. 11.11**). Moderately trained women performed one bout of maximal cycle ergometer exercise for 60 seconds on separate days in a double-blind research design under the following conditions: (1) control, no treatment; (2) 300 $mg \cdot kg^{-1}$ body mass dose of sodium bicarbonate in 400 mL of low-calorie flavored water 90 minutes before testing; and (3) placebo of equimolar dose of sodium chloride (to maintain intravascular fluid status as in bicarbonate

TABLE 11.8 Performance Time and Acid–Base Profiles for Subjects Under Control (Placebo) and Induced Preexercise Alkalosis Conditions Immediately Before and After an 800-m Race

Variable	Condition	Pretreatment	Pre-exercise	Postexercise
pH	Control	7.40	7.39[a]	7.07[b]
	Placebo	7.93	7.40[a]	7.09[b]
	Alkalosis	7.40	7.49[a]	7.18[b]
Lactate (mmol·L^{-1})	Control	1.21	1.15[a]	12.62[b]
	Placebo	1.38	1.23[a]	13.62[b]
	Alkalosis	1.29	1.31[a]	14.29[b]
Standard HCO_3^- (mEq·L^{-1})	Control	25.8	24.5[a]	9.9[b]
	Placebo	25.6	26.2[a]	11.0[b]
	Alkalosis	25.2	33.5[a]	14.3[b]
	Control	**Placebo**	**Alkalosis**	
Performance Time (min)	2:05.8	2:05.1	2:02.9[c]	

From Wilkes D, et al. Effects of induced metabolic alkalosis on 800-m racing time. Med Sci Sports Exerc 1983;15:277.
[a]Preexercise values significantly higher than pretreatment values.
[b]Alkalosis values significantly higher than placebo and control values after exercise.
[c]Alkalosis time significantly faster than control and placebo times.

condition) 90 minutes before testing. Exercise capacity represented total work accomplished during the ride. The figure's inset box shows that total work performed and peak power output reached higher levels with pre-exercise bicarbonate treatment than with either control or placebo conditions. The bicarbonate treatment also produced a higher level of blood lactate in the immediate and 1-minute postexercise periods, which explained the greater anaerobic exercise capacity. Similar benefits of induced alkalosis occur in short-term anaerobic performance using exogenous **sodium citrate** as the alkalinizing agent.[76,126]

Augmented anaerobic energy transfer during exercise probably explains the ergogenic effect of pre-exercise alkalosis.[82,161] More than likely, increased extracellular buffering from exogenous bicarbonate or citrate facilitates coupled transport of lactate and H^+ across the muscle cell membrane during anaerobic exercise.[91,182] This delays the fall in intracellular pH and its subsequent negative effects on muscle function. Nearly 3 seconds represents a dramatic improvement in 800-m race time; it transposes to a distance of about 19 m at race pace, bringing a last place finisher to first place!

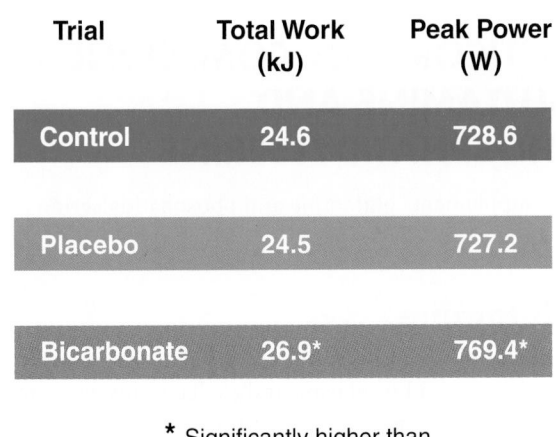

Trial	Total Work (kJ)	Peak Power (W)
Control	24.6	728.6
Placebo	24.5	727.2
Bicarbonate	26.9*	769.4*

* Significantly higher than either control or placebo

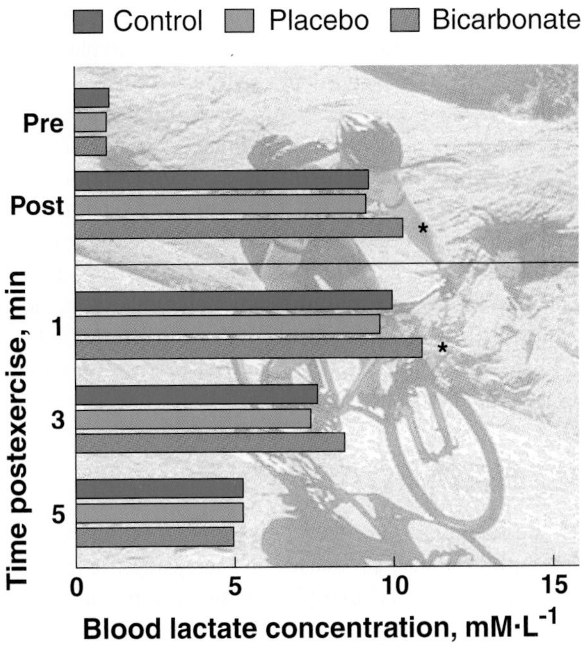

FIGURE 11.11. Bicarbonate loading and its effects on total work, peak power output, and postexercise blood lactate levels in moderately trained women. (From McNaughton LR, et al. Effect of sodium bicarbonate ingestion on high intensity exercise in moderately trained women. *J Strength Cond Res* 1997;11:98.)

Effects Related to Dosage and Degree of Exercise Anaerobiosis

The interaction between bicarbonate dosage and the cumulative anaerobic nature of the exercise influences the ergogenic effects of pre-exercise alkalosis. Doses of at least 0.3 $g{\cdot}kg^{-1}$ (ingested about 1–2 h precompetition) facilitate H^+ efflux from the cell. This enhances a single maximal effort of 1 to 2 minutes duration,[121,127] including longer term arm or leg exercise that exhausts within 6 to 8 minutes.[165] Even long-term bicarbonate ingestion (0.5 $g{\cdot}kg^{-1}$ body mass) for 5 days added to the normal diet raised plasma pH and increased performance in a 60-second maximal effort. No ergogenic effect emerges for typical resistance training exercises (e.g., squat, bench press), perhaps because of the generally lower absolute anaerobic metabolic load compared with continuous, maximal, whole-body activities. Bicarbonate loading with all-out effort of less than 1 minute improves performance *only* with both short- and longer term repetitive exercise bouts that repeatedly produce high intracellular H^+ concentrations.

Inconsistencies in the research literature cloud the issue concerning the effectiveness of pre-exercise alkalosis. For example, despite dose-dependent changes in pH, base excess, and HCO_3^- after ingestion of sodium citrate, no effect occurred on measures of performance in a bicycling time trial, even when the simulated race contained a multiple-sprint component.[170]

High-Intensity Endurance Performance

Pre-exercise alkalosis does not benefit low-intensity, aerobic exercise because pH and lactate remain near resting levels. In contrast, some research indicates benefits in prolonged aerobic exercise of higher intensity. More specifically, race times of trained male cyclists were better after consuming sodium citrate (0.5 $g{\cdot}kg^{-1}$ body mass) before a 30-km time trial than in placebo trials.[159] Despite the relatively small anaerobic component in intense aerobic exercise compared with short-term, all-out exercise, ingesting a buffering agent before exercise facilitates lactate and hydrogen ion efflux. This maintains pH closer to normal resting levels to improve muscle function in prolonged effort.

Persons who bicarbonate load often experience abdominal cramps and diarrhea about 1 hour after ingestion. This adverse effect would surely minimize any potential ergogenic benefit. Substituting the buffering agent sodium citrate (0.4–0.5 $g{\cdot}kg^{-1}$) for sodium bicarbonate can reduce or eliminate adverse gastrointestinal effects.

PHOSPHATE LOADING

The rationale concerning pre-exercise phosphate supplementation (**phosphate loading**) focuses on increasing the levels of extracellular and intracellular phosphate. This may in turn accomplish the following:

1. Increase the potential for ATP phosphorylation
2. Increase aerobic exercise performance and myocardial functional capacity
3. Augment peripheral oxygen extraction in muscle tissue by stimulating red blood cell glycolysis and subsequent elevation of erythrocyte 2,3-diphosphoglycerate (2,3-DPG)

The compound 2,3-DPG, produced within the red blood cell during anaerobic glycolytic reactions, binds loosely with subunits of hemoglobin to reduce oxygen affinity. Additional oxygen then releases to the tissues for a given decrease in the cellular oxygen pressure.

Despite the theoretical rationale for ergogenic effects with phosphate loading, benefits have not consistently emerged. Some studies show improvement in $\dot{V}O_{2max}$ and arteriovenous oxygen difference following phosphate loading, whereas others report no effects on aerobic metabolism and cardiovascular function.[109,119]

The major reasons for the inconsistencies in research findings include variations in exercise mode and intensity, dosage and duration of supplementation, standardization of pretest diets, and subjects' fitness level. In one study, subjects with low and high aerobic capacities consumed a drink containing either 22.2 g of dibasic calcium phosphate or a calcium carbonate placebo.[63] Each subject then pedaled a cycle ergometer for 20 minutes at an exercise intensity equivalent to 70% $\dot{V}O_{2max}$, followed by a 30-minute rest and then an incremental ride to exhaustion. For high- and low-fitness groups, no differences occurred for any of the variables measured, including erythrocyte 2,3-DPG, submaximal or maximal oxygen consumption, exercise time to exhaustion, and plasma lactate in submaximal exercise.

Little reliable scientific evidence exists to recommended exogenous phosphate as an ergogenic aid. On the negative side, excess plasma phosphate stimulates secretion of **parathormone**, the parathyroid hormone. Excessive hormone production accelerates the kidneys' excretion of phosphate and facilitates reabsorption of calcium salts from bones to cause loss of bone mass.

ANTICORTISOL COMPOUNDS: GLUTAMINE AND PHOSPHATIDYLSERINE

The supplements glutamine and phosphatidylserine produce an anticortisol effect.

Glutamine

Glutamine, a nonessential amino acid, is the most abundant amino acid in plasma and skeletal muscle. It accounts for more than one half of the muscles' free amino acid pool. Glutamine exerts many regulatory functions, one of which provides an anticatabolic effect and augments protein synthesis. Glutamine supplementation effectively counteracts the decline in protein synthesis and muscle wasting from repeated glucocorticoid use. In one study of female rats, infusing glutamine for 7 days inhibited the downregulation of myosin (muscle contractile protein) synthesis and atrophy in skeletal muscle that normally accompanies chronic glucocorticoid administration.[77]

PHYSIOLOGY OF CORTICOTROPHIN-RELEASING FACTOR

The hypothalamus secretes corticotrophin-releasing factor as a normal response to emotional stress, trauma, infection, surgery, and physical exertion such as resistance training. This releasing factor, in turn, stimulates the anterior pituitary gland to secrete adrenocorticotropic hormone (ACTH), which induces the adrenal cortex to release the glucocorticoid hormone cortisol (hydrocortisone). Cortisol decreases amino acid transport into the cell; this depresses anabolism and stimulates protein breakdown to its building-block amino acids in all cells except liver cells. The circulation delivers these "liberated" amino acids to the liver for synthesis to glucose (gluconeogenesis). Cortisol also serves as an insulin antagonist by inhibiting glucose uptake and oxidation. A prolonged, elevated serum concentration of cortisol (usually from therapeutic exogenous glucocorticoid intake in drug form) leads to excessive protein breakdown, tissue wasting, and negative nitrogen balance. The potential catabolic effect of cortisol has convinced many bodybuilders and other strength and power athletes to use supplements thought to inhibit the body's normal cortisol release. They believe that blunting cortisol's normal rise following exercise augments muscular development with resistance training by attenuating catabolism. In this way, muscle tissue synthesis progresses unimpeded in recovery.

Increasing glutamine availability by supplementation modulates glucose homeostasis during and after exercise in a direction that facilitates postexercise recovery.[86] It also promotes muscle glycogen accumulation in human muscle in recovery, perhaps by serving as a gluconeogenic substrate in the liver.[197] The practical application of these findings for promoting glycogen replenishment in recovery or enhancing glycogen accumulation in the pre-exercise period requires further research. The potential anticatabolic and glycogen-synthesizing effects of exogenous glutamine have promoted speculation that glutamine supplementation might benefit responses to resistance training. Daily glutamine supplementation (0.9 g·kg^{-1} lean tissue mass) during 6 weeks of resistance training in healthy young adults did not affect muscle performance, body composition, or muscle protein degradation compared with a placebo.[29]

IS CORTISOL RELEASE REALLY "BAD"?

Research must determine if the normal release and rise in serum cortisol with intense training counteracts muscular growth and development and recovery and repair. One could argue that cortisol release with exercise represents an appropriate and beneficial response to physiologic function and overall good health. It also remains unclear whether a supplement-induced decrease in cortisol output with resistance training translates into greater improvements in muscular strength and size.

Immune Response

Glutamine plays an important role in normal immune function through its use as metabolic fuel by disease-fighting cells that defend against infection. Glutamine plasma concentrations decrease following prolonged high-intensity exercise, so a glutamine deficiency has been linked to the immunosuppression caused by strenuous exercise.[20,143,162,216] Chapter 7 discusses glutamine and the immune response in regard to supplementation and the incidence and severity of upper respiratory tract infections.

Phosphatidylserine

Phosphatidylserine (PS), a glycerophospholipid typical of a class of natural lipids, constitutes the structural components of biologic membranes. This mainly pertains to the internal layer of all cell plasma membranes. Through its potential for modulating functional events in the plasma membrane (e.g., number and affinity of membrane receptor sites), PS might modify the neuroendocrine response to stress. In one study, healthy men consumed 800 mg of PS derived from bovine cerebral cortex daily for 10 days.[132] Three 6-minute intervals of cycle ergometer exercise of increasing intensity induced physical stress. Compared with the placebo condition, the PS treatment diminished ACTH and cortisol release without affecting growth hormone release. These results confirmed earlier findings that a single intravenous PS injection counteracted hypothalamic–pituitary–adrenal axis activation with exercise.[133] Ten days of supplementation with 750 mg of soybean-derived phosphatidylserine did not attenuate the cortisol response, perceived muscle soreness, or markers of muscle damage and lipid peroxidation following exhaustive intermittent running compared to a glucose polymer placebo.[104] Supplementation increased cycle time to exhaustion but did not affect oxygen kinetics, serum cortisol, substrate oxidation, or mood state during the exercise.[103] The physiologic mechanism for any ergogenic effect remains unknown.

Soybean lecithin provides most of the PS used for supplementation by athletes, yet research showing physiologic effects have used bovine-derived PS. Subtle differences in the chemical structure of these two forms of PS may create differences in physiologic action, including the potential for ergogenic effects.

β-HYDROXY-β-METHYLBUTYRATE

β-Hydroxy-β-methylbutyrate (HMB), a bioactive metabolite generated from the breakdown of the essential branched-chain amino acid leucine, may decrease protein loss during stress by inhibiting protein catabolism. A marked decrease in protein breakdown and a slight increase in protein synthesis occurred in muscle tissue of rats and chicks (in vitro) exposed to

HMB.[150] Data also suggest an HMB-induced increase in fatty acid oxidation in vitro in mammalian muscle cells exposed to HMB.[34] The body synthesizes between 0.3 and 1.0 g of HMB daily, of which about 5% derives from dietary leucine catabolism. Because of its possible nitrogen-retaining effects, many resistance-trained athletes supplement directly with HMB to prevent or slow muscle damage and depress muscle breakdown or proteolysis associated with intense physical effort.

Research has studied the effects of exogenous HMB on skeletal muscle's response to resistance training.[61,90,145,152] For example, young adult men participated in two randomized trials. In *study 1*, 41 subjects received 0, 1.5, or 3.0 g of HMB (calcium salt of HMB mixed with orange juice) daily at two protein levels, either 115 or 175 g per day for 3 weeks. The men lifted weights for 1.5 hours, 3 days a week for 3 weeks. In *study 2*, subjects consumed either 0 or 3.0 g HMB a day and lifted weights for 2 to 3 hours, 6 days a week for 7 weeks. In the first study, HMB supplementation depressed the exercise-induced rise in muscle proteolysis as reflected by urine 3-methylhistidine and plasma creatine phosphokinase (CPK) levels during the first 2 weeks of training. These biochemical indices of muscle damage ranged between 20 and 60% lower in the HMB-supplemented group. This group lifted more total weight than the unsupplemented group during each training week (**FIG. 11.12A**), with the greatest effect in the group receiving the largest HMB supplement. Specifically, muscular strength increased 8% for the unsupplemented group, whereas it increased 13% for the 1.5-g HMB per day group and 18.4% for the 3.0-g HMB per day group. Additional protein (not indicated in graph) provided no augmenting effect on any of the measurements. The lack of effect with additional protein should be viewed in proper context because the group consuming the "lower" protein quantity (115 g daily) received the equivalent of about twice the protein RDA. Other investigators have replicated the finding of reduced signs and symptoms of exercise-induced muscle damage following resistance exercise with HMB supplementation.[158,193,207]

In *study 2*, subjects who received the HMB supplement had higher FFM than unsupplemented subjects at 2 and 4 to 6 weeks of training (**FIG. 11.12B**). However, at the last measurement during training, the difference between groups decreased to the point at which no statistical significance between pretraining baseline values occurred.[62]

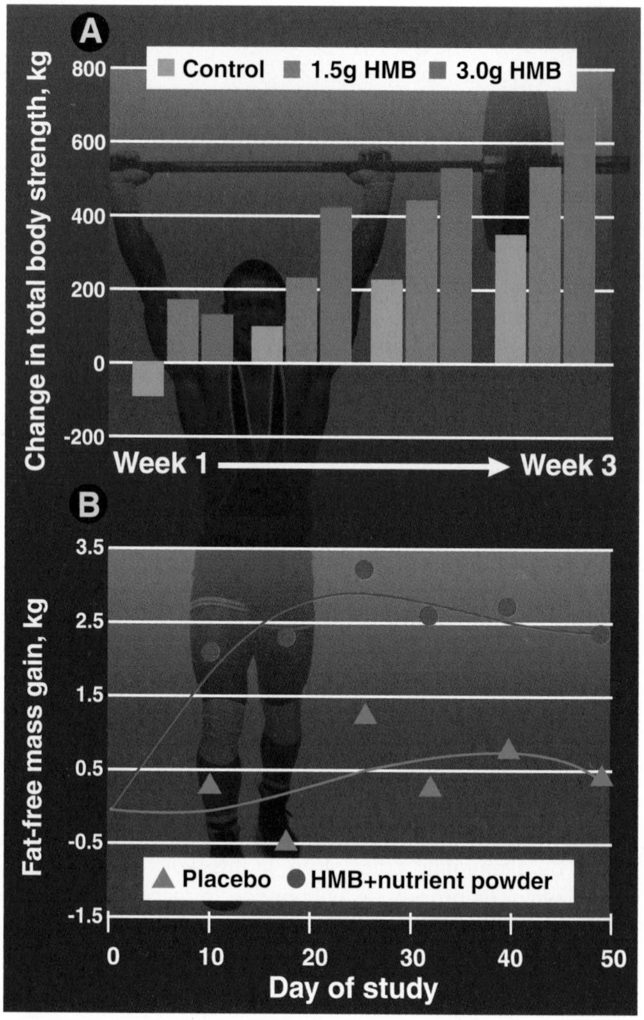

FIGURE 11.12. A. Change in muscle strength (total of upper and lower body exercises) during *study 1* from week 1 to week 3 in subjects supplemented with β-hydroxy-β-methylbutyrate (HMB). Each grouping of bars represents one complete set of upper and lower body workouts. **B.** Total-body electrical conductivity assessed change in fat-free body mass during *study 2* for a control group that received a carbohydrate drink *(placebo)* and an HMB group that received 3 g of calcium (Ca)-HMB per day mixed in a nutrient powder *(HMB + nutrient powder)*. (From Nissen S, et al. Effect of leucine metabolite β-hydroxy-β-methylbutyrate on muscle metabolism during resistance-exercise training. *J Appl Physiol* 1996;81:2095.)

Mechanism of Action

The mechanism for HMB's action on muscle metabolism, strength improvement, and body composition remains unknown. Researchers speculate that this metabolite inhibits normal proteolytic processes that accompany intense muscular overload. While the results appear to demonstrate an ergogenic effect of HMB supplementation, it remains to be shown just what component of the FFM (protein, bone, water) HMB affects. Furthermore, the data in **FIGURE 11.12B** indicate potentially transient body composition benefits of supplementation that plateau and tend to revert toward the unsupplemented state as training progresses. Additional studies must verify the present findings and assess the long-term effects of HMB supplements on body composition, training responsiveness, and overall health and safety.

Not all research shows beneficial effects of HMB supplementation with resistance training.[160,177] One study evaluated the effects of varied amounts of HMB (approximately 3 vs 6 g·d^{-1}) on muscular strength during 8 weeks of resistance training in untrained young men.[61] The study's primary finding indicated that HMB supplementation, regardless of dosage, produced *no difference* in most of the strength data (including

1-RM strength) compared with placebo treatment. Increases in training volume remained similar among groups. Lower levels of CPK in both HMB-supplemented groups in recovery indicate some potential effect of HMB in inhibiting muscle breakdown with resistance training. HMB supplementation with a dosage as high as 6 $g{\cdot}d^{-1}$ during 8 weeks of resistance training does not appear to cause adverse effects on hepatic enzyme function, blood lipid profile, renal dynamics, or immune function.[62] Age does not affect responsiveness to HMB supplementation.[201]

A NEW TWIST: HORMONAL BLOOD BOOSTING

To eliminate the cumbersome and lengthy process of blood doping, endurance athletes now use recombinant **epoetin (EPO)**, a synthetic form of **erythropoetin**. This hormone produced by the kidneys regulates red blood cell production within the marrow of the long bones, including the resynthesis and proper functioning of several erythrocyte membrane proteins involved in facilitating lactate exchange. Exogenous epoetin, commercially available since 1988, has proven clinically useful in combating anemia in patients with severe renal disease. Normally, a decrease in red blood cell concentration or decline in the pressure of oxygen in arterial blood—as in severe pulmonary disease or on ascent to high altitude—releases EPO to stimulate erythrocyte production. The 5 to 12% increase in hemoglobin and hematocrit (% red blood cells in 100 mL of blood) that typically occurs following a 6-week EPO treatment improves endurance exercise performance. Unfortunately, if self-administered in an unregulated and unmonitored manner—simply injecting the hormone requires much less sophistication than procedures for blood doping—hematocrit can increase by more than 60%. This dangerously high hemoconcentration and corresponding increase in

OTHER MEANS TO ENHANCE OXYGEN TRANSPORT

New classes of substances may emerge to enhance aerobic exercise performance.[171] These doping threats include artificial oxygen-carrying perfluorocarbon emulsions with the ability to dissolve significant quantities of oxygen and carbon dioxide and solutions formulated from either bovine or human hemoglobin that also improve oxygen transport and delivery to muscle. Despite their potential benefits in clinical use, these substances exhibit potentially lethal side effects that include increased systemic and pulmonary blood pressure, renal toxicity, and impaired immune function.

Additional Resources:

Speiss BD. Perfluorocarbon emulsions as a promising technology: a review of tissue and vascular gas dynamics. *J Appl Physiol* 2009;106:1444.

Castro CI, Briceno JC. Perfluorocarbon-based oxygen carriers: review of products and trials. *Artif Organs* 2010;34:622. Review.

ACCUSATIONS AND DISAPPOINTMENTS

The cycling world was rocked when reports in the popular press including "those in the know" have suggested that since at least 1903 many forms of doping (alcohol, cocaine, nitroglycerine, strychnine, ether, high-potency pain killers, amphetamines, cortisone), have occurred in longer duration cycling races, including the Tour de France (http://en.wikipedia.org/wiki/Doping_at_the_Tour_de_France). In 1978, Belgian rider Jean-Luc van den Broucke, when found positive of steroid use, said the following:

> In the Tour de France, I took steroids. That is not a stimulant, just a strengthener. If I hadn't, I would have had to give up.... On the first rest day, before we went into the Pyrenees, I had a first hormone injection. I had another one on the second day, at the start of the last week. You can't call that medically harmful, not if it's done under a doctor's control and within reason. There was a mass of steroids used in the Tour, everyone will admit that. How can we stay at the top otherwise? Even at Munich [at the world track championship] it was used a lot. I hope the riders will get together next season and take action. Who can ride classics and long-distance Tours the whole year through without strengtheners?*

Lance Armstrong, one of the greatest cyclists of all time who won seven consecutive Tour de France competitions, has been implicated for taking illegal drugs by cycling team member Floyd Landis who accused Armstrong of doping in 2002 and 2003. Landis also maintains that he witnessed Armstrong receiving multiple blood transfusions and dispensing testosterone patches to his teammates on the United States Postal Service Team. Landis tested positive for a high testosterone-to-epitestosterone ratio (more than twice what the WADA rules permit). In 2010, Landis admitted to taking EPO, testosterone, hGH, and blood transfusions. Another Armstrong teammate, Tyler Hamilton, detailed what he told a Los Angeles grand jury and charged that team and world cycling officials helped keep Armstrong's doping a secret. Hamilton claims he saw Armstrong receive a blood transfusion during the 2000 Tour and inject EPO during the 1999 Tour and before the 2000 and 2001 Tours.

> "I saw him inject it more than one time like we all did, like I did many, many times," Hamilton said. "He was the leader of the team. He doped himself like everybody else, being part of the culture of the sport."

Hamilton also said this about Armstrong:

> "He took what we all took, really, they're no different than anyone else in the peloton. There was EPO, testosterone and I did see a blood transfusion... Team doctors helped

*Soetaert E. De biecht van Jean-Luc van den Broucke. Het Volk, Belgium, 18 October 1978.

Armstrong with doping schedules that enabled him to evade doping tests and that Armstrong once sent him a package with EPO when doctors said his blood was too clean."

Another Armstrong ex-teammate, George Hincapie, swore under oath to a grand jury that he and Armstrong supplied each other with EPO (erythropoetin), a banned endurance booster, and spoke of using testosterone. He returned his 2004 Olympic gold medal to the US Anti-Doping Agency after admitting he took performance-enhancing drugs along with Lance Armstrong.

On February 4, 2012 Federal prosecutors cancelled its nearly two-year investigation of the Lance Armstrong doping case without disclosing the reasons. Several days later, the court of Arbitration for Sport in Lausanne, Switzerland stripped Alberto Contadone of his 2010 Tour de France and 12 other victories since then for testing positive for the banned substance clen buterol.

blood viscosity increases the likelihood for stroke, heart attack, heart failure, and pulmonary edema. Unfortunately, EPO use has become prevalent in national and international cycling competition, allegedly contributing to at least 18 deaths attributed to heart attacks among competitive world-class bicyclists. Blood hematocrit levels serve as a surrogate marker for EPO abuse.

During the 1997 and 1998 competitive seasons, Tour de France officials spot-checked the hematocrits of riders, suspending for 2 weeks any rider with an abnormally high value. This resulted in suspension of 12 riders during 1997 and 6 riders midway through the 1998 competitive season. The International Cycling Union has set a hematocrit threshold of 50% for males and 47% for females, whereas the International Skiing Federation uses a hemoglobin concentration of 18.5 $g \cdot dL^{-1}$ as the disqualification threshold. Hematocrit cutoff values of 52% for men and 48% for women (roughly three standard deviations above the mean normal value) represent "abnormally high" or extreme values in triathletes.[148] The use of a hematocrit level cutoff raises the unanswered question concerning the number of disqualified "clean" cyclists. Estimates place this number at between 3 and 5%, due mainly to factors that affect normal variation in hematocrit such as genetics, posture, altitude training, and hydration level.[7,26]

The medical community's concern centers on an anomaly in iron metabolism frequently observed among elite international cyclists where their serum iron levels exceed 500 $ng \cdot L^{-1}$ (compared to normal levels of 100 $ng \cdot L^{-1}$). The elevated iron level results from regular injections of supplemental iron to support the increased synthesis of red blood cells induced by repeated EPO use. Chronic iron overload increases the risk of liver dysfunction among these athletes.

IN THE FUTURE

As long as winning remains the top priority, persons will experiment with substances to improve exercise and sports performance and the response to training. Realistically, we see little hope for curbing this trend. Quite the contrary! Just when we believed things were getting better in terms of detection, one rider in the 2011 Tour de France was disqualified for steroid use, followed by more revelations that led to the disqualification of an entire team! To add further uncertainty about doping violations (**http://sportslawnews.wordpress.com/2011/10/17/double-jeopardy-cas-201102422-usoc-v-ioc/**), a legal case has been brought against the International Olympic Committee by one of those affected athletes. LaShawn Merritt (2008 Olympic Trials champion; 2007 World Outdoor 400 m silver medalist and 4 × 400 m gold medalist; 2-time USA Outdoor runner-up), who was prevented by the rule from representing the United States at the 2012 London Olympics. Merritt previously had tested positive in an out-of-competition test for *ExtenZe* (a male performance product containing the banned substance DHEA); the doping panel accepted that the substance was used inadvertently and that there was no intention of doping, yet Merritt still has been banned from competition.

We hope for optimism and decry presenting a negative perspective, but at this time, we can offer little in constructive comment on how to stem the onslaught of commercial exploitation. The quest for an ergogenic boost in athletics had its roots 2500 years ago in the ancient Olympic Games. Perhaps the new generation of testing equipment can stay one step ahead of the abusers, but this seems doubtful. Increased legal statutes and penalties can curb the abuse, but drug enforcement remains difficult. Maintaining stricter laws at the local, state, and national levels may provide some relief, but thus far, additional vigilance by law enforcement has not curbed the problem. Perhaps a clearer identification of the characteristics of at-risk athletes and a vigorous education about drug abuse (coupled with a focus on improving the person's decision-making skills and substituting more healthful alternatives) beginning in the early school years and continuing through college offers some limited hope for future generations. We certainly hope so.

SUMMARY

1. Ergogenic aids consist of substances or procedures that improve physical work capacity, physiologic function, or athletic performance.
2. Anabolic steroids, pharmacologic agents commonly used as ergogenic aids, function similarly to the hormone testosterone. Research findings often are inconsistent, and the precise mechanism(s) of action unclear.
3. Negative side effects of anabolic steroid use in males include at least nine deleterious effects: infertility, reduced sperm concentrations, decreased testicular volume, gynecomastia, connective tissue damage that decreases the tensile strength and elastic compliance of

SUMMARY *(continued)*

tendons, chronic stimulation of the prostate gland, injury and functional alterations in cardiovascular function and myocardial cell cultures, possible pathologic ventricular growth and dysfunction, and increased blood platelet aggregation that can compromise cardiovascular system health and function and increase risk of stroke and acute myocardial infarction.

4. Unique negative side effects of anabolic steroid use in females include virilization (more apparent than in men), deepened voice, increased facial and body hair (hirsutism), altered menstrual function, dramatic increase in sebaceous gland size, acne, decreased breast size, and enlarged clitoris. The long-term effects of steroid use on reproductive function remain unknown.
5. The β_2-adrenergic agonists clenbuterol and albuterol increase skeletal muscle mass and slow fat gain in animals to counter the effects of aging, immobilization, malnutrition, and tissue-wasting pathology. A negative finding showed hastened fatigue during short-term, intense muscle actions.
6. Debate exists whether administration of exogenous growth hormone to normal, healthy people augments increases in muscle mass when combined with resistance training.
7. DHEA levels decrease steadily throughout adulthood, prompting many persons (including large numbers of athletes) to supplement with this hormone in the hope of optimizing training and countering the effects of aging.
8. No data support ergogenic effect of DHEA supplements on young adult men and women.
9. Research findings generally indicate *no effect* of androstenedione supplementation on basal serum concentrations of testosterone or training response in terms of muscle size and strength and body composition.
10. Little credible evidence exists that amphetamines ("pep pills") aid exercise performance or psychomotor skills any better than an inert placebo. Side effects of amphetamines include drug dependency, headache, dizziness, confusion, and upset stomach.
11. Caffeine can exert an ergogenic effect in extending aerobic exercise duration by increasing fat use for energy, thus conserving glycogen reserves. These effects become less apparent in persons who maintain a high-carbohydrate diet or habitually use caffeine.
12. No compelling scientific evidence exists to conclude that ginseng supplementation offers positive benefit for physiologic function or performance during exercise. Accumulating evidence indicates significant health risk accompany ephedrine use.
13. Consuming ethyl alcohol produces an acute anxiolytic effect because it temporarily reduces tension and anxiety, enhances self-confidence, and promotes aggression. Other than the antitremor effect, alcohol conveys no ergogenic benefits and likely impairs overall athletic performance (ergolytic effect).
14. Increasing the body's alkaline reserve before anaerobic exercise by ingesting buffering solutions of sodium bicarbonate or sodium citrate improves performance. Buffer dosage and the cumulative anaerobic nature of the exercise interact to influence the ergogenic effect of bicarbonate (or citrate) loading.
15. Little scientific evidence exists to recommend exogenous phosphates as an ergogenic aid.
16. An objective decision about the potential benefits and risks of glutamine, phosphatidylserine, and HMB to provide a "natural" anabolic boost with resistance training for healthy persons awaits further research.
17. Erythropoietin (EPO), a hormone produced by the kidneys that regulates red blood cell production within the marrow of the long bones, increases hemoglobin and hematocrit to improve endurance performance. Significant risks accompany its unsupervised use.
18. Antidoping efforts by major sports (e.g., baseball, football, track and field, cycling) are attempting to level the playing field by use of high-technology methods to detect anabolic steroid abuse, as well as other ergogenic substances that may boost individual athletic performance.

thePoint *Visit* **thePoint.lww.com/MKKSEN4e** *to view the following animations related to content presented in Chapter 11:* ***Endocrine gland stimulation****;* ***Insulin functions****;* ***Hormonal control****; and* ***Oxygen transport.***

TEST YOUR KNOWLEDGE ANSWERS

1. **False:** Ancient athletes of Greece reportedly used hallucinogenic mushrooms for ergogenic purposes, while Roman gladiators ingested the equivalent of "speed" to enhance performance in the Circus Maximus. Athletes of the Victorian era routinely used chemicals such as caffeine, alcohol, nitroglycerine, heroin, cocaine, and the rat poison strychnine for a competitive edge.
2. **True:** A "placebo effect" refers to improved performance due to psychological factors in that the person performs at a higher level simply because of the suggestive power of believing that a substance or procedure should work.
3. **False:** Anabolic steroids function in a manner similar to testosterone, the chief male hormone. Prolonged high dosages of anabolic steroids often impair normal testosterone endocrine function, cause infertility, reduce sperm concentrations (azoospermia), decrease

testicular volume, induce connective tissue damage, increase prostate size, cause injury and alterations in cardiovascular function and myocardial cell cultures, produce possible pathologic ventricular growth and dysfunction when combined with resistance training, impair cardiac microvascular adaptations, and diminish myocardial blood supply, leading to stroke and acute myocardial infarction.

4. **False:** Little scientific evidence supports claims about the effectiveness or anabolic qualities of andro-type compounds. Research findings show that androstenedione (1) elevates plasma testosterone concentrations, (2) exerts no favorable effect on muscle mass, (3) does not favorably affect muscular performance, (4) does not favorably alter body composition, (5) provides no beneficial effects on muscle protein synthesis or tissue anabolism, and (6) impairs the blood lipid profile in apparently healthy men.

5. **True:** The following reasons argue against amphetamine use by athletes: It leads to physiologic or emotional drug dependency; it induces headache, tremulousness, agitation, insomnia, nausea, dizziness, and confusion, all of which negatively affect sports performance requiring rapid reaction and judgment; taking larger doses eventually requires more of the drug to achieve the same effect because drug tolerance increases with prolonged use; it aggravates or even precipitates cardiovascular and mental disorders; it suppresses normal mechanisms for perceiving and responding to pain, fatigue, or heat stress; and it can produce unwanted weight loss, paranoia, psychosis, repetitive compulsive behavior, and nerve damage.

6. **False:** Drinking 2.5 cups of regularly percolated coffee about 1 hour before exercising extends endurance in strenuous aerobic exercise under laboratory conditions, as it does in higher intensity, shorter duration effort. An ergogenic effect even occurs with caffeine ingestion in the minutes just before exercising. Elite distance runners who consume 10 mg of caffeine per kilogram of body mass immediately before a treadmill run to exhaustion improve performance time by 1.9% compared with placebo or control conditions.

7. **False:** An increasing belief in the potential for selected foods to promote health has led to coining the term *functional food.* Beyond meeting three basic nutrition needs (survival, hunger satisfaction, and preventing adverse effects), functional foods comprise those foods and their bioactive components (e.g., olive oil, soy products, omega-3 fatty acids) that promote well-being, health, and optimal body function or reduce disease risk. Examples include many polyphenolic substances (simple phenols and flavonoids found in fruits and vegetables), carotinoids, soy isoflavones, fish oils, and components of nuts that possess antioxidant and other properties that decrease risk of vascular diseases and cancers. Primary targets for this expanding branch of food science include gastrointestinal functions, antioxidant systems, and macronutrient metabolism.

8. **False:** Many commercial weight-loss products have contained combinations of ephedra and caffeine, supposedly designed to accelerate metabolism. No evidence exists that the initial weight loss obtained with high doses of ephedrine plus caffeine lasts beyond 6 months. In 2003, the FDA ordered that a prominent warning label be emblazoned on the front of all ephedra products listing death, heart attack, or stroke as possible consequences of use. In addition, a recent evaluation of more than 16,000 adverse reactions showed "five deaths, five heart attacks, 11 cerebrovascular accidents, four seizures, and eight psychiatric cases as 'sentinel events' associated with prior consumption of ephedra or ephedrine." In December 2003, the FDA banned the use of ephedra as a dietary supplement.

9. **False:** Alcohol's effect on rehydration has been studied following exercise-induced dehydration of about 2% of body mass. Increases in plasma volume in recovery compared with the dehydrated state averaged 8.1% when the rehydration fluid contained no alcohol, but only 5.3% for the beverage with 4% alcohol content. The bottom line is that alcohol-containing beverages impede rehydration.

10. **True:** Many resistance-trained athletes supplement directly with HMB to prevent or slow muscle damage and depress muscle breakdown (proteolysis) associated with intense physical effort. Subjects who received an HMB supplement showed higher FFM mass than unsupplemented subjects. Not all research has shown beneficial effects of HMB supplementation with resistance training. Furthermore, available data indicate potentially transient body composition benefits of supplementation that revert toward the unsupplemented state as training progresses. Additional studies must verify beneficial findings and assess the long-term effects of HMB supplements on body composition, training responsiveness, and overall health and safety.

Key References

Alaranta A, et al. Self-reported attitudes of elite athletes towards doping: differences between types of sport. *Int J Sports Med* 2006;27:842.

Bahrke MS, et al. Is ginseng an ergogenic aid? *Int J Sport Nutr Exerc Metab* 2009;19:298.

Bishop D, Claudius B. Effect of induced metabolic alkalosis on prolonged intermittent-sprint performance. *Med Sci Sports Exerc* 2005;37:759.

Burke LM, et al. Effect of alcohol intake on muscle glycogen storage after prolonged exercise. *J Appl Physiol* 2003;95:983.

Cafri G, et al. Pursuit of muscularity in adolescent boys: relations among biopsychosocial variables and clinical outcomes. *J Clin Adolesc Psychol* 2006;35:282.

Chester N, et al. Physiological, subjective and performance effects of pseudoephedrine and phenylpropanolamine during endurance running exercise. *Int J Sports Med* 2003;24:3.

Cordaro FG, et al. Selling androgenic anabolic steroids by the pound: identification and analysis of popular websites on the Internet. *Scand J Med Sci Sports* 2011;21: e247.

ElSayed MS, et al. Interaction between alcohol and exercise: physiological and haematological implications. *Sports Med* 2005;35:257.

Franke WW, Berendonk B. Hormonal doping and androgenization of athletes: a secret program of the German Democratic Republic government. *Clin Chem* 1997;43:1262.

Green GA, et al. Analysis of over-the-counter dietary supplements. *Clin J Sports Med* 2001;11:254.

Higgins JP, et al. Energy beverages: content and safety. *Mayo Clin Proc* 2010;85:1033B.

Ivy JL, et al. Improved cycling time-trial performance after ingestion of a caffeine energy drink. *Int J Sport Nutr Exerc Metab* 2009;19:61C.

Jacobs I, et al. Effects of ephedrine, caffeine, and their combination on muscular endurance. *Med Sci Sports Exerc* 2003;35:987.

Kanayama G, et al. Body image attitudes toward male roles in anabolic-androgenic steroid users. *Am J Psychiatry* 2006;163:697.

Keisler BD, Armsey TD. Caffeine as an ergogenic aid. *Curr Sports Med Rep* 2006;5:215.

Kingsley MI, et al. Effects of phosphatidylserine on oxidative stress following intermittent running. *Med Sci Sports Exerc* 2005;37:1300.

Maughan RJ. Contamination of dietary supplements and positive drug tests in sport. *J Sport Sci* 2005;23:883.

McCormick C, et al. Clenbuterol and formoteral decrease force production in isolated intact mouse skeletal muscle fiber bundles through a beta2-adrenorectptor-independent mechanisms. *J Appl Physiol* 2010;109:1716.

Nieman DC, Bishop NC. Nutritional strategies to counter stress to the immune system in athletes, with special reference to football. *J Sports Sci* 2006;24:763.

Noakes TD. Tainted glory-doping and athletic performance. *N Engl J Med* 2004;351:847.

Portal S, et al. Effect of HMB supplementation on body composition, fitness, hormonal profile and muscle damage indices. *J Pediatr Endocrinol Metab* 2010;23:641.

Trabulo D, et al. Caffeinated energy drink intoxication. *Emerg Med J* 2011;28:712.

Van Montfoort MC, et al. Effects of ingestion of bicarbonate, citrate, lactate, and chloride on sprint running. *Med Sci Sports Exerc* 2004;36:1239.

Villareal DT, Holloszy J. Effect of DHEA on abdominal fat and insulin action in elderly women and men. *JAMA* 2004;292:2243.

Zanchi NE, et al. HMB supplementation: clinical and athletic performance-related effects and mechanisms of action. *Amino Acids* 2011;40:1015.

thePoint *Visit* **thePoint.lww.com/MKKSEN4e** *for a list of the references cited in this chapter, including additional, relevant references.*

CHAPTER 12

Nutritional Ergogenic Aids Evaluated

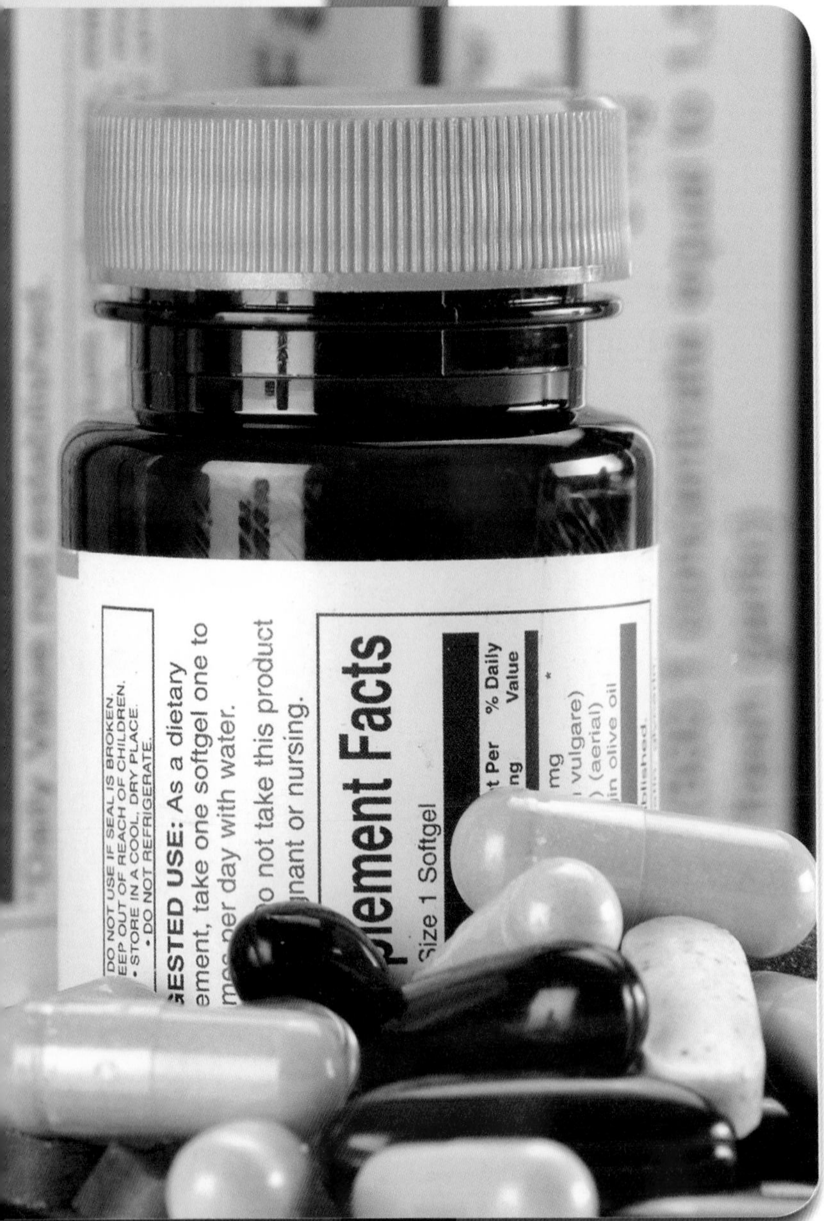

OUTLINE

- Modification of Carbohydrate Intake
- Amino Acid Supplements and Other Dietary Modifications for an Anabolic Effect
- L-Carnitine
- Chromium
- Coenzyme Q_{10} (Ubiquinone)
- Creatine
- Ribose: The Next Creatine?
- Inosine and Choline
- Lipid Supplementation with Medium-Chain Triacylglycerols
- (−)-Hydroxycitrate: A Potential Fat Burner?
- Vanadium
- Pyruvate
- Glycerol
- Nutritional Ergogenic Resources

TEST YOUR KNOWLEDGE

Select true or false for the 10 statements below, then check out the answers at the end of the chapter. Retake the test after you've read the chapter; you should achieve 100%	True	False
1. Reduced levels of muscle glycogen induce fatigue in intense aerobic exercise.	❍	❍
2. It is possible to modify nutrition to "superpack" muscle with glycogen and thereby delay the onset of fatigue in prolonged intense marathon running.	❍	❍
3. Amino acid supplements augment muscular strength and size with resistance training.	❍	❍
4. L-Carnitine supplementation aids endurance athletes by enhancing fat burning and sparing liver and muscle glycogen; it also promotes fat loss in body builders.	❍	❍
5. Chromium, the second largest selling mineral supplement in the United States, is a well-documented "fat burner" and "muscle builder."	❍	❍
6. Creatine supplementation improves performance in short-duration, intense exercise.	❍	❍
7. Limited research indicates a potential for exogenous pyruvate as a partial replacement for dietary carbohydrate to augment endurance exercise performance and to promote fat loss.	❍	❍
8. The hyperhydration effect of glycerol supplementation reduces overall heat stress during exercise, lowers heart rate and core temperature, and enhances endurance performance under heat stress.	❍	❍
9. Because of its role in electron transport–oxidative phosphorylation, athletes supplementing with coenzyme Q_{10} (CoQ_{10}) improve aerobic capacity and exercise cardiovascular dynamics.	❍	❍
10. Well-designed research clearly indicates that supplementation with (−)-hydroxycitrate (HCA) facilitates the rate of fat oxidation at rest and during moderate-intensity exercise to effectively act as an antiobesity agent and ergogenic aid.	❍	❍

Chapter 11 highlighted that physically active individuals often resort to using banned pharmacologic and chemical agents to augment training and gain a competitive edge; they also focus on gaining a performance-enhancing advantage by consuming specific foods and food components in their daily diet. This chapter focuses on popular nutritional ergogenic aids and their impact on exercise performance and training.

MODIFICATION OF CARBOHYDRATE INTAKE

Exercise performance benefits from increased carbohydrate intake before, during, and following intense aerobic exercise and arduous training. Vigilance and mood also improve with a carbohydrate beverage administered during a day of sustained aerobic activity interspersed with rest.[114] Carbohydrate loading represents one of the more popular nutritional modifications to increase glycogen reserves. Judicious adherence to this dietary technique improves specific exercise performance, yet some aspects of carbohydrate loading could prove detrimental.

Nutrient-Related Fatigue in Prolonged Exercise

Glycogen stored in the liver and active muscle supplies most of the energy for intense aerobic exercise. Prolonging such exercise reduces glycogen reserves and causes lipid catabolism to supply a progressively greater percentage of energy from liver and adipose tissue fatty acid mobilization. Exercise that severely lowers muscle glycogen precipitates fatigue. This occurs even though active muscles have sufficient oxygen and unlimited potential energy from stored fat. Ingesting a glucose and water solution near the point of fatigue allows exercise to continue, but for all practical purposes, the muscles' "fuel

WHAT'S INSIDE YOUR HEAD MAY MATTER

Research firmly establishes the importance of muscle and liver glycogen to sustain a high level of prolonged endurance exercise, but what about the role of the brain's glycogen content in resisting fatigue when glucose supply from the blood becomes inadequate (a condition called hypoglycemia)? To investigate the effects of prolonged exercise that induces hypoglycemia and muscle glycogen depletion on brain glycogen content, male Wistar rats ran at moderate intensity on a treadmill for 30- to 120-minute durations. High-power microwave irradiation then measured their brain glycogen levels, which remained unchanged from resting levels at the end of 30 to 60 minutes of running. Following the 120-minute run, brain glycogen levels decreased by between 36% and 60% in five discrete brain loci. Brain glycogen levels in all five regions after running correlated positively with the respective blood and brain glucose levels. These findings with animals support the hypothesis that a decrease in brain glycogen content may link in some manner to central fatigue in prolonged exercise.

Source: Matsui T, et al. Brain glycogen decreases during prolonged exercise. *J Physiol* 2011;589:3383.

CARBOHYDRATE AND SURGICAL OUTCOMES

Successful operative outcomes often depend on an optimal nutritional state, which is often compromised by preoperative dietary restrictions. Consuming carbohydrate-containing drinks up to 2 hours before surgery provides an effective way to minimize insulin resistance, improve patient comfort, and reduce length of hospital stays. Preoperative carbohydrate loading now serves as a strategy to reduce postoperative stress and speed the recovery process—shorter postoperative hospital stays, faster return to normal functions, and a reduced occurrence of surgical complications. Further benefits to surgical outcome include the supplemental use of the so-called *immunonutrients* such as omega-3 fatty acids, arginine, glutamine, and nucleotides to boost the immune system, improve wound healing, and reduce markers of inflammation. The bottom line is that good preoperative nutrition improves postoperative outcomes.

Source: Kratzing C. Pre-operative nutrition and carbohydrate loading. *Proc Nutr Soc* 2011;70:311.

tanks" read empty. A corresponding decrease in exercise power output occurs from the slower rate of fat's mobilization and catabolism compared with carbohydrate.

In the late 1930s, Swedish exercise physiologists reported a startling research finding—athletes' endurance performance improved markedly when they consumed a carbohydrate-rich diet days before exercising.[31] Conversely, switching to a high-fat diet markedly lowered glycogen reserves and reduced capacity in intense aerobic exercise (see Fig. 5.6 and Chapters 1 and 5). In a classic series of later experiments, endurance capacity tripled for subjects fed a high-carbohydrate diet compared with a high-fat diet of similar energy content.[11] Because carbohydrate represents the important energy substrate during 1 to 2 hours of intense exercise, researchers began to investigate additional relatively "simple" ways to elevate the body's glycogen reserves.

Enhanced Glycogen Storage: Carbohydrate Loading

Combining a specific dietary regimen with exercise produces considerable "packing" of muscle glycogen, a procedure termed **carbohydrate loading** or **glycogen supercompensation**. Endurance athletes often use carbohydrate loading before competition because it increases muscle glycogen more than maintaining a diet high in carbohydrate. Normally, each 100-g of muscle contains about 1.7 g of glycogen; carbohydrate loading packs up to 5 g of glycogen per 100 g of skeletal muscle.

Classic Loading Procedure

TABLE 12.1 indicates that the classic two-stage dietary plan to achieve the supercompensation effect first reduces the muscle's glycogen content with prolonged exercise about 6 days before competition. Glycogen supercompensation occurs *only* in the specific muscles depleted by exercise, so athletes must fully engage the muscles involved in their sport during the depletion phase. Preparing for a marathon requires a 15- or 20-mile run, whereas for swimming and bicycling, each activity requires approximately 90 minutes of moderately intense submaximal exercise. The athlete then maintains a low, 60 to 100 g per day carbohydrate diet for several additional days to further deplete glycogen stores. Glycogen depletion increases

TABLE 12.1 Two-Stage Dietary Plan to Increase Muscle Glycogen Storage

Stage 1—Depletion	Day 1: Exhausting exercise performed to deplete muscle glycogen in specific muscles Days 2, 3, 4: Low-carbohydrate food intake (high percentage of protein and lipid in the daily diet)
Stage 2—Carbohydrate loading	Days 5, 6, 7: High-carbohydrate food intake (normal percentage of protein in the daily diet)
Competition day	Follow high-carbohydrate precompetition meal

UNIQUE DESCRIPTIVE TERM

Of the hundreds of thousands of runners who attempted to race a major marathon over the past three decades, more than two fifths experienced severe and performance-limiting depletion of physiologic carbohydrate reserves, and thousands dropped out before reaching the finish lines (approximately 1%–2% of those who started). Marathon runners use the term "**hitting the wall**" (endurance cyclists use *bonking*) to describe the sensations of fatigue and discomfort in the active muscles associated with severe glycogen depletion. Factors for success include muscle mass distribution (relatively large leg muscles), high liver and muscle glycogen densities, running speed as a fraction of aerobic capacity, and low oxygen cost of running at a particular speed (economy of effort). Successful runners possess large aerobic capacities and store enough liver and muscle glycogen to fuel marathon runs at paces that challenge the current world record of 2:03:59 for men and 2:15:25 for women without depleting carbohydrate below a critical level. Runners with lower aerobic capacities or a relatively small leg muscle mass must run at slower paces or refuel during the race to avoid "hitting the wall."

Source: Rapoport BI. Metabolic factors limiting performance in marathon runners. *PLoS Comput Biol* 2010;10:6.

formation of intermediate forms of the glycogen-storing enzyme **glycogen synthetase** within the muscle fibers. This enzyme facilitates the conversion of glucose to glycogen by changing short polymers of glucose into long polymers for glycogen storage in the biochemical process of glycogenesis. The highest concentration of glycogen synthetase occurs within 1 hour following moderately intense exercise at about 60% $\dot{V}O_{2max}$. Then at least 3 days before competing, the athlete switches to a high 400- to 700-g daily carbohydrate diet and maintains this regimen up to the precompetition meal. The supercompensation diet should also contain adequate protein, minerals, and vitamins and abundant water. For athletes who follow the classic loading procedure, the supercompensated muscle glycogen levels remain stable in a resting, nonexercising individual for at least 3 days if the diet contains about 60% of calories from carbohydrate.[59]

The trained state facilitates both the rate and the magnitude of glycogen replenishment. For sports competition and exercise training, a diet containing between 60 and 70% of calories as carbohydrates generally provides adequate muscle and liver glycogen reserves. This high carbohydrate content ensures about twice the level of muscle glycogen obtained with consumption of a typical diet. Consequently, for well-nourished, physically active individuals, the supercompensation effect remains relatively small. During intense training, individuals who do not increase daily caloric and carbohydrate intakes to meet increased energy demands may experience chronic muscle fatigue and staleness associated with reduced glycogen reserves.

Individuals should learn all they can about carbohydrate loading before trying to manipulate their diet and exercise habits to achieve a supercompensation effect. If a person decides to supercompensate after weighing the pros and cons (see pages 397–398), the new food regimen should progress in stages during training and not be attempted for the first time a few days before competition. For example, a runner should start with a long run followed by a high-carbohydrate diet. The runner should keep a detailed log of how the dietary manipulation affects performance and note subjective feelings during exercise depletion and

Connections to the Past

Frederick Gowland Hopkins (1861–1947)

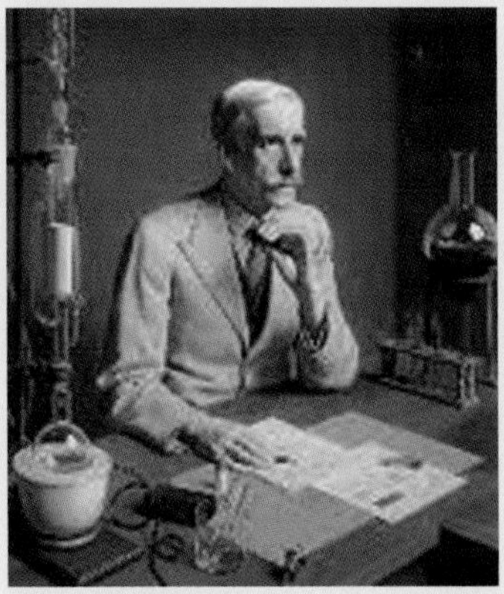

Hopkins did not rise to prominence in the early 20th century by following normal academic channels. He had many interests including invertebrates. At age 17, when he finally left school, he published a paper in *The Entomologist* on the bombardier beetle. Soon after, he began work for an insurance company and then a railroad, and he eventually enrolled in the Royal School of Mines and assisted in a private chemistry laboratory. Hopkins qualified for membership in the Institute of Chemistry by attending lectures at London's University College. Hopkins both produced pioneering studies in nutritional biochemistry and collaborated with physiologist Walter Morley Fletcher (mentor to A.V. Hill) to study muscle chemistry. Their classic 1907 paper in experimental physiology employed new methods to isolate lactic acid in muscle. Prior studies of stimulated muscle showed large concentrations of lactic acid in both stimulated and nonexercised muscle. Fletcher and Hopkins' chemical methods reduced the muscle's enzyme activity prior to analysis to isolate the reactions. They found that a muscle contracting under low oxygen conditions produced lactic acid at the expense of glycogen.

thePoint

Visit **thePoint.lww.com/MKKSEN4e** *to find more details about how this Nobel Prize recipient pioneered studies in nutritional biochemistry and experimental physiology.*

Additional Insights

Probiotics: Empty Promises or the Real Deal?

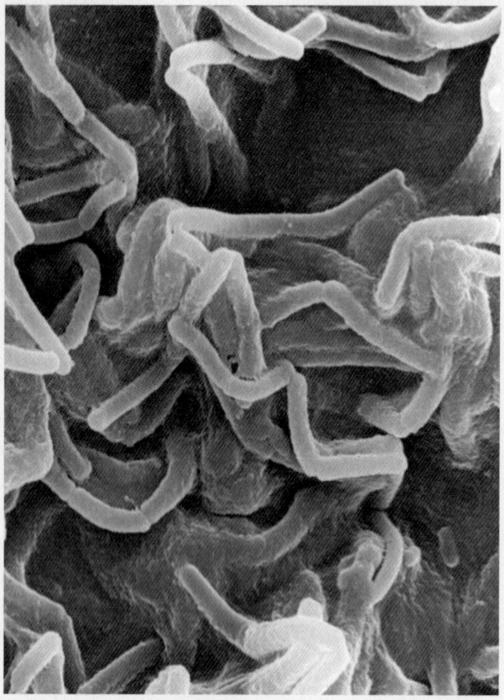

The history of health claims for live microorganisms in food (initially lactic acid bacteria) traces back to antiquity. A version of the Old Testament (Genesis 18:8) writes that Abraham owed his longevity to the consumption of sour milk. Roman physicians often prescribed fermented milk products to alleviate gastroenteritis. From the dawn of microbiology, researchers have attributed many health effects to shifts in the intestinal microbial balance. Reports since the 1800s have touted the many benefits of fermented foods with added live cultures (e.g., lactic acid bacteria, lactobacilli, bifidobacteria, *Lactobacillus acidophilus*). The idea at the time, which still prevails, was that these substances beneficially improved the body's intestinal microbial balance by inhibiting pathogens and toxin-producing bacteria and fostering the growth of beneficial bacterial flora.

The term *probiotic*, from the Greek *for life*, was coined in 1953 by German bacteriologist Werner Kollath (1892–1970). The following represents the most recent and accepted definition of probiotic: "A preparation of or a product containing viable, defined microorganisms in sufficient numbers, which alter the microflora (by implantation or colonization) in a compartment of the host and by that exert beneficial health effects in this host." Alleged health benefits of probiotics include:

1. Lower the frequency and duration of diarrhea associated with antibiotics (Clostridium difficile), rotavirus infection, chemotherapy, and to a lesser extent, traveler's diarrhea
2. Stimulate humoral and cellular immunity
3. Decrease unfavorable metabolites (e.g., the colon's ammonium and procarcinogenic enzymes)
4. Reduce untoward effects in lactose-intolerant individuals

Less convincing evidence of the health effects of probiotics include:

5. Reduction of *Helicobacter pylori* infection
6. Reduction of allergic symptoms
7. Relief from constipation
8. Relief from irritable bowel syndrome
9. Beneficial effects on mineral metabolism, particularly bone density
10. Colon cancer prevention
11. Reduce cholesterol and triacylglycerol plasma concentrations

Live probiotic cultures often are available in fermented dairy products and probiotic-fortified foods. The following are examples of the most common marketed strains of probiotics, some of which can be found in different foods, tablets, capsules, and powders:

1. Bifidobacterium
2. *Lactobacillus acidophilus*
3. *Lactobacillus casei*
4. *Bifidobacterium animalis*
5. *Bifidobacterium breve*
6. *Bifidobacterium infantis*
7. *Escherichia coli*
8. *Saccharomyces boulardii*

Of interest to athletes, coaches, exercise scientists, and sports nutritionists is the potential for probiotic supplements to modulate the intestinal microbial flora and provide a practical means to enhance gut and immune function. Any nutritional practice that upgrades immune function following exercise would certainly benefit individuals exposed to high levels of physical and environmental stressors. Limited data exist concerning potential benefits of probiotic supplementation in exercise. One study evaluated the effect of *Lactobacillus rhamnosus* and *Lactobacillus paracasei* on oxidative stress in athletes during a 4-week period of intense physical activity. Results demonstrated that intense physical activity induced oxidative stress and that probiotic supplementation increased plasma antioxidant levels, thus neutralizing reactive oxygen species with the two *Lactobacillus* strains that exerted strong antioxidant activity. The researchers concluded: "Athletes and all those exposed to oxidative stress may benefit from the ability of these probiotics to increase antioxidant levels and neutralize the effects of reactive oxygen species." Future studies must address issues of dose–response under various exercise conditions, probiotic species-specific effects, and mechanisms of action in affecting exercise performance.

Sources:

Martarelli D, et al. Effect of a probiotic intake on oxidant and antioxidant parameters in plasma of athletes during intense exercise training. *Curr Microbiol* 2011;62:1689.

Rijkers GT, et al. Health benefits and health claims of probiotics: bridging science and marketing. *Br J Nutr* 2011;24:1.

West NP, et al. Probiotics, immunity and exercise: a review. *Exerc Immunol Rev* 2009;15:10.

Related References

Hamilton-Miller JM, et al. Some insights into the derivation and early uses of the word 'probiotic.' *Br J Nutr* 2003;90:845.

Ohigashi S, et al. Functional outcome, quality of life, and efficacy of probiotics in postoperative patients with colorectal cancer. *Surg Today* 2011;419:1200.

Prakash S, et al. Gut microbiota: next frontier in understanding human health and development of biotherapeutics. *Biologics* 2011;5:71.

Schrezenmeir J, de Vrese M. Probiotics, prebiotics, and synbiotics-approaching a definition. *Am J Clin Nutr* 2001;73(2 Suppl):361S.

Wallace TC, Mackay D. The safety of probiotics: considerations following the 2011 U.S. Agency for Health Research and Quality Report. *J Nutr* 2011;141:1923.

Weichselbaum E. Potential benefits of probiotics: main findings of an in-depth review. *Br J Community Nurs* 2010;15:110.

replenishment phases. With positive results, the runner should repeat the entire series of depletion, low-carbohydrate diet, and high-carbohydrate diet but maintain the low-carbohydrate diet for only 1 day. If no adverse effects appear, the low-carbohydrate diet should gradually extend to a maximum of 4 days.

Sample Diets to Achieve the Supercompensation Effect: **TABLE 12.2** gives meal plans for carbohydrate depletion (stage 1) and carbohydrate loading (stage 2) preceding an endurance event.

Limited Applicability

Carbohydrate loading benefits only intense aerobic activities that last more than 60 minutes, unless the person begins competing in a relative state of glycogen depletion. In contrast, less than 60 minutes of intense exercise requires only normal carbohydrate intake and glycogen reserves. For example, carbohydrate loading did not benefit trained runners in a 20.9-km (13-mile) run compared with a run following a low-carbohydrate diet. Similarly, no ergogenic effect emerged in time trial performance, heart rate, and rating of perceived exertion (RPE) for endurance-trained cyclists in a 100-km trial that simulated continuous changes in exercise intensity typical of competition.[22] In addition, ingesting 40 g of carbohydrate immediately before exercise did not benefit a 30-minute maximal cycling performance of trained cyclists.[131] Variations in carbohydrate percentage between 40 and 70% for an isocaloric diet produced no effect on intense exercise of either 10 or 30 minutes in duration.[134] Furthermore, anaerobic power output for 75 seconds or repetitive power performance did not improve when pre-exercise dietary manipulation increased muscle glycogen above normal levels.[69,73] A 2-day maintenance on a high-carbohydrate diet (61% carbohydrate) or a low- to moderate-carbohydrate diet (31% carbohydrate) produced no effect on intermittent anaerobic exercise consisting of five 20-second bouts interspersed with a 100-second recovery period followed by a sixth 30-second bout to exhaustion.[116] Ergogenic benefits did emerge for high-carbohydrate versus low-carbohydrate intakes when performing *multiple bouts* of short-term sprints.[6]

Negative Aspects of Carbohydrate Loading

The effect of extra weight may negate any potential benefits from increased glycogen storage. Each gram of stored glycogen requires the addition of 2.7 g of water bound to the molecule. This makes this storage form of carbohydrate a heavy fuel compared with equivalent energy stored as lipid. The added body mass in the carbohydrate-loaded state often makes the exerciser feel "heavy" and uncomfortable; any extra load also directly adds to the energy cost of weight-bearing running, race-walking, or cross-country skiing activities. Every 11 g of newly stored glycogen stores an additional 1 oz (28.4 g) of water, which means that only 1 oz of additional stored glycogen stores an additional 3 oz (85.2 g) of water, not a trivial amount of weight in terms of additional exercise energy cost. Under normal conditions, total muscle glycogen stores typically average about 400 g, although in trained subjects with a large muscle mass and after a high-carbohydrate meal, this may increase up to 900 g.[92] An additional 500 g of glycogen (17.7 oz) above the normal storage quantity would add 1350 g of water or approximately 48 oz, an amount equivalent to 3 lb added to the individual's body weight! Just adding 100 g to each shoe during jogging or running increases oxygen consumption (and calorie burn) approximately 1%, so adding 3 lb of water from glycogen loading seems fairly substantial in comparison. On the positive side, water liberated during glycogen breakdown aids in temperature regulation, which provides positive benefits during exercise in the heat.

The classic model for supercompensation poses a potential hazard for individuals with specific health problems. A severe, long-term carbohydrate overload interspersed with

TABLE 12.2 Sample Meal Plan for Carbohydrate Depletion and Carbohydrate Loading Diets Preceding an Endurance Event

Meal	Stage 1—Depletion	Stage 2—Carbohydrate Loading
Breakfast	0.5 cup fruit juice 2 eggs 1 slice whole-wheat toast 1 glass whole milk	1 cup fruit juice 1 bowl hot or cold cereal 1–2 muffins 1 tbsp butter Coffee (cream/sugar)
Lunch	6 oz hamburger 2 slices bread Salad (normal size) 1 tbsp mayonnaise and salad dressing 1 glass whole milk	2–3 oz hamburger with bun 1 cup juice 1 orange 1 tbsp mayonnaise Pie or cake (8-inch slice)
Snack	1 cup yogurt	1 cup yogurt, fruit, or cookies
Dinner	2–3 pieces of chicken, fried 1 baked potato with sour cream 0.5 cup vegetables Iced tea (no sugar) 2 tbsp butter	1–1.5 pieces of chicken, baked 1 baked potato with sour cream 1 cup vegetables 0.5 cup sweetened pineapple Iced tea (sugar) 1 tbsp butter
Snack	1 glass whole milk	1 glass chocolate milk with 4 cookies

During stage 1, the intake of carbohydrate approaches approximately 100 g, 400 kcal; in stage 2, the carbohydrate intake increases to 400 to 625 g or about 1600 to 2500 kcal.

periods of high lipid or high protein intake can increase blood cholesterol and urea nitrogen levels. This could negatively affect individuals susceptible to type 2 diabetes and heart disease or those with muscle enzyme deficiencies (e.g., McArdle disease, or glycogen storage disease type V, first described in 1951 by Dr. Brian McArdle of Guy's Hospital, London) or renal disease. High lipid intake causes gastrointestinal distress plus poor recovery from the exercise depletion sequence of the loading procedure. During the low-carbohydrate phase, marked ketosis can occur among individuals who exercise while carbohydrate-depleted. Failure to eat a balanced diet often produces mineral and vitamin deficiencies, particularly of the water-soluble vitamins, which then require supplementation. The glycogen-depleted state certainly reduces one's capability to train hard, possibly resulting in a detraining effect during the loading period. Adverse alterations in mood state also appear in individuals who consume low-carbohydrate diets while they train. Dramatically reducing dietary carbohydrate for 3 or 4 days sets the stage for lean tissue loss because muscle protein serves as gluconeogenic substrate to maintain blood glucose levels in the glycogen-depleted state.

Modified Loading Procedure

Following the less stringent modified dietary protocol outlined in **FIGURE 12.1** minimizes or eliminates many of the negative outcomes of the classic glycogen-loading sequence. This 6-day protocol does not require prior exercise to exhaustion. The athlete exercises at about 75% of $\dot{V}O_{2max}$ (85% of maximum heart rate) for 1.5 hours and then, on successive days, gradually reduces or tapers exercise duration. During the first 3 days, carbohydrates supply about 50% of total calories. Three days before competition, the diet's carbohydrate content then increases to 70% of total energy intake. This causes glycogen reserves to accumulate to about the *same level* as the classic protocol. The modified approach to carbohydrate loading increases the glycogen-storing enzyme glycogen synthetase without requiring the dramatic glycogen depletion with exercise and diet required by the classic loading procedure.[91,196]

MUSCLE GLYCOGEN SUPERCOMPENSATION ENHANCED BY PRIOR CREATINE SUPPLEMENTATION

A synergy exists between glycogen storage and creatine supplementation. For example, preceding a glycogen loading protocol with a 5-day creatine loading protocol (20 $g \cdot d^{-1}$) produced 10% more glycogen packing in the vastus lateralis muscle than achieved with glycogen loading alone.[150] More than likely, increases in creatine and cellular volume with creatine supplementation facilitate subsequent storage of muscle glycogen.

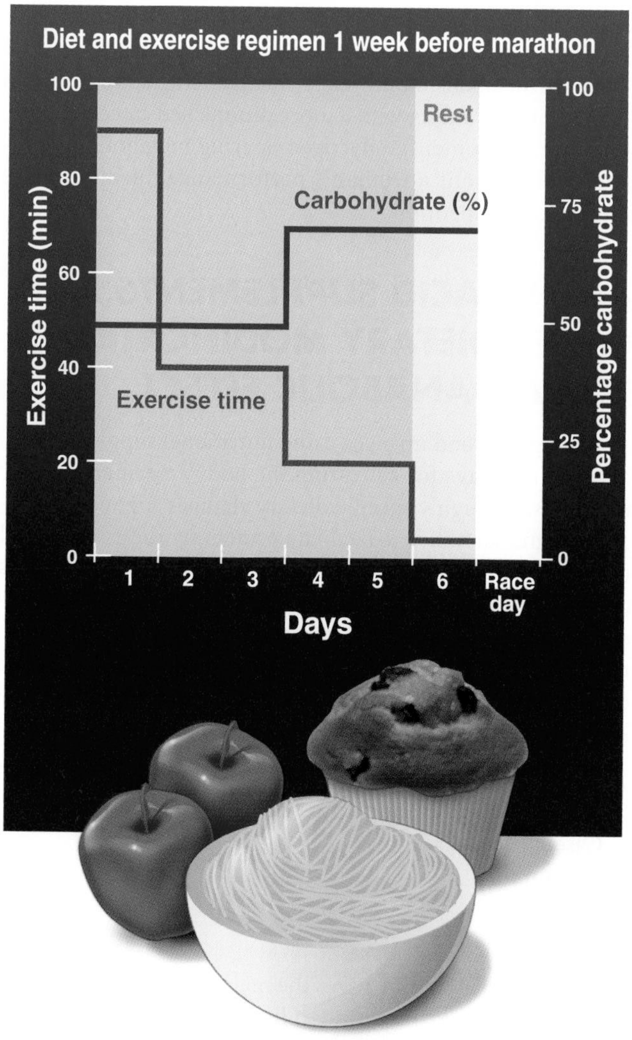

FIGURE 12.1. The modified carbohydrate-loading approach. Recommended combination of diet and exercise for overloading muscle glycogen stores in the week before an endurance contest. Time devoted to exercise becomes gradually reduced during the week, while the diet's carbohydrate content increases for the last 3 days. (From Sherman WM, et al. Effect of exercise-diet manipulation on muscle glycogen and its subsequent utilization during performance. *Int J Sports Med* 1981;2:114.)

Rapid Loading Procedure: A 1-Day Requirement

The 2 to 6 days required to achieve supranormal muscle glycogen levels represent a limitation of typical carbohydrate loading procedures. Research has evaluated whether a shortened time period that combines a relatively brief bout of intense exercise with only 1 day of high-carbohydrate intake achieves the desired loading effect. Endurance-trained athletes cycled for 150 seconds at 130% of $\dot{V}O_{2max}$ followed by 30 seconds of all-out cycling. In the recovery period, the men consumed 10.3 $g \cdot kg^{-1}$ body mass of high-glycemic carbohydrate foods. Biopsy data presented in **FIGURE 12.2** indicated that carbohydrate levels increased in all muscle fiber types of the vastus lateralis muscle from a 109.1 $mmol{\cdot}kg^{-1}$ preloading average to 198.3 $mmol{\cdot}kg^{-1}$ after only 24 hours. This 82% increase in glycogen storage equaled or exceeded values reported by others using a 2- to 6-day regimen. The short-duration loading procedure benefits individuals who wish to continue normal training without the time required and potential negative aspects of other loading protocols.

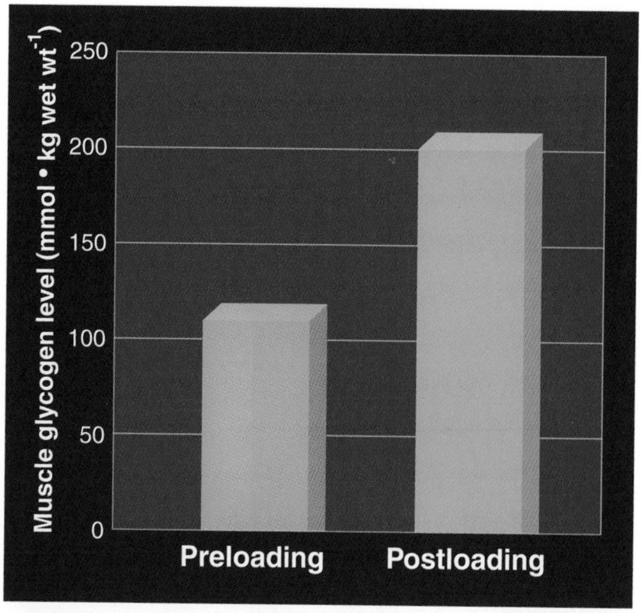

FIGURE 12.2. Muscle glycogen concentration of the vastus lateralis before (preloading) and after 180 seconds of near-maximal intensity cycling exercise followed by 1 day of high carbohydrate intake (postloading). (From Fairchild TJ, et al. Rapid carbohydrate loading after short bout of near maximal-intensity exercise. *Med Sci Sports Exerc* 2002;34:980.)

Gender Differences in Glycogen Supercompensation and Glucose Catabolism During Exercise

Gender-related differences in muscle glycogen supercompensation remain controversial. One study reported a relatively small 13% increase in the muscle glycogen content of women when they switched from a mixed diet to a high-carbohydrate diet.[186] Other research also indicated that women stored less glycogen than men when dietary carbohydrate increased from 60 to 75% of total energy intake.[168] This increase in carbohydrate intake as a percentage of total calories represents *significantly less total carbohydrate intake* relative to lean body mass for women than for men. **FIGURE 12.3** illustrates that equalizing daily carbohydrate intake for endurance-trained men and women at 12 $g \cdot kg^{-1}$ of lean body mass for 3 consecutive days produced no gender differences in glycogen loading. These and other findings[169] support the notion that men and women possess an equal capacity to accumulate muscle glycogen when fed comparable amounts of carbohydrate relative to their lean body mass.

Gender differences exist in carbohydrate metabolism during exercise before and after endurance training. During submaximal exercise at equivalent percentages of $\dot{V}O_{2max}$ (i.e., same relative workload), women derive a smaller proportion of total energy

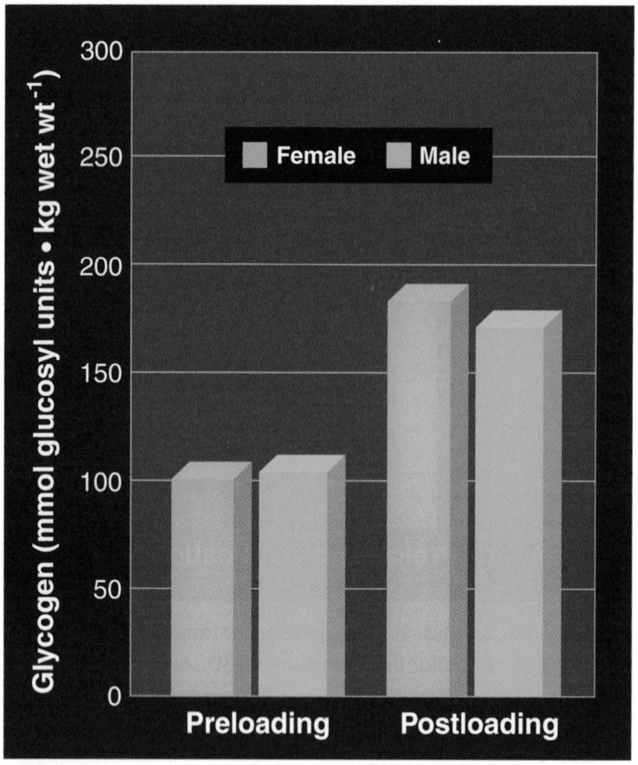

FIGURE 12.3. Muscle glycogen concentrations pre- and postcarbohydrate loading in exercise-trained men and women. (From James AP, et al. Muscle glycogen supercompensation: absence of a gender-related difference. *Eur J Appl Physiol* 2001;85:533.)

from carbohydrate oxidation than men.[85] This gender difference in substrate oxidation does not persist into recovery.[79]

With similar endurance training protocols, both women and men decrease glucose use during a given submaximal power output.[34,54] At the same relative workload after training, women show an exaggerated shift toward fat catabolism, whereas men do not.[85] This suggests that endurance training induces greater glycogen sparing at a given percentage of maximal effort for women. Gender differences in exercise substrate metabolism may reflect sympathetic nervous system adaptation to training with a more diminished catecholamine response for women. A glycogen-sparing metabolic adaptation could benefit a woman's performance during intense endurance competition.

AMINO ACID SUPPLEMENTS AND OTHER DIETARY MODIFICATIONS FOR AN ANABOLIC EFFECT

An emerging trend involves using nutritional supplements as a legal alternative for activating the body's normal anabolic mechanisms. Highly specific dietary changes supposedly create a hormonal milieu to facilitate protein synthesis in skeletal muscle. Moreover, many different nutritional compounds can decrease the breakdown of body tissues. These substances, known as "anticatabolic" compounds, slow the breakdown mostly of cellular protein, thus tilting the metabolic balance toward increased tissue building. The most commonly marketed anticatabolic dietary supplements include:

1. Alpha-ketoglutarate
2. Branched-chain amino acids (BCAA)
3. Casein protein
4. Glutamine
5. Leucine
6. Whey protein

TABLE 12.3 briefly summarizes the major claims of six anticatabolic nutritional compounds, all of which have been tested with human subjects.

More than 100 companies in the United States manufacture and/or market alleged ergogenic protein and/or amino acid supplements. Many athletes and fitness enthusiasts use these supplements believing they boost the body's natural

TABLE 12.3 Major Claims of six commonly marketed nutritional compounds

Claims	Effectiveness	Comments/Concerns
Alpha-ketogluterate: Spares glutamine (thus sparing muscle tissue), the largest source of the body's glutamine	Moderate to high	Well tolerated, but long-term safety unclear
Branched-chain amino acids (BCAAs): Stimulated protein synthesis to spare muscle	Moderate to high	Safe
Casein protein: Helps decrease protein breakdown; increases protein synthesis	Moderate to high	May increase blood cholesterol
Glutamine: Involved in energy metabolism to spare protein breakdown	High	Requires high doses; safe
Leucine: Helps spare muscle tissue	Moderate	Safe
Whey protein: Sources of essential amino acids; decreases protein catabolism, spares protein	High	Safe

production of the anabolic hormones testosterone, growth hormone (GH), and insulin-like growth factor 1 (IGF-1) to increase muscle size and strength and decrease body fat. The rationale for trying nutritional ergogenic stimulants comes from clinical use of amino acid infusion or ingestion in protein-deficient patients to regulate anabolic hormones.

Research on healthy subjects does not provide convincing evidence for an ergogenic effect of a general dietary increase of oral amino acid supplements on hormone secretion, training responsiveness, or exercise performance. For example, in studies with appropriate design and statistical analysis, supplements of arginine, lysine, ornithine, tyrosine, and other amino acids, either singly or in combination, produced no effect on GH levels,[52,167] insulin secretion,[21,52] diverse measures of anaerobic power,[51] or all-out running performance at $\dot{V}O_{2max}$.[164] For older men, protein supplementation before and after resistance training provided no additional effect on gains in muscle mass and strength.[24] Elite junior weightlifters who supplemented regularly with 20 amino acids did not improve physical performance or resting or exercise-induced responses of testosterone, cortisol, or GH.[56] The indiscriminate use of amino acid supplements at dosages considered pharmacologic rather than nutritional increases risk of direct toxic effects or creation of an amino acid imbalance.[119]

Prudent Means to Possibly Augment an Anabolic Effect

Manipulation of exercise and nutritional variables in the immediate pre-exercise and postexercise periods can impact responsiveness to resistance training via mechanisms that alter nutrient availability, circulating metabolites and hormonal secretions, interactions with receptors on target tissues, and gene translation and transcription.[184] With resistance training, muscle enlargement or hypertrophy occurs from shifts in the body's normal dynamic state of protein synthesis and degradation to greater tissue synthesis. The normal hormonal milieu (e.g., insulin and GH levels) in the immediate period following resistance exercise stimulates the muscle fiber's anabolic processes while inhibiting muscle protein degradation. Specific dietary modifications that increase amino acid transport into muscle, raise energy availability, or increase anabolic hormone levels would theoretically augment the training effect by increasing the rate of anabolism and/or depressing catabolism. Either effect should create a positive body protein balance to improve muscular growth and increase strength.

Carbohydrate–Protein Supplementation Immediately in Recovery Augments Hormonal Response to Resistance Exercise

Studies of hormonal dynamics and muscle protein anabolism indicate a transient but potential ergogenic effect (up to fourfold increase in protein synthesis[141]) of carbohydrate and/or protein supplements consumed *before*[171,194] or *immediately after*[102,103,142,146] resistance exercise workouts. This effect of carbohydrate–protein supplementation in resistance exercise may prove effective to improve net protein balance at rest and for repair and synthesis of muscle proteins following aerobic exercise.[112,113] It also may blunt the loss in muscle strength during the initial high-volume stress of resistance training, possibly by reducing muscle damage by maintaining an anabolic environment.[106]

Drug-free male weightlifters with at least 2 years of resistance training experience consumed carbohydrate and protein supplements immediately following a standard resistance training workout.[30] Treatment included either (1) placebo of pure water or a supplement of (2) carbohydrate (1.5 g · kg^{-1} body mass), (3) protein (1.38 g · kg^{-1} body mass), or (4) carbohydrate plus protein (carbohydrate, 1.06 g · kg^{-1} body mass; protein, 0.41 g · kg^{-1} body mass) consumed immediately following and then 2 hours after the training session. Compared with the placebo condition, each supplement produced a hormonal environment in recovery conducive to protein synthesis and muscle tissue growth (elevated plasma concentrations of insulin and GH). Subsequent research from the same laboratory showed that protein–carbohydrate supplementation before and after resistance training favorably altered metabolic and hormonal responses to 3 consecutive days of intense resistance training.[105] Changes in the immediate recovery period included increased concentrations of glucose, insulin, GH, and IGF-1 and decreased blood lactate concentration. Such data provide indirect evidence for a possible training benefit of increasing carbohydrate and/or protein intake immediately after a resistance training workout.

Postexercise Glucose Augments Protein Balance after Resistance Training: Research with postexercise glucose ingestion complements the previously described studies of carbohydrate/protein supplementation following resistance training.[152] Healthy men familiar with resistance training performed unilateral knee extensor exercise consisting of eight sets of 10 repetitions at 85% of maximum strength (one-repetition maximum) in a placebo-controlled, randomized, double-blind trial. Immediately following the exercise session and 1 hour later, subjects received either a carbohydrate supplement (1.0 g · kg^{-1} body mass) or a NutraSweet placebo. Measurements consisted of urinary 3-methylhistidine (3-MH) excretion to indicate muscle protein degradation, vastus lateralis muscle incorporation rate for the amino acid leucine (L-[l-^{13}C]) to indicate protein synthesis, and urinary nitrogen excretion to reflect protein breakdown. **FIGURE 12.4** shows that glucose supplementation reduced myofibrillar protein breakdown reflected by decreased excretion of both 3-MH and urinary urea. Glucose supplementation did not significantly increase leucine incorporation into the vastus lateralis over the 10-hour postexercise period. Any beneficial effect of glucose supplementation immediately following resistance

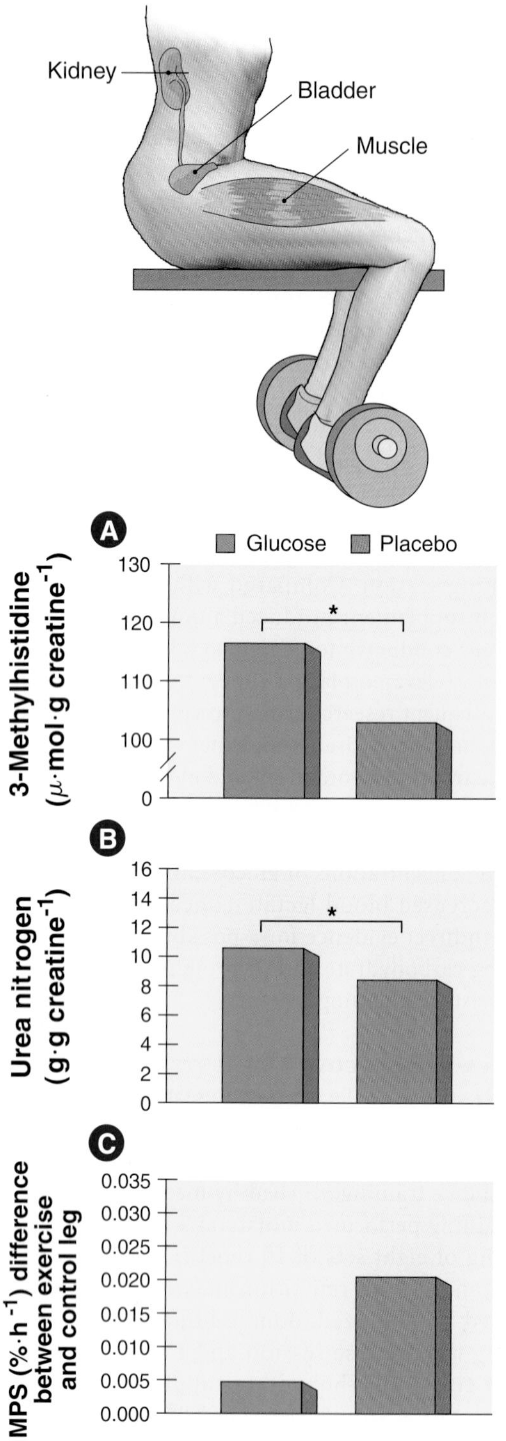

FIGURE 12.4. The effects of glucose (1.0 g · kg^{-1} body mass) versus NutraSweet placebo ingested immediately after exercise and 1 hour later on protein degradation reflected by 24-hour urinary output of **(A)** 3-methylhistidine and **(B)** urea nitrogen, and **(C)** the rate of muscle protein synthesis *(MPS)* measured by vastus lateralis muscle incorporation rate for the amino acid leucine (L-[I-^{13}C]). *Bars* for MPS indicate difference between exercise and control leg for glucose and placebo conditions. *Significantly different from placebo condition. (From Roy BD, et al. Effect of glucose supplement timing on protein metabolism after resistance training. *J Appl Physiol* 1997;82:1882.)

exercise most likely results from increased insulin release. This hormone would enhance a positive muscle protein balance in recovery.

Dietary Lipid Affects Hormonal Milieu

The diet's lipid content modulates resting neuroendocrine homeostasis in a direction that may modify tissue synthesis. Research evaluated the effects of an intense resistance exercise bout on postexercise plasma testosterone, an anabolic and anticatabolic hormone released by the testes' Leydig cells.[183] In agreement with prior research, testosterone levels significantly increased 5 minutes postexercise. A more impressive finding revealed a close association between the individual's regular dietary nutrient composition and resting plasma testosterone levels. **TABLE 12.4** shows that dietary macronutrient amount and composition (protein, lipid, saturated fatty acids, monounsaturated fatty acids, polyunsaturated unsaturated fatty acid/saturated fatty acid ratio, and protein-to-carbohydrate ratio) correlated with pre-exercise testosterone concentrations. More specifically, dietary lipid and saturated and monounsaturated fatty acid levels best predicted

TABLE 12.4 Association (Correlations) Between Pre-exercise Testosterone Concentration and Selected Nutritional Variables

Nutrient	Correlation with Testosterone[a]
Energy (kJ)	−0.18
Protein (%)[b]	−0.71*
CHO (%)	−0.30
Lipid (%)	0.72*
SFA (g·1000 kcal·d^{-1})	0.77†
MUFA (g·1000 kcal·d^{-1})	0.79†
PUFA (g·1000 kcal·d^{-1})	0.25
Cholesterol (g·1000 kcal·d^{-1})	0.53
PUFA/SFA	−0.63‡
Dietary fiber (g·1000 kcal·d^{-1})	−0.19
Protein/CHO	−0.59‡
Protein/lipid	0.16
CHO/lipid	0.16

From Volek JS, et al. Testosterone and cortisol in relationship to dietary nutrients and resistance exercise. J Appl Physiol 1997;82:49.

[a] *Correlation coefficients, Pearson product-moment correlations.*

[b] *Nutrient percentage values expressed as percentage of total energy per day.*

*$P \le .01$. †$P \le .005$. ‡$P \le .05$.

CHO, cholesterol; MUFA, monounsaturated fatty acids; PUFA, polyunsaturated fatty acids; SFA, saturated fatty acids.

testosterone concentrations at rest—lower levels of each of these dietary components related to lower testosterone levels. These findings agree with previous studies that showed that a low-fat diet of about 20% fat produced lower testosterone levels than a diet with a higher 40% lipid content.[140,145,170]

Interestingly, the data in Table 12.4 also show that the diet's protein percentage correlated *inversely* with testosterone levels (higher protein levels related to *lower* testosterone levels). Because many resistance-trained athletes consume considerable dietary protein, the implications of this association for exercise training remain unresolved. Also, if low dietary lipid levels decrease resting levels of testosterone, then individuals consuming low-fat diets (e.g., vegetarians and many dancers, gymnasts, and wrestlers) may experience a diminished training response. Athletes who show reduced plasma testosterone with overtraining might benefit from changing their diet's macronutrient composition in the direction of higher lipid intake.

L-CARNITINE

L-Carnitine (L-3-hydroxytrimethylamminobutanoate), a short-chain carboxylic acid containing nitrogen and stereoisomer of carnitine, is a vitamin-like compound with well-established functions in intermediary metabolism. It is found mostly in meat and dairy products. (*Note:* DL-Carnitine is toxic and should never be consumed.) The liver and kidneys synthesize L-carnitine from methionine and lysine, with about 95% of the total 20 g (120 mmol) of carnitine located within muscle cells. Vital to normal metabolism, carnitine facilitates the influx of long-chain fatty acids into the mitochondrial matrix as part of the carnitine–acyl-coenzyme A (CoA) transferase system. The system causes activated acyl groups to reversibly transfer between coenzyme A and carnitine (see Chapter 4). The fatty acid components then enter β-oxidation during mitochondrial energy metabolism as follows:

$$\text{Carnitine} + \text{acyl-CoA} \leftrightarrow \text{acylcarnitine} + \text{CoA}$$

This reaction enables the acyl components of long-chain fatty acyl-CoA (carbon chain lengths ≥10) to cross the mitochondrial membrane as substrate for oxidation. This carnitine-dependent process represents an important rate-limiting step in fatty acid oxidation. Intracellular carnitine helps to maintain the acetyl-CoA/CoA ratio within the cell. Optimizing this ratio augments skeletal muscle energy metabolism by limiting inhibition of the pyruvate dehydrogenase enzyme; this effect facilitates conversion of pyruvate (and lactate) to acetyl-CoA, particularly in type I, slow-twitch muscle fibers.[29,55] Theoretically, enhanced carnitine function could inhibit lactate accumulation and enhance exercise performance.[35,94] The box titled "Potential Mechanisms for a Beneficial Effect of Carnitine Supplementation on Exercise Performance in Healthy Humans" outlines the potential mechanisms by which carnitine supplementation could enhance exercise performance.

POTENTIAL MECHANISMS FOR A BENEFICIAL EFFECT OF CARNITINE SUPPLEMENTATION ON EXERCISE PERFORMANCE IN HEALTHY HUMANS

- Enhance muscle fatty acid oxidation
- Decrease muscle glycogen depletion
- Shift substrate use in muscle from fatty acid to glucose
- Replace muscle carnitine redistributed into acylcarnitine
- Activate pyruvate dehydrogenase via lowering of acetyl-CoA content
- Improve muscle fatigue resistance
- Replace carnitine lost during training

From Brass EP. Supplemental carnitine and exercise. *Am J Clin Nutr* 2000;72(Suppl):618S.

A COMPOUND FOR ALL

Marketers of L-carnitine target endurance athletes who believe this "metabolic stimulator" enhances fat burning and spares glycogen. Not surprisingly, the alleged fat-burning benefits of carnitine also appeal to body builders as a practical way to reduce body fat.

Rate of Fatty Acid Oxidation Affects Aerobic Exercise Intensity

During prolonged aerobic exercise, plasma free fatty acids (FFAs) often rise to a greater extent than required by the actual energy expenditure. The plasma lipid elevation could result from inadequate mitochondrial fatty acid uptake and oxidation because of insufficient L-carnitine concentration. Increasing intracellular L-carnitine levels through dietary supplementation should elevate aerobic energy transfer from fat breakdown while conserving limited glycogen reserves. Supplementation should prove most beneficial under conditions of glycogen depletion, which places the greatest demand on fatty acid oxidation.

Patients with progressive muscle weakness benefit from carnitine administration, yet few data suggest that healthy adults require carnitine above levels in a well-balanced diet. *Research shows no ergogenic benefits, positive metabolic alterations (aerobic or anaerobic), enhanced recovery effect, or body fat–reducing effects from l-carnitine supplementation.*[1,20,165] For example, no difference exists in muscle carnitine levels between young and middle-aged men who consume a normal carnitine intake of about 100 to 200 mg daily. For these individuals, typical variations in carnitine levels do not reflect capacity for aerobic metabolism.[163] Furthermore, no L-carnitine deficit occurs during long-term exercise or intense training.[40,84,130] The low bioavailability and rapid renal excretion of oral carnitine make it highly unlikely that supplementation affects muscle carnitine stores in healthy subjects. Taking up to 2000 mg of L-carnitine, either orally or intravenously, during aerobic exercise does not affect the fuel mixture catabolized or endurance performance, aerobic capacity, or exercise level for the onset of blood lactate accumulation.[18,185]

Short-term administration of 2000 mg of L-carnitine to endurance athletes 2 hours before a marathon and after 20 km of the run increased plasma concentrations of all carnitine fractions.[39] The carnitine increases did not affect running performance, alter metabolic mixture during the run, or enhance recovery. Even with exercise prolonged and intense enough to deplete glycogen reserves, L-carnitine supplements did not alter substrate metabolism to indicate enhanced fat oxidation.[40] Carnitine supplementation also exerts no effect on repetitive short-term anaerobic exercise. Lactate accumulation, acid–base balance, and performance in five 100-yard swims with 2-minute rest intervals did not differ between competitive swimmers who consumed 2000 mg of L-carnitine in a citrus drink twice daily for 7 days and swimmers who only consumed the citrus drink.[172]

Perhaps of Some Benefit

L-Carnitine acts as a vasodilator in peripheral tissues, possibly enhancing regional blood flow and oxygen delivery. In one study, subjects took either L-carnitine supplements (3000 mg per day for 3 weeks) or an inert placebo to evaluate the effectiveness of L-carnitine supplementation on delayed-onset muscle soreness (DOMS).[57] They then performed eccentric muscle actions to induce muscle soreness. Compared with placebo conditions, subjects receiving L-carnitine experienced less postexercise muscle pain and tissue damage as indicated by lower plasma levels of the muscle enzyme creatine kinase (CK). The vasodilation property of L-carnitine might improve oxygen supply to injured tissue and promote clearance of muscle damage by-products, thus reducing DOMS.

CHROMIUM

Chromium occurs widely in soil as chromite at a concentration that averages 250 μg · kg^{-1} of soil. Its distribution in plants ranges between 100 and 500 μg · kg^{-1} and in foodstuffs between 20 and 590 μg · kg^{-1}. This trace mineral serves as a cofactor (as trivalent chromium) for a low molecular weight protein that potentiates insulin function, although chromium's precise mechanism of action remains unclear. Insulin promotes glucose transport into cells, augments fatty acid metabolism, and triggers cellular enzyme activity to facilitate protein synthesis.

Chronic chromium deficiency increases blood cholesterol and decreases sensitivity to insulin, thus increasing the chance for developing type 2 diabetes. Some adult Americans consume less than the 50 to 200 μg of chromium each day considered the *estimated safe and adequate daily dietary intake.* This occurs largely because chromium-rich foods—brewer's yeast, broccoli, wheat germ, nuts, liver, prunes, egg yolks, apples with skins, asparagus, mushrooms, wine, and cheese—do not usually form a significant part of the regular diet. Processing also removes considerable chromium from foods, and strenuous exercise and associated high carbohydrate intake promote urinary chromium losses, thus increasing the potential for chromium deficiency.

For athletes with chromium-deficient diets, modification to increase chromium intake or prudent use of chromium supplements seems appropriate. Touted as a "fat burner" and "muscle builder," chromium represents one of the largest selling mineral supplements in the United States (second only to calcium). Used by more than 10 million people, it commands annual sales of roughly $100 million. Poor intestinal absorption of chromium in its inorganic form (chromium chloride) provides a main hindrance to effective oral chromium supplementation. Supplement intake of chromium, usually as **chromium picolinate** (picolinic acid, an organic compound in breast milk that helps transport minerals), often reaches 600 μg daily. This chelated picolinic acid combination supposedly improves chromium absorption. Millions of Americans believe the unsubstantiated claims of health food faddists, television infomercials, and exercise zealots that additional chromium promotes muscle growth, curbs appetite, fosters body fat loss, and lengthens life.

Generally, studies suggesting beneficial effects of chromium supplements on body fat and muscle mass inferred body composition modifications from changes in body weight (or unvalidated anthropometric measurements) instead of a more appropriate assessment by hydrostatic weighing or dual-energy x-ray absorptiometry (DXA). One

A NUTRITIONAL LINK TO BIGGER MUSCLES?

Advertisers target chromium supplements to body builders and other resistance-trained individuals as a safe alternative to anabolic steroids to favorably modify body composition. Chromium supplements supposedly potentiate insulin's action, thus increasing skeletal muscle's amino acid anabolism. This belief persists despite sufficient scientific evidence that chromium supplements exert no effect on glucose or insulin concentrations in nondiabetic individuals.[2]

study observed that supplementing daily with 200 μg (3.85 μmol) of chromium picolinate for 40 days produced a small increase in fat-free body mass (FFM; estimated from skinfold thickness) and a decrease in body fat in young men undergoing 6 weeks of resistance training.[48] Another study reported increased body mass without changes in muscular strength or body composition in previously untrained female college students (no change in males) receiving daily chromium supplements of 200 μg during a 12-week resistance training program compared with unsupplemented controls.[72]

Other research evaluated the effects of a daily 200-μg chromium supplement on muscle strength, body composition, and chromium excretion in untrained men during 12 weeks of resistance training.[68] Muscular strength improved 24% for the supplemented group and 33% for the placebo group. No changes occurred in any of the body composition variables. The group receiving the supplement did show higher chromium excretion than the controls after 6 weeks of training. The researchers concluded that chromium supplements provided *no ergogenic effect* on any of the measured variables.

Daily supplementation of 400 μg of chromium picolinate for 9 weeks did not promote weight loss for sedentary obese women but actually caused weight gain during the treatment period.[62] In support of chromium supplementation, greater body fat loss (no increase in FFM) occurred in subjects "recruited from a variety of fitness and athletic clubs" who consumed 400 μg daily over 90 days than in subjects receiving a placebo.[93] Hydrostatic weighing and DXA assessed body composition. The pretest versus posttest body composition data from hydrostatic weighing were not presented, and the DXA-derived analysis indicated average percentage body fat values of 42% for both control and experimental subjects, a seemingly extraordinary level of obesity for fitness club members.

Collegiate football players who received daily supplements of 200 μg of chromium picolinate for 9 weeks showed no changes in body composition and muscular strength from intense weightlifting training compared with a control group who received a placebo.[33] Similar findings of no benefit on body composition and exercise performance variables emerged from a 14-week study of National Collegiate Athletic Association Division I wrestlers who combined chromium picolinate supplementation with a typical preseason training program, compared with identical training without supplementation.[187]

Muscle mass loss commonly affects older individuals, so any potential benefit on muscle from chromium supplementation should readily emerge in this group. This did not occur for older men involved in intense resistance training. A daily high dose of 924 μg of chromium picolinate did not augment gains in muscle size, strength, or power or FFM compared with the no-supplement condition.[24] Among obese personnel enrolled in the US Navy's mandatory remedial physical conditioning program, consuming an additional 400 μg of chromium picolinate daily caused no greater loss in body weight and percentage body fat or increase in FFM than occurred in a group receiving a placebo.[173]

A comprehensive double-blind research design studied the effect of a daily chromium supplement (3.3–3.5 μmol either as chromium chloride or chromium picolinate) or a placebo for 8 weeks during resistance training in young men.[115] For each group, dietary intakes of protein, magnesium, zinc, copper, and iron equaled or exceeded recommended levels during training; subjects also maintained adequate baseline chromium intakes. Supplementation increased serum chromium concentration and urinary chromium excretion equally, regardless of its ingested form. **TABLE 12.5** shows that compared with placebo treatment, chromium supplementation did not affect training-related changes in muscular strength, physique, FFM, or muscle mass. The Federal Trade Commission (www.ftc.gov/) has ordered manufacturers of chromium supplements to cease promoting unsubstantiated weight loss and health claims (e.g., reduced body fat, increased muscle mass, increased energy level) for chromium picolinate. Companies can no longer claim benefits for this compound unless reliable research data substantiated such claims.

Not Without a Potential Down Side

Chromium competes with iron for binding to transferrin, a plasma protein that transports iron from ingested food and damaged red blood cells and delivers it to tissues in need. The chromium picolinate supplements for the group whose data appear in Table 12.5 did reduce serum transferrin (a measure of current iron intake) compared with chromium chloride or placebo treatments. However, other researchers have observed that giving middle-aged men 924 μg of supplemental chromium picolinate daily for 12 weeks did not affect hematologic measures or indices of iron metabolism or iron status.[23] Further research must determine whether chromium supplementation above recommended values adversely affects iron transport and distribution within the body. No studies have evaluated the safety of long-term supplementation with chromium picolinate or the ergogenic efficacy of supplementation in individuals with suboptimal chromium status. Concerning the bioavailability of trace minerals in the diet, excessive dietary chromium inhibits zinc and iron absorption. At the extreme, this could induce iron deficiency anemia, blunt the ability to train intensely, and negatively affect exercise performance requiring a high level of aerobic metabolism.

Further potential bad news emerges from studies in which human tissue cultures that received extreme doses of chromium picolinate show eventual chromosomal damage. Critics contend that such high laboratory dosages do

TABLE 12.5 Effects of Two Different Forms of Chromium Supplementation on Average Values for Anthropometric, Bone, and Soft Tissue Composition Measurements before and after Weight Training

	Placebo		Chromium chloride		Chromium picolinate	
	Pre	Post	Pre	Post	Pre	Post
Age (y)	21.1	21.5	23.3	23.5	22.3	22.5
Stature (cm)	179.3	179.2	177.3	177.3	178.0	178.2
Weight (kg)	79.9	80.5[a]	79.3	81.1[a]	79.2	80.5
∑ 4 skinfold thickness (mm)[b]	42.0	41.5	42.6	42.2	43.3	43.1
Upper arm (cm)	30.9	31.6[a]	31.3	32.0[a]	31.1	31.4[a]
Lower leg (cm)	38.2	37.9	37.4	37.5	37.1	37.0
Endomorphy	3.68	3.73	3.58	3.54	3.71	3.72
Mesomorphy	4.09	4.36[a]	4.25	4.42[a]	4.21	4.33[a]
Ectomorphy	2.09	1.94[a]	1.79	1.63[a]	2.00	1.88[a]
FFMFM (kg)[c]	62.9	64.3[a]	61.1	63.1[a]	61.3	62.7[a]
Bone mineral (g)	2952	2968	2860	2878	2918	2940
Fat-free mass (kg)	65.9	67.3[a]	64.0	65.9[a]	64.2	66.1[a]
Fat (kg)	13.4	13.1	14.7	15.1	14.7	14.5
Fatness (%)	16.4	15.7	18.4	18.2	18.4	17.9

From Lukaski HC, et al. Chromium supplementation and resistance training: effects on body composition, strength, and trace element status of men. *Am J Clin Nutr 1996;63:954.*

[a]*Significantly different from pretraining value*

[b]*Measured at biceps, triceps, subscapular, and suprailiac sites*

[c]*Fat-free, mineral-free mass*

not occur with supplement use in humans. Nonetheless, one could argue that cells continually exposed to excessive chromium (e.g., long-term supplementation) accumulate this mineral and retain it for years.

COENZYME Q_{10} (UBIQUINONE)

Coenzyme Q_{10} (CoQ_{10}, *ubiquinone* in oxidized form and *ubiquinol* when reduced), found primarily in meats, peanuts, and soybean oil, functions as an integral component of the mitochondrion's electron transport system of oxidative phosphorylation. This lipid-soluble natural component of all cells exists in high concentrations within myocardial tissue. CoQ_{10} has been used therapeutically to treat cardiovascular disease because of its role in oxidative metabolism and its antioxidant properties that promote scavenging of free radicals that damage cellular components.[86,178] Due to its positive effect on oxygen uptake and exercise performance in cardiac patients, some consider CoQ_{10} a potential ergogenic nutrient for endurance performance. Based on the belief that supplementation could increase the flux of electrons through the respiratory chain and thus augment aerobic resynthesis of adenosine triphosphate (ATP), the popular literature touts that CoQ_{10} supplements improve "stamina" and enhance cardiovascular function.

Supplementation with CoQ_{10} increases serum CoQ_{10} levels, but it does not improve aerobic capacity, endurance performance, plasma glucose, or lactate levels at submaximal workloads or cardiovascular dynamics compared with a placebo.[19,148,198] One study evaluated oral supplements of CoQ_{10} on the exercise tolerance and peripheral muscle function of healthy, middle-aged men.[137] Measurements included $\dot{V}O_{2max}$, lactate threshold, heart rate response, and upper extremity exercise blood flow and metabolism. For 2 months, subjects received either CoQ_{10} (150 $mg \cdot d^{-1}$) or a placebo. Blood levels of CoQ_{10} increased during the treatment period and remained unchanged in the controls. No differences occurred between groups for any of the physiologic or metabolic variables. Similarly, for trained young and older men, CoQ_{10} supplementation of 120 $mg \cdot d^{-1}$ for 6 weeks did not benefit aerobic capacity or lipid peroxidation, a marker of oxidative stress.[111] Subsequent data also indicate that CoQ_{10} supplements (60 mg daily combined with vitamins E and C) did not affect lipid peroxidation during exercise in endurance athletes.[178]

However, rats supplemented with CoQ_{10} (10 mg daily for 4 days) showed marked suppression of exercise-induced lipid peroxidation in liver, heart, and gastrocnemius muscle tissues.[49]

Future research must elucidate any potential benefits from exogenous CoQ_{10} supplementation. If benefits result, do they depend on the health status of one's cardiovascular system? On a negative note, CoQ_{10} supplementation may induce harmful effects. Increased cell damage (increased plasma CK) occurred during intense exercise in subjects receiving 60 mg of CoQ_{10} twice daily for 20 days.[120] Researchers speculate that under conditions of high proton concentrations as occur in intense aerobic exercise, CoQ_{10} supplementation augments free radical production.[42,120] If this proves true, supplementation could trigger plasma membrane lipid peroxidation and eventual cellular damage. This is indeed paradoxical in light of CoQ_{10}'s wide use as an oral antioxidant supplement.[74]

CREATINE

Meat, poultry, and fish provide rich sources of creatine; they contain approximately 4 to 5 $g \cdot kg^{-1}$ of food weight. The body synthesizes only about 1 to 2 g of this nitrogen-containing organic compound daily, primarily in the kidneys, liver, and pancreas, from the amino acids arginine, glycine, and methionine. Thus, adequate dietary creatine usually becomes important for obtaining required amounts of this compound.[195] Because the animal kingdom contains the richest creatine-containing foods, vegetarians experience a distinct disadvantage in obtaining ready sources of exogenous creatine.

Creatine supplements sold as **creatine monohydrate (CrH_2O)** come as a powder, tablet, capsule, and stabilized liquid. A person can purchase creatine over the counter or via mail order as a nutritional supplement (without guarantee of purity). Ingesting a liquid suspension of creatine monohydrate at the relatively high dosage of 20 to 30 g per day for up to 2 weeks increases intramuscular concentrations of free creatine and phosphocreatine by 10 to 30%. These levels remain high for weeks after only a few days of supplementation.[66,71,121] An athlete can supplement with creatine in international competition because international governing bodies (including the International Olympic Committee; www.olympic.org/ioc) do not consider creatine an illegal substance.

THREE IMPORTANT BENEFITS TO STRENGTH/POWER ATHLETES

Creatine supplementation at recommended levels exerts the following three positive effects in individuals involved in power-type physical activities:

1. Improves repetitive performance in muscular strength and short-term power activities
2. Augments short bursts of muscular endurance
3. Provides greater muscular overload to enhance training effectiveness

Important Component of High-Energy Phosphates

The precise physiologic mechanisms underlying the potential ergogenic effectiveness of supplemental creatine remain poorly understood. Creatine passes through the digestive tract unaltered for absorption into the bloodstream by the intestinal mucosa. Just about all ingested creatine incorporates within skeletal muscle (120–150 g total with average concentration of 125 mM [range, 90–160 mM] per kilogram of dry muscle) via insulin-mediated active transport. About 40% of the total exists as free creatine; the remainder combines readily with phosphate (in the CK reaction shown below) to form phosphocreatine (PCr). Type II, fast-twitch muscle fibers store about four to six times more PCr than ATP.[28] As emphasized in Chapter 4, PCr serves as the cells' "energy reservoir" to provide rapid phosphate-bond energy to resynthesize ATP (more rapid than ATP generated in glycogenolysis) in the reversible CK reaction:

$$\text{PCr} + \text{ADP} \xleftrightarrow{\text{creatine kinase}} \text{Cr} + \text{ATP}$$

PCr may also "shuttle" intramuscular high-energy phosphate between the mitochondria and the cross-bridge sites that initiate muscle action. Maintaining a high sarcoplasmic ATP/adenosine diphosphate (ADP) ratio by energy transfer from PCr becomes important in all-out physical effort lasting up to 10 seconds. Such short-duration exercise places considerable demands on the rate of ATP resynthesis, the breakdown of which greatly exceeds energy transfer from the intracellular macronutrients.[15] Improved energy transfer capacity from PCr also lessens reliance on energy transfer from anaerobic glycolysis with its associated increase in intramuscular H^+ and decrease in pH from lactate accumulation. Due to limited amounts of intramuscular PCr, it seems reasonable that any increase in PCr availability should have the following four effects[15,27,65]:

1. Accelerating ATP turnover rate to maintain power output during short-term muscular effort
2. Delaying PCr depletion
3. Diminishing dependence on anaerobic glycolysis with subsequent lactate formation
4. Facilitating muscle relaxation and recovery from repeated bouts of an intense, brief effort via increased rate of ATP and PCr resynthesis; rapid recovery allows continued high-level power output

A PRACTICAL FINDING

Creatine supplementation (0.3 g · kg^{-1} body weight) offered no benefit to endurance exercise performance in elderly women. Importantly, it did increase their ability to perform functional living tasks involving rapid movements of the lower body.[26]

Documented Benefits Under Certain Exercise Conditions

Creatine received notoriety as an ergogenic aid when used by British sprinters and hurdlers in the 1992 Barcelona Olympic Games. Creatine supplementation at the recommended level exerts ergogenic effects in short-duration, high-intensity exercise (5–10% improvement) without producing harmful side effects (**TABLE 12.6**). Anecdotes indicate a possible association between creatine supplementation and cramping in multiple muscle areas during competition or lengthy practice by football players. This effect may result from one or both of the following:

1. Altered intracellular dynamics from increased free creatine and PCr levels
2. An osmotically induced enlarged muscle cell volume (greater cellular hydration) caused by the increased creatine content

Gastrointestinal tract nausea, indigestion, and difficulty absorbing food have also been linked to exogenous creatine ingestion.

FIGURE 12.5 clearly illustrates the positive ergogenic effects of creatine loading on total work accomplished during repetitive sprint cycling performance. Physically active but untrained males performed sets of maximal 6-second bicycle sprints interspersed with various recovery periods (24, 54, or 84 seconds) between sprints to simulate sport conditions. Performance evaluations took place under creatine-loaded (20 g·d^{-1} for 5 days or placebo conditions. Supplementation increased muscle creatine (48.9%) and PCr (12.5%) over the placebo levels. Increased intramuscular creatine produced a 6% increase in total work accomplished (251.7 kJ presupplement vs 266.9 kJ after creatine loaded) compared with the group that consumed the placebo (254.0 kJ presupplement vs 252.3 kJ after placebo). Creatine supplements have benefited an on-court "ghosting" routine of

TABLE 12.6 Selected Studies Showing Increase in Exercise Performance Following Creatine Monohydrate Supplementation

Reference	Exercise	Protocol	Exercise Performance
1.	Cycle ergometry (140 rev·min^{-1})	Ten 6-s bouts w/1-min rest periods	Better able to maintain pedal frequency during 4–6 s of each bout
2.	Cycle ergometry (80 rev·min^{-1})	Three 30-s bouts w/4-min rest periods	Increase in peak power during bout 1 and increase in mean power and total work during bouts 1 and 2
3.	Bench press	1-RM bench press and total reps at 70% of 1-RM	Increase in 1-RM; increase in reps at 70% of 1-RM
4.	Isokinetic, unilat. knee extensions (180°·s^{-1}1)	5 bouts of 30 ext. w/1-min rest periods	Reduction in decline of peak torque production during bouts 2, 3, and 4
5.	Running	Four 300 m w/4-min rest periods; four 1000 m w/ 3-min rest periods	Improved time for final 300- and 1000-m runs; improved total time for four 1000-m runs; reduction in best time for 300- and 1000-m runs
6.	Cycle ergometry (140 rev·min^{-1})	Five 6-s bouts w/30- s recovery followed by one 10-s bout	Better able to maintain pedal frequency near the end of 10-s bout
7.	Bench press Jump squat	5 sets bench press w/2-min rest periods 5 sets jump squat w/2-min rest periods	Increase in reps completed during all 5 sets Increase in peak power during all 5 sets

From Volek JS, Kraemer WJ.Creatine supplementation: its effect on human muscular performance and body composition. J Strength Cond Res 1996;10:200.

1. Balsom PD, et al. Creatine supplementation and dynamic high-intensity intermittent exercise. *Scand J Med Sci Sports 1993;3:143.*
2. Birch R, et al. The influence of dietary creatine supplementation on performance during repeated bouts of maximal isokinetic cycling in man. *Eur J Appl Physiol 1994; 69:268.*
3. Earnest CP, et al. The effect of creatine monohydrate ingestion on anaerobic power indices, muscular strength and body composition. *Acta Physiol Scand 1995;153:207.*
4. Greenhaff PL, et al. Influence of oral creatine supplementation on muscle torque during repeated bouts on maximal voluntary exercise in man. *Clin Sci 1993;84:565.*
5. Harris RC, et al. The effect of oral creatine supplementation on running performance during maximal short-term exercise in man. *J Physiol 1993;467:74P.*
6. Soderlund K, et al. Creatine supplementation and high-intensity exercise: influence on performance and muscle metabolism. *Clin Sci 1994;87(suppl.):120.*
7. Volek JS, et al. Creatine supplementation enhances muscular performance during high-intensity resistance exercise. *J Am Diet Assoc 1997;97:765.*

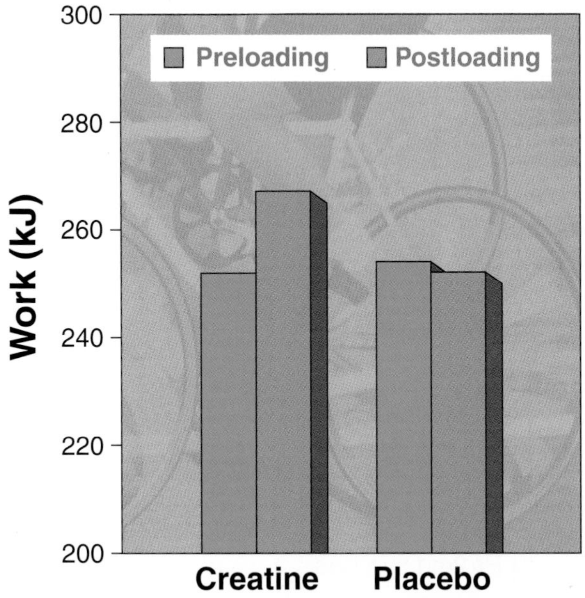

FIGURE 12.5. Effects of creatine loading versus placebo on total work accomplished during long-term (80-minute) repetitive sprint cycling performance. (From Preen CD, et al. Effect of creatine loading on long-term sprint exercise performance and metabolism. *Med Sci Sports Exerc* 2001;33:814.)

METABOLIC RELOADING OF HIGH-ENERGY PHOSPHATES

A large dose of creatine helps to replenish muscle creatine levels following intense exercise bouts.[28,65] Such metabolic "reloading" should facilitate recovery of muscle contractile capacity to enable athletes to sustain repeated bouts of exercise. Whether this potential to maintain "quality" workouts enhances the training response for strength and power athletes awaits further research.

simulated positional play of competitive squash players.[151] It augments repeated sprint cycle performance after 30 minutes of constant-load, submaximal exercise in the heat, without adversely affecting thermoregulatory dynamics.[181] These benefits to muscular performance also occur in normally active older men.[60]

FIGURE 12.6 outlines mechanisms of how elevating intramuscular free creatine and PCr with creatine supplementation might enhance exercise performance and the training response. Improved immediate anaerobic power output capacity also aids sprint running, swimming, kayaking, and cycling, and in jumping, football, and volleyball. Increased intramuscular PCr concentrations should also enable individuals to increase training intensity.

Creatine supplementation effects also occur in animals. Specifically, supplementation combined with exercise training enhanced repetitive, intense running performance of rats to a greater extent than only training or only supplementing.[17] In addition, in vitro preparations of myogenic satellite cells obtained from young adult sheep showed increased proliferation or differentiation when exposed to creatine.[179] In humans, oral creatine supplementation combined with resistance training affected cellular functional processes in a manner that increased protein deposition within the muscle's contractile mechanism.[192] This response could possibly explain any increase in muscle size and strength associated with creatine supplementation in vivo. Clinically, exogenous creatine may reduce damage when administered after traumatic head injury. It also enhances neuromuscular functions in severe diseases, including muscular dystrophy.[133]

Oral supplements of creatine monohydrate (20–25 g daily) increase muscle creatine and performance of men and women in intense exercise, particularly repeated intense muscular effort.[16,46,126,138] The ergogenic effect does not vary between vegetarians and meat eaters.[155] Even daily doses as low as 6 g for 5 days promote improvements in repeated power performance.[47] Other research evaluated the effects of a 6-day creatine supplement of 30 g daily on the exercise performance of trained runners under two conditions: four repeated 300-m runs with 4-minute recovery and four 1000-m runs with 3-minute recovery.[69] Compared with placebo treatment, creatine supplementation improved performance in both running events. The most impressive improvements occurred in repeated 1000-m runs.

For Division I American football players, creatine supplementation with resistance training increased body mass, lean body mass, cellular hydration, and muscular strength and performance.[10] Similarly, supplementation augmented muscular strength and size increases during 12 weeks of resistance training.[191] The enhanced hypertrophic response with supplementation and resistance training possibly resulted from accelerated myosin heavy chain synthesis. For resistance-trained men classified as "responders" to creatine supplementation, (i.e., an increase of $\geq$32 $mmol \cdot kg^{-1}$ dry weight muscle), 5 days of supplementation increased body weight, FFM, peak force, and total force during repeated maximal isometric bench presses.[101] For men classified as "nonresponders" to supplementation (i.e., increase of $\leq$21 $mmol \cdot kg^{-1}$ dry weight muscle), no ergogenic effect occurred.

TO LOAD QUICKLY

To rapidly "creatine load" skeletal muscle, ingest 20 g of creatine monohydrate daily for 6 days; switch to a reduced dosage of 2 g per day to keep levels elevated for up to 28 days. If rapidity of "loading" is not a consideration, supplementing 3 g daily for 28 days achieves the same high levels.

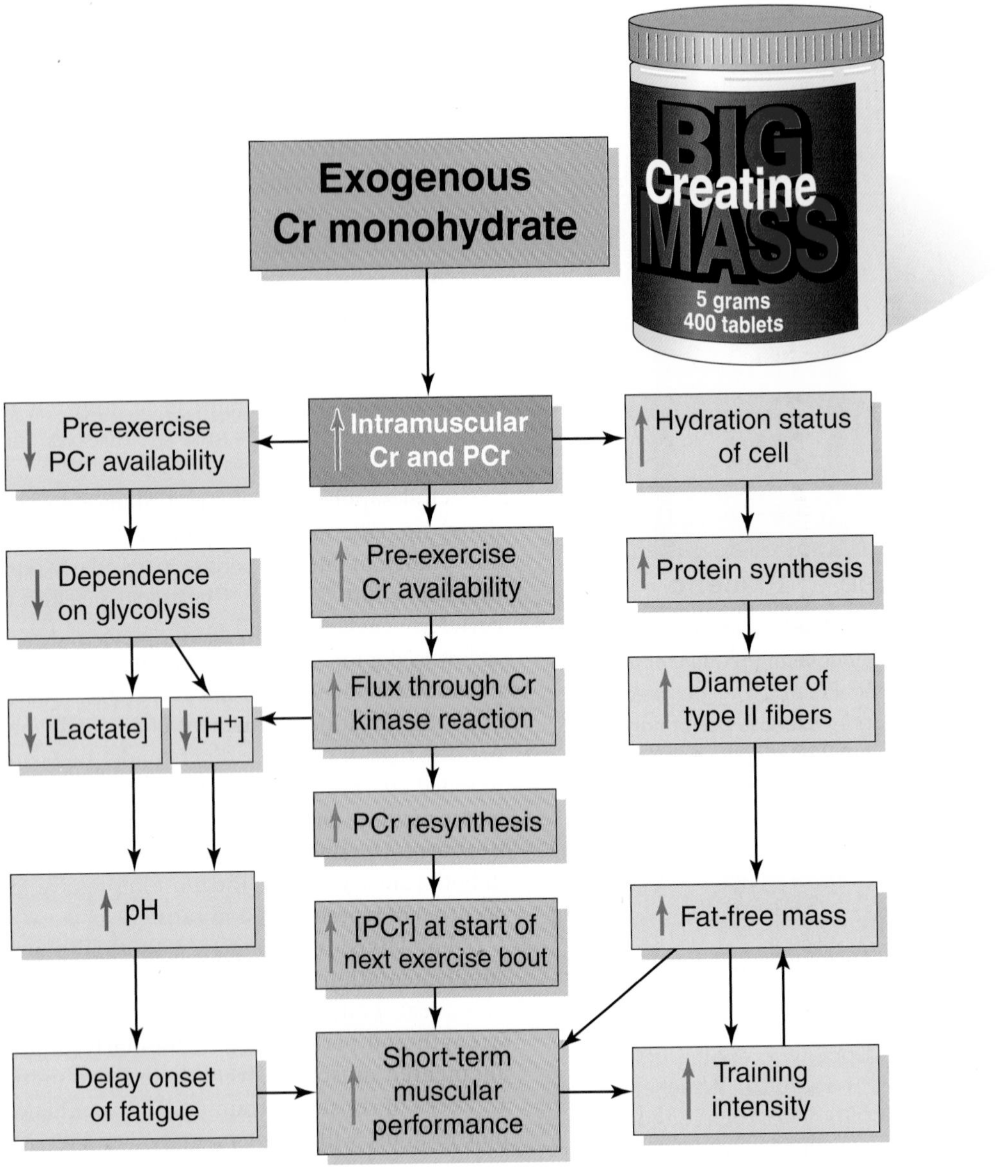

FIGURE 12.6. Possible mechanisms of how elevating intracellular creatine *(Cr)* and phosphocreatine *(PCr)* enhances intense, short-term exercise performance and the exercise-training response. (Modified from Volek JS, Kraemer WJ. Creatine supplementation: its effect on human muscular performance and body composition. *J Strength Cond Res* 1996;10:200.)

Creatine supplementation does *not* improve exercise performance that requires a high level of aerobic energy transfer[4,5,47] or cardiovascular and metabolic responses during continuous incremental treadmill running.[64] It also exerts little effect on isometric muscular strength or dynamic muscle force measured during a brief *single* movement.[9,53,143]

Age Effects Uncertain

Whether or not creatine supplementation augments the training response in older individuals remains equivocal. For 70-year-old men, a creatine supplementation loading phase ($0.3\ g \cdot kg^{-1}$ body mass for 5 days) followed by a daily maintenance phase ($0.07\ g \cdot kg^{-1}$ body mass) increased lean tissue mass, leg strength, muscular endurance, and average power of the legs during resistance training to a greater extent than a placebo.[32] Additional research shows no enhancement in resistance training response to creatine ingestion among sedentary and weight-trained older adults.[12] The investigators attributed their results to an age-related decline in creatine transport efficiency. Short-term creatine supplementation per se, without resistance training, does not increase muscle protein synthesis or FFM.[132]

Are There Risks?

Limited research exists about the potential dangers of creatine supplementation in healthy individuals, particularly the effects on cardiac muscle and kidney function (creatine degrades to creatinine before excretion in urine). Short-term use (e.g., 20 g daily for 5 consecutive days) in healthy men produced no detrimental effect on blood pressure, plasma creatine, plasma CK activity, or the renal response as measured by glomerular filtration rate and total protein and albumin excretion rates.[109,122,135] In addition, no differences emerged in healthy subjects in plasma contents and urine excretion rates for creatinine, urea, and albumin between control subjects and those who consumed creatine for between 10 months and 5 years.[136] Glomerular filtration rate, tubular reabsorption, and glomerular membrane permeability remained normal with chronic creatine use. Individuals with suspected renal malfunction should refrain from creatine supplementation because of the potential for exacerbating the disorder.[137] As a nutritional supplement, creatine requires less stringent regulations governing its manufacturing standards, purity, and reporting of adverse side effects than if classified as a drug. Clearly, more research needs to focus on the safety of long-term creatine supplementaion.[14,154]

Effects on Body Mass and Body Composition

Body mass increases of between 0.5 and 2.4 kg often accompany creatine supplementation,[65,82,123] independent of short-term changes in testosterone or cortisol concentrations.[182] In fact, short-term creatine supplementation exerts no effect on the hormonal responses to resistance training.[128] It remains unclear how much of the weight gain occurs from the following two factors, including possible unknown factors:

1. Anabolic effect of creatine on muscle tissue synthesis
2. Osmotic retention of intracellular water from increased creatine stores

Research has determined the effect of creatine supplementation plus resistance training on body composition, muscle fiber hypertrophy, and exercise performance adaptations. In one study of young adult women, creatine intake during resistance training (4 days of pretraining dose of 20 g·d^{-1} followed by 5 g·d^{-1} during training) caused greater increases in muscle strength (20–25%), maximal intermittent exercise capacity of the arm flexors (10–25%), and FFM (6%) than the placebo condition.[177] Part of the FFM increase resulted from muscle water content. Data indicate that a 2.42-kg body mass gain with creatine supplementation plus resistance/agility training partly resulted from increases in fat/bone-free body mass that did not relate to an increase in total body water.[107]

In other research, resistance-trained men matched on physical characteristics and maximal strength randomly received either a placebo or a creatine supplement. Supplementation consisted of 25 g daily followed by maintenance with 5 g daily. Both groups resistance trained for 12 weeks. **FIGURE 12.7** shows the greater training-induced increase in

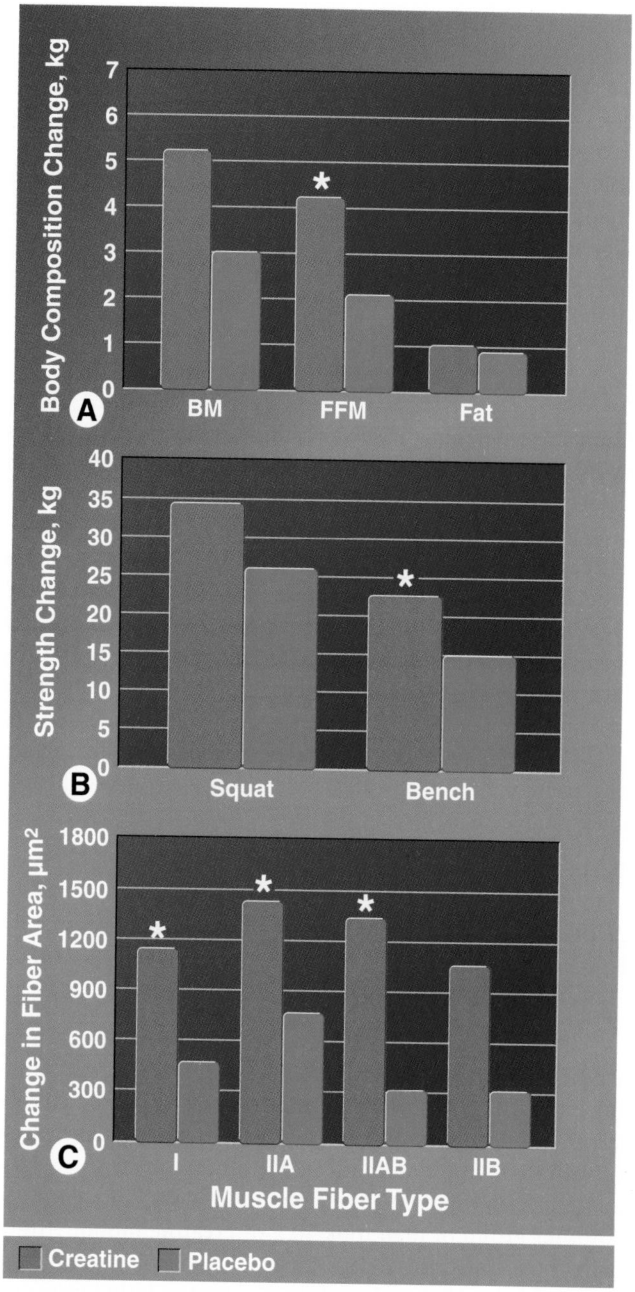

FIGURE 12.7. Effects of 12 weeks of creatine supplementation plus heavy resistance training on changes in **(A)** body mass *(BM)*, fat-free body mass *(FFM)*, and body fat, **(B)** muscular strength in the squat and bench press, and **(C)** cross-sectional areas of specific muscle fiber types. The placebo group underwent identical training and received an equivalent quantity of powdered cellulose in capsule form. *Change significantly greater than in placebo group. (From Volek JS, et al. Performance and muscle fiber adaptations to creatine supplementation and heavy resistance training. *Med Sci Sports Exerc* 1999;31:1147.)

body mass (6.3%) and FFM (6.3%) for the creatine-supplemented group than for controls (3.6% increase in body mass and 3.1% increase in FFM). Maximum bench press (+24%)

and squat strength (+32%) increases were greater in the creatine group than in controls (+16% bench press; +24% squat; **FIG. 12.7B**). Creatine supplementation induced a greater muscle fiber hypertrophy indicated by enlarged type I (35 vs 11%), IIA (36 vs 15%), and IIAB (35 vs 6%) muscle fiber cross-sectional areas (**FIG. 12.7C**). The larger average volume of weight lifted in the bench press during weeks 5 to 8 for the creatine supplement group suggests that a higher quality of training mediated more favorable adaptations in FFM, muscle morphology, and strength.

Creatine Loading

Many creatine users pursue a "loading" phase for 5 to 7 days by ingesting 20 to 30 g of creatine daily (usually in tablet form or as powder added to liquid). A maintenance phase follows the loading phase where the person supplements daily with as little as 2 to 5 g of creatine. Individuals who consume vegetarian-type diets show the greatest increase in muscle creatine because of the already low creatine content of their diets. Large increases also characterize "responders," that is, individuals with normally low basal levels of intramuscular creatine.[66]

Practical questions for the person desiring to elevate intramuscular creatine with supplementation concern the following three factors:

1. The magnitude and time course of intramuscular creatine increase
2. The dosage necessary to maintain a creatine increase
3. The rate of creatine loss or "washout" following cessation of supplementation

To provide insight into these questions, researchers studied two groups of men. In one experiment, the men ingested 20 g of creatine monohydrate (approximately 0.3 g · kg^{-1} body mass) for 6 consecutive days and then terminated supplementation. Muscle biopsies were taken before supplement ingestion and at days 7, 21, and 35. Another group of men took 20 g of creatine monohydrate daily for 6 consecutive days. Instead of discontinuing supplementation, they reduced dosage to 2 g daily (approximately 0.03 g · kg^{-1} body mass) for an additional 28 days. **FIGURE 12.8A** shows that after 6 days, muscle creatine concentration increased by approximately 20%. Without continued supplementation, muscle creatine content gradually declined to baseline in 35 days. The group that continued to supplement with reduced creatine intake for an additional 28 days maintained muscle creatine at the increased level (**FIG. 12.8B**).

For both groups, the increase in total muscle creatine content during the initial 6-day supplement period averaged 23 mmol·kg^{-1} of dry muscle, which represented about 20 g (17%) of the total creatine ingested. Interestingly, a similar 20% increase in total muscle creatine concentration occurred with only a 3-g daily supplement. This increase progressed more gradually and required 28 days in contrast to only 6 days with the 6-g supplement.

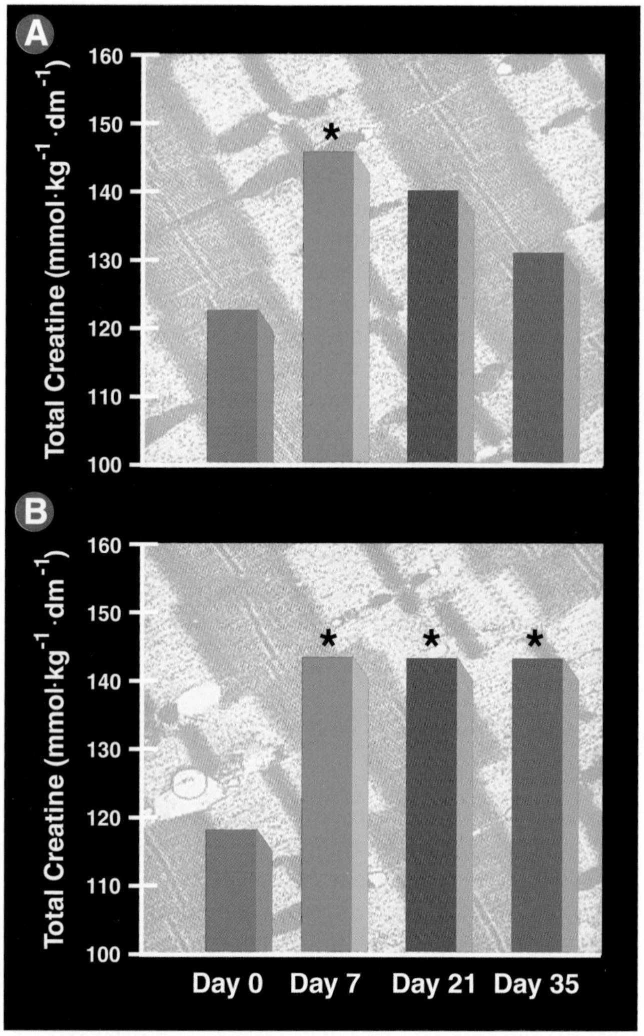

FIGURE 12.8. Muscle total creatine concentration in six men who ingested 20 g of creatine for 6 consecutive days. Muscle biopsy samples were obtained before ingestion (day 0) and on days 7, 21, and 35. **B.** Muscle total creatine concentration in nine men who ingested 20 g of creatine for 6 consecutive days and thereafter ingested 2 g of creatine daily for the next 28 days. Muscle biopsy samples were taken before ingestion (day 0) and on days 7, 21, and 35. Values refer to averages per dry muscle (dm). *Significantly different from day 0. (From Hultman E, et al. Muscle creatine loading in men. *J Appl Physiol* 1996;81:232.)

Carbohydrate Ingestion Augments Creatine Loading

Research supports the common belief among athletes that consuming creatine with a sugar-containing drink increases creatine uptake and storage in skeletal muscle (**FIG. 12.9**).[63,156] For 5 days, subjects received either 5 g of creatine four times daily, or a 5-g supplement followed 30 minutes later by 93 g of a high-glycemic simple sugar four times daily. For the creatine-only supplement group, increases occurred for muscle PCr (7.2%), free creatine (13.5%), and total creatine (20.7%). Much larger increases occurred for the

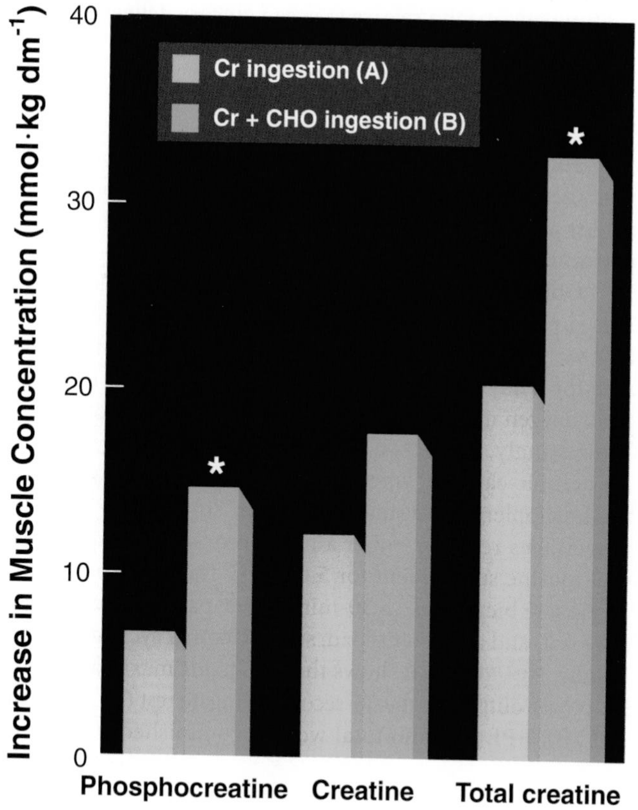

FIGURE 12.9. Increases in dry muscle *(dm)* concentrations of phosphocreatine, creatine *(Cr)*, and total Cr in group A after 5 days of Cr supplementation and in group B after 5 days of Cr plus carbohydrate *(CHO)* supplementation. Values represent averages. *Significantly greater than Cr-only supplementation. (From Green AL, et al. Carbohydrate ingestion augments skeletal muscle creatine accumulation during creatine supplementation in humans. *Am J Physiol* 1996;271:E821.)

creatine plus sugar–supplemented group (14.7% in muscle PCr, 18.1% in free creatine, and 33.0% in total creatine). Creatine supplementation alone did not affect insulin secretion, whereas adding sugar elevated plasma insulin. More than likely, greater creatine storage with a creatine plus sugar supplement results from insulin-mediated glucose absorption by skeletal muscle, which also facilitates transport of creatine into muscle fibers.

Stop Caffeine When Using Creatine

Caffeine diminishes the ergogenic effect of creatine supplementation. To evaluate the effect of pre-exercise caffeine ingestion on intramuscular creatine stores and intense exercise performance, subjects consumed either a placebo, a daily creatine supplement (0.5 g · kg^{-1} body mass), or the same daily creatine supplement plus caffeine (5 mg · kg^{-1} body mass) for 6 days.[176] Under each condition, they performed maximal intermittent knee extension exercise to fatigue on an isokinetic dynamometer. Creatine supplementation, with or without caffeine, increased intramuscular PCr by between 4 and 6%. Dynamic torque production also increased by 10 to 23% with creatine-only treatment compared with the placebo. Consuming caffeine *totally negated* creatine's ergogenic effect.

The researchers initially speculated that caffeine, through its action as a sympathomimetic agent, might facilitate the uptake and trapping of exogenous creatine by skeletal muscle, but no enhanced retention occurred. From a practical standpoint, caffeine supplements totally counteracted any ergogenic effect of muscle creatine loading. *Athletes who load creatine should refrain from caffeine-containing foods and beverages for several days before competition.*

Some Research Shows No Benefit

Not all research supports positive ergogenic results from standard creatine supplementation. For example, no effects on exercise performance, fatigue resistance, and recovery appeared for untrained subjects performing a single 15-second bout of sprint cycling[50]; trained subjects performing sport-specific physical activities such as swimming, cycling, and running[50,123,144]; trained and untrained older adults[83,193]; resistance-trained individuals[166]; or trained rowers[43] or when short-term supplementation failed to significantly increase muscle PCr.[50,123] The reason for these discrepancies could include variations in subject population, length of exercise and recovery intervals, training methods, inadequate statistical power, inappropriate or unreliable performance measures, and the degree that supplementation increases intramuscular creatine and PCr concentrations.

RIBOSE: THE NEXT CREATINE?

Ribose has emerged as a competitor to creatine as a supplement to increase power and replenish high-energy compounds following intense exercise. The body readily synthesizes ribose, and the diet provides small amounts through ripe fruits and vegetables. Metabolically, this five-carbon sugar serves as an energy substrate for ATP resynthesis. Exogenous ribose ingestion has been touted as a way to quickly restore the body's limited amount of ATP. To maintain optimal ATP levels and thus provide its ergogenic effect, recommended ribose doses range from 10 to 20 g daily. Clearly, any compound that either increases ATP levels or facilitates its resynthesis would benefit short-term, high-power requirement physical activities. A double-blind randomized study evaluated the effects of oral ribose supplementation (four doses daily at 4 g per dose) on repeated bouts of maximal exercise and ATP replenishment after intermittent maximal muscle contractions.[127] No significant difference in any measure emerged between ribose and placebo trials (e.g., intermittent isokinetic knee extension force, blood lactate, and plasma ammonia concentration). The exercise decreased intramuscular ATP and total adenine nucleotide content immediately after exercise and 24 hours later, but ribose supplementation proved ineffective in facilitating recovery of these compounds. Other researchers have demonstrated no ergogenic effects of ribose supplementation in healthy untrained or trained groups,[10,44,97,106] even though it facilitated ATP resynthesis following intense intermittent exercise training.[76]

INOSINE AND CHOLINE

Inosine

Many popular articles and advertisements tout inosine as an amino acid, when in fact it is a nucleic acid derivative found naturally in brewer's yeast and organ meats. Inosine (and choline) are not considered essential nutrients. The body synthesizes inosine from precursor amino acids and glucose. Metabolically, inosine participates in forming purines such as adenine, one of ATP's structural components. Strength and power athletes supplement with inosine believing that it increases ATP stores to improve training quality and competitive performance. Some also theorize that inosine supplementation augments red blood cell 2,3-diphosphoglycerate synthesis, thus facilitating oxygen release from hemoglobin at the tissue level. Others suggest that inosine plays an ergogenic role in one of three ways:

1. Stimulates insulin release to speed glucose delivery to the myocardium
2. Augments cardiac contractility
3. Acts as a vasodilating agent

These three assertions including anecdotal claims provide the basis for popular marketing themes that extol inosine as a supplement to boost anaerobic and aerobic exercise performance.

Objective data do not support an ergogenic role for inosine supplementation. Highly trained young and older men and women who supplemented daily with 6000 mg of inosine for 2 days failed to improve 3-mile treadmill run time, peak oxygen uptake, blood lactate level, heart rate, or RPE.[190] Interestingly, subjects could not exercise as long on a test for aerobic capacity when supplemented with inosine as in the unsupplemented state. In another study, male competitive cyclists received either a placebo or a 5000-mg per day oral inosine supplement for 5 days.[162] They then performed a Wingate bicycle test, a 30-minute self-paced bicycle endurance test, and a constant-load, supramaximal cycling sprint to fatigue. **FIGURE 12.10** shows the results for maximal anaerobic power output on the 30-second Wingate test (A) and heart rate (B), RPE (C), and total work accomplished (D) during

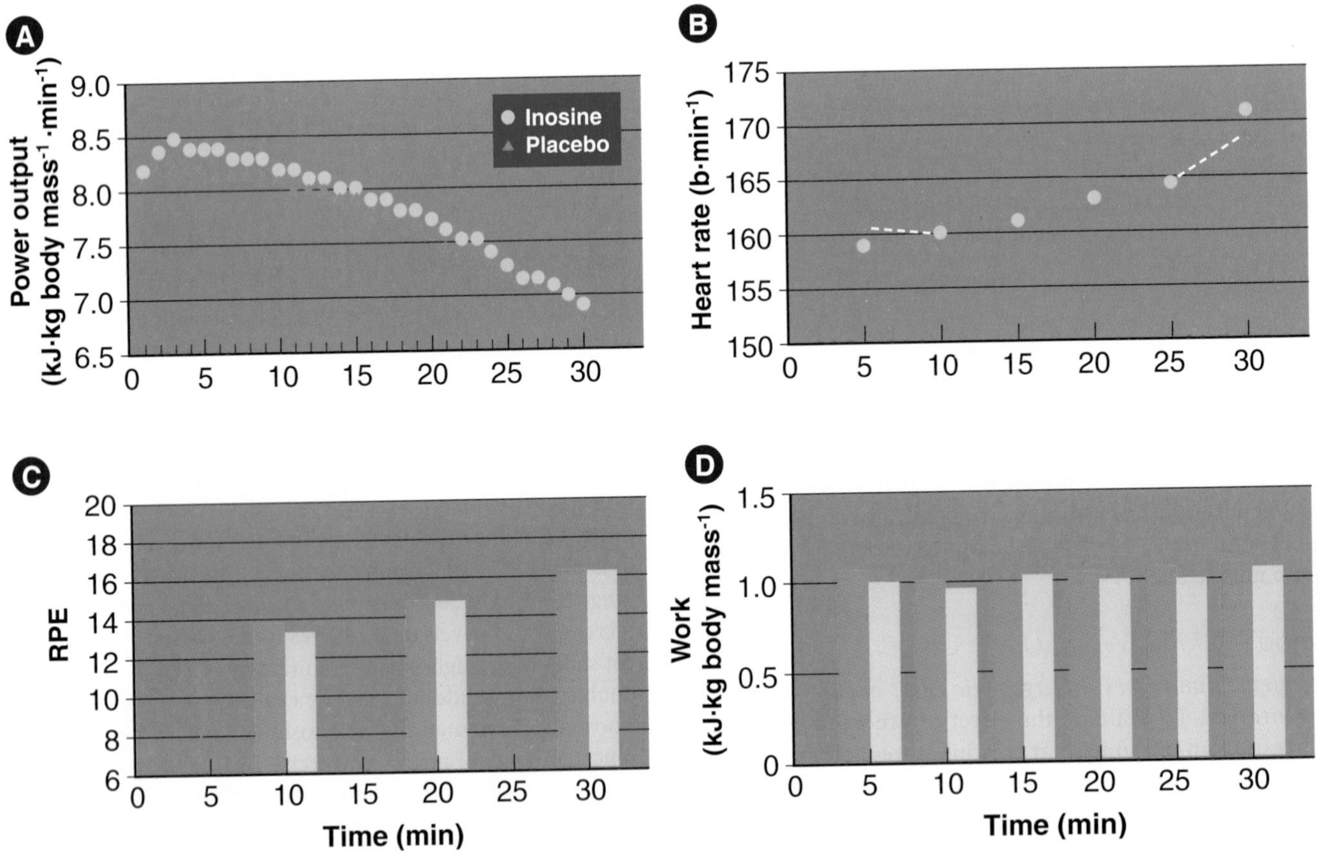

FIGURE 12.10. Maximal anaerobic power output on the 30-second Wingate test **(A)** and for heart rate **(B)**, ratings of perceived exertion *(RPE)* **(C)**, and total work accomplished **(D)** during segments of the 30-minute endurance ride for inosine and placebo trials for 10 male competitive cyclists. (From Starling RD, et al. Effect of inosine supplementation on aerobic and anaerobic cycling performance. *Med Sci Sports Exerc* 1996;28:1193.)

segments of the 30-minute endurance ride. No significant differences occurred in any of the criterion variables between placebo and supplemented conditions. In agreement with the ergolytic effect of inosine noted previously,[190] cyclists fatigued nearly 10% faster on the supramaximal sprint test when they consumed inosine than without it. Additionally, serum uric acid levels increased nearly twofold following 5 days of inosine supplementation—a level normally associated with gout, an inherited metabolic disorder characterized by recurrent acute arthritis and deposition of crystalline urate in connective tissues and articular cartilage. *These findings alone contraindicate any use of inosine supplements for possible ergogenic effects.*

Choline

All animal tissues contain choline, an important compound for normal cellular functioning. Although humans synthesize choline, it also, like inosine, must be obtained in the diet. Lecithin, a structural component of the lipoproteins and the cells' phospholipid plasma membrane, and the neurotransmitter acetylcholine, which controls skeletal muscle activation at the myoneural junction, incorporate choline into their chemical structures. Choline functions as a lipotrophic agent as part of the lecithin molecule either to depress accumulation of fat in the liver or to increase fatty acid uptake by the liver. Very low-density lipoproteins (the major transporting vehicle of triacylglycerols synthesized in the liver) also contain choline. A subpar choline intake increases the triacylglycerol content of the liver. Many foods contain ample choline; top food sources include eggs (yolk), brewer's yeast, liver (beef, pork, lamb), wheat germ, soybeans, dehydrated potatoes, oatmeal, and vegetables in the cabbage (cucurbit) family.

Inositol and choline supplements depress fat accumulation in the liver when given to animals deficient in these compounds. Supplements did not affect percentage of carcass fat of aerobically trained rats, although the supplemented animals gained less weight during the training period.[96] In addition, no depletion of plasma choline occurred with prolonged exhaustive exercise, and no ergogenic effect was noted with supplementation in humans.[189] Bodybuilders frequently take choline- and inositol-containing "metabolic optimizing powders" and "fat-burning tablets" before competition, hoping to increase their muscle mass/fat mass ratio to achieve the "cut" look. We are unaware of any research on humans that supports supplementation with inositol–choline products for such purposes.

LIPID SUPPLEMENTATION WITH MEDIUM-CHAIN TRIACYLGLYCEROLS

Do high-fat foods or supplements elevate plasma lipid levels to make more energy available during prolonged aerobic exercise? One must consider several factors to achieve such an effect. First, consuming triacylglycerols composed of predominantly long-chain fatty acids (12–18 carbons) *delays* gastric emptying. This negatively affects the rapidity of exogenous fat availability and also fluid and carbohydrate replenishment—crucial factors in intense endurance exercise. In addition, following normal digestion and intestinal absorption processes, normally a 3- to 4-hour period, long-chain triacylglycerols reassemble with phospholipids, fatty acids, and a cholesterol shell to form fatty droplets called chylomicrons. Chylomicrons then travel slowly to the systemic circulation via the lymphatic system. Once in the bloodstream, the tissues remove the triacylglycerols bound to chylomicrons. Consequently, the relatively slow rate of digestion, absorption, and oxidation of long-chain fatty acids make this energy source undesirable as a supplement to augment energy metabolism in active muscle during exercise.[41,87]

Medium-chain triacylglycerols (MCTs) provide a more rapid source of fatty acid fuel. MCTs are processed oils (primarily from lauric acids, coconut oil, and palm kernel oils) frequently produced for patients with intestinal malabsorption and tissue-wasting diseases. Marketing for the sports enthusiast hypes MCT as a "fat burner," "energy source," "glycogen sparer," and "muscle builder." Unlike longer chain triacylglycerols, MCTs contain saturated fatty acids with 8 to 10 carbon atoms along the fatty acid chain. During digestion (see Chapter 3), they hydrolyze by lipase action in the mouth, stomach, and intestinal duodenum to glycerol and medium-chain fatty acids (MCFAs). The water solubility of MCFAs enables them to move across the intestinal mucosa directly into the portal vein without the necessity of slow transport in chylomicrons by the lymphatic system as required for long-chain triacylglycerols. Once at the tissues, MCFAs readily move through the plasma membrane where they diffuse across the inner mitochondrial membrane for oxidation. They pass into the mitochondria largely independent of the carnitine–acyl-CoA transferase system, which contrasts with the relatively slower transfer and mitochondrial oxidation rate of long-chain fatty acids. Due to their relative ease of oxidation, MCTs do not usually store as body fat. Ingesting MCTs elevates plasma FFAs rapidly, so supplements of these lipids might spare liver and muscle glycogen during intense aerobic exercise.

Exercise Benefits Inconclusive

Consuming MCTs does not inhibit gastric emptying, as does consuming common fat, but conflicting research exists about their use in exercise.[3,89] In early studies, subjects consumed 380 mg of MCT oil per kilogram of body mass per hour before exercising 1 hour at between 60 and 70% of aerobic capacity.[39] Plasma ketone levels generally increased with MCT ingestion, but the exercise metabolic mixture did not change compared with a placebo trial or a trial after subjects consumed a glucose polymer. By consuming 30 g of MCTs, an estimated maximal amount tolerated in the gastrointestinal tract before exercising, MCT catabolism contributed only between 3 and 7% of the total exercise energy cost.[90]

Research has investigated the metabolic and ergogenic effects of consuming a large quantity of 86 g of MCTs (surprisingly well tolerated by subjects). Endurance-trained cyclists rode for 2 hours at 60% $\dot{V}O_{2peak}$; they then immediately performed a simulated 40-km cycling time trial. During each of three rides they drank 2 L containing either 10% glucose, 4.3% MCT emulsion, or 10% glucose plus 4.3% MCT emulsion. **FIGURE 12.11** shows the effects of the beverages on average speed in the 40-km trials. Replacing the carbohydrate beverage with only the MCT emulsion impaired exercise performance by approximately 8% (in agreement with another study[89]). The combined carbohydrate plus MCT solution consumed repeatedly during exercise produced a 2.5% improvement in cycling speed. This small ergogenic effect occurred with (1) reduced total carbohydrate oxidation at a given level of oxygen uptake, (2) higher final circulating FFA and ketone levels, and (3) lower final glucose and lactate concentrations. The small endurance enhancement with MCT supplementation probably occurred because this exogenous fatty acid source contributed to the total exercise energy expenditure and total fat oxidation.[88]

Consuming MCTs does not stimulate the release of bile, the fat-emulsifying agent from the gallbladder. Thus, cramping and diarrhea often accompany excess intake of this lipid form.[58,87] Additional research must validate the ergogenic claims for MCT, including the tolerance level for these lipids during exercise. In general, relatively small alterations in substrate oxidation occur by increasing the availability of FFAs during exercise at 65 to 90% of aerobic capacity; this likely accounts for its small effect on exercise capacity.[75]

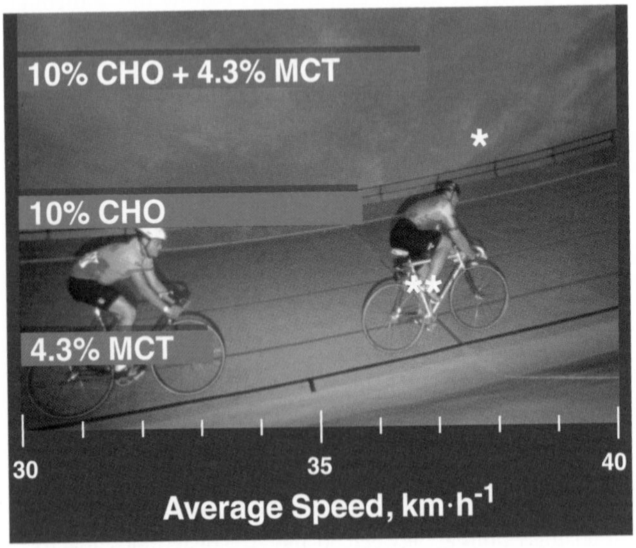

FIGURE 12.11. Effects of carbohydrate (*CHO;* 10% solution), medium-chain triglyceride (*MCT;* 4.3% emulsion), and carbohydrate + MCT ingestion during exercise on simulated 40-km time trial cycling speeds after 2 hours of exercise at 60% of peak oxygen uptake. *Significantly faster than 10% CHO trials; **significantly faster than 4.3% MCT trials. (From Van Zyl CG, et al. Effects of medium-chain triglyceride ingestion on fuel metabolism and cycling performance. *J Appl Physiol* 1996;80:2217.)

(–)-HYDROXYCITRATE: A POTENTIAL FAT BURNER?

(–)-Hydroxycitrate (HCA), a principal constituent of the rind of the fruit of *Garcinia cambogia* used in Asian cuisine, is promoted as a "natural fat burner" to facilitate weight loss and enhance endurance performance. Metabolically, HCA operates as a competitive inhibitor of citrate lyase, which catalyzes the breakdown of citrate to oxaloacetate and acetyl-CoA in the cytosol. Inhibition of this enzyme limits the pool of two-carbon acetyl compounds and thus reduces cellular ability to synthesize fat. Inhibition of citrate catabolism also slows carbohydrate breakdown, so HCA supplementation should theoretically conserve glycogen and increase lipolysis during exercise.[99,104]

Research has evaluated short-term effects of HCA ingestion on HCA availability in the plasma and fat oxidation rates at rest and during moderate-intensity exercise.[174] Endurance-trained cyclists received either a 3.1 $mL \cdot kg^{-1}$ body mass HCA solution (19 $g \cdot L^{-1}$; 6–30 times the dosage in weight-loss studies) or a placebo at 45 and 15 minutes before starting exercise (resting measure) and 30 and 60 minutes after a 2-hour exercise bout at 50% maximal working capacity. Plasma concentrations of HCA increased at rest and during exercise after supplementation, but no significant difference occurred between trials in energy expenditure or fat and carbohydrate oxidation. These findings indicate that increasing plasma HCA availability with supplementation exerts no effect on skeletal muscle fat oxidation during rest or exercise, at least in endurance-trained humans. In addition, no effects of HCA supplementation occurred for resting or postexercise energy expenditure and markers of lipolysis in healthy men[110] or for weight or fat loss in obese subjects.[77] Taken together, these findings cast serious doubt on the usefulness of large quantities of HCA as an antiobesity agent or ergogenic aid—claims frequently made by supplement purveyors.

VANADIUM

Vanadium, a trace element widely distributed in nature, comes from the bluish salt of vanadium acid and was named in 1831 for Vanadis, the Norse goddess of beauty because of how it forms multicolored compounds. This important element, without a Recommended Dietary Allowance, exhibits insulin-like properties by facilitating glucose transport and use in skeletal muscle, stimulating glycogen synthesis, and activating glycolytic reactions. In animals, vanadium supplements attenuated the effects of diabetes, perhaps by augmenting the action of available insulin.[13,125] In humans, administering 50 mg of vanadium twice daily for 3 weeks improved hepatic and skeletal muscle insulin sensitivity in patients with type 2 diabetes, partly by enhancing insulin's inhibitory effect on fat breakdown. No altered insulin sensitivity occurred in nondiabetic subjects.[67] Optimal iodine metabolism and thyroid function may also require adequate vanadium intake. Radishes (79 $\mu g \cdot 100\ g^{-1}$) are the best "natural" source of vanadium, followed by dill, olives, cereal and grain products, and dietary oils; meat, fish (particularly cod, scallops, and canned tuna), and poultry contain moderate amounts of this element.

Bodybuilders ingest vanadium supplements usually in its oxidized form as vanadyl sulfate, often combined with additional minerals or coatings, or as bis-maltolato-oxovanadium (BMOV).[197] Enthusiasts believe that vanadium provides the "pumped look" to give the appearance of muscular hypertrophy (hardness, density, and size) because of enhanced muscle glycogen storage and amino acid uptake. Research does not support an ergogenic role for vanadium supplements. Individuals should not supplement with this element because an extreme excess of vanadium becomes toxic (particularly to the liver) in mammals. In general, the documented toxic effects of vanadium compounds result in local irritation of the eyes and upper respiratory tract rather than systemic toxicity, with essentially no negative human impact coming from food.[7]

PYRUVATE

Ergogenic effects have been extolled for pyruvate, the three-carbon end-product of the cytoplasmic breakdown of glucose in glycolysis. Exogenous pyruvate, as a partial replacement for dietary carbohydrate, allegedly augments endurance exercise performance and promotes fat loss. Pyruvic acid, a relatively unstable chemical, causes intestinal distress. Consequently, various forms of the salt of this acid (e.g., sodium, potassium, calcium, or magnesium pyruvate) come as capsules, tablets, or powder. Supplement manufacturers recommend taking two to four capsules daily. One capsule usually contains 600 mg of pyruvate. The calcium form of pyruvate contains approximately 80 mg of calcium with 600 mg of pyruvate. Some advertisements recommend a dose of one capsule per 20 lb of body weight. Manufacturers also combine creatine monohydrate and pyruvate; 1 g of creatine pyruvate provides about 80 mg of creatine and 400 mg of pyruvate. Recommended pyruvate dosages range from 5 to 20 g daily. Pyruvate content in the normal diet ranges from 100 to 2000 mg daily. The largest dietary amounts occur in fruits and vegetables, particularly red apples (500 mg each), with smaller quantities in dark beer (80 $mg \cdot 12\ oz^{-1}$) and red wine (75 $mg \cdot 6\ oz^{-1}$). Therapeutic dosages to correct dietary deficiencies are much higher than what foods contain; one would have to consume about 70 apples daily to obtain a typical therapeutic dose of approximately 30 g.

Effects on Endurance Performance

Several reports indicate beneficial effects of exogenous pyruvate on endurance performance. Two double-blind, crossover studies by the same laboratory showed that 7 days of daily supplementation of a 100-g mixture of pyruvate (25 g) plus 75 g of dihydroxyacetone (DHA; another three-carbon compound of glycolysis) increased upper and lower body aerobic endurance by 20% compared with exercise with a 100-g supplement of an isocaloric glucose polymer.[160,161] The pyruvate–DHA mixture increased cycle ergometer time to exhaustion of the legs (lower body) by 13 minutes (66 vs 79 minutes), whereas upper body arm-cranking exercise time increased by 27 minutes (133 vs 160 minutes). Local muscle and overall body ratings of perceived exertion were also lower when subjects exercised with the pyruvate–DHA mixture than with the placebo condition.[149] Dosage recommendations range between a total of 2 and 5 g of pyruvate spread throughout the day and taken with meals.

Proponents of pyruvate supplementation maintain that elevations in extracellular pyruvate augment glucose transport into active muscle. Enhanced "glucose extraction" from blood provides the important carbohydrate energy source to sustain intense aerobic exercise while at the same time conserving intramuscular glycogen stores.[81] When the individual's diet contains a normal level of carbohydrate (approximately 55% of total energy), pyruvate supplementation also increases pre-exercise muscle glycogen levels.[160] Both of these effects—higher pre-exercise glycogen levels and facilitated glucose uptake and oxidation by active muscle—benefit endurance exercise similarly to the ergogenic effects of pre-exercise carbohydrate loading and glucose feedings during exercise.

Body Fat Loss

Subsequent research by the same investigators who showed ergogenic effects of pyruvate supplementation indicates that pyruvate intake also augments body fat loss when accompanied by a low-energy diet. Obese women in a metabolic ward maintained a liquid 1000-kcal daily energy intake (68% carbohydrate, 22% protein, 10% lipid). Adding 20 g of sodium pyruvate plus 16 g of calcium pyruvate (13% of energy intake) daily for 3 weeks induced greater weight loss (13.0 vs 9.5 lb) and fat loss (8.8 vs 5.9 lb) than in a control group on the same diet who received an equivalent amount of extra energy as glucose.[158] These findings complement the researchers' previous study with obese subjects that showed that adding DHA and pyruvate (substituted as equivalent energy for glucose) to a severely restricted low-energy diet facilitated weight and fat loss (without increased nitrogen loss).[157] The inhibition of weight and fat gain through dietary substitution with three-carbon compounds, originally observed in growing animals, indicated that pyruvate might cause a greater effect than DHA.[36,161] The precise role of pyruvate in facilitating weight loss remains unknown. Taking pyruvate may stimulate small increases in futile metabolic activity (metabolism not coupled to ATP production) with a subsequent wasting of energy.

Recent research indicates *no beneficial effect* of up to 2 g daily of pyruvate supplementation on measures of body composition, the metabolic response to exercise, or exercise performance.[101,175,129]

GLYCEROL

Glycerol plays four important roles in body functions and structures:

1. Component of the triacylglycerol molecule
2. Gluconeogenic substrate
3. Constituent of the cells' phospholipid plasma membrane
4. Osmotically active natural metabolite

The two-carbon glycerol molecule achieved clinical notoriety along with mannitol, sorbitol, and urea for helping to produce an osmotic diuresis. The capacity for influencing water movement within the body makes glycerol effective in reducing edema (excess accumulation of fluid) in the brain and eye. Glycerol's effect on water movement occurs because extracellular glycerol enters the tissues of the brain, cerebrospinal fluid, and eye's aqueous humor at a relatively slow rate; this creates an osmotic effect that draws fluid from these tissues.

Ingesting a concentrated mixture of glycerol plus water increases the body's fluid volume and glycerol concentrations in plasma and interstitial fluid compartments. This sets the stage for fluid excretion from increased renal filtrate and urine flow. The proximal and distal tubules reabsorb much of this glycerol, so a large fluid portion of renal filtrate also becomes reabsorbed, averting a marked diuresis. Renal reabsorption does not occur with tissue dehydrators such as mannitol and sorbitol, which produce a true osmotic diuresis.

The kidneys generally reabsorb from the renal filtrate almost all of the glycerol from food and metabolism. Normal plasma glycerol concentration at rest averages 0.05 $mmol \cdot L^{-1}$; it often rises to 0.5 $mmol \cdot L^{-1}$ during prolonged exercise with accompanying carbohydrate depletion and elevated fat catabolism. Exaggerated increases in urine glycerol concentration most likely indicate the use of exogenous glycerol, usually ingested at quantities of 1.2 $g \cdot kg^{-1}$ body mass.

When consumed with 1 to 2 L of water, glycerol facilitates water absorption from the intestine and causes extracellular fluid retention mainly in the plasma fluid compartment.[100,147,188] The hyperhydration effect of glycerol supplementation reduces overall heat stress during exercise reflected by increased sweating rate; this lowers heart rate and body temperature during exercise and enhances endurance performance under heat stress.[45,78,117]

Reducing heat stress with hyperhydration using glycerol plus water supplementation before exercise increases safety for the exercise participant. The typically recommended pre-exercise glycerol dosage of 1.0 g of glycerol per kilogram of body mass in 1 to 2 L of water lasts up to 6 hours.

Not all research demonstrates meaningful thermoregulatory, cardiovascular, or exercise performance benefits of glycerol hyperhydration over pre-exercise hyperhydration with plain water.[61,95,118] For example, exogenous glycerol diluted in 500 mL of water consumed 4 hours before exercise failed to promote fluid retention or ergogenic effects.[80] Also, no cardiovascular or thermoregulatory advantages occurred when consuming glycerol with small volumes of water during exercise.[124] Side effects of exogenous glycerol ingestion include nausea, dizziness, bloating, and light-headedness. Proponents of glycerol supplementation argue that any ban on glycerol use only increases the risk of elite athletes to heat injury, including potentially fatal heat stroke. This area clearly requires further research.

NUTRITIONAL ERGOGENIC RESOURCES

TABLE 12.7 presents a listing of Internet resources about nutritional ergogenic aids. These sites provide information about banned substances and can further help exercise/nutrition specialists make informed choices about supplement use. Athletes in particular need to know about substances marketed and promoted to gain muscle, lose fat, enhance energy, and promote exercise performance and training responsiveness.

TABLE 12.7 Internet Sites About Nutritional Ergogenic Aids

Source	URL	Comments
International Bibliographic Information on Dietary Supplements (IBIDS) Database	www.ods.od.nih.gov/Health_Information/IBIDS.aspx	Health information, news and events, research, frequently asked questions, and supplement fact sheets
FDA, CFSAN (Center for Food Safety and Applied Nutrition)	www.fda.gov/Food/DietarySupplements/default.htm	FDA gateway on information, legislation, and education for consumers. Latest updates on all matters regarding supplements.
Food and Nutrition Information Center	http://fnic.nal.usda.gov/nal_display/index.php?info_center=4&tax_level=1&tax_subject=274	US Department of Agricultural Library. Includes information about regulations, reports, and resources.
US Pharmacopeia	www.usp.org/USPVerified	The US Pharmacopeial Convention (USP) is a scientific nonprofit organization that sets standards for the quality, purity, identity, and strength of medicines, food ingredients, and dietary supplements manufactured, distributed, and consumed worldwide.

TABLE 12.7 *(Continued)* **Internet Sites About Nutritional Ergogenic Aids**

Source	URL	Comments
National Collegiate Athletic Association	http://www.ncaa.org/wps/portal/ncaahome?WCM_GLOBAL_CONTEXT=/ncaa/ncaa/academics+and+athletes/personal+welfare/health+and+safety/drug+education+programs/nutritional_supplements	All matters regarding supplements, nutritional information and videos for athlete education
American College of Sports Medicine	www.acsm.org	Articles; position stands and references
National Institutes of Health, Office of Dietary Supplements	www.health.nih.gov	Complete listings for health information from the National Institutes of Health
Consumer Laboratories	www.consumerlab.com	Reviews, product testing, quality ratings, comparisons, and expert views on supplements
Supplement Watch, Inc.	www.supplementwatch.com	Scientific product reviews, research reviews, articles, and blog about supplements
National Center for Complementary and Alternative Medicine	www.nccam.nih.gov	Health information, research, reviews, and evaluations of supplements and alternative treatments
World Anti-Doping Agency	www.wada-ama.org	Listing of banned ergogenic aids and other information for athletes and consumers
US Anti-Doping Agency	www.usantidoping.org	Listing of banned ergogenic aids and other information for athletes and consumers
PubMed	www.ncbi.nlm.nih.gov/pubmed/	Search the US National Library of Medicine on topics of choice

PERSONAL HEALTH AND EXERCISE NUTRITION 12.1

How to Identify the Metabolic Syndrome

Modification of risk factors greatly reduces the likelihood of coronary heart disease (CHD). Specifically, a major target of therapy includes a constellation of lipid and nonlipid risk factors of metabolic origin known as the *metabolic syndrome*. This syndrome closely links to the generalized metabolic disorder of *insulin resistance,* in which the normal actions of insulin are impaired. Excess body fat (particularly abdominal obesity) and physical inactivity promote the development of insulin resistance. Some individuals are genetically predisposed to this condition.

The risk factors for the metabolic syndrome are highly concordant; in aggregate, they enhance risk for CHD at any given low-density lipoprotein (LDL) cholesterol level. Diagnosis of the metabolic syndrome is made when three or more of the risk determinants shown in **TABLE 1** are present. These determinants include a combination of categorical and borderline risk factors that can be readily measured.

Management of Underlying Causes of the Metabolic Syndrome

Weight reduction and increased physical activity represent the first-line therapy for the metabolic syndrome. Weight reduction facilitates the lowering of LDL cholesterol and reduces all of the risk factors of the syndrome. Regular physical activity reduces very low-density lipoprotein (VLDL) levels, raises high-density lipoprotein (HDL) cholesterol, and in some persons lowers LDL cholesterol. It also can lower blood pressure, reduce insulin resistance, and favorably influence overall cardiovascular function.

Student Activity

Select two influential "older" family members to determine their extent of metabolic syndrome.

TABLE 1 Clinical Identification of the Metabolic Syndrome

Risk Factor	Defining Level
Abdominal obesity[a]	Waist girth[b]
Men	>102 cm (>40 in)
Women	>88 cm (>35 in)
Triacylglycerols	≥150 mg·dL^{-1}
HDL cholesterol	
Men	<40 mg·dL^{-1}
Women	<50 mg·dL^{-1}
Blood pressure	≥130/≥85 mm Hg
Fasting glucose	≥110 mg · dL^{1}

From Third Report of the National Cholesterol Education Program (NCEP) Expert Panel on Detection, Evaluation, and Treatment of High Blood Cholesterol in Adults (Adult Treatment Panel III). National Heart, Lung, and Blood Institute. NIH publ. no. 01-3670, May 2001.

[a]Overweight and obesity are associated with insulin resistance and the metabolic syndrome. However, the presence of abdominal obesity is more highly correlated with the metabolic risk factors than is an elevated body mass index (BMI). Therefore, the simple measure of waist girth is recommended to identify the body weight component of the metabolic syndrome.

[b]Some males can develop multiple metabolic risk factors when the waist girth is only marginally increased (e.g., 94–102 cm [37–39 in]). Such patients may have a strong genetic contribution to insulin resistance. They would benefit from changes in life habits, similar to men with larger increases in waist girth.

Metabolic Syndrome	Family Member 1	Family Member 2 Factors
Overweight or obese	Yes ❑ No ❑	Yes ❑ No ❑
Diagnosed with prediabetes or diabetes	Yes ❑ No ❑	Yes ❑ No ❑
Takes medication for high blood pressure	Yes ❑ No ❑	Yes ❑ No ❑
Generally physically active most days of the week	Yes ❑ No ❑	Yes ❑ No ❑
Takes medication for high cholesterol and/or elevated triacylglycerols	Yes ❑ No ❑	Yes ❑ No ❑
Extra weight around waist or BMI >30kg·m^{-2}	Yes ❑ No ❑	Yes ❑ No ❑

With regard to the metabolic syndrome, what do you conclude about family members 1 and 2?

____

____

____

What recommendations would you make for both individuals?

____

____

____

SUMMARY

1. Carbohydrate loading generally increases endurance in prolonged submaximal exercise. A modification of the classic loading procedure provides for the same high level of glycogen storage without dramatic alterations in one's diet and exercise routine. A 1-day rapid loading procedure produces nearly as high glycogen storage as the more prolonged loading techniques.
2. Men and women achieve equal supramaximal muscle glycogen levels when fed comparable amounts of carbohydrate in relation to their lean body mass.
3. Many resistance-trained athletes supplement their diets with amino acids, either singly or in combination to create a hormonal milieu to facilitate protein synthesis in skeletal muscle. Research shows no benefit of such general supplementation on levels of anabolic hormones or measures of body composition, muscle size, or exercise performance.
4. Carbohydrate–protein supplementation immediately in recovery from resistance training produces a hormonal environment conducive to protein synthesis and muscle tissue growth (elevated plasma concentrations of insulin and growth hormone).
5. Long-term exercise or intense training does not adversely affect intracellular carnitine levels. This explains why most research with carnitine supplementation fails to show an ergogenic effect, positive metabolic alterations, or body fat reductions.
6. Many tout chromium supplements (usually as chromium picolinate) for their fat-burning and muscle-building properties. For individuals with adequate dietary chromium intakes, research fails to show any beneficial effect of chromium supplements on training-related changes

in muscular strength, physique, fat-free body mass, or muscle mass.

7. Excess chromium can adversely affect iron transport and distribution in the body. Prolonged excess may even contribute to chromosomal damage.

8. Athletes supplement with coenzyme Q_{10} (CoQ_{10}) to improve aerobic capacity and cardiovascular dynamics. CoQ_{10} supplements in healthy individuals provide no ergogenic effect on aerobic capacity, endurance, submaximal exercise lactate levels, or cardiovascular dynamics.

9. In supplement form, creatine increases intramuscular creatine and phosphocreatine, enhances short-term anaerobic power output capacity, and facilitates recovery from repeated bouts of intense effort.

10. Creatine loading occurs by ingesting 20 g of creatine monohydrate for 6 consecutive days. Reducing intake to 2 g daily then maintains elevated intramuscular levels.

11. Consuming creatine with a glucose-containing drink increases creatine uptake and storage in skeletal muscle. More than likely, this results from insulin-mediated glucose uptake by skeletal muscle, which facilitates creatine uptake.

12. Limited research indicates no effect of inosine supplements on physiologic or performance measures during aerobic or anaerobic exercise. A decidedly negative effect includes an increase in serum uric acid levels after only 5 days of supplementation.

13. Choline forms part of the cells' phospholipid plasma membrane; it is also a constituent of the neurotransmitter acetylcholine. Bodybuilders frequently supplement with choline to enhance fat metabolism and achieve the "cut look." Research does not support such effects.

14. Some believe that consuming medium-chain triacylglycerols (MCTs) enhances fat metabolism and conserves glycogen during endurance exercise. Ingesting about 86 g of MCT enhances performance by an additional 2.5%.

15. Increasing plasma (–)-hydroxycitrate (HCA) availability via supplementation exerts no effect on skeletal muscle fat oxidation at rest or during exercise. These findings cast doubt on the usefulness of HCA, even when provided in large quantities as an antiobesity agent or ergogenic aid.

16. Vanadium exerts insulin-like properties in humans. No research documents an ergogenic effect, and extreme intake produces toxic effects.

17. Pyruvate supplementation purportedly augments endurance performance and promotes fat loss. A definitive conclusion concerning pyruvate's effectiveness requires verification by other investigators.

18. Pre-exercise glycerol ingestion promotes hyperhydration, which supposedly protects the individual from heat stress and heat injury during high-intensity exercise.

thePoint *Visit* **thePoint.lww.com/MKKSEN4e** *to view the following animations related to content presented in Chapter 12:* ***Glycogen synthesis*** *and* ***Metabolism of amino acids.***

TEST YOUR KNOWLEDGE ANSWERS

1. **True:** Glycogen stored in the liver and active muscle supplies most of the energy for intense aerobic exercise. Reduced glycogen reserves allow fat catabolism to supply a progressively greater percentage of energy from fatty acid mobilization from the liver and adipose tissue. Exercise that severely lowers muscle glycogen precipitates fatigue, even though the active muscles have sufficient oxygen and unlimited use of potential energy from stored fat. This occurs because the aerobic breakdown of FFAs progresses at about 50% the rate of glycogen breakdown. Ingesting a glucose and water solution near the point of fatigue allows exercise to continue, but for all practical purposes, the muscles' "fuel tank" reads empty.

2. **True:** A particular combination of diet plus exercise significantly "packs" muscle glycogen, a procedure termed *carbohydrate loading* or *glycogen supercompensation.* Endurance athletes often use carbohydrate loading for competition because it increases muscle glycogen even more than a high-carbohydrate diet. Normally, each 100 g of muscle contains about 1.7 g of glycogen; carbohydrate loading packs up to 5 g of additional glycogen.

3. **False:** Research on healthy subjects does not provide convincing evidence for an ergogenic effect of oral amino acid supplements on hormone secretion, training responsiveness, or exercise performance. For example, in studies with appropriate design and statistical analysis, supplements of arginine, lysine, ornithine, tyrosine, and other amino acids, either singly or in combination, produced no effect on GH levels, insulin secretion, diverse measures of anaerobic power, or all-out running performance at $\dot{V}O_{2max}$.

4. **False:** Vital to normal metabolism, carnitine facilitates the influx of long-chain fatty acids into the mitochondrial matrix as part of the carnitine–acyl-CoA transferase system. Theoretically, enhanced carnitine function could inhibit lactate accumulation and enhance exercise performance. Increasing

intracellular L-carnitine levels through dietary supplementation should elevate aerobic energy transfer from fat breakdown while conserving limited glycogen reserves. Research shows no ergogenic benefits, positive aerobic or anaerobic metabolic alterations, or body fat–reducing effects from L-carnitine supplementation.

5. **False:** For individuals with adequate dietary chromium intakes, research fails to show any beneficial effect of chromium supplements on training-related changes in muscular strength, physique, fat-free body mass, or muscle mass. Excess chromium can possibly adversely affect iron transport and distribution in the body. Prolonged excess may damage chromosomes.

6. **True:** Creatine monohydrate supplementation at the recommended level (20–25 $g \cdot d^{-1}$) exerts ergogenic effects in short-duration, high-intensity exercise (5–10% improvement) without producing harmful side effects. Anecdotes indicate a possible association between creatine supplementation and cramping in multiple muscle areas during competition or lengthy practice by football players.

7. **True:** Several reports indicate beneficial effects of exogenous pyruvate on endurance performance. Two double-blind crossover studies by the same laboratory showed that 7 days of daily supplementation of a 100-g mixture of pyruvate (25 g) plus 75 g of dihydroxyacetone (DHA; another three-carbon compound of glycolysis) increased upper and lower body aerobic endurance by 20% compared with exercise with a 100-g supplement of an isocaloric glucose polymer. Proponents of pyruvate supplementation maintain that elevations in extracellular pyruvate augment glucose transport into active muscle. Enhanced "glucose extraction" from blood provides the important carbohydrate energy source to sustain high-intensity aerobic exercise while at the same time conserving intramuscular glycogen stores. Subsequent research by the same investigators also indicates that exogenous pyruvate intake augments body fat loss when accompanied by a low-energy diet. Until additional studies from independent laboratories reproduce existing findings for exercise performance and body fat loss, one should view with caution conclusions about the effectiveness of pyruvate supplementation.

8. **False:** Not all research demonstrates meaningful thermoregulatory or exercise performance benefits of glycerol hyperhydration over pre-exercise hyperhydration with plain water. Side effects of exogenous glycerol ingestion include nausea, dizziness, bloating, and light-headedness.

9. **False:** CoQ_{10} functions as an integral component of the mitochondrion's electron transport system of oxidative phosphorylation. The popular literature touts CoQ_{10} supplements to improve "stamina" and enhance cardiovascular function based on the belief that supplementation could increase the flux of electrons through the respiratory chain and thus augment aerobic resynthesis of adenosine triphosphate. Although positive benefits have been reported for cardiac patients, CoQ_{10} supplements in healthy individuals provide no ergogenic effect on aerobic capacity, endurance, submaximal exercise lactate levels, or cardiovascular dynamics. On the negative side, supplementation could trigger plasma membrane lipid peroxidation and eventual cellular damage.

10. **False:** Plasma concentrations of HCA increase at rest and during exercise after supplementation, but no effect emerges in energy expenditure or in fat and carbohydrate oxidation. Consequently, increasing plasma HCA availability with supplementation does not influence skeletal muscle fat oxidation during rest or exercise. In addition, no effects of HCA supplementation occurred for resting or postexercise energy expenditure and markers of lipolysis in healthy men, or weight or fat loss in obese subjects. Taken together, these findings cast serious doubt on the usefulness of large quantities of HCA as an antiobesity agent or ergogenic aid—claims frequently made by supplement purveyors.

Key References

Bergstrom J, et al. Diet, muscle glycogen and physical performance. *Acta Physiol Scand* 1967;71:140.

Bishop D. Dietary supplements and team-sport performance. *Sports Med* 2010;40:995.

Costill DL, et al. Effects of repeated days of intensified training on muscle glycogen and swimming performance. *Med Sci Sports Exerc* 1988;20:249.

Fleck SJ, et al. Anaerobic power effects of an amino acid supplement containing no branched amino acids in elite competitive athletes. *J Strength Cond Res* 1995;9:132.

Green AL, et al. Carbohydrate ingestion augments skeletal muscle creatine accumulation during creatine supplementation in humans. *Am J Physiol* 1996;271:E821.

Hargreaves M, et al. Effect of muscle glycogen availability on maximal exercise performance. *Eur J Appl Physiol* 1997;75:188.

Hawley JA. Effect of increased fat availability on metabolism and exercise capacity. *Med Sci Sports Exerc* 2002;34:1485.

Horton TJ, et al. Fuel metabolism in men and women during and after long-duration exercise. *J Appl Physiol* 1998;85:1823.

Ivy JL. Effect of pyruvate and dehydroxyacetone on metabolism and aerobic endurance capacity. *Med Sci Sports Exerc* 1998;6:837.

Jenkins RR. Exercise, oxidative stress, and antioxidants: a review. *Int J Sports Nutr* 1993;3:356.

Jeukendrup AE, Aldred S. Fat supplementation, health, and endurance performance. *Nutrition* 2004;20:678.

Jeukendrup AE, et al. Nutritional considerations in triathlon. *Sports Med* 2005;35:163.

Kraemer WJ, et al. Hormonal responses to consecutive days of heavy-resistance exercise with or without nutritional supplementation. *J Appl Physiol* 1998;85:1544.
Kreider RB, et al. Effects of creatine supplementation on body composition, strength, and sprint performance. *Med Sci Sports Exerc* 1998;30:73.
Levenhagen DK, et al. Postexercise protein intake enhances whole-body and leg protein accretion in humans. *Med Sci Sports Exerc* 2002;34:828.
Maughan RJ. Creatine supplementation and exercise performance. *Int J Sport Nutr* 1995;5:94.
Ostojic SM, Ahmetovic Z. The effect of 4 weeks treatment with a 2-gram daily dose of pyruvate on body composition in healthy trained men. *Int J Vitam Nutr Res* 2009;79:173.
Palmer GS, et al. Carbohydrate ingestion immediately before exercise does not improve 20 km time trial performance in well trained cyclists. *Int J Sports Med* 1998;19:415.
Pitsiladis YP, Maughan RJ. The effects of alterations in dietary carbohydrate intake on the performance of high-intensity exercise in trained individuals. *Eur J Appl Physiol* 1999;79:433.
Rasmussen BB, Phillips SM. Contractile and nutritional regulation of human muscle growth. *Exerc Sport Sci Rev* 2003;31;127.
Rennie MJ, Tipton KD. Protein and amino acid metabolism during and after resistance exercise and the effects of nutrition. *Annu Rev Nutr* 2000;20:457.
Roy BD, et al. Macronutrient intakes and whole body protein metabolism following resistance exercise. *Med Sci Sports Exerc* 2000;32:1412.
Starling RD, et al. Relationships between muscle carnitine, age and oxidative status. *Eur J Appl Physiol* 1995;71:143.
Warber JP, et al. The effect of choline supplementation on physical performance. *Int J Sport Nutr Exerc Metab* 2000;10:170.
Willoughby DS, Rosene J. Effects of oral creatine and resistance training on myogenic regulatory factors expression. *Med Sci Sports Exerc* 2003;35:923.

thePoint *Visit* **thePoint.lww.com/MKKSEN4e** *for a list of the references cited in this chapter, including additional, relevant references.*

Body Composition, Weight Control, and Disordered Eating Behaviors

PART 6

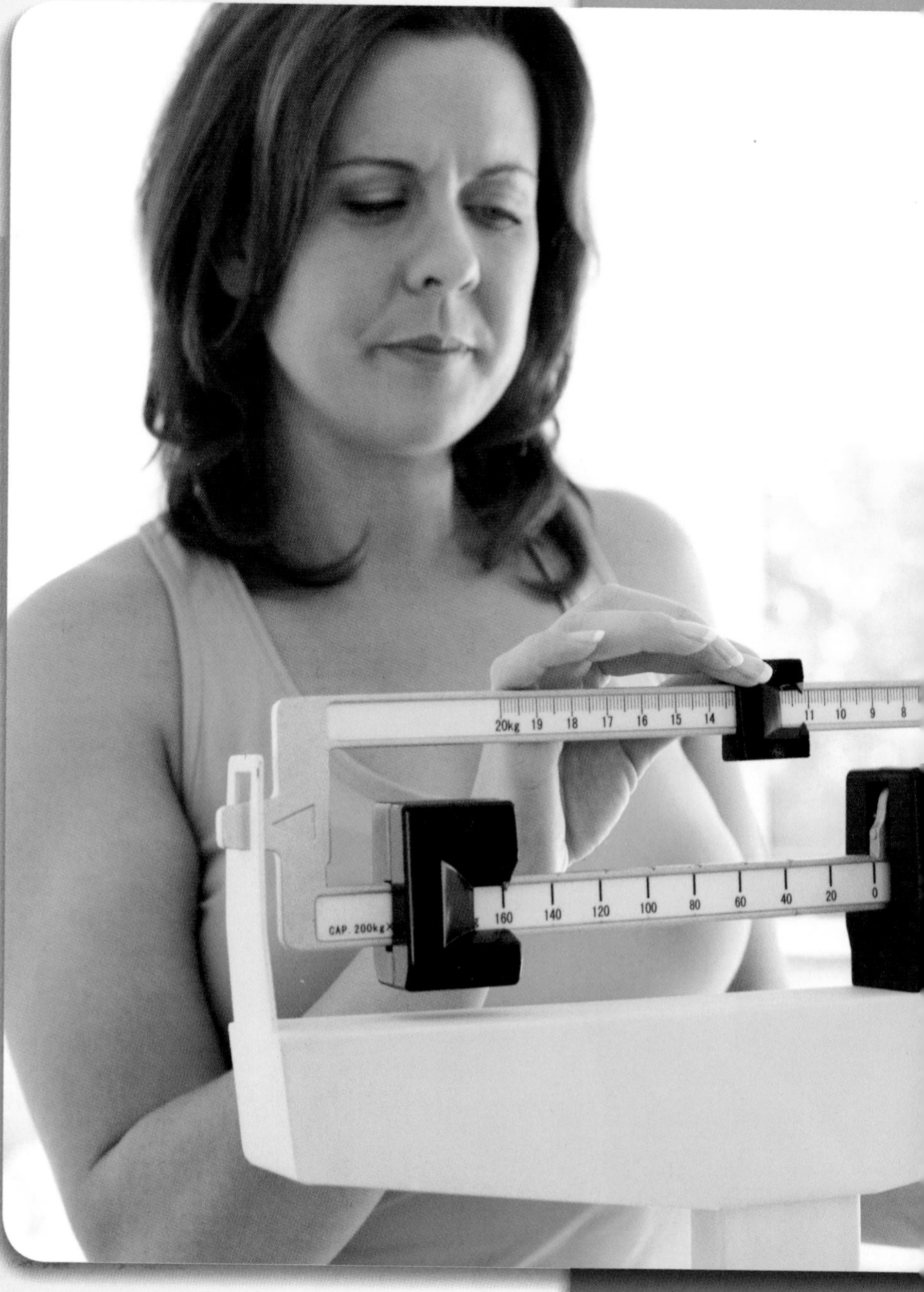

CONTENTS

CHAPTER 13

Body Composition Assessment and Sport-Specific Observations

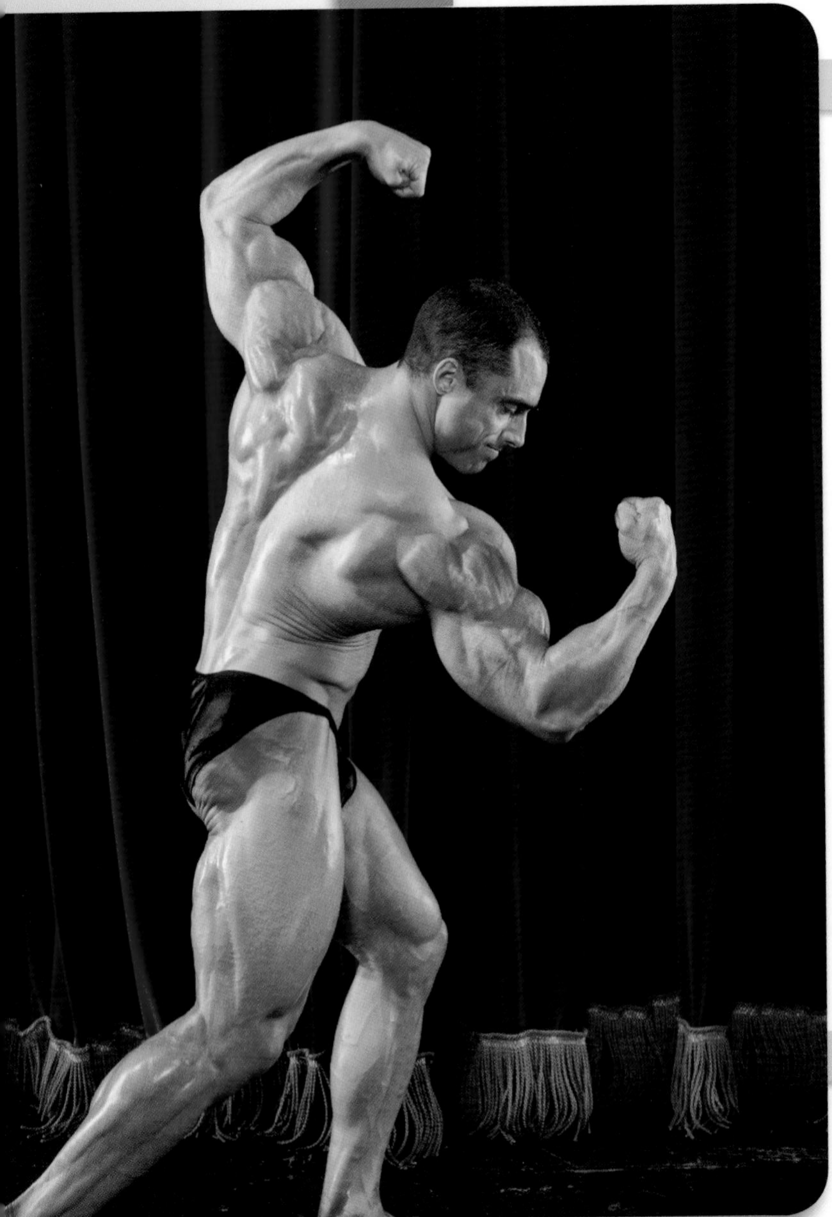

OUTLINE

Assessment of Body Composition

- Body Composition Assessment Procedures
- Body Composition Definitions: Overweight, Overfatness, and Obesity
- Composition of the Human Body
- Leanness, Exercise, and Menstrual Irregularity: An Inordinate Focus on Body Weight
- Common Laboratory Methods to Assess Body Composition
- Hydrostatic Weighing (Archimedes' Principle)
- Skinfold Measurements
- Girth Measurements
- Regional Fat Distribution: Waist Girth and Waist-to-Hip Ratio
- Bioelectrical Impedance Analysis
- Computed Tomography, Magnetic Resonance Imaging, and Dual-Energy X-Ray Absorptiometry
- BOD POD
- Estimating Body Fat Among Athletic Groups
- Average Values for Body Composition in the General Population
- How to Determine Goal Body Weight

Physique of Champion Athletes

- Elite Athletes
- Percentage Body Fat Grouped by Sport Category
- Other Longitudinal Trends in Body Size

TEST YOUR KNOWLEDGE

Select true or false for the 10 statements below, then check out the answers at the end of the chapter. Retake the test after you've read the chapter; you should achieve 100%!

	True	False
1. The fundamental importance of the body mass index (BMI) allows classification of persons by level of body fat and total muscle mass.	❍	❍
2. A male with a stature of 175.3 cm and body mass of 97.1 kg would classify as obese.	❍	❍
3. Men and women of superior athletic status generally possess similar values for body composition, particularly percentage body fat.	❍	❍
4. Total body fat exists in two storage sites called subcutaneous and intra-abdominal.	❍	❍
5. Archimedes' fundamental discovery explained the concept of specific gravity.	❍	❍
6. A male with a body density of 1.0725 has a body fat content of 15% of body mass and a fat mass of 7.5 kg.	❍	❍
7. A female with a waist girth of 38 in falls just below the threshold value for increased health risk for major diseases.	❍	❍
8. The average percentage body fat is 15% for college-age men and 25% for women.	❍	❍
9. A 120-kg (265-lb) shot-put athlete with 24% body fat who wishes to attain a body fat level of 15% must lose 40 lb of fat.	❍	❍
10. Among female athletes, bodybuilders possess the lowest percentage body fat.	❍	❍

The accurate appraisal of body composition plays an important role in a comprehensive program of total nutrition and physical fitness for six important reasons:

1. Provides a starting point to base current and future decisions about weight loss and weight gain
2. Provides realistic goals about how to best achieve an "ideal" balance between the body's fat and nonfat compartments
3. Relates to general health status, thus serving an important role in formulating short *and* long-term health and fitness goals
4. Monitors changes in the body's fat and fat-free components during exercise regimens of different durations and intensities and rehabilitation programs that use different modalities and treatment practices
5. Delivers an important message about the potential need to alter lifestyle, particularly to increase the quantity and quality of physical activity beginning in early adulthood and continuing throughout the life span independent of trying to gain or reduce excess body weight
6. Allows sports nutritionists (and dieticians, personal trainers, coaches, athletic trainers, physical therapists, chiropractors, physicians, and exercise leaders) to interact with the persons they deal with to provide quality information intimately related to nutrition, weight control, exercise, training, and rehabilitation

ASSESSMENT OF BODY COMPOSITION

The sections that follow discuss the advantages and limitations of the diverse techniques currently used to assess the composition of the human body.

BODY COMPOSITION ASSESSMENT PROCEDURES

Weight-for-Height Tables

The weight-for-height tables first proposed in 1943 by the Metropolitan Life Insurance Company and revised in 1983 serve as statistical landmarks based on the average ranges of body mass related to stature in which men and women age 25 to 59 years have the lowest mortality rate. They were originally called "desirable" weight tables, but the phrase "ideal weight" gradually became commonly associated with these tables, even though the word "ideal" was not used in the original or updated publications. More recent weight-for-height tables were published by the National Institutes of Health (www.nhlbi.nih.gov/guidelines/obesity/bmi_tbl.htm). Weight-for-height tables *do not* consider specific causes of death or disease status before death (morbidity). Many versions of the tables unfortunately recommend different "desirable" weight ranges, with some considering frame size, age, and sex, whereas others do not. **TABLE 13.1A** and **B** shows examples of two weight-for-height standards; Table 13.1A gives suggested body weights for adults with adjustment for age. Table 13.1B presents sex-specific standards proposed by the Metropolitan Life Insurance Company with consideration for bony frame size. **TABLE 13.1C** presents a convenient method to estimate sex-specific frame size using elbow breadth (measured with a micrometer-type caliper) and height. The proper scientific terms expressed in SI units for *height* and *weight* are *stature* (centimeters) and *mass* (kilograms); in most cases, we have changed *weight* to *mass* and *height* to *stature.*

Limitations of Weight-for-Height Tables

The actuarial-based weight-for-height tables assess the extent of "overweightness" from sex and bony frame size. Such tables do not, however, provide reliable information about the relative *composition* of the human body. The popular weight-for-height tables have limited value as a standard to evaluate physique status because "overweight" and "overfat" often describe different aspects of body composition for physically active men and women. Competitive athletes clearly illustrate this point; many possess high muscularity and exceed the average weight for their sex and height but otherwise possess a lean body composition. For example, most power and strength athletes (e.g., bodybuilders, American footballers, field athletes) weigh more than the average weight-for-height standards of life insurance company statistics; the "extra" weight is due simply to additional muscle mass. According to Table 13.1A, for example, the desirable body mass for a 24-year-old professional football player who is 6 ft 2 in (188 cm) and 255 lb (116 kg) ranges between 148 lb (67.3 kg) and 195 lb (88.6 kg). Similarly, a young adult male of the same stature should weigh on average 187 lb (85 kg). Using either criterion, the player's "overweight" means he should reduce body mass at least 27 kg to the upper limit of the desirable weight range for a man of his stature. He must reduce an additional 3.6 kg to match his "average" American male counterpart. If the player followed these guidelines, he certainly would jeopardize his football career and possibly overall health. Some larger-sized persons are indeed "overweight," yet they may fall within a normal range for body fat without need to reduce weight. The football player's total fat content equaled only 12.7% of body mass (compared with 15.0% body fat for untrained young men), even though he weighed 31 kg more than the average.

In the early 1940s, Navy physician and medical researcher Dr. Albert Behnke (1919–1990) was first to assess the body composition of 25 professional football players using methods other than weight-for-height tables. When he applied standards based on height and weight, 17 players failed to qualify for military service because their "overweight" status incorrectly indicated excessive fatness.[10] Carefully evaluating each player's body composition from body density (discussed on p. 441) indicated the excess weight consisted primarily of muscle mass not fat mass. These observations clearly specified that the term "overweight" refers only to body mass greater than some standard, usually the average body mass for a given stature. Being above some "average," "ideal," or "desirable" body mass based on weight-for-height tables should not dictate whether someone should reduce weight. A more desirable strategy, particularly for physically active persons, evaluates body composition by more sophisticated techniques reviewed in this chapter.

The Body Mass Index: A Better Use for Mass and Stature

Clinicians and researchers use the body mass index (BMI), derived from body mass related to stature squared, to evaluate the "normalcy" of body size.

$$\text{BMI} = \text{Body mass, kg} \div \text{Stature, m}^2$$

The BMI was originally derived in 1832 by the Belgian mathematician, astronomer, and statistician Adolphe Quetelet (1796–1874). Quetelet applied his passionate interest in probability calculus to study physical characteristics and social aptitudes. He utilized the BMI to explain his observations of the Belgian population that body mass increased in relation to the square of stature. From 1832 to 1972, this index was termed the "Quetelet Index." In 1972, Ancel B. Keys (1904–2004), an American scientist who studied the influence of diet on health, first used the term "body mass index" to refer to the Quetelet Index, which he discovered as the best proxy for body fat percentage among ratios of body mass and stature.

TABLE 13.1 Weight-for-Height Tables and Determination of Frame Size

A. *Suggested Body Weights for Adults, with Recommended Adjustment for Age based on National Institutes of Health Recommendations*[a]

Height[b]	Weight (lb)[c] 19–34 years	35 years
5′0″	97–128	108–138
5′1″	101–132	111–143
5′2″	104–137	115–148
5′3″	107–141	119–152
5′4″	111–146	122–157
5′5″	114–150	126–162
5′6″	118–155	130–167
5′7″	121–160	134–172
5′8″	125–164	138–178
5′9″	129–169	142–183
5′10″	132–174	146–188
5′11″	136–179	151–194
6′0″	140–184	155–199
6′1″	144–189	159–205
6′2″	148–195	164–210
6′3″	152–200	168–216
6′4″	156–205	173–222
6′5″	160–211	177–228
6′6″	164–216	182–234

[a]*The lower weights more often apply to women who have less muscle and bone.*

[b]*Without shoes.*

[c]*Without clothes.*

B. *1983 Sex-Specific Standards Proposed by the Metropolitan Life Insurance Company*[d]

Men

Height	Small Frame	Weight (lb)[d] Medium Frame	Large Frame
5′2″	128–134	131–141	138–150
5′3″	130–136	133–143	140–153
5′4″	132–138	135–145	142–156
5′5″	134–140	137–148	144–160
5′6″	136–142	139–151	146–164
5′7″	138–145	142–154	149–168
5′8″	140–148	145–157	152–172
5′9″	142–151	148–160	155–176
5′10″	144–154	151–163	158–180
5′11″	146–157	154–166	161–184
6′0″	149–160	157–170	164–188
6′1″	152–164	160–174	168–192
6′2″	155–168	164–178	172–197
6′3″	158–172	167–182	176–202
6′4″	162–176	171–187	181–207

Women

Height	Small Frame	Weight (lb)[d] Medium Frame	Large Frame
4′10″	102–111	109–121	118–131
4′11″	103–113	111–123	120–134
5′0″	104–115	113–126	122–137
5′1″	106–118	115–129	125–140
5′2″	108–121	118–132	128–143
5′3″	111–124	121–135	131–147
5′4″	114–127	124–138	134–151
5′5″	117–130	127–141	137–155
5′6″	120–133	130–144	140–159
5′7″	123–136	133–147	143–163
5′8″	126–139	136–150	146–167
5′9″	129–142	139–153	149–170
5′10″	132–145	142–156	152–173
5′11″	135–148	145–159	155–176

From Statistical Bulletin, Metropolitan Life Insurance Company, New York City.

[d]*Weights at ages 25–59 years based on lowest comparative mortality.*

Weight in pounds according to fra me size for men wearing indoor clothing weighing 5 lb, shoes with 1-in heels; for women, indoor clothing.

(continued)

TABLE 13.1 (*continued*) **Weight-for-Height Tables and Determination of Frame Size**

C. *How to Determine Frame Size from Elbow Breadth Based on Height.*

The person's right arm extends forward perpendicular to the body, with arm bent so angle at the elbow forms 90°, with fingers pointing up and palm turned away from body. The greatest breadth across the elbow joint is measured with a sliding caliper along the axis of the upper arm. This records as elbow breadth. The table gives the ***elbow breadth*** *measurements for medium-framed men and women of various heights. Smaller measurements indicate a small frame size; higher measurements indicate a large frame size.*

Men		Women	
Height in 1″ Heels	Medium-Framed Elbow Breadth	Height in 1″ Heels	Medium-Framed Elbow Breadth
5′2″–5′3″	2′1/2″–2′7/8″	4′10″–4′11″	2′1/4″–2′1/2″
5′4″–5′7″	2′5/8″–2′7/8″	5′0″–5′3″	2′1/4″–2′1/2″
5′8″–5′11″	2′3/4″–3′	5′4″–5′7″	2′3/8″–2′5/8″
6′0″–6′3″	2′3/4″–3′1/8″	5′8″–5′11″	2′3/8″–2′5/8″
>6′4″	2′7/8″–3′1/4″	>6′0″	2′1/2″–2′3/4″

Current classification standards for overweight and obese discussed on page 432 assume the relationship between BMI and percentage body fat remains independent of age, gender, ethnicity, and race. For example, Asians have greater body fat content than Caucasians at a given BMI level and thus show greater risk for fat-related illness such as obesity and type 2 diabetes. Hispanic American women also have a higher body fat percentage at a given BMI than European American and African American women.[58]

The importance of this easily obtained index illustrated in the bottom table of **FIGURE 13.1** lies not in predicting overfatness but rather in its curvilinear relationship to all-cause mortality; this means that as BMI increases, so does the risk for cardiovascular complications, including hypertension, stroke, type 2 diabetes, and renal disease.[19] The classification schema at the bottom of the figure indicates level of risk with each 5-unit increase in BMI. The lowest health risk category occurs for persons with BMIs between 20 and 25, whereas the highest risk category includes persons whose BMIs exceed 40. For women, the desirable BMI ranges between 21.3 and 22.1; the corresponding desirable range for men is 21.9 to 22.4. An increased incidence of high blood pressure, obesity, diabetes, and coronary heart disease occurs when the BMI exceeds 27.8 for men and 27.3 for women.

Sample Computation of Body Mass Index

Male:

Stature = 175.3 cm, 1.753 m (69 in)
Body mass = 97.1 kg (214.1 lb)
BMI = $97.1 \text{ kg} \div (1.753 \text{ m})^2$
= $97.1 \div 3.073$
= $31.6 \text{ kg} \cdot \text{m}^{-2}$

In this example, the BMI falls above the threshold of the upper range of BMI values, which places the person in the obese classification.

LACK OF SLEEP AND BODY MASS INDEX INCREASE

Lack of nightly sleep may have a positive association with an increased BMI. This seems paradoxical because sleep remains the quintessential sedentary behavior, and people with minimal physical activity patterns do indeed have larger BMIs. The National Sleep Foundation (www.sleepfoundation.org) states that sleep duration has been steadily decreasing over the past century. Subjects who slept 5 to 6 h a night gained an average of 4.4 lb more over the course of 6 years than subjects who slept 7 to 8 h a night. In 1024 participants in the population-based Wisconsin Sleep Cohort Study (www.wisconsinsleep.org/WisconsinStudyDocumentsApneaRisk.htm), an inverse correlation was found between sleep duration and BMI in persons sleeping less than 8 h nightly. Explanations include nocturnal snacking or that people with diminished sleep feel too tired to exercise. Short sleepers had 15% higher serum levels of the orexigenic (appetite-stimulating) gut peptide ghrelin and 16% lower levels of leptin. Orexigenic medications increase appetite and therefore enhance food consumption. Scientists generally believe that neurohormonal links exist between appetite and sleep. Mice with genetic destruction of orexin neurons (neurons that control sleep and appetite) become heavier than controls by 10 to 12 weeks of age, although they consume less food than controls and gain weight from reduced energy output. Higher levels of orexin may help to defend against negative energy balance.

St-Onge MP, et al. Gender differences in the association between sleep duration and body composition: the Cardia Study. *Int J Endocrinol* 2010;2010:726071.

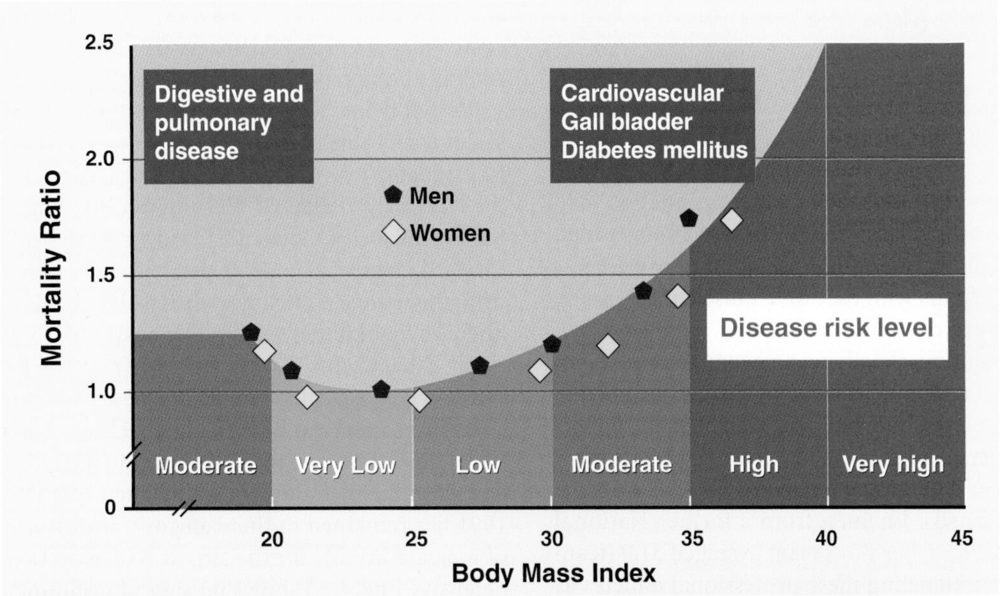

Body Mass Index ($kg \cdot m^2$)*

Height (in)	19	20	21	22	23	24	25	26	27	28	29	30	35	40
	Body weight (pounds)													
58	91	96	100	105	110	115	119	124	129	134	138	143	167	191
59	94	99	104	109	114	119	124	128	133	138	143	148	173	198
60	97	102	107	112	118	123	128	133	138	143	148	153	179	204
61	100	106	111	116	122	127	132	137	143	148	153	158	185	211
62	104	109	115	120	126	131	136	142	147	153	158	164	191	218
63	107	113	118	124	130	135	144	146	152	158	163	169	197	225
64	110	116	122	128	134	140	145	151	157	163	169	174	204	232
65	114	120	126	132	138	144	150	156	162	168	174	180	210	240
66	118	124	130	136	142	148	155	161	167	173	179	186	216	247
67	121	127	134	140	146	153	159	166	172	178	184	191	223	254
68	125	135	138	144	151	158	164	171	177	184	190	197	230	262
69	128	135	142	149	155	162	169	176	182	189	196	203	236	270
70	132	139	146	153	160	167	174	181	188	195	202	207	243	278
71	136	143	150	157	165	172	179	186	193	200	208	215	250	286
72	140	147	154	162	169	176	183	191	199	206	213	221	258	294
73	144	151	159	166	174	182	189	197	204	212	219	227	265	302
74	148	155	163	171	178	186	194	202	210	218	225	233	272	311
75	152	160	168	176	184	192	200	208	216	224	232	240	280	319
76	156	164	172	180	189	197	205	213	221	230	238	246	287	328

***The intersection of weight and height provides the BMI ($kg \cdot m^2$). For an exact calculation of BMI, follow these steps:**

Step 1. Multiply body weight (lb) by 0.45 to convert to kilograms
Step 2. Multiply height (in) by 0.0254 to convert to meters
Step 3. Multiply answer in step 2 by itself to obtain height in square meters (m^2)
Step 4. To compute BMI, divide step 1 result (mass, kg) by step 3 result (m^2)

FIGURE 13.1. Curvilinear relationship based on American Cancer Society data between all-cause mortality and body mass index. (Modified from Bray GA. Pathophysiology of obesity. *Am J Clin Nutr* 1992;55:488S.)

Limitations of Body Mass Index for Physically Active Persons

As with weight-for-height tables, the BMI fails to consider the body's fat distribution, referred to as *fat patterning*. Also, increased bone, muscle mass, and quantity of plasma volume induced by exercise training, each or in combination, can increase the numerator (mass) of the BMI equation. A high BMI could lead to an incorrect interpretation of overfatness in relatively lean persons with excessive muscle mass due to genetic makeup or exercise training.

The possibility of misclassifying someone as overweight or "overfat" by BMI applies particularly to large-sized males, particularly field athletes, bodybuilders, weightlifters, upper-weight-class wrestlers, and professional football players (particularly offensive and defensive linemen). For example, the BMI for seven defensive linemen from a former National Football League (NFL) Super Bowl team averaged 31.9 (team BMI = 28.7), clearly signaling these professional athletes as overweight and placing them in the moderate category for mortality risk. Their body fat content, 18.0% for the linemen and 12.1% for the team, did not indicate excessive fatness, suggesting a misclassification when using BMI as a standard.

Interestingly, the trend for excessively large BMIs still applies to offensive and defensive linemen on the 2011 Super Bowl teams (**TABLE 13.2**). The data for the 2007 teams shown for comparison illustrate that over 5 years the trend for "largeness" continues. The Green Bay Packers offensive and defensive linemen are the heaviest ever to play on a Super Bowl team and possess the largest BMI of any group of players. The players from the 2007 and 2011 teams classify as obese. Note that this group of players has about twice the body weight of Behnke's reference man discussed on pages 434 and 435. By any standard including the BMI for the reference man, they classify as "obese" (overfat) with a relative "overweight" that exceeds 100 pounds! Although their levels of body fat most likely exceed the "normal" value of 15% for the reference man, their large body size undoubtedly includes a much larger than average lean mass component.

Misclassification of body weight relative to body fat also applied to the typical NFL player from 1920 to 1996. **FIGURE 13.2** displays the average BMI for all 53,333 NFL roster players at 5-year intervals between 1920 and 1996. Average body fat content during the late 1970s through the 1990s fell below the range typically associated with normal males (see Table 13.10). The teams whose players had body fat evaluated by hydrostatic weighing (see page 443) included the NFL New York Jets, Washington Redskins, New Orleans Saints, and Dallas Cowboys. On average, all players from 1960 forward classify as overweight based on weight-for-height using insurance company statistics. Up to 1989, the BMI for linebackers, skill players, and defensive backs represents the "low" category for disease risk, whereas the BMI for offensive and defensive linemen places these players at "moderate" risk. Thereafter, the BMI for linebackers changed from the low to moderate category, whereas the BMI for offensive and defensive linemen quickly approached "high" risk and since 1991 has remained in that category. Unfortunately, the rate of increase in BMI for the largest NFL players (offensive and defensive linemen) shows no sign of declining, as indicated by the 2011 Super Bowl offensive and defensive linemen.

The extent of "largeness" is not limited to just professional players—it also includes Division I collegiate football athletes from Big Ten Conference teams, Division II and III schools, and high school All-Americans. If such findings can be generalized, a common trend in almost all levels of collegiate football—including top high school linemen—is the rising preponderance of players heavier than 300 pounds. This certainly does not bode well from a future health standpoint because these large-size athletes often carry their excess weight well into their after-sport work years.

BODY COMPOSITION DEFINITIONS: OVERWEIGHT, OVERFATNESS, AND OBESITY

Considerable confusion surrounds the precise meaning of the terms **overweight**, **overfat**, and **obesity**. Research and contemporary discussion among diverse disciplines emphasizes the need to distinguish between these terms to ensure consistency in use and interpretation. The term **overweight** simply refers to

TABLE 13.2 Comparison of the Average Body Mass, Stature, and BMI for the 2007 and 2011 NFL Super Bowl Offensive and Defensive Linemen[a]

Variable	Indianapolis Colts, 2007	Chicago Bears, 2007	Pittsburg Steelers, 2011	Green Bay Packers, 2011	Reference Man[b]
Body mass (lbs)	301.3	302.2	310.1	313.7	154
Stature (in)	75.1	75.9	76.4	75.2	68.5
BMI (kg/m^2)	37.5	37.0	37.3	39.0	20.1
BMI classification[c]	Obese	Obese	Obese	Obese	Very low

[a] *From 2006 and 2010 team rosters.*

[b] *Behnke's reference man data from Figure 13.4.*

[c] *Obese = BMI >30.0; normal weight = BMI 22.0–25.9.*

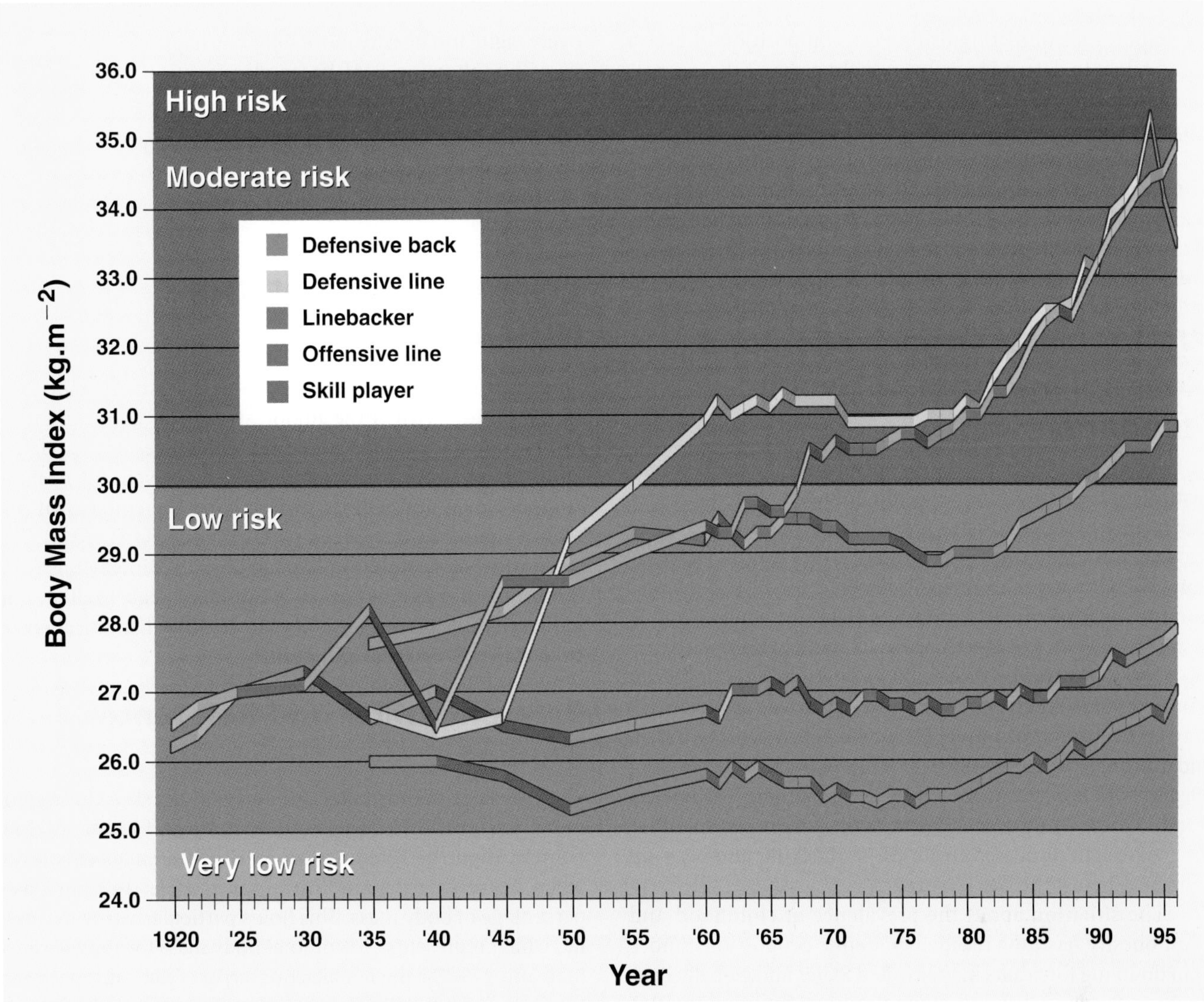

FIGURE 13.2. Body mass index (BMI) for all roster players in the National Football League between 1920 and 1996 (N = 53,333). Categories include offensive and defensive linemen, linebackers, skill players (quarterbacks, receivers, backfield), and defensive backs. The four horizontal bands of color refer to Bray's classification in Figure 13.1 for relative disease risk levels. According to the 1998 federal guidelines for identification, evaluation, and treatment of overweight and obesity, offensive and defensive linemen from 1980 to present would classify as obese. (Data courtesy of F. Katch.)

a body weight that exceeds some average for stature and perhaps age, usually by some standard deviation unit or percentage. This condition frequently accompanies an increase in body fat, but not always (e.g., power athletes and body builders), and may or may not coincide with the comorbidities of glucose intolerance, insulin resistance, dyslipidemia, and hypertension (e.g., physical fit overfat men and women).

When better methods besides height and weight determine body composition, as described in subsequent sections, one can more accurately place an person's body fat level on a continuum from low to high, independent of body mass or stature. **Overfat** then would refer to a condition in which body fat exceeds an age- and/or gender-appropriate average by a predetermined amount. In most situations, "overfatness" represents the correct term when assessing person and group body fat levels.

The term **obesity** refers to the overfat condition that accompanies a constellation of comorbidities that include one or all of the following nine components of the "obese syndrome":

1. Glucose intolerance
2. Insulin resistance
3. Dyslipidemia
4. Type 2 diabetes
5. Hypertension
6. Elevated plasma leptin concentrations
7. Increased visceral adipose tissue
8. Increased coronary heart disease risk
9. Increased cancer risk

Research suggests that excess body fat, not excess body weight per se, explains the relationship between above-average body weight and disease risk,[3,96] emphasizing the importance of distinguishing the composition of excess body weight to determine an overweight person's disease risk. Likewise, many persons are not overfat but may exhibit obese correlates.

We urge caution in using the term obesity (instead of overfatness) to describe cases of excessive body weight. We acknowledge that these terms often are used interchangeably in the allied health professions when a more specific categorization seems preferred and justified.

World Health Organization and National Institutes of Health Standards

In 1998, a 24-member expert panel convened by the National Institutes of Health (NIH; www.nih.gov) and National Heart, Lung, and Blood Institute (NHLBI; www.nhlbi.nih.gov) adopted the single standards of the World Health Organization (WHO; www.who.int) and lowered the BMI demarcation for "overweight" (the preobese state) for adults from 27 to 25. **FIGURE 13.3** shows the current standards for identifying obesity (defined by BMI ≥ 30.0) for six heights (from 5 ft 6 in to 6 ft 3 in). Persons with a BMI of 30 average about 30 lb overweight. For example, a man 6 ft 0 in weighing 221 lb and a woman weighing 186 lb at 5 ft 6 in both have a BMI of 30, and both are approximately 30 lb overweight. The revised standards currently place 65% of adult Americans in either the overweight or obese categories—a shocking number—up from 56% in just the last 15 years![38,77]

The situation about the prevalence of childhood and adult obesity has now reached epidemic proportions, more than doubling for adults in the United States and globally over the past 30 years. For the first time, overweight persons (BMI >25) outnumber those of desirable body weight! In terms of ethnicity and gender, significantly more black, Mexican, Cuban, and Puerto Rican men and women classify as overweight compared with white counterparts, and overweight and obesity may account for 14% of all cancer deaths in men and 20% in women. We discuss the worldwide prevalence of overweight and obesity more fully in Chapter 14.

The following BMI-based classification can determine the adequacy of one's body weight:

Normal Weight: BMI ≤ 25.0
Overweight: BMI 25.0–29.9
Obese: BMI ≥ 30.0

COMPOSITION OF THE HUMAN BODY

One approach to body composition assessment views the human body with three major structural components—muscle, fat, and bone. Marked sex differences in the relative amounts of these parameters make a convenient basis to compare men and women by applying the concept of reference standards developed by Dr. Behnke (**FIG. 13.4**). The standards incorporate the average physical dimensions from thousands of persons measured in large-scale civilian and military anthropometric surveys to create a theoretical **reference man** and **reference woman**.[9]

Reference Man and Reference Woman

The reference man is taller and heavier, his skeleton weighs more, and he has a larger muscle mass and lower total fat content than the reference woman. Differences exist even when expressing the amount of fat, muscle, and bone as a percentage of body mass. This holds particularly true for body fat, which represents 15% of total body mass for the reference man and 27% for the female counterpart. The concept of reference standards does not mean that men and women should strive to achieve this body composition or that the reference man and reference woman are, in fact, "average," "normal," or "healthy." Instead, the model provides a useful frame of reference for statistical comparisons and interpretations of data from other studies of diverse groups of athletes, persons

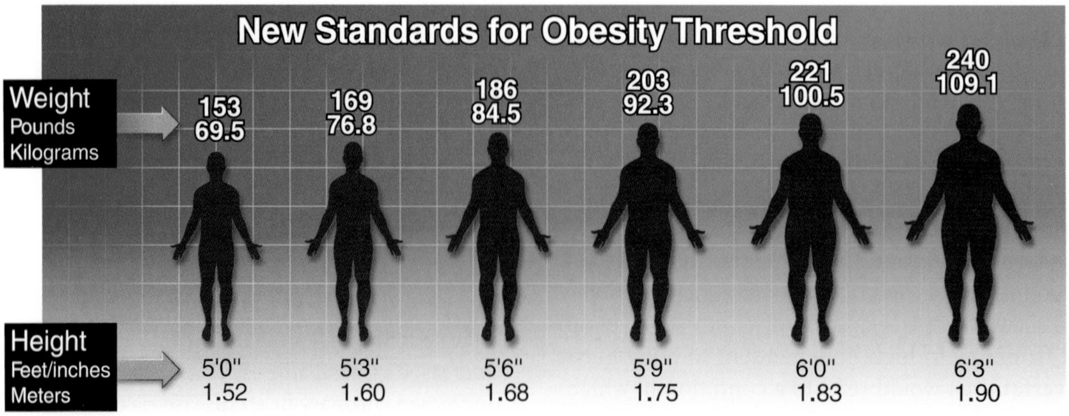

FIGURE 13.3. New standards for the threshold of obesity.

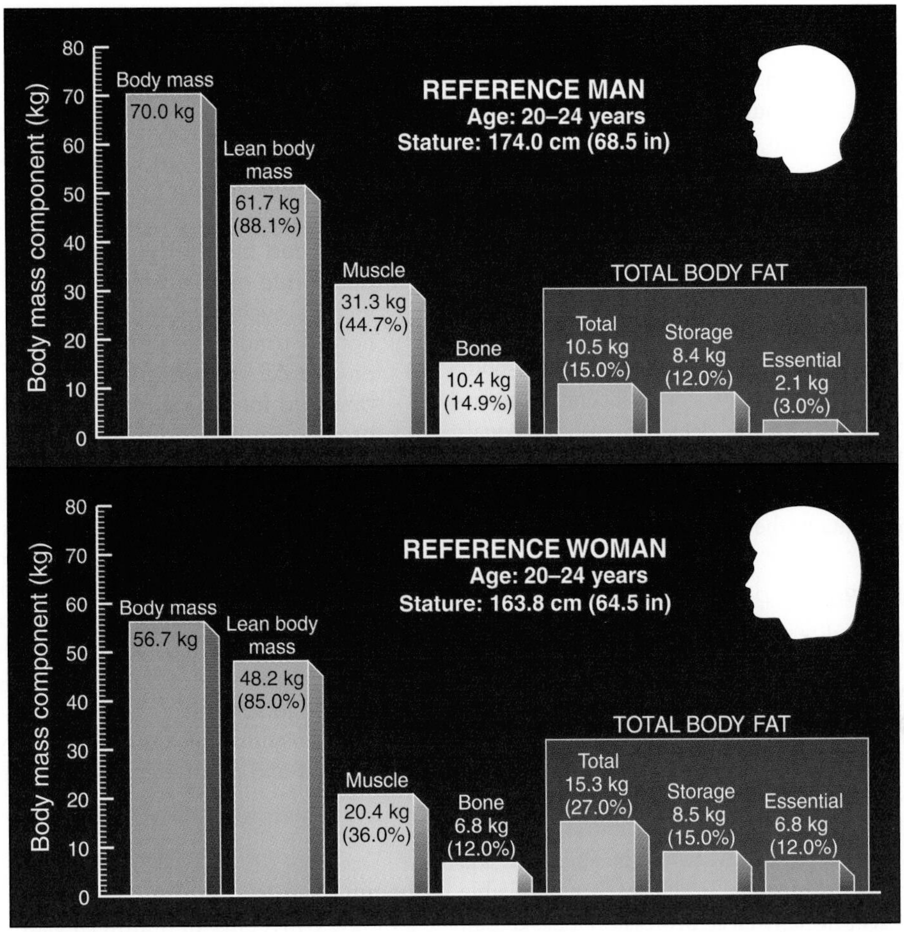

FIGURE 13.4. Behnke's theoretical model for the reference man and reference woman. Values in parentheses represent the specific value expressed as a percentage of total body mass.

involved in physical training programs, and the underweight and obese.

Essential and Storage Fat

In the reference model, total body fat exists in two storage sites or depots called essential fat and storage fat.

Essential Fat

Essential fat consists of the fat stored in the marrow of bones, heart, lungs, liver, spleen, kidneys, intestines, muscles, and lipid-rich tissues of the central nervous system. *Normal physiologic functioning requires this fat.* In the female, essential fat includes additional **sex-specific essential fat**. Researchers believe that sex-specific essential fat serves biologically important childbearing and other hormone-related functions. **FIGURE 13.5** partitions the distribution of body fat for the reference woman. As part of the 5 to 9% sex-specific fat reserves, breast fat probably contributes no more than 4% of body mass for women whose body fat content varies from 14 to 35% of body mass.[71] This means that sites other than the breasts (lower body region, including the pelvis, hips, and thighs) furnish a large proportion of sex-specific essential fat. Essential body fat apparently represents a biologically established range limit below which encroachment impairs health status.

Storage Fat

This major fat depot consists of fat accumulation in adipose tissue, and contains about 83% pure fat in addition to 2% protein and 15% water within its supporting structures. Storage fat includes the visceral fatty tissues that protect the various organs within the thoracic and abdominal cavities and the larger subcutaneous fat tissue volume deposited beneath the skin's surface. The reference man and reference woman have similar percentages of storage fat—approximately 12% of body mass in men and 15% in women.

Fat-Free Body Mass and Lean Body Mass (Men)

The terms *fat-free body mass* and *lean body mass* refer to specific entities. Lean body mass (LBM) contains the small percentage of essential fat stores equivalent to approximately 3% of body mass. In contrast, fat-free body mass (FFM) represents the body devoid of *all* extractable fat. Behnke points out that FFM refers to an in vitro entity appropriate to carcass analysis. In contrast, the LBM represents an in vivo entity that remains relatively constant in its content of water, organic matter, and minerals throughout the adult's life span. *In normally hydrated, healthy adults, FFM and LBM differ only in the "essential" lipid-rich stores in bone marrow, brain, spinal cord, and internal organs.* Thus, LBM calculations include the small quantity of essential fat, whereas FFM computations exclude "total" body fat (FFM = body mass − fat mass).

Figure 13.4 reveals that LBM in men and the **minimal body mass** in women consist chiefly of essential fat (plus sex-specific fat for females), muscle, water, and bone. Whole-body density of the reference man with 12% storage fat and 3% essential fat equals 1.070 g · cm^{-3}, and the density of his FFM equals 1.094 g · cm^{-3}. If the reference man's total body fat percentage equals 15.0% (storage plus essential fat), the density of a hypothetical "fat-free" body attains the upper limit of 1.100 g · cm^{-3}.

Upper Limit for Fat-Free Body Mass

The FFM for Japanese elite sumo wrestlers (*seki-tori*) averages 109 kg.[76] These athletes share the distinction of being among the world's largest athletes with some American professional football players who weigh 159 kg (350 lb) or more. It seems unlikely that athletes in this weight range would possess less than 15% body fat; the FFMs of the largest football players at 15% body fat theoretically would correspond to 135 kg. At 20% body fat, the FFM would be about 127 kg. But this value remains hypothetical in the absence of reliable data. Even for an exceptionally large professional basketball player (body mass, 138.3 kg [305 lb], and stature, 210.8 cm [83 in]), percentage body fat is unlikely to be less than 10% of body mass. Thus, fat mass equals 13.8 kg and FFM equals 114.2 kg—perhaps an upper limit FFM value for an athlete of such dimensions. The body composition of an exceptionally large professional football player (NFL Oakland Raiders; unpublished data, Dr. Robert Girandola, Department of Kinesiology, University of Southern California) determined by repeated trials of underwater weighing exceeds values for FFM presented in the research literature. The player whose body fat content assessed using this valid criterion method equaled 11.3% (body mass, 141.4 kg; stature, 193 cm; BMI, 38.4 kg · m^{-2}) had a FFM of 125.4 kg, the uppermost value we have ever seen reported through October 2011.

SARCOPENIC OBESITY: A GROWING CONCERN

Sarcopenic obesity refers to decreases in muscle mass and increases in fat mass with aging. Inflammatory cytokines (e.g., protein and peptide signaling compounds that allow intercellular communication) produced mostly by visceral fat in adipose tissue accelerate muscle breakdown, which maintains the vicious cycle that initiates and sustains the condition. A random sample of 378 men and 493 women age 65 years and older from Tuscany, Italy were assessed for anthropometry, handgrip strength, and proinflammatory cytokine markers. Participants were cross-classified by sex-specific tertiles of waist circumference and grip strength and obesity defined as a BMI greater than 30. After adjusting for age, sex, education, smoking history, physical activity, and history of comorbid diseases, components of sarcopenic obesity were associated with elevated cytokines. The findings suggest that obesity directly affects inflammation, which negatively affects muscle strength that contributes to sarcopenic obesity. These results suggested that proinflammatory cytokines may impact the development and progression of sarcopenic obesity.[114]

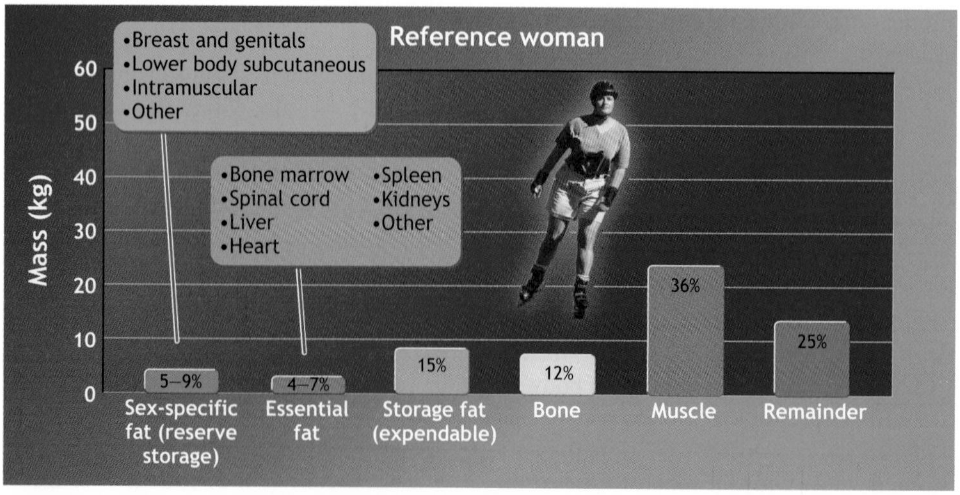

FIGURE 13.5. Theoretical model for body fat distribution for a reference woman whose body mass equals 56.7 kg (stature = 163.8 cm) and body fat equals 23.6%. (From Katch VL, et al. Contribution of breast volume and weight to body fat distribution in females. *Am J Phys Anthropol* 1980;53:93.)

Minimal Standards for Leanness

A biologic lower limit seems to exist beyond which a person's body mass cannot decrease without impairing health status or altering normal physiologic functions.

Men

To calculate the lower fat limit in men (i.e., the LBM), subtract storage fat from body mass. For the reference man, LBM (61.7 kg) includes approximately 3% (2.1 kg) essential body fat. Encroachment into this reserve may impair normal physiologic function and capacity for vigorous exercise.

Low body fat values exist for world-class male endurance athletes and some conscientious objectors to military service who voluntarily reduce body fat stores with prolonged semi-starvation.[73] The low fat levels of marathon runners, ranging from 1 to 8% of body mass, likely reflect the combined effect of self-selection into the sport and adaptations to the severe training for distance running that often exceeds 100 miles weekly at relatively intense training speeds. A low body fat level reduces the energy cost of weight-bearing exercise; it also provides a more effective gradient to dissipate metabolic heat generated during intense physical activity.

TABLE 13.3 presents data on the physique status and body composition of selected professional athletes classified as "underfat" and "overweight." Striking differences occur between these groups in body size, percentage body fat, FFM, lean-to-fat ratio, and various girth measures. The defensive and offensive backs in football are "underfat" compared with the reference man (or any other nonathletic standard), whereas the linemen and shot putters are clearly "overweight" for their stature. Body mass relative to stature (mass per unit size) for these athletic men represents the 90th percentile for nonathletic males.

Women

In contrast to the lower limit of body mass for the reference man, which includes about 3% essential fat, the lower limit for the reference woman includes about 12% essential fat. This theoretical lower limit termed *minimal body mass* equals 48.5 kg for the reference woman. Generally, body fat percentages for the leanest women in the population do not fall

TABLE 13.3 Physique and Body Composition of "Underfat" Professional Football Players and "Overweight" Offensive and Defensive Professional Football Linemen and Shot Putters

	Four Defensive Backs (All-Pro)				Offensive Back, All-Pro	Defensive Linemen, Dallas 1977	Offensive Linemen, Dallas 1977	Shot-Putters, Olympics
Variable	1	2	3	4	(N = 1)	(N = 510)	(N = 5)	(N = 13)
Age, years	27.1	30.2	29.4	24.0	32	31	29	24
Stature (cm)	184.7	181.9	187.2	181.5	184.7	193.8	197.6	187.0
Mass (kg)	87.9	87.1	88.4	88.9	90.6	116.0	116.5	112.3
Relative fat (%)	3.9	3.8	3.8	2.5	1.4	18.6	13.2	14.8
Absolute fat (kg)	3.4	3.3	3.4	2.2	1.3	21.6	15.4	16.6
Fat-free body mass (kg)	84.5	83.8	85.0	86.7	89.3	94.4	101.1	95.7
Lean/fat ratio	24.85	25.39	25.00	39.41	68.69	4.37	6.57	5.77
Girths (cm)								
Shoulders	122.1	119.0	120.5	117.2	121.8	129.5	122.5	133.3
Chest	101.6	101.0	99.5	107.5	102.0	116.5	109.9	118.5
Abdomen (avg)	81.8	85.5	81.0	82.6	81.7	102.0	97.0	100.3
Buttocks	98.0	99.0	101.9	102.0	96.5	112.8	111.5	112.3
Thigh	61.0	61.0	58.5	64.0	63.2	66.2	69.3	69.4
Knee	39.5	41.3	41.1	38.0	41.0	44.8	45.8	42.9
Calf	37.6	38.8	38.8	37.8	41.3	43.5	42.4	43.6
Ankle	21.8	23.1	23.5	22.4	22.7	25.8	25.7	24.7
Forearm	31.8	29.1	31.1	31.8	33.5	33.5	34.8	33.7
Biceps	38.0	35.8	37.1	37.7	40.4	41.5	41.7	42.2
Wrist	18.5	17.2	17.4	17.5	18.0	19.3	19.3	18.9

From Katch FI, Katch VL. The body composition profile: techniques of measurement and applications. *Clin Sports Med* 1984;3:30.

below 10 to 12% of body mass. This value probably represents the lower limit of fatness for most women in good health. *Behnke's theoretical concept of minimal body mass in women, which incorporates about 12% essential fat, corresponds to the LBM in men that includes 3% essential fat.*

UNDERWEIGHT AND THIN: The terms *underweight* and *thin* at times describe different physical conditions. Measurements in our laboratories have focused on the structural characteristics of apparently "thin" women.[92] Subjects were initially screened subjectively as appearing thin or "skinny." Each of the 26 women then underwent a thorough anthropometric evaluation that included measurement of skinfolds, circumferences, bone diameters, and percentage body fat and FFM from hydrostatic weighing.

Unexpectedly, the women's body fat averaged 18.2%, only about 7 percentage points below the average value of 25 to 27% typical for young adult women. Another striking finding included equivalence in four trunk and four extremity bone-diameter measurements in comparisons among the 26 thin-appearing women, 174 women who averaged 25.6% fat, and 31 women who averaged 31.4% body fat. *Thus, appearing thin or skinny did not necessarily correspond to a diminutive frame size or an excessively low percentage body fat.*

LEANNESS, EXERCISE, AND MENSTRUAL IRREGULARITY: AN INORDINATE FOCUS ON BODY WEIGHT

In 1967, professional models weighed only 8% less than the average American woman; today, their weight averages 23% lower. In January 2007, the Council of Fashion Designers of America (CFDA; www.cfda.com) formulated guidelines as part of a new health initiative that targeted its models to emulate a healthy lifestyle, rather than one that promotes eating disorders. These nonbinding guidelines include the following:

1. Keep models younger than age 16 off the runway, and disallow models younger than 18 to work at fittings or photo shoots past midnight.
2. Educate those in the industry to identify the early warning signs of eating disorders (see chapter 15).
3. Require models identified with eating disorders to receive professional help, and allow those models to continue only with approval from that professional.
4. Develop workshops on the causes and effects of eating disorders, and raise awareness of the effects of smoking and tobacco-related disease.
5. Provide healthy meals and snacks during fashion shows while prohibiting alcohol and smoking.

The CFDA, in contrast to the fashion industry in Italy, does not mention the applicability of a BMI under 18.5 as a screening tool to determine the degree of underweight established by the WHO. Some organizations (e.g., American Academy of Eating Disorders: **www.aedweb.org**) have called for even stricter guidelines than the WHO to target two distinct populations of young women: models and the millions of girls worldwide who try to emulate them.

As we discuss in Chapter 15, eating disorders and unrealistic weight goals have become common among females of all ages, particularly among athletes for whom the "norm" fosters striving for excessive leanness as a prerequisite for success. Physically active women, particularly participants in the "low-weight" or "appearance" sports such as distance running, bodybuilding, figure skating, diving, ballet, and gymnastics, increase their chances of these three maladies:

1. Delayed onset of menstruation after age 16 years
2. Irregular menstrual cycle or oligomenorrhea
3. Complete cessation of menses or amenorrhea

Amenorrhea occurs in 2 to 5% of women of reproductive age in the general population, but reaches 10 to 15% among athletes and as high as 40% in some athletic groups. As a group, ballet dancers remain exceptionally lean, with a greater incidence of menstrual dysfunction and eating disorders and a higher mean age at menarche than age-matched, nondancer females. One third to one half of female athletes in endurance-type sports experience some menstrual irregularity. In premenopausal women, menstrual irregularity or absence of menstrual function increases risk of bone loss and musculoskeletal injury in vigorous exercise.[7,47]

Leanness Not the Only Factor

For any given person, the lean-to-fat ratio plays a key role in normal menstrual function. Potential causes of menstrual dysfunction include the complex interplay of physical, nutritional, genetic, hormonal, fat distribution, psychosocial, and environmental factors.[88] For physically active women, an intense exercise bout triggers the release of an array of hormones, some with antireproductive properties. When injuries in young amenorrheic ballet dancers prevent them from exercising regularly, normal menstruation resumes even though body weight remains low.[196] *Primary predisposing factors for reproductive endocrine dysfunction that affect physically active women include nutritional inadequacy and an exercise-induced energy deficit with intense training. Proper nutrition that emphasizes the maintenance of energy balance can prevent or reverse athletic amenorrhea without requiring the athlete to reduce exercise training volume or exercise intensity.*

In all likelihood, 13 to 17% body fat (determined by a valid method to assess body fat) represents the minimal fat level for regular menstrual function. The effects and risks of sustained amenorrhea on the reproductive system remain unknown. A gynecologist/endocrinologist should evaluate failure to menstruate or cessation of the normal cycle because it may reflect pituitary or thyroid gland malfunction or premature menopause.[6,87] As noted previously in Chapter 2, prolonged menstrual dysfunction profoundly diminishes the density of the bone mass, which usually is not regained if and when menstruation resumes.

COMMON LABORATORY METHODS TO ASSESS BODY COMPOSITION

Two general approaches determine the fat and fat-free components of the human body:

1. Direct measurement by chemical analysis of the animal carcass or human cadaver
2. Indirect estimation by hydrostatic weighing, simple anthropometric measurements, or other noninvasive procedures

Direct Assessment

One direct technique of body composition assessment literally dissolves the body in a chemical solution to determine the fat and fat-free components of the mixture. The other technique involves the physical dissection of fat, fat-free adipose tissue, muscle, and bone. Considerable research exists on the direct chemical assessment of body composition in various animal species, but relatively few studies have directly determined human fat content. These analyses are time consuming and tedious, require specialized laboratory equipment, and involve ethical questions and legal problems in obtaining cadavers for research purposes.

PERSONAL HEALTH AND EXERCISE NUTRITION 13.1

How to Predict Percentage Body Fat from Body Mass Index

Body weight adjusted for height squared, referred to as BMI (in $kg \cdot m^{-2}$), in excess of 25 and 30 indicates overweight and obesity, respectively. The assumption underlying BMI guidelines lies in its supposed close association with body fatness and consequent morbidity and mortality. Several formulae predict percentage body fat (%BF) from BMI, which may provide a better indication of morbidity and mortality than BMI alone.

Measurement Variables

The following variables predict percentage body fat (%BF) from BMI:

- 1.00 ÷ BMI
- Age in years
- Sex: male, female
- Race: white, African American, Asian

Equation

Predict %BF with the following equation:

$$\%BF = 63.7 - [864 \times (1.00 \div BMI)] - (12.1 \times sex) + (0.12 \times age) + [129 \times Asian \times (1 \div BMI)] - (0.091 \times Asian \times age) - (0.030 \times African\ American \times age)$$

where sex = 1 for male and 0 for female; Asian = 1 for Asians and 0 for other races; African American = 1 for African Americans and 0 for other races; age in years; and BMI = body weight in kg ÷ stature in m^2

Examples

Example 1. African American male; age 30 years; BMI = 25

$$\%BF = 63.7 - [864 \times (1.00 \div BMI)] - (12.1 \times sex) + (0.12 \times age) + [129 \times Asian \times (1 \div BMI)] - (0.091 \times Asian \times age) - (0.030 \times African\ American \times age)$$
$$= 63.7 - (864 \times 0.04) - (12.1 \times 1) + (0.12 \times 30) + (129 \times 0 \times 0.04) - (0.091 \times 0 \times 30) - (0.030 \times 1 \times 30)$$
$$= 63.7 - (34.56) - (12.1) + (3.6) + (0) - (0) - (0.9)$$
$$= 19.7\%$$

Example 2. Asian female; age 50 years; BMI = 30

$$\%BF = 63.7 - [864 \times (1.00 \div BMI)] - (12.1 \times sex) + (0.12 \times age) + [129 \times Asian \times (1 \div BMI)] - (0.091 \times Asian \times age) - (0.030 \times African\ American \times age)$$
$$= 63.7 - (864 \times 0.0333) - (12.1 \times 0) + (0.12 \times 50) + (129 \times 1 \times 0.0333) - (0.091 \times 1 \times 50) - (0.030 \times 0 \times 50)$$
$$= 63.7 - (28.80) - (0) + (6.0) + (4.295) - (4.55) - (0)$$
$$= 40.7\%$$

Using the same computational strategies for Examples 1 and 2, compute the body fat percentage for examples 3 and 4 shown below.

Example 3. Asian male; age 70 years; BMI = 28

Example 4. White male; age 55 years; BMI = 24.5

thePoint *Visit* **thePoint.lww.com/MKKSEN4e** *to review the correct calculations for examples 3 and 4.*

Accuracy

The correlation coefficient between predicted %BF (using the above formulae) and measured %BF (using a four-compartment model to estimate body fat) is r = 0.89 with a standard error for estimating an person's %BF equal to ± 3.9% body fat units. This compares favorably with other body fat prediction methods that use skinfolds and girths.

Predicted Percentage Fat at Given Critical BMI Values

TABLE 1 presents predicted %BF values for different threshold BMI values for men and women of different ethnicity. These data provide an approach for developing healthy percentage body fat ranges from BMI guidelines.

TABLE 1 Predicted Percentage Body Fat by Sex and Ethnicity Related to BMI Healthy Weight Guidelines

	Women			Men		
Age and BMI	African Americans	Asians	White	African Americans	Asians	White
20–39 years						
BMI <18.5	20%	25%	21%	8%	13%	8%
BMI ≥25	32%	35%	33%	20%	23%	21%
BMI ≥30	38%	40%	39%	26%	28%	26%
40–59 years						
BMI <18.5	21%	25%	23%	23%	13%	11%
BMI ≥25	34%	36%	35%	35%	24%	23%
BMI ≥30	39%	41%	42%	41%	29%	29%
60–79 y						
BMI <18.5	23%	26%	25%	11%	14%	13%
BMI ≥25	35%	36%	38%	23%	24%	25%
BMI ≥30	41%	41%	43%	29%	29%	31%

From Gallagher D, et al. Healthy percentage body fat ranges: an approach for developing guidelines based on body mass index. *Am J Clin Nutr* 2000;72:694.

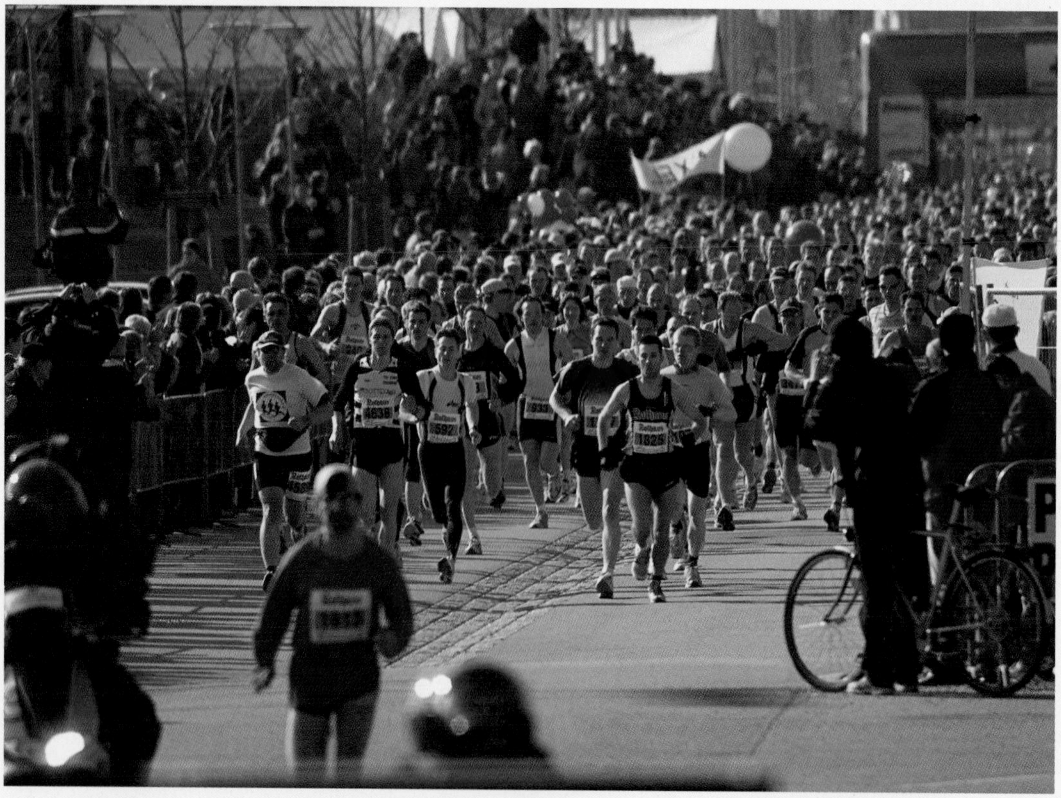

DELAYED ONSET OF MENSTRUATION AND CANCER RISK

The delayed onset of menarche in chronically active young females may offer positive health benefits.[56] Female athletes who start training in high school or earlier show a lower lifetime occurrence of cancers of the breast and reproductive organs and non–reproductive system cancers than less active counterparts. Even among older women, regular exercise protects against reproductive cancers. Women who exercise an average of 4 h a week after menarche reduce breast cancer risk by 50% compared with age-matched inactive women. One proposed mechanism for reduced cancer risk links less total estrogen production (or a less potent estrogen form) over the athlete's lifetime with fewer ovulatory cycles because of the delayed onset of menstruation. Lower body fat levels in physically active persons also may contribute to lowered cancer risk because peripheral fatty tissues convert androgens to estrogen.

Direct assessment of body composition indicates that the compositions of skeletal mass and lean and fat tissues remain relatively stable despite considerable person differences. The assumed constancy of these tissues enables researchers to develop mathematical equations to predict the body's fat percentage.

Indirect Assessment

Different indirect procedures commonly assess body composition. One involves Archimedes' principle applied to hydrostatic weighing (also referred to as *densitometry* or *underwater weighing*). This method computes percentage body fat from whole-body density (the ratio of body mass to body volume). Other popular procedures to predict body fat use skinfold thickness and girth measurements, x-ray, total-body electrical conductivity or impedance, ultrasound, computed tomography, dual-energy x-ray absorptiometry, air plethysmography, and magnetic resonance imaging.

HYDROSTATIC WEIGHING (ARCHIMEDES' PRINCIPLE)

The Greek mathematician and inventor Archimedes (287–212 BC) discovered a fundamental principle currently applied to evaluate human body composition. An itinerant scholar of that time described the interesting anecdote surrounding the event:

> King Hieron of Syracuse suspected that a pure gold crown crafted for a temple had been altered by substitution of silver for gold. The King directed Archimedes to devise a method for testing the crown for its gold content without dismantling or melting it. Archimedes pondered over this problem for many weeks without succeeding, until one day he stepped into a bath filled to the top with water and observed the overflow. He thought about this for a moment, and then, wild with joy, jumped from the bath and ran naked through the streets of Syracuse shouting eureka, eureka, I have discovered a way to solve the mystery of the King's crown.

Archimedes reasoned that a substance such as gold must have a volume in proportion to its mass, and the way to measure the volume of an irregularly shaped object like a crown required submersion in water with collection of the overflow. Archimedes took lumps of gold and silver, each having the same mass as the crown, and submerged each in a container full of water. To his delight, he discovered the crown displaced more water than the lump of gold and less than the lump of silver. This could only mean the crown consisted of *both* silver and gold as the King suspected.

Essentially, Archimedes evaluated the specific gravity of the crown (ratio of the crown's mass to the mass of an equal volume of water) compared to the specific gravities of gold and silver. Archimedes probably also reasoned that an object submerged or floating in water becomes buoyed up by a counterforce equaling the weight of the volume of water it displaces. This buoyant force helps to support an immersed object against the downward pull of gravity. Thus, an object is said to lose weight in water. The object's loss of weight in water equals the weight of the volume of water it displaces, so specific gravity refers to the ratio of the weight of an object in air divided by its *loss* of weight in water. The loss of weight in water equals the weight in air minus the weight in water:

Specific gravity = Weight in air ÷ Loss of weight in water

In practical terms, suppose a crown weighed 2.27 kg in air and 0.13 kg less (2.14 kg) when weighed underwater (**FIG. 13.6**). A specific gravity value of 17.5 is obtained by dividing the weight of the crown (2.27 kg) by its loss of weight in water (0.13 kg). This ratio differs considerably from the specific gravity of gold with a value of 19.3, so we too can conclude: "Eureka, the crown is a fraud!" The physical principle Archimedes discovered allows us to apply water submersion (underwater weighing or hydrodensitometry) to determine the body's volume. Dividing a person's body mass by body volume yields body density (Density = Mass ÷ Volume) and from this a reasonably valid estimate of percentage body fat.

Computing Body Density

Consider a 50-kg person who weighs 2 kg when submerged in water. According to Archimedes' principle, loss of weight in water of 48 kg equals the weight of the displaced water. This is analogous to submerging in a tub of water, where the rise in water equals the volume of the submerged body. The volume of water displaced can be computed from standard chemistry tables because chemistry tables list the density of water at any temperature. In the example, 48 kg of water equals 48 L or 48,000 cm^{-3} (1 g of water = 1 cm^{-3} by volume at 39.2°F). Measuring the person at the cold-water temperature of 39.2°F

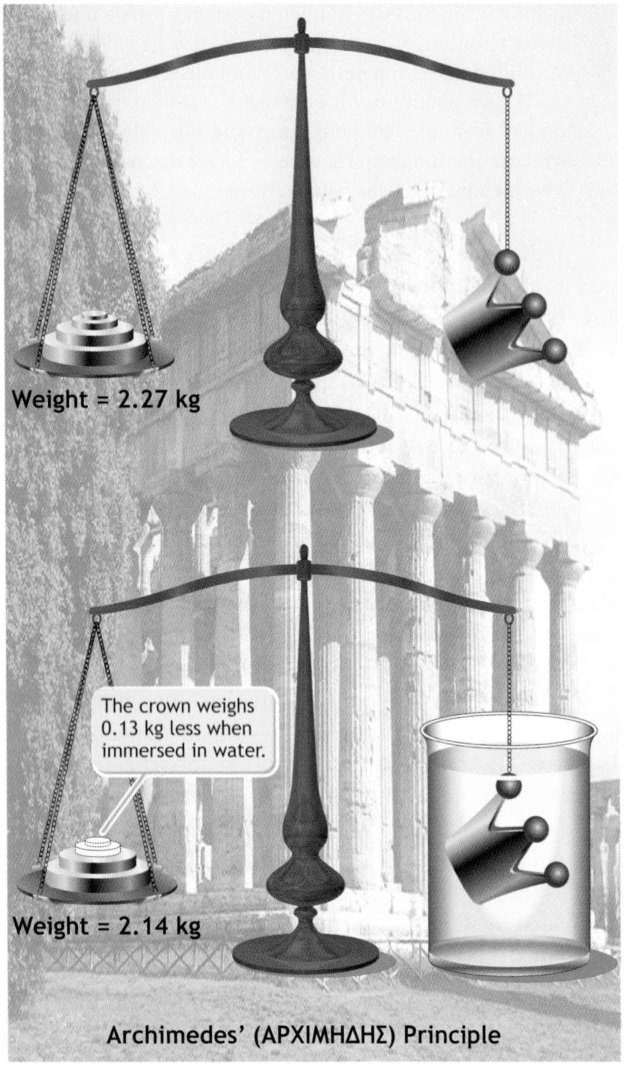

FIGURE 13.6. Archimedes' principle of buoyant force to determine the volume and subsequently the specific gravity of the king's crown.

requires no density correction for water. In practice, researchers use warmer water and apply the appropriate density value for water at the particular temperature. The density of this person, computed as mass ÷ volume, equals 50,000 g (50 kg) ÷ 48,000 cm^{13}, or 1.0417 g · cm^{-3}. The next step estimates percentage of body fat and the mass of fat and fat-free tissues.

Computing Percentage Body Fat and Mass of Fat and Fat-Free Tissues

An equation that incorporates whole-body density can estimate the body's fat percentage. This equation is derived from the premise that the densities of fat mass (all extractable lipid from adipose and other body tissues) and FFM (remaining lipid-free tissues and chemicals, including water) remain relatively constant (fat tissue, 0.90 g · cm^{-3}; fat-free tissue, 1.10 g · cm^{-3}). These consistencies remain even with large variations in total body fat and the fat-free tissue components of bone and muscle. The assumed densities for the components of the FFM at a body temperature of 37°C (98.6°F) are as follows: water, 0.9937 g · cm^{-3} (73.8% of FFM); minerals, 3.038 g · cm^{-3} (6.8% of FFM); and protein, 1.340 g · cm^{-3} (19.4% of FFM). The following equation, derived by Berkeley scientist Dr. William Siri (1919–2004), computes percentage body fat by incorporating the measured value of whole-body density:

Siri Equation

$$\text{Percentage body fat} = 495 \div \text{Body density} - 450$$

To estimate percentage body fat, substitute the body density value of 1.0417 g · cm^{-3} for the subject in the previous example in the Siri equation as follows:

$$\text{Percentage body fat} = 495 \div 1.0417 - 450 = 25.2$$

Compute mass of body fat by multiplying body mass by percentage fat:

$$\begin{aligned}\text{Fat mass (kg)} &= \text{Body mass (kg)} \times (\text{Percentage fat} \div 100)\\ &= 50\text{ kg} \times 0.252\\ &= 12.6\end{aligned}$$

Compute FFM by subtracting the mass of fat from body mass:

$$\begin{aligned}\text{FFM (kg)} &= \text{Body mass (kg)} - \text{Fat mass (kg)}\\ &= 50\text{ kg} - 12.6\text{ kg}\\ &= 37.4\end{aligned}$$

In this example, 25.2% or 12.6 kg of the 50 kg body mass consists of fat, with the remaining 37.4 kg representing the FFM.

Possible Limitations of Hydrostatic Weighing

The generalized density values for fat-free (1.10 g · cm^{-3}) and fat (0.90 g · cm^{-3}) tissues represent averages for young and middle-aged adults. These assumed "constants" vary among persons and groups, particularly the density and chemical composition of the FFM. Such variation limits the accuracy of predicting percentage body fat from whole-body density. More specifically, a significantly larger average density of the FFM exists for blacks (1.113 g · cm^{-3}) and Hispanics (1.105 g · cm^{-3}) than whites (1.100 g · cm^{-3}).[48,103,126] Consequently, using the existing equations formulated on assumptions for whites to calculate body composition from whole-body density of blacks or Hispanics *overestimates* the FFM and *underestimates* percentage body fat. The following modifications of the Siri equation compute percentage body fat from body density measures for blacks[144]:

Modification of Siri's equation for blacks:

$$\text{Percentage body fat} = [(4.858 \div \text{Body density}) - 4.394] \times 100$$

Applying constant density values for the fat and fat-free tissues to growing children or aging adults can introduce errors in predicting body composition. For example, the water and mineral contents of the FFM continually change during the growth period and the well-documented demineralization of osteoporosis with aging. Reduced bone density

TABLE 13.4 Percentage (%) Body Fat Estimated from Body Density (BD) Using Age- and Sex-Specific Conversion Constants to Account for Changes in the Density of the Fat-Free Body Mass as the Child Matures

Age (years)	Boys	Girls
7–9	% Fat = (5.38/BD – 4.97) × 100	% Fat = (5.43/BD – 5.03) × 100
9–11	% Fat = (5.30/BD – 4.89) × 100	% Fat = (5.35/BD – 4.95) × 100
11–13	% Fat = (5.23/BD – 4.81) × 100	% Fat = (5.25/BD – 4.84) × 100
13–15	% Fat = (5.08/BD – 4.64) × 100	% Fat = (5.12/BD – 4.69) × 100
15–17	% Fat = (5.03/BD – 4.59) × 100	% Fat = (5.07/BD – 4.64) × 100

From Lohman T. Applicability of body composition techniques and constants for children and youth. *Exerc Sports Sci Rev* 1986;14:325.

reduces the density of the fat-free tissue of young children and the elderly below the assumed constant of 1.10 g · cm^{-3}, thus overestimating percentage body fat. For boys and girls, researchers have modified equations to predict body fat from whole-body density to adjust for density changes in FFM during childhood and adolescence (**TABLE 13.4**).

Adjustments for Large Musculoskeletal Development: Chronic resistance training changes the density of the FFM, thus altering body fat estimation from whole-body density determinations.

Based on the revised densities of the FFM (1.089 g · cm^{-3}) and fat mass (0.9007 g · cm^{-3}), researchers recommend modifying Siri's equation for more accurate appraisal with resistance-trained white males:

Modification for resistance-trained white males:
Percentage body fat = (521 ÷ Body density) – 478

Measuring Body Volume by Hydrostatic Weighing

Hydrostatic weighing, illustrated in **FIGURE 13.7**, shows common applications of Archimedes' principle to determine body volume. We have used different variations of underwater weighing configurations depending on equipment availability. In each case, the principle of measurement remains the same. An accurate measure of water displaced requires an autopsy scale (or electronic scale) sensitive to at least ± 10 g. Body volume computes as the difference between body mass measured in air (M_a) and body weight measured during water submersion (W_w); *weight* is the correct term, because the body's mass remains unchanged under water. *Body volume equals loss of weight in water with the appropriate temperature correction for water density.*

VARIATIONS WITH MENSTRUATION

Normal fluctuations in body mass (chiefly body water) related to the menstrual cycle generally do not affect body density and body fat assessed by hydrostatic weighing. However, some females experience noticeable increases in body water (>1.0 kg) during menstruation. Water retention of this magnitude affects body density and introduces a small error in computing percentage body fat.

Examples of Calculations

Data for two professional football players, an offensive guard and a quarterback, illustrate the sequence of steps to compute body density, percentage body fat, mass of fat, and FFM.

	Offensive Guard	Quarterback
Body mass	110 kg	85 kg
Underwater weight	3.5 kg	5.0 kg
Residual lung volume	1.2 L	1.0 L
Water temperature	0.996	0.996 correction factor

The loss of body weight in water equals body volume, so the body volume of the offensive guard becomes 110 kg – 3.5 kg = 106.5 kg or 106.5 L; body volume for the quarterback (85 kg – 5.0 kg) equals 80.0 kg or 80 L. Dividing body volume by the water temperature correction factor of 0.996 increases body volume slightly for both players (106.9 L for the guard and 80.3 L for the quarterback). By subtracting residual lung volume, the body volume of the offensive guard then becomes 105.7 L (106.9 L – 1.2 L) and for the quarterback 79.3 L (80.3 L – 1.0 L).

Body density computes as mass ÷ volume. Body density for the offensive guard becomes 110 kg ÷ 105.7 L = 1.0407 kg · L^{-1}, or 1.0407 g · cm^{-3}. The corresponding density for the quarterback is 85.0 kg ÷ 79.3 L = 1.0719 kg · L^{-1}, or 1.0719 g · cm^{-3}.

From the Siri equation, percentage body fat computes as follows:

Offensive guard:

$$495 \div 1.0407 - 450 = 25.6\%$$

Quarterback:

$$495 \div 1.0719 - 450 = 11.8\%$$

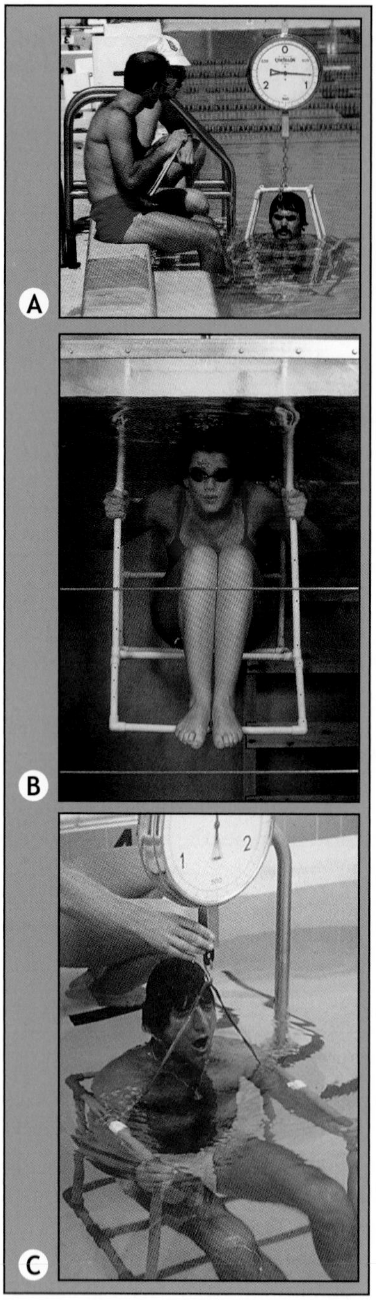

FIGURE 13.7. Measuring body volume by underwater weighing in **(A)** swimming pool, **(B)** stainless steel tank in the laboratory, and **(C)** therapy pool at a professional football training facility.

Total mass of body fat calculates as follows:
Offensive guard:

$$110 \text{ kg} \times 0.256 = 28.2 \text{ kg}$$

Quarterback:

$$85 \text{ kg} \times 0.118 = 10.0 \text{ kg}$$

FFM computes as follows:
Offensive guard:

$$110 \text{ kg} - 28.2 \text{ kg} = 81.8 \text{ kg}$$

Quarterback:

$$85 \text{ kg} - 10.0 \text{ kg} = 75.0 \text{ kg}$$

Body composition analysis illustrates that the offensive guard possesses more than twice the percentage body fat of the quarterback (25.6 vs 11.8%) and almost three times as much total fat (28.2 vs 10.0 kg). In contrast, the guard's FFM, which largely indicates muscle mass, exceeds the quarterback's FFM.

SKINFOLD MEASUREMENTS

Simple anthropometric procedures validly predict body fatness. The most common of these procedures measures skinfolds. The rationale for using skinfolds to estimate body fat comes from the relationships among three factors:

1. Fat in the adipose tissue deposits directly beneath the skin called subcutaneous fat
2. Internal fat stores
3. Whole-body density

Caliper and Measurement Sites

By 1930, a special pincer-type caliper accurately measured subcutaneous fat at selected body sites. The three calipers shown in **FIGURE 13.8** operate on the same principle as a micrometer that measures distance between two points. The most common anatomic sites for skinfold measurement

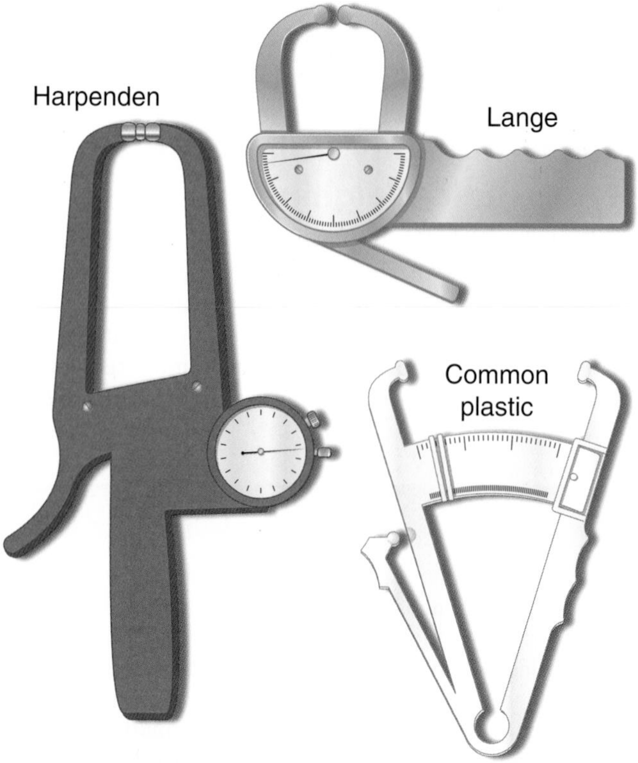

FIGURE 13.8. Common calipers for skinfold measurements. The Harpenden and Lange calipers provide constant tension at all jaw openings.

include the triceps, subscapular, suprailiac, abdominal, and upper thigh sites displayed in **FIGURE 13.9**. For added accuracy, the tester takes a minimum of two or three measurements at each site on the right side of the body with the subject standing, with the average representing the skinfold score. The five sites are measured at the following anatomic locations:

1. **Triceps**: Vertical fold at the posterior midline of the upper arm, halfway between the tip of the shoulder and tip of the elbow; elbow remains in an extended, relaxed position
2. **Subscapular**: Oblique fold, just below the bottom tip of the scapula
3. **Suprailiac (iliac crest)**: Slightly oblique fold, just above the hipbone (crest of ileum); the fold follows the natural diagonal line
4. **Abdominal**: Vertical fold 1 in to the right of the umbilicus
5. **Thigh**: Vertical fold at the midline of the thigh, two thirds of the distance from the middle of the patella (kneecap) to the hip

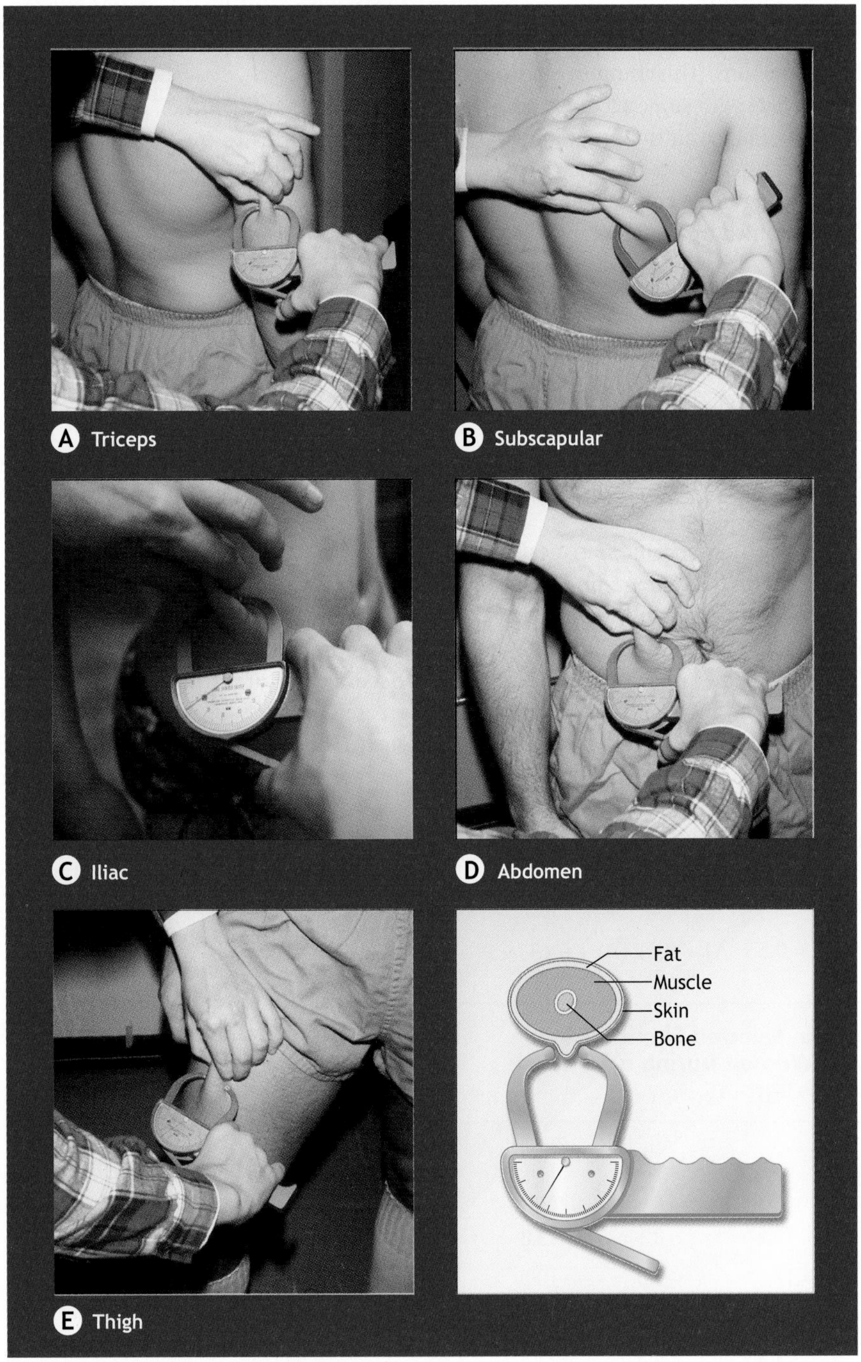

FIGURE 13.9. Anatomic location of five common skinfold sites: **A.** Triceps. **B.** Subscapular. **C.** Iliac (suprailiac). **D.** Abdomen. **E.** Thigh. The *lower right* shows a schematic diagram for use of a skinfold caliper. Note the compression of a double layer of skin and underlying tissue during the measurement. Except for subscapular and suprailiac sites measured diagonally, take measurements in the vertical plane.

Other sites often include the following:

- **Chest**: Diagonal fold with its long axis directed toward the nipple, on the anterior axillary fold, as high as possible
- **Biceps**: Vertical fold at the posterior midline of the upper arm
- **Midaxillary**: Vertical fold on the midaxillary line at the level of the sternum's xiphoid process

Usefulness of Skinfold Scores

Skinfold measurements provide consistent and meaningful information concerning body fat and its distribution. We recommend two options to use skinfolds:

Options One: Compute the sum of the skinfold scores to indicate relative fatness among persons. This "sum of skinfolds" and person skinfold values reflect with some accuracy body fat changes "before" and "after" an intervention program. Evaluate these changes on either an absolute or a percentage basis.

One can draw the following three conclusions from the skinfold data in **TABLE 13.5** obtained from a 22-year-old female college student before and after a 16-week exercise program:

1. Largest changes in skinfold thickness occurred at the suprailiac and abdominal sites.
2. Triceps skinfold showed the largest percentage decrease, and the subscapular skinfold showed the smallest percentage decrease.
3. Total skinfold reduction at the five sites equaled 16.6 mm, or 12.6% below the "before" condition.

Option Two: Incorporate population-specific statistical equations to predict body density or percentage body fat. The equations prove accurate for subjects similar in age, gender, training status, fatness, and race to the group for whom they were derived.[15,60,67,104,139] When meeting these criteria, predicted percentage body fat for an person usually ranges between 3 and 5% body fat units of the value computed using hydrostatic weighing or another valid criterion method.

We have developed the following equations to predict body fat from triceps and subscapular skinfolds in young women and men[67–70]:

Young women, age 17 to 26 years:

$$\text{Percentage body fat} = 0.55\ (A) + 0.31\ (B) + 6.13$$

TABLE 13.5 Changes in Selected Skinfolds for a Young Woman During a 16-Week Exercise Program

Skinfolds	Before (mm)	After (mm)	Absolute Change (mm)	Percentage Change (mm)
Triceps	22.5	19.4	-3.1	-13.8
Subscapular	19.0	17.0	-2.0	-10.5
Suprailiac	34.5	30.2	-4.3	-12.8
Abdomen	33.7	29.4	-4.3	-12.8
Thigh	21.6	18.7	-2.9	-13.4
Sum	**131.3**	**114.7**	**-16.6**	**-12.6**

Young men, age 17 to 26 years:

$$\text{Percentage body fat} = 0.43\ (A) + 0.58\ (B) + 1.47$$

In both equations, A = triceps skinfold (mm) and B = subscapular skinfold (mm).

We computed the "before" and "after" percentage body fat of the woman who participated in the 16-week physical conditioning program (Table 13.5). Body fat equals 24.4% by substituting the pretraining values for triceps (22.5 mm) and subscapular (19.0 mm) skinfolds into the equation:

$$\begin{aligned}\text{Percentage body fat} &= 0.55\ (A) + 0.31\ (B) + 6.13\\ &= 0.55\ (22.5) + 0.31\ (19.0) + 6.13\\ &= 12.38 + 5.89 + 6.13\\ &= 24.4\%\end{aligned}$$

Substituting the posttraining values for triceps (19.4 mm) and subscapular (17.0 mm) skinfolds produced a body fat value of 21.1%:

$$\begin{aligned}\text{Percentage body fat} &= 0.55\ (A) + 0.31\ (B) + 6.13\\ &= 0.55\ (19.4) + 0.31\ (17.0) + 6.13\\ &= 10.67 + 5.27 + 6.13\\ &= 22.1\%\end{aligned}$$

Percentage body fat determined before and after a physical conditioning or weight-loss program proves useful to assess body composition alterations, often independent of body weight changes.

Skinfolds and Age

In young adults, subcutaneous fat constitutes approximately one half of the body's total fat, with the remainder being visceral and organ fat. As persons age, a proportionately greater quantity of fat deposits internally than subcutaneously. Thus, the same skinfold score reflects *greater* total percentage body fat for an older age group. By around age 45 years or earlier, a noticeable deposit of fat accumulates around the midabdominal area. (Performing crunches or sit-ups ad nauseam does not seem to substantially reduce this fat pad.) *For this reason, we recommend using age-adjusted generalized equations to predict body fat from skinfolds or girths in children and in older men and women.*[59,60,136]

For both fatter and leaner white and African American children, the following two skinfold equations best predict percentage body fat[16]:

$$\text{Percentage body fat} = 9.02 + 1.09\ (\text{biceps, mm}) + 0.42\ (\text{calf, mm})$$

$$\text{Percentage body fat} = 8.596 + 0.81\ (\text{biceps, mm}) + 0.40\ (\text{triceps, mm}) + 0.30\ (\text{subscapular, mm})$$

User Beware

The person taking skinfold measurements must develop expertise with the proper measurement techniques. Also, skinfold thickness in extremely obese persons frequently exceeds the width of the caliper's jaws. It often becomes difficult to determine which prediction equation to use because of lack of standards to judge the results of different investigators.

A prediction equation developed by one researcher (that shows high validity for the sample measured) may produce large prediction errors when applied to skinfolds from a dissimilar group. What this means is that two testers who measure skinfolds at the same site on the same person often obtain disparate results. Two different personal trainers or sports nutritionists who take "before" and "after" skinfolds can obtain values that just do not seem to "make sense." One would be hard pressed to tell a client how a posttest measurement measured by one person can actually *increase* with a 20-lb weight *decrease* compared to the original value taken by a different person! The take home message that we cannot overemphasize is that the same tester must take all of the measurements before, during, and after an experimental treatment. This could be a weight-loss program, a fitness training program, or during a competitive sport season. The same applies to two persons who take skinfolds over a span of months or years for purposes of classifying or tracking changes in a person's body fat percentage. In addition, selected skinfold prediction equations using three or seven skinfold sites may not be valid to track body composition changes (relative and absolute fat mass, FFM) prior to athletic competition in highly trained athletes.[121]

GIRTH MEASUREMENTS

The girth technique provides a valuable way to assess body composition with minimal expense and training. The technique requires the tester to apply a linen or plastic measuring tape lightly to the skin surface so the tape remains taut but not tight. This avoids skin compression that produces lower than normal scores. As with skinfolds, the tester should take duplicate measurements at each site and average the scores to increase the dependability of the scores. **FIGURE 13.10** displays common anatomic landmarks for taking girths for anthropometric measurement and to predict body fatness.

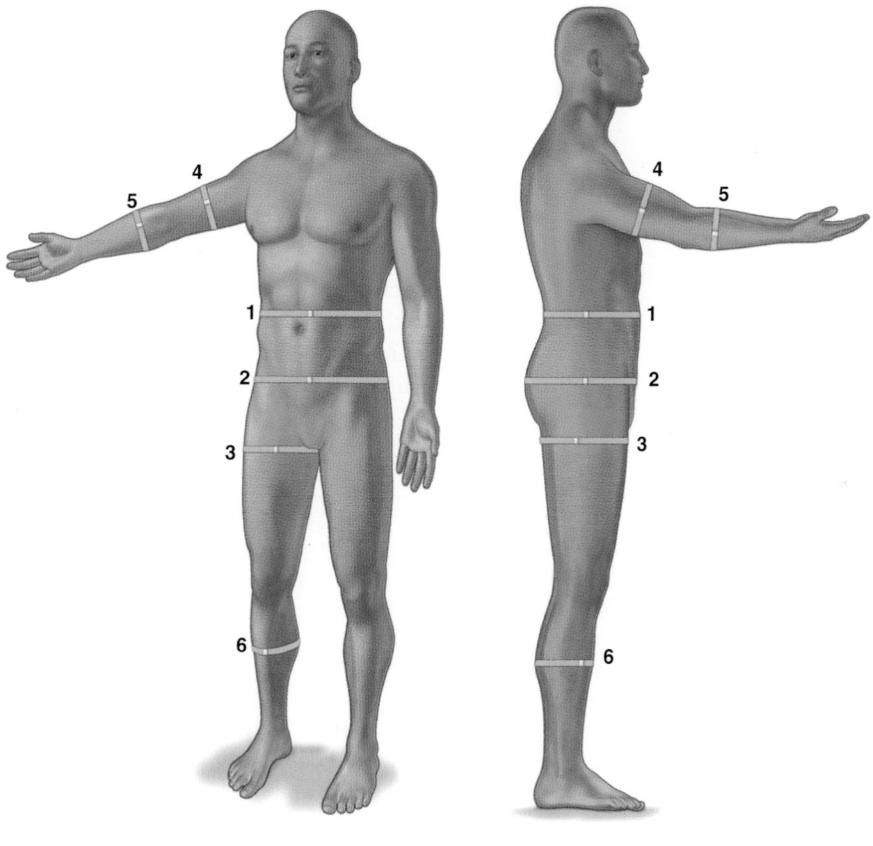

1. **Abdomen:** 1 in above the umbilicus
2. **Buttocks:** Maximum protrusion of buttocks with the heels together
3. **Right thigh:** Upper thigh, just below the buttocks
4. **Right upper arm (biceps):** Palm up, arm straight and extended in front of the body; taken at the midpoint between the shoulder and the elbow
5. **Right forearm:** Maximum girth with the arm extended in front of the body
6. **Right calf:** Widest girth midway between the ankle and knee

FIGURE 13.10. Landmarks for measuring various girths at six common anatomic sites.

Usefulness of Girth Measurements

The equations and constants presented in Appendix D for young and older men and women predict an person's body fat within ± 2.5 to 4.0% of the value from hydrostatic weighing, provided the person resembles the original validation group. Such relatively small prediction errors make the equations particularly useful to those without access to laboratory facilities. Do not use the equations to predict fatness in persons who appear excessively thin or fat or who participate regularly in strenuous sports or resistance training. Along with predicting percentage body fat, girths can analyze patterns of body fat distribution, including changes in fat distribution during

PERSONAL HEALTH AND EXERCISE NUTRITION 13.2

Predicting Percentage Body Fat of Hispanics

Hispanics represent the second largest minority population in the United States, yet little validated research exists on body composition prediction equations for this group. The available research suggests the density of the fat-free body mass of Hispanic women differs from their white counterparts.

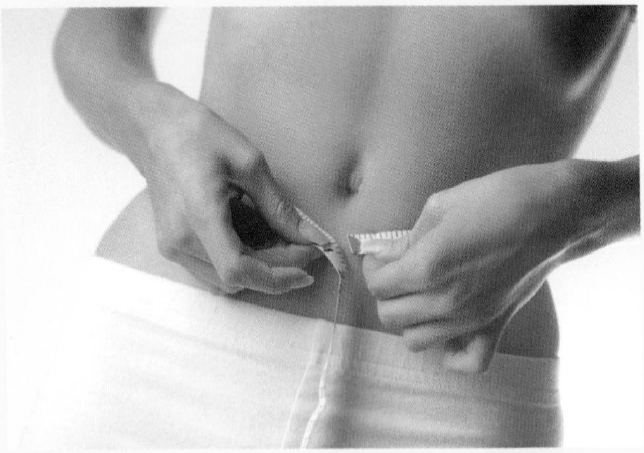

Variables

The generalized skinfold equations of Jackson and colleagues[59,60] have been used successfully with Hispanic men and women. The seven skinfold measurements for men and women are listed below and include the five skinfold sites listed in **FIGURE 13.9**. For both males and females, the chest skinfold is the diagonal fold, midway between the upper armpit and the nipple. The midaxillary skinfold is the horizontal fold directly below the armpit.

1. Abdomen
2. Thigh
3. Triceps
4. Subscapular
5. Suprailiac
6. Midaxillary
7. Chest

Equations

For both men and women: Db = body density in $g \cdot cm^{-3}$; Σ7SKF comprises chest + abdomen + thigh + triceps + subscapular + suprailiac + midaxillary skinfolds in mm.

Men (ages 18–61 years):

$$Db = 1.112 - (0.00043499 \times \Sigma 7SKF) + [0.00000055 \times (\Sigma 7SKF)^2] - (0.00028826 \times age)$$

To convert Db to %BF:

$$\%BF = 495 \div Db - 450$$

Women (ages 18–55 years):

$$Db = 1.0970 - (0.00046971 \times \Sigma 7SKF) + [0.00000056 \times (\Sigma 7SKF)^2] - (0.00012828 \times age)$$

To convert Db to %BF:

$$\%BF = 487 \div Db - 441$$

Examples

Example 1. Hispanic male, age 24 years

Skinfold data: chest = 15.0 mm; abdomen = 33.0 mm; thigh = 21.0 mm; triceps = 18 mm; subscapular = 19 mm; suprailiac = 30 mm; midaxillary = 12.0 mm

$$\begin{aligned} Db &= 1.112 - (0.00043499 \times \Sigma 7SKF) + [0.00000055 \times (\Sigma 7SKF)^2] - (0.00028826 \times age) \\ &= 1.112 - (0.00043499 \times 148) + (0.00000055 \times 21{,}904) - (0.00028826 \times 24) \\ &= 1.112 - 0.064378 + 0.012047 - 0.0069182 \\ &= 1.0528\ g \cdot cm^{-3} \\ \%BF &= 495 \div Db - 450 \\ &= 495 \div 1.0528 - 450 \\ &= 20.2 \end{aligned}$$

Example 2. Hispanic female, age 30 years

Skinfold data: chest = 12.0 mm; abdomen = 30.0 mm; thigh = 18.0 mm; triceps = 20.0 mm; subscapular = 16.0 mm; suprailiac = 30 mm; midaxillary = 15.0 mm

$$\begin{aligned} Db &= 1.0970 - (0.00046971 \times \Sigma 7SKF) + [0.00000056 \times (\Sigma 7SKF)^2] - (0.00012828 \times age) \\ &= 1.0970 - (0.00046971 \times 141) + (0.00000056 \times 19{,}881) - (0.00012828 \times 30) \\ &= 1.0970 - 0.066229 + 0.011133 - 0.003848 \\ &= 1.0381\ g \cdot cm^{-3} \\ \%BF &= 487 \div Db - 441 \\ &= 487 \div 1.0381 - 441 \\ &= 28.2 \end{aligned}$$

weight loss. Specific equations based on girths also accurately estimate the body composition of obese adults.[135,147] Not surprisingly, equations that use the more labile sites of fat deposition (e.g., waist and hips instead of upper arm or thigh in females and abdomen in males) provide the greatest accuracy for predicting *changes* in body composition.[41]

Predicting Body Fat from Girths

From the appropriate tables in Appendix D, substitute the corresponding constants A, B, and C in the formula shown at the bottom of each table. This requires one addition and two subtraction steps. The following five-step example shows how to compute percentage body fat, fat mass, and FFM for a 21-year-old man who weighs 79.1 kg:

Step 1. Measure upper arm, abdomen, and right forearm girths with a cloth tape to the nearest tenth of an inch (0.24 cm): upper arm = 11.5 in (29.2 cm); abdomen = 31.0 in (78.7 cm); right forearm = 10.7 in (27.3 cm).

Step 2. Determine the three constants A, B, and C corresponding to the three girths from Appendix D: constant A corresponds to 11.5 in = 42.56; constant B corresponds to 31.0 in = 40.68; constant C corresponds to 10.7 in = 58.37.

Step 3. Compute percentage body fat by substituting the appropriate constants in the formula for young men shown at the bottom of Chart 1 in Appendix D.

$$\begin{aligned}\text{Percentage fat} &= \text{Constant A} + \text{Constant B} - \text{Constant C} - 10.2\\ &= 42.56 + 40.68 - 58.37 - 10.2\\ &= 83.24 - 58.37 - 10.2\\ &= 24.87 - 10.2\\ &= 14.7\%\end{aligned}$$

Step 4. Calculate the mass of body fat as follows:

$$\begin{aligned}\text{Fat mass} &= \text{Body mass} \times (\%\ \text{fat} \div 100)\\ &= 79.1\ \text{kg} \times (14.7 \div 100)\\ &= 79.1\ \text{kg} \times 0.147\\ &= 11.63\ \text{kg}\end{aligned}$$

Step 5. Calculate FFM as follows:

$$\begin{aligned}\text{FFM} &= \text{Body mass} - \text{Fat mass}\\ &= 79.1\ \text{kg} - 11.63\ \text{kg}\\ &= 67.5\ \text{kg}\end{aligned}$$

REGIONAL FAT DISTRIBUTION: WAIST GIRTH AND WAIST-TO-HIP RATIO

Measures of waist girth and the ratio of waist girth to hip girth provide an important indication of disease risk. **FIGURE 13.11** shows two types of regional fat distribution. The increased health risk from fat deposition in the abdominal area (called central or android-type obesity), particularly internal visceral deposits, may result from this tissue's active lipolysis with catecholamine stimulation. Fat stored in this region shows greater metabolic responsiveness than fat in the gluteal and femoral regions (called peripheral or gynoid-type obesity). Increases in central fat more readily support processes that associate with heart disease.

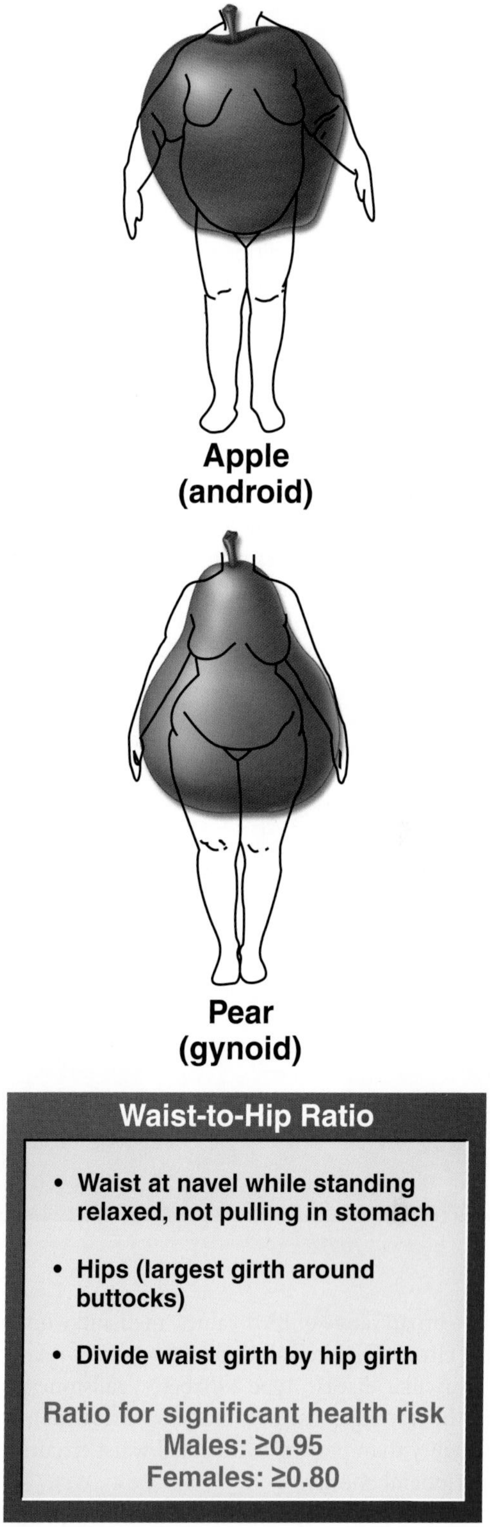
Apple
(android)
Pear
(gynoid)
Waist-to-Hip Ratio
• Waist at navel while standing relaxed, not pulling in stomach
• Hips (largest girth around buttocks)
• Divide waist girth by hip girth
Ratio for significant health risk
Males: ≥0.95
Females: ≥0.80

FIGURE 13.11. Male (android pattern) and female (gynoid pattern) fat patterning, including waist-to-hip girth ratio threshold for significant health risk.

ETHNIC GROUP INFLUENCES DIABETES RISK

The high-fat and refined carbohydrate content of the Puerto Rican diet plus their sedentary lifestyle has turned Puerto Ricans into the second largest ethnic group (Native American Pima tribe is the first) in US jurisdictions afflicted with type 2 diabetes. Twenty-five percent of Puerto Ricans between ages 45 and 74 are diabetics. Fifty percent of Hispanic women and 40% of Hispanic men will develop diabetes at some point in their life. Economic, social, and nutritional changes (overnutrition and improper nutrition) over the past 20 to 30 years combined with a decline in regular physical activity link closely to the creeping epidemic of obesity, which increases diabetes risk approximately 10-fold. The figure here illustrates that not all fat is created equal, and that different forms of excess storage fat (subcutaneous, visceral, and retroperitoneal) in the abdominal region significantly contributes to diabetes risk in addition to other negative alterations in the metabolic profile.

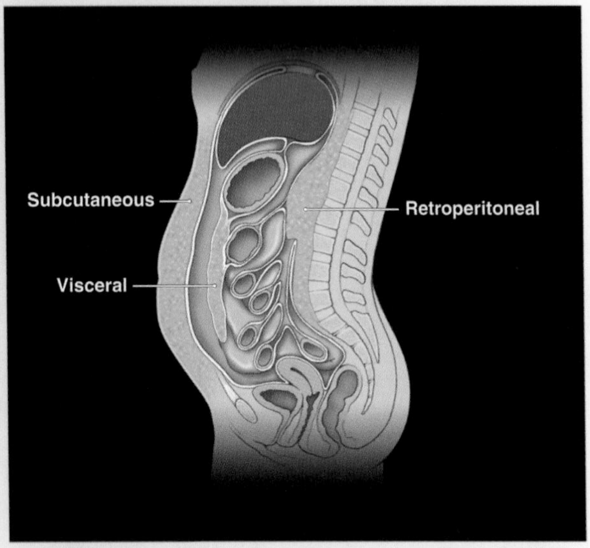

Over a broad range of BMI values, men and women with high waist circumference values possess greater relative risk for cardiovascular disease, type 2 diabetes, gallstones, cancer, cataracts (the leading cause of blindness worldwide), and all-cause mortality than persons with small waist circumference or with peripheral obesity.

For men, the percentage of visceral fat increases progressively with age, whereas this fat deposition in women begins to increase at the onset of menopause. The waist-to-hip ratio poorly captures the specific effects of each girth measure. Waist and hip circumferences reflect different aspects of body composition and fat distribution. Each has an independent and often opposite effect on cardiovascular disease risk. Waist girth reflects central fat deposition and provides a reasonable indication of the accumulation of intra-abdominal (visceral) adipose tissue. This currently makes waist girth the trunk measure of clinical choice to evaluate health risks when more precise assessments are impractical.[65,97,120]

VARIATIONS IN VISCERAL ADIPOSE TISSUE AND WAIST CIRCUMFERENCE

Physical fitness, age, and gender alter the relation between waist circumference and abdominal adipose tissue, with men having more visceral adipose tissue than women at any waist circumference. For a given waist circumference, visceral adipose tissue also increases with age, whereas it decreases with improved physical fitness.[82,103]

TABLE 13.6 presents classification guidelines and associated disease risk for overweight and obesity based on BMI or waist girth. Men with a waist girth of 102 cm (40.2 in) or larger and women with a waist girth larger than 88 cm (36.6 in) maintain a high risk for various diseases. Waist girths of 90 cm (35.4 in) for men and 83 cm (32.7 in) for women correspond to a BMI threshold of overweight (BMI $\geq$ 25), whereas waist girths of 100 cm (39.4 in) for men and 93 cm (36.6 in) for women reflect the obesity cutoff (BMI $\geq$ 30).[96]

Documentation of a strong effect of regular exercise on reducing waist girth selectively in men may partially explain why physical activity reduces disease risk more effectively in men than in women. Both physical activity and energy intake selectively predict waist-to-hip ratio in men but not in women.

A RISKY PLACE TO STORE EXCESS BODY FAT

Central excess fat deposition, independent of excess fat storage in other anatomic areas, reflects an altered metabolic profile that increases risk of the following eight conditions:

1. Hyperinsulinemia (insulin resistance)
2. Glucose intolerance
3. Type 2 diabetes
4. Endometrial cancer
5. Hypertriglyceridemia
6. Hypercholesterolemia and negatively altered lipoprotein profile
7. Hypertension
8. Atherosclerosis

In addition to the impact of excess abdominal fat and alterations in the metabolic profile, recent research has focused on neuropeptide-adipose tissue communication and how such interactions affect intra-abdominal fat tissue physiology and disease state in that anatomic region (e.g., Crohn's disease).

Karagiannides I, et al. Neuropeptide - adipose tissue communication and intestinal pathophysiology. *Curr Pharm Des* 2011;17:1576.

Karagiannides I, Pothoulakis C. Neuropeptides, mesenteric fat, and intestinal inflammation. *Ann N Y Acad Sci* 2008;1144:127.

Additional Insights
Waist Girth and Health Risk with Normal Body Mass Index

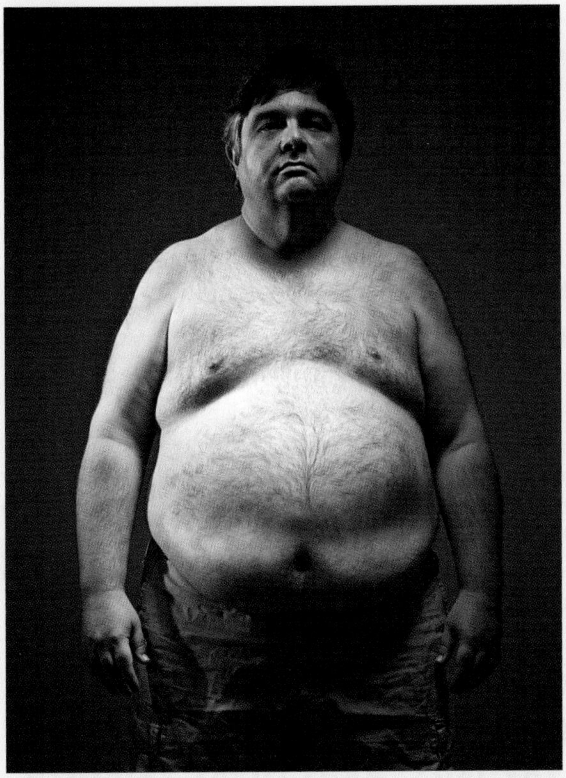

Many persons believe that a large waist girth is not a risk to good health as long as one's body mass index (BMI) falls within the normal range (BMI 18.5–24.9)—that is, the person does not classify as overweight (BMI 25.0–29.9) or obese (BMI ≥30.0). Now the issue has been clarified. Researchers at the American Cancer Society examined the association between waist circumference and overall mortality among 48,000 men and 56,343 women age 50 and older who had participated in the Cancer Prevention Study II Nutrition Cohort. Waist girth closely relates with the fatty tissue surrounding abdominal organs, which may be a greater health risk than subcutaneous fat. Over the 14-year study period, 9315 of the men and 5332 of the women died. The data analysis was adjusted for BMI and other risk factors associated with disease. Waist girths exceeding 47 in in men and 43 in in women associated with approximately twice the likelihood of dying during the study period. The surprising finding, however, was that a larger waistline was linked to greater mortality regardless of BMI levels, even for men and women who classified normal in terms of BMI. For men who were not overweight, an additional 3.9 in on the waistline increased death risk by 16% compared to counterparts with the same BMI but a slimmer waist girth. For normal-weight women, an extra 3.9 in on the waist increased risk by 25%. Death from respiratory disease associated to the greatest extent with excess waist girth, followed by cardiovascular disease and then cancer.

Current clinical guidelines from the National Institutes of Health recommend that waist circumference be used to identify disease risk *only* in persons who classify as overweight or obese by BMI. These guidelines do not recommend weight loss for normal-weight persons with large waist girths unless they have two or more cardiovascular risk factors. More than one half of US men age 50 to 79 have a waist girth considered "abdominally obese" (≥40.1 in), whereas 70% of women in this age category have an "abdominally obese" waist girth (≥34.6 in). The researchers concluded, "Regardless of body weight, avoiding gains in waist circumference may reduce risk of premature mortality. Even if you have not had a noticeable weight gain, if you notice your waist size increasing, that's an important sign it's time to eat better and start exercising more."

Sources:

Jacobs EJ, et al. Waist circumference and all-cause mortality in a large US cohort. *Arch Intern Med* 2010;170:1293.

Related References

Kanhai DA, et al. The risk of general and abdominal adiposity in the occurrence of new vascular events and mortality in patients with various manifestations of vascular disease. *Int J Obes (Lond)*; in press.

Lee JS, et al. Survival benefit of abdominal adiposity: a 6-year follow-up study with dual x-ray absorptiometry in 3,978 older adults. *Age (Dordr)*; in press.

RISK NOT LIMITED TO ADULTS

For children and adolescents, central body fat distribution associates with higher blood cholesterol, triacylglycerol, and insulin levels and lower high-density lipoprotein cholesterol, in addition to higher blood pressure and increased left ventricular wall thickness.

BIOELECTRICAL IMPEDANCE ANALYSIS

A small alternating current flowing between two electrodes passes more rapidly through hydrated fat-free body tissues and extracellular water than through fat or bone tissue. This occurs because of the greater electrolyte content (lower electrical resistance) of the fat-free component. Impedance to

TABLE 13.6 Classifications of Overweight and Obesity by BMI, Waist Circumference, and Associated Disease Risk

Classification	BMI, kg·m^{-2}	Disease Risk[a] Relative to Normal Weight and Normal Waist Circumference	
		Men ≤102 cm Women ≤88 cm	**Men >102 cm Women >88 cm**
Normal weight	18.5–24.9	NR	NR
Overweight	25.0–29.9	Increased	High
Obese	30 to >40	High to very high	Very high to extremely high

[a]Disease risk for type 2 diabetes, hypertension, and cardiovascular disease. NR indicates no risk assigned at these BMI levels.

electric current flow relates to total body water content and in turn relates to FFM and percentage body fat.

With **bioelectrical impedance analysis (BIA)**, a person lies on a flat nonconducting surface. Injector or source electrodes attach on the dorsal surfaces of the foot and wrist, and detector or sink electrodes attach between the radius and ulna at the styloid process and at the ankle between the medial and lateral malleoli (**FIG. 13.12**). A painless, localized electric current (about 800 μ at a frequency of 50 kHz) is introduced, and the impedance (resistance) to current flow is determined between the source and detector electrodes. Conversion of the impedance value to body density—adding body mass and stature, gender, age, and sometimes race, level of fatness, and several girths to the equation—computes percentage body fat from the Siri equation or another similar density conversion equation.

Influence of Hydration and Ambient Temperature

Hydration level, even small changes that occur with exercise, affects BIA accuracy and may give inaccurate information about a person's body fat content. Hypohydration and hyperhydration alter normal electrolyte concentrations, which in turn affect current flow independent of a real change in body composition. For example, a loss of body water through prior exercise sweat loss or voluntary fluid restriction decreases the impedance measure. This *lowers* the estimate of percentage body fat, whereas hyperhydration produces the opposite effect (*higher* fat estimate).

Skin temperature, influenced by ambient conditions, also affects whole-body resistance and thus the BIA prediction of body fat. A *lower* predicted body fat value occurs in a warm environment (less impedance to electrical flow) than in a cold one.[5,22]

Even with normal hydration and environmental temperature, body fat predictions prove less satisfactory than hydrostatic weighing. BIA tends to *overpredict* body fat in lean and athletic subjects and *underpredict* body fat in obese subjects. BIA often predicts body fat less accurately than girths and skinfolds. In contrast to skinfold and girth measurements, conventional BIA technology cannot assess regional fat distribution.

At best, BIA provides a noninvasive, safe, and relatively easy and reliable means to assess total body water. Proper BIA use requires that experienced personnel make measurements under strictly standardized conditions, particularly those related to electrode placement and subject's body position, hydration status, previous food and beverage intake, skin temperature, and recent physical activity. Fatness-specific BIA equations exist for obese and nonobese American Indian, Hispanic, and white men and women.[125,126] Menstrual cycle does not affect body composition assessment by BIA.[89]

Applicability of Bioelectrical Impedance Analysis in Sports and Exercise Training

The BIA technique cannot detect small changes in body composition. For example, sweat-loss dehydration or reduced glycogen reserves and associated loss of glycogen-bound water from prior exercise increase body resistance or impedance to electrical current flow. Increased impedance underestimates FFM and overestimates percentage body fat measured by BIA. The tendency to overestimate body fat becomes more pronounced among black athletes.[52,116]

COMPUTED TOMOGRAPHY, MAGNETIC RESONANCE IMAGING, AND DUAL-ENERGY X-RAY ABSORPTIOMETRY

Computed tomography (CT) and **magnetic resonance imaging (MRI)** produce images of body segments. The CT scan provides pictorial and quantitative information for total tissue area, total fat and muscle area, and thickness and volume of tissues within an organ.[42,92]

FIGURE 13.13A–C shows CT scans of the upper legs and a cross section at the midthigh in a professional walker who completed an 11,200-mile walk around the 50 United States in 50 weeks. Total cross section of muscle increased significantly, and subcutaneous fat decreased correspondingly in the midthigh region in the "after" scans.

Studies have demonstrated the efficiency of CT scans to evaluate the relationship between skinfolds and girths measured at the abdominal region and total adipose tissue volume measured from single or multiple pictorial "slices" through the abdominal region. Surprisingly, almost no relationship exists between "external" (subcutaneous) abdominal fat and "internal" (visceral) abdominal fat depots in men and women. Thus, a person with a large, external abdominal fat pad does not necessarily have a thick layer of fat within the abdominal cavity.

The newer technology of MRI provides a rapid, safe technique to obtain accurate information about the body's tissue compartments. **FIGURE 13.13D** displays a color-enhanced MRI transaxial image of the midthigh of a 30-year-old male middle-distance runner. Computer software subtracts fat and bony

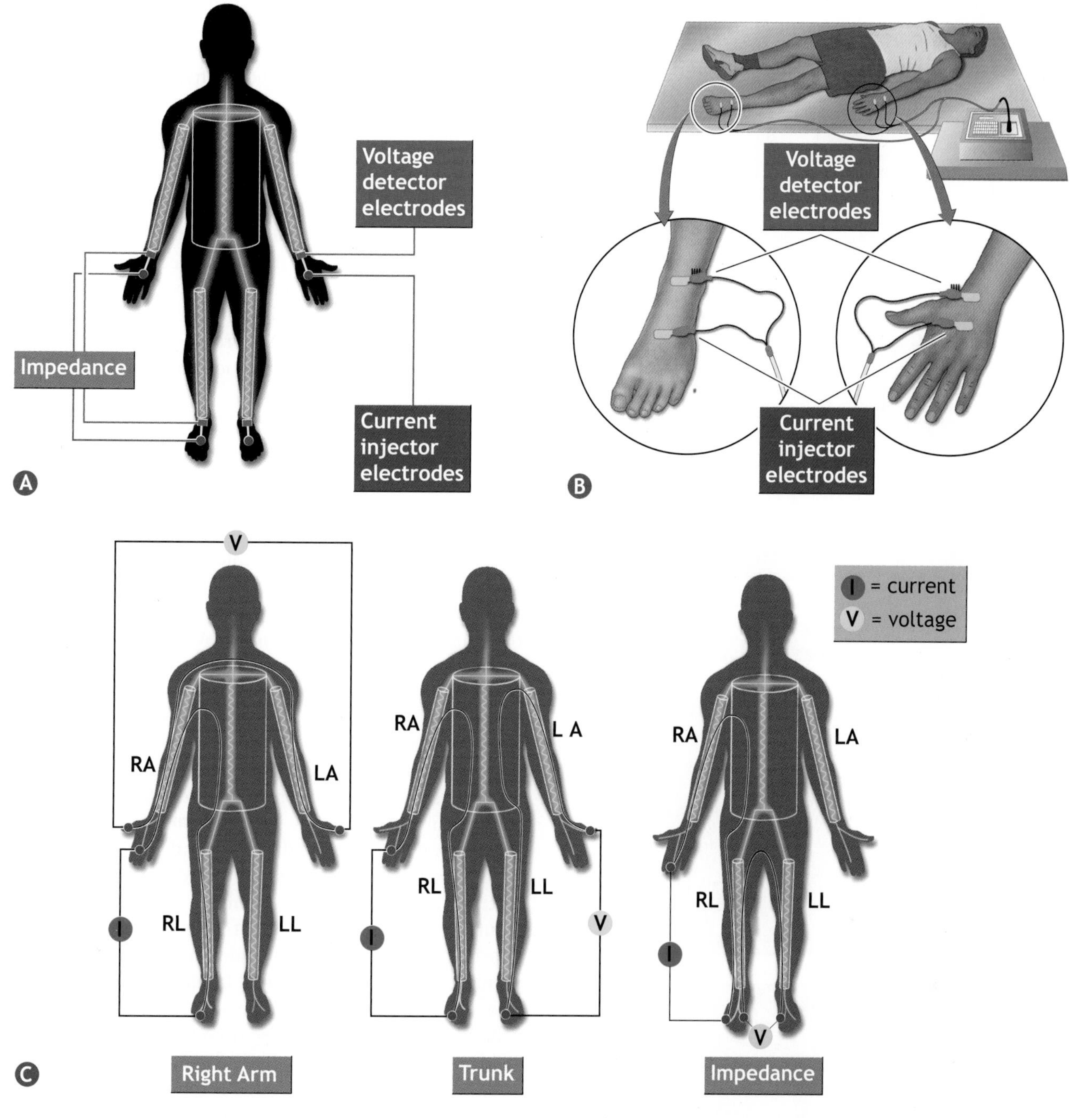

FIGURE 13.12. Body composition assessment by bioelectrical impedance analysis. **A.** Four-surface electrode technique that applies current via one pair of distal (injection) electrodes while the proximal (detector) electrode pair measures electrical potential across the conducting segment. **B.** Standard placement of electrodes. **C.** Proper body position during whole-body impedance measurement.

tissues (*lighter-colored areas*) to compute thigh muscle cross-sectional area (*blue area*). With MRI, electromagnetic radiation (not ionizing radiation as in CT scans) in a strong magnetic field excites the hydrogen nuclei of the body's water and lipid molecules. The nuclei then project a detectable signal that rearranges under computer control to visually depict the body tissues. MRI effectively quantifies total and subcutaneous adipose tissue in persons of varying degrees of body fatness. Combined with muscle mass analysis, MRI can assess changes in a muscle's lean and fat components following resistance training or during different stages of growth and aging,[62] and even changes in muscle volume during and following spaceflight.[80]

Dual-energy x-ray absorptiometry (DXA), another high-technology procedure, reliably quantifies fat and nonbone regional LBM. This includes the mineral content of the body's deeper bony structures and muscle mass. DXA can also assess spinal osteoporosis and related bone disorders.[17,108] For body composition analysis, DXA does not require the assumptions about the biologic constancy of the fat and fat-free components inherent with hydrostatic weighing.

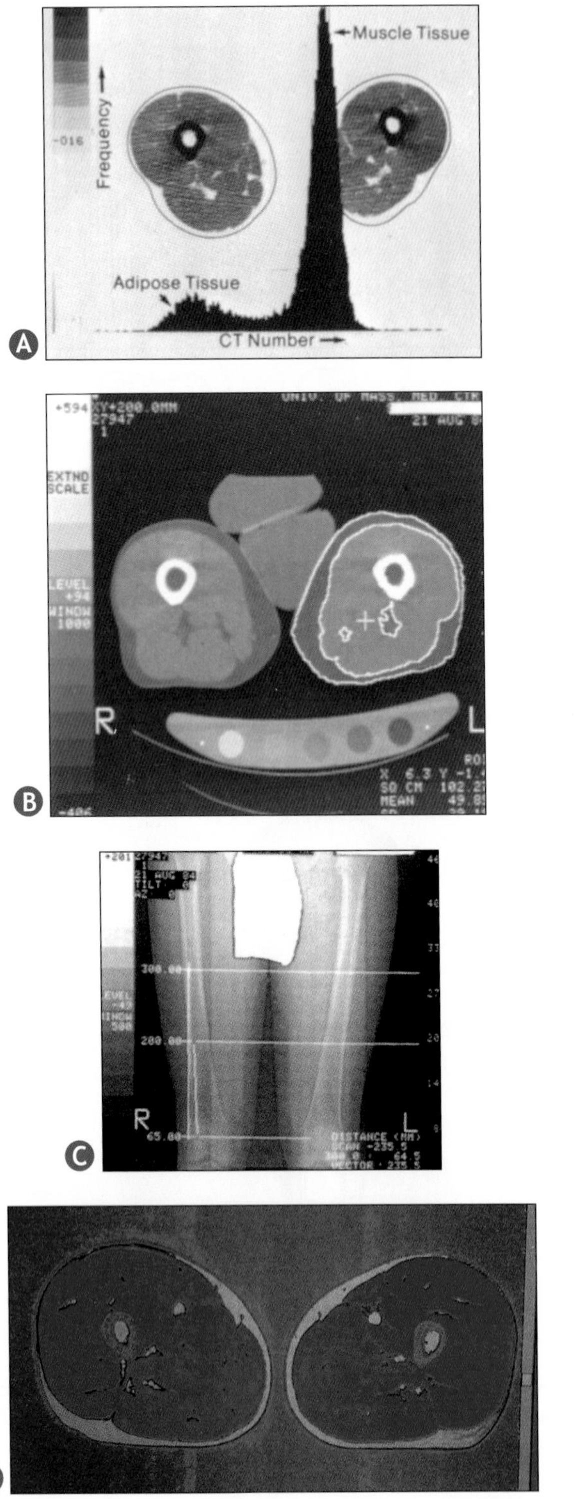

FIGURE 13.13. Computed tomography (CT) and magnetic resonance imaging (MRI) scans. **A.** Plot of pixel elements (CT scan) illustrating the extent of adipose and muscle tissue in a thigh cross section. The two other views show a cross section of the midthigh **(B)** and an anterior view of the upper leg **(C)** before a 1-year walk across the United States in a champion walker. **D.** MRI scan of the midthigh of a 30-year-old male middle-distance runner. (CT images courtesy of Dr. Steven Heymsfeld, St. Luke's Roosevelt Hospital Center, New York, NY; MRI scan courtesy of J. Staab, Department of the Army, USARIEM, Natick, MA.)

With DXA, two distinct low-energy, short exposure x-ray beams with low radiation dosage penetrate bone and soft tissue to a 30-cm depth. An entire DXA scan takes approximately 12 min. Computer software reconstructs the attenuated x-ray beams to produce an image of the underlying tissues and quantify the following:

1. Bone mineral content
2. Total fat mass
3. FFM

Analyses also can include selected trunk and limb regions for detailed study of tissue composition and possible relation to disease risk, including the effects of exercise training and detraining.[11,84,89] DXA provides a sensitive noninvasive tool to asses body composition and body composition changes in diverse populations.

BOD POD

A procedure to estimate body volume has been perfected in groups ranging from infants to the elderly to collegiate wrestlers and exceptionally large athletes such as professional football and basketball players.[26,36,138] The method has adapted air displacement plethysmography first reported in the late 1800s and in the 1950s using helium as the gas displaced. The subject sits inside a small chamber (marketed commercially as **BOD POD**; Cosmed. www.cosmed.com/). Measurement requires 2 to 5 min, and reproducibility of test scores within and across days is high ($r \geq 0.90$).

After being weighed to the nearest 5 g on an electronic scale, the subject sits comfortably in the 750-L volume, dual-chamber fiberglass shell shown in **FIGURE 13.14A**. The molded front seat separates the unit into front and rear chambers. The electronics include pressure transducers, breathing circuit, and an air circulation system. To ensure measurement accuracy, the person wears a tight-fitting swimsuit. Body volume becomes the chamber's initial volume minus the reduced chamber volume with the subject inside. The subject breathes into an air circuit for several breaths to assess thoracic gas volume, which when subtracted from measured body volume yields actual body volume. Body density computes as body mass (measured in air) ÷ body volume (measured in BOD POD). The Siri equation converts body density to percentage body fat. **FIGURE 13.14B** shows the relationship between percentage body fat assessed by hydrostatic weighing versus percentage body fat by BOD POD. A difference of only 0.3% (0.2% fat units) occurred between body fat determined by hydrostatic weighing and BOD POD; the validity correlation was $r = 0.96$ between the two methods.

ESTIMATING BODY FAT AMONG ATHLETIC GROUPS

Accurate body composition assessment enhances precision in determining a competitor's appropriate body weight for sports with specific weight classifications or that emphasize a "required" physical appearance. Valid body composition

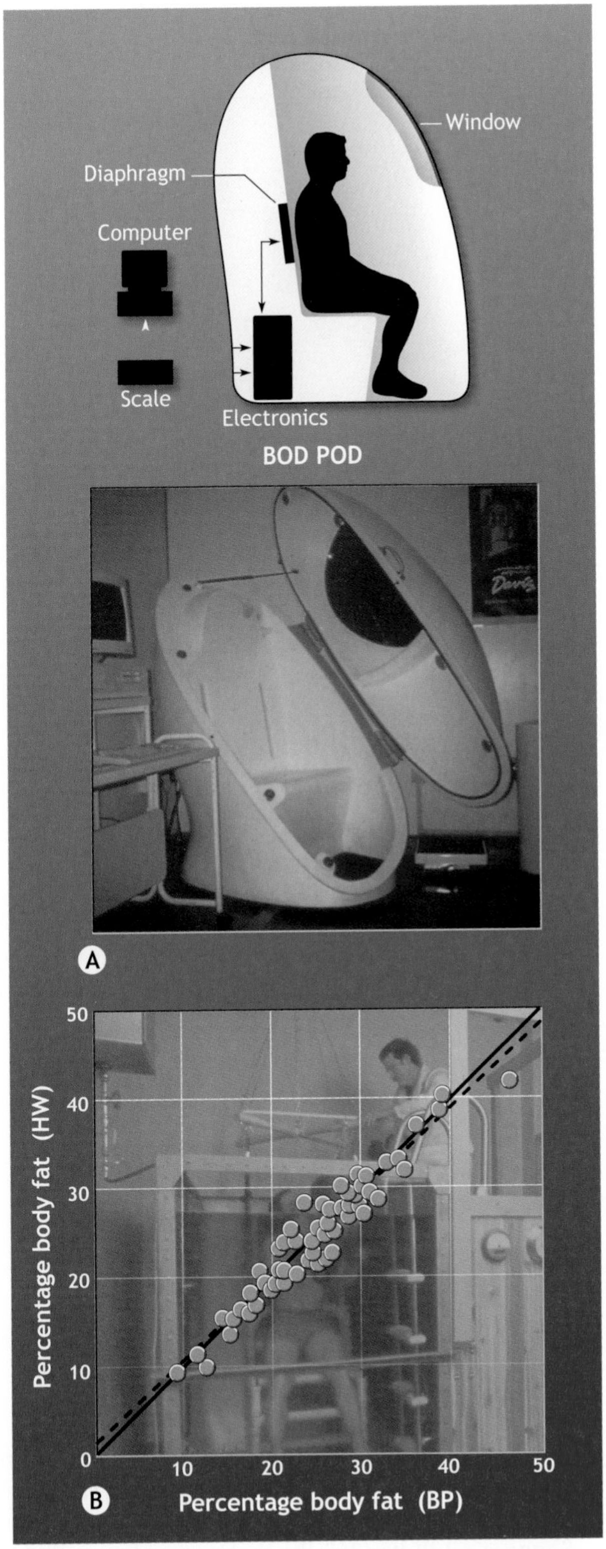

FIGURE 13.14. A. BOD POD to measure human body volume. (Photo courtesy of Dr. Megan McCrory, Purdue University, West Lafayette, IN.) **B.** Regression of percentage body fat assessed by hydrostatic weighing (HW) versus percentage body fat assessed by BOD POD (BP). (Data from McCrory MA, et al. Evaluation of a new air displacement plethysmograph for measuring human body composition. *Med Sci Sports Exerc* 1995;27:1686.)

appraisal also provides an important first step to *identify* potential eating disorders and *formulate* and *assess* nutritional information during counseling.

Skinfolds and girth measurements and BIA have estimated body density and percentage body fat for diverse athletic groups. Generalized equations using these methods apply to athletes in all sports, with sport-specific equations available for ballet dancers, wrestlers, and football players. Additional equations for wrestlers and high school female gymnasts appear in Chapter 14. When sport-specific equations are unavailable, population-based generalized equations (accounting for age and sex) provide an acceptable alternative to estimate body fat.[25,53,59,133]

AVERAGE VALUES FOR BODY COMPOSITION IN THE GENERAL POPULATION

TABLE 13.7 lists average values for percentage body fat in samples of men and women throughout the United States. Values representing ± one standard deviation provide some indication of the variation or spread from the average; the column headed "68% Variation Limits" indicates the range for percentage body fat that includes one standard deviation or 68 of every 100 persons measured. As an example, the average percentage body fat of 15.0% for young men from the New York sample includes the 68% variation limits that range between 8.9 and 21.1% fat. Interpreting this statistically, for 68 of every 100 young men measured, percentage fat ranges between 8.9 and 21.1%. Of the remaining 32 young men, 16 possess more than 21.1% body fat, whereas 16 others have a body fat percentage below 8.9%. *Percentage body fat for young adult men averages between 12 and 15%; the average fat value for women falls between 25 and 28%.* For comparative purposes, see the inset tables in **FIGURE 13.16** for percentage body fat values for various groups of male and female athletes.

Percentage body fat usually increases in adult men and women as they age. Persons who maintain a vigorous physical activity profile throughout life slow the "average" or "normal" age-related fat accretion. Age-related body composition changes could occur because the aging skeleton becomes demineralized and porous, decreasing bone density and reducing body density. In contrast, remaining physically active maintains or increases bone mass while preserving muscle mass. Reduced physical activity provides another plausible reason for the relative increase in body fat with age. A sedentary lifestyle increases storage fat and reduces muscle mass, even if the daily caloric intake remains essentially unaltered.

HOW TO DETERMINE GOAL BODY WEIGHT

Excess body fat detracts from good health, physical fitness, and athletic performance. No one really knows the optimum body fat or body mass for a particular persons. Inherited genetic

TABLE 13.7 Average Values of Percentage Body Fat for Younger and Older Women and Men from Selected Studies

Study	Age Range (y)	Stature (cm)	Mass (kg)	% Fat	68% Variation Limits
Younger women					
North Carolina, 1962	17–25	165.0	55.5	22.9	17.5–28.5
New York, 1962	16–30	167.5	59.0	28.7	24.6–32.9
California, 1968	19–23	165.9	58.4	21.9	17.0–26.9
California, 1970	17–29	164.9	58.6	25.5	21.0–30.1
Air Force, 1972	17–22	164.1	55.8	28.7	22.3–35.3
New York, 1973	17–26	160.4	59.0	26.2	23.4–33.3
North Carolina, 1975	–	166.1	57.5	24.6	–
Army Recruits, 1986	17–25	162.0	58.6	28.4	23.9–32.9
Massachusetts, 1998	17–31	165.2	57.8	21.8	16.7–27.9
Older women					
Minnesota, 1953	31–45	163.3	60.7	28.9	25.1–32.8
	43–68	160.0	60.9	34.2	28.0–40.5
New York, 1963	30–40	164.9	59.6	28.6	22.1–35.3
	40–50	163.1	56.4	34.4	29.5–39.5
North Carolina, 1975	33–50	–	–	29.7	23.1–36.5
Massachusetts, 1993	31–50	165.2	58.9	25.2	19.2–31.2
Younger men					
Minnesota, 1951	17–26	177.8	69.1	11.8	5.9–11.8
Colorado, 1956	17–25	172.4	68.3	13.5	8.3–18.8
Indiana, 1966	18–23	180.1	75.5	12.6	8.7–16.5
California, 1968	16–31	175.7	74.1	15.2	6.3–24.2
New York, 1973	17–26	176.4	71.4	15.0	8.9–21.1
Texas, 1977	18–24	179.9	74.6	13.4	7.4–19.4
Army recruits, 1986	17–25	174.7	70.5	15.6	10.0–21.2
Massachusetts, 1998	17–31	178.1	76.4	12.9	7.8–19.0
Older men					
Indiana, 1966	24–38	179.0	76.6	17.8	11.3–24.3
	40–48	177.0	80.5	22.3	16.3–28.3
North Carolina, 1976	27–50	–	–	23.7	17.9–30.1
Texas, 1977	27–59	180.0	85.3	27.1	23.7–30.5
Massachusetts, 1993	31–50	177.1	77.5	19.9	13.2–26.5

factors greatly influence body fat distribution and affect the long-term determination of body size.[13,14] Women and men who exercise on a regular basis through their younger and middle years have lower percentage body fat values than the population average. In contact sports and activities that emphasize muscular power, successful performance usually requires a larger than normal body mass with minimal body fat. In contrast, success in weight-bearing endurance locomotor activities requires a lighter body mass and less body fat. For these persons, attaining a low body weight must not compromise lean tissue mass and energy reserves. *Proper assessment of body composition, not body weight, determines a physically active person's ideal body weight. For athletes, this* **goal body weight** must coincide with optimizing sport-specific measures of physiologic function and exercise capacity.

Suppose a 120-kg (265-lb) shot-put athlete with 24% body fat wishes to know how much fat weight to lose to attain a body fat composition of 15%. Compute a goal body weight based on the desired body fat level as follows:

Goal body weight = Fat-free body mass ÷ (1.00 – % fat desired)

Fat mass = 120 kg × 0.24
= 28.8 kg

Fat-free body mass = 120 kg – 28.8 kg
= 91.2 kg

Goal body weight = 91.2 kg ÷ (1.00 – 0.15)
= 91.2 kg ÷ 0.85
= 107.3 kg (236.6 lb)

Desirable fat loss weight = Present body weight – Goal body
= 120 kg – 107.3 kg
= 12.7 kg (28.0 lb)

If this athlete reduced 12.7 kg of body fat, his new body weight of 91.2 kg would contain fat equal to 15% of body mass. These calculations assume no change in FFM during weight loss. Moderate caloric restriction plus increased daily energy expenditure through regular exercise induce fat loss and conserve lean tissue. Chapter 14 discusses prudent yet effective approaches to lose body fat.

Connections to the Past

Archibald Vivian (A.V.) Hill (1886–1977)

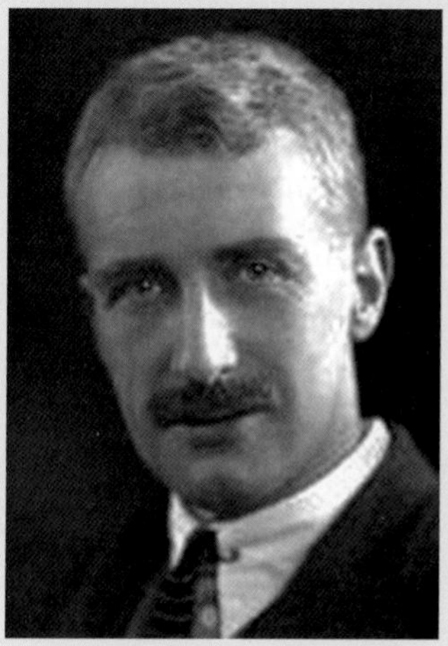

A.V. Hill, a brilliant student at Trinity and Kings Colleges, Cambridge, England, completed a double major in mathematics and the natural sciences (chemistry, physics, and physiology). His interest in physiology attracted the notice of two eminent physiologists at Trinity, Walter Morley Fletcher (1873–1933) and Sir Frederick Gowland Hopkins (1861–1947; Nobel Prize in Physiology or Medicine, 1923; see p. 395). They convinced Hill to pursue advanced studies in physiology rather than mathematics. Hill's early experiments researched the effects of electrical stimulation on nerve function, the mechanical efficiency of muscle actions, energy processes in muscle during recovery, the interaction between oxygen and hemoglobin, and quantitative aspects of drug kinetics on muscle. Hill applied his background in mathematics to explain the results of his experiments. Later, Hill devised mathematical models describing heat production in muscle and applied kinetic analysis to explain the time course of oxygen uptake during both exercise and recovery. Hill combined aspects of physics and biology, a discipline he championed as biophysics.

During World War I, Hill directed a laboratory and published technical reports on antiaircraft defense. After the war, Hill achieved international acclaim for research in muscle physiology. The 1922 Nobel Prize in Physiology or Medicine was divided equally between Hill "for his discovery relating to the production of heat in the muscle" and Otto Fritz Meyerhoff for his discovery of the "fixed relationship between the consumption of oxygen and the metabolism of lactic acid in the muscle."

thePoint *Visit* **thePoint.lww.com/MKKSEN4e** *for more details about Hill's crucial discoveries about chemical and mechanical events in muscle contraction.*

SUMMARY

1. Standard weight-for-height tables reveal little about an person's body composition. Studies of athletes clearly show that overweight does not coincide with excessive body fat.
2. Body mass index (BMI) relates more closely to body fat and health risk than simply body mass and stature. BMI fails to consider the body's proportional composition.
3. For the first time in the United States, overweight persons (BMI 25–29) outnumber persons of desirable weight.
4. Total body fat consists of essential fat and storage fat. Essential fat contains fat present in bone marrow, nerve tissue, and organs; it is not a labile energy reserve, but instead an important component for normal biologic functions. Storage fat represents the energy reserve that accumulates mainly as adipose tissue beneath the skin and in visceral depots.
5. Storage fat averages 12% of body mass for men and 15% of body mass for women. Essential fat averages 3% of body mass for men and 12% for women. The greater

SUMMARY *(continued)*

essential fat for women probably relates to childbearing and hormonal functions.

6. A sumo wrestler has the largest fat-free body mass (FFM) reported in the literature (121.3 kg); this value most likely represents the upper limit for male athletes. Estimates place the upper limit for FFM for athletic women at 80 kg (176 lb).
7. Menstrual dysfunction often occurs in athletes who train hard and maintain low body fat levels. The precise interaction among the physiologic and psychological stress of intense training and competition, hormonal balance, energy and nutrient intake, and body fat remains unknown.
8. The most popular indirect methods to assess body composition include hydrostatic weighing and prediction methods based on skinfolds and girths. Hydrostatic weighing determines body density with subsequent estimation of percentage body fat. Subtracting fat mass from body mass yields FFM.
9. Part of the error inherent in predicting body fat from whole-body density lies in the correctness of assumptions concerning the densities of the body's fat and fat-free components. These densities differ from assumed constants because of race, age, and athletic experience.
10. Common body composition assessments use prediction equations from relationships among selected skinfolds and girths and body density and percentage fat. These equations show population specificity because they most accurately predict body fat with subjects similar to those who participated in the equations' original derivation.
11. Hydrated fat-free body tissues and extracellular water facilitate electrical flow compared with fat tissue, because of the greater electrolyte content of the fat-free component. Bioelectrical impedance analysis (BIA) applies this fact to assess body composition.
12. Computed tomography (CT), magnetic resonance imaging (MRI), and dual-energy x-ray absorptiometry (DXA) indirectly assess body composition. Each has a unique application and special limitations for expanding knowledge of the compositional components of the live human body and its changes with regular exercise training.
13. The BOD POD air displacement method offers promise for body composition assessment because of the high reliability of body volume scores and relatively high validity.
14. Data from healthy young adults indicate that the average male possesses approximately 15% body fat and women possess about 25%. These values often provide a frame of reference for evaluating the body fat of person athletes and specific athletic groups.
15. Goal body weight computes as FFM ÷ (1.00 – desired % body fat).

PHYSIQUE OF CHAMPION ATHLETES

Body composition differs considerably between athletes and nonathletes. Pronounced differences in physique also exist among sports participants of the same sex, including Olympic competitors, track and field specialists, wrestlers, football players, and highly proficient adolescent competitors. We now take a closer look at examples of the physiques of elite athletes by selected sport category and competition level.

ELITE ATHLETES

Different anthropometric methodologies have quantified physique status. Visual appraisal often describes persons as small, medium, or large or thin (ectomorphic), muscular (mesomorphic), or fat (endomorphic). This approach, termed *somatotyping,* describes body shape by placing a person into a category such as thin or muscular. Visual appraisal does not quantify body dimensions such chest or shoulder size, or how biceps development compares with thighs or calves. Somatotyping has provided a valuable adjunct in the analysis of physique status of world-class athletes.[21,31] The remainder of this chapter focuses on body fat and FFM components of body composition.

Olympic and Elite Athletes

Early studies of Olympic competitors revealed that physique related to a high level of sports achievement.[29,74] Also of interest are the body size differences among different groups of athletes within a particular sport. **FIGURE 13.15** *(top)* compares the body mass, stature, chest girth, and upper and lower limb lengths for 12 male swimmers rated "best" in the 200 + 400-m freestyle with measures of less successful counterparts. The bottom of the figure also compares selected body size variables between the "best" 50-, 100-, and 200-m breaststroke female swimmers and other swimmers. The best male swimmers are heavier and taller and have larger

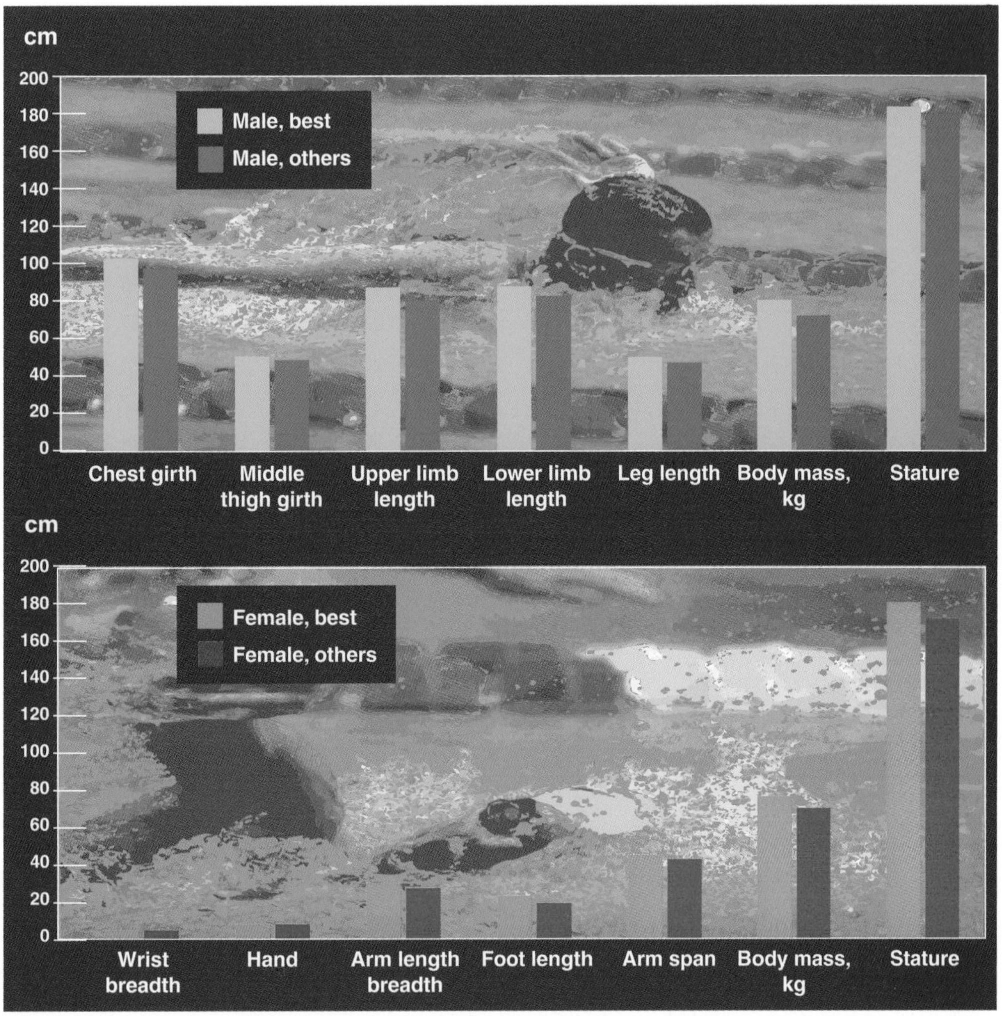

FIGURE 13.15. *Top.* Comparison of 200 + 400-m freestyle male swimmers for body mass, stature, chest girth, arm span (actual values divided by 4), and upper and lower limb lengths, categorized as best performers (top 12 ranks) with those of remaining competitors. *Bottom.* Comparison of differences in body size variables between the best 50-, 100-, and 200-m female breaststroke swimmers (top 12 ranks) and the rest of the competitors. Data on the *y* axis is in centimeters for all data except body mass (kilograms). (Modified from Mazza JC, et al. Absolute body size. In: Carter JE, Ackland TR, eds. *Kinanthropometry in Aquatic Sports: A Study of World Class Athletes.* Human kinetics sport science monograph series, vol 5. Champaign, IL: Human Kinetics, 1994.)

chest, upper arm, and thigh girths and larger upper and lower limb lengths than counterparts not ranking among the top 12. The best female breaststroke swimmers are taller and heavier, but also possess larger arm spans, foot and arm lengths, and hand and wrist breadth than less successful competitors.

Gender Differences

Male basketball players, rowers, and weight-throwers are taller and heavier than female counterparts; they also possess the largest FFM and percentage body fat.

For aquatic athletes, skinfolds at most sites are generally larger in females than in males. A swimmer's morphology influences the horizontal components of lift and drag. Selected anthropometric variables play important roles in propulsive and resistive forces acting on the swimmer that affect forward movement. The combined influence of stroke length and stroke frequency on swimming velocity also relates to a swimmer's overall body size and shape. In well-trained freestyle swimmers, arm length, leg length, and hand and foot size—factors governed largely by genetics—influence stroke length and stroke frequency.

TABLE 13.8 presents scarce anthropometric comparisons between male and female Olympians in five different sports including swimming assessed at the 1976 Montreal Summer Olympics.

Ratio of Fat-Free Body Mass to Fat Mass: **FIGURE 13.16** compares the ratios of FFM to fat mass (FFM/FM) derived from data in the world literature among male and female competitors. The inset tables present their

TABLE 13.8 Selected Anthropometric Measurements in Males and Females Who Competed in Five Different Sports at the Montreal Olympic Games

	Canoe		Gymnastics		Rowing		Swimming		Track	
Measurement[a]	M	F	M	F	M	F	M	F	M	F
Stature, cm	185.4	170.7	169.3	161.5	191.3	174.3	178.6	166.9	179.1	168.5
Upper extremity L[a]	82.4	76.0	76.0	72.2	85.2	76.0	80.2	74.7	80.9	74.8
Lower extremity L[a]	88.0	81.8	78.9	76.5	91.7	82.3	84.1	78.1	86.9	80.3
Biacromial D	41.4	36.8	39.0	35.9	42.5	37.4	40.8	37.1	40.2	36.3
Billiac D	28.1	27.3	25.8	25.0	30.2	28.2	27.9	26.7	27.1	27.2
Arm relaxed G	32.2	27.6	30.7	24.3	31.7	27.6	30.6	27.3	29.1	24.5
Arm flexed G	35.3	29.6	33.9	25.9	34.9	29.3	33.3	28.2	32.2	26.4
Forearm G	29.3	25.4	27.5	23.2	30.3	25.5	27.4	23.9	27.9	23.3
Chest G	102.6	88.9	95.1	83.5	103.7	89.6	98.6	88.0	94.3	83.8
Waist G	80.6	69.8	72.8	63.2	84.0	70.8	79.3	69.4	77.7	67.4
Thigh G	54.6	54.0	51.0	49.9	60.2	57.5	55.4	52.8	55.0	53.9
Calf G	37.5	34.9	34.7	33.3	39.3	37.0	36.9	34.0	37.6	34.9

[a]L, length; D, diameter; G, girth; all values are in centimeters.

Adapted from Carter JE, et al. Anthropometry of Montreal Olympic athletes. In: Carter JEL, ed. Physical structure of Olympic athletes. Part 1: The Montreal Olympic Games Anthropological Project. Basal: Karger, 1982.

average body mass, percentage body fat, fat weight, and FFM. Appendix E presents additional body composition data from various studies of male and female athletes. Such data help to evaluate typical variation in body fat within and between diverse athletic groups. Male marathon runners and gymnasts have the largest FFM/FM, whereas American football offensive and defensive lineman and shot putters show the smallest ratios. Among women, bodybuilders have the largest FFM/FM values (equal to those of men), whereas the smallest ratios emerge for field event participants. Surprisingly, female gymnasts and ballet dancers rank about intermediate compared with other female sport participants.

PERCENTAGE BODY FAT GROUPED BY SPORT CATEGORY

FIGURE 13.17 presents six classifications of sports activities based on common characteristics and performance requirements, with percentage body fat rankings within each category for male and female competitors (where applicable). This provides an overview of percentage body fat of athletes within a broad grouping of relatively similar sports. The sports nutritionist should find such information useful in counseling athletes in different sports to appreciate the extent of variability in body fat percentage so as to counter any belief that they need conform to a specific body fat percentage for success.

RACIAL DIFFERENCES IN PHYSIQUE AFFECT ATHLETIC PERFORMANCE

Black sprinters and high jumpers have longer limbs and narrower hips than white counterparts.[173] From a mechanical perspective, a black sprinter with leg and arm size identical to a white sprinter would have a lighter, shorter, and slimmer body to propel. This might confer a more favorable power-to-body mass ratio at any given body size. Greater power output provides an advantage in jumping and sprint running events, where generating rapid energy for short durations is crucial to success. This advantage diminishes somewhat in the various throwing events. Compared with whites and blacks, Asian athletes have short legs relative to upper torso components, a dimensional characteristic beneficial in short and longer distance races and in weightlifting. In fact, successful weightlifters of all races (compared with other athletic groups) have relatively short arms and legs for their stature.

Field Event Athletes

FIGURE 13.18 shows body composition obtained by densitometry and anthropometry—ranked from high to low in percentage body fat, fat weight, FFM, and lean-to-fat ratio—for the 10 top American athletes in the discus, shot put, javelin, and hammer throw 2 years before the 1980 Moscow

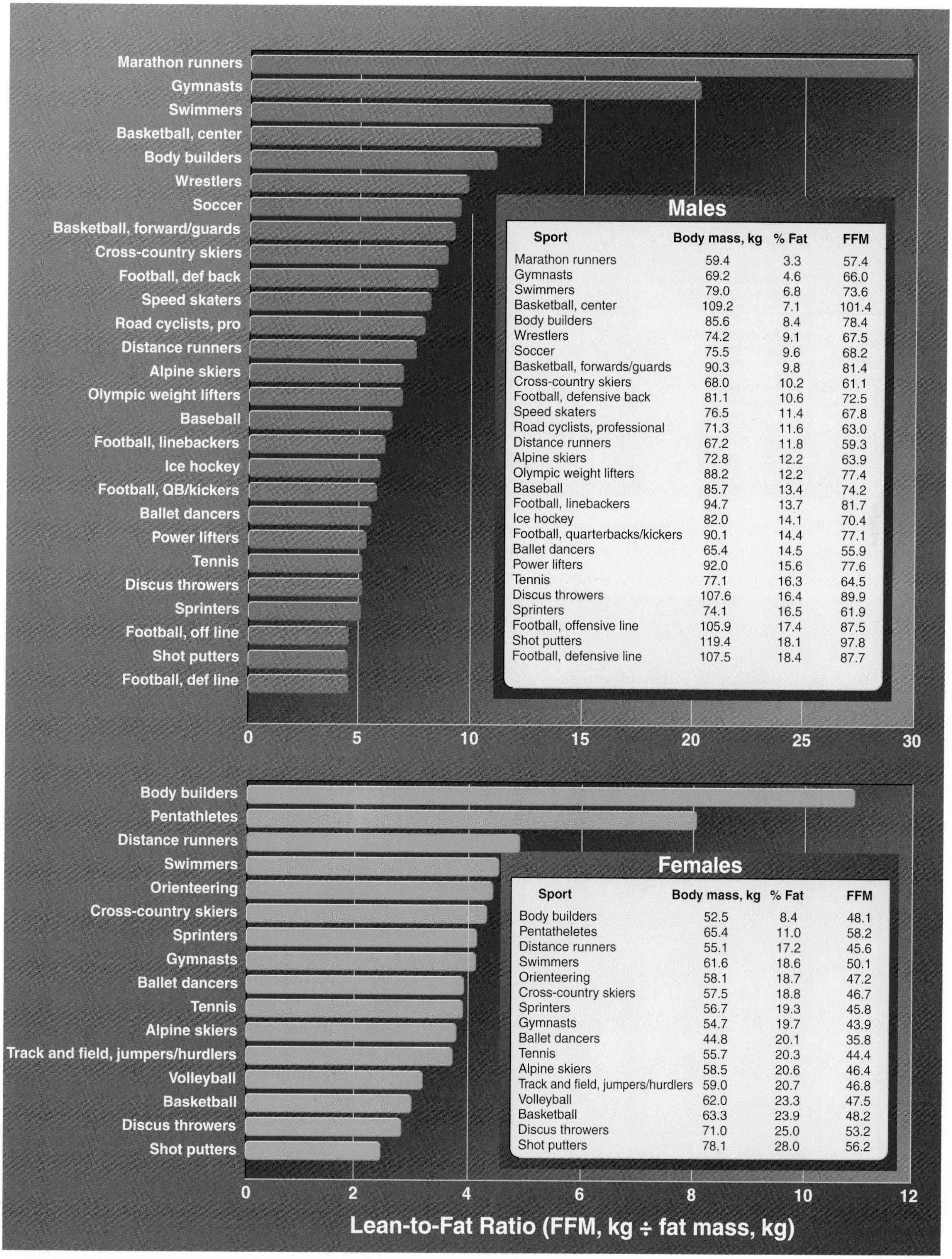

Males

Sport	Body mass, kg	% Fat	FFM
Marathon runners	59.4	3.3	57.4
Gymnasts	69.2	4.6	66.0
Swimmers	79.0	6.8	73.6
Basketball, center	109.2	7.1	101.4
Body builders	85.6	8.4	78.4
Wrestlers	74.2	9.1	67.5
Soccer	75.5	9.6	68.2
Basketball, forwards/guards	90.3	9.8	81.4
Cross-country skiers	68.0	10.2	61.1
Football, defensive back	81.1	10.6	72.5
Speed skaters	76.5	11.4	67.8
Road cyclists, professional	71.3	11.6	63.0
Distance runners	67.2	11.8	59.3
Alpine skiers	72.8	12.2	63.9
Olympic weight lifters	88.2	12.2	77.4
Baseball	85.7	13.4	74.2
Football, linebackers	94.7	13.7	81.7
Ice hockey	82.0	14.1	70.4
Football, quarterbacks/kickers	90.1	14.4	77.1
Ballet dancers	65.4	14.5	55.9
Power lifters	92.0	15.6	77.6
Tennis	77.1	16.3	64.5
Discus throwers	107.6	16.4	89.9
Sprinters	74.1	16.5	61.9
Football, offensive line	105.9	17.4	87.5
Shot putters	119.4	18.1	97.8
Football, defensive line	107.5	18.4	87.7

Females

Sport	Body mass, kg	% Fat	FFM
Body builders	52.5	8.4	48.1
Pentatheletes	65.4	11.0	58.2
Distance runners	55.1	17.2	45.6
Swimmers	61.6	18.6	50.1
Orienteering	58.1	18.7	47.2
Cross-country skiers	57.5	18.8	46.7
Sprinters	56.7	19.3	45.8
Gymnasts	54.7	19.7	43.9
Ballet dancers	44.8	20.1	35.8
Tennis	55.7	20.3	44.4
Alpine skiers	58.5	20.6	46.4
Track and field, jumpers/hurdlers	59.0	20.7	46.8
Volleyball	62.0	23.3	47.5
Basketball	63.3	23.9	48.2
Discus throwers	71.0	25.0	53.2
Shot putters	78.1	28.0	56.2

FIGURE 13.16. Comparison of the lean-to-fat ratios among male and female competitors in diverse sports. Values are based on the average body mass and percentage body fat for each sport from various studies in the literature. The lean-to-fat ratio equals FFM (kg) ÷ fat mass (kg). The values in the inset tables represent averages for body composition if the literature contained two or more citations about a specific sport.

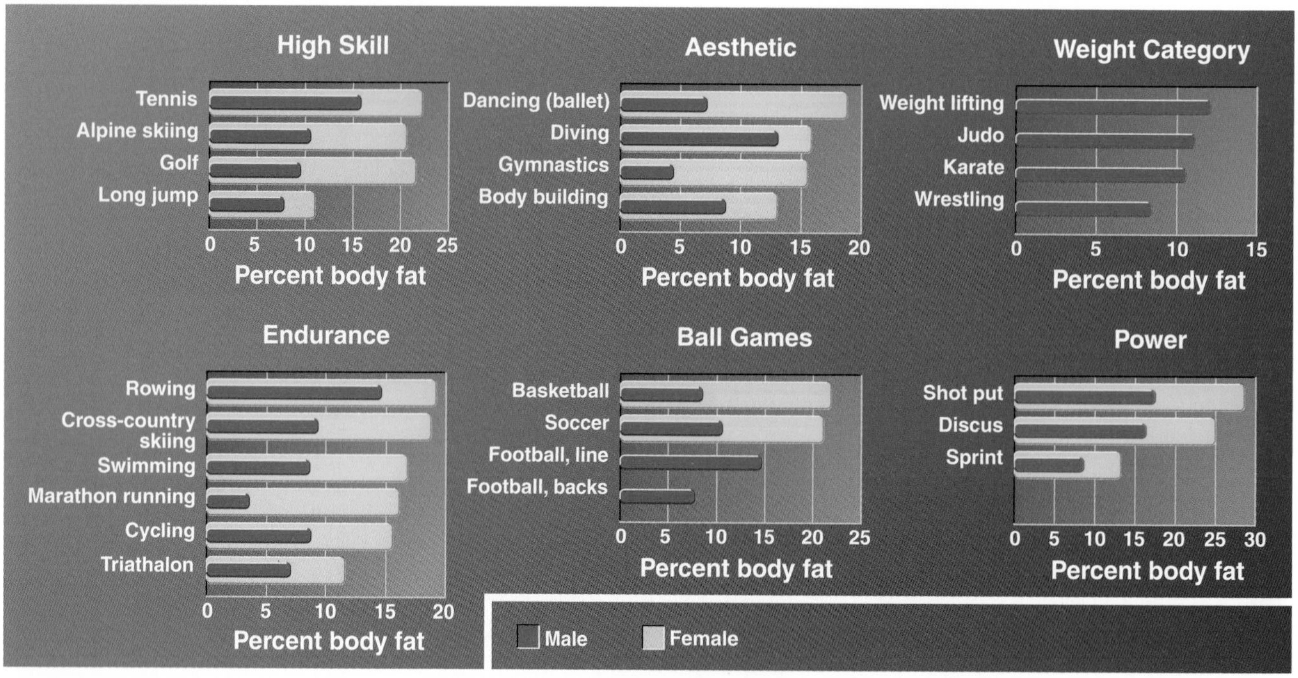

FIGURE 13.17. Percentage body fat in athletes grouped by sport category. Value for males is displayed within the bar *(red)* when a corresponding value exists for females *(yellow)*. Values for percentage body fat represent averages from the literature.

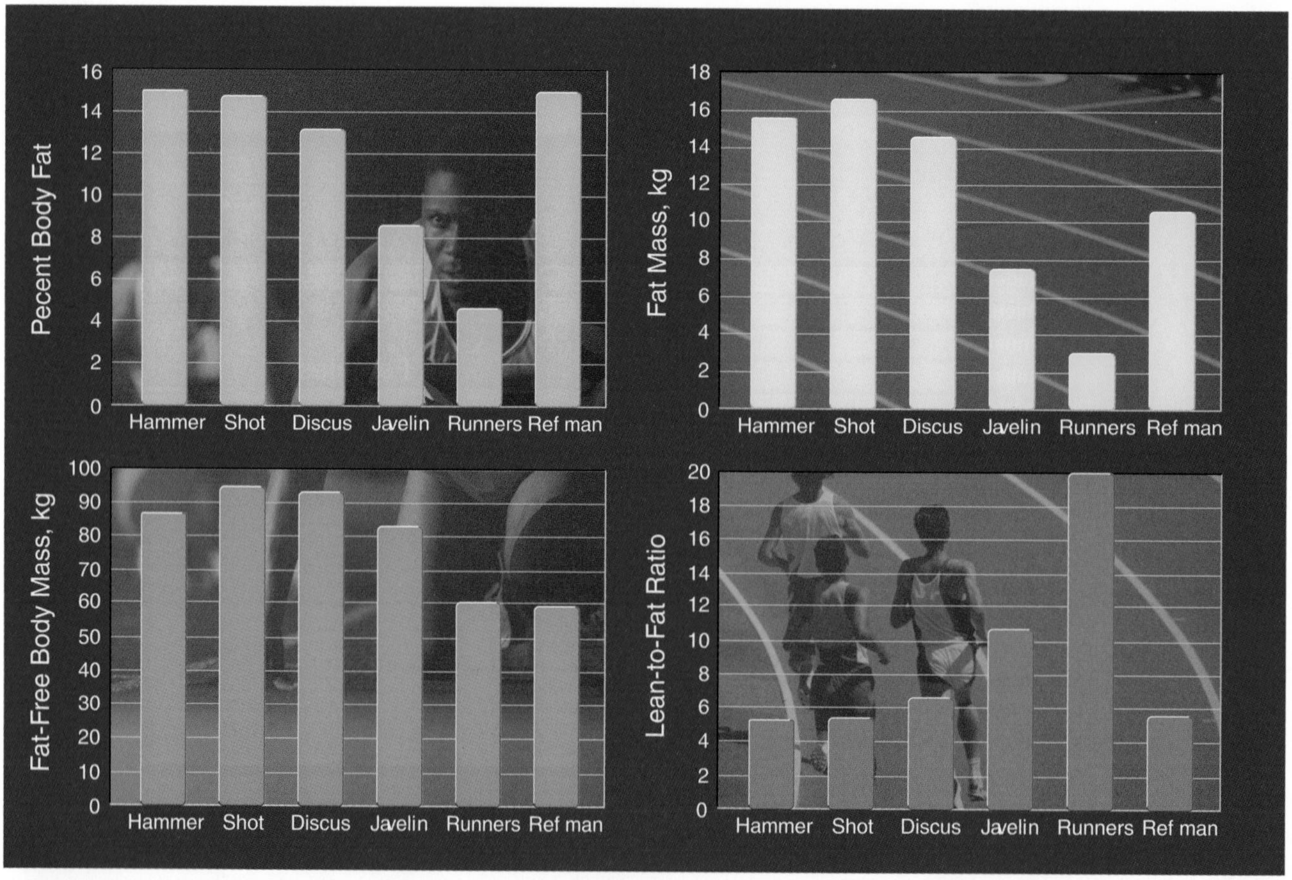

FIGURE 13.18. Body composition (determined by hydrostatic weighing) of the 10 top American male athletes in the discus, shot put, javelin, and hammer throw. (Data collected by two of the textbook authors [FK and VK] at a 1978 US Olympic thrower's minicamp at the University of Houston, Houston, TX. Data include gold medalist Wilkins [discus] and world record holder Powell [discus]). Data for the international elite middle- and long-distance runners from Pollock ML, et al. Body composition of elite class distance runners. *Ann NY Acad Sci* 1977;301:361. Reference man *[Ref man]* data from Behnke model.

TABLE 13.9 Skinfold and Girth Anthropometry of the Top 10 American Athletes in the Discus, Shot Put, Javelin, and Hammer Throw

Measurement[a]	Discus	Shot Put	Javelin	Hammer	Runners	Ref Man
Body mass, kg	108.2	112.3	90.6	104.2	63.1	70.0
Stature, cm	191.7	187.0	186.0	187.3	177.0	174.0
Skinfolds, mm						
Triceps	13.0	15.0	11.9	12.7	5.0	–
Scapular	18.0	23.8	12.5	21.5	6.4	–
Iliac	24.5	29.6	17.0	27.4	4.6	–
Abdomen	25.6	31.4	18.4	29.1	7.1	–
Thigh	16.4	15.7	13.3	17.3	6.1	–
Girths, cm						
Shoulders	129.8	133.3	121.5	127.4	106.1	110.8
Chest	113.5	118.5	104.6	111.3	91.1	91.8
Waist	94.1	99.1	86.6	94.8	74.6	77.0
Abdomen	97.5	101.5	87.8	98.0	74.2	79.8
Hips	110.4	112.3	102.0	108.7	87.8	93.4
Thighs	66.3	69.4	61.5	67.3	51.9	54.8
Knees	41.5	42.9	40.0	41.0	36.2[b]	36.6
Calves	42.6	43.6	39.5	41.5	35.4	35.8
Ankles	25.4	24.9	24.1	24.3	21.0	22.5
Biceps	41.8	42.2	37.7	39.9	28.2	31.7
Forearms	33.1	33.7	30.8	32.4	26.4	26.4
Wrists	18.7	18.9	18.2	18.4	16.0	17.3
Diameters, cm						
Biacromial	44.5	43.8	43.2	44.8	39.5	40.6
Chest	33.1	33.7	30.8	32.6	31.3	30.0
Bi-iliac	31.3	31.2	29.6	30.4	28.0	28.6
Bitrochanter	35.5	34.9	33.7	34.8	32.2	32.8
Knee	10.2	10.5	10.0	10.2	9.5	9.3
Wrist	6.3	6.2	6.0	6.2	5.6	5.6
Ankle	7.6	7.6	7.5	7.4	–	7.0
Elbow	7.6	7.6	7.6	7.2	–	7.0

[a]*Details about measurement procedures from Katch FI, Katch VL. The body composition profile: techniques of measurement and applications. Clin Sports Med, 1984;3:31. Data correspond to the athletic groups presented in Fig. 13.18.*

Olympics. For comparison, data include international elite middle- and long-distance runners and Behnke's reference man. **TABLE 13.9** lists the corresponding data for girth and skinfold anthropometry. Shot putters clearly possessed the largest overall size (body mass and girths), followed by athletes in discus, hammer, and javelin.

Female Endurance Athletes

Female long-distance runners of national and international caliber averaged 15.2% body fat (hydrostatic weighing), similar to high school cross-country runners[17] and elite Kenyan female endurance runners who averaged 16.0% body fat,[12] but considerably lower than the 26% typically reported for sedentary females of the same age, stature, and body mass. Compared with other female athletic groups, runners have relatively less fat than collegiate basketball players (20.9%),[123] competitive gymnasts (15.5%),[124] younger distance runners (18%),[74] swimmers (20.1%),[65] and tennis players (22.8%).[65]

Interestingly, the runners' average body fat equaled the 15% value generally reported for nonathletic males and close to the quantity of essential fat proposed by Behnke's model for the reference woman. The 6 to 9% body fat levels of several apparently healthy runners fall within the range reported for elite male endurance athletes. The leanest women in the population

BENEFITS OF A LEAN PHYSIQUE

A lean physique most likely influences success in distance running. This makes sense for several reasons: First, effective heat dissipation during running maintains thermal balance—excess fat thwarts heat dissipation. Second, excess body fat represents "dead weight"; it adds directly to exercise energy cost without providing propulsive energy.

based on Behnke's reference standards have essential fat equal to 12 to 14% of body mass. The relatively high body fat (35.4%) of one of the best runners suggests that other factors must override limitations to distance running imposed by excess fat.

Male Endurance Athletes

Male elite middle- and long-distance runners and marathoners typically maintain extremely low body fat values (3–5% of body mass). Such competitors represent the lower end of the lean-to-fat continuum for elite athletes.

For body dimension and structure, male distance runners generally have smaller girths and bone diameters than untrained males. Structural differences, particularly bone diameters, reflect a "genetic" influence similar to the distinct anthropometric characteristics of aquatic athletes (**FIG. 13.15**). The best long-distance runners possess a slight build, not only in stature but also in skeletal dimensions. The prime ingredients for a champion blend a genetically optimal physique profile with a lean body composition, a highly developed aerobic system, and a proper psychological attitude for prolonged, intensive training.

Triathletes

The triathlon combines continuous endurance performance in swimming, bicycling, and running. The extreme of triathlon requirements, the ultra-endurance Ironman competition (www.ironman.com), requires competitors to swim 3.9 km (2.4 miles), bicycle 180.2 km (112 miles), and run a standard 42.2 km (26.2 miles) marathon. The serious triathlete's training averages nearly 4 h daily, covering a total of 280 miles a week by swimming 7.2 miles at about a 30:00 per mile pace, bicycling 227 miles at about 19.0 mph, and running 45 miles close to a 7:30 per mile pace.[52] In an early study, percentage body fat of six male and three female triathletes ranged between about 5.0 and 12.0% for men and between 7.0 and 17.0% for women. Body fat averaged 7.1% for the top 15 male finishers. Contemporary triathletes possess a relatively low body fat content and high aerobic capacity comparable to other athletes in single endurance sports.[101] In general, male triathletes possess aerobic capacities similar to highly trained competitive swimmers; $\dot{V}O_{2max}$ values for females cluster at the upper range for top-class endurance runners.

Swimmers Versus Runners

Male and female competitive swimmers generally have more body fat than distance runners. Speculation suggests that the cool water of the training environment produces lower core temperatures than with equivalent-intensity land exercise. A lower core temperature may prevent the decreased appetite that often accompanies intense training on land, despite swim training's significant energy requirement.

Limited evidence indicates similar daily energy intakes for male collegiate swimmers (3380 kcal) and distance runners (3460 kcal), which balances training energy expenditure. In contrast, female swimmers averaged a higher daily energy intake (2490 kcal) compared with their running counterparts (2040 kcal).[62] However, the swimmers had a higher estimated daily energy expenditure than did the runners. The swimmers' energy expenditure even surpassed energy intake, placing them in a slightly *negative* energy balance. Thus, a positive energy balance (intake greater than output) does not explain typically higher percentage body fat levels in male (12%) and female (20%) swimmers than in male (7%) and female (15%) runners. Subsequent research from the same laboratory evaluated energy expenditure and fuel use of swimmers and runners during each form of training (45 min at 75–80% $\dot{V}O_{2max}$) and 2 h of recovery.[39] Differences in hormonal response and substrate catabolism between the two exercise modes probably accounts for body fat differences between groups. Thus, the small differences between activities in energy expenditure, substrate use, and hormone levels would *not* account for body fat differences.

American Football Players

The first detailed body composition analyses of American professional football players in the 1940s clearly demonstrated the inadequacy of determining a person's "optimal" body mass from weight-for-height standards.[146] The players as a group had body fat content that averaged only 10.4% of body mass, while FFM averaged 81.3 kg (179.3 lb). Certainly these men were heavy but not fat. The heaviest lineman weighed 118 kg (260 lb, 17.4% body fat, 215 lb FFM), whereas the lineman with the most body fat (23.2%) weighed 115.4 kg (252 lb). Body mass of a defensive back with the least fat (3.3%) was 82.3 kg (182 lb) with a FFM of 79.6 kg (175 lb).

TABLE 13.10 presents a clearer picture for body mass, stature, percentage body fat, and FFM of college and professional players grouped by position. The *Pro, older* group consists of 25 players from the 1942 Washington Redskins, the first professional players measured for body composition by hydrostatic weighing. The *Pro, modern* group consists of 164 players from 14 teams in the NFL (69% veterans, 31% rookies). Some 107 members of the 1976 to 1978 Dallas Cowboys and New York Jets make up the third group. Four groups of collegiate players include candidates for spring practice at St. Cloud State College in Minnesota, the University of Massachusetts (UMass), and Division III Gettysburg College and teams from the University of Southern California (USC), 1973 to 1977, national champions and participants in two

TABLE 13.10 Body Compositions of Collegiate and Professional Football Players Grouped by Position

Position[a]	Level	N	Stature (cm)	Mass (kg)	Body Fat (%)	FFM (kg)
Defensive backs	St. Cloud[b]	15	178.3	77.3	11.5	68.4
	U Mass[c]	12	179.9	83.1	8.8	76.8
	USC[d]	15	183.0	83.7	9.6	75.7
	Gettysburg[e]	16	175.9	79.8	13.6	68.9
	Pro, modern[f]	26	182.5	84.8	9.6	76.7
	Pro, older[g]	25	183.0	91.2	10.7	81.4
Offensive backs and receivers	St. Cloud	15	179.7	79.8	12.4	69.6
	U Mass	29	181.8	84.1	9.5	76.4
	USC	18	185.6	86.1	9.9	77.6
	Gettysburg	18	176.0	78.3	12.9	68.2
	Pro, modern	40	183.8	90.7	9.4	81.9
	Pro, older	25	183.0	91.7	10.0	87.5
Linebackers	St. Cloud	7	180.1	87.2	13.4	75.4
	U Mass	17	186.1	97.1	13.1	84.2
	USC	17	185.6	98.8	13.2	85.8
	Gettysburg	—	—	—	—	—
	Pro, modern	28	188.6	102.2	14.0	87.6
Offensive linemen and tight ends	St. Cloud	13	186.0	99.2	19.1	79.8
	U Mass	23	187.5	107.6	19.5	86.6
	Gettysburg	15	182.6	110.4	26.2	81.0
	USC	25	191.1	106.5	15.3	90.3
	Pro, modern	38	193.0	112.6	15.6	94.7
Defensive linemen	St. Cloud	15	186.6	97.8	18.5	79.3
	U Mass	8	188.8	114.3	19.5	91.9
	USC	13	191.1	109.3	14.7	93.2
	Gettysburg	11	178.0	99.4	21.9	77.6
	Pro, modern	32	192.4	117.1	18.2	95.8
	Pro, older	25	185.7	97.1	14.0	83.5
All positions	St. Cloud	65	182.5	88.0	15.0	74.2
	U Mass	91	184.9	97.3	13.9	83.2
	USC	88	186.6	96.6	11.4	84.6
	Gettysburg	60	178.0	90.6	18.1	73.3
	Pro, modern	164	188.1	101.5	13.4	87.3
	Pro, older	25	183.1	91.2	10.4	81.3
	Dallas-Jets[h]	107	188.2	100.4	12.6	87.7

[a] *Grouping according to Wilmore JH, Haskel WL. Body composition and endurance capacity of professional football players. J Appl Physiol 1972;33:564.*
[b] *Data from Wickkiser JD, Kelly JM. The body composition of a college football team. Med Sci Sports 1975;7:199.*
[c] *UMass data from Coach Robert Stull and F Katch, University of Massachusetts. Data collected during spring practice, 1985; %fat by densitometry.*
[d] *USC data from Dr. Robert Girandola, University of Southern California, Los Angeles, 1978, 1993.*
[e] *Data courtesy of Dr. Kristin Steumple, Department of Exercise and Sport Science, Gettysburg College, Gettysburg, PA, 2000.*
[f] *Data from Wilmore JH, et al. Football pros' strengths—and CV weakness—charted. Phys Sportsmed 1976;4:45.*
[g] *Data from Dr. A. R. Behnke.*
[h] *Data from Katch FI, Katch, VL. Body composition of the Dallas Cowboys and New York Jets football teams, unpublished, 1978.*

Rose Bowls. Body composition measurements for this data set included hydrostatic weighing with correction for measured residual lung volume.

One would generally expect modern-day professional players to have a larger body size at each position than a representative collegiate group. Although this occurred for comparison with the St. Cloud and UMass players, the USC players generally maintained a physique similar to modern professionals. With the exception of defensive linemen, the USC players at each position showed nearly the same fat content as current professionals. No USC player possessed more than 4.4 kg less FFM than that of the professionals at each position. The average defensive lineman in the NFL outweighed his USC counterpart in FFM by only 1.8 kg. Total body mass of the professional linemen significantly exceeded that of USC counterparts, primarily because professionals possessed 18.2% body fat versus the collegians' 14.7%. These data suggest that elite college and professional players maintain similar body size and body composition.

As a group, professional players of 75 years ago had lower body fat (10.4%), shorter stature, and lighter total body mass and FFM than contemporary professionals. The exceptions, defensive and offensive backs and receivers, were almost identical to more current players in body size and composition. The biggest differences in physique emerged for defensive linemen; modern players were 6.7 cm taller, 20 kg heavier, and 4.2 percentage points of body fat fatter and had 12.3 kg more FFM. Obviously, "bigness" was not an important factor in line play during the 1940s. To illustrate this point, the *top* of **FIGURE 13.19** shows the average body weight for all roster players in the NFL (N = 51,333) over a 76-year period. From 1920 to 1985, offensive linemen were the heaviest; this changed beginning with the 1990 season, when defensive linemen achieved the same body mass as the offensive linemen and then surpassed them. While the body mass for offensive linemen appeared to level off at nearly 280 lb, defensive linemen continued to increase in weight, particularly from 1990 to 1996. At this time, they weighed an average of 16 lb more or double the weight gain for offensive linemen for the comparable period. On average, offensive linemen were 1.3 lb heavier per year from 1920 to 1996. At this rate of increase, they should attain a weight of 320 lb by the year 2012 (at an average height of 6 ft 8 in)! At this size, their BMI equals 35.6, classifying them as high for disease risk (**FIG. 13.1**).

The body weight of offensive and defensive linemen for each of the NFL teams during the 1994 season (*bottom* of **FIG. 13.19**) ranged from heaviest (Kansas City Chiefs; Super Bowl 1970) to lightest (San Francisco 49ers; Super Bowls 1990 and 1995). For the 1994 season (the date of the comparison in the bottom figure), the average body weight of the winning Dallas Cowboys Super Bowl offensive line ranked fifth highest of 28 teams.

Even more eye opening was the body size of the 2010 Super Bowl teams' 28 offensive and defensive linemen (Indianapolis Colts and Chicago Bears). BMI averaged 38.3 (body mass, 139.2 kg; stature, 194.7 cm), the largest yet reported for Super Bowl teams. The inset figure shows the number of 2011 Super Bowl offensive and defensive linemen that exceeded 300 pounds, including averages for body weight, stature, and BMI. There is no reason to believe these results will be curtailed in the near future, and in fact, a 10% increase within the next decade seems entirely plausible Research must determine whether such relatively homogenous groups of elite, physically active, overweight men experience greater morbidity and mortality than normal-weight peers. Figure 13.20 illustrates the increasing number of player exceeding 300 pounds in 10-year intervals from 1970 to 2010 with projected numbers (1000) for the year 2020.

A Worrisome Trend Among Less Skilled and Younger Players

Exceptionally high BMIs also occur at less elite levels of collegiate competition. The average BMIs of 33.1 for the Division III 1999 Gettysburg offensive line (N = 15) (29.9 for 2000 offensive line, N = 13)[128] and 31.7 for other National Collegiate Athletic Association (NCAA) Division III America football linemen (N = 26; 1994–1995) raise similar concerns about potential health risks for such large young men (stature, 1.84 m; body mass, 107.2 kg).[113] At the high school level, The BMI of *Parade Magazine's* (www.parade.com) All-America football teams increased dramatically beginning in the early 1970s through 1989 and then further increased in rate of gain to the year 2006. The plot in **FIGURE 13.21** shows a clear shift at 1972 in the slope of the regression line (*yellow line*) relating BMI to year of competition compared with age-matched persons from large-scale epidemiologic normative data (*red line*). Particularly disturbing are the most recent 2011 data for the high school offensive and defensive linemen whose BMI averaged 34.2 (stature, 195.0 cm; mass, 129.9 kg). These values for stature and body mass for the high school players now are *almost identical* to the average values for the 2011 National Champion BCS (Bowl Championship Series) teams (University of Oregon and Auburn University; BMI, 33.8) and 2011 Super Bowl teams (Pittsburg Steelers and Green Bay Packers)! Such data are consistent with data from current NFL offensive and defensive linemen that indicate that over 60% of players are considered obese based on BMI classification. The implications for the student athlete linemen's health risks (e.g., high blood pressure, insulin resistance, type 2 diabetes) and long-term outlook are not encouraging.[80]

THE INTERACTION OF ENHANCED TRAINING AND PERFORMANCE-ENHANCING DRUGS

The shift toward a higher BMI among high school football players probably relates to two factors: (1) improved nutrition and training and/or (2) the emerging prevalent use among high school athletes of performance-enhancing drugs such as anabolic steroids and human growth hormone.

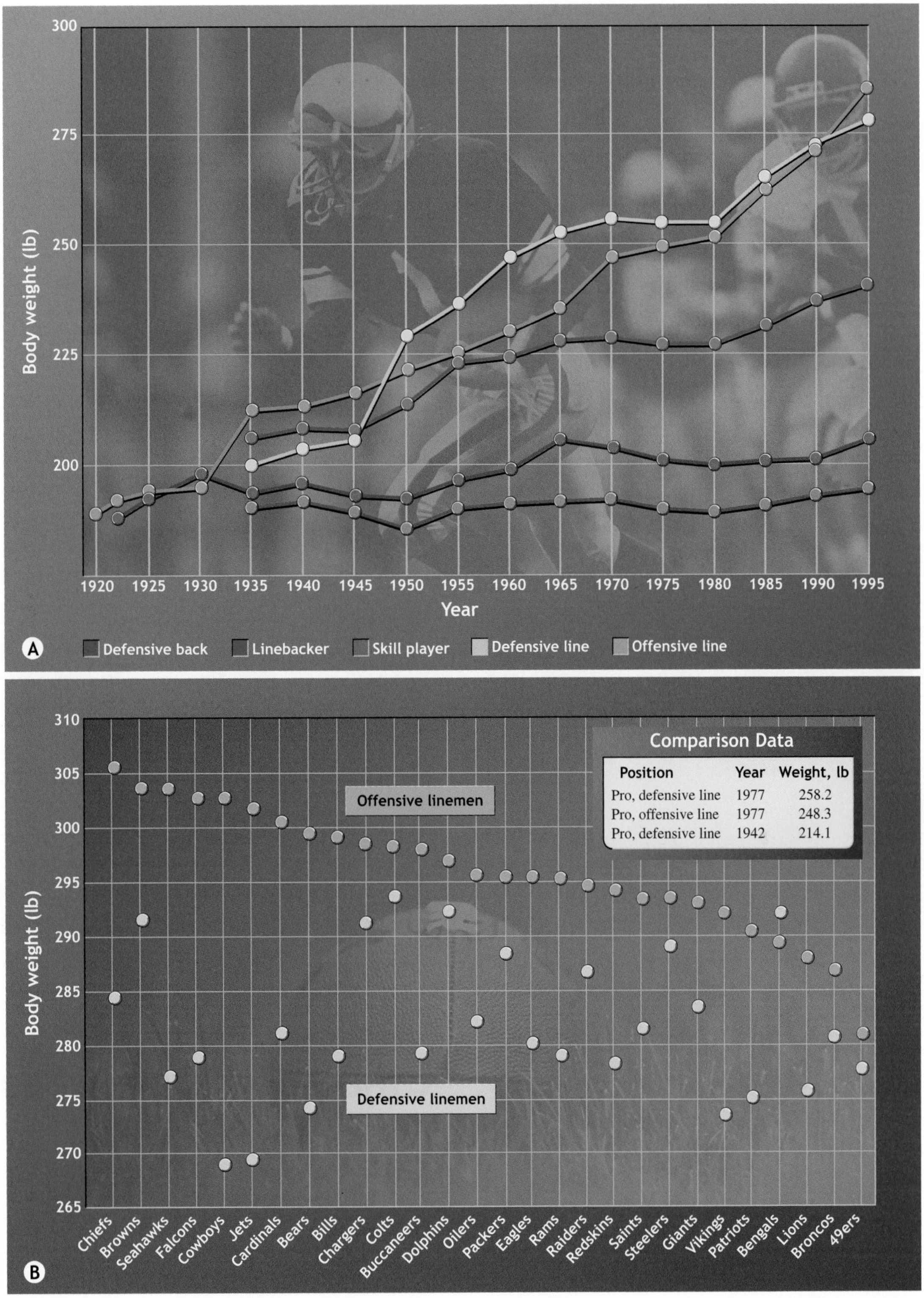

FIGURE 13.19. **A.** Average body weights by position for all roster players in the NFL between 1920 and 1995. **B.** Average body weights of all roster offensive and defensive linemen in the NFL in 1994. Team rankings progress from the heaviest to lightest body weight for the team's offensive linemen. (From active team rosters for 28 NFL teams as of the first regular season weekend, September 4–5, 1994.) Comparisons of body weight data for the professional offensive and defensive line (1977) shown in the inset box combine data for the New York Jets and Dallas Cowboys football teams (collected by textbook authors FK and VK). The 1942 data were provided by Dr. Albert Behnke from his pioneering studies of the Washington Redskins. (Data courtesy of the National Football League public relations department.)

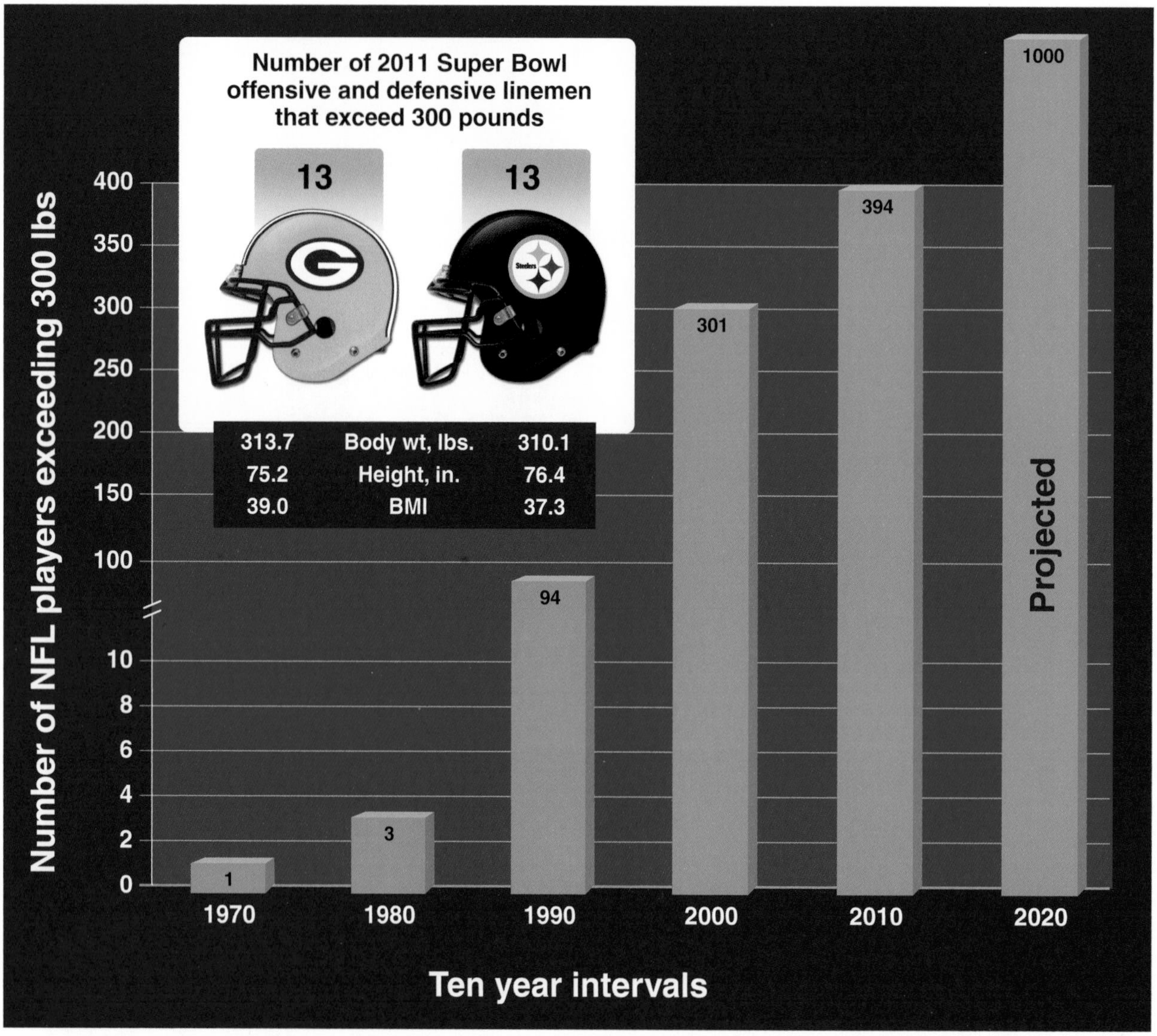

FIGURE 13.20. Number of NFL players exceeding 300 pounds in 10-year intervals from 1970 to 2010 including a projected value for the year 2010. The inset figure shows the number of 2011 Super Bowl offensive and defensive linemen that exceeded 300 lb, including averages for body weight, stature, and body mass index.

Professional Golfers

Limited data exist on the body composition of professional golfers, although height and weight for 2005 tour Professional Golfers' Association (PGA) and Champions Tour players were available from popular golf magazines. **TABLE 13.11** lists the height, weight, and BMI for the Champions Tour and PGA Tour champions, including 19 of the 2011 top 20 PGA players. Data for Behnke's reference man are included for comparison. Interestingly, little difference in the physical characteristics and BMI exists for the three groups of PGA players. The projected mortality ratio for these high-skill performers based on BMI displayed in **FIGURE 13.1** rates as very low. This contrasts to the high school and professional football players who classify as obese and fall in the high range for mortality risk. For the obese NFL players, one half fall in the severely obese range (BMI that reaches 35), and those with a BMI above 40 classify as morbidly obese.

OTHER LONGITUDINAL TRENDS IN BODY SIZE

To expand upon longitudinal trends in body size for elite athletes, we determined stature and body mass for two groups of professional athletes: (1) all National Basketball Association (NBA) players from 1970 to 1993 (number ranged from 156 to 400) and (2) professional Major League Baseball (MLB) players from 28 teams during the 1986, 1988, 1990, 1992, and 1995 seasons (5031 roster players).

For the NBA players (**FIG. 13.22A**), average body mass increased by 3.8 lb (1.7 kg) or 1.8% during the 23-year interval. Stature increased more slowly; it changed by only 1 in, or less than 1%, over the same interval. The NBA players' BMI during this time remained within a narrow range of 0.8 BMI units from 23.6 to 24.4. The MLB players (shown in *red* in the same figure) reveal slightly higher mean values than do

TABLE 13.11 Comparison of Height, Body Weight, and BMI for 2005 Champions Tour and PGA Golf Tour Champions and 2011 Top 20 PGA Players

Group[a]	Height (cm)	Weight (kg)	BMI
PGA Tour (*N* = 33)	182.0	84.1	25.4
Champions Tour (*N* = 18)	181.0	85.8	26.2
PGA Tour 2011[b] (*N* = 19)	184.0	81.2	24.0
Behnke reference man	174.0	70.0	23.1

[a] ***Source:*** PGA TOUR Annual 2006, published by Boston Hannah International, www.bostonhannah.com

[b] *2011 players: Casey, Donald, Els, Fowler, Furyk, D. Johnson, Kuchar, McDonwell, Michelson, Oglivy, Poulter, Rose, Schwartzel, Scott, Stricker, Watney, Watson, Wilson, Woods.*

the basketball players. Compared with American professional and collegiate football players, baseball and basketball athletes have maintained BMIs within guidelines considered relatively healthful for minimizing mortality and disease risk.

One might question whether gross body size reflected by BMI relates to sports performance variables. For example, the graphs in **FIGURE 13.22B** show the BMI of National and American League Cy Young award winners and their earned run average over the 5-year comparison period. This comparison, while of interest, fails to delineate a clear relation between BMI and performance among the best pitchers in baseball.

Wrestlers

Wrestlers represent a unique athletic group who train intensely and attempt to keep a low body weight with as high a fat-free mass as possible. The NCAA introduced rule changes for the 1998–1999 season in response to the deaths of three collegiate wrestlers in 1997 from excessive weight loss (largely from dehydration) to discourage dangerous weight-cutting practices and increase safe participation.[102] Another rule change included measures of urine specific gravity (ratio of the density of urine to the density of water) to assess hydration status to ensure euhydration of wrestlers at weight certification. Athletes with a urine specific gravity of 1.020 or less are considered euhydrated, whereas those with specific gravity in excess of 1.020 cannot have their body fat assessed to determine minimum competitive wrestling weight for the season. Urine specific gravity reflects hydration status, but it does lag behind true hydration status in periods of rapid body fluid turnover during acute dehydration.

Weightlifters and Bodybuilders

Men

Resistance-trained athletes, particularly bodybuilders, Olympic weightlifters, and power weightlifters, exhibit remarkable muscular development and FFM and a relatively lean physique. Percentage body fat from underwater weighing averaged 9.3% in bodybuilders, 9.1% in power weightlifters, and 10.8% in Olympic weightlifters.[72] Considerable leanness exists for each group of athletes, even though height-for-weight tables classify up to 19% of these athletes as overweight. Groups did not differ in skeletal frame size, FFM, skinfolds, and bone diameters. The only differences occurred for shoulders, chest, biceps (relaxed and flexed), and forearm girths, with bodybuilders larger at each site. Bodybuilders exhibited nearly 16 kg more muscle than predicted for their size; power weightlifters, 15 kg; and Olympic weightlifters, 13 kg.

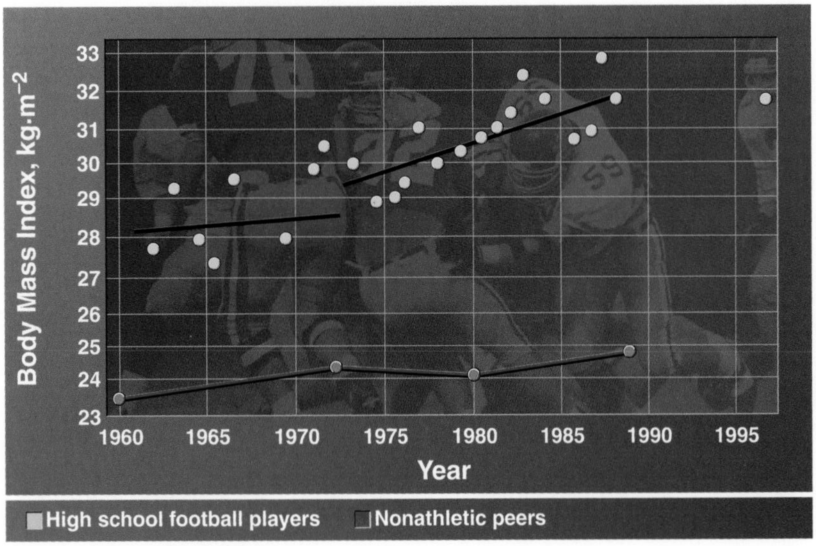

FIGURE 13.21. Body mass index (BMI) of *Parade Magazine's* All-America high school football players from 1960 to 2011. Comparison data are available for similar-age high school students from 1960 to 1995. The 2006 data included 18 linemen who ranged in body mass from 104.3 to 153.3 kg and in stature from 188.0 to 203.2 cm. The 2011 lineman with the highest BMI of 38.7 weighed 153.3 kg (338 lb; stature = 198.1 cm; 6 ft 8 in).

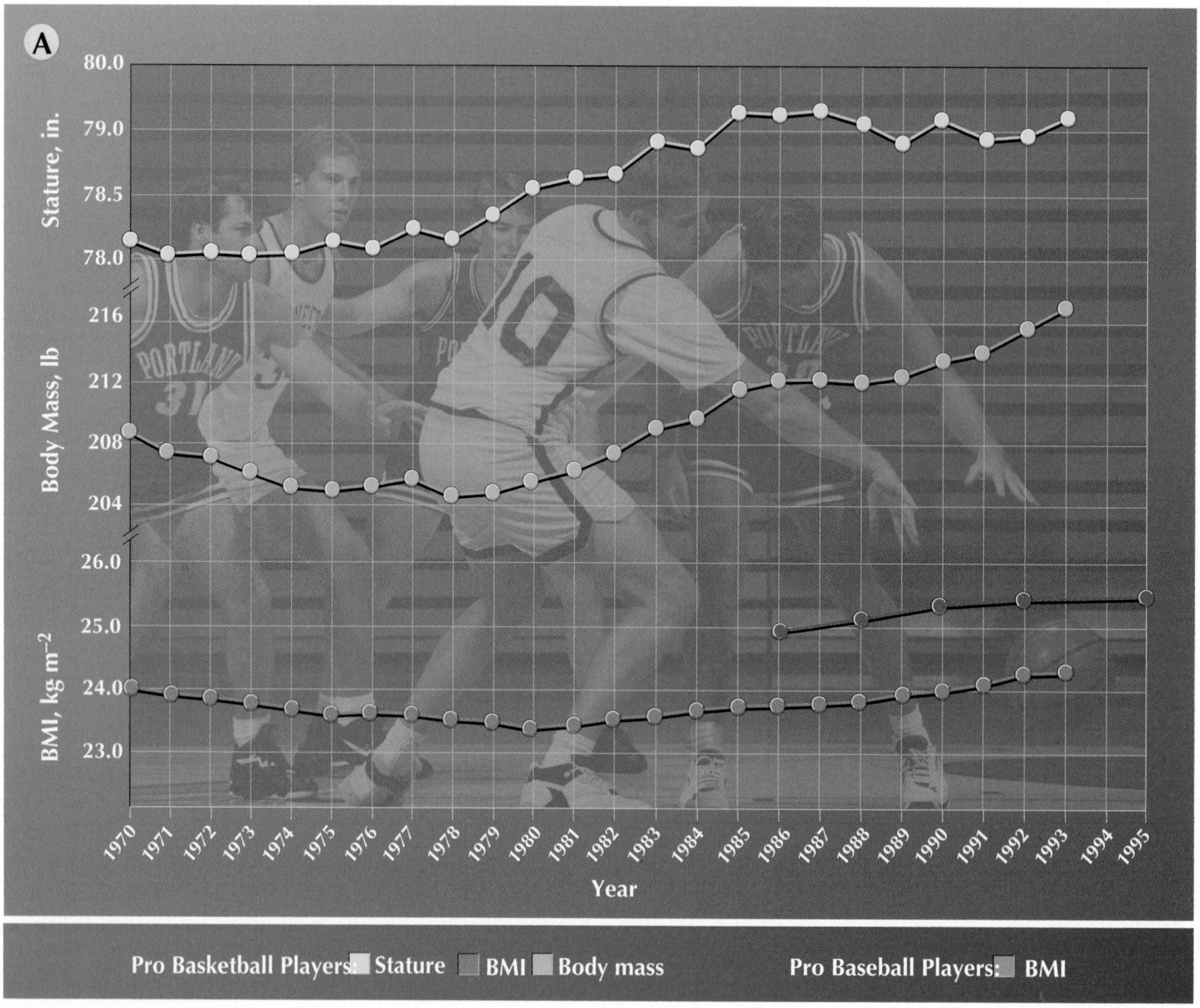

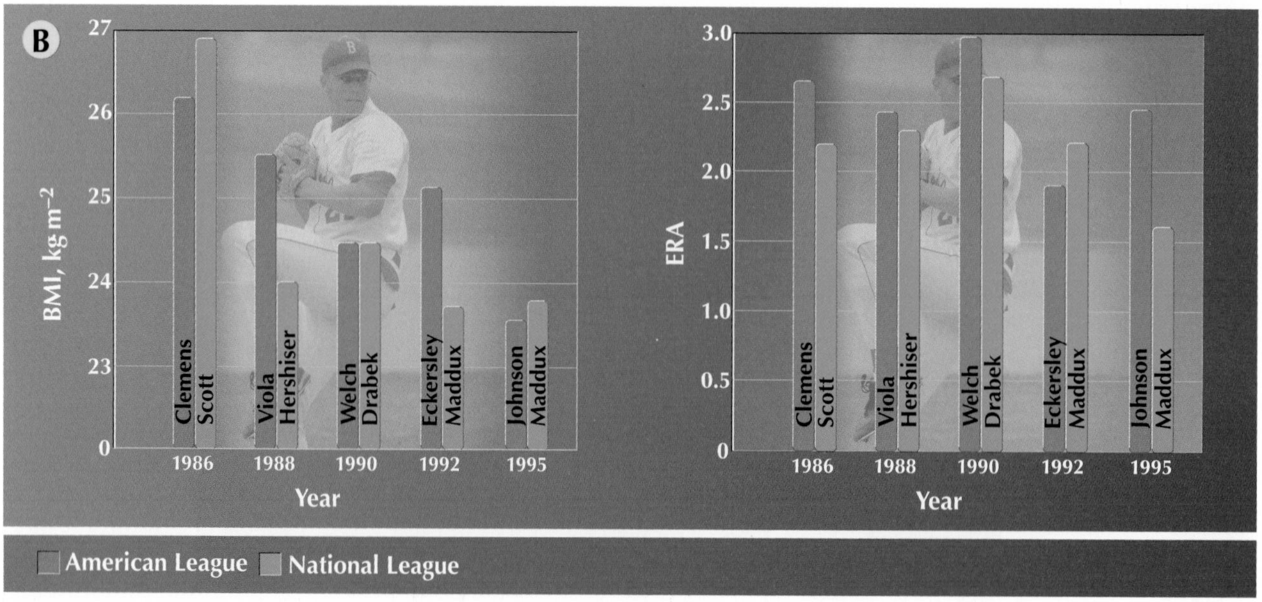

FIGURE 13.22. A. Body mass index (BMI), body mass, and stature of professional National Basketball Association (NBA) players (1970–1993) and BMI of Major League Baseball (MLB) players (1986–1995). **B.** BMI for American League and National League Cy Young award winners (best baseball pitcher) along with corresponding earned run average (ERA). (Data for NBA players from team rosters, compiled by F. Katch; MLB data from team rosters courtesy of Major League Baseball.)

Women

Bodybuilding gained widespread popularity among women in the United States during the late 1970s. As women aggressively undertook the vigorous demands of resistance training, competition became more intense, and the level of achievement increased significantly. Bodybuilding success depends on a slim and lean appearance, with a well-defined yet enlarged musculature. These requirements raise interesting questions about the women's body composition. How lean do competitors become, and does a relatively large muscle mass accompany their low body fat levels?

Scarce data exist about the body composition of "lean" competitive or professional female athletes. Limited data are available on the body composition of 10 competitive female bodybuilders who averaged 13.2% body fat (range, 8.0–18.3%) and 46.6 kg of FFM.[53] Except for champion gymnasts, who also average about 13% body fat, bodybuilders were 3 to 4% shorter, were 4 to 5% lighter, and had 7 to 10% less total fat mass than other competitive female athletes. *Women probably can alter muscle size to the same relative extent as males, at least when scaled to body size.* The larger hip size in women probably relates to greater fat stores in this location.

A REMARKABLE PHYSIQUE CHARACTERISTIC

A most striking compositional characteristic of the female bodybuilder is her dramatically large FFM/FM ratio of 7:1, which nearly doubles the 4.3:1 ratio for other female athletic groups. This difference presumably occurred without steroid use (assessed by questionnaire). Interestingly, 8 of the 10 bodybuilders reported normal menstrual function despite relatively low body fat.

SUMMARY

1. Body composition assessment reveals that athletes generally have physique characteristics unique to their specific sport. Field event athletes have relatively large fat-free body mass (FFM) and high percentage body fat; distance runners have the lowest FFM and fat mass.
2. Champion performance blends physique characteristics with highly developed physiologic support systems.
3. Male and female triathletes possess the body composition and aerobic capacity most similar to elite bicyclists.
4. American football players and strength and power athletes are among the heaviest of all athletes, yet they maintain a relatively lean body composition. At the highest levels of competition, collegiate and professional football players attain similar body size and body composition.
5. Competitive male and female swimmers generally have higher body fat levels than distance runners, probably from self-selection related to economically exercising in the different environments rather than real metabolic effects caused by the environments.
6. The FFM/FM ratio of female bodybuilders significantly exceeds the FFM/FM ratios of other elite female athletes.
7. Female bodybuilders can probably alter muscle size to almost the same *relative* extent as male bodybuilders.

TEST YOUR KNOWLEDGE ANSWERS

1. **False:** The importance of the BMI is not that it predicts body fat level (although it moderately relates to this variable), but rather its curvilinear relationship to all-cause mortality ratio. As BMI increases, so does the risk for cardiovascular complications including hypertension and stroke, diabetes, and renal disease. The lowest health risk category includes persons with BMIs between 20 and 25, and the highest risk category includes persons whose BMI exceeds 40.
2. **True:** His BMI = 31.6 kg/m^2 [97.1 ÷ (1.753)^2], which exceeds the upper range of BMI values (BMI: normal weight, <25.0; overweight, 25.0–29.9; obese, ≥30.0). This classifies him as obese.
3. **False:** In the general population, the average man is taller and heavier, his skeleton weighs more, and he has a larger muscle mass and lower total fat content than the typical woman. Differences exist even when expressing the amount of fat, muscle, and bone as a percentage of body mass. This holds particularly true for body fat, which represents 15% of total body mass for the man and 27% for his female counterpart. These differences in body composition emerge in comparisons among elite athletes in diverse sports. Among the leanest male competitors such as elite marathon runners, body fat levels range between 3 and 5%, whereas for female counterparts, percentage body fat rarely falls below 12 to 15%. This higher level of body fat among females across the entire fitness spectrum most likely relates to sex-specific essential

fat that serves biologically important childbearing and other hormone-related functions.

4. **False:** The two main locations or depots for body fat deposition include essential fat and storage fat. Essential fat comprises fat stored in the marrow of bones, heart, lungs, liver, spleen, kidneys, intestines, muscles, and lipid-rich tissues of the central nervous system. In the female, essential fat also includes additional sex-specific essential fat. Storage fat consists of fat accumulation in adipose tissue. This includes the visceral fatty tissues that protect the various internal organs within the thoracic and abdominal cavities and the larger subcutaneous fat tissue volume deposited beneath the skin's surface.

5. **True:** Archimedes showed that an object submerged or floating in water becomes buoyed up by a counterforce equal to the weight of the volume of water it displaces. This buoyant force helps to support an immersed object against gravity's downward pull. Thus, an object is said to *lose* weight in water. The object's loss of weight in water equals the weight of the volume of water it displaces; specific gravity thus refers to the *ratio* of the weight of an object in air divided by its loss of weight in water.

6. **False:** From the Siri equation, percentage body fat computes as follows: 495 ÷ 1.0719 – 450 = 11.8%. Total mass of body fat equals 85 kg × 0.118 = 10.0 kg.

7. **False:** Men with a 102-cm (40-in) or larger waist and women with waist girth larger than 88 cm (35 in) maintain a high risk for various diseases. Waist girths of 90 cm for men and 83 cm for women correspond to a BMI threshold of overweight (BMI, 25), whereas girths of 100 cm for men and 93 cm for women reflect the obesity cutoff (BMI = 30).

8. **True:** Based on an average computed from data in diverse studies, percentage body fat for young adult men averages between 12 and 15%, whereas the average fat value for women ranges between 25 and 28%.

9. **False:** Given the data, desirable fat loss computes as follows:

   Fat mass = 120 kg × 24% (0.24) body fat = 28.8 kg

   Fat-free body mass = 120 kg – 28.8 kg = 91.2 kg

   Goal body weight = 91.2 kg ÷ (1.00 – 0.15) = 91.2 kg ÷ 0.85 = 107.3 kg (236.6 lb)

   Desirable fat loss = 120 kg – 107.3 kg = 12.7 kg (28.0 lb)

10. **True:** The body composition for 10 competitive female bodybuilders averaged 13.2% body fat (range, 8.0–18.3%) and 46.6 kg of FFM. Except for champion gymnasts, who also average about 13% body fat, bodybuilders were 3 to 4% shorter, were 4 to 5% lighter, and possessed 7 to 10% less total fat mass than other top female athletes. The bodybuilders' most striking compositional characteristic is a dramatically large FFM/FM ratio of 7:1, nearly double the 4.3:1 ratio for other female athletic groups.

Key References

Beals KA, Manore MM. Behavioral, psychological, and physical characteristics of female athletes with subclinical eating disorders. *Int J Sport Nutr Exerc Metab* 2000;10:128.

Behnke AR, Wilmore JH. *Evaluation and Regulation of Body Build and Composition.* Englewood Cliffs, NJ: Prentice Hall, 1974.

Bouchard C, et al. Inheritance in the amount and distribution of human body fat. *Int J Obes* 1988;12:205.

Brandon LJ. Comparison of existing skinfold equations for estimating body fat in African American and white women. *Am J Clin Nutr* 1998;67:1115.

Eliakim A, et al. Assessment of body composition in ballet dancers: correlation among anthropometric measurements, bio-electrical impedance analysis, and dual-energy x-ray absorptiometry. *Int J Sports Med* 2000;21:598.

Fernáandez JR, et al. Is percentage body fat differentially related to body mass index in Hispanic Americans, African Americans, and European Americans? *Am J Clin Nutr* 2003;77:71.

Flegal KM, et al. Prevalence and trends in obesity among US adults, 1999-2000. *JAMA* 2002;288:1723.

Jackson AS, et al. Generalized equations for predicting body density of women. *Med Sci Sports* 1980;12:175.

Jackson AS, Pollock ML. Generalized equations for predicting body density of men. *Br J Nutr* 1978;40:497.

Katch FI, et al. Effects of physical training on the body composition and diet of females. *Res Q* 1969;40:99.

Katch FI, Katch VL. Measurement and prediction errors in body composition assessment and the search for the perfect prediction equation. *Res Q Exerc Sport* 1980;51:249.

Katch FI, McArdle WD. Prediction of body density from simple anthropometric measurements in college-age men and women. *Hum Biol* 1973;45:445.

Katch FI, McArdle WD. Validity of body composition prediction equations for college men and women. *Am J Clin Nutr* 1975;28:105.

Katch VL, et al. Contribution of breast volume and weight to body fat distribution in females. *Am J Phys Anthropol* 1980;53:93.

Keys A, et al. *The Biology of Human Starvation.* Minneapolis: University of Minnesota Press, 1950.

Loucks AB. Energy availability, not body fatness, regulates reproductive unction in women. *Exerc Sport Sci Rev* 2003;31:144.

Mei Z, et al. Validity of body mass index compared with other body-composition screening indexes for the assessment of body fatness in children and adolescents. *Am J Clin Nutr* 2002;75:978.

National Task Force on the Prevention and Treatment of Obesity. Obesity, overweight and health risk. *Arch Intern Med* 2000;160:898.

Schrager MA, et al. Sarcopenic obesity and inflammation in the CHIANTI Study. *J Appl Physiol* 2007;102:919.

Silva AM, et al. Are skinfold-based models accurate and suitable for assessing changes in body composition in highly trained athletes? *J Strength Cond Res* 2009;6:1688.

Stuempfle KJ, et al. Body composition relates poorly to performance tests in NCAA Division III football players. *J Strength Cond Res* 2003;17:238.

Tran ZV, Weltman A. Generalized equation for predicting body density of women from girth measurements. *Med Sci Sports Exerc* 1989;21:101.

van der Ploeg GE, et al. Use of anthropometric variables to predict relative body fat determined by a four-compartment body composition model. *Eur J Clin Nutr* 2003;57:1009.

Welham WC, Behnke AR. The specific gravity of healthy men. *JAMA* 942;118:498.

Weltman A, et al. Accurate assessment of body composition in obese males. *Am J Clin Nutr* 1988;48:1179.

thePoint *Visit* **thePoint.lww.com/MKKSEN4e** *for a list of the references cited in this chapter, including additional, relevant references.*

CHAPTER 14

Energy Balance, Exercise, and Weight Control

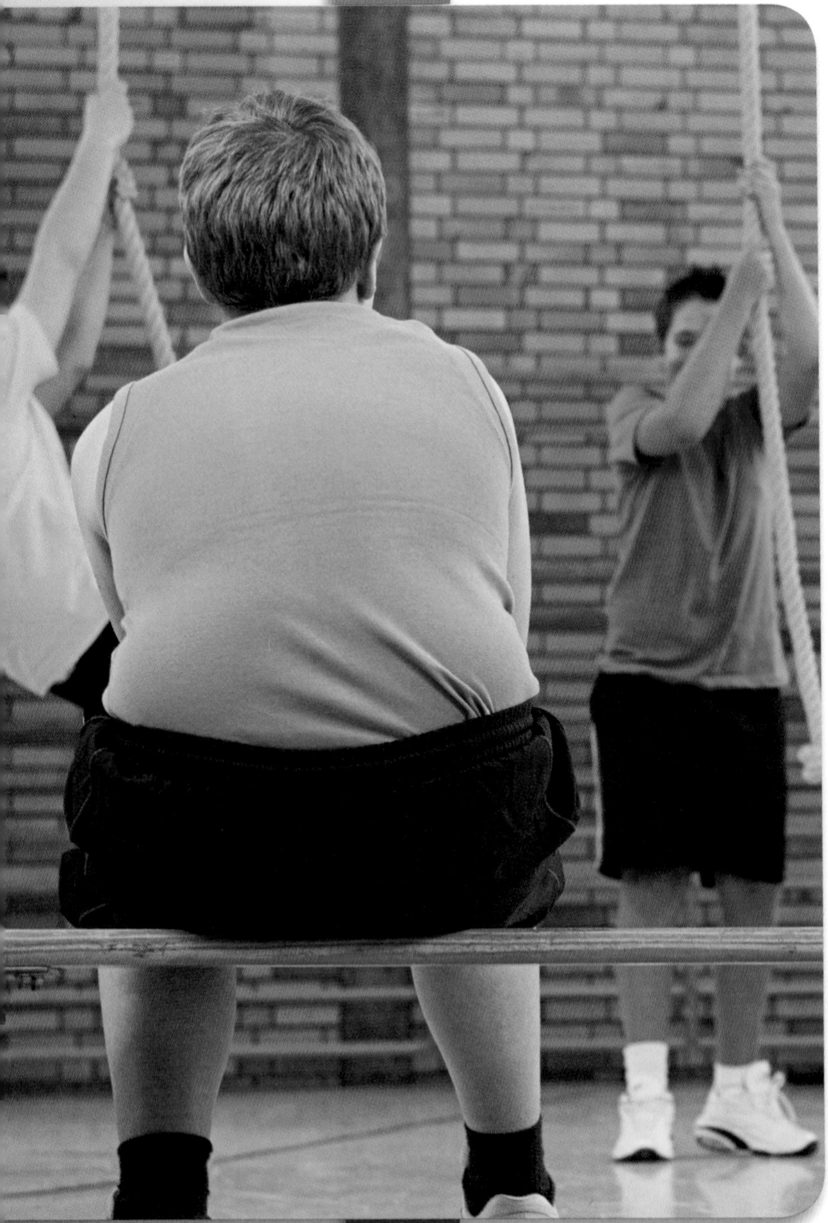

OUTLINE

- A National Concern
- Global Obesity Epidemic
- Health Risks and Financial Impact of Obesity
- Increased Physical Activity Modifies Age-Related Increases in Body Mass and Body Fat
- Genetics Plays a Role in Body Weight Regulation
- Physical Activity: A Crucial Component in Weight Control
- Weight Loss: A Unique Dilemma for the Competitive Athlete
- Applying the Energy Balance Equation to Weight Loss
- Dieting to Tip the Energy Balance Equation
- The Appropriate Diet Plan: Well Balanced but Less of It
- Maximizing Dieting's Chances for Success
- Regular Exercise for Weight Control
- Maximizing Success by Increasing Physical Activity: Modifying Behaviors
- Strategies for Alternative Exercise Behaviors
- The Ideal: Food Restriction Plus Increased Physical Activity
- Does Selective Exercise "Spot Reduction" Work?
- Possible Gender Differences in Physical Activity Effects on Weight Loss
- Effects of Diet and Physical Activity on Body Composition During Weight Loss
- Weight Loss Recommendations for Wrestlers and Other Power Athletes
- Appropriate Weight Gain for the Physically Active person

TEST YOUR KNOWLEDGE

Select true or false for the 10 statements below, then check out the answers at the end of the chapter. Retake the test after you've read the chapter; you should achieve 100%!	True	False
1. A global obesity epidemic currently exists.	❍	❍
2. No "racial" differences exist in the prevalence of obesity; overfatness does not discriminate.	❍	❍
3. Dietary approaches offer the best defense against regaining lost body weight.	❍	❍
4. Weight gain is an inevitable consequence of aging.	❍	❍
5. The most prudent approach to weight control combines moderate food restriction with increased daily physical activity.	❍	❍
6. The body reduces basal energy expenditure during weight loss by food restriction.	❍	❍
7. Very low-calorie diets (VLCDs) offer the best and fastest method to successfully induce weight loss.	❍	❍
8. Simply stated, excessive food intake produces weight gain.	❍	❍
9. Increasing regular physical activity improves one's health status but does little for weight control because of the few number of calories expended during most physical activities.	❍	❍
10. One must engage in aerobic exercises for weight loss; weight/resistance exercises offer little value as they burn few calories.	❍	❍

The daily calorie intake of persons in the United States above age 19 years averages 1785 kcal for women and 2640 kcal for men. On an annual basis, this translates into a food intake of about 741 kg (1633 lb) (2008 latest data: www.ers.usda.gov/Data/FoodConsumption/) that includes approximately 14.5 kg of eggs, 121 kg of dairy products including fluid milk and related products, 89 kg of flour and cereal products, 49 kg of red meats (33 kg of poultry), 7.2 kg of fish and shellfish, 15 kg of cheese, 62 kg of caloric sweeteners, 40 kg of fats and oils, 155 kg of fruits and vegetables, 50 L of soft drinks, 34 L of wine, 83 L of beer, and 14 L of liquor! From age 21 to 50 years, consuming this amount of food yearly amounts to approximately 24 tons, or a total caloric input of 14 million calories! It is little wonder that just a slight increase (or decrease) in food consumption, even without any change in energy output, can dramatically change a person's body weight, typically by 0.5 to 1 lb yearly. This means that for a person age 21 in 2012 who weighs 150 lb, the weight gain of 1 lb a year would bring the new body weight to 179 lb at age 50 in 2041!

Physically active men and women often consume 50% more of many of the previously mentioned categories of foods, yet have better control of their yearly weight as they age. When calories from food exceed daily energy requirements, the excess calories store mainly as fat in adipose tissue. For example, eating an extra 2 oz of roasted peanuts daily theoretically would produce a weight gain of about 7.3 kg (16 lb) in only 1 year. Energy output must balance energy input to prevent this caloric disparity. Unfortunately, most of the time, this does not occur. This has led to a national and global crisis in excess caloric consumption and a frightening epidemic of overweightness and overfatness (obesity).

A random-digit telephone survey of nearly 110,000 US adults found that nearly 70% struggle to either lose weight (29% men and 40% women) or just maintain it.[112] Only one fifth of the 45 to 50 million Americans trying to lose weight follow the recommended combination of eating fewer calories and engaging in at least 150 min of weekly moderate physical activity. Those attempting weight loss spent over $80 billion in 2011 on weight-reduction products and services, often engaging in potentially harmful dietary practices and drug use while ignoring sensible approaches to weight loss maintenance. More than 2 million Americans collectively spend $150 million or more on over-the-counter appetite-suppressing diet pills that line the shelves of drugstores, health food and fitness centers, and supermarkets, not to mention sales via television and radio marketing, mail order, and the Internet.

JUST A FEW EXTRA POUNDS MAY SHORTEN LIFE

It's not just the body mass index (BMI) classification of obesity that raises the risk of premature death. One of the largest studies to date indicates that merely being overweight also carries significant health risks. The latest research with about 1.5 million healthy white adults found that those who were classified as overweight by BMI were 13% more likely to die during a 5- to 28-year follow-up period than counterparts whose weight was in an ideal range. For those classified as obese, the increased risk of dying prematurely ranged from 44 to 88%.[12]

A NATIONAL CONCERN

Despite the upswing in attempts at weight loss, Americans have become more overweight than a generation ago, with obesity increasing in all regions of the United States.[86,133] **FIGURE 14.1** shows the 2008 state-by-state prevalence of adult and childhood obesity in the United States. *Current classification by the National Heart, Lung, and Blood Institute (www.nhlbi.nih.gov) defines "overweight" as a BMI of 25 to 29.9 and "obesity" as a BMI equal to or greater than 30.* These standards place the prevalence of overweight and obesity in adults at about 130 million Americans or 65% of the population (including 35% of college students), up from 56% in 1982. Currently, more than 4 million persons exceed 300 lb, and more than 500,000 people (mostly males) exceed 400 lb—with the average adult woman now weighing an unprecedented 165 lb! Researchers maintain that if this trend continues, 70 to 75% of the US adult population may reach overweight or obesity status by the year 2020, with essentially the entire adult population becoming overweight within three generations.[22] Overweight occurrence particularly affects women and minority groups (Hispanic, African American, Pacific Islander). The major increase occurs from a near doubling of the obesity component to nearly one in three Americans over the past two decades.

FIGURE 14.2 displays the 2009 state-specific percentages of US adults categorized as obese (lower right panel), white non-hispanic and black race (upper 2 panels) or Hispanic ethnicity (lower left panel). For the total population of US adults, the prevalence of obesity varied from 18.6 to 34.4% among states. Obesity prevalence was 36.8% for non-Hispanic blacks and 30.7% for Hispanics. Further analysis about obesity prevalence indicated that those who did not graduate from high

COLORADO: THE ONLY STATE WITH AN ADULT OBESITY FATNESS RATE BELOW 20%

The most recent data on adult and childhood obesity rates in the United States present more disappointing news about the war on obesity ("*F as in Fat: How Obesity Threatens America's Future 2011*." Trust for America's Health and the Robert Wood Johnson Foundation. Visit www.healthyamericans.org/report/88/ for an interactive state-by-state review of adult and childhood obesity rates). The following summarizes the 2011 major findings for adults:

- Adult obesity rates increased in 16 states in 2010. No state decreased. Northeastern and Western states continue to have the lowest obesity rates, with 38 states exceeding 25%.
- Twelve states have obesity rates above 30% (Al, AR, KY, LA, MS, MI, MS, OK, SC, TN, TX, WV). Four years ago, only one state exceeded 30%. Mississippi had the highest rate of obesity at 34.4%. Colorado was the only state with a rate below 20% (19.8%).
- Obesity rates rose for a second year in a row in six states (IL, KY, MA, MO, RI, and TX) and for a third year in a row in five states (FL, KS, ME, OK, and VT).
- Obesity and obesity-related diseases (diabetes and hypertension) continue to remain the highest in the South.
- Except for Michigan, the South hosts the top 10 most states with the highest rates of obesity and overweight. Nine of 10 states with the highest diabetes and physical inactivity rates are in the South, as are the 10 states with the highest rates of hypertension.
- The number of adults who report they do not engage in any physical activity rose in 14 states in the past year. California and Texas declined in adult physical inactivity levels.
- Obesity increased in nine states for men and in 10 states for women, and decreased for women in one state (NV). Those who did not graduate high school have the highest rate of obesity (32.8%). Those who graduated high school but did not go on to college or a technical school have the second highest obesity rate (30.4%).
- Households with less than $15,000 annual income have a 33.8% obesity rate, followed by

households with annual incomes between $15,000 and $25,000 (31.8%), $25,000 and $35,000 (29.7%), and $35,000 and $50,000 (29.5%). Households with incomes above $50,000 have a 24.6% obesity rate.

school (32.9%), and persons age 50 to 59 years (31.1%) and 60 to 69 years (30.9%) were disproportionally affected. By state, obesity prevalence ranged from 18.6% in Colorado to 34.4% in Mississippi; only Colorado (lower right panel shown in blue) and the District of Columbia (19.7%; not shown) had prevalences of less than 20%; nine states had prevalence rates that exceeded 30% (Alabama, Arkansas, Kentucky, Louisiana, Mississippi, Missouri, Oklahoma, Tennessee, and West Virginia)! Similar statistics for obesity prevalence exist worldwide.

Disturbingly Prevalent Among Children

A 2009 report, "How Obesity Policies Are Failing in America," from the Trust for Americans Health (http://healthyamericans.org/reports/obesity2009/), provides further alarming data and trends regarding current strategies including school nutrition and physical activity policies to battle the obesity epidemic. The inset table of Figure 14.1 adds the prevalence of childhood obesity to the accumulating data on adults, with Mississippi (32.5%), Alabama (31.2%), West Virginia (31.1%), and Tennessee (30.2) showing prevalence rates above 30%. Eight of the 10 states

A SIGNIFICANT AND EXPENSIVE RISK TO HEALTH

The Centers for Disease Control and Prevention (CDC; www.cdc.gov/) ranks obesity as a close second to cigarette smoking as the leading cause of preventable death in America. Fourteen percent of the money spent on healthcare for American men age 50 to 69 went to obesity-related complications. If the body mass of the nation continues to increase at the current rate, obesity will account for about one in five healthcare dollars spent on middle-aged Americans by the year 2020.

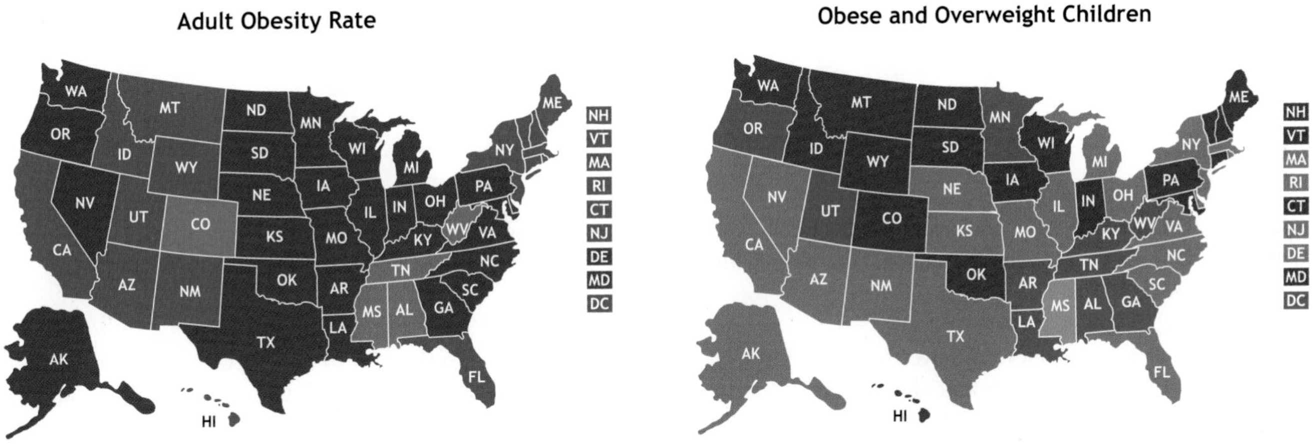

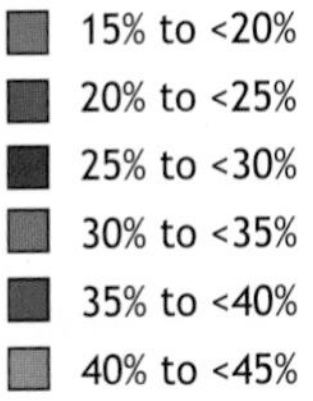

Note: 1 = Highest rate of adult obesity. Rankings are based on combining three years of data (2006-2008) from the U.S. Centers for Disease Control and Prevention's Behavioral Risk Factor Surveillance System to "stabilize" data for comparison purposes. This methodology, recommended by the CDC, compensates for any potential anomalies or usual changes due to the specific sample in any given year in any given state. Additional information about methodologies and confidence interval appears at http://healthyamericans.org/reports/obesity2009/. Adults with a BMI of 30 or higher are considered obese.

Top Ten Rank	Childhood Obesity Highest To Lowest Rankings by State	Percentage Obese
1.	Mississippi	32.5%
2.	Alabama	31.2%
3.	West Virginia	31.1%
4.	Tennessee	30.2%
5.	South Carolina	29.7%
6.	Oklahoma	29.5%
7.	Kentuncy	29.0%
8.	Louisiana	28.9%
9.	Michigan	28.8%
10.	Arkansas, Ohio	28.6%

FIGURE 14.1. Prevalence of adult and childhood obesity in the United States 2006–2008. Top 10 ranking for children is by percentage. (Adapted from Trust for America's Health. F as in fat 2009: how obesity policies are failing America. Available at: http://healthyamericans.org/reports/obesity2009/. Accessed October 30, 2011.)

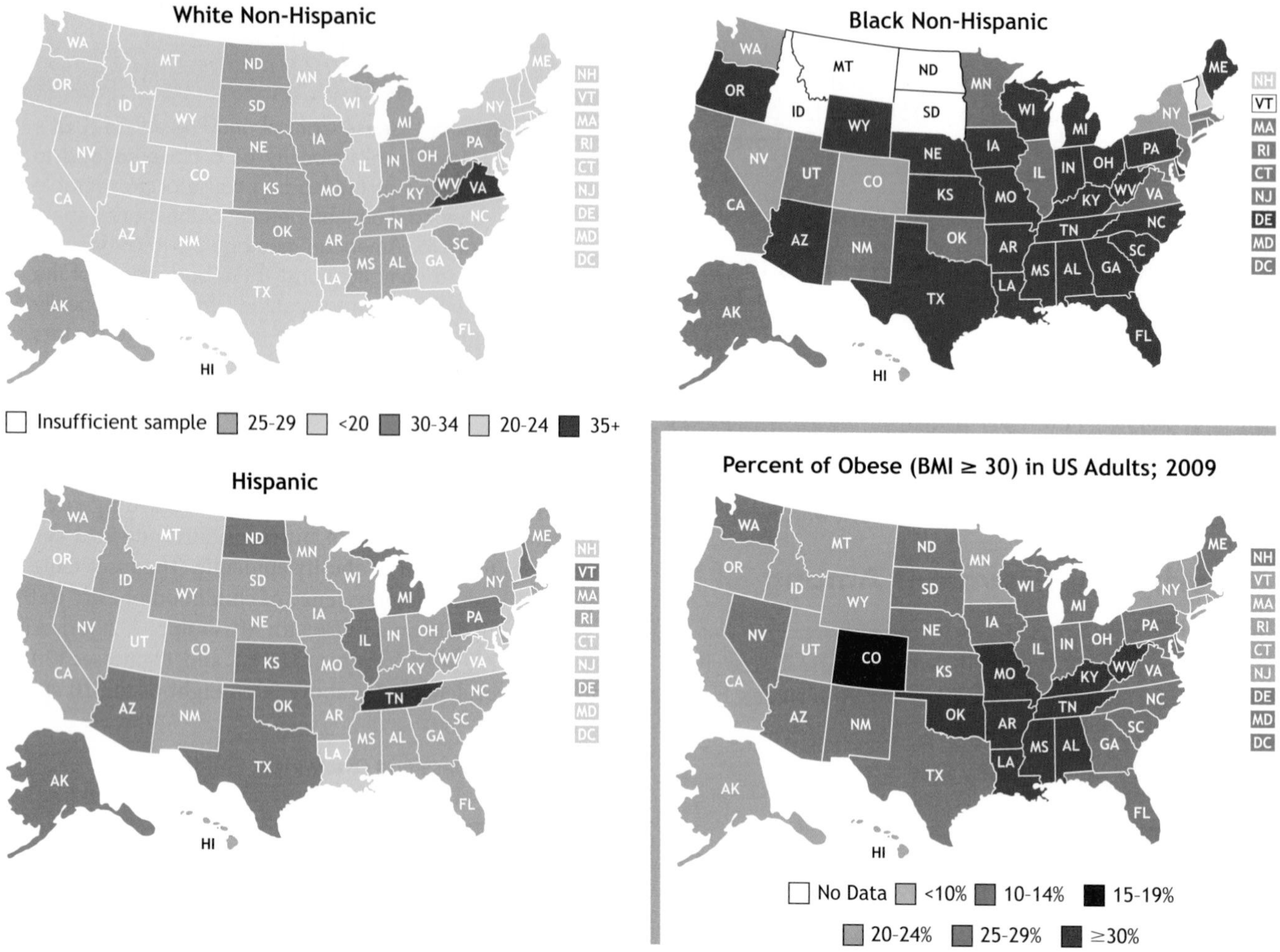

FIGURE 14.2. State-specific percentages of US adults categorized as obese by black/white race or Hispanic ethnicity. (From Centers for Disease Control and Prevention. U.S. obesity trends. Available at: **http://www.cdc.gov/obesity/data/trends.html**. Accessed Nov 8, 2011.)

with the highest rates of obese and overweight children were in the South. Childhood obesity rates have more than tripled since 1980.[94]

A MYPLATE FOR THE UNDER-2 SET?

Currently, one in five preschoolers (2–5 years old) are overweight or obese, and the majority of these children do not outgrow their baby fat. A June 2011 report from the Institute of Medicine (IOM; www.iom.edu/) claims that extra pounds early in life can lead to lasting harmful effects on health as children grow. Recommendations call for better guidelines to help parents and caregivers know how much toddlers should eat as they progress from baby food to more solid food items. Whereas babies drink milk only until they are full, children as young as 2 or 3 are sensitive to portion size: The larger the portion, the more they will eat. Also recommended is assurance that preschoolers get at least 15 min of physical activity for every hour spent in child care.

According to the World Health Organization (WHO; www.who.int/), the number of overweight children younger than the age of 5 in 2010 was estimated to be more than 43 million. Almost 35 million of these children live in developing countries.

A child or adolescent with a high BMI percentile ranking shows a considerable risk of being overweight or

INCREASED CALORIE INTAKE AND A DEPRESSED ENERGY OUTPUT SPELL TROUBLE

By 2025, nearly 75% of the American population will classify as overweight, with about one third classified as obese. More than likely, a sedentary lifestyle and ready availability of tasty, fatty, and calorie-rich foods served in increasingly "supersized" portions remain prime culprits for expressing unhealthy patterns of preexisting susceptible genes in the fattening of Western civilization.[97]

obese at age 35, and that risk increases with the youth's age.[46,50,124,125] More than 60% of children between ages 5 and 10 years exhibit at least one risk factor for cardiovascular disease. Excessive fatness in youth represents even more of an adult health risk than obesity begun in adulthood. Overweight children and adolescents, regardless of final body weight as adults, exhibit greater risk for a broad range of illnesses as adults than children who maintain a normal body weight.[14,32,49]

GLOBAL OBESITY EPIDEMIC

Obesity represents a complex condition with serious social and psychological dimensions that impacts all age and socioeconomic groups and threatens to overwhelm both developed and developing countries. The WHO's latest global data updated in March 2011 indicate the following grim statistics:

1. Worldwide obesity has more than doubled since 1980.
2. In 2008, 1.5 billion adults age 20 and older were overweight. Of these, over 200 million men and nearly 300 million women were obese. This means that more than one in 10 of the world's adult population was obese.
3. Sixty-five percent of the world's population lives in countries where overweight and obesity kill more people than underweight.
4. By 2015, approximately 2.3 billion adults will be overweight and more than 700 million will be obese.

The WHO posits that increased consumption of more energy-dense, nutrient-poor foods with high levels of sugar and saturated fats and reduced physical activity have led to obesity rates that have risen threefold or more since 1980 in some areas besides North America—the United Kingdom, Eastern Europe, the Middle East, the Pacific Islands, Australia, and China.[93]

CALORIC INTAKE CONTINUES TO INCREASE

Adult women now eat 335 more calories daily than in 1970, whereas the daily intake for men has increased by 168 calories. In 2000, this translated to an average yearly increase of 278 lb of food per capita intake. On the surface, some of this increase seems desirable because it includes increased vegetable intake. Nevertheless, nearly one third of the vegetables comprised iceberg lettuce, French fries, and potato chips. The grain component of this increase consisted of processed flour-based items such as pasta, tortillas, and hamburger buns, not the fiber-rich whole-grain breads and cereals recommended. Highly processed, low-fiber carbohydrates have the equivalent nutritional value of table sugar.

TABLE 14.1 lists the global prevalence of adult obesity in 153 countries through 2010. The country of Papua New Guinea has the highest rates of adult obesity—74.8% for men and 79.5% for women. The United States ranks 18th overall. Worldwide, women in 84 countries have lower obesity rates than the rate in the state of Colorado in the United States! The most underdeveloped countries in the world have obesity prevalence rates below 3% (e.g., Eritrea, Ethiopia, Madagascar, Central African Republic, Democratic Republic of the Congo, Malawi, Rwanda, Zambia). Besides having a poor standard of living with less than modest economic resources, these countries have a high infant mortality rate and generally lower adult life expectancy. Most of these countries also have a high prevalence of foodborne or waterborne diseases, bacterial diarrhea, hepatitis A, and typhoid fever.

Connections to the Past

Claude Bernard (1813–1878)

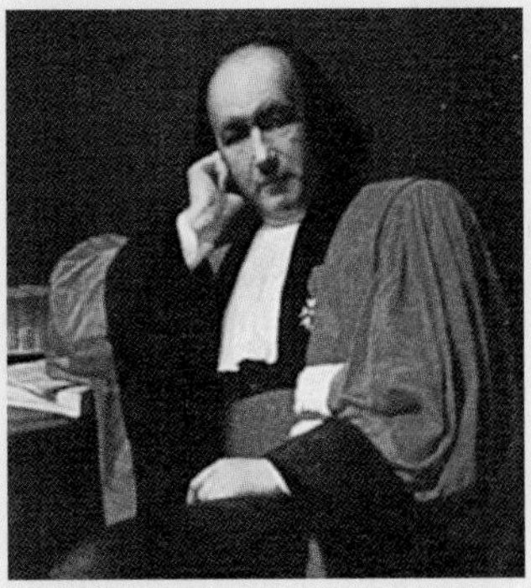

Claude Bernard, generally acclaimed as the greatest physiologist of all time, succeeded François Magendie (1783–1855) as Professor of Medicine at the Collège de France. Bernard interned in medicine and surgery before serving as laboratory assistant (*préparateur*) to Magendie in 1839. Three years later, he followed Magendie to the Hôtel-Dieu hospital in Paris. For the next 35 years, Bernard discovered fundamental properties about physiology. He participated in the explosion of scientific knowledge in the mid-19th century. Bernard indicated his single-minded devotion to research by producing an MD thesis (1843) on gastric juice and its role in nutrition ("Du Sac Gastrique et de Son Rôle dans la Nutrition"). Ten years later, he received the Doctorate in Natural Sciences for his study entitled, "*Recherches sur une Nouvelle Fonction du Foie, Consideré Comme Organe Producteur de Matière Sucrée Chez l'Homme et les Animaux*" ("Research on a New Function of the Liver as a Producer of Sugar in Man and Animals"). Prior to this seminal research, scientists assumed that only plants could synthesize sugar and that sugar within animals must be derived from ingested plant matter. Bernard disproved this notion by documenting the presence of sugar in the hepatic vein of a dog whose diet lacked carbohydrate.

thePoint *Visit thePoint.lww.com/MKKSEN4e for more details about Bernard's seven crucial discoveries that impacted medicine, nutrition, and exercise science.*

TABLE 14.1 Global Prevalence Estimates of Adult Obesity in 2012 by Country (Percentage of Adult Population with Body Mass Index [BMI] of 30 or Higher, Ranked from Highest to Lowest Percentage of the Adult Female Population)[a]

Rank	Country	Male %	Female %	Rank	Country	Male %	Female %
1	Tonga	46.6	70.3	26	Bahamas	13.9	28
2	Samoa	32.9	63	27	South Africa	8.8	27.4
3	Nauru	55.7	60.5	28	Guyana	14.3	26.9
4	Kuwait	36.4	47.9	29	Venezuela	25	26.4
5	Niue	15	46	30	England	26	26
6	Qatar	34.6	45.3	31	New Zealand	24.7	26
7	French Polynesia	36.3	44.3	32	Israel	19.9	25.7
8	Saudi Arabia	26.4	44	33	Greece	27.9	25.6
9	Palestine	23.9	42.5	34	Bosnia & Herzegovina	17	25
10	Cook Island	40.6		35	Australia	25.6	24
11	Egypt	18.2	39.5	36	Jamaica	7.6	23.9
12	Panama	27.9	36.1	37	Poland	20.8	23.8
13	USA	35.5	35.8	38	Oman	16.7	23.8
14	Paraguay	22.9	35.7	39	Cyprus	26.6	23.7
15	Mexico	24.2	34.5	40	Lesotho		23.7
16	Seychelles	14.7	34.2	41	Canada	27.6	23.5
17	Bahrain	23.3	34.1	42	Ireland (Northern)	25	23
18	UAE	17.1	31.4	43	Croatia	21.6	22.7
19	Marshall Islands	21	31	44	Tunisia	6.7	22.7
20	Barbados	10	31	45	Czech Republic	23.9	22.3
21	Turkey (Urban)	16.5	29.4	46	Italy	18	22
22	Chile	19.6	29.3	47	Morocco	8.2	21.7
23	Jordan		28.7	48	Russia	10.3	21.6
24	St Lucia	8.4	28.7	49	Spain	24.4	21.4
25	Scotland	26.6	28.1	50	Algeria	8.8	21.4

[a] Please note not all surveys are age standardised and due to varying methodologies are not always directly comparable. Prevalence's are based on the best available data for the country, in some circumstances the data may be based on sub national surveys. Sources and references are available from IASO www.iaso.org. © International Association for the Study of Obesity, London – January 2012

HEALTH RISKS AND FINANCIAL IMPACT OF OBESITY

Excess body fat represents the second leading cause of preventable death in America (cigarette smoking ranks first), with the cost of obesity-related diseases exceeding $140 billion annually in the year 2010. One trip to the doctor annually made by 25% of the total obese American population costs more than $810 million based on an average doctor visit charge of $60. Even more disconcerting, the estimated number of annual deaths attributed to obesity per se ranges between 280,000 and 325,000.[23,37,87]

On a positive note, increasing physical activity exerts a considerable influence in reducing risk for cardiovascular disease and has a more moderate effect on type 2 diabetes risk. In essence, increased adiposity and reduced physical activity strongly and independently predict death risk by these two conditions.[60] These consequences heighten a sedentary, overweight person's risks of poor health at any given level of excess weight. Unfortunately, the increasing prevalence of obesity has slowed the decline in coronary heart disease among middle-aged women.[59] Obese and overweight persons with two or more heart disease risk factors should reduce excess weight. Overweight persons without other risk factors should at least maintain their current body weight. Even a modest weight reduction improves insulin sensitivity and the blood lipid profile and prevents or delays the onset of diabetes in high-risk persons.[48] Epidemiologic evidence also indicates that excess body weight carries an independent and powerful risk for congestive heart failure. In terms of cancer risk, maintaining a BMI below 25 could prevent one of every six cancer deaths in the United States (14% in men and 20% in women), or about 90,000 deaths yearly.[23]

TWELVE SPECIFIC HEALTH RISKS OF EXCESSIVE BODY FAT

1. Abnormal plasma lipid and lipoprotein levels
2. Endometrial, breast, prostate, and colon cancers
3. Enormous psychological burden and social stigmatization and discrimination
4. Gallbladder disease
5. Hypertension, stroke, and deep vein thrombosis
6. Impaired cardiac function from increased mechanical work and autonomic and left ventricular dysfunction
7. Increased insulin resistance in children and adults and type 2 diabetes (80% of these patients are overweight)
8. Menstrual irregularities
9. Osteoarthritis, degenerative joint disease, and gout
10. Problems receiving anesthetics during surgery
11. Renal disease
12. Sleep apnea, mechanical ventilatory constraints (particularly in exercise), and pulmonary disease from impaired function because of added effort to move the chest wall

EXCESS BODY WEIGHT LINKED TO DIVERSE CANCERS

In addition to endometrial cancer, extra pounds now link to occurrence of postmenopausal breast cancer and cancers of the colon, esophagus, kidney, and pancreas. A likely association also exists for leukemia, lymphoma, and ovarian, cervical, gallbladder, liver, and aggressive prostate cancer.

Related healthcare costs of obesity by insurance status also have soared (win.niddk.nih.gov/statistics/&#econ).

1. **For each obese beneficiary:**
- Medicare pays $1723 more than it pays for normal-weight beneficiaries.
- Medicaid pays $1021 more than it pays for normal-weight beneficiaries.
- Private insurers pay $1140 more than they pay for normal-weight beneficiaries.

2. **For each obese patient:**
- Medicare pays $95 more for an inpatient service, $693 more for a non-inpatient service, and $608 more for prescription drugs in comparison with normal-weight patients.
- Medicaid pays $213 more for an inpatient service, $175 more for a non-inpatient service, and $230 more for prescription drugs in comparison with normal-weight patients.
- Private insurers pay $443 more for an inpatient service, $398 more for a non-inpatient service, and $284 more for prescription drugs in comparison with normal-weight patients.

FIGURE 14.3 depicts the powerful effect of excess body weight in predicting death at older age. The most profound effect occurs for persons with a BMI that exceeds 30 (gold line). Overweight but not obese, nonsmoking men and women in their mid-30s to mid-40s die at least 3 years sooner than normal-weight counterparts—a risk as damaging to life expectancy as cigarette smoking.[96] Obese persons can expect an approximately 7-year decrease in longevity. In industrialized nations, economic factors operate to counter the advice of most health professionals to eat less and increase the time devoted to more vigorous physical activities of daily living. Food continues to become cheaper and more fat laden, while most occupations have decreased their exertional demands.

LIFESTYLE MODIFICATION AMONG PATIENTS WITH PREDIABETES COULD SAVE BILLIONS

Even a modest sustained weight reduction in overweight and obese prediabetic persons would profoundly limit the incidence of type 2 diabetes and save Medicare between $1.8 and $2.3 billion over a 10-year period. Estimated savings would be $3.0 to $3.7 billion if equally overweight people at risk for cardiovascular disease (those with hypertension and dyslipidemia) also enrolled in community-based lifestyle interventions geared toward weight loss and increased physical activity. This would translate to lifetime Medicare savings of approximately $7 to $15 billion, depending on how broadly program eligibility was defined and actual levels of program participation. Successful adoption of such programs would extend benefits beyond diabetes prevention to reduce risk of heart disease, cancer, musculoskeletal problems, and perhaps cognitive decline.

Thorpe KE, Yang Z. Enrolling people with prediabetes ages 60-64 in a proven weight loss program could save medicare $7 billion or more. *Health Aff (Millwood)* 2011;30:1673.

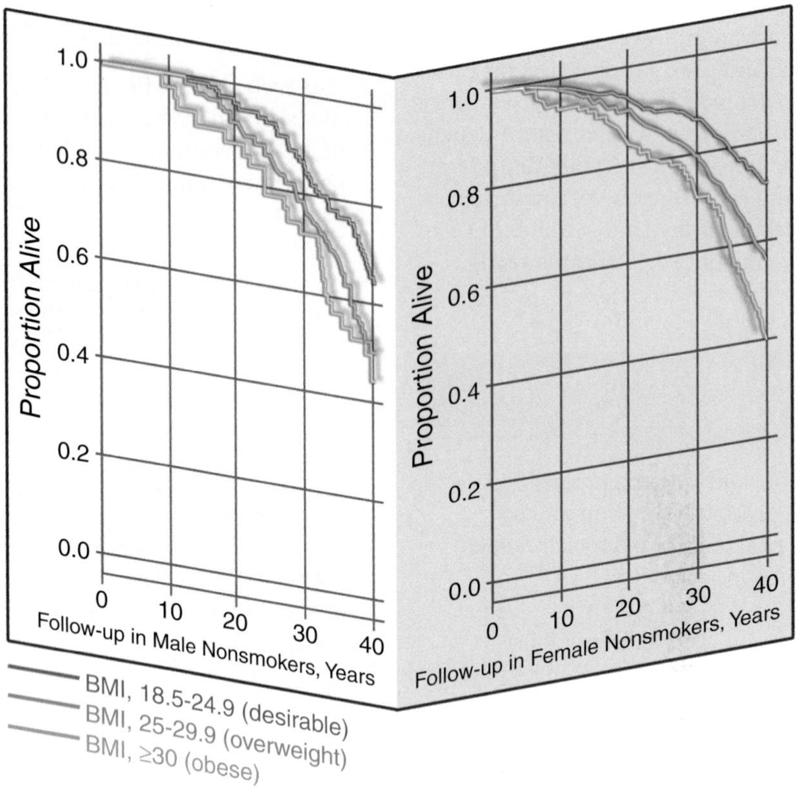

FIGURE 14.3. Survival estimates for groups of women and men categorized by body mass index (BMI). (From Peeters A, et al. Obesity in adulthood and its consequences for life expectancy. *Ann Intern Med* 2003;138:24.)

INCREASED PHYSICAL ACTIVITY MODIFIES AGE-RELATED INCREASES IN BODY MASS AND BODY FAT

Maintaining an increased level of physical activity modifies age-related increases in body weight and body fat. Prospec - tive 7-year survey data from male and female runners who maintained detailed records of body weight and abdominal and hip girths during 7 years of continuous run training confirmed that persons who accumulated more running miles ≥ 48 km · wk^{-1} or 29.8 miles · wk^{-1}) reduced the normal aging tendency to gain body weight (and increase BMI) and body fat more than less physically active runners (≤ 24 km · wk^{-1} or 14.9 miles · wk^{-1}).[145] For example, the yearly gain in body weight for men between the ages of 18 and 24 years who exceeded 48 km · wk^{-1} was 0.83 kg compared to a gain of 1.56 kg for the same age group of men who ran less than 24 km · wk^{-1}. For female counterparts, the change in body weight over a 7-year interval was about three times less (0.39 kg · y^{-1}) in women who exceeded running 48 km · wk^{-1} than women who ran less distance (0.91 kg · y^{-1}). Supportive data[130,131,143] indicate that increased physical activity maintained over protracted time periods is more important as an independent factor to minimize the increase in body weight that occurs normally with aging. This contrasts with simply reducing body weight repeatedly over a short time span of weeks or even a year to normalize any excess weight accumulation. The public health message seems clear—increased *regular* physical activity as a lifestyle choice, not chronic dieting and/or short-term exercise, should become the important consideration in a healthful prescription for weight control and good health.

GENETICS PLAYS A ROLE IN BODY WEIGHT REGULATION

Body weight status should be viewed as the end result of complex interactions between one's genes and environmental influences, rather than simply the consequence of psychological factors that affect eating behaviors. Research with twins, adopted children, and specific segments of the population attribute up to 80% of the risk of becoming obese to genetic factors.[15,16,42]

In our modern scientific era, molecular geneticists are determined to unravel intimate secrets of subcellular function related to obesity, trying to answer a seemingly simple question: Why have so many people become so fat, and what can be done to resolve the problem? British researchers in December 2009 provided clear evidence of a biological mechanism that helps to explain why some people are more susceptible to gaining weight in a world dominated by high-calorie food

PHYSICAL ACTIVITY AND DECREASED MORTALITY: A LITTLE IS GOOD BUT MORE MAY BE BETTER

The largest prospective cohort of US adults (527,265 men and women age 50 to 71 years) enrolled in the NIH-AARP Diet and Health Study (www.dietandhealth.cancer.gov) examined the relationship between physical activity and overall mortality. Results showed that persons who vigorously exercised a minimum of 20 min 1 to 3 times a month, 1 to 2 times weekly, 3 to 4 times a week, or 5 or more times per week showed a lower mortality relative risk (more frequent physical activity more effective) compared with those who rarely exercised. These findings indicate that vigorous physical activity reduces the risk of premature mortality for women and men. (Data courtesy of Dr. Michael Leitzmann, U.S. National Cancer Institute.) Additional supportive data for lower mortality risk with higher levels of occupational physical activity come from a 24-year follow-up analysis of 47,405 Norwegian men and women.[62]

and a sedentary lifestyle. The experiment turned the spotlight on the protein-coding gene *FTO*, which affects a person's risk of becoming obese or overweight. The *FTO* gene exists in two varieties, and all persons inherit two copies of the gene. Children who inherited two copies of one variant were 70% more likely to be obese than those who inherited two copies of the other variant. Fifty percent of children who inherited one copy of each *FTO* variant had a 30% greater obesity risk. The groundbreaking part of the study involved a subgroup of 76 children whose metabolism was monitored for 10 days and who ate special test meals at school. The available food was measured before and after consumption to see how much was consumed. Interestingly, the FTO variant did not depress metabolism but instead increased the tendency to eat more high-calorie foods in the test meals. In each case, the extra weight was explained entirely by more body fat, not increased muscle mass or structural differences like being taller.

BIOCHEMICALS THAT INFLUENCE EATING BEHAVIORS: SIGNALS THAT TRAVEL AMONG THE DIGESTIVE TRACT, ADIPOSE TISSUE, AND EATING CONTROL CENTERS

Leptin: Produced by adipocytes. Normal levels signal the hypothalamus to maintain food intake so body weight remains stable. Below-normal leptin levels signal the brain to increase appetite so that body fat levels increase. Leptin also elevates metabolic rate.

Peptide YY3-36 (PYY): Produced by intestinal cells in response to food intake. It then travels to the hypothalamus to inhibit the urge to eat. Overweight persons normally make less of this satiety signal than persons of normal body weight.

Neuropeptide Y: A transmitter protein of the nervous system that stimulates food intake and regulates metabolism and fat synthesis.

Ghrelin: Exerts effects opposite of leptin. A powerful appetite-stimulating hormone (also slows energy output) produced in the stomach and small intestine. Only known natural appetite stimulant made outside the brain. Drugs that block this hormone would not only stimulate weight loss but also increase energy expenditure.

Melanocortin-4: Possibly supplies the signal to stop eating. About 10% of obese patients show genetic mutations in the gene that regulates this compound.

CB(1) Cannabinoid Receptors: Signaling mechanism in the gut that responds to oral sensory signals that drive dietary fat intake. The endocannabinoid system plays central and peripheral roles in regulating food intake, energy balance, and reward. Such a powerful regulatory influence over fat intake by providing positive feedback control of fat intake that encourages people to seek more fatty foods (while not responding to carbohydrate or protein surges) could be a target for future antiobesity drugs such as rimonabant (also known as SR141716; trade names include Acomplia, Bethin, Monaslim, Remonabent, Riobant, Slimona, Rimoslim, and Zimulti).

NOT SIMPLY A LACK OF WILLPOWER

The linkage of genetic and molecular abnormalities to obesity allows researchers to view overfatness as a disease rather than a psychological flaw. Athletes in body weight–related sports who have a genetic propensity to accumulate fat must constantly battle to achieve (and maintain) an optimal body weight and body composition for competitive performance.

Genetic makeup does not necessarily cause obesity, but it does lower the threshold for its development; it contributes to differences in weight gain for persons fed identical daily caloric excess. **FIGURE 14.4** summarizes findings from a large number of persons representing nine different types of backgrounds. Genetic factors determined about 25% of the transmissible variation among people in percentage body fat and total fat mass, whereas the largest transmissible variation related to a cultural effect. *In an obesity-producing environment (sedentary and stressful with easy access to calorie-dense food), the genetically susceptible person gains weight.*

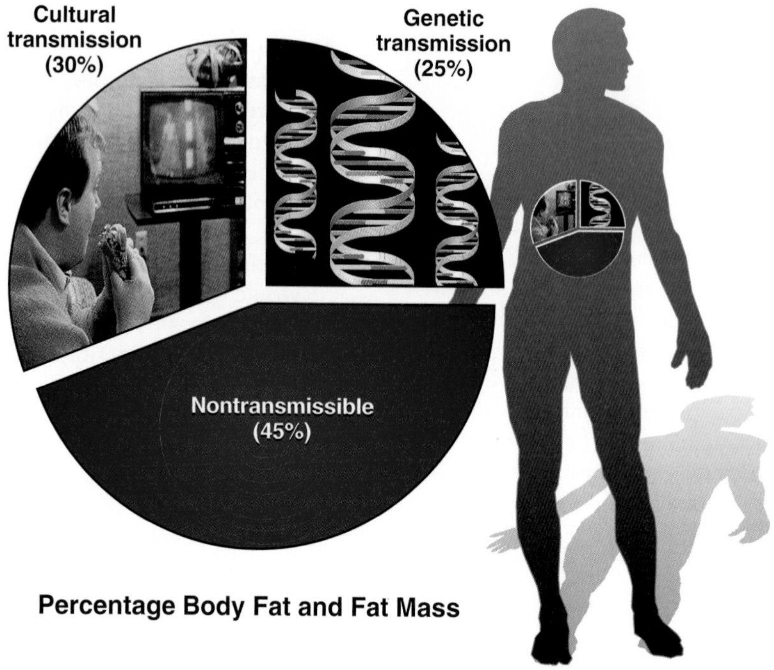

FIGURE 14.4. Total transmissible variance for body fat. Total body fat and percentage body fat determined by hydrostatic weighing. (Data from Bouchard C, et al. Inheritance of the amount and distribution of human body fat. *Int J Obes* 1988;12:205.)

Racial Factors Contribute

The greater prevalence of obesity among black women (about 50%) compared with white women (33%) frequently has been attributed to racial differences in food and exercise habits and cultural attitudes toward body weight. Studies of obese women whose weight averaged 224 lb show that small differences in resting metabolism also contribute to the racial differences in obesity.[43,64] On average, black women burned nearly 100 fewer calories each day during rest than white counterparts; the slower rate of processing calories persists even after adjusting for differences in body mass and body composition. The greater energy economy of black women during exercise and throughout the day reflects an inherited trait because it persists both before and after weight loss.[135] This "racial" effect, which also exists among children and adolescents,[118,123] predisposes a black female to gain weight and more readily regain it after weight loss. A 100-kcal reduction in daily metabolism translates to nearly 1 lb of body fat gained each month. Such data suggest that black female athletes with weight problems may experience greater difficulty achieving and maintaining a goal body weight for competition than an overweight white counterpart.

A Mutant Gene and Leptin

Researchers have linked human obesity to a mutant gene. Studies at the University of Cambridge in England identified a specific defect in two genes that control body weight. Two cousins from a Pakistani family in England inherited a defect in the gene that synthesizes leptin, a crucial body weight–regulating protein hormone produced by adipose tissue and released into the bloodstream that acts on the hypothalamus. Congenital absence of leptin produced continual hunger and marked obesity in these children. The second genetic defect observed in an English patient affected the body's response to leptin's "signal." This triggering signal largely determines how much one eats, how much energy one expends, and ultimately how much one weighs.

The genetic model in **FIGURE 14.5** proposes that the *ob* gene normally becomes activated in adipose tissue (and perhaps muscle tissue), where it encodes and stimulates production of a body fat–signaling, hormonelike protein (***ob* protein** or **leptin**), which then enters the bloodstream. This satiety signal molecule travels to the arcuate nucleus, a collection of specialized neurons in the mediobasal hypothalamus that controls appetite and metabolism and develops soon after birth. Normally, leptin blunts the urge to eat when caloric intake maintains ideal fat stores.[28] Leptin may affect certain neurons in the hypothalamic region that stimulates the production of chemicals that suppress appetite and/or reduce the levels of neurochemicals that stimulate appetite.[98] Such mechanisms would explain how body fat remains intimately "connected" via a physiologic pathway to the brain to regulate energy balance. In essence, leptin availability (or its lack) affects the neurochemistry of appetite and the brain's dynamic "wiring" to possibly impact appetite and obesity in adulthood.

Gender, hormones, pharmacologic agents, and the body's current energy requirements also affect leptin production. Neither short- nor long-term exercise meaningfully affects leptin, independent of the effects of exercise on total adipose tissue mass. Importantly, leptin alone does not

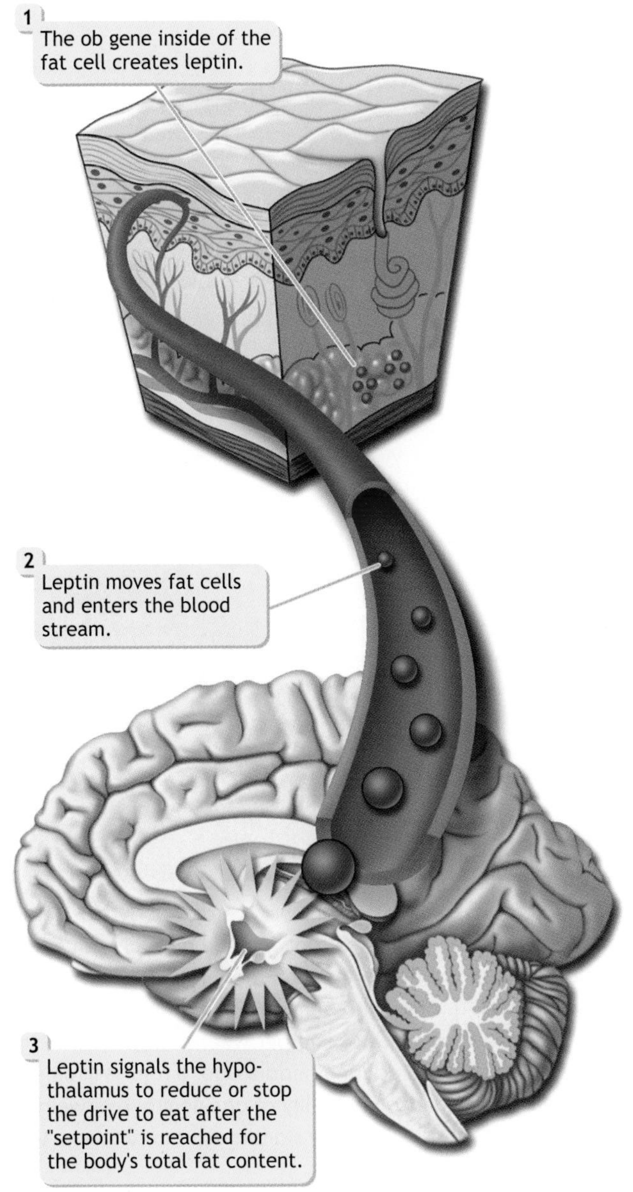
1
The ob gene inside of the fat cell creates leptin.
2
Leptin moves fat cells and enters the blood stream.
3
Leptin signals the hypo-thalamus to reduce or stop the drive to eat after the "setpoint" is reached for the body's total fat content.

FIGURE 14.5. Genetic model for obesity. A malfunction of the satiety gene affects production of the satiety hormone leptin. Underproduction of leptin disrupts proper function of the hypothalamus (Step #3), the center that regulates the body's fat level. (Model based on research conducted at Rockefeller University, New York, NY.)

determine obesity or fully explain why some people eat whatever they want and gain little weight, while others become overfat at the same caloric intake.

The linkage of genetic and molecular abnormalities to obesity allows researchers to view overfatness as a disease instead of a psychological flaw. Early identification of one's genetic predisposition toward obesity makes it possible to begin diet and exercise interventions before obesity sets in and fat loss becomes exceedingly difficult. Pharmaceutical companies continue their attempt to synthesize compounds that produce satiety or impact the resting rate of fat catabolism. These chemicals would control weight with a smaller caloric intake and fewer feelings of hunger and deprivation that often accompany conventional food restriction plans.[27]

PHYSICAL ACTIVITY: A CRUCIAL COMPONENT IN WEIGHT CONTROL

The standard dietary approach to weight loss (dieting) that decreases caloric intake below the requirement for current weight maintenance generally helps overweight or overfat patients lose about 0.5 kg · week. Success at preventing weight regain, however, remains relatively poor, averaging between 5 and 20%. Weight-loss professionals now argue that regular physical activity, through either recreation or occupation, effectively contributes to preventing weight gain and thwarts the tendency to regain lost weight.[55,63,75,138] For example, persons who maintain weight loss over time show greater muscle strength and engage in more physical activity than counterparts who regained lost weight.[106] Variations in physical activity alone accounted for more than 75% of the regained body weight. Such findings point to the need to identify and promote strategies that increase regular physical activity. Current national guidelines by the Surgeon General (**www.surgeongeneral.gov/**) and Institute of Medicine of the National Academy of Sciences (**www.iom.edu/**) both recommend a minimum of 30 to 60 min of moderate physical activity daily. We endorse an increase to at least 75 min of total daily exercise (preferably 90 min over and above that required during "normal" living) to combat the prevalence of obesity in the US population.

Older men and women who maintain active lifestyles thwart the "normal" pattern of fat gain in adulthood. Middle-aged male distance runners remain leaner than sedentary counterparts.[140] Time spent in physical activity inversely relates to body fat level in young and middle-aged men who exercise regularly. Surprisingly, no relationship emerged between the runners' body fat level and caloric intake. Thus, the greater level of body fat among active middle-aged men compared with younger, more active counterparts resulted from less vigorous training, not greater energy intake.

From age 3 months to 1 year, the total energy expenditure of infants who later became overweight averaged 21% less than infants with normal weight gain.[102,105] For children age 6 to 9 years, percentage body fat inversely related to physical activity level in boys but not in girls.[9] Overfat preadolescent children generally spend less time in physical activity or engage in lower-intensity physical activity than normal-weight peers.[26,29,101] By the time young girls reach adolescence, many do no leisure-time physical activity. For girls, the decline in time spent in physical activity averaged nearly 100% among blacks and 64% among whites between ages 9 or 10 and 15 or 16.[70] By age 16 or 17, 56% of the black girls and 31% of the white girls reported no leisure-time physical activity. The 24-h energy expenditure of young-adult Native Americans inversely related to body weight changes over a 2-year period.[45] A four times greater risk of gaining more than 7.5 kg occurred in persons with low rather than high 24-h energy expenditures.

Benefits of Increased Energy Output with Aging

Maintaining a lifestyle that includes a regular but constant level of endurance-type exercise attenuates but does not fully forestall the tendency to add weight through middle age. Sedentary men and women who begin an exercise regimen lose weight and body fat compared with those who remain sedentary; those who stop exercising gain more body weight compared to those who continue to remain physically active. Moreover, the amount of weight change is proportional to the change in exercise dose.[136] **FIGURE 14.6** displays the association between distance run and BMI and waist circumference in all age categories. Active men typically remained leaner than sedentary counterparts for each age group; men who ran longer distances each week weighed less than those who ran shorter distances. The typical man who maintained a constant weekly running distance through middle age gained 3.3 lb, and waist size increased about three fourths of an inch, regardless of distance run. Such findings suggest that by age 50, a physically active man can expect to weigh about 10 lb more (with a 2-in larger waist) than he weighed at age 20 despite maintaining a constant level of increased physical activity. To counter weight gain in middle age, one should gradually increase the amount of weekly exercise by the equivalent of running 1.4 miles extra per week for each year of age starting at about age 30. One can achieve the same effect without additional exercise by modestly reducing energy (food) intake while making more nutritious food selections.

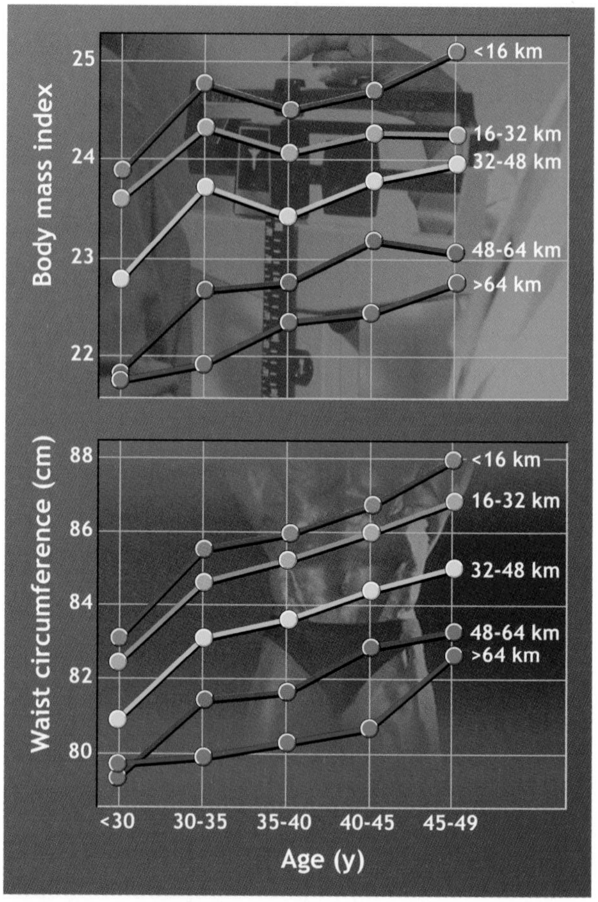

FIGURE 14.6. Relationship among average body mass index (*top*) and waist circumference (*bottom*) and age for men who maintained constant weekly running for varying distances (<16 to >64 km · wk^{-1}). Men who annually increase their running distance by 1.39 miles (2.24 km) per week compensate for the anticipated weight gain during middle age. (From Williams PT. Evidence for the incompatibility of age-neutral overweight and age-neutral physical activity standards from runners. *Am J Clin Nutr* 1997;65:1391.)

WEIGHT LOSS: A UNIQUE DILEMMA FOR THE COMPETITIVE ATHLETE

For many "overweight" athletes whose competitive careers have ended, achieving a lighter body weight and favorable body composition (combined with proper nutritional practices) offers overall health benefits. For the athlete currently competing, successful performance depends on achieving an "ideal" body mass and body composition.[57] In figure skating, ballet dancing, springboard diving, gymnastics, and bodybuilding, success often requires a predefined "lean aesthetic look." To complicate matters, the relatively low intensity of training in some of these sports contributes little to fat loss.

Reduced Body Size Affects Exercise Performance

In weight-bearing competitive racewalking, running, cross-country skiing, and ice skating, energy cost relates directly to body mass.[144] Consequently, achieving the lightest body weight without compromising physiologic function and metabolic capacity should improve performance. In weight-supported sports such as swimming, body weight reduction may not have as dramatic an effect on performance, although a smaller body size should reduce the drag forces that impede movement through the water.

A reasonable approach to enhance performance for some athletes should involve reducing body weight, particularly fat mass. Pole vaulters and jumpers who reduce body weight without compromising skill and power-output capacity achieve greater ease in overcoming gravity's downward pull. The same holds true for runners, skaters, cyclists, and others who compete at high movement velocities. Not only does the resistance of gravity diminish with a lighter body weight, but also the impeding effects of the drag force created by air (or water) are reduced with a smaller body frontal surface area.

A Prudent Approach Most Effective

A person can reduce body weight in a relatively short time by restricting food and fluid intake and sweating excessively. Body weight loss in this situation occurs mainly from water loss and depletion of liver and muscle glycogen reserves. Longer term attempts at weight loss through semistarvation increase risks of depressing resting metabolism (making continued weight loss more difficult) and increasing loss of lean tissue, glycogen stores, and muscular strength and power. Severe dehydration in trying to "make weight" also places these persons at risk for heat injury. Combining moderate food restriction with additional daily physical activity offers the greatest flexibility for achieving fat loss, yet remaining well nourished for training and peak performance.

The potential to improve competitive performance with weight loss assumes that any lost weight does not adversely affect skill, strength, or power capacity. If these important determinants of performance deteriorate, the athlete does worse, not better. The weight loss program must not adversely affect daily training. One should view weight loss from a longer term perspective, because body fat's contribution to an energy deficit increases as the duration of weight loss progresses. No more than 1 or 2 lb (about 1% of body mass) should be lost per week to minimize adverse effects on fat-free body mass (FFM), nutrient status, overall health, and exercise performance. Food composition tables, Internet nutritional tables (e.g., **www.nal.usda.gov/fnic/foodcomp/search/**), or appropriate computer software (e.g., **http://fnic.nal.usda.gov/**) should assess the diet's nutrient status to ensure maintenance of the predetermined daily caloric deficit and recommended carbohydrate, protein, and micronutrient intake. Concurrently, body composition evaluation can regularly assess the compositional characteristics of the weight lost.

APPLYING THE ENERGY BALANCE EQUATION TO WEIGHT LOSS

Guidelines for weight loss generally come from studies of sedentary, overly fat persons. Although precise recommendations do not exist for physically active men and women or competitive athletes, the current understanding of prudent body fat loss should also apply to these persons. As discussed in Chapter 7 and illustrated in Figure 7.1, the human body functions in accord with the established laws of thermodynamics. If total daily food calories exceed daily energy expenditure, excess calories accumulate as fat in adipose tissue.[139] Conversely, if energy expenditure exceeds the energy from food intake, body weight decreases.

Three methods unbalance the energy balance equation to produce weight loss:

1. Reduce caloric intake below daily energy requirements
2. Maintain daily caloric intake and increase energy expenditure through additional physical activity
3. Decrease daily caloric intake and increase daily energy expenditure

When considering the sensitivity of overall energy balance, note that if daily energy intake exceeds output by only 100 kcal, the surplus calories consumed in a year equal 36,500 kcal (365 × 100 kcal). Each pound (454 g or 0.45 kg) of body fat consists of about 87% lipid (454 g × 0.87 = 395 g × 9 kcal · g^{-1} = 3555 kcal [usually rounded to 3500 kcal] per 0.45 kg). This caloric excess would theoretically cause a yearly gain of about 4.7 kg (10.3 lb) of body fat. In contrast, if daily food intake decreases by 100 kcal, and energy expenditure increases by 100 kcal (e.g., by jogging 1 extra mile each day), then the yearly caloric deficit equals about 9.5 kg (21 lb) of body fat.

A Prudent Recommendation

The objective of weight-loss therapy has changed dramatically over the past 20 years. The prior typical approach assigned a goal body weight that coincided with an "ideal" weight based on body stature and mass. Achievement of goal body weight heralded the weight-loss program's success.

Currently, the WHO, the Institute of Medicine, and the National Heart, Lung, and Blood Institute (**www.nhlbi.nih.gov**) recommend that an overweight person reduce initial body weight by 5 to 15%. This more realistic weight loss diminishes weight-related comorbidities and complications from hypertension, type 2 diabetes, and abnormal blood lipids and often exerts a positive effect on social–psychological complications. Setting the initial weight loss goal beyond the 5 to 15% recommendation often gives patients an unrealistic and probably unattainable target in light of current treatment methods.[17]

DIETING TO TIP THE ENERGY BALANCE EQUATION

Many people incorrectly believe that only calories from dietary lipids increase body fat. These persons reduce lipid intake (generally a good idea) but often disproportionately increase carbohydrate and protein intakes so total caloric intake remains unchanged or even increases. *Weight loss occurs whenever energy output exceeds energy intake regardless of the diet's macronutrient mixture, reaffirming the first law of thermodynamics.*

A prudent dietary-only approach to weight loss unbalances the energy balance equation by reducing daily energy intake 500 to 1000 kcal below daily energy expenditure. Moderately reduced food intake produces greater body fat loss relative to the energy deficit than more severe energy restriction that exacerbates loss of lean tissue. In addition, persons poorly tolerate a prolonged caloric restriction of more than 1000 kcal daily; this form of semistarvation increases the chances for poor nourishment, lean tissue loss, and depletion of liver and muscle glycogen reserves. *Total energy intake, not diet composition, determines the effectiveness of weight loss with reduced-energy diets.*

Suppose an overly fat man who consumes 3800 kcal daily and maintains body mass of 80 kg wishes to reduce 5 kg by dieting. He maintains his activity level but decreases food intake to create a daily caloric deficit of 1000 kcal. Thus, instead of consuming 3800 kcal, he takes in only 2800 kcal daily. In 7 days, the accumulated deficit equals 7000 kcal, or the energy equivalent of 0.9 kg (2 lb) of body fat. Actually, he would lose considerably more than 0.9 kg during the first week because initially the body's glycogen stores make up a substantial portion of the energy deficit. Stored glycogen contains fewer calories per gram and considerably more water than stored fat. For this reason, short periods of caloric restriction often encourage the dieter but produce a large percentage of water and carbohydrate loss per unit weight loss and only a small decrease in body fat. As weight loss progresses, a larger proportion of body fat contributes to the energy deficit created by food restriction. To reduce body fat by an additional 1.4 kg, the dieter must maintain the reduced caloric intake of 2800 kcal for another 10.5 days; at this point, body fat theoretically decreases at a rate of 0.45 kg every 3.5 days.

Weight Loss Results Not Always Predictable

The mathematics of weight loss through caloric restriction seems straightforward, but the results do not always follow. One assumes that daily energy expenditure remains relatively unchanged throughout the dieting period. Some dieters experience lethargy (often related to depletion of the body's glycogen stores), which decreases daily energy expenditure. The energy cost of physical activity also decreases proportionately with body weight reduction. This shrinks the energy output side of the energy balance equation. As we discuss in the next section, the body also "defends" itself against a depressed caloric intake by reducing resting metabolism, which further blunts the weight-loss effort.

Set-Point Theory: A Case Against Dieting

One can reduce large amounts of weight in a relatively short time simply by not eating. But success remains short-lived, and eventually the urge to eat wins out and the lost weight returns. Some argue that the reason for this failure lies in a genetically determined "set point" that differs from what the dieter expects. The proponents of a **set-point theory** maintain that all persons, fat or thin, have a well-regulated internal control mechanism located deep within the lateral hypothalamus that tightly maintains a preset level of body weight and/or body fat. In a practical sense, this represents a person's body weight when not counting calories. Regular exercise and antiobesity drugs may lower a person's pre-established set point, whereas dieting exerts no effect (**www.fda.gov**). Each time body fat decreases below the person's set point, internal adjustments and regulatory mechanisms resist the change and attempt to conserve and/or replenish body fat. For example, resting metabolism slows, and the person becomes obsessed with food, unable to control the urge to eat. Even when a person overeats to gain weight above the normal level, the body resists this change by increasing resting metabolism and altering brain chemistry to cause the person to lose interest in food.

Resting Metabolism Decreases: Resting metabolism often decreases when dieting.[77,137] This hypometabolic response to caloric deficit often exceeds the decrease attributable to the loss of body mass or FFM. An overly reduced metabolism characterizes those persons who attempt to reduce weight, whether they dieted previously or whether they are obese or lean. Depressed metabolism conserves energy, causing the diet to become less effective despite restricted caloric intake. This produces a weight-loss plateau at which further weight loss becomes considerably less than predicted from the mathematics of the restricted energy intake.

FIGURE 14.7 depicts the body's defense against deviations in body weight. This classic study carefully monitored body mass, resting oxygen uptake (minimal energy requirement), and caloric intake of six obese men for 31 days. During the prediet period, body mass and resting oxygen uptake stabilized with a daily food intake of 3500 kcal. When the men then switched to 450-kcal low-calorie diet, body mass and resting metabolism decreased, and the percentage decline in metabolism exceeded the body mass decrease. The dashed line represents the expected weight loss from the 450-kcal diet. The decline in resting metabolism (*middle figure*) conserved energy, causing the diet to become progressively less effective. More than half of the total weight loss occurred over the first 8 days of dieting; the remaining weight loss occurred during the final 16 days. A plateau in the theoretical weight-loss curve often frustrates and discourages dieters, causing them to abandon the program.

Further disconcerting news awaits those desiring permanent fat loss. When obese persons lose weight, adipocytes increase their level of the fat-storing enzyme lipoprotein lipase.[69] Unfortunately, this adaptation facilitates body fat synthesis, and the fatter the person before weight loss, the greater is the lipoprotein lipase production with weight loss. This observation supports the existence of a feedback mechanism between the brain and body fat levels and helps explain the great difficulties obese persons encounter in maintaining weight loss.[56,147]

The set-point theory delivers unwelcome news to those with a set point tuned "too high." Fortunately, regular exercise may lower the set-point level. Concurrently, regular exercise conserves and even increases FFM, marginally raises resting metabolism (if FFM increases), and alters metabolism to facilitate fat breakdown.[77,128] These healthful adaptations all augment the weight-loss effort. Food intake declines initially with regular exercise for overly fat men and women. Eventually, as an active lifestyle continues and body fat reserves decrease, caloric intake balances daily energy requirements and body mass stabilizes at a new, lower level.

PERSONAL HEALTH AND EXERCISE NUTRITION 14.1

How to Predict Percentage Body Fat from Girths for Overly Fat Men and Women

Estimating percentage body fat (%BF) in the overly fat by skinfold prediction becomes problematic because of difficulty securing accurate and repeatable measurements owing to an extensive mass of subcutaneous fat. In addition, with increasing levels of body fatness, the proportion of subcutaneous fat to total body fat changes, thereby affecting the relationship between skinfolds and body density (Db). The following four factors limit skinfold use with the overly fat population:

1. Difficulty of site selection and palpation of body landmarks
2. Skinfold thickness may exceed caliper jaw aperture
3. Variability in adipose tissue composition affects skinfold compressibility
4. Poorer objectivity in skinfold measures as body fat increases

Predicting Percentage Body Fat

Use the following equations to predict %BF in obese (>30%BF) women (age 20–60 years) and obese (>20%BF) men (age 24–68 years).

Women

%BF = 0.11077 (ABDO) – 0. 17666 (HT) + 0.14354 (BW) + 51.03301

Men

%BF = 0.31457 (ABDO) – 0.10969 (BW) + 10.8336

where ABDO = the average of (1) waist girth (taken horizontally at the level of the natural waist—narrowest part of the torso, as seen from the anterior) and (2) abdomen girth (taken horizontally at the level of the greatest anterior extension of the abdomen, usually, but not always, at the level of the umbilicus). Duplicate measurements are taken and averaged. BW = body weight in kilograms; and HT = stature in centimeters.

Examples

1. **Overly Fat Woman**

   Data: waist girth = 115 cm;
   abdomen girth = 121 cm; HT = 165.1 cm;
   BW = 97.5 kg

   %BF = 0.11077 (ABDO) – 0.17666 (HT) + 0.14354 (BW) + 51.03301
   = 0.11077 [(115 + 121)/2] – 0.17666 (165.1) + 0.14354 (97.5) + 51.03301
   = 13.07 – 29.17 + 13.995 + 51.03301
   = 48.9

2. **Overly Fat Man**

   Data: waist girth = 131 cm;
   abdomen girth = 136 cm; BW = 135.6 kg
   %BF = 0.31457 (ABDO) – 0.10969 (BW) + 10.8336
   = 0.31457 [(131.0 + 136.0)/2] – 0.10969 (135.6) + 10.8336
   = 41.995 – 14.873 + 10.8336
   = 37.9

Tran ZV, Weltman A. Predicting body composition of men from girth measurements. *Hum Biol* 1988;60:167.
Weltman A, et al. Accurate assessment of body composition in obese females. *Am J Clin Nutr* 1988;48:1179.

Some research challenges the argument that persons who lose weight necessarily maintain the initial depressed metabolism that predisposes them to weight regain.[134] Energy restriction produces a transient state of hypometabolism if the dieter maintains a negative energy intake. This adaptive downregulation in resting metabolism does not necessarily persist if persons lose weight but then re-establish (at their lower body weight) a balance in which energy intake equals energy expenditure.

Weight Cycling: Going No Place Fast

The futility of repeated cycles of weight loss and weight gain referred to as the **yo-yo effect** emerged from food efficiency studies that evaluated weight loss–weight gain related to ingested calories in animals. Considerable debate exists on this subject,[53,89,146] but weight regain may occur more readily with repeated cycles of weight loss. For example, animals require twice the time to lose the same weight during a second period of caloric restriction and only one-third the time to regain it.[20]

Overfatness raises the risk of heart disease, yet failure to keep off the lost weight may pose an additional risk. Repeated bouts of weight loss–weight regain increase the likelihood of death from a heart attack. The risk averaged almost 70% more for weight regainers than those who maintained body weight.[65] In contrast, data from 6500 originally healthy Japanese American men revealed no ill effects from

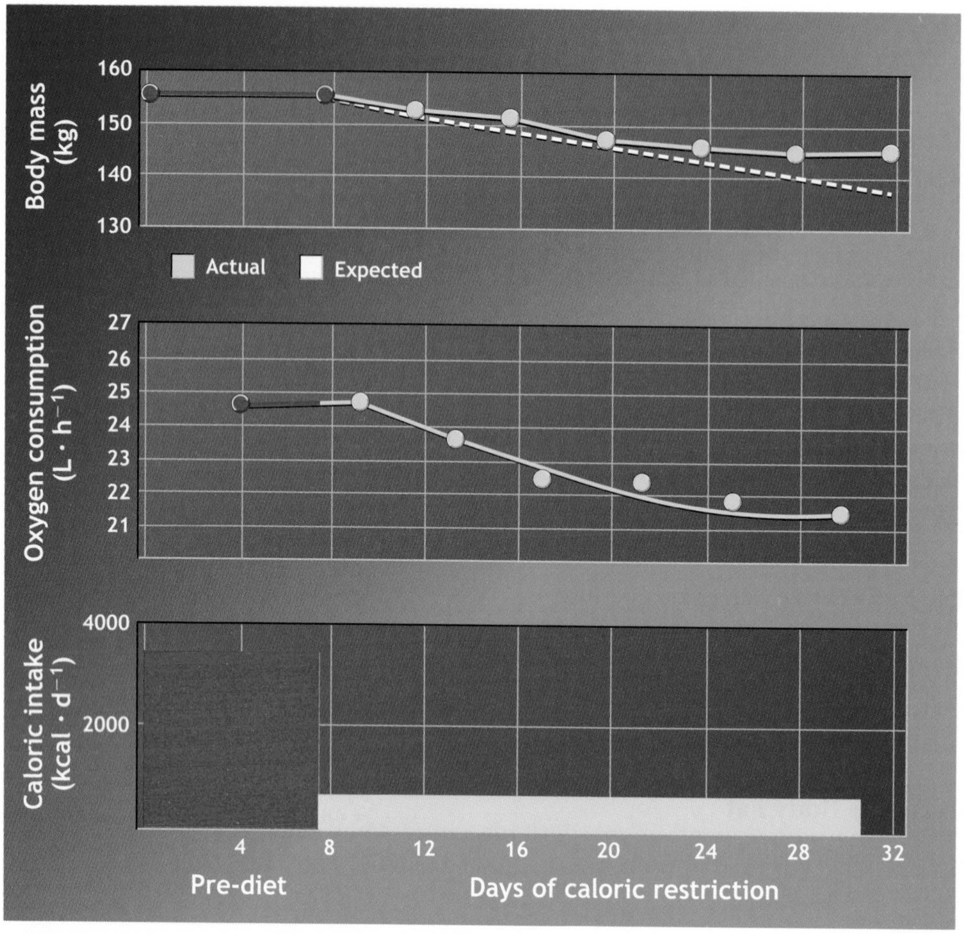

FIGURE 14.7. Results of a classic study of the effects of two levels of caloric intake on body mass and resting oxygen consumption. Failure of the actual weight loss to keep pace with that predicted on the basis of food restriction (*dashed line*) often leaves the dieter frustrated and discouraged. (Adapted from Bray G. Effect of caloric restriction on energy expenditure in obese subjects. *Lancet* 1969;2:397.)

a repeated cycle of weight loss and regain.[61] The periods of rapid weight loss and regain common in dieters did not increase hypertension risk any more than the increased risk from being overweight or gaining weight in the first place.[21] Also, repeated cycles of dieting did not induce adverse psychological effects for stress level, anxiety, anger, and depression.[114]

From a public health perspective, the risks from overfatness and obesity far exceed those for weight cycling. The obese should not use potential hazards of yo-yo dieting as an excuse to abandon efforts to reduce excess body fat. In particular, this weight loss approach should include efforts to dramatically increase "extra" physical activities of daily living and sports and recreational activities.

Negative Consequences of Dieting Extremes

Professional organizations have voiced strong opposition to certain dietary practices, particularly extremes of fasting and low-carbohydrate, high-fat, and high-protein diets. These practices remain troublesome to professionals in sports medicine and exercise physiology because of reports documenting that physically active persons often exhibit bizarre and pathogenic weight-control behaviors and disordered eating patterns. Imprudent eating behaviors negatively affect body composition, energy reserves, and psychological and physical well-being (see Chapter 15).

Low-Carbohydrate Ketogenic Diets

Ketogenic diets emphasize carbohydrate restriction while generally ignoring total calories and the diet's cholesterol and saturated fat content. Billed as a "diet revolution" and championed by the late Dr. Robert C. Atkins (1930–2003), the diet was first promoted in the latter part of the 19th century and has appeared in various forms since then. Long disparaged by the medical establishment, advocates maintain that restricting daily carbohydrate intake to 20 g or less for the initial 2 weeks, with some liberalization afterward, causes the body to mobilize considerable fat for energy. This generates excess plasma ketone bodies—by-products of incomplete fat breakdown from inadequate carbohydrate catabolism; ketones supposedly suppress appetite. Theoretically, the ketones lost in the urine represent unused energy that should further facilitate weight loss. Some advocates claim that urinary energy loss becomes so great that dieters can eat all they want as long as they restrict carbohydrates.

The singular focus of the low-carbohydrate diet craze may eventually reduce caloric intake, despite claims that dieters need not consider calorie intake as long as lipid represents the excess. Initial weight loss also may result largely from dehydration caused by an extra solute load on the kidneys that increases water excretion. Water loss does *not* reduce body fat. Low-carbohydrate intake also sets the stage for lean tissue loss because the body recruits amino acids from muscle to maintain blood glucose via gluconeogenesis—an undesirable side effect for a diet designed to induce body fat loss.

Perhaps Not as Bad as Previously Thought: Three clinical trials compared the Atkins-type, low-carbohydrate diet with traditional low-fat diets for weight loss.[44,110,148] The low-carbohydrate diet was more effective in achieving a modest weight loss for severely overweight persons. Some measures of heart health also improved as reflected by a more favorable lipid profile and glycemic control in those who followed the low-carbohydrate diet for up to 1 year. Such findings add a measure of credibility to low-carbohydrate diets and challenge conventional wisdom concerning the potential dangers from consuming a high-fat diet.

Importantly, Atkin's-type, high-fat, low-carbohydrate diets require systematic long-term evaluation (up to 5 years) for safety and effectiveness, particularly related to the blood lipid profile. The diet, which places no limit on the amount of meat, fat, eggs, and cheese a person consumes, poses nine potential health hazards:

1. Raises serum uric acid levels
2. Potentiates development of kidney stones
3. Alters electrolyte concentrations to initiate cardiac arrhythmias
4. Causes acidosis
5. Aggravates existing kidney problems from the extra solute burden in the renal filtrate
6. Depletes glycogen reserves, contributing to a fatigued state
7. Decreases calcium balance and increases risk for bone loss
8. Causes dehydration
9. Retards fetal development during pregnancy from inadequate carbohydrate intake

For endurance athletes who train at or above 70% of maximum effort, switching to a high-fat diet is ill advised because the physically active body needs to maintain adequate blood glucose and glycogen packed in the active muscles and liver storage depots. Fatigue during intense exercise of more than 60 min in duration occurs more rapidly when athletes regularly consume high-fat meals than carbohydrate-rich meals (see Chapter 12).

The South Beach Diet: A More Modest Approach

Similar to the Atkins diet, the South Beach diet strictly limits intake of bread, potatoes, and other carbohydrates while permitting consumption of higher fat red meat, cheese, and eggs. Advocates argue that most carbohydrate foods in the US diet are of the high-glycemic variety that digest and absorb rapidly and raise blood glucose levels.

> **BODY WEIGHT STIGMA: NO BENEFIT BUT THE OPPOSITE EFFECT**
>
> Stigmatizing overweight people by making them feel "bad" about themselves and their condition represents an unacceptable and ineffective form of motivation to lose weight that actually contributes to unhealthy behaviors that add to the problem of obesity. Surprisingly, family members and healthcare professionals represent the most common sources of weight stigmatization.

The first 2 weeks of the diet (phase 1) focus on stabilizing blood glucose by consuming only foods with the lowest glycemic indexes. Fiber-rich carbohydrates and unsaturated fatty acids are gradually reintroduced in phase 2 until desired weight is reached and then maintained in phase 3. If weight gain occurs, the person returns to phase 1. In essence, the effectiveness of the South Beach diet hinges on whether it reduces caloric intake, mainly by reducing cravings induced by dramatic swings in blood insulin. With the exception of the extreme nature of phase 1, the South Beach diet appears more modest than its Atkins counterpart because it offers more variety and promotes more healthful foods.

High-Protein Diets

Low-carbohydrate, high-protein diets may shed pounds in the near term, but their long-term success remains questionable, and they may even pose health risks. Such diets have been commercially extolled as "last-chance diets." Earlier versions consisted of protein in liquid form advertised as "miracle liquid." Unknown to the consumer, the liquid protein mixture often contained a blend of ground-up animal hooves and horns, with pigskin mixed in a broth with enzymes and tenderizers to "predigest" it. Such collagen-based blends produced from gelatin hydrolysis (supplemented with small amounts of essential amino acids) often failed to contain the highest quality amino acid mixture and lacked required vitamins and minerals, particularly copper. A negative copper balance coincides with electrocardiographic abnormalities and rapid heart rate.[38] Protein-rich foods often contain high levels of saturated fat that promote heart disease and type 2 diabetes risk. Diets excessively high in animal protein increase urinary excretion of oxalate, a compound that combines primarily with calcium to form kidney stones.[103] High levels of urinary calcium with these diets also indicate decreased calcium balance and increased risk for bone loss. The diet's safety improves by adding high-quality protein with ample carbohydrate, essential fatty acids, and micronutrients.

Some "experts" claim that extremely high protein intake suppresses appetite through reliance on fat mobilization and subsequent ketone formation. In addition, the elevated thermic effect of dietary protein, with a relatively low coefficient of digestibility particularly for plant protein, ultimately reduces the net calories available from ingested protein compared with a well-balanced meal of equivalent caloric value (see Chapter 6). This point has some validity, but one must consider other factors when formulating a sound weight-loss program, particularly for the physically active person. A high-protein diet has the potential for these five deleterious outcomes:

1. Strain on liver and kidney function and accompanying dehydration
2. Electrolyte imbalance
3. Glycogen depletion
4. Lean-tissue loss
5. Kidney stones and reduced calcium absorption

Semistarvation Diets

Physically active persons often "starve" themselves to lose weight. A therapeutic fast or **very low-calorie diet (VLCD)** may benefit severe clinical obesity where body fat exceeds 40 to 50% of body mass.[89,116] The diet provides between 400 and 800 kcal daily as high-quality protein foods or liquid meal replacements. Dietary prescriptions usually last up to 3 months but only as a "last resort" before undertaking more extreme medical approaches for morbid obesity that include various surgical treatments (collectively called *bariatric surgery*: www.asmbs.org/). Surgical treatments that considerably reduce stomach size and reconfigure the small intestine induce a sustained weight loss, but they generally are prescribed for patients with a BMI of at least 40, or a BMI of 35 when accompanied by other obesity-related medical conditions.[39]

Dieting with VLCDs requires close supervision, usually in a hospital setting. Proponents maintain that severe food restriction breaks established dietary habits, which in turn improves the long-term prospects for success.[18] These diets also may depress appetite to help compliance. Daily medications that accompany a VLCD include calcium carbonate for nausea, bicarbonate of soda and potassium chloride to maintain consistency of body fluids, mouthwash and sugar-free chewing gum for bad breath (from a high level of ketones from fatty acid catabolism), and bath oils for dry skin. *For most persons, semistarvation does not compose an "ultimate diet" or proper approach to weight loss.* A VLCD provides inadequate carbohydrate, causing liver and muscle glycogen storage depots deplete rapidly. This impairs physical tasks that require either intense aerobic effort or shorter duration anaerobic power output. The continuous nitrogen loss with fasting and resulting weight loss reflects an exacerbated lean tissue loss, which may occur disproportionately from critical organs like the heart.[92] The success rate remains poor for prolonged fasting.

TABLE 14.2 summarizes the principles and main advantages and disadvantages of popular dietary approaches to weight loss. Although proposed over 30 years ago, the basic principles espoused in the table still hold true. Most diets induce weight loss during the first several weeks, but body water makes up much of the lost weight. In addition, considerable lean tissue loss occurs with dieting alone, particularly in the early phase of a VLCD.

THE APPROPRIATE DIET PLAN: WELL BALANCED BUT LESS OF IT

A calorie-counting approach to weight loss should provide an appropriate dietary plan that contains all the essential nutrients. If one maintains a caloric deficit, diet composition exerts little effect on the magnitude of weight lost. Weight-loss diets should contain the recommended micronutrients and protein, with reduced cholesterol, saturated fat, and essentially no *trans* fatty acids. For the physically active person, the remainder should consist predominantly of unrefined, fiber-rich, complex carbohydrates. Calories do count; the trick lies in keeping within the daily limit specified by the rate of fat loss desired.[19]

Two factors largely determine one's daily energy expenditure:

1. Resting energy requirement
2. Energy expended in daily physical activities

Weight loss occurs if a true caloric deficit exists and energy output *exceeds* energy input. Short periods of caloric restriction often encourage the dieter, but do not produce the desired decrease in body fat. Instead, the lost weight consists largely of water and carbohydrate per unit of body weight lost. As weight loss progresses, a larger proportion of body fat provides energy to make up the caloric deficit created by food restriction.

MAXIMIZING DIETING'S CHANCES FOR SUCCESS

We usually eat for two reasons. First, we consume food because of true physiologic hunger. This maintains the energy and building blocks to power the body's vital processes and sustain life. Second, we eat to satisfy appetite, which in America usually "turns on" at least three times daily. Human eating behavior intimately ties to both external (environmental) cues and internal (physiologic) cues that signal a real need to eat. External "food cues" include the sight of food; its packaging, display, and advertising; the time and physical environment for eating; and the taste, smell, color, texture, and mainly portion size, which has increased steadily over the past 30 years.

TABLE 14.2 Principles and Main Advantages and Disadvantages of Some Popular Weight Loss Methods

Method	Principle	Advantages	Disadvantages	Comments
Surgical procedure	Alteration of the gastrointestinal tract changes capacity or amount of absorptive surface	Caloric restriction less necessary	Risks of surgery and postsurgical complications can include death	Radical procedures include stapling of the stomach and removal of a section of the small intestine (a jejunoileal bypass)
Fasting	No energy input, ensures negative energy balance	Rapid weight loss (which may be a disadvantage); reduced exposure to temptation	Ketogenic; a large portion of weight loss comes from lean body mass; nutrients lacking	Medical supervision mandatory and hospitalization recommended
Protein-sparing modified fast	Same as fasting except protein or protein with carbohydrate intake presumably helps preserve lean body mass	Same as in fasting	Ketogenic; nutrients lacking; some unconfirmed deaths have been reported, possibly from potassium depletion	Medical supervision mandatory; popular presentation in Lin's "The Last Chance Diet"
One food–centered diets	Low-caloric intake favors negative energy balance	Being easy to follow, initial psychological appeal	Being too restrictive means that nutrients are probably lacking; repetitious nature may cause boredom	No food or food combination known to "burn off" fat; examples include the grapefruit diet and the egg diet
Low-carbohydrate/high-fat diets	Increased ketone excretion removes energy-containing substances from the body; fat intake is often voluntarily decreased; a low-calorie diet results	Inclusion of rich foods may have psychological appeal; initial rapid loss of water may be an incentive	Ketogenic; high fat intake contraindicated for heart disease and diabetes patients; nutrients lacking	Popular versions have been offered by Taller and Atkins; some called "Mayo," "Drinking Man's," and "Air Force" diets
Low-carbohydrate/high-protein diets	Low-caloric intake favors negative energy balance	Initial rapid water loss an incentive; increased thermic effect of protein	Expense and repetitious nature may make diet difficult to sustain	Emphasizing meats makes the diet high in lipid; Pennington diet an example
High-carbohydrate/low-fat diets	Low-caloric intake favors negative energy balance	Wise food selections can make the diet nutritionally sound	Initial water retention may be discouraging	Pritikin diet is an example

Modified and reprinted with permission from Reed PB. Nutrition: An Applied Science. *Copyright 1980 by West-Publishing Co. All rights reserved.*

Personal Assessment: The Important First Step

Accurately assessing food intake and energy expenditure provides the framework for unbalancing the energy balance equation to favorably modify body mass and body composition.

Estimates of caloric intake from carefully obtained records of daily food intake (refer to Appendix F) usually fall within an acceptable level of accuracy of 10% of the actual number of calories consumed. For example, suppose the caloric value of daily food intake directly measured in the bomb calorimeter averages 2130 kcal. With a careful 3-day dietary history to estimate caloric intake, the daily value falls between about 1920 and 2350 kcal.

Careful record keeping of food intake accomplishes two goals:

1. Provides the dieter with an objective list of the foods actually consumed (rather than a "guesstimate" of food intake)
2. Triggers the awareness of current eating habits and food preferences, an important aspect of the weight-control process

Psychological Factors Influence Eating Behaviors

Depression, frustration, boredom, "uptight" or anxious feelings, guilt, sadness, and anger often trigger the urge to eat. A dieter must learn to make accurate appraisals of eating behavior, not only the quantity and frequency of eating, but also specific circumstances linked to food intake. Self-analysis requires keen awareness of all aspects of food consumption. Once accomplished, a new set of desirable eating responses can substitute for previously learned "undesirable" behaviors.

How to Modify Eating Behaviors

The first step in eating behavior modification involves describing the various eating behaviors of the person desiring to lose weight, not immediately changing the diet. The person keeps meticulous records and answers the following eight questions:

1. When were meals eaten?
2. In what place were meals eaten?
3. What was the mood, feeling, or psychological state during the meal?
4. How much time was spent eating?
5. What activities were engaged in during the meal (e.g., watching television, driving a car, reading, during or after a workout)?
6. Who was present during the meal?
7. What food was eaten?
8. How much food was eaten?

This time-consuming and often annoying record keeping provides objective information concerning one's personal eating behaviors and reveals certain recurring patterns associated with eating. The basic idea is to identify the patterns. Consider these five patterns related to eating behavior:

1. Eating candy often accompanies feelings of depression.
2. Snacking occurs while watching television.
3. Hunger becomes prevalent at a particular time of day or after physical activity.
4. An ice cream binge usually takes place after an argument.
5. Breakfast and lunch are never eaten at the kitchen table.

SUBSTITUTES FOR UNDESIRABLE EATING BEHAVIORS

Established Behavior Patterns	Replacement Behavior
Eating candy while driving	Singing along with the radio
Eating snacks while watching television	Sewing, painting, or writing letters
Feeling hungry at 4:00 PM	Going for a walk at 4:00 PM
Eating ice cream after an argument	Doing 20 repetitions of an exercise
Never eating breakfast or lunch at the kitchen table	Eating breakfast and lunch only at the kitchen table
Visiting the kitchen during television commercials	Jogging in place; doing sit-ups
Food shopping on the way home before dinner	Do all food shopping after eating and buy only what is on the list

With clear patterns identified, the next step is to substitute *alternative* behaviors to replace undesirable ones.

Substitute Alternative Eating Behaviors Many acceptable behaviors can replace an established set of undesirable ones. The box below lists some existing behaviors associated with overeating and possible substitute more desirable behaviors. Many of these recommended substitutions have been promulgated for the general population, but they also apply to recreational and competitive athletes. The major aim of this approach creates new, more positive associations to replace inappropriate eating behavior patterns.

Upgrading Control of Eating Behaviors

1. **Make the act of eating a ritual**. Limit eating to one place in the house. No matter what foods you eat, follow a set routine. For example, use a place mat, set the table with silverware, and use the same dishes at each meal. Do this for main meals and snacks. One dieter who continually snacked between meals curbed this habit by dressing up in formal attire for each meal and snack—snacking between meals soon stopped. To discourage eating bread, take only one slice at a time and toast it before eating it. For each slice, get up from the table, unwrap the loaf and take out a slice, rewrap the loaf and replace it in the cupboard, toast the slice, and return to the table to eat it. Following an inconvenient routine to obtain some "special" food item often suppresses desire for the food.
2. **Use smaller dishes**. The impetus to finish a meal may not be the food per se, but the desire to view an empty plate or glass. Also, try to always leave some food on the plate.
3. **Eat slowly**. Fight the tendency to eat too rapidly by taking more time at meals. Cut food into smaller pieces and chew each piece 10 to 15 times before swallowing. Also, place the knife, spoon, or fork back on the table after each two or three bites, and allow a 1- or 2-min rest pause between mouthfuls.
4. **Reduce the lipid content of meals**. Simple modifications in food selection within the same food category dramatically affect the meal's caloric density. The box "Sixteen-Item Checklist for Cutting Down on Dietary Lipid" presents a convenient checklist for cutting down on the intake of dietary lipid; **TABLE 14.3** provides appropriate low-calorie substitutions within various food categories.
5. **Follow a food plan**. Following a highly structured daily food plan (what, when, and where food will be eaten) reduces the risk of eating high-calorie "impulse" foods.

Develop New Techniques to Control Food Consumption

Many useful techniques can control eating behaviors once undesirable environmental cues and associated behaviors have been identified and replaced or modified. Delaying, substituting, and avoiding represent three behavioral strategies for interrupting poor eating behaviors:

1. **Delaying**. Add time or steps between the links in the behavior chain:
   - Slow down the eating pace.
   - Take a roundabout way to the kitchen.

TABLE 14.3 Substituting Foods with Lower Calorie Content

Type of Food	Select Most Often	Select Moderately	Select Least Often
Animal protein	Lean cuts of beef/pork Salmon, halibut (broiled) Canned tuna in water Poultry (without skin) Egg Crab	Untrimmed beef/pork Canned tuna in oil Poultry (with skin) Lobster, shrimp Canadian bacon	Fatty beef/lamb/pork Luncheon meats/hot dogs Fried chicken Fried fish Liver, kidneys
Dairy	Nonfat yogurt Nonfat milk (or ½%) Nonfat dry milk Nonfat frozen yogurt	Reduced-fat and part-skim cheeses Low-fat cottage cheese Low-fat milk Low-fat yogurt 95% fat-free frozen yogurt	Whole-milk cheese (cheddar, muenster) Whole milk Sour cream, ice cream Cream, half-and-half
Vegetable protein	Dried beans and peas (kidney, lima, and soy beans; lentils; split peas) Tofu (bean curd)	Raw or dry-toasted nuts and seeds Peanut and other butters (moderate amounts)	Oil-processed nuts and seeds
Vegetables	Raw, fresh vegetables Fresh or frozen, slightly cooked vegetables	Canned vegetables Canned tomatoes or vegetable juice	Vegetables in cream or butter sauces Fried vegetables
Fruits	Fresh, raw fruit Dried fruit Frozen and fresh fruit juices	Canned fruit packed in juice Canned fruit juices Frozen fruit	Fruit-flavored beverages Canned fruit packed in syrup Avocados Olives
Grain products	Shredded wheat, oats Whole-grain cereals Whole-grain breads Brown rice Wheat bran, oat bran Bagels Fig bars	Refined cereals Enriched white breads Refined pastas White rice Granolas Toast with margarine Plain cookies	Cookies, cakes, pies Sweetened cereals Tortilla chips Oil-processed crackers Cream-filled doughnuts Croissants, doughnuts
Other	Popcorn (air-popped)	Low-fat salad dressing Low-fat mayonnaise Pretzels	Fat-rich salad dressing Mayonnaise Gravies, cream sauces Potato chips

From Wardlaw GM, et al. Contemporary Nutrition Issues and Insights. 2nd ed. St. Louis, MO: Mosby, 1992.

- Purchase single-portion packages of snacks.
- Put off unplanned eating as long as possible—mail a letter, read a book, mow the lawn, or do sit-ups or push-ups.

2. **Substituting**. Break the behavior chain with activities incompatible with eating:
   - Pleasant activities—read, go for a walk, listen to music, do hobbies, surf the Internet
   - Required activities—plan the budget, pay bills, do errands, clean the house
3. **Avoiding**. Keep yourself out of situations in which food is visible or easily accessible:
   - Stay out of the kitchen or other areas associated with eating.
   - Do not combine eating with other activities such as reading, television watching, driving, or working out.
   - When finished eating, remove dishes and food from the table.
   - Scrape excess food directly into the trash.

REGULAR PHYSICAL ACTIVITY FOR WEIGHT CONTROL

A sedentary lifestyle consistently emerges as an important factor in weight gain for children, adolescents, and adults.

Weight Gain: Not Simply a Problem of Gluttony

Conventional wisdom views excessive food intake as the prime cause of the overly fat condition. Most persons believe that the only way to reduce unwanted body fat entails caloric restriction by dieting. This overly simplistic strategy partly accounts for the dismal success in maintaining weight loss over the long term, refocusing debate on the contribution of food intake alone to obesity.

Per capita caloric intake in the United States has not increased enough to totally account for the steady rise in the

SIXTEEN-ITEM CHECKLIST FOR CUTTING DOWN ON DIETARY LIPID

1. Substitute cold cuts with 1 g of fat per 1-oz serving for regular bologna, salami, or pickled beef.
2. Substitute frozen yogurt or sherbet with 4 g or less of fat per 4-oz serving for high-fat ice cream.
3. Substitute air-popped popcorn and pretzels for party chips.
4. Substitute whole-grain breads and crackers for croissants and corn bread.
5. Substitute a variety of cereals for high-fat granola preparations.
6. Substitute cheese with less than 4 to 5 g of fat per ounce for high-fat cheeses.
7. Substitute egg whites for egg yolks, or use a dehydrated egg substitute.
8. Substitute light or fat-free mayonnaise for regular mayonnaise.
9. Substitute 2% or 1% milk for whole milk.
10. Substitute a variety of herbs or use low-calorie salad dressings or salsa instead of oil-rich or creamy salad dressings.
11. Avoid frozen vegetables in rich sauces.
12. Buy beef and pork with words "round" or "lean" in the name.
13. Buy low-fat cake mixes.
14. Do not add oil or butter to water when cooking pasta, macaroni, or oatmeal.
15. Make hamburgers from ground round or ground sirloin.
16. Substitute two egg whites for one whole egg in baking.

US body weight over the last century, a weight gain equivalent to 30 lb for a 6-foot-tall man. Only in the past decade has daily energy intake increased above the level reported in the early part of the 20th century. The observation that overly fat persons often eat the same or even less than thinner people holds true for a large number of overly fat adults over a broad age range as they become less active and slowly add weight. Excess weight gain often parallels reduced physical activity rather than increased caloric intake. Approximately 27% of US adults engage in no daily physical activity, and another 28% do not regularly take part in physical activity. Among active endurance-trained men, body fat inversely relates to energy expenditure (low body fat, high energy expenditure and vice versa); no relationship emerges between body fat and food intake.[84] Surprisingly, physically active people who eat the most generally weigh the least and exhibit the highest levels of physical fitness.

Excessive food intake does not fully explain the rise in body weight among children.[120] Overfat infants do not characteristically consume more calories than recommended dietary standards. For children age 4 to 6 years, a reduced level of physical activity primarily accounted for their daily energy expenditure being 25% lower than the energy intake recommendation for this age.[24] More specifically, 50% of boys and 75% of girls in the United States fail to engage in even moderate physical activity three or more times weekly. Children age 6 to 17 years have consumed 4% fewer calories over the past 30 years, yet the prevalence of childhood obesity continues to increase dramatically.[25,117] In contrast, physically active children tend to be leaner than less active counterparts. For preschool children, no relationship emerged between total energy intake or the fat, carbohydrate, and protein composition of the diet and percentage body fat.[7] Time-in-motion photography to document activity patterns of elementary school students showed that overweight children remained less physically active than their normal-weight peers; excess body weight did not relate to food intake. Overly fat high school girls and boys actually consumed fewer calories than their nonobese peers.[67,107] Excessive fatness and incidence of type 2 diabetes relate directly to the number of hours spent watching television (a consistent marker of physical inactivity) among persons of all ages.[4,8] For example, 3 h of television viewing a day led to a twofold increase in overfatness and a 50% increase in type 2 diabetes.[60] Each 2-h · day increment of television watching coincided with a 23% increase in overfatness and a 14% rise in diabetes risk. Family structure (e.g., with or without siblings and number of siblings, one-parent vs two-parent families) also influences children's physical activity and television viewing time.[9] Excessive television watching, playing video games, and otherwise remaining physically inactive particularly characterizes minority teens.[47,106] Minimizing time devoted to these behaviors helps to combat fat accumulation in childhood.

Effectiveness of Increasing Energy Expenditure

Regular physical activity plays a central role in mitigating weight gain. Men and women of all ages who maintain a physically active lifestyle (or become involved in regular exercise programs) maintain a more desirable level of body composition than less active counterparts. For overweight adult women, a dose-response relationship exists between the amount of physical activity and long-term weight loss. Overfat adolescents and adults improve body composition and visceral fat distribution from regular moderate physical activity or more vigorous exercise that improves cardiovascular fitness.[80,83] For overfat boys and girls, the most favorable body composition changes occur either with low-intensity, long-duration activity, aerobic exercise combined with high-repetition resistance training, or exercise programs combined with a behavior modification component.[51,80] For those who lose weight, regular exercise facilitates weight-loss maintenance more effectively than programs relying solely on dieting.[1,3,142] This positive effect occurs partly because regular exercise counteracts the typical postdiet decline in fat oxidation in those who lose weight by only energy restriction.[127]

Additional Insights

Can Exercise Really Benefit a Weight-Loss Program?

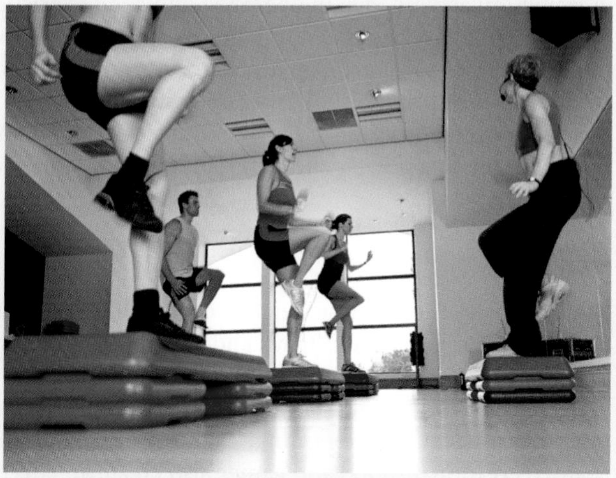

Some truth exists to the notion that one must perform an extraordinary amount of exercise to reduce body fat. Just to lose 0.45 kg (1 lb) of body fat, a person has to chop wood for 10 h, golf for 20 h, perform mild calisthenics for 22 h, play ping-pong for 28 h or volleyball for 32 h, or run 35 miles. Understandably, such a commitment seems overwhelming to the person whose long-range plans are to reduce weight by 10 or 15 kg or more. If the person walked an extra 3.5 miles (about 350 kcal) 2 days a week (700 kcal), it would take about 5 weeks or 10 walking days to lose 0.45 kg of body fat, the equivalent of about 3500 kcal. Assuming one continued to walk year-round, walking 2 days a week reduces body fat by 4.5 kg during the year provided food intake remains fairly constant. Exercise produces cumulative calorie-expending effects; a 0.45-kg body fat loss occurs when the caloric deficit equals 3500 kcal, regardless of whether the deficit occurs rapidly or systematically over time.

Two misconceptions attempt to counter the exercise approach to weight loss.

Misconception 1: Exercise and Food Intake

Sedentary people often do not balance between energy intake and energy expenditure. Failure to accurately regulate energy balance at the lower end of the physical activity spectrum contributes to the unacceptable "creeping obesity" observed in highly mechanized and technically advanced societies. In contrast, regular exercisers maintain appetite control within a reactive zone where food intake more readily matches daily energy expenditure.

In considering the effects of exercise on appetite and food intake, one must distinguish exercise mode and duration and the participant's body fat status. Lumberjacks, farm laborers, and endurance athletes consume about twice the daily calories as sedentary persons. More specifically, marathon runners, cross-country skiers, and cyclists consume about 4000 to 5000 kcal daily, yet they are the leanest people in the population. Obviously, their large caloric intake meets the energy requirements of training while maintaining a relatively lean body composition.

For the overweight person, the extra energy required for exercise more than offsets moderate physical activity's small compensatory appetite-stimulating effect. To some extent, the large energy reserve of the overfat person makes it easier to tolerate weight loss with exercise without the obligatory increase in caloric intake typically observed for leaner counterparts. *In essence, a weak coupling exists between the short-term energy deficit induced by exercise and energy intake. Increased physical activity by overweight, sedentary persons does not necessarily alter physiologic needs and automatically produce compensatory increases in food intake to balance additional energy expenditure.*

Misconception 2: Caloric Stress of Physical Activity

This common misconception concerns the contribution to weight loss of the calories burned in typical exercise. Some argue correctly that it requires an inordinate amount of short-term exercise to lose just 0.45 kg of body fat. Consequently, a 2- or 3-month exercise regimen produces only a small fat loss in an overfat person. From a different perspective, if one played golf (no cart) for 2 h daily (350 kcal) twice weekly (700 kcal), it would take about 5 weeks to reduce 0.45 kg of body fat. Assuming the person plays year-round, golfing 2 days a week produces a 4.5-kg yearly fat loss provided food intake remains relatively constant. Even an activity as innocuous as chewing gum burns an extra 11 kcal each hour, a 20% increase over normal resting metabolism. *Simply stated, the calorie-expending effects of exercise add up. A caloric deficit of 3500 kcal equals a 0.45-kg body fat loss, whether the deficit occurs rapidly or systematically over time.*

Related References

Cook CM, Schoeller DA. Physical activity and weight control: conflicting findings. *Curr Opin Clin Nutr Metab Care* 2011;14:419.

Dietz WH. Reversing the tide of obesity. *Lancet* 2011;378:744.

Hetherington MM, Regan MF. Effects of chewing gum on short-term appetite regulation in moderately restrained eaters. *Appetite* 2011;57:475.

Josse AR, et al. Increased consumption of dairy foods and protein during diet- and exercise-induced weight loss promotes fat mass loss and lean mass gain in overweight and obese premenopausal women. *J Nutr* 2011;141:1626.

Kreider RB, et al. A structured diet and exercise program promotes favorable changes in weight loss, body composition, and weight maintenance. *J Am Diet Assoc* 2011; 111:828.

Levine J, et al. The energy expended in chewing gum. *N Engl J Med.* 1999;341:2100.

Steig AJ, et al. Exercise reduces appetite and traffics excess nutrients away from energetically efficient pathways of lipid deposition during the early stages of weight regain. *Am J Physiol Regul Integr Comp Physiol* 2011;301:R656.

Even for currently active persons, additional physical activity unbalances the energy balance equation for weight loss, favorably alters body composition and body fat distribution,[74,108] and further improves physical fitness.[13,108,126] Additional spin-off from regular physical activity includes the following four benefits[52,76,81]:

1. Slowing of the age-related loss in muscle mass
2. Improvement in obesity-related comorbidities
3. Decreased mortality
4. Beneficial effects on existing chronic diseases

The Recovery Afterglow

During low-to-moderate physical activity as performed by most persons, recovery metabolism—the so-called "recovery afterglow"—contributes minimally to total energy expenditure because recovery usually occurs rapidly. In addition, regular activity causes faster adjustments in postexercise energetics, thus reducing the total recovery oxygen consumption.[113] *Calories burned during physical activity represent the most important factor in total exercise energy expenditure, not calories expended during recovery.*

The Ideal: Conserve Lean and Reduce Fat

Regular physical activity with or without dietary restriction protects against weight gain and favorably changes body mass and body composition. This occurs because exercise training enhances fat mobilization from adipose depots and increases fat breakdown by active muscle.[82] Exercise retains skeletal muscle protein by maintaining positive nitrogen balance while simultaneously retarding protein breakdown. The protein-sparing effect of regular activity partly explains why more of the weight lost comes from fat in a program that uses physical activity than in one using only food restriction. Persons with the largest amount of excess fat lose body weight and fat more readily with exercise than their leaner counterparts.[10] Even without dietary restrictions, exercise provides positive "spin-off" to favorably alter body composition by reducing body fat and maintaining or even increasing FFM.

Best Types of Physical Activities for Weight Loss

When using exercise to lose weight, consider the **FITT** acronym: **F**requency, **I**ntensity, **T**ime, and **T**ype of exercise. Ideal aerobic activities having moderate-to-high caloric cost include brisk walking and hiking, running, rope skipping, stair stepping, circuit resistance training, cycling, and swimming. Many recreational sports and games also create an effective caloric deficit for weight loss, but precise quantification and regulation of energy expenditure remain difficult with these activities. **TABLE 14.4** lists the "top 12" physical activities for energy expenditure. No selective effect exists for running, walking, or bicycling; each effectively burns sufficient calories to favorably alter body composition. When using low-impact walking as the sole means of physical activity, energy expenditure increases by adding hand-held weights or adopting race-walking techniques. An extra 300-kcal caloric expenditure induced by moderate jogging daily for 30 min theoretically produces a 0.45-kg fat loss in about 12 days, or a yearly caloric deficit equivalent to the energy in 13.6 kg of body fat.

TABLE 14.4 Top 12" Exercises Ranked by Relative Strenuousness (Kilocalories Expended per Minute)

Rank	kcal · min^{-1}	Activity
1	25.9	Roller skating, V-Skate technique, 11.2 mph, trained athletes
2	23.3	In-line skiing, double-pole technique, 11.2 mph, trained athletes
3	22.0	Skiing, cross-country, hard snow, uphill (5° grade), maximum effort, trained
4	19.3	Swimming, Mini-Gym Swim Bench, 45 strokes · min^{-1} (freely chosen)
5	18.2	Rowing, mechanically braked rowing ergometer; stroke rate = 28–32 per min, 1750 kg · m · min^{-1}, athletes
6	18.1	Rowing, "all out" for 6 min on a rowing ergometer
7	18.0	Running, 10.9 mph (5.5 min · mile pace^{-1})
8	18.0	Race walking, competition, 8.5 mph, men
9	17.2	Marathon running, 5:03 min · mile pace^{-1}, trained
10	17.1	Running, shallow water (1.3-m depth), no vest, maximal effort
11	17.0	Forestry, ax chopping, fast
12	16.0	Skin diving, vigorous

Data from Katch FI, et al. Calorie Expenditure Charts. Ann Arbor, MI: Fitness Technologies Press, 1996. Used with permission. All rights reserved.

TABLE 14.5 Changes in Body Composition After 12 Weeks of Either Resistance Training or Endurance Training

Variable	Controls		Resistance Trained		Endurance Trained	
	Before Treatment	After Treatment	Before Treatment	After Treatment	Before Treatment	After Treatment
Relative body fat (%)	20.1 ± 8.5	20.2 ± 8.5	21.8 ± 6.2	18.7 ± 6.6[a]	18.4 ± 7.9	16.5 ± 6.4[a]
Fat mass (kg)	16.2 ± 10.8	16.3 ± 10.5	17.2 ± 7.6	14.8 ± 6.2[a]	14.4 ± 7.9	12.8 ± 7.1[a]
Fat-free body mass (kg)	64.3 ± 5.4	64.4 ± 6.6	61.9 ± 8.3	64.4 ± 9.0[a]	64.1 ± 8.2	64.7 ± 8.6
Total body mass (kg)	80.5 ± 8.1	80.7 ± 8.5	79.1 ± 8.3	79.2 ± 7.6	78.5 ± 8.2	77.5 ± 7.9

All values are means ± SD.
[a] Significant difference between measurements before and after testing (P ≤.05).
From Broeder CE, et al. Assessing body composition before and after resistance or endurance training. *Med Sci Sports Exerc* 1997;29:705.

Resistance Training: Resistance training provides an important adjunct to aerobic training to promote weight loss and weight maintenance. The energy expended in circuit resistance training—continuous exercise using low resistance and high repetitions—averages about 9 kcal a minute. Consequently, this exercise mode burns substantial calories during a typical 30- to 60-min workout. Even conventional resistance training that involves less total energy expenditure affects muscular strength and FFM more positively during weight loss than programs that rely solely on food restriction.[11,129] Persons who maintain high muscular strength levels tend to gain less weight than weaker counterparts. In addition, standard resistance training performed regularly reduces coronary heart disease risk, improves glycemic control, favorably modifies the lipoprotein profile, and increases resting metabolic rate (if FFM increases).[36,99,100,119] **TABLE 14.5** illustrates the effects of 12 weeks of either endurance training or resistance training on nondieting young men. Endurance training reduced percentage body fat by reducing fat mass (−1.6 kg; no change in FFM), while resistance training decreased body fat mass (−2.4 kg) and increased the FFM (+2.4 kg). Conserving and/or increasing FFM maintains a higher level of resting metabolism independent of age, [33,79,109] but this level is relatively slight. Some estimates indicate that the average pound of resting muscle burns 6 cal a day, which is only marginallly higher per day than the 2 cal burned by a pound of fat. Thus, if you work out and lose 30 lb of fat and add 10 lb of muscle, the fat loss indicates that you are burning 60 (30 × 2) *fewer calories* daily at rest. The gain in muscle burns 120 (20 × 6) cal, a daily net increase of 60 cal, albeit a positive but relatively minor contributor to the weight loss effort. For athletes, on the other hand, maintaining FFM during weight reduction counters the potential negative effects of weight loss on exercise performance.

USE IT OR LOSE IT

A meta-analysis that examined the overall value of progressive resistance exercise among healthy aging adults showed that this form of activity helps older adults build muscle mass and increase strength to function better in daily life. Sedentary adults, with an average age of 50, added 2.4 lb of lean muscle and increased overall strength by up to 30% after 18 to 20 weeks of resistance training. The amount of weight lifted and frequency and duration of the training sessions interact in a dose-response manner to facilitate changes. Sedentary adults above age 50 typically lose up to 0.4 lb of muscle each year.

Peterson MD, Gordon PM. Resistance exercise for the aging adult: clinical implications and prescription guidelines. *Am J Med* 2011;124:194.

A Dose-Response Relationship

Some persons believe that light aerobic physical activity induces more effective weight loss because fat contributes a greater percentage of total calories burned in exercise compared with more intense physical activity in which carbohydrate represents the primary fuel. Fat combustion does provide a greater percentage of the total energy metabolism during light versus intense aerobic exercise (see Chapter 5). A larger *total quantity* of fat combustion occurs in higher intensity aerobic exercise performed for an equivalent duration. *The total number of calories expended to create the exercise energy deficit, not the percentage mixture of macronutrients oxidized, determines the effectiveness of physical activity to promote weight loss.*

A direct dose-response relationship exists between time spent moving in an activity and weight lost. The person who walks burns considerably more calories simply by extending the duration of the walk (e.g., 30 min increased to 75 min). Also, a linear relationship exists between the energy cost of weight-bearing walking exercise and body weight[141]; this means the overweight person expends considerably more calories walking than does someone of average body weight.

MAXIMIZING SUCCESS BY INCREASING PHYSICAL ACTIVITY: MODIFYING BEHAVIORS

A person burns additional calories through increased physical activity simply by extending exercise duration, even if done at a low intensity. Another effective calorie-burning strategy replaces daily periods of inactivity with additional physical activity that requires greater energy expenditure.

Describe the Behavior for Modification

Any hope of changing the profile of physical activity depends on an accurate appraisal of daily activities. The first step in exercise behavior modification determines the daily pattern of activity, including the minimal requirements of sleeping, eating, going to the bathroom, and bathing. The next step substitutes more strenuous activities for those that rate low in energy expenditure. Appendix F illustrates a physical activity profile from daily records of time spent in various activities for 3 consecutive days. The records should describe the activity, the duration, and estimated energy requirements.

Substitute Alternative Behaviors

Various options exist to increase energy expenditure within the time allotted to daily routines. The important consideration involves determining when and how to make changes with alternative exercise behaviors.

Maximize Success

Four techniques can help to maximize success when using exercise for weight loss:

1. **Progress slowly**. Add additional exercise gradually.
2. **Include variety**. Rather than performing the same exercise repeatedly in a given time, vary the exercise mode and number of repetitions. For a competitive athlete, the added physical activity for weight loss need not be in the specific sport?
3. **Become goal oriented**. Set a specific and realistic goal for increasing physical activity. Three general ways to add additional exercise using goal-oriented behavior include the following:
   a. Exercise for a certain length of time?
   b. Continue to exercise until you reach a predetermined number of repetitions or distance?
   c. Manipulate exercise duration and repetitions or distance?
   d. **Be systematic**. Set aside certain times during the day to exercise. Do not allow outside factors (e.g., watching television, shopping, housework) to interfere with daily physical activity. Once you commit to the exercise routine, do not allow outside influences to cancel or postpone the activity.

STRATEGIES FOR ALTERNATIVE EXERCISE BEHAVIORS

1. When driving to school, work, or the gym, park one-half mile away and walk the remaining distance; brisk walking to and from the car each day, 5 days a week, burns the caloric equivalent of about 3.2 kg of body fat in 1 year.
2. When taking public transportation, depart several stops early and walk the remaining distance.
3. When traveling relatively short distances, walk, jog, or bicycle instead of driving.
4. Skip the restaurant for lunch; instead, "brown bag" it and then participate in some form of physical activity for 15 to 30 min.
5. Wake up an hour early and take a brisk walk, cycle, row, rollerblade, or swim before breakfast.
6. Replace the cocktail hour or evening beer with 20 min of exercise.
7. Replace 15-min coffee breaks with 15-min exercise breaks.

STRUCTURED ASSISTANCE MAY PROVE USEFUL FOR SUCCESSFUL WEIGHT LOSS

Effective approaches for weight loss are required to combat the increase prevalence of overweight and obesity in primary medical care and community settings. The usefulness of a commercial provider of weight loss services (Weight Watchers) versus the standard treatment in primary care practices in Australia, Germany, and the United Kingdom was evaluated in 772 overweight and obese adults in a randomized controlled trial. Participants received either 12 months of standard care (defined by national treatment guidelines) or 12 months of free membership to the commercial program. Two hundred and thirty of the participants (61%) completed the commercial program and 214 participants (54%) completed standard care. Weight loss after 12 months was 5.06 kg for the commercial program participants versus 2.25 kg for those receiving standard care. The researchers concluded: "Referral by a primary health-care professional to a commercial weight loss program that provides regular weighing, advice about diet and physical activity, motivation, and group support can offer a clinically useful early intervention for weight management in overweight and obese people that can be delivered at large scale."

Jebb SA, et al. Primary care referral to a commercial provider for weight loss treatment versus standard care: a randomized controlled trial. *Lancet* 2011;378:1485.

8. Walk up and down several flights of stairs after each hour at work or school.
9. Sweep the sidewalks in front of your house, apartment, or dorm.
10. Allow time for exercise when going on a family outing. Get out of the car before reaching your destination; let a friend or family member drive the rest of the way while you walk or jog.
11. Instead of eating at an intermission at sporting events, walk around the stadium or arena; at the airport, stadium, mall, or train station, climb up and down stairs instead of using an elevator or escalator.
12. Replace outside help by undertaking the following tasks yourself:
    - Garden
    - Mow the lawn
    - Paint
    - Wash and wax the car
    - Rake leaves
    - Shovel snow
13. Run in place, jump rope, jog up and down stairs, or perform vigorous calisthenics during television commercials.

THE IDEAL: FOOD RESTRICTION PLUS INCREASED PHYSICAL ACTIVITY

Among lifetime members of a commercial weight-loss organization that promotes prudent caloric restriction, behavior modification, group support, and moderate physical activity, over one half maintained their original weight loss goal after 2 years, and more than one third had done so after 5 years.[85] Combinations of increased physical activity and dietary restraint with more unrefined, low-glycemic carbohydrates and less lipids offer considerably more flexibility for achieving a negative caloric balance than either exercise alone or diet alone.[35,88,101] Body fat losses of up to 2 lb (0.9 kg) each week fall within acceptable limits, but a steady 0.5- to 1.0-lb a week loss is more desirable.

Set a Realistic Target Time

Suppose 20 weeks represents the target time to achieve a 9 kg (20 lb) fat loss. With this goal, the weekly energy deficit must average 3500 kcal, or a daily average of 500 kcal (3500 kcal ÷ 7 days). By dieting, the person reduces daily caloric intake by 500 kcal for 5 months (3500-kcal weekly deficit) to achieve the desired 9-kg fat loss. Instead, if the dieter performed an additional one-half hour of moderate physical activity equivalent to 350 "extra" kcal 3 days a week, then the weekly caloric deficit increases by 1050 kcal (3 days × 350 kcal · exercise session^{-1}). Consequently, weekly food intake could decrease to only 2400 kcal (about 350 kcal · day^{-1}) instead of 3500 kcal to achieve the desired 0.45-kg weekly fat loss. Increasing the number of weekly activity days from 3 to 5 requires reducing daily food intake by only 250 kcal. If the duration of the 5-day · week^{-1} extra activity sessions lengthens from 30 min to 1 h, then the desired weight loss occurs without reducing food intake because the extra physical activity produces the entire 3500-kcal deficit.

If intensity of the 1-h exercise performed 5 days · week^{-1} increased by only 10% (cycling at 22 mph instead of 20 mph; running a mile in 9 min instead of 10 min; swimming each 50 yards in 54 s instead of 60 s), the number of weekly exercise calories burned increases by 350 kcal (3500 kcal a week × 10%). This new weekly deficit of 3850 kcal, or 550 kcal a day, would then permit the "dieter" to increase daily food intake by 50 kcal and still lose a pound of fat each week, a clear example of "eat more, weigh less!"

The effective use of physical activity by itself or in combination with mild dietary restriction unbalances the energy balance equation to produce meaningful weight loss. This coordinated approach should reduce feelings of intense hunger and psychological stress more than weight loss exclusively by caloric restriction. Prolonged dieting increases the chances of developing a variety of nutritional deficiencies that hinder exercise training and competitive sports performance. Combining exercise with weight loss produces desirable reductions in blood pressure at rest and in situations that typically elevate blood pressure such as intense physical activity and emotional distress.[115]

> **A REALITY CHECK**
>
> Regardless of the approach to weight loss, a statement from the National Task Force on the Prevention and Treatment of Obesity best sums up the difficulty in solving the overly fat condition on a long-term basis: "Obese individuals who undertake weight loss efforts should be ready to commit to lifelong changes in their behavioral patterns, diet, and physical activity."[90]

DOES SELECTIVE EXERCISE "SPOT REDUCTION" WORK?

The notion of exercise spot reduction comes from the belief that increasing a muscle's activity facilitates fat mobilization from adipose tissue in close proximity to the active muscle. In theory, exercising a specific body area should selectively reduce more fat from that area than if different muscle groups exercised at the same caloric intensity. Advocates of selective exercise spot reduction recommend large numbers of sit-ups and alternate leg lifts and side-bends for a person with excessive abdominal fat. Proponents of spot reduction promise aesthetic and health risk benefits, yet laboratory research evidence generally does not support its effectiveness.

To examine the claims for spot reduction, researchers compared the girths and subcutaneous fat stores of the right and left forearms of high-caliber tennis players.[51] As expected, the girth of the dominant or playing arm exceeded that of the nondominant arm because of modest muscular hypertrophy from the exercise overload from years of practice with the specific arm and shoulder musculature. Measurements of skinfold thickness indicated that many years of playing tennis on a regular basis did not reduce subcutaneous fat in the playing arm. Another relatively short-duration experiment evaluated fat biopsy specimens from the abdominal, subscapular, and buttock sites before and after 27 days of sit-up exercise training.[68] The daily number of sit-ups increased from 140 at the end of the first week to 336 on day 27. Despite this impressive amount of localized "spot" exercise, adipocytes in the abdominal region were no smaller than in unexercised buttocks or subscapular control regions. Both of these studies serve as examples (one for chronic specific training and one for acute training) to demonstrate that selective exercise training does not "sculpt" the intended anatomic area.

Undoubtedly, a negative energy balance created through regular exercise reduces total body fat because exercise stimulates mobilization of fatty acids through hormones that impact fat depots throughout the body. Body areas of greatest body fat concentration and/or lipid-mobilizing enzyme activity supply the greatest amount of this energy. The bottom line is that selective exercise does not cause significantly more fatty acid release from the fat pads directly over the active muscles.

Where on the Body Does Fat Loss Occur?

Changes in body fat and fat distribution in obese women at successive 2.3-kg (5-lb) increments of weight loss over a 14-week period addressed the frequently asked question, "Where on the body does fat loss occur when weight is lost?" Caloric restriction and a 45-min, 3-day · week^{-1} exercise program affected weight loss.[71] **FIGURE 14.8** displays the changes in body composition, skinfolds, and girths in the three subgroups that reduced body mass by 2.3, 4.5, and 9.1 kg. A 4.5-kg weight loss produced approximately twice as much change in overall body composition as a loss of 2.3 kg (*top graph*). The corresponding change in body composition almost tripled when weight loss doubled from 4.5 to 9.1 kg. Skinfolds (*middle graph*) and girths (*bottom graph*) in the trunk region decreased about twice as much as those in the extremities. Decreases in body fat with exercise training and/or caloric restriction preferentially occur in upper body subcutaneous fat and deep abdominal fat rather than the more "resistant" fat depots in gluteal and femoral regions.[30,72,91]

POSSIBLE GENDER DIFFERENCES IN PHYSICAL ACTIVITY EFFECTS ON WEIGHT LOSS

An interesting question concerns the possibility of a gender difference in the responsiveness of weight loss to regular exercise.[74,135] A meta-analysis of 53 research studies on this topic concluded that men generally respond more favorably than women to the effects of exercise on weight loss.[10] One possible explanation involves gender differences in body fat distribution and gender-related differences from an increased energy intake in response to exercise and a lower energy expenditure in exercise for women compared to men.[34] The mobilization capacity of triacylglycerols for energy depends on anatomic location. Fat distributed in the upper body and abdominal regions (central fat) shows an active lipolysis to sympathetic nervous system stimulation and preferentially mobilizes fat for energy from these areas during exercise.[5,111,132] The greater distribution of upper body adipose tissue in men than in women may contribute to their greater sensitivity to lose fat with regular exercise. The final answer to this intriguing question awaits further research.

EFFECTS OF DIET AND PHYSICAL ACTIVITY ON BODY COMPOSITION DURING WEIGHT LOSS

The box "Eight Benefits of Adding Exercise to Dietary Restriction for Weight Loss" summarizes the benefits of physical activity for weight loss. Addition of physical activity to a weight-loss program favorably modifies the composition of the weight lost in the direction of greater fat loss. In a pioneering study in this area, three groups of adult women maintained a 500-kcal daily caloric deficit during 16 weeks of weight loss.[149] The diet group reduced daily food intake by

EIGHT BENEFITS OF ADDING EXERCISE TO DIETARY RESTRICTION FOR WEIGHT LOSS

1. Increases the overall size of the energy deficit
2. Facilitates fat mobilization and oxidation, especially from visceral adipose tissue depots
3. Increases the relative loss of body fat by preserving the fat-free body mass
4. By conserving and even increasing the fat-free body mass, blunts the drop in resting metabolism that frequently accompanies weight loss
5. Requires less reliance on caloric restriction to create energy deficit
6. Contributes to the long-term success of the weight loss effort
7. Provides unique and significant health-related benefits
8. May provide moderate suppression of appetite

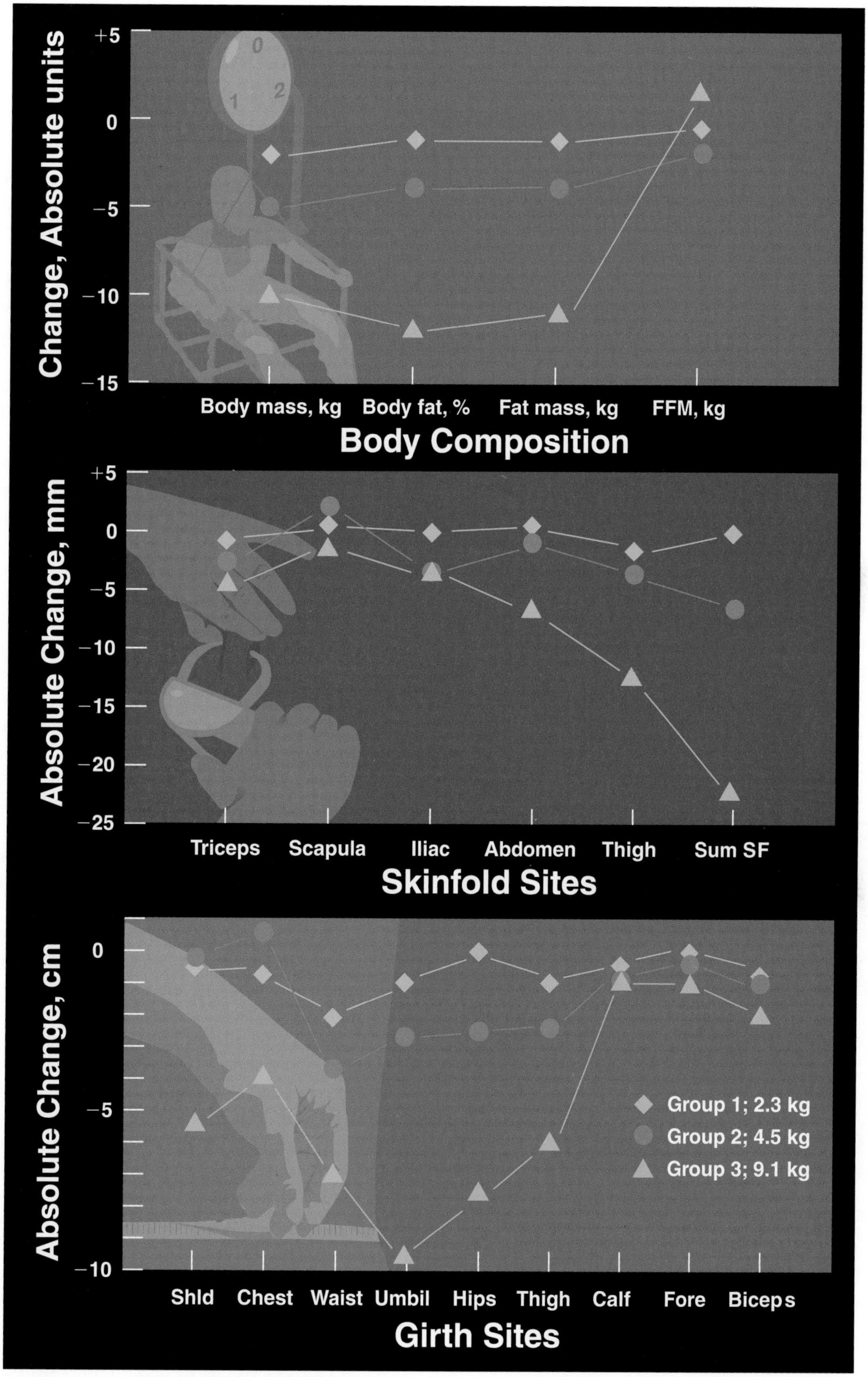

FIGURE 14.8. Changes in body composition (*top*), skinfold (*middle*), and girths (*bottom*) with specified amounts of weight loss. Abbreviations for girths: *Shld*, shoulders; *umbil*, umbilicus abdomen; *Fore*, forearm; *SF*, skinfolds. Figures 13.9 and 13.10 illustrate the anatomic sites for skinfold and girth measurement. (Data from King AC, Katch FL. Changes in body density, fatfold, and girths at 2.3-kg increments of weight loss. *Hum Biol* 1986;58:708.)

500 kcal, whereas women in the exercise group maintained daily energy intake but increased energy output by 500 kcal with a supervised walking and overall physical conditioning program. The women using diet plus exercise created the daily 500-kcal deficit by reducing food intake by 250 kcal and increasing exercise energy output by 250 kcal. No difference emerged among the three groups for weight loss; each group lost approximately 5 kg. This finding highlights that a caloric deficit reduces body weight regardless of the method used to create the energy imbalance. An interesting observation for weight loss concerned FFM. The exercise group increased FFM by 0.9 kg and the combination group by 0.5 kg, but the dieters lost 1.1 kg of lean tissue! For body fat reduction, combining diet and exercise proved most effective.

FIGURE 14.9 displays body composition changes for 40 overfat women placed into one of four groups: (1) control, with no exercise and no diet; (2) diet only, no exercise (DO); (3) diet plus resistance exercise (D + E); and (4) resistance exercise only, no diet (EO). The exercise groups trained 3 days a week for 8 weeks. They performed 10 repetitions for each of three sets of eight strength exercises. Body mass decreased for the DO (−4.5 kg) and D + E (−3.9 kg) groups, compared with the EO (+0.5 kg) and control (−0.4 kg) groups. Importantly, FFM increased significantly for the EO group (+1.1 kg), whereas the DO group lost 0.9 kg of FFM. Clearly, augmenting a calorie restriction program with resistance exercise training preserves FFM compared with dietary restriction alone.

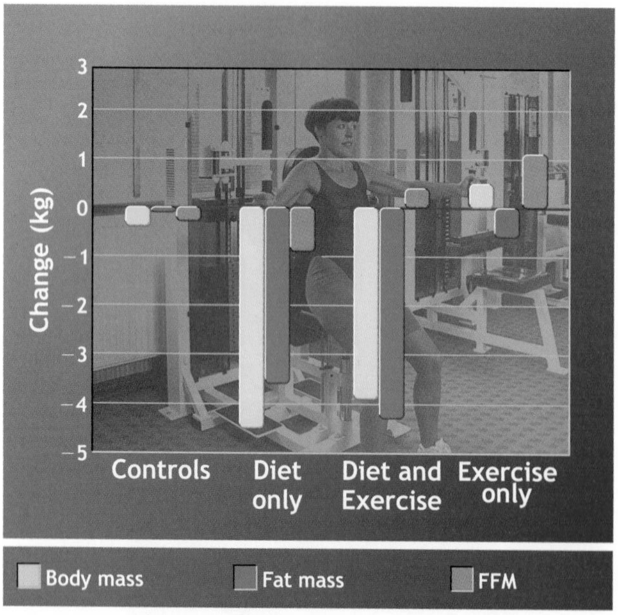

FIGURE 14.9. Changes in body composition with combinations of resistance exercise and/or diet in obese females. (From Ballor DL, et al. Resistance weight training during caloric restriction enhances lean body weight. *Am J Clin Nutr* 1988;47:19.)

WEIGHT LOSS RECOMMENDATIONS FOR WRESTLERS AND OTHER POWER ATHLETES

Weightlifters, gymnasts, and some track and field athletes require large muscular strength and power in relation to body mass. These athletes often must lose body fat without negatively impacting exercise performance. For them, an increase in relative muscular strength (strength per pound of body weight) and short-term power output capacity should improve competitive performance. The following discussion focuses on wrestlers but applies to all physically active persons who desire to reduce body fat without negatively affecting health, safety, and exercise capacity.

To reduce injury and medical complications from short and longer term periods of weight loss and dehydration, the American College of Sports Medicine (ACSM; **www.acsm.org**), National Collegiate Athletic Association (NCAA; **www.ncaa.org**), and the American Medical Association (AMA; **www.ama-assn.org**) recommend assessing each wrestler's body composition. The National Federation of State High School Associations (**www.nfhs.org**) required the adoption of weight certification beginning with the 2005 season. This assessment takes place several weeks before the competitive season to determine a **minimal wrestling weight** based on percentage body fat.[121] Five percent body fat (determined using hydrostatic weighing or population-specific skinfold equations) represents the lowest acceptable level for safe wrestling competition.[26,95] For wrestlers under 16 years of age (272,890 participants in 10,363 schools during the 2009–2010 season), 7% body fat level represents the recommended lower limit. The hydrostatic weighing or skinfold assessment of body fat recommended by the NCAA has recently been cross-validated by the more rigorous four-component body composition assessment and found acceptable in terms of accuracy and precision.[26] Importantly, percentage body fat must be determined in the euhydrated state (normal state of body water content), because dehydration of between 2 and 5% body weight through fluid restriction and exercise in a hot environment (techniques commonly used by wrestlers) violates the assumptions necessary for accurate and precise prediction of minimal wrestling weight. The most significant changes in weight classes in high school wrestling in 23 years occurred in the 2011 to 2012 season. The Wrestling Rules Committee of the National Federation of State High School Associations (**www.nfhs.org/content.aspx?id=5159**) approved an upward shift of the weight classes, beginning with the 103-lb class moving to 106 lb, which resulted in new weights for 10 of the 14 classes. The 14 weight classes (in pounds) for 2011 to 2012 are as follows: 106, 113, 120, 126, 132, 138, 145, 152, 160, 170, 182, 195, 220, and 285.

TABLE 14.6 Using Anthropometric Equations to Predict a Minimal Wrestling Weight and to Select a Competitive Weight Class

A. To predict body density (BD), use one of the following equations: (For each skinfold, record the average of at least three trials in mm.)

1. Lohman equation[a]
   BD = 1.0982 – (0.00815 × [triceps + subscapular + abdominal skinfolds]) + (0.00000084 × [triceps + subscapular + abdominal skinfolds]^2)
2. Katch and McArdle equation[b]
   BD = 1.09448 – (0.00103 × triceps skinfold) – (0.00056 × subscapular skinfold) – (0.00054 × abdominal skinfold)
3. Behnke and Wilmore equation[c]
   BD = 1.05721 – (0.00052 × abdominal skinfold) + (0.00168 × iliac diameter) + (0.00114 × neck circumference) + (0.00048 × chest circumference) + (0.00145 × abdominal circumference)
4. Thorland equation[d]
   BD = 1.0982 – (0.000815 × [triceps + abdominal skinfolds]) + (0.00000084 × [triceps + abdominal skinfolds])

B. To determine fat percentage, use the Brožek equation: % Fat = [4.570 % BD – 4.142] × 100

C. To determine fat-free weight and to identify a minimum weight class, follow the examples below:

1. Jonathan, a 15-year-old wrestler who weighs 132 lb, has a body density of 1.075 g · cc^{-1} and hopes to compete in the 119-lb weight class.
2. Jonathan's percentage fat is (4.570 ÷ 1.075 – 4.142) × 100 = 10.9%
3. Jonathan's fat weight and fat-free weight are:
   a. 132.0 lb × 0.109 = 14.4 lb fat weight
   b. 132.0 lb – 14.4 lb fat = 117.6 lb fat-free weight

D. To calculate a minimal wrestling weight:

1. Realize that the recommended minimum body weight for those 15 years and younger contains 93% (0.93) fat-free weight and 7% (0.07) fat.
2. Divide the wrestler's calculated fat-free weight by the greatest allowable fraction of fat-free weight to estimate minimal wrestling weight: 117.6 ÷ (93/100) = 117.6 ÷ 0.93 = 126.5 lb.

E. To allow for a 2% error, perform the following calculations:

1. 126.5 minimal weight × 0.02 = 2.5 lb error allowance
2. 126.5 l – 2.5 lb = 124.0 lb minimum wrestling weight

F. Conclusion: Jonathan cannot wrestle in the 119-lb weight class; rather he must compete in the 125-lb class.

G. The 2010 revised NCAA minimal wrestling strategy can be accessed at his website: http:// fs.Ncaa.org/Docs/rules/wrestling/2010/WM_preseason_mailing.pdf. The same guidelines apply to 2011-2012.

From Tipton CM. Making and maintaining weight for interscholastic wrestling.Gatorade Sports Science Exchange. 1990;2(22).

[a]Lohman TG. Skinfolds and body density and their relationship to body frames: a review. Hum Biol 1981;53:181.

[b]Katch FI, McArdle WD. Prediction of body density from simple anthropometric measurements in college-age men and women. Hum Biol 1973;145:445.

[c]Behnke AR, Wilmore JH. Evaluation and regulation of body build and composition. Englewood Cliffs, NJ: Prentice Hall, 1974.

[d]Thorland W, et al. New equations for prediction of a minimal weight in high school wrestlers. Med Sci Sports Exerc 1989;21:S72.

TABLE 14.6 outlines a practical application to determine minimal wrestling weight and an appropriate competitive weight class. The ACSM also recommends that weight loss, if warranted, should progress gradually and not exceed a 1- to 2-lb loss a week. The athlete also should continue to consume a nutritious, well-balanced diet.

Adolescent Female Gymnasts

As with wrestlers, coaches must consider a safe minimal competitive body weight for female gymnasts; golfers; swimmers and divers; volleyball, softball, and soccer players; cheerleaders; dancers; and track and field competitors, many of whom adopt disordered eating behaviors to achieve weight loss (see Chapter 15). Based on a cross-validation analysis of 11 skinfold equations for predicting percentage body fat, the following equation most accurately estimates body composition in female high school gymnasts.[40,58,122]

Female High School Gymnasts

% Body Fat = [457 ÷ 1.0987 – 0.00122 (Σ triceps, subscapular, suprailiac skinfolds in mm) + 0.00000263 (Σ triceps, subscapular, suprailiac skinfolds in mm)^2] – 414.2

This prediction equation can assess body composition in the preseason (1 standard error of estimate equals ± 2.4% body fat); for female gymnasts, body weight should contain no less than 14 to 16% body fat.

TABLE 14.7 presents general guidelines and recommendations for athletes who wish to lose weight (specifically body fat) without jeopardizing health, safety, and exercise capacity and training responsiveness. These recommendations were originally formulated for athletes in the high-power sports, but they also apply to other athletes.

TABLE 14.7 Recommendations to High-Power Athletes Who Want to Reduce Excess Body Weight

Many athletes will lose weight one way or another in an attempt to increase relative strength and power for their sport. These recommendations help the athlete lose weight in a way that minimizes health risks and maximizes sport performance and training.

1. **Arrange for qualified personnel (exercise physiologist, nutritionist, physician, or athletic trainer) to do the following:**
   a. Determine % body fat and fat-free body mass.
   b. Calculate minimal weight at 5% fat (males) or 12% (females). The textbook authors recommend 16 to 17% fat.

   The difference between present weight and minimal weight is the amount of weight that can be lost.
2. **Begin weight loss early, before the competitive season begins and progress slowly to maximize fat loss and minimize muscle and water loss; maximum rate of weight loss. should be 0.5–1.0 kg (1–2 lb) . week^{-1}.**
3. **Increase energy expenditure by doing aerobic training at least twice per week before and early in the competitive season.**
4. **Decrease the intake of calories by reducing dietary lipid, protein, and carbohydrate, but DO NOT totally eliminate any one of these three. Consume at least 1500 calories . day^{-1} to prevent vitamin and mineral deficiencies. Specific recommendations include:**
   a. Cut out desserts, butter and margarine, sauces, gravy, and dressings.
   b. Eat foods high in complex carbohydrates (fruits, vegetables, whole-grain cereals).
   c. Grill, bake, broil, or boil food; do not fry.
5. **Weigh in before and after each practice session to keep track of body water loss. Specifically:**
   a. Do not restrict water during intense training, especially in hot training environments.
   b. Consume water, sports drinks, or other fluids after practice to restore at least 80% of the weight lost in a practice session.
   c. Drink fluids low in calories (e.g., skim milk rather than whole milk).

Based in part on recommendations from the National Athletic Trainer's Association position statement on safe weight loss and maintenance practices in sport and exercise (*J Athl Train* 2011;46:322); American Dietetic Association (*J Am Diet Assoc* 2009;109:509); and American College of Sports Medicine (*Med Sci Sports Exerc* 2009;41:709. Review).

APPROPRIATE WEIGHT GAIN FOR THE PHYSICALLY ACTIVE PERSON

Gaining weight to enhance body composition and exercise performance in activities requiring muscular strength, power, or aesthetic appearance poses a unique dilemma not easily resolved. Most persons focus on weight loss to reduce excess body fat and improve overall health and appearance. Weight (fat) gain per se occurs all too readily by tilting the body's energy balance to favor greater caloric intake. *Weight gain for physically active persons should represent muscle mass and accompanying connective tissue.* Generally, this form of weight gain occurs if increased caloric intake—carbohydrates for adequate energy and protein sparing plus protein's amino acid building blocks for tissue synthesis—accompanies a resistance training program.

Persons attempting to increase muscle mass often easily fall prey to health food and diet supplement manufacturers who market "high-potency, tissue-building" substances, such as chromium, boron, vanadyl sulfate, β-hydroxymethyl β-butyrate, and numerous protein and amino acids mixtures, none of which reliably increase muscle mass. Of the hundreds of products marketed in the health and bodybuilding literature to enhance exercise performance, most focus on augmenting muscular development. Chapters 11 and 12 discuss the efficacy of many of these compounds and chemicals. Commercially prepared mixtures of powdered protein, predigested amino acids, or special high-protein "cocktails" do not promote muscle growth any more effectively than protein consumed in a well-balanced diet.[27] If an athlete experiences difficulty achieving the recommended protein intake through normal food intake—because of lifestyle, eating habits, and time requirements of training and competition—then high-quality protein supplements should prove beneficial.

Increase the Lean, Not the Fat

Endurance training usually increases FFM only slightly, but the overall effect reduces body weight from the calorie-burning and possible appetite-depressing effects of this training form. In contrast, heavy muscular overload through resistance training, supported by adequate energy and protein intake (with sufficient recovery), greatly increases muscle mass and strength.[66,78] Adequate energy intake during such training ensures that no catabolism of the protein available for muscle growth occurs from an energy deficit. Intense aerobic training should not coincide with resistance training designed to increase muscle mass.[54,73] More than likely, the added energy and perhaps protein demands of concurrent aerobic and resistance training impose a limit on muscle growth with resistance training. A prudent recommendation increases daily protein intake to about 1.6 g · kg^{-1} body mass during the resistance-training period. Diverse sources of plant and animal proteins should be consumed; relying solely on animal protein (high in saturated fatty acids and cholesterol) potentially increases heart disease risk.

If all calories consumed in excess of the energy requirement of resistance training sustained muscle growth, then 2000 to 2500 extra kcal could supply each 0.5-kg increase in lean tissue. In practical terms, 700 to 1000 kcal added to the well-balanced daily meal plan supports a weekly 0.5- to 1.0-kg gain in lean tissue plus the additional energy needs for training. The ideal situation presupposes that all extra calories synthesize lean tissue.

How Much Lean Tissue Gain Should Be Expected?

A 1-year program of intense resistance training for young, athletic men can increase body mass by about 20%, mostly from lean tissue accrual. The rate of lean tissue gain rapidly plateaus as training progresses beyond the first year. For athletic women, first-year gains in lean tissue mass average 50 to 75% of the absolute values for men, probably from the women's smaller initial lean body mass. Individual differences in the daily quantity of nitrogen incorporated into body protein (and protein incorporated into muscle) also limit and explain differences among persons in muscle mass increases with resistance training. Regularly monitoring body mass and body fat verifies whether the combination of training and additional food intake increases lean tissue and not body fat.

FIGURE 14.10 presents eight specific factors that affect the responsiveness of lean tissue synthesis to resistance training. Persons with relatively high androgen/estrogen ratios and greater percentages of fast-twitch muscle fibers probably increase lean tissue to the greatest extent in response to resistance training. Muscle mass increases occur most readily at the start of training in persons with the largest relative FFM (i.e., FFM corrected for stature and body fat).[129]

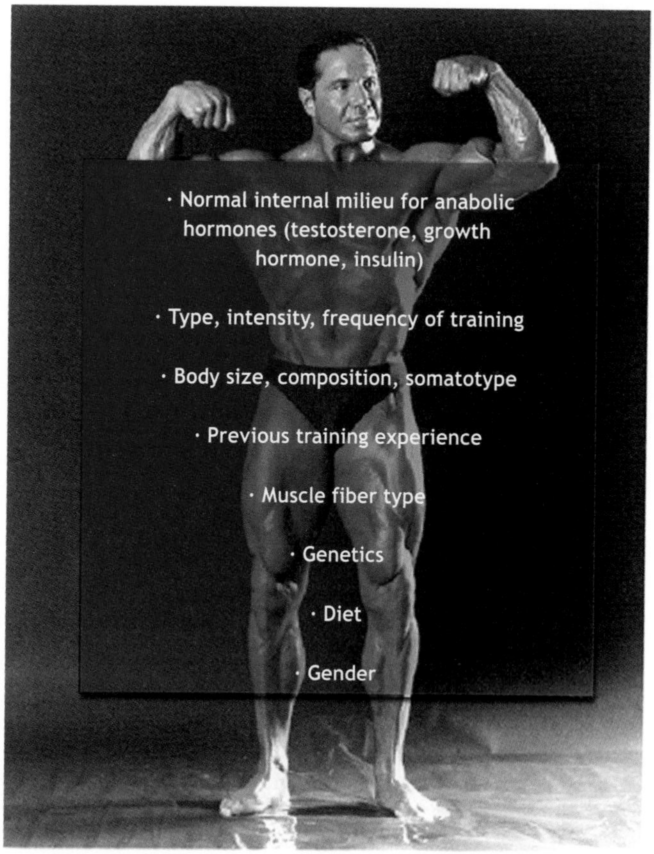

FIGURE 14.10. Specific factors affecting the magnitude of lean tissue synthesis with resistance training. (Photo courtesy of Bill Pearl.)

PERSONAL HEALTH AND EXERCISE NUTRITION 14.2

Weight Loss and Exercise Prescription

About 300,000 adult Americans die each year from obesity-related diseases. Heart disease, high blood pressure, and type 2 diabetes directly link to excess body weight and insufficient aerobic exercise.[31] Regular aerobic exercise reduces risks of some diseases by 50% or more.

Exercise prescription for weight loss in overweight persons emphasizes frequency and duration that progresses to 45 to 60 min each day. Exercise intensity becomes a consideration only when the person achieves sufficient weight loss and a fitness level suitable for cardiovascular conditioning.

Exercise Prescription

Initial focus of a prudent exercise prescription for weight loss centers on progressively increasing exercise volume (and thus caloric expenditure) with relatively low-intensity physical activity. Walking or running energy expenditure proportionally increases with speed. For example, a 70-kg person walking at 3.5 mph (17 min · mile pace^{-1}) burns about 3.3 net kcal · min^{-1}, that is, calories above the resting level. If the same person runs at 7 mph (8.5 min · mile pace^{-1}), the net calories burned are four times greater. For each mile covered, the runner burns twice as many calories as the walker and covers each mile twice as fast. This accounts for the fourfold greater rate of energy expenditure. These calculations are based on net energy expenditure values—the energy expenditure due to the exercise itself—in contrast to gross energy expenditure, which includes the resting value. The resting energy expenditure should not be counted toward weight (fat) loss because these calories are burned whether or not the person exercises.

Interestingly, nearly the same energy expenditure occurs for running and walking a given distance (about 100 kcal · mile^{-1} for a 70-kg person); this refers to the gross energy expenditure and not net values. Because walkers take longer to cover a mile than runners, they burn more calories associated with the resting component, which results in similar total kcal per mile. For weight-loss purposes, however, consider only the net caloric expenditure in exercise. Thus, one must evaluate the payoff between increasing speed of walking/running and increasing exercise duration (and/or frequency) to increase total net energy expenditure. In practice, prudent exercise for the untrained, overweight person emphasizes duration and frequency, particularly in the early stages of the program.

Subject Data and History

Female; single with no children; cigarette smoker (10 years); secretary in big office; family history of diabetes (father, type 2 diabetes) and heart disease (mother, grandmother)

Age: 35 years

Body weight: 199 lb (90.3 kg)

Height: 5 ft 6 in (1.676 m)

BMI: 32.1

Percentage body fat: 37%

Fat weight (FW): 73.6 lb (33.4 kg)

Fat-free body mass (FFM): 125.44 lb (56.9 kg)

Physical examination: Knee problems make walking/running difficult; no other obvious medical problems.

Exercise experience: Has not exercised for past 10 years except for occasional weekend biking, which she enjoys; she dislikes walking/running/swimming; sedentary throughout life; family of nonexercisers.

Laboratory data:

- Normal lipid profile
- Normal blood glucose
- Daily caloric intake of about 3200 kcal
- High lipid intake (>38% of total kcal)
- Normal blood pressure

General impressions: Obese female with four risk factors (sedentary; obesity; smoking; family history of heart disease). Person needs lifestyle modification.

Case Questions

1. Give a preliminary assessment.
2. Recommend a body weight goal.
3. Formulate a prudent exercise prescription.

thePoint *Visit* thePoint.lww.com/MKKSEN4e *to find suggested answers to these Case Questions.*

SUMMARY

1. Slight but prolonged caloric excesses produce substantial weight gain. To prevent such a caloric disparity, energy output must balance energy input.
2. Nearly 70% of Americans struggle to lose weight (29% of men and 40% of women), yet only one-fifth use the recommended combination of eating fewer calories and exercising regularly.
3. Almost 65% of the US population classify as either overweight (BMI 25.0–29.9) or obese (BMI ≥30). Of this total, 30.5% classify as obese. The obesity epidemic contributes significantly to the rising tide of type 2 diabetes, cancer, and cardiovascular disease.
4. Among US youth, obesity has more than doubled in the last 15 years, with an ever-widening gap between the weights of persons deemed overly fat and those considered thin. Excessive body fatness becomes particularly prevalent among poor and minority children.
5. Genetic factors probably account for 25 to 30% of excessive body fat accumulation.
6. Genetic predisposition does not necessarily cause obesity, but given the right environment, the genetically susceptible person gains body fat. Substantial alterations in the population's gene pool (which require many thousands of years) cannot explain the dramatic worldwide obesity epidemic.
7. A defective gene for adipocyte leptin production and/or hypothalamic leptin insensitivity (plus defects in production and/or sensitivity to other chemicals) causes the brain to assess adipose tissue status improperly. This creates a chronic state of positive energy balance.
8. The standard dietary approach to weight loss that decreases caloric intake below the requirement for current weight maintenance generally helps obese patients to lose about 0.5 kg · week^{-1}. Success in preventing weight regain is relatively poor, averaging between 5 and 20% of those who lose weight. Typically, one third to two thirds of the lost weight returns within a year, and almost all of it returns within 5 years.
9. Reducing body fat generally improves exercise performance because it directly increases relative (per unit

body size) muscular strength and power and aerobic capacity. Reduced drag force, which impedes forward movement in air and water, also represents a positive effect of weight loss on exercise performance.

10. Three methods unbalance the energy balance equation to produce weight loss: (1) reduce energy intake below daily energy expenditure, (2) maintain normal energy intake and increase energy output, and (3) decrease energy intake and increase energy expenditure.
11. A caloric deficit of 3500 kcal, created through either diet or exercise, represents the calories in 0.45 kg (1.0 lb) of adipose tissue.
12. Appropriate modification of eating and exercise behaviors increases one's chance for successful weight loss.
13. Prudent dieting effectively promotes weight loss. Disadvantages of extremes of semistarvation include loss of fat-free mass (FFM), lethargy, possible malnutrition, and depressed resting metabolism (as long as one maintains an energy deficit).
14. Repeated cycles of weight loss–weight regain (yo-yo effect) may increase the body's ability to conserve energy, thus making weight loss with subsequent dieting less effective. The risks from obesity far exceed those from weight cycling.
15. Daily energy expenditure consists of the sum of resting metabolism, thermogenic influences (particularly the thermic effect of food), and energy generated during physical activity. Physical activity most profoundly affects the variability among humans in daily energy expenditure.
16. The calories burned in exercise accumulate. Regular extra physical activity creates a considerable energy deficit over time.
17. The precise role of exercise in appetite suppression or stimulation remains unclear, but moderate increases in physical activity may blunt appetite and depress energy intake of a previously sedentary, overweight person. Most athletes eventually consume enough calories to counterbalance training's added caloric expenditure.
18. Combining exercise with caloric restriction offers a flexible and effective means for weight loss. Exercise enhances fat mobilization and catabolism. Regular aerobic exercise retards lean tissue loss; resistance training increases the FFM.
19. Rapid weight loss during the first few days of a caloric deficit mainly reflects loss of body water and stored glycogen; greater fat loss occurs per unit of weight lost as caloric restriction continues.
20. Selective exercise of specific body areas proves no more effective for localized fat loss than more general physical activity. Areas of greatest fat concentration and/or lipid-mobilizing enzyme activity supply the most energy for exercise, regardless of the area exercised.
21. Differences in body fat distribution partially explain the gender difference in exercise-induced weight loss. Fat deposited in the upper body and abdominal regions (male pattern obesity) responds readily to neurohumoral stimulation and preferentially mobilizes in exercise compared with fat deposited in gluteal and femoral regions (female pattern obesity).
22. Wrestlers undergo severe training and repeated bouts of short-term weight loss. Wrestlers should be discouraged from drastically reducing body fat if it brings them below 5%.
23. A total of 700 to 1000 extra kcal per day supports a weekly 0.5- to 1.0-kg gain in lean tissue and the energy requirements of resistance training. Person physiologic variations and training factors affect gains in muscle mass.

thePoint *Visit* **thePoint.lww.com/MKKSEN4e** *to view the following animations related to content presented in Chapter 14:* ***Muscle contraction; Muscle contraction type;*** *and* ***Sliding filament theory.***

TEST YOUR KNOWLEDGE ANSWERS

1. **True:** The World Health Organization, International Obesity Task Force, and other major healthcare organizations have declared a global obesity epidemic. Obesity now represents the second leading cause of preventable deaths in the United States at a total yearly cost of $160 billion, or approximately 10% of the US healthcare expenditures. Overweight, but not obese, nonsmoking men and women in their mid-30s to mid-40s die at least 3 years sooner than normal-weight counterparts, a risk just as damaging to life expectancy as cigarette smoking. Obese persons can expect about a 7-year decrease in life expectancy.
2. **False:** Greater prevalence of obesity occurs among black women (about 50%) than among white women (33%). Studies of obese black and white women show small differences in resting metabolism; on average, black women burn nearly 100 fewer calories each day during rest than whites. This slower rate of processing calories persists even after adjusting for differences in body mass and body composition. The greater energy economy of black women during exercise and throughout the day most likely reflects an inherited trait, as it persists both before and after weight loss. This effect, which also exists among children and adolescents, predisposes a black female to gain weight and regain it following weight loss.

3. **False:** The standard dietary approach to weight loss that decreases caloric intake below the requirement for current weight maintenance generally helps obese patients lose about 0.5 kg · $week^{-1}$. Success at preventing weight regain is relatively poor, averaging between 5 and 20%. Regular physical activity, through either recreation or occupation, effectively contributes to preventing weight gain and thwarts the tendency to regain lost weight.

4. **False:** Older men and women who maintain active lifestyles impede the "normal" pattern of fat gain observed in most adults. Research shows that time spent in physical activity inversely relates to body fat level in young and middle-aged men who exercise regularly. The greater level of body fat among active middle-aged men compared with younger, more active counterparts resulted from less vigorous training, not greater energy intake.

5. **True:** Combining moderate food restriction with additional daily physical activity offers the greatest flexibility for achieving fat loss. This combination also enables the persons to remain well nourished for exercise training and peak performance.

6. **True:** Resting metabolism decreases when food restriction progressively produces weight loss. This hypometabolism often exceeds the decrease attributable to the loss of body mass or fat-free body mass. Depressed metabolism conserves energy, causing the diet to become less effective despite a restricted caloric intake. This produces a weight-loss plateau at which further weight loss becomes considerably less than predicted from the mathematics of the restricted energy intake.

7. **False:** For most persons, semistarvation with a very low-calorie diet (VLCD) does not compose an "ultimate diet" or the proper approach to weight control. Because a VLCD provides inadequate carbohydrate, the glycogen storage depots in the liver and muscles deplete rapidly. This impairs physical tasks requiring either high-intensity aerobic effort or shorter duration anaerobic power output. The continuous nitrogen loss with fasting and resulting weight loss reflects an exacerbated lean tissue loss, which may occur disproportionately from critical organs like the heart. The success rate remains poor for prolonged VLCD use.

8. **False:** Excess weight gain often parallels reduced physical activity rather than increased caloric intake. Approximately 27% of US adults engage in no daily physical activity, and another 28% do not regularly take part in physical activity. Among active endurance-trained men, body fat inversely relates to energy expenditure (low body fat, high energy expenditure and vice versa); no relationship emerges between body fat and food intake. Surprisingly, physically active people who eat the most generally weigh the least and exhibit the highest levels of fitness. Also, excessive food intake does not fully explain the rise in obesity among children. Obese infants do not characteristically consume more calories than recommended dietary standards. For children ages 4 to 6 years, a reduced level of physical activity primarily accounts for their 25% lower daily energy expenditure than the energy expenditure recommendation for this age.

9. **False:** Regular physical activity can play a singularly important role in protecting against weight gain. Men and women of all ages who maintain a physically active lifestyle (or become involved in regular exercise regimens) maintain a more desirable level of body composition. For overweight adult women, a dose-response relationship exists between the amount of exercise and long-term weight loss.

10. **False:** Resistance training provides an important adjunct to aerobic training in programs of weight loss and weight maintenance. The energy expended in circuit resistance training (continuous exercise using low resistance and high repetitions) averages about 9 kcal a minute. This exercise mode, therefore, can "burn" substantial calories during a typical 30- to 60-min workout. Even conventional resistance training that involves less total energy expenditure affects muscular strength and fat-free body mass during weight loss more positively than programs that rely solely on food restriction.

Key References

Bagley S, et al. Family structure and children's television viewing and physical activity. *Med Sci Sports Exerc* 2006;38:910.

Berrington A, et al. Body mass index and mortality among 1.46 million white adults. *N Engl J Med* 2010;363:2211.

Bouchard C, et al. The response to long term feeding in identical twins. *N Engl J Med* 1990;322:1477.

Bouchard C, et al. The response to exercise with constant energy intake in identical twins. *Obes Res* 1994;2:400.

Calle EE, et al. Overweight, obesity, and mortality from cancer in a prospectively studied cohort of U.S. adults. *N Engl J Med* 2003;348:1625.

Clark RR, et al. Minimum weight prediction methods cross-validated by the four-component model. *Med Sci Sports Exerc* 2004;36:639.

Dietz WH, Robinson TN. Overweight children and adolescents. *N Engl J Med* 2005;352:2100.

Donnelly JE, Smith BK. Is exercise effective for weight loss with ad libitum diet? Energy balance, compensation, and gender differences. *Exerc Sport Sci Rev* 2005;33:169.

Finkelstein EA, et al. Annual medical spending attributable to obesity: payer- and service-specific estimates. *Health Aff* 2009;28:w831

Foster GD, et al. A randomized trial of a low-carbohydrate diet for obesity. *N Engl J Med* 2003;348:2082.

Guo SS, et al. Predicting overweight and obesity in adulthood from body mass index values in childhood and adolescence. *Am J Clin Nutr* 2002;76:653.

Gwinup G, et al. Thickness of subcutaneous fat and activity of underlying muscles. *Ann Intern Med* 1971;74:408.

Hansen RD, Allen BJ. Habitual physical activity, anabolic hormones, and potassium content of fat-free mass in post menopausal women. *Am J Clin Nutr* 2002;75:314.

Heitmann BL, Garby L. Composition (lean and fat tissue) of weight changes in adult Danes. *Am J Clin Nutr* 2002;75:834.

Hirsch J, et al. Diet composition and energy balance in humans. *Am J Clin Nutr* 1998;67(Suppl):551S.

Hortobagyi T, et al. Comparison of four methods to assess body composition in black and white athletes. *Int J Sports Nutr* 1992;2:60.

Housh TJ, et al. Validity of skinfold estimates of percent fat in high school female gymnasts. *Med Sci Sports Exerc* 1996;28:1331.

Iversen SG, et al. Occupational physical activity, overweight, and mortality: a follow-up study of 47,405 Norwegian women and men. *Res Q Exerc Sport* 2007;78:151.

Katch FI, et al. Effects of situp exercise training on adipose cell size and adiposity. *Res Q Exerc Sport* 1984;55:242.

Keogh JB, et al. Long-term weight maintenance and cardiovascular risk factors are not different following weight loss on carbohydrate-restricted diets high in either monounsaturated fat or protein in obese hyperinsulinaemic men and women. *Br J Nutr* 2007;97:405.

King AC, Katch FI. Changes in body density, fatfolds and girths at 2.3 kg increments of weight loss. *Hum Biol* 1986;58:708.

Oppliger RA, et al. NCAA rule change improves weight loss among national championship wrestlers. *Med Sci Sports Exerc* 2006;38:963.

Wang Y, Beydoun MA. The obesity epidemic in the United States: gender, age, socioeconomic, racial/ethnic, and geographic characteristics: a systematic review and meta-regression analysis. *Epidemiol Rev* 2007;29:6.

Williams PT. Maintaining vigorous activity attenuates 7-yr weight gain in 8340 runners. *Med Sci Sports Exer* 2007;39:801.

Williams PT, Thompson PD. Dose-dependent effects of training and detraining on weight in 6406 runners during 7.4 years. *Obesity* (Silver Spring) 2006;14:1975.

thePoint *Visit* thePoint.lww.com/MKKSEN4e *for a list of the references cited in this chapter, including additional, relevant references.*

CHAPTER 15

Disordered Eating

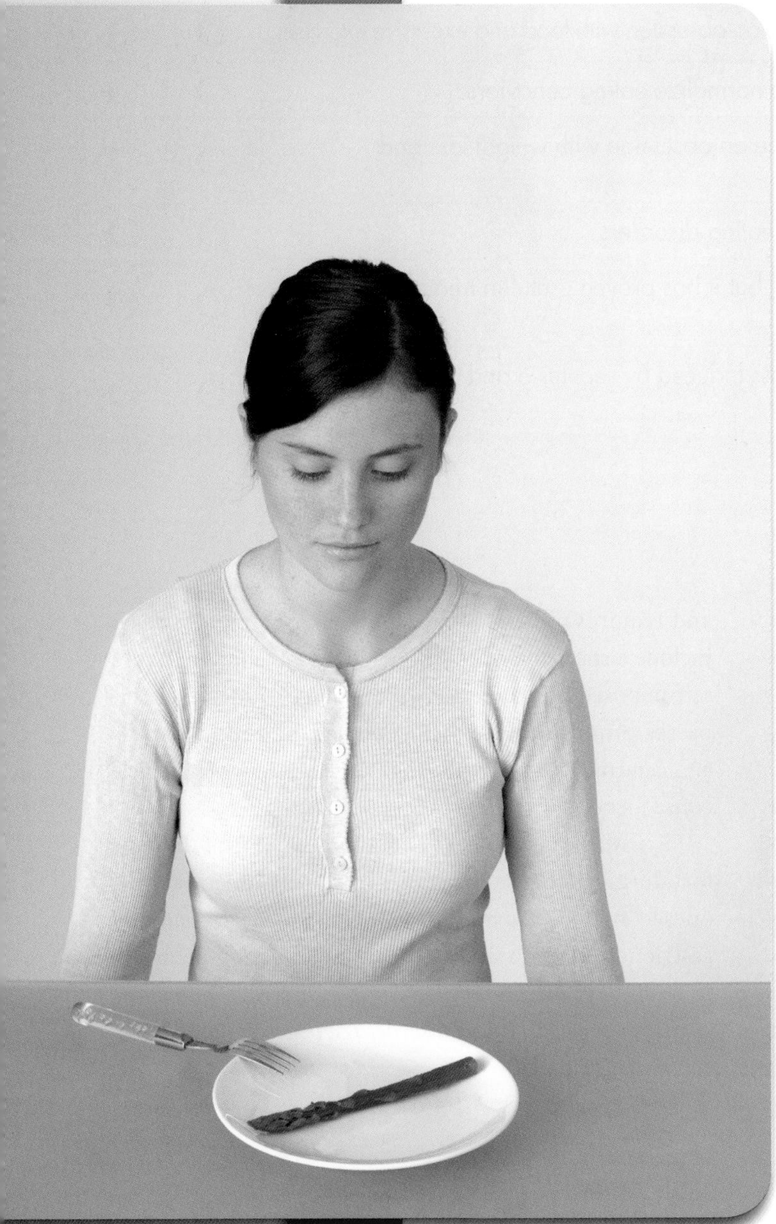

OUTLINE

- Eating Disorders Versus Disordered Eating
- An Inordinate Focus on Body Weight
- Muscle Dysmorphia: "The Adonis Complex"
- The Exercise Addict
- Clinical Eating Disorders
- Cause or Effect? The Role of Sport in Eating Disorders
- Eating Disorders Affect Exercise Performance
- Eating Disorders Affect Bone Mineral Density
- Management of Eating Disorders in Athletes
- Common Sense Guidelines for Coaches and Trainers Concerning Eating Disorders
- Therapeutic Methods to Treat Eating Disorders
- Athletics Must Change from Within
- Future Research

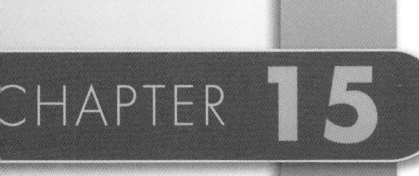

TEST YOUR KNOWLEDGE

Select true or false for the 10 statements below, then check out the answers at the end of the chapter. Retake the test after you've read the chapter; you should achieve 100%!	True	False
1. The Miss America contestants serve as a prime example of the perfect reference woman for body fat and body mass.	❍	❍
2. In general, athletes are at no greater risk for disordered eating behaviors than nonathletes.	❍	❍
3. A unique subclass of disordered eating behaviors most likely exists among female athletes.	❍	❍
4. Disordered eating behaviors do not appear to afflict men.	❍	❍
5. Two major characteristics of anorexia nervosa include an obsession with food and excessive exercise.	❍	❍
6. The primary goal in treating anorexia nervosa is to normalize eating behaviors.	❍	❍
7. Two major characteristics of bulimia nervosa include an obsession with weight loss and excessive exercise.	❍	❍
8. Forced hospitalization is the primary treatment for eating disorders.	❍	❍
9. Exercise is not useful for treating anorexia nervosa, but it has proven useful in treating bulimia nervosa.	❍	❍
10. Muscle dysmorphia refers to severe muscle weakness induced by repetitive and compulsive purging behaviors.	❍	❍

Eating disorders and *disordered eating* do not describe the same phenomenon. Anorexia nervosa and bulimia nervosa represent *eating disorder* illnesses that seriously interfere with daily activities. In contrast, *disordered eating* represents a temporary or mild change in eating *behaviors*. Often, disordered eating patterns occur following either an illness or stressful event or are related to a dietary change intended to improve health or appearance. Disordered eating activities rarely persist and usually do not require professional intervention; in contrast, continued disordered eating behaviors often lead to a diagnosed eating disorder.

For those with an eating disorder, the focus on food becomes a source of consistent stress and anxiety and requires professional intervention. Eating disorders include a spectrum of emotional illnesses that range from self-imposed starvation to chronic binge eating. These illnesses produce severe distortions of the eating process and can trigger life-threatening physical and psychological consequences.

Many people have eaten to the point of discomfort during a Thanksgiving or Christmas dinner. Stuffing oneself at a holiday meal or going on an occasional food restriction plan does not constitute an eating disorder. According to the *Manual of Clinical Dietetics*, *"a defining characteristic of an eating disorder is a persistent inability to eat in moderation."*

EATING DISORDERS: A CONTINUUM

The American Psychiatric Association's *Diagnostic and Statistical Manual of Mental Disorders* (DSM-IV) places eating disorders into three categories, with small but significant areas of overlap.[23] These categories form a continuum with self-starvation at one end and compulsive overeating at the other end (**FIG. 15.1** and **TABLE 15.1**). A diagnosis of an eating disorder not otherwise specified (EDNOS) usually comprises disorders not diagnosed as anorexia, bulimia, or binge-eating disorders.

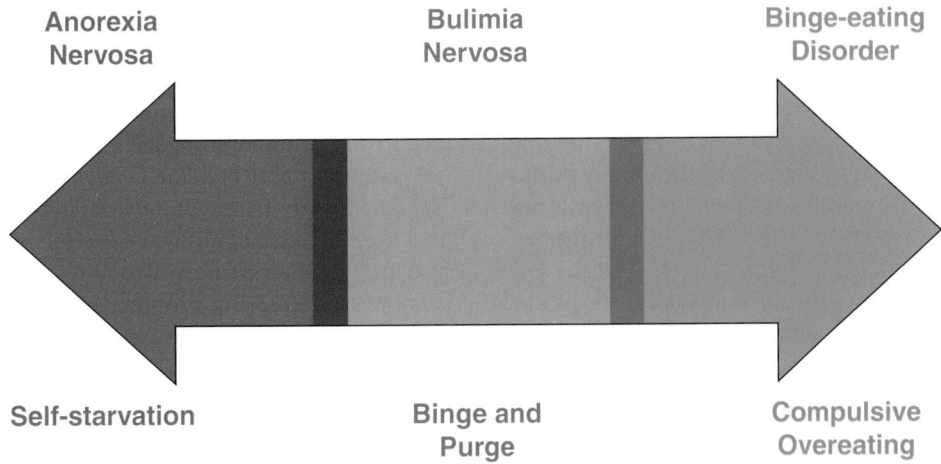

FIGURE 15.1. The continuum of eating disorders.

This DSM-IV scheme for classifying eating disorders poorly reflects clinical reality because at least one half of the cases seen in clinical practice relate to EDNOS or combination of conditions. The changes proposed for the next version, DSM-V, hopefully will address this apparent shortcoming.

Anorexia nervosa occurs at the self-starvation end of the continuum. Anorexia, a self-imposed starvation syndrome triggered by multiple factors, includes a severely distorted body image. Anorectics are at never-ending war with their bodies, and even when they are dangerously underweight, they continue to severely restrict food intake (the major symptom of anorexia nervosa).

Binge eating or compulsive overeating lies at the opposite end of the continuum of eating disorders. People with this disorder chronically consume massive quantities of food and are typically overfat; however, not all overfat people binge eat. The diagnosis of binge-eating disorder is based on a person having an average of two binge-eating episodes a week for 6 continuous months. Bulimia nervosa occurs in the middle of the eating disorder continuum. These persons compulsively gorge themselves and then purge to eliminate the ingested food.

History

Anorexia nervosa, while considered a relatively recent disorder, has a history that dates back many centuries.[16,63,82] Examples of self-starvation appeared in the Hellenistic era (circa 323–146 BC). Holy or saintly anorexics abused their bodies, rejected marriage, and sought religious asylum, where unfortunately, many perished. During the Victorian era (reign of Queen Victoria from 1837 to 1901), large numbers of mothers and daughters avoided food for fear of giving the impression that their physical appetite was linked to their appetite for sex. It was commonly believed that women who consumed too much food had a greater sexual appetite!

TABLE 15.1 Distinguishing Characteristics of Eating Disorders

Factor	Anorexia Nervosa	Bulimia Nervosa	Binge-Eating Disorder
Body weight	Below normal (<85% of recommended weight)	Usually normal	Above normal
Binge eating	Possible	Yes, at least twice for 3 months	Yes, at least twice for 6 months
Purging	Possible	Yes, at least twice for 3 months	No
Restrict food intake	Yes	Yes	Yes
Body image	Dissatisfaction with body and distorted image of body size	Dissatisfaction with body and distorted image of body size	Dissatisfaction with body
Fear of being fat	Yes	Yes	Not excessive
Self-esteem	Low	Low	Low
Menstrual abnormalities	Absence of at least 3 consecutive periods	No	No

Richard Morton (1637–1698) generally receives credit for the first medical description in 1689 of a wasting (anorectic) disease often associated with tuberculosis.[63] In the early 1800s, scattered reports appeared in the English medical literature concerning eating disorders, and two neurologists in 1873 separately described the condition now called **anorexia nervosa**. Well-published French physician Ernest Charles Lasègue (1816–1883; student with aspiring physician Claude Bernard (see Chapter 14, p. 479) at the Faculté de Médecine in Paris, wrote of women's refusal of food "that may be indefinitely prolonged," and Sir William Gull (1816–1890; physician to Queen Victoria of England) studied women who refused food. Gull is credited as the first person to "officially" use the term anorexia nervosa instead of anorexia hysteria coined by Lasègue. A publication by Lasègue in an 1870 French medical journal chronicled cases of "anorexia hysteria." The photos below may be the first photographs published in 1900 that depicted the condition in young French girls.

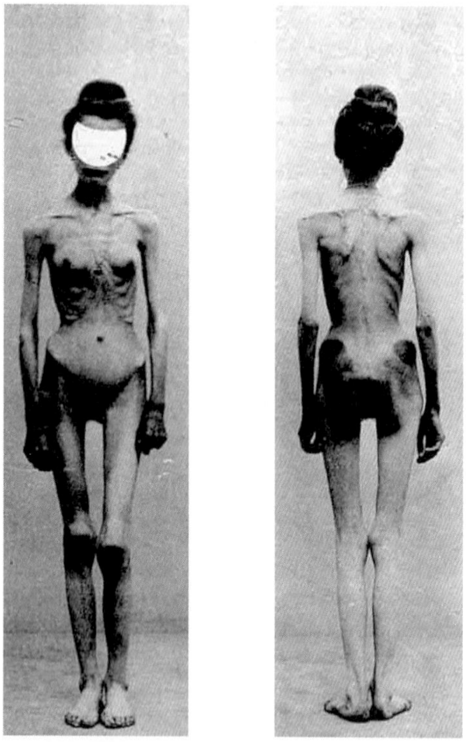

It was not until the early 1970s that the American media began to write about eating disorders. Beginning in 1974, articles described how young women refused to eat but without really explaining the seriousness of the illness. In 1983, the popular folksinger Karen Carpenter died of anorexia nervosa, bringing intense media scrutiny about the history and seriousness of eating disorders in general, and anorexia nervosa in particular. This watershed event prompted other actresses and public figures to speak out about their battles to achieve thinness.

The first published photo of a female suffering from anorexia nervosa was presented at the annual meeting of the New Hampshire Medical Society at Manchester, NH, on May 17, 1932, and published that same year in the *New England Journal of Medicine* (**FIG. 15.2**). Before the common usage of the term "anorexia nervosa," the disease was known as "long-term fasting" or "self-starvation."

In 1978, noted Hungarian psychologist Hilde Bruch (1904–1984) published *The Golden Cage*, a book based on 70 cases mostly from young women's testimonials during her three decades of clinical experience in treating eating disorders.[15] Interestingly, Bruch claimed the disease had become an increasing problem in American colleges and universities. Research now confirms this supposition, particularly in women's individual sports (e.g., gymnastics, swimming and diving, dance) where thinness and "looking good" remain a premium (see Chapter 14). Fortunately, many private and public science-oriented organizations have focused research efforts devoted to the causes and etiology of eating disorders.

Prevalence and Incidence of Eating Disorders

The term *prevalence* of eating disorders refers to the estimated population of people afflicted with an eating disorder at any given time. The term *incidence* refers to the annual diagnosis rate or number of new cases diagnosed yearly. These two statistics differ; a short-lived disease such as the flu can have high annual incidence but low prevalence, and a lifelong disease such as diabetes can have a low annual incidence but high prevalence.

Over a lifetime, an estimated 0.5 to 3.7% of females suffer from anorexia nervosa and 1.1 to 4.2% suffer from bulimia nervosa.[25,35] Community surveys estimate that between 2 and 5% of Americans experience binge-eating disorder in any 6-month period.[37] The mortality rate among people with anorexia nervosa averages 0.6% a year or approximately 5.6% per decade—about 12 times higher than the annual death rate from all causes of death among females age 15 to 24 years in the general population.[41]

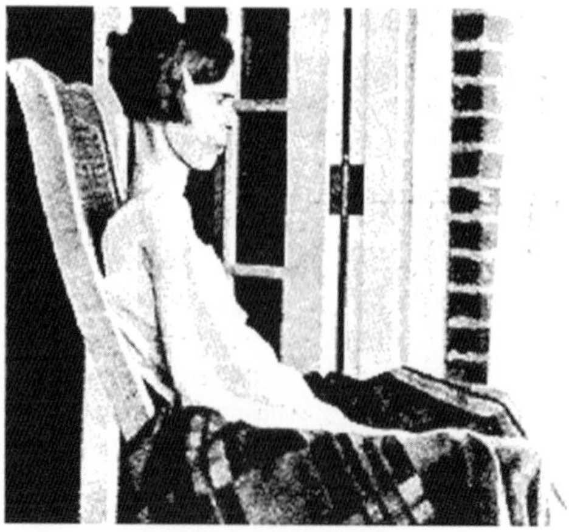

FIGURE 15.2. The first published photo of an anorectic in an American medical journal. (From Clow FE. Fasting girls. *N Engl J Med* 1932;207(14):813.)

STATISTICS ABOUT EATING DISORDERS

A. Prevalence

1. Eight million Americans have an eating disorder—seven million women and one million men.
2. One in 200 American women suffers from anorexia.
3. Two to three in 100 American women suffers from bulimia.
4. Nearly one-half of all Americans personally know someone with an eating disorder. (Note: One in five Americans suffers from mental illnesses.)
5. Males represent an estimated 10 to 15% of people afflicted with anorexia or bulimia.

B. Mortality Rates

1. Eating disorders have the highest mortality rate of any mental illness.
2. A study by the National Association of Anorexia Nervosa and Associated Disorders reported that 5 to 10% of anorexics die within 10 years after contracting the disease; 18 to 20% of anorexics will be dead after 20 years; and only 30 to 40% ever fully recover.
3. The mortality rate associated with anorexia nervosa is 12 times higher than the death rate of all causes of death for females age 15 to 24 years.
4. Twenty percent of people who suffer from anorexia prematurely die from complications related to their eating disorder, including suicide and heart problems.

Source: South Carolina Department of Mental Health. Eating disorder statistics. Available at: www.state.sc.us/dmh/anorexia/statistics.htm. Accessed August 8, 2011.

TABLE 15.2 Prevalence of Unhealthy and Extreme Weight Reduction Practices Among Teenage Girls

Behavior (monthly)	Prevalence (%)
No dairy[a]	16
No meats[a]	18
No starchy foods[a]	13
Slimming biscuit use	15
Slimming drink use	11
Skipping meals	46
Fad dieting	14
"Crash" dieting[b]	22
Fasting[b]	21
Diet pills	5
Diuretic use[b]	2
Laxative use[b]	5
Cigarette use[b]	12

[a] *These foods are eliminated and not compensated for with a balanced diet (e.g., a balanced vegetarian diet).*

[b] *Extreme dieting is defined as "crash" dieting, fasting, or use of diet pills, diuretics, laxatives, and cigarettes.*

From Grigg M, et al. Disordered eating and unhealthy weight-reduction practices among adolescent females. *Prevent Med 1996;25:745.*

AN INORDINATE FOCUS ON BODY WEIGHT

Among 3000 middle-school children studied for body image and dietary practices, 55% of eighth-grade girls believed they were fat (13% actually were), and 50% had dieted. For the boys, 28% considered themselves fat (13% actually were), and 15% had dieted. Among 869 Australian schoolgirls age 14 to 17 years, 335 reported at least one disordered eating behavior, whereas monthly bingeing occurred in 8% and vomiting in 27%.[35] **TABLE 15.2** lists the prevalence of monthly unhealthy and extreme weight reduction practices of these teenage girls. Of the group, 57% practiced "unhealthy dieting" and 36% practiced dieting behaviors considered extreme, such as crash dieting, fasting, and use of diet pills, diuretics, laxatives, and cigarettes.

Disordered eating behaviors generally affect females between the ages of 15 and 35, although women in the United States in their 30s to 50s may account for up to one third of eating disorder patients. The prevalence in the general population ranges from 1 to 5% of female high school and college students to as high as 12 to 15% of women in medical and graduate schools.[25,39,40,66] Thin body preoccupation and social pressure in adolescent girls represent important risk factors for the development of eating disorders.[58] Childhood traits reflecting obsessive–compulsive personality also appear to be important risk factors.[1] Adolescent girls who experience physical and sexual dating violence show a relatively high rate of abnormal weight control behaviors that include laxative use and/or vomiting.[72,82] Contrary to the conventional belief of many health professionals, African American women are not immune from eating disorders. A survey of African American college women found a prevalence of eating disorders similar to that among white peers; 2% had a full-blown eating disorder, and 23% showed some eating disorder symptoms. Cultural differences in the view of attractiveness—thin African American women are often considered unattractive—often causes some African American women to gain weight by binge eating.[64]

FIGURE 15.3 displays the relationship between teenage girls' actual body weight classification (determined by body mass index [BMI]) and perceived body weight. Regardless of objective weight categorization, 47% of all girls actively tried to lose weight, including 19% of underweight girls and 56% of normal-weight girls. When asked to categorize their current weight, 63% considered themselves overweight, yet only

Additional Insights

A Little Excess Weight May Not Be So Bad Above Age 70

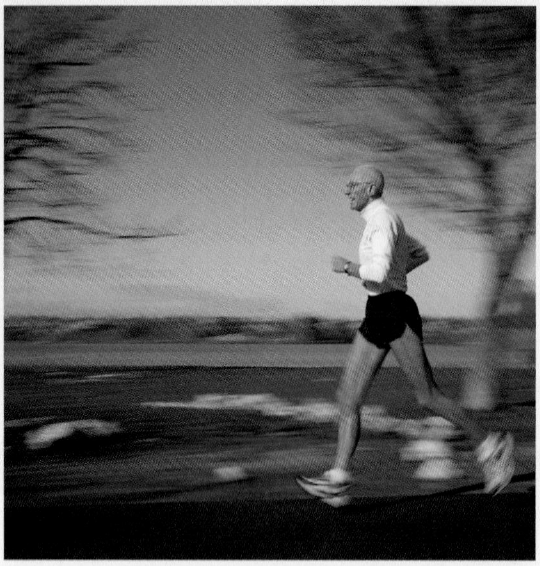

Recommendations about body weight and health may change as one ages. Two long-running Australian studies of 9240 men and women age 70 to 75 found that being classified overweight by BMI classification (originally developed on studies of younger and middle-aged adults) associated with a 13% *lower* all-cause mortality risk, whereas normal-weight and obese persons had a slightly higher risk of death from all causes. Even after controlling for early mortality, the overweight persons were still at lowest risk of death. These findings are consistent with the following observation; *weight loss in the elderly associates with an increased mortality risk, supporting the claim that BMI thresholds for overweightness and obesity may be overly restrictive for older persons.* The findings, however, should not be taken as an excuse for the elderly to continue to be physically inactive, particularly because a self-described sedentary lifestyle doubled mortality risk for women and increased risk by 28% for men.

These intriguing findings of beneficial effects of some excess weight in the elderly are in line with a controversial 2007 study by US Centers for Disease Control and Prevention and National Cancer Institute researchers that showed that overweight adults were at a reduced rate of dying from lung disease, infection, and Alzheimer disease. One hypothesis maintains that the availability of a modestly larger nutritional and metabolic fat reserve with aging provides some benefit in warding off and/or recovery from serious illness. According to the lead author of the Australian research: *"Our study suggests that those people who survive to age 70 in reasonable health have a different set of risks and benefits associated with the amount of body fat compared to younger individuals. Overweight older people are not at greater mortality risk, and there is little evidence that dieting in the group confers any benefit."*

Source: Flicker L, et al. Body mass index and survival in men and women aged 70 to 75. *J Am Geriatr Soc* 2010;58:234.

Related References

Calle EE, et al. Overweight, obesity, and mortality from cancer in a prospectively studied cohort of U.S. adults. *N Engl J Med* 2003;348:1625.

Dall TM, et al. Weight loss and lifetime medical expenditures: a case study with TRICARE prime beneficiaries. *Am J Prev Med* 2011;40:338.

Flicker L, et al. Body mass index and survival in men and women aged 70 to 75. *J Am Geriatr Soc* 2010;58:234.

Hotchkiss JW, Leyland AH. The relationship between body size and mortality in the linked Scottish Health Surveys: cross-sectional surveys with follow-up. *Int J Obes* 2011;35:838.

Paganini-Hill A. Lifestyle practices and cardiovascular disease mortality in the elderly: the Leisure World Cohort Study. *Cardiol Res Pract* 2011;35:838.

Power BD, et al. Body adiposity in later life and the incidence of dementia: the Health in Men Study. *PLoS One* 2011;6:e17902.

Singh PN, et al. Does excess body fat maintained after the seventh decade decrease life expectancy? *J Am Geriatr Soc* 2011;59:1003.

16% actually were; 28% seemed "just right" (55% were of normal weight), and 9% concluded they were underweight (30% actually were). Such findings take on additional significance because previous attempts at dieting often develop into a fully developed eating disorder.

Miss America and BMI—Undernourished Role Models?

In 1967, only an 8% difference in body weight existed between professional models and the average American woman. Today, a model's body weight is an average of 23 lb below the national average for women (5 ft 11 in, 117 lb vs 5 ft 4 in, 140 lb). This makes the BMI of most fashion models lower than all but 2% of American women. A focus on thinness has become particularly apparent among Miss America contestants.

Many consider Miss America beauty pageant contestants to possess the ideal combination of beauty, grace, and talent. Each competitor survives the rigors of state and local contests, thus satisfying judges that finalists have "ideal qualities" worthy of role-model status. To some extent, the consummate image of the Miss America physique shapes society's generalized "ideal" for female size and shape. The contest, televised worldwide to millions of viewers, reinforces

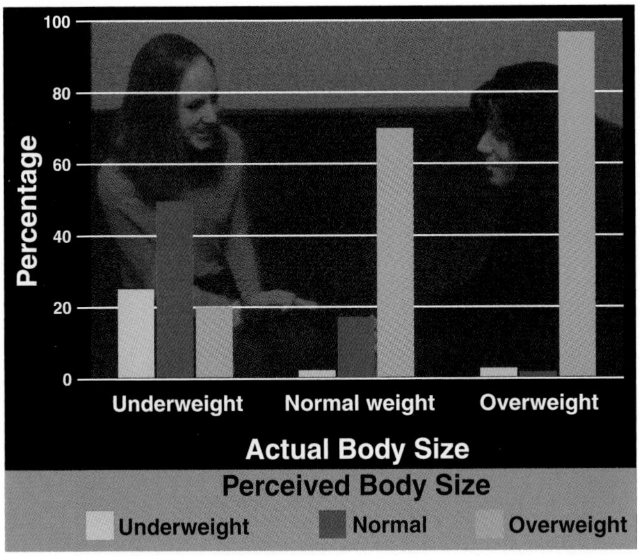

FIGURE 15.3. Perception of current body weight and actual body weight classification determined by BMI in 851 teenage girls. (From Grigg M, et al. Disordered eating and unhealthy weight reduction practices among adolescent females. *Prevent Med* 1996;25:745.)

BIGGER MODELS? SLIM CHANCE!

Recent deaths of several high-profile models (a 22-year-old popular Uruguayan model suffered a heart attack believed to be the result of a 10-year struggle with anorexia nervosa; a 21-year-old Brazilian, 5-ft 7-in model who weighed only 88 lb died during a runway shoot) have caused some clothes designers to require that models submit proof they do not suffer from eating disorders.

The Council of Fashion Designers of America (CFDA) recently recommended that model agencies (1) do not hire women under age 16, (2) supply their models with healthy snacks backstage at shoots, and (3) provide them with nutrition and fitness education. But the CFDA failed to endorse recommendations by nutritionists and scientists that any model with a BMI below 18.5 not be allowed to walk the runway. In the fashion industry, thin remains in; fashion ideals are set by the highest social classes and fashion magazine editors, who believe that clothes on skinny girls (size 2–4) look better. The industry preys on women who fantasize that they might look like a model if they wear the clothes. Even though more than half of American women wear a size 14 or larger, they want to be smaller or at least try to look that way, and the fashion industry promotes this dream. Twenty years ago, a current size 2 dress was a size 6, and a current size 8 was a size 12. This size distortion, which occurs only with women's clothing, is designed to sell more cloths to women who desire to be smaller when in reality they are actually considerably larger.

this notion. However, does such an image project or reinforce an unhealthful message to those who attempt to emulate these women?

FIGURE 15.4 shows the BMIs of Miss America contestants from available data between 1922 and 1999 (excluding 1927–1933, when the pageant was not held). The body weights and different girths for Miss America were published by the pageant organizers for the years 1921 to 1986. Since 1987, the Miss America organization ceased reporting contestant measurement data. We were able to obtain at least some of the weights and heights for several recent winners by scouring archived local newspapers.

The *lower horizontal dashed line* designates the World Health Organization (WHO; **www.who.int/**) cutoff for undernutrition established at a BMI of 18.5.[100] The *upper horizontal line* represents the BMI for Behnke's standard for the reference woman (see **FIG. 13.5**; stature, 1.638 m; body mass, 56.7 kg; BMI, 21.1). The downward slope of the regression line from 1922 to 1999 shows a clear tendency for relative undernutrition from the mid-1960s to approximately 1990. Using the WHO cutoff, the BMIs of 30% (n = 14) of the 47 Miss America winners fell below 18.5. Raising the BMI cutoff to 19.0 adds another 18 women, or a total of 48% of the winners with undesirable values. Approximately 24% of the BMIs of contest winners ranged between 20.0 and 21.0, and no winner after 1924 had a BMI greater than 21!

Interestingly, 1965 was the last year that we could locate girth measurements from official press releases or newspaper coverage of the contest. We compared the percentage difference between Miss America girth averages with corresponding values for the reference woman (*bottom row* of *right inset table*). For the average bust, waist, and hip values (35.1 in, 24.0 in, and 35.4 in, respectively), Miss America's bust measurement exceeded the reference woman's measurement by 2.6 in (8%), but the waist value was 7% below (−1.8 in) and the hip value decreased 5% below (−1.7 in) the reference woman's measurements. Unfortunately, no contemporary BMI data exist from 1966 to 2012 to compare the "modern" Miss America's physique status with historical data. If the Miss America contest indeed serves as a subtle promoter of the "ideal" female size and shape, then the more recent message delivered to impressionable teenagers overemphasizes that "thin is in" regardless of the potential negative nutritional and long-term health implications.[29]

Female Athletes at Greater Risk

Most studies documenting disordered eating behaviors among athletes rely on anonymous self-report surveys or inventories, with relatively little data from in-depth interviews. Generalizations come mainly from "snapshots" of small numbers of high school and college athletes in specific sports without considering the athletes' skill level, experience, and achievement status. Notwithstanding these limitations in research strategy, female athletes clearly face a unique set of circumstances that make them particularly vulnerable to

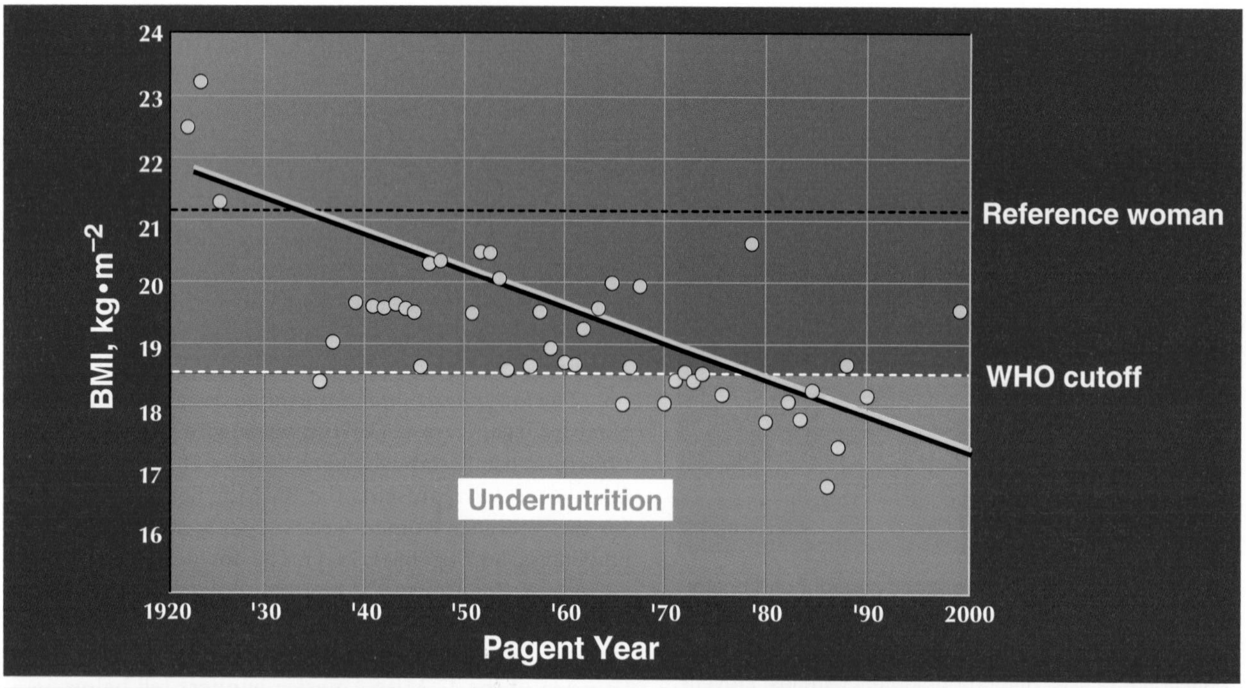

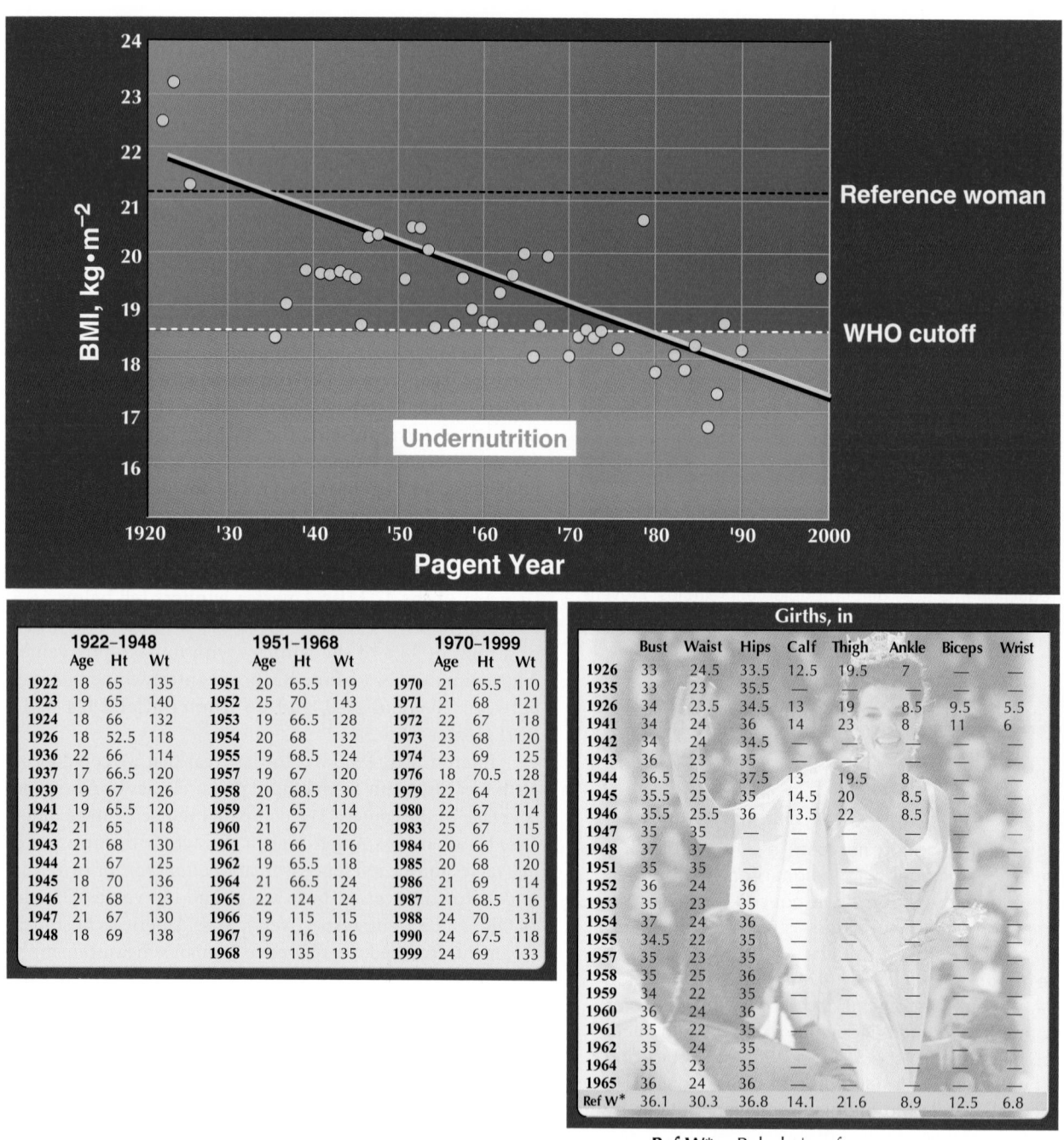

	1922–1948				1951–1968				1970–1999		
	Age	Ht	Wt		Age	Ht	Wt		Age	Ht	Wt
1922	18	65	135	**1951**	20	65.5	119	**1970**	21	65.5	110
1923	19	65	140	**1952**	25	70	143	**1971**	21	68	121
1924	18	66	132	**1953**	19	66.5	128	**1972**	22	67	118
1926	18	52.5	118	**1954**	20	68	132	**1973**	23	68	120
1936	22	66	114	**1955**	19	68.5	124	**1974**	23	69	125
1937	17	66.5	120	**1957**	19	67	120	**1976**	18	70.5	128
1939	19	67	126	**1958**	20	68.5	130	**1979**	22	64	121
1941	19	65.5	120	**1959**	21	65	114	**1980**	22	67	114
1942	21	65	118	**1960**	21	67	120	**1983**	25	67	115
1943	21	68	130	**1961**	18	66	116	**1984**	20	66	110
1944	21	67	125	**1962**	19	65.5	118	**1985**	20	68	120
1945	18	70	136	**1964**	21	66.5	124	**1986**	21	69	114
1946	21	68	123	**1965**	22	124	124	**1987**	21	68.5	116
1947	21	67	130	**1966**	19	115	115	**1988**	24	70	131
1948	18	69	138	**1967**	19	116	116	**1990**	24	67.5	118
				1968	19	135	135	**1999**	24	69	133

Girths, in

	Bust	Waist	Hips	Calf	Thigh	Ankle	Biceps	Wrist
1926	33	24.5	33.5	12.5	19.5	7	—	—
1935	33	23	35.5	—	—	—	—	—
1926	34	23.5	34.5	13	19	8.5	9.5	5.5
1941	34	24	36	14	23	8	11	6
1942	34	24	34.5	—	—	—	—	—
1943	36	23	35	—	—	—	—	—
1944	36.5	25	37.5	13	19.5	8	—	—
1945	35.5	25	35	14.5	20	8.5	—	—
1946	35.5	25.5	36	13.5	22	8.5	—	—
1947	35	35	—	—	—	—	—	—
1948	37	37	—	—	—	—	—	—
1951	35	35	—	—	—	—	—	—
1952	36	24	36	—	—	—	—	—
1953	35	23	35	—	—	—	—	—
1954	37	24	36	—	—	—	—	—
1955	34.5	22	35	—	—	—	—	—
1957	35	23	35	—	—	—	—	—
1958	35	25	36	—	—	—	—	—
1959	34	22	35	—	—	—	—	—
1960	36	24	36	—	—	—	—	—
1961	35	22	35	—	—	—	—	—
1962	35	24	35	—	—	—	—	—
1964	35	23	35	—	—	—	—	—
1965	36	24	36	—	—	—	—	—
Ref W*	36.1	30.3	36.8	14.1	21.6	8.9	12.5	6.8

Ref W* = Behnke's reference woman;
stature = 163.8 cm, body mass = 56.7 kg

FIGURE 15.4. BMI of 47 Miss America pageant contestants from 1922 to 1999. The top horizontal dashed black line represents the BMI for Behnke's reference woman (21.1 kg · m^{-2}). The bottom horizontal dashed white line designates the World Health Organization's (WHO) BMI demarcation for undernutrition (18.5 kg · m^{-2}). The *left inset table* shows the available data for age, height (in), and weight (lb) for the contest winners. The *right inset table* shows selected girths for 24 Miss America winners from 1926 to 1965. (Height and body weight presented in this figure were tracked down by the textbook authors from yearly stories about the pageant in the winner's hometown papers and from published interviews with the winners in local and national newspapers following a pageant.)

disordered eating behaviors. These behaviors flourish when strong negative aesthetic connotations about excess body fat blend with the athlete's belief that *any* body fat dooms success. Thirty years ago, female gymnasts weighed about 21 lb more than today's counterparts.

Clinical observations indicate a prevalence between 15 and 70% for eating disorders among athletes, with some groups at higher risk than others. More specifically, eating disorders and unrealistic weight goals (and general dissatisfaction with one's body) occur most frequently among

PERSONAL HEALTH AND EXERCISE NUTRITION 15.1

How to Calculate Recommended (Optimal) Body Weight

A major objective in determining a person's body composition relates to recommending an "optimal" body weight (OBW). Usually this refers to a recommended weight for health considerations, occupational and sport performance requirements, or simply aesthetics (self-assessment based on appearance). OBW computation is based on comparison with an optimal percentage body fat (OPT%BF). Determining OPT%BF becomes subjective because no absolute standards by age, fitness, ethnicity, or any other variable are available. Several body composition reference classifications can serve as guidelines for setting OPT%BF levels for different ages (**TABLE 1**). Selecting the OPT%BF should reflect the person's current percentage body fat and his or her personal objectives.

TABLE 1 Body Composition Classification by Age According to Percentage Body Fat from Typical Data in the Research

Age, y	Below Average	Average	Above Average
Males			
≤19	12–17	17–22	22–27
20–29	13–18	18–23	23–28
30–39	14–19	19–24	24–29
40–49	15–20	20–25	25–30
≥50	16–20	21–26	26–31
Females			
≤19	17–22	22–27	27–32
20–29	18–23	23–28	28–33
30–39	19–24	24–29	29–34
40–49	20–25	25–30	30–35
≤50	21–26	26–31	31–36

Procedures

1. Determine body weight (BW) in kilograms and %BF using available valid techniques (see Chapters 13 and 14).
2. Calculate body fat weight (FW) in kilograms:

$$FW = BW \times \%BF$$

where %BF is expressed in decimal form (e.g., 23.0% = 0.23)

3. Determine fat-free body mass (FFM) in kilograms:

$$FF = BW - FW$$

4. Select an optimal body weight (OBW) expressed in decimal form (e.g., 15.0% = 0.15).
5. Compute OBW in kilograms:

$$OBW = FFM \div (1.00 - OPT\%BF)$$

Example Calculations

1. Data: Female; age 19 years; body weight = 66.0 kg; %BF from hydrostatic weighing = 30.0% (decimal form = 0.30); OPT%BF chosen = 25.0% (0.25)
2. Calculate FW in kilograms:

$$\begin{aligned} FW &= BW \times \%BF \\ &= 66.0 \text{ kg} \times 0.30 \\ &= 19.8 \text{ kg } (43.7 \text{ lb}) \end{aligned}$$

3. Determine FFM in kilograms:

$$\begin{aligned} FFM &= BW - FW \\ &= 66.0 \text{ kg} - 19.8 \text{ kg} \\ &= 46.2 \text{ kg } (101.9 \text{ lb}) \end{aligned}$$

4. Select OPT%BF expressed in decimal form:

$$\%BF = 0.25$$

5. Compute OBW in kg:

$$\begin{aligned} OBW &= FFM \times (1.00 - \%BF) \\ &= 46.2 \text{ kg} \times (1.00 - 0.25) \\ &= 61.6 \text{ kg } (135 \text{ lb}) \end{aligned}$$

Computing Recommended Fat Loss

From the above calculations, the amount of fat loss in kilograms required to reach OBW (at the chosen OPT%BF of 25.0%) computes as:

$$\begin{aligned} \text{Fat loss} &= BW - OBW \\ &= 66.0 \text{ kg} - 61.6 \text{ kg} \\ &= 4.4 \text{ kg } (9.7 \text{ lb}) \end{aligned}$$

female athletes in the aesthetic sports such as ballet, bodybuilding, diving, figure skating, cheerleading, and gymnastics, in which success often coincides with extreme leanness.[13,34,38,46,70,90–92] An inordinate preoccupation with eating also occurs among adolescent female swimmers.[9,26,97,98] Controversy exists as to the prevalence of eating disorders among endurance runners,[20] but recent data show a nearly 26% prevalence of eating disorders as indicated by elevated scores on the Eating Disorders Inventory.[21] Coaches often compound the problem.[84] Sixty-seven percent of female collegiate gymnasts reported that their coaches said they weighed too much, and 75% of these athletes used weight-loss strategies involving vomiting, laxatives, or diuretic use.[80,81] Weight reduction attempts averaged 85% in female and 93% in male weight-class athletes.[30] Between 27 and 37% of women in aesthetic, endurance, and weight-class

RISK FACTORS FOR DISORDERED EATING AMONG ATHLETES

1. Pressure to optimize performance and/or modify appearance
2. Psychological factors, such as low self-esteem, poor coping skills, perceived loss of control, perfectionism, obsessive–compulsive traits, depression, anxiety, and history of sexual/physical abuse
3. Underlying chronic diseases related to caloric use (e.g., diabetes)

sports experienced menstrual disorders, compared with only 5% in other sports. Unfortunately, reducing body weight considerably below normal levels also coincides with inadequate nutrientintake.[53]

Among athletes classified "at risk" for developing an eating disorder, 92% met the criteria for anorexia nervosa, bulimia nervosa, or anorexia athletica (see next section).[79] Eighty-five percent of the athletes dieted compared with 27% of controls. Adolescent dancers and figure skaters exhibited more frequent patterns of disordered eating than other athletic groups and nonathletes.[14] In a survey of female college athletes, 14% of the women reported self-induced vomiting, whereas 16% indicated laxative use for weight control.[81] Among female college gymnasts, all were trying to diet and 25% reported self-induced vomiting.[80] Other studies also indicate that female gymnasts exhibit a high incidence of disordered eating behaviors, yet prevalence rates did not differ from age-matched, nonathletic controls.[67,71,74,97]

Preoccupation with body weight and associated eating disorders among female gymnasts during college abate considerably after retirement from the sport.[68] **TABLE 15.3** presents data on eating disorder symptoms from former college gymnasts approximately 15 years after competition. These women scored below published average values (*norms*) for each variable measured. Nonathletic controls and gymnasts scored similarly on all variables except asceticism and body dissatisfaction, on which gymnasts scored significantly lower. The former gymnasts also maintained nutrient intakes within the recommended range and possessed greater bone mineral density at multiple body sites than controls.[53] One must determine if findings from former gymnasts of 15 to 25 years ago apply to contemporary gymnasts, for whom exaggerated leanness and small body structure now seem to play a more important part in competitive success.

TABLE 15.4 summarizes a sample of findings from 23 studies of eating patterns of athletes. In general, the incidence of eating disorders is greater among athletes than in nonathletic comparison groups or the general population. Future research should investigate the extent to which eating disorders permeate the competitive athletic scene among junior and senior high school female participants.

A study in conjunction with the National Collegiate Athletic Association clearly shows a greater prevalence of eating disorders among female athletes than male counterparts.[45] Among women, 1.1% met the clinical diagnostic criteria for bulimia nervosa; none met the criteria for anorexia nervosa, but 9.2% showed subclinical bulimia and subclinical anorexia. For the male athletes, none met the diagnostic criteria for anorexia, bulimia, or subclinical anorexia, and only 0.01% presented with subclinical bulimia. It is difficult to determine the actual prevalence because eating disorders go mostly unreported to coaches, parents, or allied-health practitioners.

TABLE 15.3 Eating Disorders Inventory Scores from Normative Data (Norms), Former Gymnasts, and Control Subjects

	Norms (*n* = 205)	Gymnasts (*n* = 22)	Controls (*n* = 22)
Drive for thinness	5.5	3.3	4.0
Bulimia	1.2	0.6	1.0
Body dissatisfaction	12.2	7.9	14.1[a]
Ineffectiveness	2.3	1.2	2.3
Perfectionism	6.2	5.0	4.3
Interpersonal distrust	2.0	1.6	2.5
Interoceptive awareness	3.0	0.9	1.4
Maturity fears	2.7	1.8	2.0
Asceticism	3.4	2.4	4.5[a]
Impulse regulation	2.3	0.7	0.9
Social insecurity	3.3	1.4	3.1

[a] *Significantly different from gymnasts ($P \leq 0.05$).*

From O'Connor PJ, et al. Eating disorder symptoms in former female college gymnasts: relations with body composition. Am J Clin Nutr 1996;64:840.

Anorexia Athletica

The cluster of personality traits among athletes often shares a commonality with patients with clinical eating disorders. The same traits that make an athlete excel in sports—compulsive, driven, dichotomous thinker, perfectionist, competitive, compliant and eager to please ("coachable"), and self-motivated—increase risk for developing an eating disorder.[42,73,86] More than likely, the greatest risk exists for persons whose normal, genetically determined body size and shape deviate from the "ideal" imposed by the sport. The term **anorexia athletica** describes the continuum of subclinical eating behaviors of physically active persons who fail to meet the criteria for a true eating disorder, but who exhibit at least one unhealthy weight control method or disordered eating pattern.[3,67,68] This includes fasting, vomiting (termed "instrumental vomiting" when used to make weight), and use of diet pills, laxatives, or diuretics (water pills).

A study of Norwegian elite female athletes age 12 to 35 years examined risk factors and triggers for eating disorders.[93] **TABLE 15.5** lists the criteria to identify anorexia athletica.

TABLE 15.4 Summary of Selected Studies of Eating Disorders in Athletes

Study (ref. #)	Sport	Subjects	Measures[a]	Outcome
10	Female and male athletes from 8 sports	695 athletes (55% female) from 8 sports. Mean age, 19 y (range, 16–25)	41-item questionnaire mailed to coaches in 21 colleges in the midwest; coaches administered it to athletes	59% lost weight by "excessive" exercise, 24% by consuming less than 600 kcal/d, 12% by fasting, 11% by using fad diets, 6% by vomiting, 4% by using laxatives, and 1% by using enemas; relatively few gender differences, but trend for males to use exercise and females to use dieting to lose weight
11	Female athletes from 7 sports	79 female athletes in sports emphasizing leanness (ballet, bodybuilding, cheerleading, gymnastics) or sports with no emphasis (swimming, track and field, volleyball); 101 nonathlete controls	EDI	No overall differences between athletes and controls; athletes in sports emphasizing leanness had a higher percentage of elevated scores than athletes in other sports
13	Ballet dancers	55 female dancers in national and regional companies	EAT-26	33% had anorexia or bulimia in the past; 50% of amenorrheic subjects reported anorexia compared with 13% of women with normal cycles
22a	Various sports	64 female athletes in "thin-build" sports (e.g., gymnastics); 62 females in "normalbuild" sports (e.g., volleyball); 64 female univ. student controls	EDI	Overall EDI scores not different among groups; athletes in thin-build sports had greater weight concerns, more body dissatisfaction, and more dieting than normal-build athletes and controls, even though body weights were lower
26	Swimmers	487 girls and 468 boys, ages 9–18, at a competitive swimming camp	Questionnaire on dieting and weight-control practices	15.4% of the girls (24.8% of the postmenarchal girls) and 3.6% of boys used pathogenic weight loss techniques; girls were more likely than boys to perceive themselves heavier than they were
28	Wrestlers, swimmers, Nordic skiers	26 male wrestlers, 21 male swimmers, and cross-country skiers	EAT-40, restraint questionnaire, body image assessment	Higher EAT scores in wrestlers due to higher scores on weight fluctuation and dieting; no overall differences in estimates of body size; a small subsample of wrestlers who scored high on restraint and EAT scores had distortions of body size
28a	Dancers	21 female university dancers and 29 female university controls	EAT-40	33% of dancers and 14% of controls scored in the range symptomatic of anorexia on the EAT; difference in overall EAT scores not significant
31a	Ballet dancers	10 female ballet dancers with stress fractures, 10 dancers without fractures, and 10 nondancer controls	EAT-26, structured interview on DSM-III criteria for eating disorders	Nonsignificant trend for stressfracture dancers to have higher EAT scores than other 2 groups; greater incidence of eating disorders in stressfracture group
34	Ballet dancers	35 female ballet students ages 11–14, followed 2–4 y	EDI	At follow-up, 26% of subjects had anorexia nervosa and 14% had bulimia nervosa or a "partial syndrome"; the "drive for thinness" and "body dissatisfaction" scales of the EDI predicted eating disorders at follow-up
38	Ballet dancers	55 white and 11 black female dancers in national and regional companies (mean age, 24.9 y)	EAT-26	15% of white dancers reported anorexia and 19% report bulimia; none of the black dancers reported anorexia or bulimia
38a	Ballet dancers	32 female ballet dancers from 4 national US companies, 17 dancers from national company in China (mean age, 24.6 y)	Variation in EAT-26, subjects given description of eating disorders and asked if they had the problem	American dancers from lessselected companies had more eating problems, more anorectic behaviors and more female obesity than the highly selected American or Chinese dancers
43a	Majorettes	11 varsity majors	24-h dietary recall on eating and weight practices; no standardized measures	Based on clinical observations, all subjects had distorted body image due to low weight standards. Subjects reported eating and drinking little for several days prior to weighings, high levels of exercise and using sauna, diet pills, and diuretics

(continued)

TABLE 15.4 (continued) Summary of Selected Studies of Eating Disorders in Athletes

Study (ref. #)	Sport	Subjects	Measures[a]	Outcome
Unpublished data	Runners	4551 (1911 females, 2640 males) respondents to survey in *Runners World* magazine	EAT-26 questions on eating and diet concerns	Mean EAT score = 9.0 for males, 14.1 for females; 8% of males and 24% of females scored 20 on EAT; 15% of males who ran 45 mi/wk scored 20, compared with 7% of males who ran less; 24% of females who ran 40 mi/wk scored 20, compared with 23% of those who ran less
50	Jockeys	10 male jockeys from England (mean age, 22.9 y; mean weight, 108.5 lb)	EDI, EAT-26	Poor response rate to full battery of tests (from 58 stables, only 10 subjects responded); mean EAT score was 14.9, higher than expected in young males; most reported food avoidance, saunas, and laxative abuse; diuretics and appetite suppressants were used; binges were common, but vomiting was unusual
53a	Athletes from unspecified sports	126 female athletes from unspecified sports, 590 students from other groups (e.g., sororities, classes)	EDI questionnaire with eating disorder diagnosis questions	Athletes had generally lower scores on all eating disorders measures than other groups, but statistical tests not performed
58	Female athletes from different sports	87 female athletes from track, swimming, gymnastics, and ballet; 41 females with eating disorders, 120 female high school and junior high controls	Self-reports of dieting, vomiting, and eating disorders	Frequent dieting, vomiting, and self-reported anorexia more common in athletes than normal controls but less common than eating disorders subjects, but no statistical comparisons performed
70	Obligatory runners and weightlifters	15 males and 15 females in each of 3 groups; obligatory runners, obligatory weightlifters, and sedentary controls	Body size estimation 3 subscales on EDI	Runners and weightlifters had more eating disturbances than controls; females had more eating pathologies than males
80	Gymnasts	42 female college gymnasts	Questionnaire on dieting and weight control practices	All subjects were dieting (50% for appearance, 50% for performance); 62% used at least 1 pathogenic weight method (e.g., vomiting, diet pills, fasting); 66% were told they were too heavy by coaches
81	Varsity level female athletes from 10 sports	182 female varsity athletes	Questionnaire on dieting and weight control practices	32% engaged in at least 1 pathogenic weight-control practice; the percentages were 14% for vomiting, 16% for laxatives, 25% for diet pills, 5% for diuretics, 20% for regular binges, and 8% for excessive weight loss
81a	Ice skaters	17 male (mean age, 21.1 y) and 23 female (mean age, 17.6 y) figure skaters from mid-Atlantic training facility	EAT-40	Mean EAT scores were 29.3 for women and 10 for men; 48% of the women and no man had EAT scores in anorectic range (>30)
86a	Wrestlers	63 male college wrestlers and 378 high school wrestlers	Questionnaire on dieting and weight control practices	63% of college and 43% of high school wrestlers were preoccupied with food during the season (19% and 14% in the off-season); 41% of college and 29% of high school wrestlers reported eating out of control between matches; 52% of college and 26% of high school wrestlers reported fasting at least once a week
97	Female athletes from 7 sports	82 female athletes from gymnastics, crosscountry, basketball, golf, volleyball, swimming, and tennis; 52 nonathlete controls	EAT-40, EDI	None of athletes scored in disturbed range; no overall differences between athletes and controls; cross-country runners showed less and gymnasts showed more eating disturbance than controls, but only on selected scales
97a	Runners	125 female distance runners, 25 nonrunning controls	EAT-26, EDI	No greater incidence of eating problems in runners than in controls; elite runners more likely than other runners to have problems

From Brownell KD, Rodin J. Prevalence of eating disorders in athletes. In: Brownell KD, et al., eds. Eating, body weight and performance in athletes. Philadelphia: *Lea & Febiger*, 1992.

[a] *EAT-40, Eating Attitudes Test containing 40 questions in which subjects rate how well a statement applies to them on a 6-point scale; EAT-26, 26-question modification of EAT-40; EDI, Eating Disorder Inventory containing 64 questions with 8 subscales to assess behaviors and attitudes related to body image, eating behaviors, and dieting.*

TABLE 15.5 Criteria for Identifying Anorexia Athletica

Common Features	Anorexia Athletica
Weight loss[a]	+
Delayed puberty[b]	(+)
Menstrual dysfunction[c]	(+)
Gastrointestinal complaints	+
Absence of medical illness or affective disorder explaining the weight reduction	+
Disturbance in body image	(+)
Excessive fear of becoming obese	+
Purging[d]	(+)
Bingeing[d]	(+)
Compulsive exercising[d]	(+)
Restricted caloric intake[e]	+

+, criteria that all athletes had to meet; (+), anorexia athletica athletes met one or more of the listed criteria.

[a] Greater than 5% expected body weight.

[b] No menstrual flow at age 16 (primary amenorrhea).

[c] Primary amenorrhea, secondary amenorrhea, or oligomenorrhea.

[d] Defined in DSM-III-R(1).

[e] Use of diets at or below 1200 kcal for unspecified durations.

Based on the Eating Disorder Inventory (EDI), 117 of 522 athletes classified as "at risk." Follow-up with this subgroup revealed a significant incidence of anorexia nervosa (n = 7), bulimia nervosa (n = 42), and anorexia athletica (n = 43). **TABLE 15.6** provides selected characteristics for sport-specific groupings from the 92 athletes with eating disorders; characteristics included weekly training volume and percentage of each athletic subgroup with high inventory scores. Interestingly, the athletes traced their eating disorder to one of three causes: (1) prolonged periods of dieting and fluctuations in body weight (37%), (2) new coach (30%), and (3) injury or illness (23%). All of the athletes and controls (athletes without eating disorders) dieted to enhance performance. Sixty-seven percent of athletes with an eating disorder dieted on their coach's recommendation, whereas 75% of control athletes dieted because of a coach's influence. This latter finding reveals that most female athletes, whether or not they engaged in disordered eating behaviors, remained impressionable to an authority figure, attempting to please coaches by following through on their recommendations.

For many athletes, disordered eating patterns coincide with their competitive season and abate when the season ends. For them, the preoccupation with body weight may not reflect true underlying pathology, but rather a desire to achieve optimum physiologic function and competitive status.[22] For a small number of athletes, the season never "ends," and they develop a clinical eating disorder.

TABLE 15.6 Characteristics of the Eating-Disordered Athlete Representing the Different Sport Groups

Thirty control subjects represented a random sample of athletes without elevated scores on the Eating Disorder Inventory (EDI) who were matched on age, community of residence, and sport. At-risk subjects were classified by EDI scores above the mean for anorectic patients on the "Drive for thinness" and "Body dissatisfaction" subscales of the EDI.

Sport Groups[a]	N	Age (y[b])	BMI	Training Volume (km·wk^{-1})	High EDI[c] (%)
Technical sports	13	19 (14–30)	21 (17–26)	14 (12–19)	21
Endurance sports	24	22 (15–28)	20 (15–22)	21 (19–26)	20
Aesthetic sports	22	17 (12–24)	18 (15–21)	18 (17–23)	40
Weight-dependent sports	11	21 (15–23)	21 (17–23)	14 (11–16)	37
Ball game sports	21	20 (17–27)	21 (19–27)	15 (12–17)	14
Total sample	92	20 (13–28)	21 (15–27)	17 (12–26)	22
Athletic controls	30	20 (13–28)	22 (18–24)	15 (10–22)	0

*[a] **Technical:** alpine skiing, bowling, golf, high jump, horseback riding, long jump, rifle shooting, sailing, sky diving; **endurance:** biathlon, cross-country skiing, cycling, middle-distance and long-distance running, orienteering, race walking, rowing, speed skating, swimming; **aesthetic:** diving, figure skating, gymnastics, rhythmical gymnastics, sports dance; **weight dependent:** judo, karate, wrestling; **ball games:** badminton, bandy (land hockey on ice), basketball, soccer, table tennis, team handball, tennis, volleyball, underwater rugby.*

[b] Values for age, BMI, and training volume are given as means with ranges in parentheses.

[c] Based on N = 522.

From Sundgot-Borgen J. Eating disorders in female athletes. Sports Med 1994;17:176.

Eating Disorders Also Afflict Men

Most people consider eating disorders a "female problem," yet an increasing number of men share this affliction. The question remains unanswered whether this increased number results from an actual increase in disease incidence or because more men with the condition now seek treatment. In one New York hospital treatment center, the percentage of male patients admitted with eating disorders rose steadily from 4% in 1988 to 13% in 1995. Men currently represent 6 to 10% of persons with eating disorders, with the greatest prevalence among models, dancers, men abused during childhood, and gays (**www.something-fishy.org/cultural/issuesformen.php**).

Body weight–dependent wrestling, horse racing, lightweight rowing, distance running, and bodybuilding potentially create conditions to develop patterns of disordered eating, particularly purging.[6,28,50] Of 25 lower-weight-category collegiate wrestlers (BMI, 21.1) and 59 lightweight rowers (BMI, 21.0), 52% reported bingeing; 8% of the rowers and 16% of the wrestlers showed pathologic EDI profiles.[96] The 52% rate for bingeing behavior represents approximately twice the incidence in the normal male population. A survey of Michigan high school wrestlers showed that 72% engaged in at least one potentially harmful weight loss practice over the season, regardless of grade or success level.[51] Fasting and various dehydration methods provided the primary methods for rapid weight loss. Wrestlers who lost weight each week were the most likely to binge eat. Fifty percent of the wrestlers lost more than 5 lb, and 27% lost 10 lb. Two percent of the wrestlers reported weekly use of laxatives, diet pills, or diuretics, and another 2% used vomiting to lose weight. With the changes in rules governing weight loss of wrestlers during the season, these practices are likely to become less prevalent.

Overemphasis on Healthy Eating: "Orthorexia Nervosa"

From 1970 to 1990, nutritional science assumed center stage in America's consciousness, and a new era of nutrition awareness and "negative" nutrition advertising emerged. Food journalists, marketers, and large food-producing companies introduced the concept of "good" and "bad" foods. Bad foods were to be avoided based on studies showing that foods high in saturated fat and cholesterol were related to heart disease; sugary foods supposedly increased the probabilities of developing type 2 diabetes and dental carries; excess salt increased blood pressure; and artificial flavors and coloring increased the risk of developing certain types of cancers. In 1977, the US Dietary Goals for Americans were developed, including the first publication 3 years later of the *Dietary Guidelines for Americans*, both of which conveyed the message not to eat certain foods, or to eat them "sparingly." The American Heart Association and the American Cancer Society also published dietary recommendations with a similar message—"avoid bad foods." This trend has accelerated in the last few years, and the public has become bombarded with messages that tell us to "eat better", "eat the right way", "eat healthy", and "eat well". Even the *eatright* program of the American Dietetic Association (**www.eatright.org**) emphasizes the same message.

An overemphasis on eating right can result in persons becoming so obsessed with healthy foods that they exhibit a disordered eating behavior termed **orthorexia nervosa**. This condition, first described in 1977 begins with keen interest in healthful eating.[12] The person may choose to stop eating red meat, but eventually eliminates all meat, then all processed foods, and will eventually eat only specific foods that are prepared in highly specific ways. Reliance on this attitude and out-of-the-ordinary dietary restrictions seem normal to many; bookstore shelves are replete with books recommending these types of nutritional behaviors.

Orthorexia nervosa represents a form of obsessive-compulsive disorder, and the fact that it is based on an obsessive fixation on food, just as with anorexia nervosa or bulimia nervosa, places it in the disordered eating category. A person with orthorexia nervosa spends the same time and energy thinking about food as someone with bulimia or anorexia. They may not focus on calories, but instead dwell on the overall "health benefits"—how the food was processed, prepared, and grown. Orthorexia is now believed to be its own condition, but not yet described in DSM-IV.

While orthorexia does not pose the same health threats as anorexia or bulimia, it may lead to more serious disorders. Many believe that the severe restrictive nature of orthorexia could easily morph into anorexia. The limited diet of those persons increases the risk of malnourishment and could facilitate bingeing, and later purging out of guilt—paving the way toward bulimia. Several character traits of people with anorexia and orthorexia are quite similar (e.g., low self-esteem, poor coping skills, perceived loss of control, perfectionism, obsessive–compulsive traits).

The first published study of orthorexia nervosa in 2004 determined the disorder's prevalence. In a survey of 400 students, 28 (6.9%) exhibited orthorexic behavior—a higher percentage than anorexia and bulimia combined. The condition was more prevalent among men than women.[24]

MUSCLE DYSMORPHIA: "THE ADONIS COMPLEX"

Muscle dysmorphia represents a psychological condition that has been conceptualized as an eating disorder and subsequently as a type of body dysmorphic disorder (the common feature considered to have a psychogenic basis of presenting physical symptoms indicative of a medical condition, but not fully explained by a general medical condition). This coincides with a change in the way many men view the ideal male physique. Austrian, French, and American men project the "ideal" man's body as possessing about 28 lb more muscle than their own.[78] This mismatched perception coincides with the increased number of men who use anabolic steroids, experience eating disorders, and suffer from body obsession. An important component of body obsession relates to **muscle dysmorphia**, or the "Adonis complex," the pathologic preoccupation with muscle size and overall muscularity. These persons view themselves as small and frail, when in reality, many are large and muscular.

In many ways, muscle dysmorphia and anorexia nervosa share common traits, such as a history of depression and anxiety, hyperculturalization of body image, unrealistic shame about one's body, and self-destructive behaviors. Both anorectic and dysmorphic groups act on their bodies for acceptance and use their bodies as a way to control their lives. They often endanger their health by excessive exercising, bingeing-and-purging rituals, steroid abuse, and inordinate reliance on nutritional and dietary supplements to try to alter their appearance.[7,8,59] A large number of these men binge eat or inordinately focus on consuming low-fat, high-protein diets.

No formal diagnostic criteria exist to identify a person at risk for muscle dysmorphia. The box "Signs and Symptoms of Muscle Dysmorphia" proposes some characteristic features exhibited by those with the disorder.

THE EXERCISE ADDICT

To some extent, cultural influences create similarities between anorexia nervosa and addictive exercise behaviors. Approximately 50% of women with eating disorders compulsively overexercise. Someone who exercises excessively—referred to as an **exercise addict** or exercise dependent—often does whatever it takes to make additional time to exercise. A rigid daily schedule of working out often takes place at the expense of family, career, and interpersonal relationships. Sense of worth becomes inextricably tied to volume of exercise accomplished. Disruption of the daily exercise routine often triggers conventional withdrawal symptoms that include anxiety, restlessness, and mood swings, traits that diminish only when exercise resumes. Typical regimens for the exercise-dependent person include early morning and afternoon runs, an aerobics class in the evenings, and participation in two or more aerobics classes on weekends. Missing a planned exercise session often produces extreme frustration, culminating in food restraint. Eventually, life becomes unmanageable from a fanatical drive to exercise or a relentless pursuit to achieve a high fitness level. Compulsive exercisers often display the same psychological characteristics as bulimics and anorectics. Some clinicians, therefore, see the need to include *exercise addiction* as a separate diagnostic category. Inclusion might help to identify potentially harmful psychological behaviors associated with an eating disorder.

FIGURE 15.5 compares scores for exercise dependence among female dancers, marathon and ultramarathon runners, and field hockey players. The key comparison variable, the negative addiction scale, reflects an inordinate level of exercise dependence. It consists of 14 equally weighted motivational, emotional, and behavioral components of running behavior. Dancers and runners scored significantly higher on exercise dependence than field hockey participants, with dancers achieving the highest scores. The researchers concluded that exercise-dependent athletes, particularly dancers, manifest a number of self-destructive behaviors. These findings highlight the need to carefully monitor females who participate in sports with above-normal levels of addictive exercise behavior (see **FIG. 15.9**). Compulsive exercise behavior, coupled with preoccupation to achieve an "ideal physique" for competition, should serve

SIGNS AND SYMPTOMS OF MUSCLE DYSMORPHIA

- Preoccupation with the idea that body is not sufficiently lean and muscular. Behaviors associated with this preoccupation include frequent weighing; constant checking of appearance in mirrors/windows; persistent criticism of body weight, size, and/or shape; wearing baggy clothing to camouflage the body; or, conversely, modifying clothing to accentuate muscularity (such as adding extra buttons to make a shirt sleeve look tighter).
- Preoccupation with muscularity causes clinically significant distress or impairment of social, occupational, or other important areas of life functioning (e.g., personal relationships), as demonstrated by at least two of the following:
  1. Frequently gives up important social, occupational, or recreational activities because of a compulsive need to maintain exercise and dietary regimens.
  2. Avoids situations where the body would be exposed to others (e.g., at the beach or swimming pool) or endures such situations only with marked distress or intense anxiety.
  3. Preoccupation about the inadequacy of body size or muscularity causes significant distress or impairment in social, occupational, or other important areas of life.
  4. Continues to exercise, diet, or use performance-enhancing drugs/supplements despite knowledge of adverse physical and/or psychological consequences.
- Engages in excessive exercise, demonstrates preoccupation with food, follows strict dietary regimens (e.g., avoiding specific foods or groups of foods, maintaining excessively low-fat or high-protein diets), or abuses steroids and/or dietary supplements, particularly those aimed at increasing body size (e.g., creatine, ⊠-hydroxy-⊠-methylbutyrate [HMB], dehydroepiandrosterone [DHEA], androstenedione) and/or decreasing body fat (ephedrine, ma huang, guarana).

From Pope HG Jr, et al. Muscle dysmorphia: an unrecognized form of body dysmorphic disorder. *Psychosomatics* 1997;38:548.

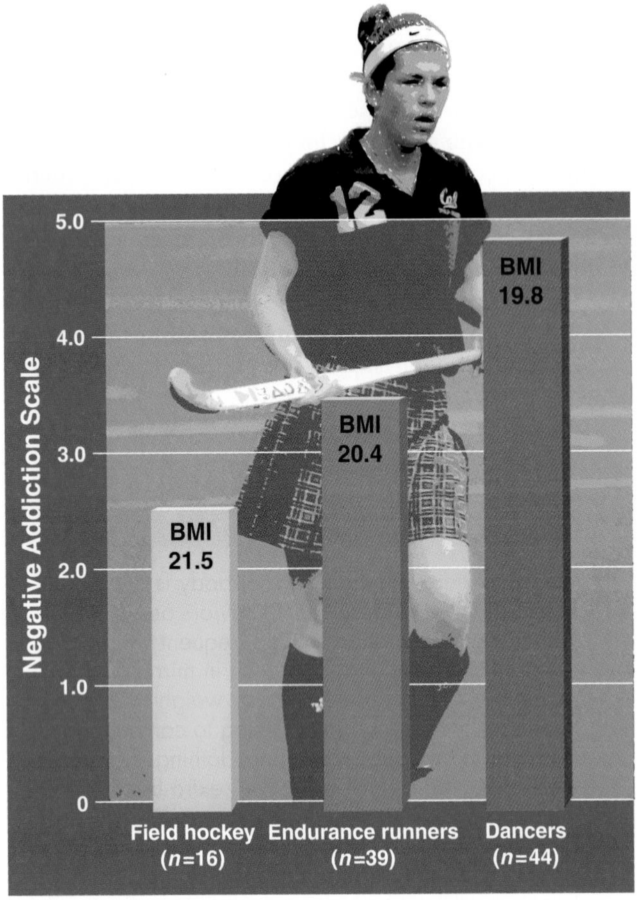

FIGURE 15.5. Comparison of exercise dependence scores among collegiate female ballet and modern dancers, marathon and ultramarathon (>50-mile distances) runners, and field hockey athletes. The dancers scored significantly higher than the runners; the field hockey athletes scored significantly lower in exercise dependence than both of these groups. Interestingly, the dancers had the lowest mean BMI (19.8), followed by the runners (20.4) and field hockey athletes (21.5). Self-destructive behaviors included perseverance in training despite serious injury, prioritization of physical activity over other responsibilities, and significant mood disturbances. (From Sachs ML, Pearman D. Running addiction: a depth interview examination. *J Sport Behav* 1979;2:143.)

as a "wake-up call" to seek professional counseling and/or clinical intervention.

Not Simply an Athletic Problem

One of our laboratories administered the 26-point, forced-choice items of the Eating Attitudes Test (EAT-26) to evaluate eating behaviors in women (nonathletes) enrolled at a university-sponsored fitness center (see p. 529). An EAT score of 20 or higher identifies persons with one of the following conditions: (1) an eating disorder that meets strict diagnostic criteria; (2) a "partial syndrome" indicating marked dietary restriction, weight preoccupation, bingeing, vomiting, and other symptoms of clinical significance, but failing to meet all diagnostic criteria for an eating disorder; and (3) "obsessive dieters" or "weight-preoccupied" persons who express concerns about weight and shape but do not present the abnormal concerns of those with the "partial syndrome." Of the 100 women, 24 scored higher on EAT (average score, 30.5; BMI, 22.2) than the remaining 76 women, whose score averaged 6.8 (BMI, 22.4).

Women with high EAT scores focused more on extreme exercise behaviors. A disturbing aspect concerns the relatively large percentage of "nonathlete" women with either high or low EAT scores who display compulsive exercise behaviors similar to those of gymnasts, dancers, and others preoccupied with eating and weight management. The exercise addict syndrome probably affects many college-age women and is not just a characteristic unique to competitive athletes.

CLINICAL EATING DISORDERS

Psychiatrists traditionally limit the definition of eating disorders to behaviors that produce negative health effects or drive a person to seek treatment. Anorexia nervosa, bulimia nervosa, and binge eating represent the three eating disorders included in the DSM-IV, the American Psychiatric Association's official roster of psychiatric illnesses.[23]

Anorexia Nervosa

Anorexia nervosa, originally described in ancient writings, represents an unhealthy physical and mental state. This "nervous loss of appetite," particularly common and increasing in prevalence among adolescent girls and young women, is characterized by four factors:

1. Distortions of body image
2. Crippling obsession with trying to obtain a smaller body size
3. Preoccupation with dieting and thinness
4. Refusal to eat enough food to maintain a minimally normal body weight

A relentless pursuit of thinness (present in about 1–2% of the general population) culminates in severe undernutrition, altered body composition characterized by depletion of fat and fat-free body mass (FFM), and cessation of menstruation (amenorrhea). Body weight decreases below normal for age and stature. Anorexia nervosa represents the third most common medical illness in girls age 15 to 19 years. Persons with anorexia actually perceive themselves as fat despite their obvious emaciation. Such distorted perceptions and persistent disturbance in eating behavior frequently persist into recovery, despite improvement in eating behavior and psychological symptoms to produce extreme feelings of vulnerability and personal inadequacy.[48] *Denial and secrecy become a large part of the problem.* Many anorectics do not believe they suffer from starvation—they do eat, but consume far less food than adequate to maintain energy balance.[47,52]

PERSONAL HEALTH AND EXERCISE NUTRITION 15.2

Eating Attitudes Test (EAT-26) for Eating Disorders

The Eating Attitudes Test (EAT-26) was the screening instrument used in the 1998 National Eating Disorders Screening Program and is probably the most widely used standardized measure of symptoms and concerns characteristic of eating disorders.

The EAT-26 alone does not yield a specific diagnosis of an eating disorder. Neither the EAT-26 nor any other screening instrument has been established as highly efficient as the sole means for identifying eating disorders. However, studies have shown that the EAT-26 can be an efficient screening instrument as part of a two-stage screening process in which those who score at or above a cutoff score of 20 are referred for a diagnostic interview. If you score above 20 on the EAT-26, please contact your doctor or an eating disorders treatment specialist for a follow-up evaluation.

Age: ____ **Sex:** ____ **Height:** ____ **feet** ____ **inches**

Current Weight: ____ **Highest Weight:** ____ **Lowest Adult Weight:** ____

Education: if currently enrolled in college/university, are you a:

☐ Freshman ☐ Sophomore ☐ Junior ☐ Senior ☐ Grad Student

If not enrolled in school, level of education completed:

☐ Jr. High/Middle School ☐ High School ☐ College ☐ Post College

Ethnic/Racial Group:

☐ African American ☐ Asian American ☐ European American ☐ Hispanic American ☐ Indian ☐ Other

Do you participate in athletics at any of the following levels:

☐ Intramural ☐ Intercollegiate ☐ Recreational ☐ High School

PLEASES CHECK A RESPONSE FOR EACH OF THE FOLLOWING STATEMENTS:

	Always	Usually	Often	Sometimes	Rarely	Never
1. Am terrified about being overweight.	3	2	1	0	0	0
2. Avoid eating when I am hungry.	3	2	1	0	0	0
3. Find myself preoccupied with food.	3	2	1	0	0	0
4. Have gone on eating binges that I feel I may not be able to stop.	3	2	1	0	0	0
5. Cut my food into small pieces.	3	2	1	0	0	0
6. Aware of the calorie content of foods I eat.	3	2	1	0	0	0
7. Particularly avoid food with a high carbohydrate content (bread, rice, potatoes, etc.).	3	2	1	0	0	0
8. Feel that others would prefer I ate more.	3	2	1	0	0	0
9. I vomit after eating.	3	2	1	0	0	0
10. Feel extremely guilty after eating.	3	2	1	0	0	0
11. Am preoccupied with a desire to be thinner.	3	2	1	0	0	0
12. Think about burning up calories when I exercise.	3	2	1	0	0	0
13. Other people think I'm too thin.	3	2	1	0	0	0
14. Am preoccupied with the thought of having fat on my body.	3	2	1	0	0	0
15. Take longer than others to eat my meals.	3	2	1	0	0	0

	Always	Usually	Often	Sometimes	Rarely	Never
16. Avoid foods with sugar in them.	3	2	1	0	0	0
17. Eat diet foods.	3	2	1	0	0	0
18. Feel that food controls my life.	3	2	1	0	0	0
19. Display self-control around food.	3	2	1	0	0	0
20. Feel that others pressure me to eat.	3	2	1	0	0	0
21. Give too much time and thought to food.	3	2	1	0	0	0
22. Feel uncomfortable after eating sweets.	3	2	1	0	0	0
23. Engage in dieting behavior.	3	2	1	0	0	0
24. Like my stomach to be empty.	3	2	1	0	0	0
25. Have the impulse to vomit after meals.	3	2	1	0	0	0
26. Enjoy trying new rich foods.	3	2	1	0	0	0

PLEASE RESPOND TO EACH OF THE FOLLOWING QUESTIONS:

1. Have you gone on eating binges and you feel that you may not be able to stop? (Eating much more than most people would eat under the circumstances.)

   ☐ No ☐ Yes, If YES, on average, how many times per month in the last 6 months? ____________

2. Have you ever made yourself sick (vomited) to control your weight or shape?

   ☐ No ☐ Yes, If YES, on average, how many times per month in the last 6 months? ____________

3. Have you ever used laxatives, diet pills, or diuretics (water pills) to control your weight or shape?

   ☐ No ☐ Yes, If YES, on average, how many times per month in the last 6 months? ____________

4. Have you ever been treated for an eating disorder?

   ☐ No ☐ Yes, If YES, when? ____

5. Have you recently thought of or attempted suicide?

   ☐ No ☐ Yes, If YES, when? ____

Scoring System for the EAT-26

Responses for each item (No. 1–26) are weighted from 0 to 3, with a score of 3 assigned to the responses farthest in the "symptomatic" direction, a score of 2 for the immediately adjacent response, a score of 1 for the next adjacent response, and a score of 0 assigned to the three responses farthest in the "asymptomatic" direction.

Total Score: Add the values circled for questions 1–26 above:

TOTAL ________________________

Items are assigned to three subscales as follows:

Dieting subscale items: 1, 6, 7, 10, 11, 12, 14, 16, 17, 22, 23, 24, 25

Subscale Score: ____________

Bulimia and Food Preoccupation subscale items: 3, 4, 9, 18, 21, 26

Subscale Score: ____________

Oral Control subscale items: 2, 5, 8, 13, 15, 19, 20

Subscale Score: ____________

To determine subscale scores, add together all item scores for that particular subscale.

Fast Track for Screening

- The EAT-26 should not be used alone as a diagnostic instrument, but can be the first step in a two-stage process in which high scorers are interviewed.
- A cutoff score of 20 on the EAT-26 is approximate for many purposes: This score identifies approximately 15% of college and high school females, 10 to 40% of whom may be suspected as having clinically significant eating disorders.
- Cutoff scores may be adjusted to be higher or lower, depending on the purpose of screening.
- Addition of selected items from a measure such as the EDI-2 Symptom Checklist (Garner, 1991) may improve the discrimination of the EAT-26 and add information relevant to diagnosis.

Eating Disorders Teleconference: Presented by America's Continuing Education Network (850) 784-9942 and endorsed by the American Academy of Child & Adolescent Psychiatry and the National Mental Health Association.

Compulsive exercise behaviors go hand-in-hand with anorexia nervosa.[18,98] Rather than starve or vomit, the anorectic fanatically expends as many calories as possible through physical activity. A common misconception about anorectics concerns their state of hunger. In reality, they often remain continually hungry; their ability to overcome the urge to eat provides a sense of self-power and control, which is self-assuring. If untreated, between 6 and 21% of anorectics die prematurely from suicide, heart failure, or infections. In about one third of patients, the disease becomes chronic, marked by frequent relapses that often require hospitalization.[76] **TABLE 15.7** lists the clinical criteria for diagnosing anorexia nervosa.

Weight gain becomes a primary goal in the treatment of anorexia nervosa. Interestingly, when patients regain weight through hospitalization or outpatient supervision, most of the weight is gained in the trunk region rather than the extremities, with up to 70% of the regained weight as fat.[44,69,102] For example, at the end of treatment that produced an 11.9-kg weight gain (pretreatment fat, 9.8%; posttreatment fat, 22.6%), the ratio of FFM to fat mass averaged 3.4:1, with fat representing 55% of the gained weight.[79]

A 9-month longitudinal study serially assessed body composition in ambulatory anorectic women.[36] Patients exhibited an abnormal body composition during times of low body weight and after weight gain compared with a control group of normal-weight women. At low body weight, anorectic women possessed trunk fat as a percentage of total body fat similar to controls, but extremity fat percentage remained lower than in controls. After a modest 4.1-kg weight gain, the percentage of extremity fat changed little, but trunk fat percentage increased significantly. In contrast to results with other groups of women, estrogen therapy provided no protection against the gain in trunk fat with spontaneous weight gain in anorectic women. Researchers do not know why anorexia nervosa patients with the most distress about weight gain in recovery (particularly abdominal fat) have the highest ratio of truncal fat to peripheral fat or gain the greatest quantity of truncal fat when they regain weight.[61]

TABLE 15.7 DSM-IV Clinical Criteria for Anorexia Nervosa (Code No. 307.1)

1. Refusal to maintain body weight at or above a minimally normal weight for age and height (e.g., weight loss leading to maintenance of body weight less than 85% of expected or failure to make expected weight gain during period of growth, leading to body weight less than 85% of expected).
2. Intense fear of gaining weight or becoming fat, even though underweight.
3. Disturbance in the way one's body weight or shape is experienced, undue influence of body weight or shape on self-evaluation, or denial of the seriousness of the current low body weight.
4. In postmenarchal females, amenorrhea, that is, the absence of at least three consecutive menstrual cycles. A woman is considered to have amenorrhea if her periods occur only following hormone (e.g., estrogen) administration.

Specify type:

1. *Restricting type:* During the current episode of anorexia nervosa, the person has not regularly engaged in binge-eating or purging behavior (i.e., self-induced vomiting or the misuse of laxatives, diuretics, or enemas).
2. *Binge-eating/purging type:* During the current episode of anorexia nervosa, the person has regularly engaged in binge-eating or purging behavior (i.e., self-induced vomiting or the misuse of laxatives, diuretics, or enemas).

Eating disorders criteria–DSM-IV: Selected Portions of the Diagnostic and Statistical Manual of Mental Disorders, Fourth Edition, relating to Eating Disorders. Copyright © 2000 American Psychiatric Association.

Adolescent girls hospitalized with anorexia nervosa had significant body wasting as indicated by extremely low body fat and a low FFM as reflected by total body nitrogen (**TABLE 15.8**).[49] Triceps skinfold thickness provided the most significant anthropometric predictor of percentage

TABLE 15.8 Comparison of Body Compositions of Female Adolescents with Anorexia Nervosa and Healthy Controls

	Age, y	Body Weight, kg	BMI	%Fat	%TBN	FFM, kg	Trunk Fat, kg	Leg Fat, kg
Anorexia nervosa	15.5	40.2	15.3	13.8	73	34.5	2.1	2.6
Healthy controls	15.1	57.3	21.2	26.3	75	41.2	6.6	7.1

FFM, fat-free body mass; %TBN, percentage total body nitrogen predicted for age.

From Kerrvish KP, et al. Body composition in adolescents with anorexia nervosa. *Am J Clin Nutr* 2002;75:31.

body fat. This skinfold measure explained 68% of the variation in body fat, while body weight accurately indicated total body nitrogen and thus protein depletion in these patients.

Physical Consequences of Anorexia Nervosa

Death often results from prolonged starvation in about 7% of anorectic patients over a 10-year period; 18 to 20% die within 30 years. A range of other profound physical ailments also occur, including cardiac abnormalities (e.g., arrhythmias, heart block), electrolyte disturbances, impaired kidney function, decreased bone mineral density, gastrointestinal dysfunction (e.g., bleeding, ulceration, bloating, constipation), and anemia. Many effects such as depressed basal metabolic rate (BMR) and leptin concentrations, not fully explained by body composition changes,[77] reflect predictable outcomes from energy conservation as the body defends against prolonged caloric deprivation. **FIGURE 15.6** depicts anorexia nervosa's potential physical and medical consequences.

Common Signs and Symptoms: Anorexia nervosa usually begins with a normal attempt to lose weight through dieting. As dieting progresses, the person continues to eat less until the person consumes practically no food. Food restriction eventually becomes an obsession, and the anorectic achieves no satisfaction with any amount of weight loss. The person denies the accompanying extreme emaciation as weight loss progresses. Some anorectic persons cannot ignore the intense hunger accompanying near-total food deprivation; this causes episodes of bingeing and subsequent purging. The warning signs listed in **TABLE 15.9** can help coaches and trainers identify athletes with anorexia nervosa.

Bulimia Nervosa

The term *bulimia,* literally meaning "ox hunger," refers to "gorging" or "insatiable appetite." At one time, some believed that **bulimia nervosa** reflected a manifestation of anorexia nervosa owing to similarities and overlap in the two conditions. For example, some anorectics experience bulimic episodes, while some bulimics experience episodes of anorexia. Based on more careful examination of the disorders, bulimia nervosa emerged in the late 1970s as a separate eating disorder classification. The disease, far more common than anorexia nervosa, is characterized by frequent episodes of binge eating, followed by purging, laxative abuse, fasting, or extreme exercise and intense feelings of guilt or shame. Approximately 2 to 4% of adolescents and adults in the general population (mainly female, including about 5% of college women) are bulimic. A large percentage of the total is obese and enrolled in self-help or commercial weight-loss programs. A sex difference probably exists in the emotional triggers for overindulgence in food. Compared with men, women with a weight problem exhibit greater binge eating during periods of negative emotions—anxiety, frustration, depression, or anger.[94]

Unlike the continual semistarvation with anorexia nervosa, bulimia nervosa includes binge eating of calorically dense food—often at night and usually between 1000 and 10,000 calories within several hours. Fasting, self-induced vomiting, taking laxatives or diuretics, or compulsively exercising solely to avoid weight gain takes place after the binge episode.[32,56]

Anorectics revel in their sense of control over eating, while striving toward a perceived level of physical perfection. In contrast, bulimics lose control; they recognize their impulsive behavior as abnormal. Eating extreme quantities of food often becomes a means to reduce stress, and purging provides the only way to regain control for their inability to stop eating voluntarily. Considerable variation exists in the type of food consumed during binge episodes. Some bulimics, who often attempt dieting with healthful eating, binge on large quantities of unhealthful, "forbidden" foods (cookies, chips, and chocolates). Others binge on food consumed regularly but in extreme quantities. Some bulimics even overeat lower-calorie, diet-type foods, while others purge after every meal, regardless of what or how much they eat. *Bulimics span the gamut between normal body weight and overweight (or a history of overweight); this represents a striking difference between anorectics and bulimics.* While obvious physical characteristics exist for anorexia nervosa, many bulimic characteristics remain behavioral.

Most persons with bulimia nervosa meet standards for major depressive disorders—loss of interest, low mood, shortened attention span, disrupted sleep patterns, and

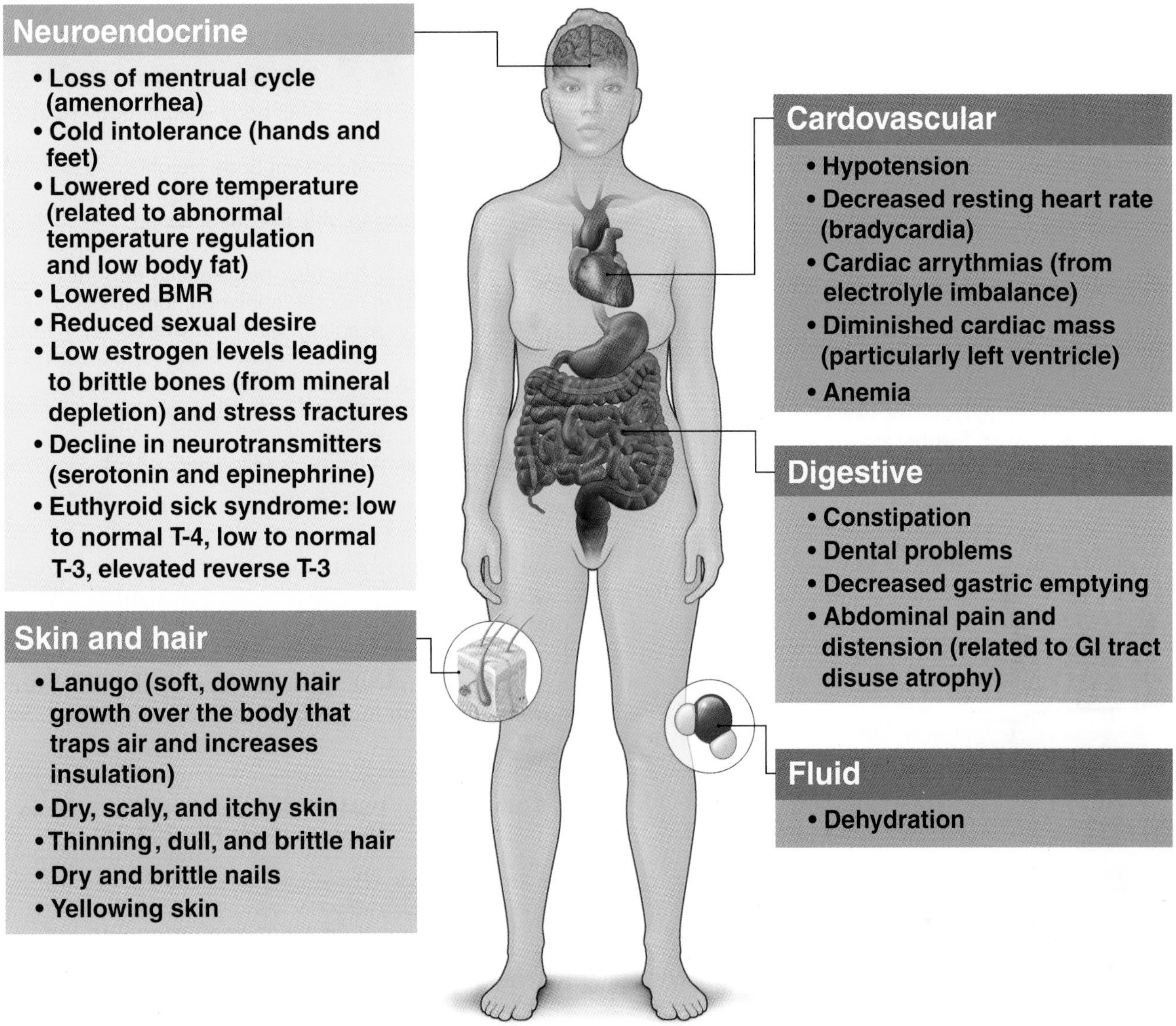
Neuroendocrine
• Loss of mentrual cycle (amenorrhea)
• Cold intolerance (hands and feet)
• Lowered core temperature (related to abnormal temperature regulation and low body fat)
• Lowered BMR
• Reduced sexual desire
• Low estrogen levels leading to brittle bones (from mineral depletion) and stress fractures
• Decline in neurotransmitters (serotonin and epinephrine)
• Euthyroid sick syndrome: low to normal T-4, low to normal T-3, elevated reverse T-3
Skin and hair
• Lanugo (soft, downy hair growth over the body that traps air and increases insulation)
• Dry, scaly, and itchy skin
• Thinning, dull, and brittle hair
• Dry and brittle nails
• Yellowing skin
Cardovascular
• Hypotension
• Decreased resting heart rate (bradycardia)
• Cardiac arrythmias (from electrolyle imbalance)
• Diminished cardiac mass (particularly left ventricle)
• Anemia
Digestive
• Constipation
• Dental problems
• Decreased gastric emptying
• Abdominal pain and distension (related to GI tract disuse atrophy)
Fluid
• Dehydration

FIGURE 15.6. Physical and medical consequences of anorexia nervosa.

suicidal thoughts. Bulimics also abuse alcohol and drugs at a higher rate than the general population. **TABLE 15.10** lists the DSM-IV clinical criteria for diagnosing bulimia nervosa.

Physical Consequences of Bulimia Nervosa

FIGURE 15.7 depicts the diverse physical symptoms and disorders suffered by persons with bulimia nervosa.

PURGING AND CALORIES: YOU CAN'T EXPEL THE TOTAL

A study that measured the amount and caloric value of food from a binge that remained in the stomach after vomiting found that, on average, 1209 kcal were retained after a binge meal that contained 3530 kcal

Danger Signals and Indications: Difficulty exists in diagnosing bulimia nervosa because there are few noticeable, outward signs. In public, bulimics remain conscious of what and how much they eat and generally never eat to excess. For the most part, they express feelings of perfectionist behavior, depression, low self-esteem, being out of control, and dissatisfaction with body size and shape. Often, those closest to the bulimic remain unaware of the problem. Another disturbing aspect of bulimia nervosa concerns substance abuse. In a comparison of women with anorexia nervosa and women with bulimia nervosa, the bulimics abused alcohol, amphetamines, barbiturates, marijuana, tranquilizers, and cocaine to a greater extent.[99] Independent of the diagnosis of either anorexia or bulimia, (1) the magnitude of caloric restriction predicted amphetamine use, (2) severity of binge eating predicted tranquilizer use, and (3) severity of purging predicted alcohol, cocaine, and cigarette use.

TABLE 15.9 Common Signs and Symptoms of Anorexia Nervosa

General	• Appetite loss • Fatigue • Inability to exercise (due to fatigue and weakness) • Impaired memory • Anxiety • Depression
Skin	• Dry • Cool • Mottled/blue • Bruises • Self-inflicted cuts • Scalp hair loss • Lanugo (baby) hair
Abdominal	• Heartburn • Nausea • Pain • Cramping • Constipation • Early satiety • Vomiting, bloating
Musculoskeletal	• Aching joints/muscles • Fractures of spine, hip, wrist
Mouth	• Sores • Cracking around lips • Tooth decay • Gum disease • Parotid gland enlargement • Adenopathy • Bad breath
Circulatory	• Cool • Blue feet and hands • Low blood pressure • Dizziness • Fainting • Dehydration • Shortness of breath • Swelling
Reproduction	• Infertility • Oligomenorrhea • Amenorrhea • Decreased libido
Urinary	• Frequency, especially at night • Diminished urine output

WARNING SIGNS OF BULIMIA NERVOSA

- Excessive concern about body weight, body size, and body composition
- Frequent gain and loss in body weight
- Frequent visits to the bathroom following meals
- Fear of not being able to control eating
- Eating when depressed
- Compulsive dieting after binge-eating episodes
- Severe shifts in mood (depression, loneliness)
- Secretive binge eating, but never overeating in front of others
- Frequent criticism of one's body size and shape
- Experiencing personal or family problems with alcohol or drugs
- Irregular menstrual cycle (oligomenorrhea)

Binge-Eating Disorder

Binge-eating disorder (BED), first described in 1959 by researcher and psychiatrist Dr. Albert Stunkard (1922–), identified specific eating behavior patterns in a subgroup of obese patients undergoing treatment to lose weight.[88] He termed the disorder "night eating syndrome." The affliction is characterized by recurrent episodes of binge eating. These occur often without subsequent purging or abusing laxatives to compensate for overeating common to bulimia nervosa and anorexia nervosa. Psychiatrists define the disorder as episodes of binge eating at least twice a week for at least 6 months and that cause significant emotional distress. Persons with BED eat more rapidly than normal until they can no longer consume additional food. Such

TABLE 15.10 DSM-IV Clinical Criteria for Bulimia Nervosa (Code No. 307.15)

1. Recurrent episodes of binge eating. An episode of binge eating is characterized by both of the following: (1) Eating, in a discrete period of time (e.g., within any 2-h period), an amount of food that is definitely larger than most people would eat during a similar period of time and under similar circumstances. (2) A sense of lack of control over eating during the episode (e.g., a feeling that one cannot stop eating or control what or how much one is eating).
2. Recurrent inappropriate compensatory behavior in order to prevent weight gain, such as self-induced vomiting; misuse of laxatives, diuretics, enemas, or other medications; fasting or excessive exercise.
3. The binge eating and inappropriate compensatory behaviors both occur, on average, at least twice a week for 3 months.
4. Self-evaluation is unduly influenced by body shape and weight.
5. The disturbance does not occur exclusively during episodes of anorexia nervosa.

Specify type:

1. *Purging type:* During the current episode of bulimia nervosa, the person has regularly engaged in self-induced vomiting or the misuse of laxatives, diuretics, or enemas.
2. *Nonpurging type:* During the current episode of bulimia nervosa, the person has used inappropriate compensatory behaviors, such as fasting or excessive exercise, but has not regularly engaged in self-induced vomiting or the misuse of laxatives, diuretics, or enemas.

Eating disorders criteria–DSM-IV: Selected Portions of the Diagnostic and Statistical Manual of Mental Disorders, Fourth Edition, relating to Eating Disorders. Copyright © 2000 American Psychiatric Association.

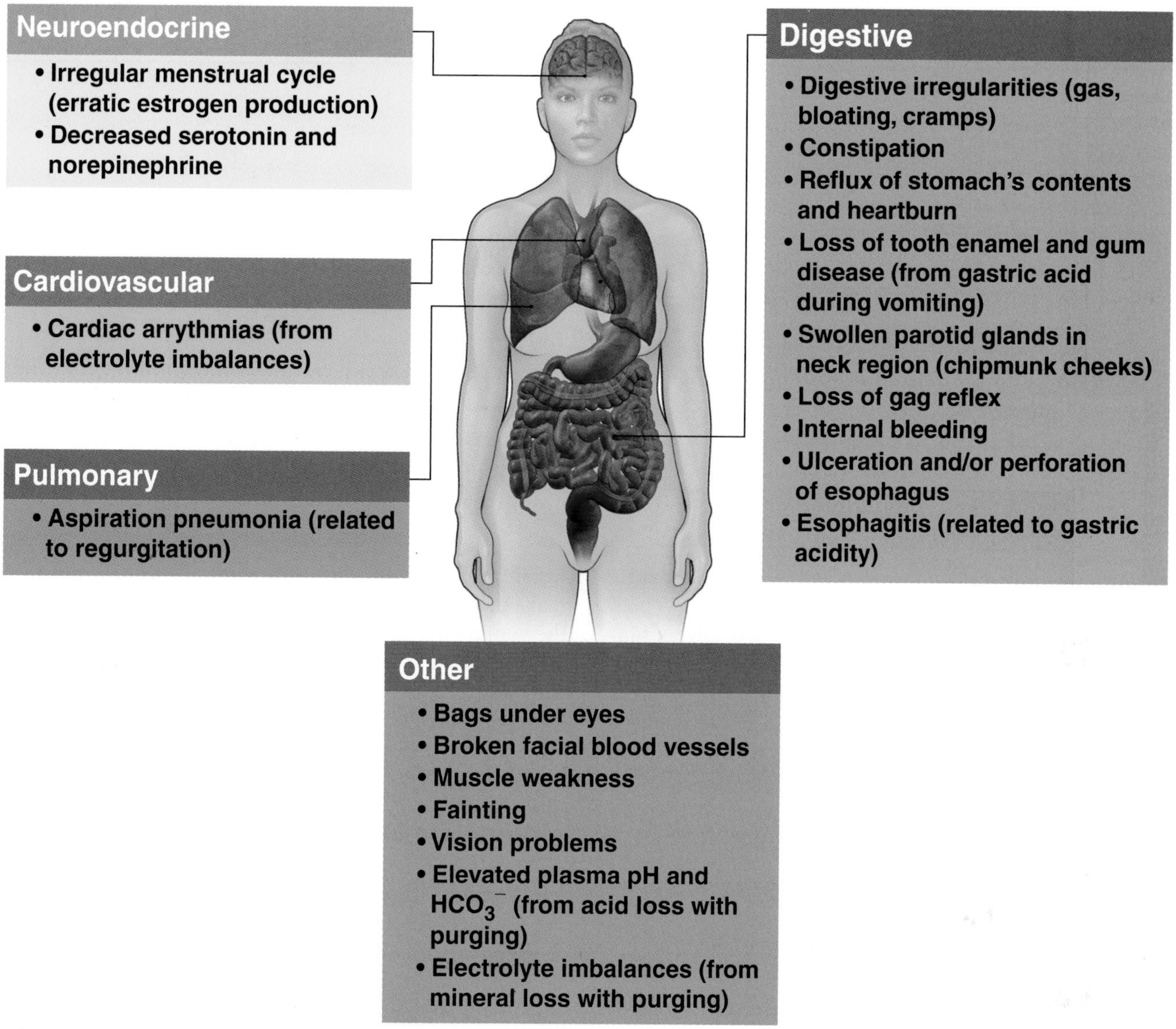
Neuroendocrine
• Irregular menstrual cycle (erratic estrogen production)
• Decreased serotonin and norepinephrine
Cardiovascular
• Cardiac arrythmias (from electrolyte imbalances)
Pulmonary
• Aspiration pneumonia (related to regurgitation)
Digestive
• Digestive irregularities (gas, bloating, cramps)
• Constipation
• Reflux of stomach's contents and heartburn
• Loss of tooth enamel and gum disease (from gastric acid during vomiting)
• Swollen parotid glands in neck region (chipmunk cheeks)
• Loss of gag reflex
• Internal bleeding
• Ulceration and/or perforation of esophagus
• Esophagitis (related to gastric acidity)
Other
• Bags under eyes
• Broken facial blood vessels
• Muscle weakness
• Fainting
• Vision problems
• Elevated plasma pH and HCO_3^- (from acid loss with purging)
• Electrolyte imbalances (from mineral loss with purging)

FIGURE 15.7. Physical and medical consequences of bulimia nervosa.

high levels of food intake exceed the physiologic drive of hunger. Binge eating, undertaken in private because of embarrassment, occurs with feelings of guilt, depression, or self-disgust. Binge eaters suffer greater self-anger, shame, lack of control, and frustration than nonbingeing obese persons.[19,31,43] They also experience relatively higher rates of sexual abuse and physical abuse and bullying by peers than the general population.[87] Studies in the early 1980s identified BED in 20 to 50% of obese patients.[56] Not only did these persons exhibit difficulties with binge eating, but they also regained lost weight faster than obese non–binge eaters, and they more likely failed in treatment.[57] As an outgrowth of these early clinical observations, diagnostic criteria developed in the early 1990s helped to identify BED (**TABLE 15.11**).

A feature distinguishing BED from anorexia nervosa and bulimia nervosa is that persons seeking treatment for BED are often overweight or obese. Approximately 2% of the US population (1–2 million people) and about 30% of Americans treated for obesity experience BED,[65] although incidence rate decreases on the basis of personal interview rather than questionnaire to assess its prevalence.[88] Current research does not support earlier beliefs that minorities were somehow "protected" from BED.[83] For example, comparisons between Caucasian and minority females showed similar scores on measures of eating disorder symptomology and general psychopathology.[54]

Ten to 15% of mildly obese people who enroll in self-help or commercial weight loss programs meet the criteria for BED. Those with body weight in excess of 20% of ideal weight exhibit the highest prevalence of BED and develop their obesity at a younger age than their non–binge-eating obese counterparts. Women experience BED at a 50% higher rate than do men. Women also report greater binge-eating episodes in response to negative emotions such as anxiety, anger and frustration, and depression. Men and women presenting for BED treatment score similarly on measures of eating disturbance, body shape and weight concerns, interpersonal

TABLE 15.11 DSM-IV Eating Disorders Not Otherwise Specified (Code No. 307.50)

Includes disorders of eating that do not meet the criteria for any specific eating disorder. Examples include:

1. For females, all of the criteria for anorexia nervosa are met except that the person has regular menses.
2. All of the criteria for anorexia nervosa are met except that, despite significant weight loss, the person's current weight is in the normal range.
3. All of the criteria for bulimia nervosa are met except that the binge eating and inappropriate compensatory mechanisms occur at a frequency of less than twice a week or for duration of less than 3 months.
4. The regular use of inappropriate compensatory behavior by an person of normal body weight after eating small amounts of food (e.g., self-induced vomiting after the consumption of two cookies).
5. Repeatedly chewing and spitting out, but not swallowing, large amounts of food.
6. Binge-eating disorder: recurrent episodes of binge eating in the absence of the regular use of inappropriate compensatory behaviors characteristic of bulimia nervosa.

problems, and self-esteem; men experience more psychiatric disturbance and less emotional eating.[85]

The causes of BED remain unknown. Up to 50% of bingers suffer depression, which may contribute to the disorder. Persons with BED experience higher lifetime rates of major depression, panic disorder, bulimia nervosa, borderline personality disorder, and avoidant personality disorder.[101] Moderately obese men and women with BED experience greater relative risk for psychiatric disorders than their obese counterparts without the disorder.[102]

BED Treated by Exercise plus Behavior Therapy Intervention

To investigate the role of exercise and behavior therapy in treating BED, two groups of women participated in identical exercise programs for 6 months.[55] One group also received behavior therapy with the exercise program. Pretreatment and posttreatment evaluations included exercise level, binge-eating frequency, and depressive symptoms. The results favored the group receiving exercise plus behavioral treatment for BED. At posttreatment, 81% of these subjects remained free from binge-eating episodes. They also exercised more frequently each week and thus expended greater energy.

CAUSE OR EFFECT? THE ROLE OF SPORT IN EATING DISORDERS

Does dedication to training for a specific sport induce development of an eating disorder, or do persons with potentially pathologic concerns about body size and shape gravitate (self-select) to the sport? The **attraction to sport hypothesis** maintains that persons with an existing eating disorder (or at high risk for developing one) find reward by participating in aesthetic-type sports that emphasize an excessively lean appearance. When training commences early in life (as in gymnastics and ballet dancing), it becomes difficult to make the case for the attraction to the sport hypothesis (i.e., the young girls participated because of the sport's focus on leanness and appearance). For these girls, disordered eating behaviors probably develop progressively as the young athlete realizes an inherent incompatibility between the sport's body-type requirements and genetic predisposition for body size and structure. Research must determine whether the inordinate focus of many athletes on food intake and leanness reflects a continuum of graded psychological disturbance that ultimately leads to a full-blown eating disorder.

TABLE 15.12 presents a brief questionnaire to evaluate the degree of restraint a person feels over issues concerning food choices, diet planning, and body-weight maintenance. Often, persons tending toward disordered eating patterns exhibit extreme concern over what they eat and how it affects body weight. If they "give in" (because of a perceived lack of self-control) and eat "bad" foods believed to contribute to weight gain, they often reduce the resulting stress by purging or excessive exercise. The questions in **TABLE 15.12** do not determine whether or not an eating disorder exists, but raise awareness about dietary restraint patterns and behaviors that ultimately may lead to an eating disorder.

EATING DISORDERS AFFECT EXERCISE PERFORMANCE

Athletes with an eating disorder faces a paradox: Behavior necessary to achieve a body weight for success in certain sports—semistarvation, purging, excessive exercising—adversely affects health, energy reserves, and physiologic function and the ability to train and compete at an optimal level. In Chapter 14, we noted that athletes often reduce body fat to improve exercise power output relative to body mass and to reduce drag forces that impede forward movement through air and water. For persons with eating disorders, chronic restriction of energy intake (as in anorexia nervosa)

Connections to the Past

Thomas Kirk Cureton (1901–1993)

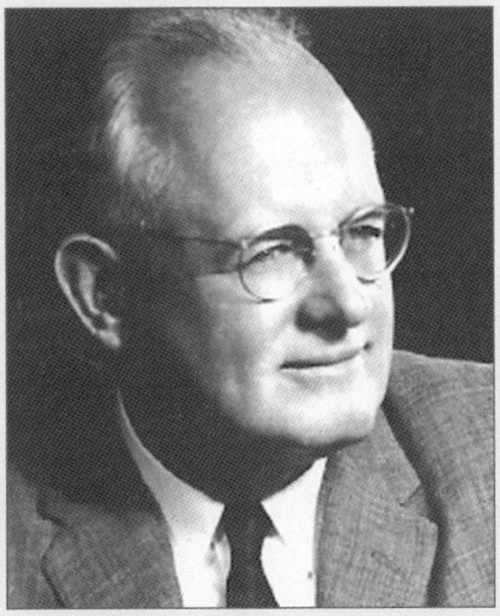

The fields of exercise physiology and exercise nutrition owe a debt of gratitude to the pioneers of the American "physical fitness" movement. Spearheading this movement was Thomas K. Cureton, PhD (one of 50 charter members of the American College of Sports Medicine [ACSM]; 1969 recipient of the prestigious ACSM Honor Award), professor of Physical Education at the University of Illinois, Champaign, IL. Cureton was a prolific and innovative physical educator and pioneer researcher in the field of physical fitness and its assessment. In 1922, Cureton attended Yale University's Sheffield Scientific School, majoring in electrical engineering and earning a BS degree in 1925. An outstanding swimmer, Cureton earned two varsity letters in intercollegiate swimming. He was introduced to physiology, exercise, and fitness training through his involvement with one of the Yale coaches who helped train members of the all-Yale varsity, heavyweight eight crew (which included Dr. Benjamin Spock [1903–1998], famous author and pediatrician) that won the Paris 1924 Olympic gold rowing medal.

Professor Cureton trained four generations of Master's and PhD degree students beginning in 1941 after an initial teaching period at Springfield College, Massachusetts that began in 1929. Cureton was mentored in his graduate studies by one of the most influential physical educators of the era, Jesse Feiring Williams, MD, ScD (1886–1966), scholar, researcher, and prolific writer at Columbia University in New York City. Williams had a strong scientific background (e.g., multiple editions of *Text-Book of Anatomy and Physiology*, and other science-based texts dealing with hygiene and physiology). Cureton earned a Master of Physical Education (MPE) degree in 1930 (thesis: "Objective Tests in Swimming"). During the early 1930s, Cureton continued to take graduate classes at Columbia University and, after graduation, was appointed Director of the Physical Sciences Curriculum and Director of Graduate Studies at Springfield College in 1937.

thePoint *Visit* **thePoint.lww.com/MKKSEN4e** *for more details on Cureton's numerous research studies and his legacy regarding the physical fitness movement worldwide.*

or reduced energy availability through purging (as in bulimia nervosa) rapidly depletes glycogen reserves. As emphasized throughout this text, the normally limited quantity of muscle and liver glycogen provides rapid energy for high-intensity anaerobic and aerobic exercise. Consequently, even short periods of disordered eating may deplete glycogen reserves, which profoundly affects capacity to train and recover. The reduced protein (and carbohydrate) intake usually accompanying an eating disorder also contributes to lean tissue loss. A subpar intake of vitamins and minerals required for energy metabolism and tissue growth and repair facilitates poor exercise performance and increases injury potential.

EATING DISORDERS AFFECT BONE MINERAL DENSITY

Dual-energy x-ray absorptiometry (DXA; see Chapter 13) has evaluated skeletal and regional body composition characteristics in anorexia nervosa. In one study, body mass averaged 44.4 kg (97.9 lb) for 10 anorectic women. **FIGURE 15.8** shows an anorectic female (*left two images*) and a typical female whose body fat percentage averaged 25% of her 56.7-kg (125-lb) body mass. Although FFM of the anorectic women approached the normal average of 43.0 kg, body fat equaled only 7.5%, a value more than three times less than that for comparison groups of typical young women. These women were anorectic for at least 1 year, and amenorrhea duration averaged 3.1 years (range, 1–8 years). The *inset table* compares regional bone mineral densities (BMD, $g{\cdot}cm^{-2}$) of anorectic women and 287 normal-weight women age 20 to 40 years. The values in the *right column* represent the percentage for BMD for the anorectic group relative to the comparison group. Total-body BMD averaged 10% lower, the BMD of the L2–L4 region of the lumbar spine averaged 27% less, and the BMD of the femoral neck averaged 13% lower than the comparable BMDs in the normal women. Spine BMD in the young anorectic group equaled the average BMD in 70-year-old women! Diminished BMD in anorexia nervosa, in addition to reduced skeletal size, may render these young women particularly vulnerable to osteoporotic fractures at a relatively young age.

MANAGEMENT OF EATING DISORDERS IN ATHLETES

Eating disorders do not just go away; there is no simple cause and no simple solution. Eating disorders represent not only a problem but also an attempted solution to a problem. In its mildest aspect, the disorder often stems from poor nutritional information. Left untreated, abnormal

TABLE 15.12 How Do You Rate in Terms of Eating Restraint?

Circle the number that best describes your feelings or behaviors related to the question.

1. **How often are you dieting?**
   0 = never
   1 = rarely
   2 = sometimes
   3 = often
   4 = always
2. **What is the maximum amount of weight (in pounds) that you have ever lost within one month?**
   0 = 0–4
   1 = 5–9
   2 = 10–14
   3 = 15–19
   4 = 20+
3. **What is the most weight (in pounds) you have ever gained within a week?**
   1 = 1.1–2.0
   2 = 2.1–3.0
   3 = 3.1–5.0
   4 = 5.1+
4. **In a typical week, how much does your weight (pounds) fluctuate?**
   0 = 0–1.0
   1 = 1.1–2.0
   2 = 2.1–3.0
   3 = 2.1–5.0
   4 = 5.1+
5. **Would a weight fluctuation of 5 lb affect the way you live your life?**
   0 = not at all
   1 = slightly
   2 = moderately
   3 = very much
6. **Do you eat sensibly in front of others and splurge alone?**
   0 = never
   1 = rarely
   2 = often
   3 = always
7. **Do you give too much time and thought to food?**
   0 = never
   1 = rarely
   2 = often
   3 = always
8. **Do you have feelings of guilt after overeating?**
   0 = never
   1 = rarely
   2 = often
   3 = always
9. **How conscious are you of what you are eating?**
   0 = not at all
   1 = slightly
   2 = moderately
   3 = extremely
10. **How many pounds over your desired weight were you at your maximum weight?**
   0 = 0–1
   1 = 1–5
   2 = 6–10
   3 = 11–20
   4 = 21+

Add up the numbers you have circled and select the category that best describes you.

0–15 Relatively unrestrained
16–23 Moderately restrained
24–35 Highly restrained

From Herman CP, Policy J. Restrained eating. In: Stunkard AJ, ed. Obesity. Philadelphia: WB Saunders, 1980.

eating behaviors often blossom into chronic eating disorders. Familial vulnerability also exists because the relatives of people with eating disorders exhibit higher risk of developing a disorder.[56] The relatives also show higher rates of depression and obsessive–compulsive disorders than the general population.

Disordered eating behaviors frequently produce nutritional problems in addition to the loss of tooth enamel from stomach acid during vomiting in bulimic patients. Effective treatment focuses primarily on the psychological realm and attempts to reverse the negative effects of disordered eating behaviors. Depending on the patient's age, disorder severity, and its affect on health and well-being, therapy takes place either on an outpatient basis or in a hospital setting. With teenage athletes, the parents must become involved. Persons with eating disorders frequently resist outside attempts at intervention and treatment. No single approach or theory has proved helpful in treating those with eating disorders. Often treatments that appear to have a high likelihood of success give opposite results.

Successful treatment usually involves a team approach using psychotherapeutic, medical, nutritional, and family support. **FIGURE 15.9** outlines an intervention model for disordered eating behaviors in an athletic setting. The process consists of four steps:

Step 1. Identify and isolate the contributing factors.
Step 2. Formulate appropriate goals for intervention and prevention.
Step 3. Formulate long-term strategies to deal with the problem.
Step 4. Initiate long-term programs to address the situation.

FIGURE 15.10 illustrates the multidisciplinary approach to manage disordered eating behaviors in athletes at the

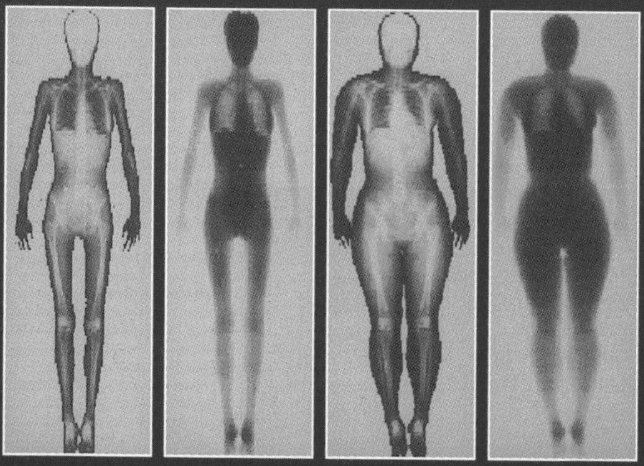

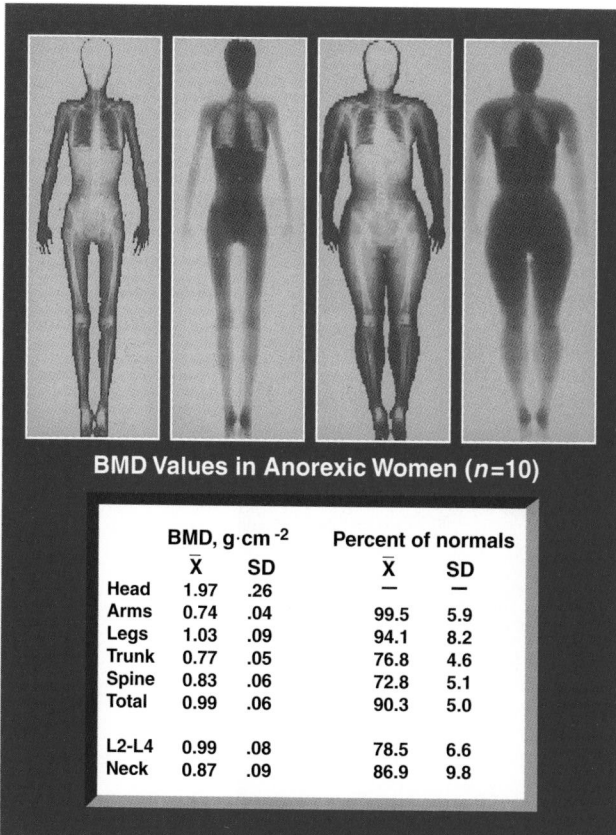

BMD Values in Anorexic Women (n=10)

	BMD, g·cm^{-2} $\bar{X}$	SD	Percent of normals $\bar{X}$	SD
Head	1.97	.26	—	—
Arms	0.74	.04	99.5	5.9
Legs	1.03	.09	94.1	8.2
Trunk	0.77	.05	76.8	4.6
Spine	0.83	.06	72.8	5.1
Total	0.99	.06	90.3	5.0
L2-L4	0.99	.08	78.5	6.6
Neck	0.87	.09	86.9	9.8

FIGURE 15.8. Example of an anorectic female (*two left images*) and a typical female (*two right images*) whose body fat percentage averages 25% of body mass of 56.7 kg (125 lb). The average anorectic subject weighed 44.4 kg (97.9 lb) and had 7.5% body fat estimated by dual-energy x-ray absorptiometry (DXA) from the fat percentages at the arms, legs, and trunk regions. The values in the right column of the *inset table* present percentage values for bone mineral density (BMD) for different regional body areas in the anorectic group compared to 287 normal females age 20 to 40 years. Photos courtesy of RB Mazes, Department of Medical Physics, University of Wisconsin, Madison, WI, and the Lunar Radiation Corporation, Madison, WI. Data from Mazes RB, et al. Skeletal and body composition effects of anorexia nervosa. Paper presented at the International Symposium On In Vivo Body Composition Studies, Toronto, Ontario, Canada, June 20–23, 1989.

University of Texas at Austin. This Division I collegiate-level athletic program prohibits coaches from weighing female athletes or talking to them about body weight or body composition; these responsibilities reside with the sports medicine staff. Three important components include the following:

1. *Education* to provide information concerning the eating disorder and its consequences
2. *Self-monitoring* to provide a clear understanding of current eating behaviors and patterns
3. *Meal planning* to help gain control of eating patterns and establish a healthful pattern of eating

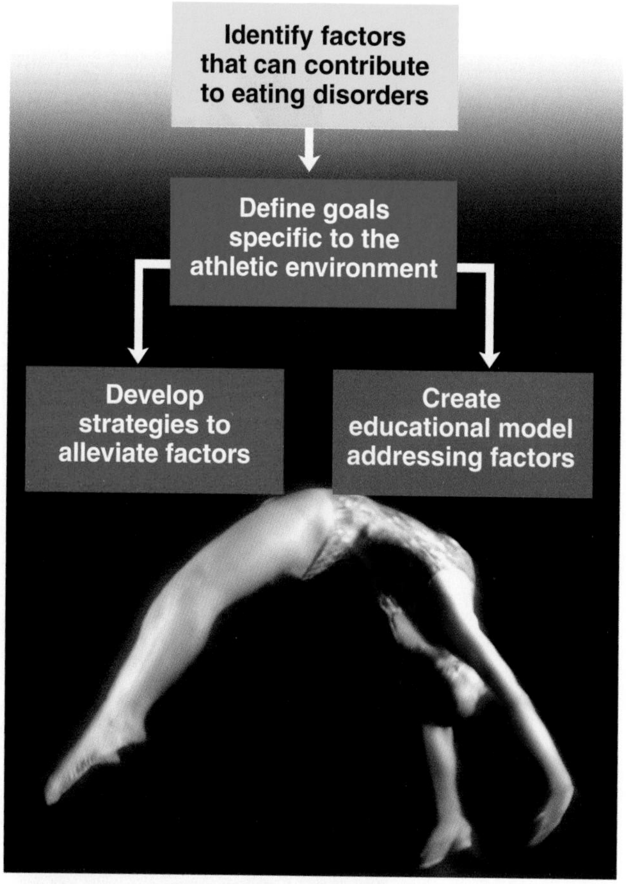

FIGURE 15.9. Model intervention for dealing with disordered eating behaviors in an athletic setting. (From Ryan R. Management of eating problems in athletic settings. In: Brownell KD, et al., eds. *Eating, Body Weight and Performance in Athletes*. Philadelphia: Lea & Febiger, 1992.)

College Women at Risk for an Eating Disorder May Benefit from Online Intervention

An Internet-based intervention program may prevent some high-risk, college-age women from developing an eating disorder.[95] Researchers conducted a randomized controlled trial of 480 women identified in preliminary interviews as at risk for developing an eating disorder. The trial included an 8-week, Internet-based, cognitive-behavioral program called "Student Bodies." The intervention aimed to reduce the participants' concerns about body weight and shape, enhance body image, promote healthy eating and weight maintenance, and increase knowledge about the risks associated with eating disorders.

The program contained reading and other assignments that included keeping an online body image journal and participation in an online discussion group moderated by clinical psychologists. Participants were interviewed immediately at the end of the online program and annually for up to 3 years to determine attitudes toward their weight and shape and to detect and measure the onset of eating disorders.

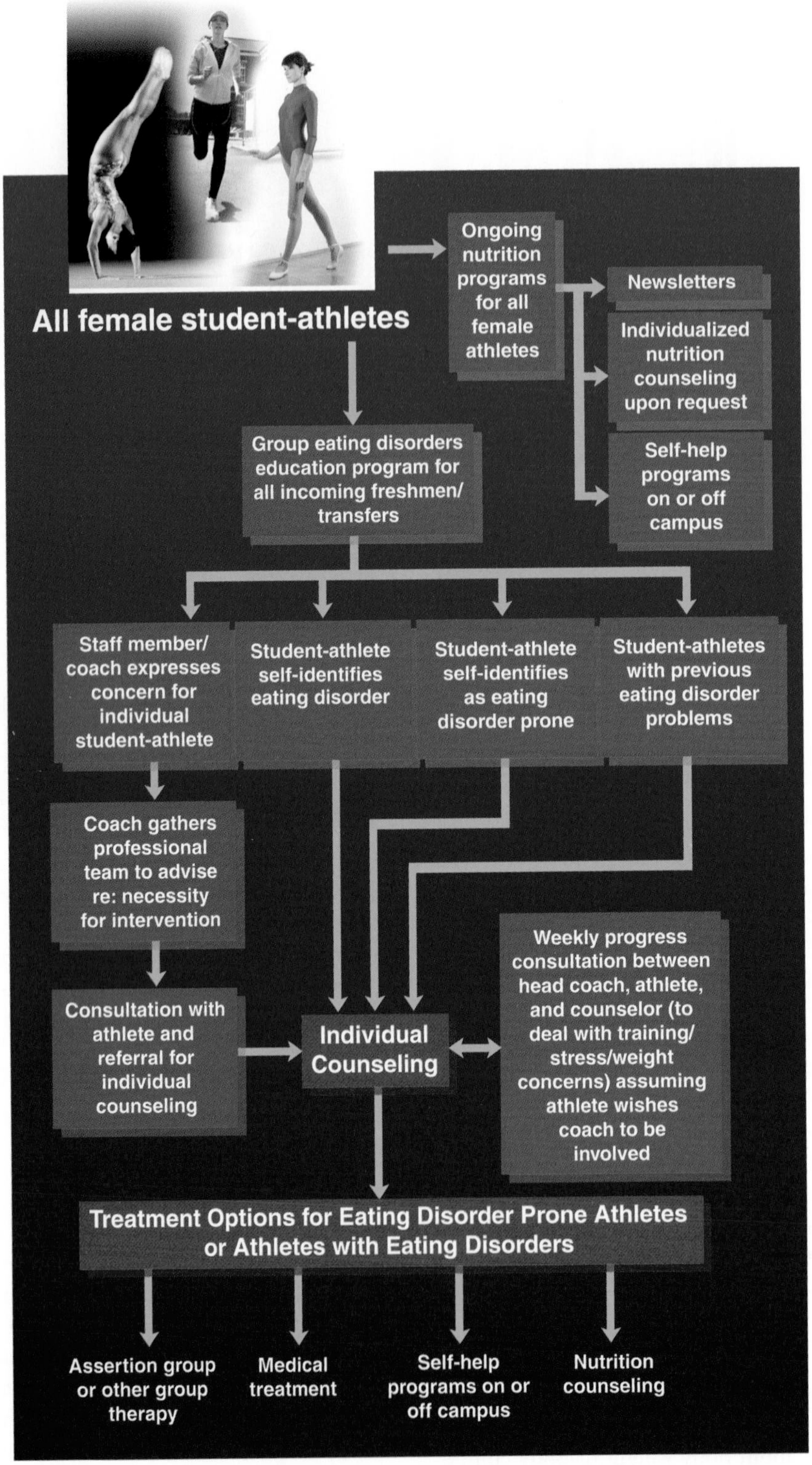

FIGURE 15.10. Flow chart to prevent eating disorders and provide services for athletes who suffer from eating disorders. (From Ryan R. Management of eating problems in athletic settings. In: Brownell KD, et al., eds. *Eating, Body Weight and Performance in Athletes*. Philadelphia: Lea & Febiger, 1992.)

The intervention achieved greatest success among overweight women with BMIs of 25 or greater at the start of the program. For these women in the intervention group, none developed an eating disorder after 2 years, whereas 11.9% of the women with comparable baseline BMIs in the control group developed an eating disorder.

The program helped women who exhibited symptoms of an eating disorder at the start of the program such as self-induced vomiting; laxative, diet pill, or diuretic use; or excessive exercise. Of those with these characteristics in the intervention group, 14% developed an eating disorder within 3 years in contrast to 30% with these characteristics in the control group. The intervention enabled high-risk women to become less concerned about their weight and shape, while helping them to better understand healthier eating and nutrition practices. This study was the first to show that eating disorders can be prevented among high-risk groups and provided additional evidence that an inordinate focus on body weight and shape are causal risk factors leading to an eating disorder. Interestingly, the rate at which the women stayed with the program remained high—nearly 80% of the online program's web pages were read—suggesting the participants were motivated to succeed.

COMMON SENSE GUIDELINES FOR COACHES AND TRAINERS CONCERNING EATING DISORDERS

Coaches and athletic trainers should play an important role in the lives of athletes with symptoms of disordered eating. Follow these 10 common sense guidelines whenever possible—they can make a difference.

1. Do not urge athletes to eat, do not watch them eat, refrain from discussing food, and forego discussions about body weight. Becoming involved with coaches concerning food and body weight provides a way for the athlete to "manipulate" the coaching and training staff; it refocuses attention on concerns the athlete feels about food or body weight.
2. Stay free from guilt about the athlete's attitudes and behaviors toward food or body weight. Solving an eating disorder ultimately remains the athlete's responsibility; your role provides support to the athlete (and parent) and, if appropriate, encourages counseling. Coaches and trainers should not permit concerns about food and body size to go unnoticed—they must exercise professional judgment in offering advice about external counseling.
3. Coaches and trainers should *not* counsel athletes about eating disorders. Reserve that role for a psychologist, psychiatrist, or other trained specialist.
4. Do not focus extra attention on the athlete with an eating disorder. This exacerbates the condition and does little to resolve issues concerning food or body weight.
5. Be prepared to "ignore" the athlete in matters of food or body weight; do not become so involved that teammates notice that the athletes receives "extra" attention about an eating disorder.
6. Refrain from telling the athlete about "successful" athletes or friends who overcame an eating disorder. Do not ask questions such as: "How are you feeling?" "How is your weight today?" "Did you eat a good breakfast?" "Are you getting enough to eat?"
7. Trust the athlete to develop their own standards and values rather than insisting the athlete emulate yours.
8. Encourage the athlete to develop initiative, become self-sufficient, and make decisions. Give choices, but not solutions to problems. This encourages independence and autonomy.
9. Show extreme patience when dealing with athletes who exhibit symptoms of disordered eating. No quick cures or fixes exist, so do not expect them.
10. Never give up on an athlete who displays symptoms of disordered eating. Be firm but fair; be tolerant but decisive, and show respect, not contempt or disapproval.

THERAPEUTIC METHODS TO TREAT EATING DISORDERS

Various therapeutic methods treat eating disorders to give patients a sense of balance, purpose, and future. One approach, **cognitive-behavioral therapy**, particularly effective in treating bulimia nervosa, focuses on teaching the patient to identify, monitor, and modify dysfunctional attitudes, core beliefs, and eating habits to lessen binges and "retrain" normal hunger and satiety responses.[27,89,93] An important component of this therapeutic approach teaches persons to change misconceptions and reasoning errors and develop coping strategies to modify dysfunctional responses to stressful situations.

Interpersonal psychotherapy helps the patient and family examine interpersonal relationships to positively affect problem areas. The therapist emphasizes the importance of body fat for return of menses and normalization of reproductive functions. For younger patients, the therapist stresses the effects of low body weight on maturation, growth, and bone mass. Paradoxically, the therapist needs to recognize that a normalization of body fat may increase the patient's fat phobia, which initially led her to pursue extreme thinness.

Pharmacologic treatment (e.g., Prozac [fluoxetine] and other antidepressants) helps some persons. Trials of diverse classes of psychotropic medications to improve mood and augment weight gain in patients with anorexia nervosa have generally showed little effect.[2,61] Psychiatrists have recently prescribed two drugs, Zonegran (zonisamide) and Topamax (topiramate), approved to treat epilepsy and migraine headaches, for persons whose overeating meets the criteria for BED. These drugs require careful use but do help to reduce the frequency of binges for a subset of patients.[62] Widespread use of such pharmacologic treatment requires further research.

No one best treatment presently exists; combined multifaceted, multidisciplinary approaches using persons with expertise in areas of psychiatry, eating disorders, body image issues, medicine, and nutrition often work best. Improvement occurs slowly, with relapses and setbacks being common. Achieving success often remains difficult in three types of situations:

1. Persons with eating disorders of long duration
2. Patients who have previously failed treatment
3. Persons with a history of disturbed family relationships and poor individual adjustment

New Findings Link Brain Chemicals and Eating Disorders

Several new lines of research suggest disturbances in one or more brain chemical pathways relate to the pathogenesis and pathophysiology of anorexia nervosa and bulimia nervosa.[4,5,75] For example, amphetamine-induced dopamine release has been shown to increase anxiety in persons recovered from anorexia nervosa,[5] and the serotonin (5-HT) pathways is now known to contribute to the modulation of a range of behaviors common in persons with eating disorders.[4,75] New technology using brain imaging with radioligands (a radioactive biochemical used in the diagnosis or study of the receptor systems of the body) offers the potential for understanding this previously inaccessible brain 5-HT neurotransmitter function and its dynamic relationship to human behaviors.

Recent studies using 5-HT–specific radioligands have consistently shown 5-HT(1A) and 5-HT(2A) receptor and 5-HT transporter alterations within the cortical and limbic structures of anorexics and bulimics, which may relate to anxiety, behavioral inhibition, and body image distortions.[4,75] These disturbances are present when subjects are ill and persist after recovery, suggesting that these may be traits that are independent of the state of the illness. Clearly, a better understanding of neurobiology will likely yield possible chemical intervention therapies for persons with eating disorders.

Physical Activity May Prove Beneficial to Treat Bulimia Nervosa

Researchers evaluated 16 weeks of regular physical activity versus an equivalent time of nutritional counseling or cognitive-behavioral therapy in treating bulimia nervosa.[93] Normal-weight female patients with bulimia randomly received either treatment or control conditions; a second control group contained healthy women. Nutritional counseling educated patients about sound principles of nutrition, nutritional needs, and the relationship between dieting and overeating. Meal-planning techniques established and maintained regular eating patterns. Cognitive-behavioral therapy focused on enabling patients to (1) identify feelings and events related to bingeing episodes and how such episodes affected emotional status, (2) identify and modify core beliefs that influence bulimic behavior, (3) apply behavior modification techniques to combat bulimic behavior and develop more healthful strategies to deal with disturbing thoughts and emotions, and (4) develop general problem-solving skills.

Exercise consisted of a 1-h weekly group session of moderate physical activities to promote physical fitness, reduce feelings of fatness and bloating associated with eating, foster a more positive body image, and prevent bingeing and purging. These subjects were also urged to exercise at least 35 min twice a week on their own. **FIGURE 15.11** compares the different treatments with respect to the EDI subscales of "Body dissatisfaction," "Bulimia," and "Drive for thinness" before and

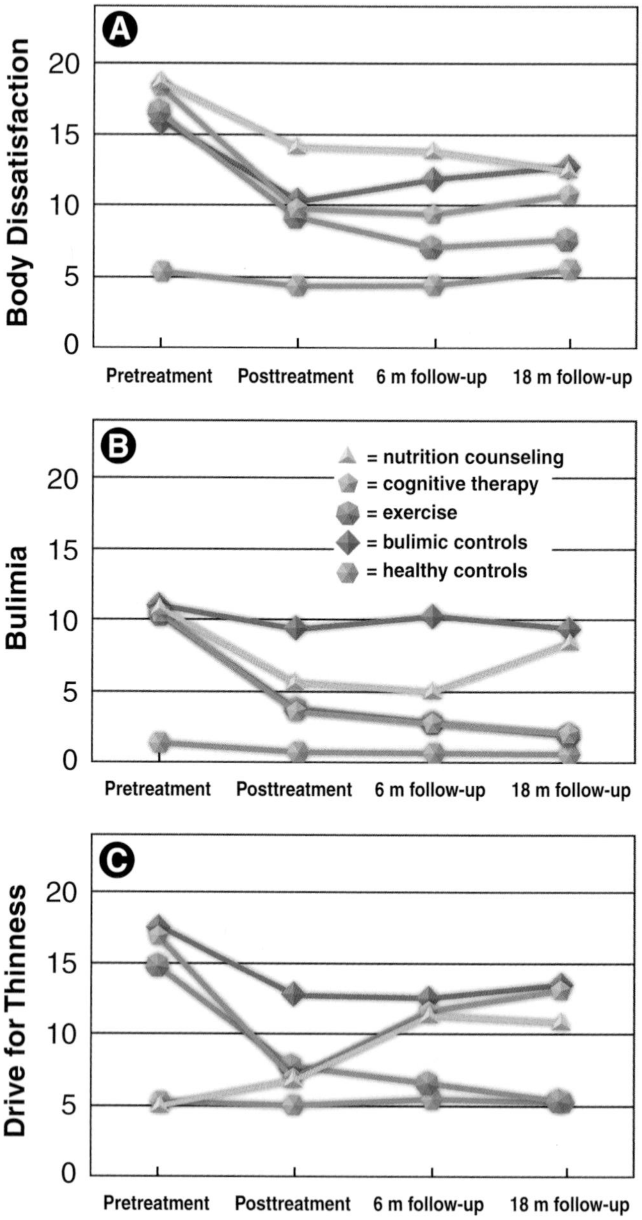

FIGURE 15.11. Exercise, cognitive therapy, and nutritional counseling in treating bulimia nervosa. **A.** Mean scores on the Eating Disorders Index "Body dissatisfaction" subscale at pretreatment, posttreatment, and 6- and 18-month follow-ups. **B.** Mean scores on the Eating Disorders Index "Bulimia" subscale. **C.** Mean scores on the Eating Disorders Index "Drive for thinness" subscale. From Sundgot-Borgen J, et al. The effect of exercise, cognitive therapy, and nutritional counseling in treating bulimia nervosa. *Med Sci Sports Exerc* 2002;34:190.

after treatment and at 6- and 18-month follow-ups. Nutritional counseling proved no more effective than cognitive-behavioral therapy. More striking was the superior effect of regular physical activity compared with cognitive-behavioral therapy in reducing the pursuit of thinness, feelings of body dissatisfaction, and frequency of bingeing, purging, and laxative abuse. The augmented self-regulation with physical activity may result from the effects of exercise on reducing bulimic patients' bodily tensions and improving their stress tolerance.

ATHLETICS MUST CHANGE FROM WITHIN

The following quote highlights the proactive role professionals in exercise nutrition, sports medicine, and athletics play in affecting the negative potential for certain sports to contribute to disordered eating among participants[33]:

"Finally, it is important to comment briefly on the need for reflection regarding the evolving aesthetic ideals for weight and shape in some sports. Particularly in those where the premium is placed on appearance and where adjudicators prevail (diving, figure skating, gymnastics and dance), questions should be raised from within the sports community regarding the potentially destructive standards for shape and weight. When these standards seriously compromise the health and well being of all but the small minority who are constitutionally gaunt, it is a matter for sincere concern for all of those involved with the sport."

FUTURE RESEARCH

Future research should include more focused and careful investigations with large representative samples, better measurement tools, and a longitudinal approach should provide a clearer understanding of the actual scope of disordered eating among athletes in general and specific athletic groups in particular (see the box in next column.[17]) Appropriate research design becomes crucial in determining whether a cause-and-effect relationship exists between athletic participation and disordered eating. Better profiling of men and women with the greatest likelihood of encountering problems requires knowledge of the following seven factors:

1. Role and interaction of sport-specific risk
2. Age risk
3. Gender risk
4. Training risk
5. Skill level and proficiency risk
6. Genetic risk
7. Psychosocial risk

Intensive education must focus on upgrading the knowledge of the coaching staff. These professionals need to maintain continual vigilance for signs and symptoms of eating disorders among their athletes.

TEN AREAS FOR FUTURE RESEARCH ABOUT EATING AND WEIGHT CONTROL BEHAVIORS IN ATHLETES

1. Carry out large-scale, epidemiologic studies using consistent measures to define the prevalence of eating disorders in various athletic populations.
2. Studies on prevalence should have the proper control groups. These should include athletes from sports with equivalent training but less emphasis on weight.
3. Examine both anorexia nervosa and bulimia nervosa, in addition to the range of behaviors and attitudes associated with eating disturbances.
4. Identify sports that bring the greatest risk for eating and weight problems.
5. Identify the psychological predisposing factors that place individual athletes at risk.
6. Identify the physiological factors that place an individual athlete at risk. Examples might be genetic predisposition to be heavy, low metabolic rate, and extreme energy efficiency.
7. Examine sex differences in the prevalence and development of eating disorders. This would involve studies of males and females in sports in which weight is emphasized (e.g., gymnastics, figure skating, and distance running).
8. Within sports, study athletes at varying levels of training and proficiency.
9. Study young athletes early in their training to identify early risk factors.
10. Validate self-report measures with athletes and identify the conditions under which self-reports of eating disturbances are most likely to be accurate.

From Brownell KD, Rodin J. Prevalence of eating disorders in athletes. In: Brownell KD, et al., eds. Eating, Body Weight and Performance in Athletes. Philadelphia: Lea & Febiger, 1992.

FIGURE 15.12 provides an overview of general and sport-specific factors that can lead to eating disorders in athletes. Parents, coaches, athletic trainers, and teammates should look for the seven "high-risk" factors. *We recommend that coaches tilt the balance between good health and athletic success in the direction of good health.*

Coaches should formulate prudent and realistic perceptions about what constitutes desirable (acceptable) body size and body shape. Advising an athlete without objective information about body composition (e.g., realistic target body fat levels, desirable FFM and lean/fat ratio, healthy BMI, and appropriate appraisals of body image and current eating behaviors) often provides the blueprint for disaster. In gymnastics and classical ballet, achieving extremes of thinness should not become a goal, even when considering the participant's health and safety. Of course, this approach requires rearrangement of priorities concerning aesthetic and performance parameters. The perpetual struggle to emulate an ideal that rewards thinness often forms the root cause of impending acute and chronic eating disorder medical problems.

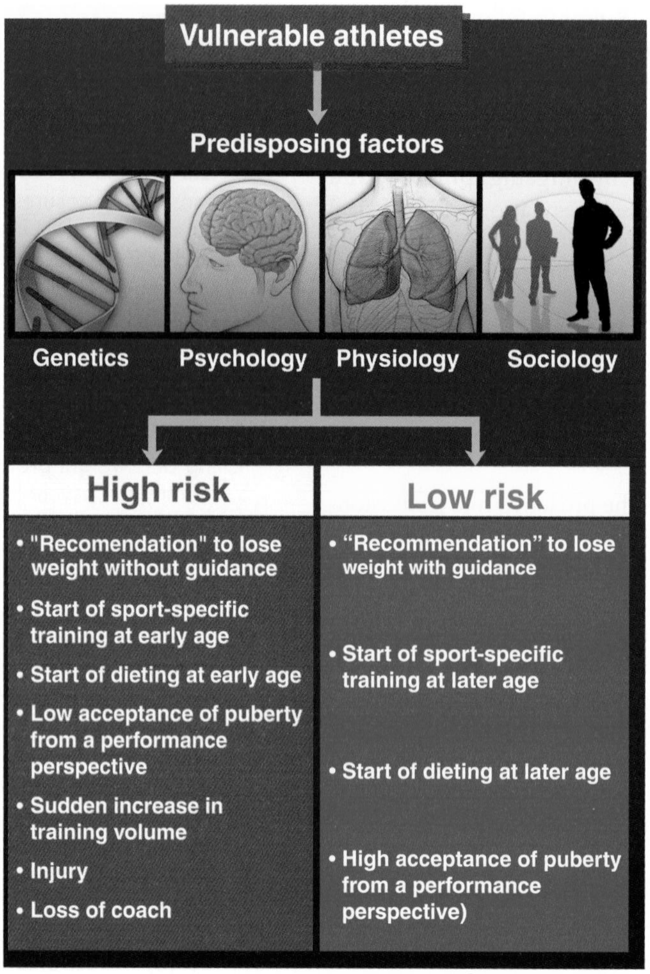

FIGURE 15.12. General and sport-specific factors that lead to eating disorders in athletes. (Modified from Sundgot-Borgen J. Eating disorders in female athletes. *Sports Med* 1994;17:176.)

SUMMARY

1. Eating disorders describe a broad spectrum of complex behaviors, core attitudes, coping strategies, and conditions that share the commonality of an emotionally based, inordinate, and pathologic focus on body shape and body weight. An estimated 8 million people in the United States exhibit eating disorders, with approximately 90% being women.
2. One in 200 American women suffers from anorexia, and two to three in 100 American women suffer from bulimia.
3. Miss America contestants exhibit an image of extreme thinness. Thirty percent of contestant winners fall below the World Health Organization's cutoff for undernutrition (BMI <18.5). Raising the BMI cutoff to 19.0 adds another 18 women or a total of 48% of the winners with undesirable values. Approximately 24% of contest winners' BMIs ranged between 20.0 and 21.0, and no winner after 1924 had a BMI that equaled the BMI of the reference woman.
4. Athletes face a unique set of circumstances that makes them vulnerable to eating disorders. These behaviors flourish when the strong negative aesthetic connotations associated with excess body fat blend with the athlete's belief that any body fat spells doom for success.
5. Estimates of the prevalence of eating disorders range between 15 and 62% among female athletes, with the greatest prevalence among athletes in the aesthetic sports (ballet, bodybuilding, diving, figure skating, cheerleading, and gymnastics) where success often coincides with extreme leanness.
6. Anorexia athletica describes the continuum of subclinical eating behaviors of physically active persons who fail to meet the criteria for a true eating disorder but exhibit at least one unhealthy method of weight control.
7. Unhealthy weight control habits include fasting, vomiting, and use of diet pills, laxatives, or diuretics.
8. An overemphasis on "eating right" can cause persons to become obsessed with healthful foods and exhibit a

disordered eating behavior termed orthorexia nervosa. This condition begins with keen interest in healthy living and eating but develops into an eating disorder.

9. Approximately 50% of women with eating disorders compulsively overexercise. The term *exercise addict* describes someone who exercises excessively often doing "whatever it takes" to make additional time in the day to exercise more.
10. Many men project the ideal male body as having about 28 lb more muscle than their own. This mismatch in perception has coincided with an increase in the number of men using anabolic steroids, experiencing eating disorders, and suffering from body obsession.
11. Body obsession encompasses a broad range of body image concerns, but an important component relates to muscle dysmorphia or a pathologic preoccupation with muscularity.
12. Anorexia nervosa, present in about 1 to 2% of the general population, is characterized by a crippling obsession with body size, a preoccupation with dieting and thinness, and a refusal to eat enough food to maintain a minimally normal body weight.
13. For anorectics, body weight decreases significantly below normal for age and stature, often leading to death.
14. Frequent episodes of binge eating followed by purging and intense feelings of guilt or shame characterize bulimia nervosa. Approximately 2 to 4% of all adolescents and adults in the general population suffer from bulimia nervosa.
15. Binge-eating disorder frequently occurs among obese patients who undergo treatment for weight loss.
16. Disordered eating behaviors—semistarvation, purging, excessive exercising—are used to achieve a body weight for success in certain "aesthetic" sports.
17. Eating disorders may be prevented among high-risk persons with an Internet-based intervention program that includes continuous monitoring and feedback.
18. Four steps constitute an intervention strategy for disordered eating behaviors in athletes: (1) identify and isolate the contributing factors, (2) formulate appropriate goals for intervention and prevention, (3) formulate long-term strategies to deal with the problem, and (4) initiate a long-term program to address the situation.
19. Cognitive-behavioral therapy, interpersonal psychotherapy, and pharmacologic treatment currently are used to treat eating disorders to give patients a sense of balance, purpose, and future. No one best treatment exists; combined approaches using persons with expertise in psychiatry, eating disorders, body image issues, medicine, and nutrition often work best.
20. New research on relationships between certain brain chemical pathways and eating disorders point to serotonin and its precursor 5-HT as possible links to the pathogenesis and pathophysiology of anorexia nervosa and bulimia nervosa.

thePoint *Visit* **thePoint.lww.com/MKKSEN4e** *to view the following animation related to content presented in Chapter 15:* ***Hormonal control.***

TEST YOUR KNOWLEDGE ANSWERS

1. **False:** In point of fact, Miss America contestants may represent an undernourished role model. The BMI of Miss America contestants generally falls below 18.5, a cutoff below the WHO standard that characterizes relative undernutrition.

2. **False:** Clinical observations indicate a prevalence of between 15 and 60% for disordered eating among athletes, with some groups at higher risk than others. More specifically, disordered eating patterns and unrealistic weight goals (and general dissatisfaction with one's body) occur most frequently among female athletes in the aesthetic sports such as ballet, body building, diving, figure skating, cheerleading, and gymnastics, in which success often coincides with extreme leanness. An inordinate preoccupation with eating also occurs among adolescent female swimmers. Controversy exists as to the prevalence of eating disorders among endurance runners.

3. **True:** The term *anorexia athletica* describes the continuum of subclinical eating behaviors of physically active persons who fail to meet the criteria for a true eating disorder, but who exhibit at least one unhealthy weight control method. This includes fasting, vomiting (termed "instrumental vomiting" when used to make weight), and use of diet pills, laxatives, or diuretics (water pills).

4. **False:** Most persons consider eating disorders a "female problem," yet an increasing number of men share this affliction. An unanswered question concerns whether this increased number results from an increase in disease incidence or because more men seek treatment. In one New York hospital treatment center, the percentage of male patients admitted with eating disorders rose steadily from 4% in 1988 to 13% in 1995. Men currently represent about 6 to 10% of persons with eating disorders, with the greatest prevalence among models, dancers, men abused during childhood, and gays.

5. **False:** Anorexia nervosa, particularly common and increasing in prevalence among adolescent girls and young women, is characterized by distortions of body image, a crippling obsession with body size, a preoccupation with dieting and thinness, and a refusal to eat enough food to maintain a minimally normal body weight. A relentless pursuit of thinness culminates in severe undernutrition, altered body composition characterized by depletion of fat and fat-free body mass, and cessation of menstruation (amenorrhea) in females. Body weight decreases below normal for age and stature.

6. **False:** Weight gain becomes a primary goal in the treatment of anorexia nervosa.

7. **False:** Bulimia nervosa, far more common than anorexia nervosa, is characterized by frequent episodes of bingeing on calorically dense food (often at night and usually between 1000 and 10,000 calories), followed within several hours by purging, laxative abuse, fasting, or extreme exercise. Intense feelings of guilt or shame accompany these behaviors.

8. **False:** The main components in treating eating disorders include education (providing information concerning the eating disorder and its consequences), self-monitoring (providing a clear understanding of current eating behaviors and patterns), and meal planning (helping to gain control of eating patterns and establish a healthful pattern of eating).

9. **True:** Exercise has proven useful to treat bulimia nervosa. Regular physical activity reduces the pursuit of thinness, feelings of body dissatisfaction, and the frequency of bingeing, purging, and laxative abuse. The augmented self-regulation may result from the effects of exercise to reduce bulimic patients' bodily tensions and improve stress tolerance.

10. **False:** Muscle dysmorphia, or the "Adonis complex," encompasses the pathologic preoccupation with muscle size and overall muscularity. These persons view themselves as small and frail when in reality many are large and muscular. In many ways, muscle dysmorphia and anorexia nervosa share common traits; these include a history of depression and anxiety, a hyperculturalization of body image, unrealistic shame about one's body, and self-destructive behaviors.

Key References

Anderluh MB, et al. Childhood obsessive-compulsive personality traits in adult women with eating disorders: defining a broader eating disorder phenotype. *Am J Psychiatry* 2003;160:242.

Bachner-Melman R, et al. How anorexic-like are the symptom and personality profiles of aesthetic athletes? *Med Sci Sports Exerc* 2006;38:628.

Bailer UF, Kaye WH. Serotonin: imaging findings in eating disorders. *Curr Top Behav Neurosci* 2011;6:59.

Bailer UF, et al. Amphetamine induced dopamine release increases anxiety in individuals recovered from anorexia nervosa. *Int J Eat Disord 2012; 45:263.*

Baum A. Eating disorders in the male athlete. *Sports Med* 2006;36:1.

Beals KA. *Disordered Eating Among Athletes: A Comprehensive Guide for Health Professionals.* Champaign, IL: Human Kinetics, 2004.

Beals KA, Hill AK. The prevalence of disordered eating, menstrual dysfunction, and low bone mineral density among US collegiate athletes. *Int J Sport Nutr Exerc Metab* 2006;16:1.

Brownell KD, Rodin J. Prevalence of eating disorders in athletes. In: Brownell KD, et al., eds. *Eating, Body Weight and Performance in Athletes.* Philadelphia: Lea & Febiger, 1992.

Bruch H. *Golden Cage: The Enigma of Anorexia Nervosa.* New York: Pocket Star, 1979.

Cobb KL, et al. Disordered eating, menstrual irregularity, and bone mineral density in female runners. *Med Sci Sports Exerc* 2003;35:711.

Friederich HC, et al. Treatment outcome in people with subthreshold compared with full-syndrome binge eating disorder. *Obesity* 2007;15:283.

Grucza RA, et al. Prevalence and correlates of binge eating disorder in a community sample. *Compr Psychiatry* 2007;48:124.

Hill AJ. Obesity and eating disorders. *Obes Rev* 2007;8(Suppl 1):151.

Hrabosky JI, et al. Overvaluation of shape and weight in binge eating disorder. *J Consult Clin Psychol* 2007;75:175.

Kerrvish KP, et al. Body composition in adolescents with anorexia nervosa. *Am J Clin Nutr* 2002;75:31.

Morton R. Origins of anorexia nervosa. *Eur Neurol* 2004;52:191.

Nichols JF, et al. Prevalence of the female athlete triad syndrome among high school athletes. *Arch Pediatr Adolesc Med* 2006;160:137.

Pernick Y, et al. Disordered eating among a multi-racial/ethnic sample of female high-school athletes. *J Adolesc Health* 2006;38:689.

Pichika R, et al. Serotonin transporter binding after recovery from bulimia nervosa. *Int J Eat Disord* 2011 Jun 13 (Epub ahead of print).

Probst M, et al. Body composition of anorexia nervosa patients assessed by underwater weighing and skinfold-thickness measurements before and after weight gain. *Am J Clin Nutr* 2001;73:190.

Striegel-Moore RH. Risk factors for eating disorders. *Ann NY Acad Sci* 1997;817:98.

Sundgot-Borgen J. Risk and trigger factors for the development of eating disorders in female elite athletes. *Med Sci Sports Exerc* 1994;26:414.

Sundgot-Borgen J, Torstveit MK. Prevalence of eating disorders in elite athletes is higher than in the general population. *Clin J Sport Med* 2004;14:25.

Sundgot-Borgen J, et al. The effect of exercise, cognitive therapy, and nutritional counseling in treating bulimia nervosa. *Med Sci Sport Exerc* 2002;34:190.

Taylor CB, et al. Prevention of eating disorders in at-risk college-age women. *Arch Gen Psychiatry* 2006;63:881.

thePoint *Visit* **thePoint.lww.com/MKKSEN4e** *for a list of the references cited in this chapter, including additional, relevant references.*

Appendix A Nutritive Values for Common Foods, Alcoholic and Nonalcoholic Beverages, and Specialty and Fast-Food Items[a]

This appendix has three parts. Part 1 lists nutritive values for common foods, Part 2 lists nutritive values for alcoholic and nonalcoholic beverages, and Part 3 presents nutritive values for specialty and fast-food items. The nutritive values of foods and alcoholic and nonalcoholic beverages, expressed in 1-ounce (28.4 g) portions, allow comparisons among different food categories. Thus, for example, the protein content of 1.55 g for 1 ounce of banana nut bread can be compared directly to the protein content of 6.28 g for 1 ounce of processed American cheese.

PART 1

Nutritive Values for Common Foods

The foods are grouped into categories and are listed in alphabetical order within each category. The categories include breads, cakes and pies, cookies, candy bars, chocolate, desserts, cereals, cheese, fish, fruits, meats, eggs, dairy products, vegetables, and typical salad bar entries. An additional section labeled Variety consists of food items such as soups, sandwiches, salad dressings, oils, some condiments, and other "goodies." The nutritive value for each food is expressed per ounce or 28.4 g of that food item. The specific values for each food include the caloric content (kcal) for 1 ounce, protein, total lipid, carbohydrate, calcium, iron, vitamin B_1, vitamin B_2, fiber content, and cholesterol.

[a] The information about the nutritive value of the foods comes from a variety of sources. This includes primarily data from Watt, BK, Merrill, AL. *Composition of Foods—Raw, Processed and Prepared*, Washington, DC: U.S. Department of Agriculture, 1963; Adams C, and Richardson, M. *Nutritive Value of Foods.* Washington, DC: Government Printing Office, 1981; Pennington JAT, and Douglass JP. Bowes & Church's Food Values of Portions Commonly Used. 18th ed. Baltimore: Lippincott Williams & Wilkins, 2005. Other sources include a comprehensive database maintained by the University of Massachusetts, the consumer relations departments of manufacturers, and journal articles that evaluated specific foods items. NA indicates data not available.

BREADS

	kcal	Protein (g)	Lipid (g)	CHO (g)	Ca (mg)	Fe (mg)	B_1 (mg)	B_2 (mg)	Fiber (g)	Cholesterol (mg)
Banana nut	91	1.55	4.00	12.7	10.0	0.470	0.054	0.046	0.66	18.3
Boston brown—canned	60	1.26	0.39	13.2	25.8	0.567	0.038	0.025	1.34	1.9
Cornmeal muffin—recipe	91	1.89	3.15	13.2	41.6	0.567	0.069	0.069	1.00	14.5
Croutons—dry	105	3.69	1.04	20.5	35.0	1.020	0.099	0.099	0.09	0
Cracked wheat	74	2.63	0.99	14.2	18.1	0.755	0.108	0.108	1.50	0
Cracked wheat—toast	88	3.00	1.17	16.9	21.6	0.899	0.100	0.128	1.82	0
French—chunk	81	2.67	1.10	14.3	31.6	0.875	0.130	0.097	0.57	0
Italian	78	2.55	0.25	16.0	4.7	0.756	0.116	0.066	0.47	0
Mixed grain	74	2.27	1.05	13.6	30.6	0.907	0.113	0.113	1.78	0
Mixed grain—toast	80	2.47	1.15	14.8	33.3	0.986	0.099	0.123	1.97	0
Oatmeal	74	2.37	1.25	13.6	17.0	0.794	0.130	0.075	1.10	0
Oatmeal—toast	80	2.47	1.36	14.8	18.5	0.863	0.110	0.081	1.20	0
Pita pocket	78	2.94	0.42	15.6	23.2	0.685	0.129	0.061	0.45	0
Pumpernickel	71	2.60	0.98	13.6	20.4	0.777	0.097	0.147	1.67	0
Pumpernickel—toast	78	2.86	1.08	15.0	22.5	0.857	0.088	0.162	1.87	0
Raisin—	77	2.15	1.12	15.0	28.4	0.879	0.093	0.176	0.68	0
Raisin—toasted	92	2.57	1.34	17.6	33.8	1.080	0.081	0.209	0.81	0
Rye—light	74	2.40	1.04	13.6	22.7	0.771	0.116	0.090	1.87	0
Rye—light—toast	84	2.73	1.18	15.5	25.8	0.876	0.107	0.103	2.15	0
Vienna	79	2.72	1.10	14.4	31.2	0.873	0.130	0.100	0.91	0
White	76	2.35	1.10	13.8	35.7	0.806	0.133	0.088	0.54	0
White—toast	84	2.67	1.26	15.7	40.6	0.915	0.121	0.103	0.64	0
Whole wheat	69	2.84	1.22	12.9	20.2	0.964	0.100	0.059	2.10	0

(continued)

BREADS (continued)

	kcal	Protein (g)	Lipid (g)	CHO (g)	Ca (mg)	Fe (mg)	B_1 (mg)	B_2 (mg)	Fiber (g)	Cholesterol (mg)
Whole wheat—toasted	79	3.42	1.47	14.4	22.5	1.090	0.090	0.066	2.74	0
Bread crumbs—dry grated	111	3.69	1.42	20.7	34.6	1.160	0.099	0.099	1.15	1.4
Bread crumbs—soft	76	2.35	1.10	13.9	35.9	0.806	0.134	0.088	0.54	0
Bread sticks wo/salt	109	3.40	0.82	21.3	7.9	0.255	0.017	0.020	0.43	0
Bread sticks w/salt	86	2.67	0.89	16.4	13.0	0.243	0.016	0.024	0.41	0

CAKES AND PIES

	kcal	Protein (g)	Lipid (g)	CHO (g)	Ca (mg)	Fe (mg)	B_1 (mg)	B_2 (mg)	Fiber (g)	Cholesterol (mg)
Cakes										
Angel food cake	67	1.71	0.09	15.2	23.5	0.123	0.014	0.057	0	0
Boston cream pie	61	0.59	1.89	10.4	6.1	0.142	0.002	0.043	0	4.7
Carrot cake	103	1.05	5.32	13.2	6.9	0.304	0.030	0.035	0	14.6
Cheesecake	86	1.54	5.45	8.1	15.9	0.136	0.009	0.037	0	52.4
Choc cupcake/choc frosting	97	1.24	3.29	16.5	16.9	0.575	0.029	0.041	0	15.2
Coffee cake	91	1.78	2.70	14.8	17.3	0.480	0.054	0.059	0	18.5
Dark fruitcake	109	1.32	4.62	16.5	27.0	0.791	0.053	0.053	0	13.2
Gingerbread cake	91	1.15	2.86	15.2	12.2	0.706	0.042	0.038	0	7.8
Pound cake	113	1.89	4.72	14.2	18.9	0.472	0.047	0.057	0	30.2
Sheet cake—plain	104	1.32	3.96	15.8	18.1	0.429	0.046	0.049	0	20.1
Sheet cake—white frosting	104	0.94	3.28	18.0	14.3	0.281	0.030	0.037	0	16.4
Sponge cake	83	2.01	1.27	16.0	10.8	0.524	0.043	0.046	0	58.8
White cake/coconut	109	1.30	4.05	17.0	13.7	0.454	0.041	0.053	0	1.2
White cake/white frosting	104	1.20	3.59	16.8	13.2	0.399	0.080	0.052	0	1.2
Yellow cake/chocolate frosting	101	1.03	4.48	15.9	9.5	0.509	0.020	0.058	0	15.6
Pies										
Apple pie	73	0.66	3.14	10.7	5.0	0.300	0.031	0.023	0	0
Apple pie—fried	85	0.73	4.67	10.7	4.0	0.312	0.030	0.020	0	4.7
Banana cream pie	46	0.90	1.85	6.7	21.0	0.156	0.022	0.042	0	2.2
Blueberry pie	68	0.72	3.05	9.9	4.7	0.377	0.031	0.025	0	0
Boston cream pie	61	0.59	1.89	10.4	6.1	0.142	0.002	0.043	0	4.7
Cherry pie	74	0.77	3.19	10.9	6.6	0.569	0.034	0.025	0	0
Cherry pie—fried	83	0.68	4.74	10.7	3.7	0.233	0.020	0.020	0	4.3
Chocolate cream pie	50	1.20	2.04	6.9	25.9	0.175	0.024	0.049	0	2.4
Coconut cream pie	57	1.03	2.79	7.2	24.0	0.198	0.021	0.042	0	2.5
Coconut custard pie	66	1.69	3.85	6.3	25.0	0.304	0.029	0.055	0	31.4
Cream pie	85	0.56	4.29	11.0	8.6	0.205	0.011	0.028	0	1.5
Custard pie	55	1.43	2.65	6.3	23.1	0.269	0.026	0.050	0	27.6
Lemon meringue pie	72	0.95	2.90	10.7	5.1	0.283	0.020	0.028	0	27.7
Mincemeat pie	70	0.65	2.13	12.8	6.9	0.360	0.028	0.024	0	0
Peach pie	73	0.63	3.14	10.9	4.8	0.340	0.031	0.028	0	0
Pecan pie	120	1.30	4.87	18.9	7.2	0.380	0.045	0.034	0	28.1
Pumpkin pie	52	1.28	2.23	7.3	30.0	0.373	0.019	0.042	0	15.5
Strawberry chiffon pie	65	0.85	3.46	8.0	7.7	0.254	0.022	0.023	0	7.1

(continued)

COOKIES

	kcal	Protein (g)	Lipid (g)	CHO (g)	Ca (mg)	Fe (mg)	B_2 (mg)	B_2 (mg)	Fiber (g)	Cholesterol (mg)
Animal cookies	120	1.90	2.89	22.0	3.0	0.918	0.080	0.130	0	0.1
Brownies w/nuts	135	1.84	8.93	15.6	12.8	0.567	0.070	0.070	0	25.5
Butter cookies	130	1.76	4.82	20.2	36.3	0.170	0.011	0.017	0	4.1
Fig bars	106	1.02	1.93	21.4	20.2	0.689	0.039	0.037	0	13.7
Lady fingers	102	2.19	2.19	18.3	11.6	0.515	0.019	0.039	0	101.0
Oatmeal raisin cookies	134	1.64	5.45	19.6	9.8	0.600	0.049	0.044	0	1.1
Peanut butter cookies	145	2.36	8.27	16.5	12.4	0.650	0.041	0.041	0	13.0
Sandwich type cookies	138	1.42	5.67	20.6	8.5	0.992	0.064	0.050	0	0
Shortbread cookies	137	1.77	7.09	17.7	11.5	0.709	0.089	0.080	0	23.9
Sugar cookies	139	1.18	7.09	18.3	29.5	0.532	0.053	0.035	0	17.1
Vanilla wafers	131	1.42	4.96	20.6	11.3	0.567	0.050	0.070	0	17.7

CANDY BARS

	kcal	Protein (g)	Lipid (g)	CHO (g)	Ca (mg)	Fe (mg)	B_1 (mg)	B_2 (mg)	Fiber (g)	Cholesterol (mg)
Almond Joy	151	1.69	7.82	18.5	2.0	0.778	0	0	0	0
Sugar-coated almonds	146	3.10	9.12	14.6	39.6	0.775	0.042	0.156	0	0
Bittersweet chocolate	141	1.90	9.73	15.7	13.0	1.040	0.015	0.050	0	0
Caramel—plain or chocolate	115	1.00	2.99	22.0	41.9	0.399	0.010	0.050	0	1.0
Chocolate candy kisses	154	2.10	8.98	15.9	52.9	0.499	0.020	0.080	0	0
Chocolate-coated almonds	161	3.92	12.70	8.0	47.8	1.090	0.052	0.186	0	0
Chocolate-covered coconut	133	0.91	7.10	17.5	8.4	0.614	0.008	0.016	0	0
Chocolate-covered mints	116	0.50	2.99	23.0	16.0	0.299	0.010	0.020	0	0
Chocolate-covered peanuts	159	5.00	11.70	9.8	32.9	0.689	0.086	0.043	0	0
Chocolate-covered raisins	111	1.06	2.71	20.6	12.2	0.663	0.034	0.025	0	0
Chocolate fudge	115	0.56	2.78	21.0	22.0	0.299	0.010	0.030	0	1.0
Chocolate fudge with nuts	114	1.06	4.99	18.8	22.0	0.299	0.016	0.030	0	7.4
English toffee	195	0.89	16.90	9.8	0	0.177	0.470	0.044	0	0
Gum drops	98	0	0.20	24.8	2.0	0.100	0	0	0	0
Hard candy	109	0	0	27.6	6.0	0.100	0	0	0	0
Jelly beans	104	0	0.10	26.4	1.0	0.299	0	0	0	0
Kit Kat	138	1.98	7.25	16.5	42.9	0.369	0.020	0.073	0	0
Krackle	149	2.00	8.09	16.9	50.0	0.400	0.017	0.075	0	0
Malted milk balls	135	2.30	6.99	17.8	62.9	0	0	0	0	0
M&M's plain chocolate	140	1.95	6.08	19.5	46.7	0.449	0.015	0.073	0	0
M&Ms peanut chocolate	144	3.23	7.25	16.5	35.4	0.402	0.016	0.056	0	0
Mars bar	136	2.27	6.24	17.0	48.2	0.312	0.014	0.093	0	0
Milk chocolate—plain	145	2.00	8.98	16.0	49.9	0.399	0.020	0.100	0	6.0
Milk chocolate w/almonds	150	2.90	10.40	15.0	60.9	0.559	0.030	0.130	0	4.5
Milk chocolate w/peanuts	155	4.89	11.70	10.0	31.9	0.679	0.112	0.065	0	3.0
Milk chocolate + rice cereal	140	2.00	6.99	18.0	47.9	0.200	0.010	0.080	0	6.0
Milky Way	123	1.53	4.25	20.3	40.6	0.232	0.013	0.070	0	6.6
Mr. Goodbar	151	3.62	9.05	13.9	39.2	0.567	0.030	0.072	0	4.2
Reese's peanut butter cup	151	3.65	9.07	13.9	21.7	0.430	0.020	0.032	0	1.6
Snickers	134	3.08	6.62	17.0	32.4	0.227	0.013	0.050	0	0
Vanilla fudge	118	0.70	3.15	22.0	29.9	0.030	0.006	0.025	0	10.0
Vanilla fudge with nuts	122	1.00	5.01	18.3	25.0	0.159	0.017	0.026	0	8.5

CHOCOLATE

	kcal	Protein (g)	Lipid (g)	CHO (g)	Ca (mg)	Fe (mg)	B_1 (mg)	B_2 (mg)	Fiber (g)	Cholesterol (mg)
Baking chocolate	145	3.49	15.00	7.5	22.0	1.900	0.015	0.099	0	0
Bittersweet chocolate	141	1.90	9.73	15.7	13.0	1.040	0.015	0.050	0	0
Milk chocolate—plain	145	2.00	8.98	16.0	49.9	0.399	0.020	0.100	0	6.0
Semi-sweet chocolate chips	143	1.17	10.20	16.2	8.5	0.967	0.017	0.023	0	0
Dark chocolate—sweet	150	1.00	9.98	16.0	7.0	0.599	0.010	0.040	0	0
Chocolate cupcake/ chocolate frosting	97	1.24	3.29	16.5	16.9	0.575	0.029	0.041	0	15.2
Chocolate candy kisses	154	2.10	8.98	15.9	52.9	0.499	0.020	0.080	0	0
Chocolate chip cookies	122	1.54	5.94	18.9	11.0	0.540	0.068	0.155	0	3.4
Chocolate coated almonds	161	3.92	12.70	8.0	47.8	1.090	0.052	0.186	0	0
Chocolate coated peanuts	159	5.00	11.70	9.8	32.9	0.689	0.086	0.043	0	0
Chocolate covered mints	116	0.50	2.99	23.0	16.0	0.299	0.010	0.020	0	0
Chocolate covered raisins	111	1.06	2.71	20.6	12.2	0.663	0.034	0.025	0	0
Chocolate cream pie	50	1.20	2.04	6.9	25.9	0.175	0.024	0.049	0	2.4
Chocolate fudge	115	0.56	2.78	21.0	22.0	0.299	0.010	0.030	0	1.0
Chocolate fudge with nuts	114	1.06	4.99	18.8	22.0	0.299	0.016	0.030	0	7.4
Cake flour-baked value	103	2.08	0.28	22.4	4.5	1.250	0.154	0.096	0	0
Reese's peanut butter cup	151	3.65	9.07	13.9	21.7	0.430	0.020	0.032	0	1.6
Chocolate pudding/recipe	42	0.88	1.25	7.3	27.3	0.142	0.005	0.039	0	4.3
Chocolate pudding instant	34	0.85	0.818	5.9	28.4	0.065	0.009	0.039	0	3.1

DESSERTS AND BREAKFAST PASTRIES

	kcal	Protein (g)	Lipid (g)	CHO (g)	Ca (mg)	Fe (mg)	B_1 (mg)	B_2 (mg)	Fiber (g)	Cholesterol (mg)
Apple brown betty	43	0.30	1.60	7.40	5.4	0.130	0.016	0.012	0	3.8
Apple cobbler	55	0.53	1.74	9.57	8.8	0.206	0.023	0.019	0	0.3
Apple crisp	53	0.33	1.93	9.09	7.4	0.278	0.018	0.013	0	0
Apple dumpling	55	0.32	2.37	8.64	7.1	0.253	0.012	0.013	0	0
Banana nut bread	91	1.60	4.00	12.70	10.0	0.470	0.054	0.046	0	18.3
Bread + raisin pudding	60	1.20	2.47	8.54	27.7	0.304	0.030	0.048	0	24.4
Cheesecake	86	1.50	5.45	8.10	15.9	0.136	0.009	0.037	0	52.4
Cherry cobbler	44	0.53	1.37	7.52	8.5	0.391	0.019	0.021	0	0.3
Cherry & cream cheese torte	79	1.28	3.96	10.00	28.5	0.266	0.015	0.052	0	11.2
Vanilla milkshake	32	0.98	0.841	5.09	34.5	0.026	0.013	0.052	0	3.2
Cream puff w/custard fill	72	1.24	4.54	6.83	16.4	0.276	0.015	0.040	0	58.8
Chocolate eclair w/custard fill	79	1.20	4.43	8.96	18.6	0.258	0.019	0.041	0	50.4
Gelatin salad	17	0.43	0	3.99	0.5	0.024	0.002	0.002	0	0
Peach cobbler	28	0.50	1.35	7.96	7.6	0.197	0.018	0.017	0	0.3
Peach crisp	34	0.31	1.06	6.18	4.8	0.203	0.010	0.010	0	0
Crepe, unfilled	49	2.06	1.32	7.07	25.0	0.475	0.045	0.070	0.21	43.0
Pancakes—plain	63	2.10	2.10	9.45	28.4	0.525	0.063	0.074	0.42	16.8
Croissant	117	2.32	6.02	13.40	10.0	1.040	0.085	0.065	0.54	6.5
Danish pastry—plain	109	1.99	5.97	12.90	29.8	0.547	0.080	0.085	0	24.4
Danish pastry w/fruit	102	1.74	5.67	12.20	7.41	0.567	0.070	0.061	0	24.4
Doughnut—cake type	119	1.33	6.75	13.90	13.0	0.454	0.068	0.068	0	11.3
Doughnut—jelly filled	99	1.48	3.84	13.00	12.2	0.349	0.052	0.044	0	0
Doughnut—yeast-raised	111	1.89	6.28	12.30	8.0	0.661	0.132	0.057	0	9.9

(continued)

DESSERTS AND BREAKFAST PASTRIES (continued)

	kcal	Protein (g)	Lipid (g)	CHO (g)	Ca (mg)	Fe (mg)	B_1 (mg)	B_2 (mg)	Fiber (g)	Cholesterol (mg)
Chocolate pudding	42	0.88	1.25	7.28	27.3	0.142	0.005	0.039	0	4.3
Tapioca pudding	38	1.43	1.44	4.85	29.7	0.120	0.012	0.052	0	27.3
Vanilla pudding	32	0.99	1.10	4.50	33.1	0.089	0.009	0.046	0	4.1
Chocolate pudding—instant	34	0.85	0.82	5.89	28.4	0.065	0.009	0.039	0	3.1
Rice pudding	33	0.86	0.86	5.80	28.6	0.107	0.021	0.039	0	3.2
Butterscotch pudding pop	47	1.19	1.29	7.80	37.8	0.020	0.015	0.055	0	0.5
Chocholate pudding pop	49	1.34	1.34	8.20	42.8	0.179	0.015	0.055	0	0.5
Vanilla pudding pop	46	1.19	1.29	7.80	37.8	0.020	0.015	0.055	0	0.5

CEREALS (WITHOUT MILK)

	kcal	Protein (g)	Lipid (g)	CHO (g)	Ca (mg)	Fe (mg)	B_1 (mg)	B_2 (mg)	Fiber (g)	Cholesterol (mg)
All-Bran	70	3.99	0.50	21.0	23.00	4.49	0.369	0.429	8.490	0
Alpha Bits	111	2.20	0.60	24.6	7.99	1.80	0.399	0.399	0.650	0
Apple Jacks	110	1.50	0.10	25.7	2.99	4.49	0.399	0.399	0.200	0
Bran Buds	73	3.95	0.68	21.6	18.90	4.52	0.371	0.439	7.860	0
Bran Chex	90	2.95	0.81	22.6	16.80	4.51	0.347	0.150	5.200	0
Buc Wheats	110	2.00	1.00	24.0	59.90	8.09	0.674	0.764	2.000	0
C.W. Post—plain	126	2.54	4.44	20.3	13.70	4.50	0.380	0.438	0.643	0
C.W. Post w/raisins	123	2.45	4.05	20.3	14.00	4.51	0.358	0.413	0.660	0
Cap'n Crunch	120	1.46	2.60	22.9	4.60	7.53	0.506	0.544	0.709	0
Cap'n Crunchberries	118	1.46	2.35	23.0	8.91	7.32	0.478	0.543	0.324	0
Cap'n Crunch—peanut butter	125	2.03	3.64	21.5	5.67	7.37	0.486	0.567	0.324	0
Cheerios	110	4.24	1.77	19.4	47.30	4.44	0.394	0.394	3.000	0
Cocoa Krispies	109	1.50	0.39	25.2	4.73	1.81	0.394	0.394	0.354	0
Cocoa Pebbles	117	1.35	1.49	24.7	5.40	1.75	0.405	0.405	0.312	0
Corn Bran	98	1.97	1.02	23.9	32.30	9.60	0.299	0.551	5.390	0
Corn Chex	111	2.00	0.10	24.9	2.99	1.80	0.399	0.070	0.499	0
Corn flakes—Kellogg's	110	2.30	0.09	24.4	1.00	1.80	0.367	0.424	0.594	0
Corn flakes—Post Toasties	110	2.30	0.09	24.4	1.00	0.70	0.367	0.424	0.594	0
Corn grits—enriched yellow dry	105	2.49	0.33	22.5	0.55	1.10	0.182	0.107	3.270	0
Corn grits—enriched ckd	17	0.41	0.06	3.7	0.12	0.18	0.028	0.018	0.527	0
Cracklin' Oat Bran	108	2.60	4.16	19.4	18.90	1.80	0.378	0.425	4.280	0
Cream of Rice	15	0.24	0.01	3.3	0.93	0.05	0.012	0	0.163	0
Cream of Wheat	16	0.42	0.07	3.4	6.27	1.27	0.028	0.008	0.395	0
Crispy Wheat 'n Raisins	99	2.00	0.46	23.1	46.80	4.48	0.396	0.396	1.320	0
Farina—cooked	14	0.41	0.02	3.0	0.49	0.14	0.023	0.015	0.389	0
Fortified Oat Flakes	105	5.32	0.41	20.5	40.20	8.09	0.354	0.413	0.827	0
40% Bran Flakes—Kellogg's	91	3.60	0.54	22.2	13.80	8.14	0.369	0.430	0.850	0
40% Bran Flakes—Post	92	3.20	0.45	22.3	12.70	4.50	0.374	0.435	3.800	0
Froot Loops	111	1.70	1.00	25.0	2.99	4.49	0.399	0.399	0.299	0
Frosted Mini-Wheats	102	2.93	0.27	23.4	9.15	1.83	0.366	0.457	2.160	0
Frosted Rice Krispies	109	1.30	0.10	25.7	1.00	1.80	0.399	0.399	0.998	0
Fruit & Fiber w/apples	90	2.99	1.00	22.0	9.98	4.49	0.374	0.424	4.190	0

(continued)

CEREALS (WITHOUT MILK) (continued)

	kcal	Protein (g)	Lipid (g)	CHO (g)	Ca (mg)	Fe (mg)	B_1 (mg)	B_2 (mg)	Fiber (g)	Cholesterol (mg)
Fruit & Fiber w/dates	90	2.99	1.00	21.0	9.98	4.49	0.374	0.424	4.190	0
Fruitful Bran	92	2.50	0	22.5	8.34	6.75	0.313	0.354	4.170	0
Fruity Pebbles	115	1.10	1.50	24.4	2.99	1.80	0.399	0.399	0.226	0
Golden Grahams	109	1.60	1.09	24.1	17.40	4.50	0.363	0.436	1.670	0
Granola—homemade	138	3.49	7.69	15.6	17.70	1.12	0.170	0.072	2.970	0
Granola—Nature Valley	126	2.89	4.92	18.9	17.80	0.95	0.098	0.048	2.960	0
Grape Nuts	100	3.28	0.11	23.2	10.90	1.22	0.398	0.398	1.840	0
Grape Nuts Flakes	102	2.99	0.30	23.2	11.00	4.49	0.399	0.399	1.900	0
Honey & Nut Corn Flakes	113	1.80	1.50	23.3	2.99	1.80	0.399	0.399	0.299	0
Honey Bran	96	2.51	0.57	23.2	13.00	4.54	0.405	0.405	3.160	0
Honey Comb	111	1.68	0.52	25.3	5.15	1.80	0.387	0.387	0.387	0
Honey Nut Cheerios	107	3.09	0.69	22.8	19.80	4.47	0.344	0.430	0.790	0
King Vitamin	115	1.49	1.62	24.0	NA	17.10	0.124	1.430	0.135	0
Kix	109	2.49	0.70	23.3	34.80	8.06	0.398	0.398	0.398	0
Life	104	5.22	0.52	20.3	99.20	7.47	0.612	0.644	0.902	0
Lucky Charms	111	2.57	1.06	23.1	31.90	4.52	0.354	0.443	0.624	0
Malt-O-Meal	14	0.43	0.03	3.1	0.59	1.13	0.057	0.028	0.354	0
Maypo—cooked	1	0.02	0.01	0.1	0.52	0.04	0.003	0.003	0.012	0
Nutri-Grain—barley	106	3.11	0.21	23.4	7.60	1.00	0.346	0.415	1.660	0
Nutri-Grain—corn	108	2.30	0.68	24.0	0.68	0.60	0.338	0.405	1.750	0
Nutri-Grain—rye	102	2.48	0.21	24.0	5.67	0.80	0.354	0.425	2.160	0
Nutri-Grain—wheat	102	2.45	0.32	24.0	7.73	0.80	0.387	0.451	1.800	0
Oatmeal—prepared	18	0.73	0.29	3.1	2.42	0.19	0.032	0.006	0.497	0
Rolled Oats	109	4.55	1.78	19.0	14.70	1.19	0.206	0.038	3.090	0
Instant Oatmeal w/apples	26	0.74	0.30	5.0	30.00	1.15	0.091	0.053	0.552	0
Instant Oatmeal w/bran & raisins	23	0.71	0.28	4.4	25.20	1.10	0.081	0.092	0.480	0
Instant Oatmeal w/maple	30	0.84	0.35	5.8	29.60	1.16	0.097	0.059	0.530	0
Instant Oatmeal w/cinnamon & spice	31	0.85	0.34	6.2	30.30	1.17	0.099	0.60	0.510	0
Instant Oatmeal w/raisins & spice	29	0.77	0.32	5.7	29.60	1.18	0.092	0.065	0.556	0
100% Bran	77	3.57	1.42	20.7	19.80	3.49	0.687	0.773	8.380	0
100% Natural	135	3.02	6.02	18.0	48.90	0.83	0.085	0.150	3.390	0
100% Natural—w/apples	130	2.92	5.32	19.0	42.80	0.79	0.090	0.158	1.300	0
100% Natural—w/raisins & dates	128	2.89	5.23	18.7	41.20	0.80	0.077	0.165	1.080	0
Product 19	108	2.75	0.17	23.5	3.44	18.00	1.460	1.720	0.369	0
Puffed Rice	111	1.79	0.20	25.5	2.03	0.30	0.030	0.028	0.227	0
Puffed Wheat	104	4.25	0.24	22.4	7.09	1.35	0.047	0.070	5.430	0
Quisp	117	1.42	2.08	23.6	8.50	5.96	0.510	0.718	0.378	0
Raisin Bran—Kellogg's	91	3.07	0.46	21.4	14.50	13.90	0.293	0.332	3.410	0
Raisin Bran—Post	86	2.68	0.55	21.4	13.70	4.56	0.373	0.430	3.190	0
Raisins, Rice & Rye	96	1.60	0.06	24.2	6.16	3.45	0.308	0.370	0.308	0
Ralston—cooked	15	0.62	0.09	3.2	1.57	0.18	0.022	0.020	0.370	0
Rice Chex	112	1.49	1.00	25.2	3.88	1.79	0.400	0.298	1.840	0
Rice Krispies	109	1.86	0.20	24.2	3.91	1.76	0.391	0.391	0.312	0
Roman Meal—dry	91	4.07	0.60	20.4	18.40	1.31	0.142	0.069	0.905	0
Roman Meal—cooked	17	0.77	0.11	3.9	3.45	0.25	0.028	0.014	0.877	0
Shredded Wheat	102	3.09	0.71	22.5	11.00	1.20	0.070	0.080	3.100	0
Shredded wheat	97	3.06	0.45	16.4	11.20	0.89	0.082	0.075	2.900	0
Special K	111	5.58	0.10	21.3	7.97	4.48	0.399	0.399	0.266	0
Sugar Corn Pops	108	1.40	0.10	25.6	0.10	1.80	0.399	0.399	0.100	0
Sugar Frosted Flakes	108	1.46	0.08	25.7	0.81	1.78	0.405	0.405	0.446	0

(continued)

CEREALS (WITHOUT MILK) (continued)

	kcal	Protein (g)	Lipid (g)	CHO (g)	Ca (mg)	Fe (mg)	B_1 (mg)	B_2 (mg)	Fiber (g)	Cholesterol (mg)
Sugar Smacks	106	2.00	0.50	24.7	2.99	1.80	0.369	0.429	0.319	0
Super Golden Crisp	106	1.80	0.26	25.6	6.01	1.80	0.344	0.430	0.430	0
Team	111	1.82	0.48	24.3	4.05	1.73	0.371	0.425	0.270	0
Total	105	2.84	0.60	22.3	172.00	18.00	1.460	1.720	2.060	0
Trix	108	1.50	0.40	24.9	5.99	4.49	0.399	0.399	0.184	0
Wheat & Raisin Chex	97	2.68	0.21	22.6	NA	4.04	0.263	0.315	1.890	0
Wheat Chex	104	2.77	0.68	23.3	11.00	4.50	0.370	0.105	2.100	0
Wheat germ—toasted	108	8.25	3.09	14.0	12.50	2.19	0.474	0.233	3.910	0
Wheat germ w/brown sugar, honey	107	6.19	2.30	17.2	8.98	1.93	0.349	0.180	3.390	0
Wheatena—cooked	16	0.58	0.13	3.4	1.28	0.16	0.002	0.006	0.385	0
Wheaties	99	2.74	0.51	22.6	43.00	4.50	0.391	0.391	2.540	0
Whole wheat berries	16	0.54	0.11	3.2	1.70	0.17	0.023	0.006	0.680	0
Whole wheat cereal—cooked	18	0.58	0.11	3.9	1.99	0.18	0.020	0.014	0.457	0

CHEESE

	kcal	Protein (g)	Lipid (g)	CHO (g)	Ca (mg)	Fe (mg)	B_1 (mg)	B_2 (mg)	Fiber (g)	Cholesterol (mg)
American—processed	106	6.28	8.84	0.45	174	0.110	0.008	0.111	0	27.0
American cheese food—cold pack	94	5.23	6.78	2.36	145	0.240	0.009	0.274	0	18.0
American cheese spread	82	5.16	6.00	2.48	159	0.090	0.014	0.380	0	16.0
Blue	100	6.09	8.14	0.66	150	0.090	0.008	0.395	0	21.0
Brick	105	6.40	8.40	0.79	191	0.130	0.004	0.159	0	27.0
Brie	95	5.87	7.84	0.13	52	0.140	0.020	0.147	0	28.0
Camembert	85	5.60	6.86	0.13	110	0.094	0.008	0.138	0	20.0
Caraway	107	7.13	8.27	0.87	191	0.100	0.009	0.196	0	25.0
Cheddar	114	7.05	9.38	0.36	204	0.197	0.008	0.106	0	29.9
Cheshire	110	6.60	8.66	1.36	182	0.060	0.013	0.198	0	28.9
Colby	112	6.73	9.08	0.73	194	0.216	0.004	0.171	0	27.0
Cottage	29	3.54	1.20	0.76	17	0.040	0.006	0.115	0	4.2
Cottage—lowfat 2%	26	3.90	0.55	1.03	20	0.045	0.007	0.052	0	2.4
Cottage—lowfat 1%	21	3.51	0.29	0.77	18	0.040	0.006	0.115	0	1.3
Cottage—dry curd	24	4.89	0.12	0.52	9	0.065	0.007	0.004	0	2.0
Cottage—w/fruit	35	2.80	0.96	3.78	14	0.031	0.005	0.115	0	3.1
Cream	99	2.10	9.87	0.75	23	0.337	0.005	0.056	0	30.9
Edam	101	7.07	7.79	0.40	207	0.125	0.010	0.274	0	25.0
Feta	75	4.49	6.19	1.16	140	0.180	0.040	0.315	0	25.0
Fontina	110	7.25	8.62	0.44	156	0.060	0.006	NA	0	32.9
Gjetost	132	2.74	8.32	12.00	113	0.130	0.009	0.170	0	25.0
Gorgonzola	111	6.99	8.98	0	149	0.120	0.010	0.512	0	25.0
Gouda	101	7.06	7.72	0.63	198	0.070	0.009	0.232	0	31.9
Gruyere	117	8.44	9.05	0.10	286	0.060	0.017	0.095	0	30.9
Liederkranz	87	4.99	7.99	0	110	0.120	0.010	0.389	0	21.0
Limburger	93	5.67	7.59	0.14	141	0.040	0.023	0.227	0	26.0
Monterey jack	106	6.93	8.56	0.19	212	0.200	0.004	0.119	0	26.0
Mozzarella—skim, low moist	80	7.60	4.67	0.89	207	0.076	0.006	0.150	0	15.0

(continued)

CHEESE (continued)

	kcal	Protein (g)	Lipid (g)	CHO (g)	Ca (mg)	Fe (mg)	B_1 (mg)	B_2 (mg)	Fiber (g)	Cholesterol (mg)
Mozzarella—whole milk, regular	80	5.50	5.75	0.63	147	0.050	0.004	0.106	0	22.0
Mozzarella—whole milk, moist	90	6.10	7.19	0.43	163	0.060	0.005	0.119	0	25.0
Muenster	104	6.40	8.42	0.32	203	0.125	0.004	0.178	0	27.0
Neufchatel	74	2.82	6.70	0.83	21	0.080	0.004	0.113	0	22.0
Parmesan—hard	111	10.00	7.30	0.91	335	0.230	0.010	0.453	0	19.0
Parmesan—grated	129	11.80	8.50	1.06	389	0.270	0.013	0.527	0	22.0
Pimento processed	106	6.26	8.82	0.49	174	0.120	0.008	0.404	0	27.0
Port du salut	100	6.73	7.99	0.16	84	0.140	0.004	0.151	0	34.9
Provolone	100	7.13	7.54	0.61	214	0.146	0.005	0.248	0	20.0
Ricotta—part skim	39	3.23	2.25	1.45	77	0.126	0.006	0.052	0	8.8
Ricotta—whole milk	49	3.19	3.68	0.86	59	0.108	0.004	0.024	0	14.3
Romano	110	9.00	7.63	1.03	301	0.230	0.010	0.339	0	28.9
Romano—grated	128	10.50	8.86	1.20	350	0.270	0.013	0.394	0	32.9
Roquefort	105	6.10	8.93	0.57	188	0.172	0.010	0.512	0	26.0
Swiss	107	8.03	7.79	0.96	272	0.050	0.006	0.074	0	26.0
Swiss processed	95	7.00	6.97	0.60	219	0.170	0.004	0.078	0	24.0

FISH

	kcal	Protein (g)	Lipid (g)	CHO (g)	Ca (mg)	Fe (mg)	B_1 (mg)	B_2 (mg)	Fiber (g)	Cholesterol (mg)
Bass—freshwater raw	32	5.36	1.05	0	22.7	0.422	0.028	0.009	0	19.3
Bluefish—baked /broiled	45	7.43	1.42	0	2.6	0.174	0.022	0.030	0	17.9
Bluefish—fried in crumbs	58	6.44	2.78	1.33	2.3	0.151	0.017	0.023	0	17
Bluefish—raw	35	5.67	1.20	0	2.0	0.136	0.016	0.023	0	16.7
Carp—raw	36	5.05	1.59	0	11.6	0.352	0.013	0.011	0	18.7
Catfish—channel—raw	33	5.16	1.20	0	11.3	0.275	0.013	0.030	0	16.4
Cod—baked w/butter	37	6.46	0.94	0	5.7	0.139	0.025	0.022	0	17.0
Cod—batter-fried	56	5.56	2.92	2.13	22.7	0.142	0.011	0.011	0	15.6
Cod—baked/broiled	30	6.46	0.24	0	4.0	0.139	0.025	0.022	0	15.6
Cod—poached	29	6.24	0.24	0	4.0	0.139	0.025	0.022	0	15.6
Cod—steamed	29	6.24	0.24	0	4.0	0.139	0.025	0.022	0	15.9
Cod—smoked	22	5.19	0.17	0	4.0	0.113	0.023	0.020	0	14.2
Cod—Atlantic—raw	23	5.05	0.19	0	4.5	0.108	0.022	0.018	0	12.2
Cod liver oil	255	0	28.40	0	0	0	0	0	0	162.0
Eel—smoked	94	5.27	7.88	0.23	26.9	0.198	0.040	0.099	0	19.8
Haddock—breaded /fried	58	5.67	3.00	2.33	11.3	0.384	0.020	0.033	0.01	18.3
Haddock—smoked	33	7.14	0.27	0	13.9	0.397	0.013	0.014	0	21.8
Haddock—raw	22	5.36	0.20	0	9.4	0.298	0.010	0.010	0	16.2
Herring—pickled	74	4.03	5.10	2.73	21.8	0.346	0.010	0.039	0	3.7
Herring—smoked/ kippered	62	6.97	3.52	0	23.8	0.428	0.036	0.090	0	22.7
Herring—canned w/liquid	59	5.64	3.86	0	41.7	0.879	0.007	0.051	0	27.5

(continued)

FISH (continued)

	kcal	Protein (g)	Lipid (g)	CHO (g)	Ca (mg)	Fe (mg)	B_1 (mg)	B_2 (mg)	Fiber (g)	Cholesterol (mg)
Mackerel—fried	49	7.00	2.35	0	4.3	0.445	0.045	0.116	0	19.8
Mackerel—Atlantic—baked/broiled	74	6.78	5.05	0	4.3	0.445	0.045	0.117	0	21.3
Mackerel—Atlantic—raw	58	5.27	3.94	0	3.4	0.462	0.050	0.088	0	19.8
Mackerel—Pacific—raw	45	6.12	2.84	0	2.3	0.567	0.043	0.096	0	22.7
Northern pike—raw	25	5.47	0.20	0	16.2	0.156	0.017	0.018	0	11.0
Ocean perch—breaded/fried	62	5.34	3.67	2.33	30.7	0.400	0.033	0.037	0.03	15.3
Pollock—baked/broiled	28	6.60	0.31	0	19.3	0.149	0.014	0.057	0	19.8
Pollock—poached	36	6.60	0.31	0	17.0	0.149	0.010	0.050	0	19.8
Salmon—broiled /baked	61	7.74	3.10	0	2.0	0.157	0.061	0.048	0	24.7
Coho salmon—steamed/poached	52	7.77	2.14	0	8.22	0.252	0.057	0.031	0	13.9
Smoked salmon—Chinook	33	5.17	1.22	0	3.0	0.240	0.007	0.029	0	6.7
Atlantic salmon—small can	36	5.05	1.62	0	3.1	0.204	0.057	0.097	0	17.0
Pink salmon—raw	33	5.64	0.98	0	11.3	0.218	0.040	0.057	0	14.7
Sardines	59	7.00	3.24	0	108.0	0.826	0.023	0.064	0	40.4
Sea trout steelhead—raw	30	4.73	1.02	0	4.8	0.077	0.023	0.057	0	23.5
Sea trout steelhead—cooked	37	6.07	1.42	0	5.7	0.088	0.024	0.064	0	32.3
Shad—baked with bacon	57	6.58	3.20	0	6.8	0.170	0.037	0.074	0	17.0
Smelt—rainbow—raw	28	4.99	0.69	0	17.0	0.255	0.016	0.034	0	19.8
Snapper—baked or broiled	36	7.46	0.49	0	11.3	0.068	0.015	0.021	0	13.3
Snapper—raw	28	5.81	0.38	0	9.1	0.051	0.013	0.017	0	10.5
Sole/flounder—baked w/ butter	40	5.34	2.00	0	5.3	0.093	0.023	0.032	0	22.7
Sole /flounder—baked/broiled	33	6.84	0.43	0	5.3	0.093	0.023	0.032	0	19.3
Sole/flounder—batter-fried	83	4.47	5.10	4.07	16.7	0.239	0.057	0.042	0.01	15.0
Sole/flounder—breaded/fried	53	4.96	2.55	2.54	11.3	0.128	0.037	0.034	0	15.0
Sole/flounder—steamed	26	5.67	0.33	0	4.5	0.079	0.017	0.027	0	14.7
Sole/flounder—raw	26	5.33	0.34	0	5.1	0.102	0.025	0.022	0	13.6
Lemon sole—raw	23	4.85	0.21	0	4.8	0.088	0.026	0.023	0	17.0
Lemon sole—fried w/ crumbs	56	4.56	3.12	2.64	26.9	0.176	0.020	0.023	0	18.4
Lemon sole—steamed	26	5.84	0.26	0	6.0	0.147	0.026	0.026	0	17.0
Swordfish—raw	34	5.61	1.14	0	1.1	0.230	0.010	0.027	0	11.0
Swordfish—broiled/baked	44	7.20	1.46	0	1.7	0.295	0.012	0.033	0	14.2
Trout—baked/broiled	43	7.47	1.22	0	24.3	0.690	0.024	0.064	0	20.7
Tuna—oil pack	56	8.26	2.34	0	3.8	0.395	0.010	0.030	0	5.0
Tuna—water pack	37	8.38	0.14	0	3.4	0.409	0.010	0.033	0	16.0
Tuna—raw	31	6.63	0.27	0	4.5	0.207	0.123	0.013	0	12.8
Whiting—flour/bread-fried	54	5.13	1.56	1.98	11.3	0.198	0.023	0.020	0	18.4

FRUITS

	kcal	Protein (g)	Lipid (g)	CHO (g)	Ca (mg)	Fe (mg)	B_1 (mg)	B_2 (mg)	Fiber (g)	Cholesterol (mg)
Apple w/peel	16	0.055	0.100	4.31	2.05	0.051	0.005	0.004	0.709	0
Apple slices w/peel—fresh	17	0.054	0.100	4.33	2.06	0.052	0.005	0.004	0.709	0
Apple juice—canned/bottled	13	0.017	0.032	3.32	1.94	0.105	0.006	0.005	0.034	0
Apple juice—frozen concentrate	47	0.144	0.105	11.60	5.78	0.258	0.003	0.015	0.089	0
Applesauce—sweetened	22	0.052	0.052	5.67	1.11	0.111	0.003	0.008	0.397	0
Apricot—fresh halves	14	0.397	0.110	3.15	4.02	0.154	0.009	0.011	0.538	0
Apricot halves—light syrup	18	0.150	0.013	4.67	3.34	0.110	0.005	0.006	0.319	0
Apricot nectar—canned	16	0.104	0.025	4.08	2.03	0.108	0.003	0.004	0.170	0
Avocado—average	46	0.563	0.340	2.10	3.07	0.284	0.030	0.035	2.720	0
Banana—fresh slices	26	0.293	0.136	6.63	1.74	0.088	0.013	0.028	0.578	0
Blackberries—canned	26	0.370	0.040	6.54	5.98	0.184	0.008	0.011	1.011	0
Blackberries—fresh	15	0.205	0.110	3.62	9.06	0.158	0.008	0.011	1.910	0
Blackberries—frozen	18	0.334	0.122	4.45	8.26	0.173	0.008	0.013	1.460	0
Blueberries—fresh	16	0.190	0.108	4.00	1.76	0.047	0.014	0.014	0.763	0
Blueberries-frozen unsweetened	14	0.119	0.181	3.46	2.19	0.051	0.009	0.010	0.658	0
Boysenberries—frozen	14	0.314	0.075	3.46	7.73	0.240	0.015	0.010	1.100	0
Sour cheeries—frozen	13	0.260	0.124	3.13	3.66	0.150	0.012	0.010	0.384	0
Sweet cherries—fresh	20	0.340	0.272	4.69	4.10	0.110	0.014	0.017	0.430	0
Sweet cherries—frozen	25	0.325	0.037	6.34	3.39	0.099	0.008	0.013	0.224	0
Cranberries—whole—raw	14	0.110	0.057	3.58	2.09	0.057	0.009	0.006	1.190	0
Cranberry/apple juice	19	0.015	0.090	4.82	2.02	0.017	0.001	0.006	0.070	0
Cranberry juice cocktail	16	0.009	0.015	4.03	0.90	0.043	0.002	0.002	0.085	0
Date—whole—each	78	0.557	0.127	20.80	9.22	0.342	0.026	0.028	2.300	0
Figs—medium—fresh	21	0.215	0.085	5.44	10.20	0.102	0.017	0.014	1.050	0
Fig—dried—each	72	0.864	0.330	18.50	40.80	0.634	0.020	0.025	3.140	0
Fruit cocktail—heavy syrup	21	0.111	0.020	5.36	1.78	0.081	0.005	0.005	0.280	0
Fruit cocktail—light syrup	16	0.114	0.020	4.23	1.80	0.082	0.005	0.005	0.284	0
Grapefruit half—pink/red	9	0.157	0.028	2.18	3.00	0.034	0.010	0.006	0.369	0
Grapefruit half—white	10	0.195	0.029	2.38	3.36	0.017	0.010	0.006	0.368	0
Grapefuit sections/fresh	9	0.179	0.028	2.29	3.33	0.025	0.010	0.006	0.370	0
Grapefruit sections—canned	17	0.160	0.028	4.38	4.02	0.114	0.010	0.006	0.313	0
Grapefruit juice—fresh	11	0.142	0.029	2.60	2.53	0.056	0.011	0.006	0.113	0
Grapefruit juice—sweetened	13	0.164	0.026	3.15	2.27	0.102	0.011	0.007	0.076	0
Grapefruit juice—unsweetened	11	0.148	0.028	2.54	1.95	0.057	0.012	0.006	0.077	0
Grapefruit juice—frozen concentrate	41	0.548	0.137	9.86	7.67	0.140	0.041	0.022	0.383	0
Grapes—Thompson	20	0.188	0.163	5.03	3.01	0.073	0.026	0.016	0.333	0
Grape juice—bottled/canned	17	0.158	0.021	4.25	2.47	0.068	0.007	0.010	0.141	0
Grape juice—frozen concentrate	51	0.184	0.088	12.60	3.68	0.102	0.015	0.026	0.492	0
Grape juice—prep frozen	15	0.053	0.026	3.62	1.13	0.029	0.004	0.007	0.142	0
Kiwi fruit	17	0.280	0.127	4.22	7.46	0.112	0.007	0.015	0.962	0
Lemon—fresh wo/peel	8	0.313	0.083	2.64	7.33	0.171	0.011	0.006	0.582	0
Lemon juice—fresh	7	0.107	0.081	2.45	2.09	0.009	0.008	0.003	0.099	0
Lemon juice—bottled	6	0.114	0.081	1.84	3.02	0.036	0.012	0.003	0.085	0
Lime—fresh	9	0.199	0.055	2.99	9.30	0.169	0.008	0.006	0.228	0
Lime juice—fresh	8	0.124	0.029	2.56	2.54	0.009	0.006	0.003	0.113	0
Lime juice—bottled	6	0.115	0.115	1.84	3.46	0.069	0.009	0.001	0.099	0

(continued)

FRUITS (continued)

	kcal	Protein (g)	Lipid (g)	CHO (g)	Ca (mg)	Fe (mg)	B_1 (mg)	B_2 (mg)	Fiber (g)	Cholesterol (mg)
Loganberries—fresh	20	0.430	0.088	3.69	8.50	0.181	0.014	0.010	1.760	0
Loganberries—frozen	16	0.430	0.089	3.68	7.33	0.181	0.014	0.010	1.760	0
Mango—fresh—slices	19	0.146	0.077	4.83	2.92	0.360	0.016	0.016	0.997	0
Mango—fresh—whole	19	0.145	0.078	4.82	2.88	0.356	0.016	0.016	1.010	0
Cantaloupe—cubes	10	0.250	0.079	2.37	3.19	0.060	0.006	0.006	0.284	0
Casaba melon—cubes	8	0.255	0.028	1.75	1.50	0.113	0.017	0.006	0.284	0
Honeydew melon—cubes	10	0.128	0.028	2.60	1.67	0.020	0.022	0.005	0.307	0
Melon balls—mixed—frozen	9	0.239	0.023	2.25	2.79	0.008	0.005	0.006	0.295	0
Mixed fruit—dried	69	0.697	0.139	18.20	10.60	0.767	0.012	0.045	1.220	0
Mixed fruit—frozen—thawed	28	0.397	0.052	6.87	2.04	0.079	0.005	0.010	0.386	0
Nectarine	14	0.267	0.129	3.34	1.25	0.044	0.005	0.012	0.554	0
Orange	13	0.266	0.035	3.33	11.30	0.029	0.025	0.011	0.680	0
Orange sections—fresh	13	0.266	0.035	3.34	11.30	0.029	0.025	0.011	0.680	0
Mandarin oranges—canned	17	0.113	0.011	4.61	2.03	0.101	0.015	0.012	0.478	0
Orange juice—fresh	13	0.199	0.057	2.95	3.09	0.057	0.025	0.008	0.113	0
Oranged juice—frozen concentrate	45	0.679	0.059	10.80	9.05	0.099	0.079	0.018	0.313	0
Orange juice—frozen	13	0.191	0.016	3.05	2.50	0.031	0.023	0.005	0.057	0
Papaya—whole fresh	11	0.173	0.040	2.78	6.71	0.028	0.008	0.009	0.482	0
Papaya—slices fresh	12	0.174	0.040	2.77	6.68	0.060	0.008	0.009	0.482	0
Papaya nectar—canned	16	0.049	0.043	4.12	2.72	0.098	0.002	0.001	0.170	0
Peaches—fresh	12	0.199	0.026	3.14	1.30	0.031	0.005	0.012	0.489	0
Peach slices—frozen/thawed	27	0.177	0.037	6.80	0.91	0.105	0.004	0.010	0.467	0
Peach halves—heavy syrup	21	0.130	0.028	5.67	1.05	0.077	0.003	0.007	0.315	0
Peach halves—light syrup	15	0.126	0.010	4.13	1.05	0.101	0.002	0.007	0.402	0
Peach halves—dried	68	0.020	0.216	17.40	8.07	1.150	0	0.060	2.330	0
Peach nectar—canned	15	0.076	0.006	3.95	1.48	0.054	0	0.004	0.170	0
Pears—Bartlett	17	0.111	0.113	4.29	3.24	0.070	0.006	0.011	0.779	0
Pear halves—heavy syrup	21	0.057	0.036	5.42	1.44	0.061	0.004	0.006	0.395	0
Pear halves—light syrup	16	0.054	0.007	4.30	1.44	0.082	0.003	0.005	0.395	0
Pear nectar—canned	17	0.030	0.003	4.47	1.25	0.073	0	0.004	0.204	0
Pineapple slices—heavy syrup	22	0.098	0.034	5.72	3.91	0.108	0.025	0.007	0.270	0
Pineapple slices—light syrup	15	0.103	0.034	3.81	3.91	0.110	0.026	0.007	0.268	0
Pineapple—frozen sweetened	24	0.113	0.029	6.29	2.55	0.113	0.028	0.009	0.496	0
Pineapple juice—frozen concentrate	51	0.369	0.029	12.60	11.00	0.255	0.065	0.017	0.255	0
Plums	16	0.223	0.176	3.69	1.29	0.030	0.012	0.027	0.550	0
Plums—canned—heavy syrup	25	0.102	0.028	6.59	2.53	0.238	0.005	0.010	0.434	0
Plums—canned—light syrup	18	0.105	0.029	4.61	2.70	0.243	0.005	0.011	0.444	0
Prunes—dried	68	0.739	0.145	17.80	14.50	0.702	0.023	0.046	2.700	0
Prune juice—bottled	20	0.172	0.009	4.95	3.43	0.334	0.005	0.020	0.310	0
Raisins—seedless	85	0.914	0.130	22.50	13.90	0.594	0.044	0.025	1.670	0
Raspberries—fresh	14	0.256	0.157	3.27	6.22	0.162	0.009	0.026	1.770	0
Raspberries—canned w/ liquid	26	0.235	0.034	6.62	2.99	0.120	0.006	0.009	1.200	0
Raspberries—frozen	29	0.197	0.044	7.42	4.30	0.184	0.005	0.013	1.300	0

(continued)

FRUITS (continued)

	kcal	Protein (g)	Lipid (g)	CHO (g)	Ca (mg)	Fe (mg)	B_1 (mg)	B_2 (mg)	Fiber (g)	Cholesterol (mg)
Rhubarb—raw—diced	6	0.253	0.056	1.29	39.50	0.062	0.006	0.009	0.737	0
Rhubarb—cooked w/sugar	33	0.111	0.013	8.85	41.10	0.060	0.005	0.006	0.624	0
Strawberries—fresh	9	0.173	0.105	2.00	4.00	0.108	0.006	0.019	0.736	0
Strawberries—frozen	10	0.120	0.030	2.59	4.38	0.213	0.006	0.010	0.736	0
Tangerine—fresh	13	0.179	0.054	3.17	4.05	0.028	0.030	0.006	0.574	0
Tangerines—canned—light syrup	17	0.127	0.028	4.61	2.03	0.105	0.015	0.012	0.453	0
Watermelon	9	0.175	0.121	2.04	2.24	0.048	0.023	0.006	0.114	0

MEATS

	kcal	Protein (g)	Lipid (g)	CHO (g)	Ca (mg)	Fe (mg)	B_1 (mg)	B_2 (mg)	Fiber (g)	Cholesterol (mg)
Beef chuck—pot roasted	108	7.20	8.64	0	3.67	0.840	0.020	0.065	0	29.0
Beef chuck—pot roasted lean	77	8.80	4.34	0	3.67	1.040	0.024	0.080	0	30.0
Beef round—pot roasted lean & fat	74	8.44	4.20	0	1.67	0.920	0.020	0.069	0	27.0
Beef round—pot roasted lean	63	8.97	2.74	0	1.33	0.980	0.021	0.074	0	27.0
Ground beef—lean	77	7.00	5.34	0	3.00	0.600	0.013	0.060	0	24.7
Ground beef—regular	82	6.67	5.94	0	3.00	0.700	0.010	0.053	0	25.3
Sirloin steak—lean	57	8.10	2.53	0	2.33	0.700	0.026	0.056	0	21.7
T-bone steak—lean & fat	92	6.80	6.97	0	2.67	0.720	0.026	0.059	0	23.7
Beef lunchmeat—thin-sliced	50	7.96	1.09	1.62	2.99	0.759	0.023	0.054	0	12.0
Beef lunchmeat—loaf/roll	87	4.06	7.42	0.82	2.99	0.659	0.030	0.062	0	18.0
Beef rib—oven roasted—lean	68	7.70	3.90	0	3.34	0.740	0.023	0.060	0	22.7
Beef round—oven roasted—lean	54	8.14	2.12	0	1.67	0.834	0.028	0.076	0	23.0
Beef rump roast—lean only	51	8.40	1.89	0	1.13	0.567	0.026	0.049	0	19.6
Beef brains—pan-fried	56	3.57	4.50	0	2.67	0.630	0.037	0.074	0	566.0
Beef heart	47	8.17	1.59	0.12	1.67	2.130	0.040	0.436	0	54.7
Beef kidney	41	7.23	0.97	0.27	5.00	2.070	0.054	1.150	0	110.0
Beef liver—fried	61	7.57	2.27	2.23	3.00	1.780	0.060	1.170	0	137.0
Beef tongue—cooked	80	6.27	5.87	0.09	2.00	0.960	0.009	0.009	0	30.4
Beef tripe—raw	28	4.14	1.12	0	36.00	0.553	0.002	0.047	0	26.9
Beef tripe—pickled	17	3.29	0.40	0	25.00	0.389	0	0.028	0	15.0
Corned beef—canned	71	7.67	4.24	0	5.67	0.590	0.006	0.042	0	24.3
Corned beef hash—canned	49	2.35	1.29	2.82	3.74	0.567	0.016	0.052	0.153	17.0
Beef—dried/cured	47	8.24	1.10	0.44	2.00	1.280	0.050	0.230	0	45.9
Beef & vegetable stew	26	1.85	1.27	1.74	3.36	0.336	0.017	0.020	0.393	8.2
Beef stew—canned	22	1.64	0.88	2.06	2.66	0.368	0.008	0.014	0.150	1.7
Burrito—beef & bean	63	3.40	2.84	6.48	26.70	0.437	0.042	0.047	0.810	8.4
Tostada w/beans & beef	49	2.72	3.06	2.98	27.50	0.319	0.012	0.036	0.583	9.1
Beef + macaroni + tomato	24	1.25	0.73	3.16	3.81	0.300	0.024	0.021	0.291	2.8
Beef enchilada	69	3.09	3.26	3.69	60.20	0.418	0.017	0.039	0.465	8.9
Frankfurter—beef	92	3.20	8.36	0.68	3.48	0.378	0.014	0.029	0	13.4
Frankfurter—beef & pork	91	3.20	8.26	0.73	2.98	0.328	0.056	0.034	0	14.4
Beef pot pie—frozen	52	1.99	2.73	4.77	2.42	0.436	0.022	0.018	0.109	5.0
Beef pie—recipe	70	2.84	4.05	5.27	3.92	0.513	0.039	0.039	0.155	5.7
Beef taco	75	4.94	4.80	3.67	30.90	0.469	0.010	0.049	0.407	16.2

(continued)

MEATS (continued)

	kcal	Protein (g)	Lipid (g)	CHO (g)	Ca (mg)	Fe (mg)	B_1 (mg)	B_2 (mg)	Fiber (g)	Cholesterol (mg)
Chicken meat—all-fried	62	8.67	2.59	0.48	4.86	0.383	0.024	0.056	0.002	26.5
Chicken meat—all-roasted	54	8.20	2.10	0	4.25	0.342	0.020	0.050	0	25.3
Chicken meat—all-stewed	50	7.74	1.90	0	4.05	0.330	0.014	0.046	0	23.5
Boned chicken w/broth	47	6.17	2.26	0	3.99	0.439	0.004	0.037	0	17.6
Chicken—dark meat—fried	68	8.22	3.30	0.74	5.06	0.423	0.026	0.070	0.002	27.3
Chicken—dark meat—roasted	58	7.76	2.75	0	4.25	0.377	0.020	0.064	0	26.3
Chicken—dark meat—stewed	55	7.37	2.55	0	4.05	0.385	0.016	0.057	0	24.9
Chicken—light meat—fried	54	9.31	1.57	0.12	4.45	0.322	0.020	0.036	0	25.3
Chicken—light meat—roasted	49	8.77	1.28	0	4.25	0.302	0.018	0.033	0	23.9
Chicken—light meat—stewed	45	8.18	1.17	0	3.64	0.265	0.012	0.033	0	21.7
Chicken breast—no skin	47	8.80	0.99	0	4.29	0.295	0.020	0.032	0	24.0
Chicken breast meat—stewed	43	8.20	0.86	0	3.58	0.250	0.012	0.034	0	21.8
Chicken drumstick—batter fried	76	6.22	4.45	2.36	4.73	0.382	0.032	0.061	0.008	24.4
Chicken drumstick—roasted	61	7.69	3.16	0	3.27	0.376	0.020	0.061	0	26.2
Chicken wing—batter-fried	92	5.64	6.19	3.10	5.79	0.365	0.030	0.043	0.012	22.6
Chicken wing—flour-fried	91	7.40	6.28	0.67	4.43	0.354	0.017	0.039	0.009	23.0
Chicken wing—roasted	83	7.48	5.53	0	4.17	0.359	0.012	0.037	0	24.2
Chicken gizzards—simmered	44	7.73	1.04	0.32	2.58	1.180	0.008	0.070	0	54.9
Chicken hearts—simmered	52	7.49	2.23	0.03	5.27	2.560	0.017	0.206	0	68.7
Chicken livers—simmered	44	6.90	1.55	0.25	4.05	2.400	0.043	0.496	0	179.0
Chicken roll—light meat	45	5.52	2.08	0..69	11.90	0.274	0.018	0.037	0	13.9
Chicken frankfurter	73	3.67	5.52	1.93	27.00	0.567	0.019	0.033	0	28.4
Chicken a la king	54	3.12	3.93	1.93	14.70	0.289	0.012	0.049	0.154	25.6
Chicken + noodles	43	2.60	2.13	3.07	3.07	0.278	0.006	0.020	0.142	12.2
Chicken chow mein	29	2.60	1.25	1.13	6.58	0.284	0.009	0.026	0.466	8.5
Chicken curry	26	2.21	1.53	0.64	2.52	0.170	0.009	0.019	0.033	5.3
Chicken frankfurter	72	3.67	5.52	1.93	27.00	0.567	0.019	0.033	0	28.4
Chicken pot pie—frozen	53	1.84	2.84	5.08	3.70	0.382	0.020	0.020	0.210	4.9
Chicken roll—light meat	45	5.52	2.08	0.69	11.90	0.274	0.018	0.037	0	13.9
Chicken salad w/celery	97	3.82	8.90	0.47	5.92	0.239	0.012	0.028	0.109	17.3
Chicken patty sandwich	79	4.48	4.06	6.10	7.95	0.338	0.052	0.047	0.244	12.3
Chicken broth—from dry	2	0.16	0.13	0.17	1.74	0.009	0	0.004	0.001	0.1
Chicken broth—from cube	2	0.11	0.04	0.18	0.04	0.014	0.001	0.003	0	0.1
Chicken noodle soup	9	0.48	0.29	1.10	2.00	0.092	0.006	0.007	0.085	0.8
Tostada w/beans/chicken	45	3.50	2.06	3.38	29.30	0.305	0.013	0.034	0.668	9.6
Chicken taco	63	5.60	3.03	3.67	31.60	0.237	0.014	0.043	0.407	16.5
Chicken enchilada	64	3.38	2.48	3.69	60.50	0.359	0.018	0.036	0.465	9.1
Turkey dark meat—roasted	53	8.10	2.05	0	9.11	0.662	0.018	0.070	0	24.0
Turkey white meat—roasted	44	8.48	0.91	0	5.47	0.380	0.017	0.037	0	19.6
Turkey breast—barbecued	40	6.39	1.40	0	2.00	0.120	0.010	0.030	0	16.0
Turkey gizzards	46	8.34	1.10	0.17	4.32	1.540	0.009	0.093	0	65.6
Turkey hearts	50	7.58	1.73	0.58	3.72	1.950	0.019	0.250	0	64.0
Turkey livers	48	6.80	1.69	0.97	3.02	2.210	0.015	0.404	0	177.0
Turkey loaf	31	6.38	0.45	0	2.00	0.113	0.011	0.030	0	11.6
Turkey roll	41	5.27	2.03	0.15	11.40	0.358	0.025	0.064	0	11.9
Turkey bologna	56	3.86	4.27	0.27	23.40	0.432	0.015	0.047	0	28.0
Turkey frankfurter	64	4.05	5.22	0.42	36.50	0.485	0.023	0.050	0	24.6
Turkey ham	36	5.37	1.49	0.42	2.49	0.776	0.020	0.075	0	15.9
Turkey pastrami	37	5.22	1.75	0.43	2.49	0.403	0.022	0.075	0	14.9
Turkey salami	55	4.62	3.89	0.15	5.47	0.463	0.029	0.075	0	22.9
Turkey pot pie—frozen	51	1.80	2.75	4.65	7.79	0.256	0.020	0.020	0.110	2.4

EGGS

	kcal	Protein (g)	Lipid (g)	CHO (g)	Ca (mg)	Fe (mg)	B_1 (mg)	B_2 (mg)	Fiber (g)	Cholesterol (mg)
Egg white, cooked	13	2.68	0	0.33	3.20	0.008	0.002	0.072	0	0
Egg yolk, cooked	108	4.76	8.73	0.07	44.40	1.620	0.044	0.121	0	355.0
Egg, fried in butter	56	3.54	3.45	0.38	15.70	0.536	0.018	0.148	0	129.0
Egg, hard cooked	40	3.52	2.79	0.34	13.80	0.474	0.014	0.132	0	113.0
Egg, poached	40	3.50	2.79	0.34	13.80	0.474	0.014	0.132	0	113.0
Egg, scrambled milk + butter	40	2.88	2.57	0.61	23.90	0.412	0.013	0.106	0	93.9
Egg raw—large	40	3.52	2.79	0.34	13.80	0.474	0.017	0.139	0	113.0
Egg white—raw	13	2.68	0	0.33	3.20	0.008	0.002	0.075	0	0
Egg yolk, raw	108	4.76	8.73	0.07	44.40	1.620	0.051	0.126	0	355.0
Egg substitute, frozen	45	3.20	3.15	0.91	20.80	0.562	0.034	0.110	0	0.5
Egg substitute, powder	125	15.60	3.66	6.12	90.70	0.879	0.062	0.493	0	162.0

DAIRY PRODUCTS

	kcal	Protein (g)	Lipid (g)	CHO (g)	Ca (mg)	Fe (mg)	B_1 (mg)	B_2 (mg)	Fiber (g)	Cholesterol (mg)
Milk—1% lowfat	12	0.93	0.30	1.36	34.9	0.014	0.011	0.047	0	1.16
Milk—2% lowfat	14	0.94	0.56	1.36	34.5	0.012	0.011	0.047	0	2.56
Milk—skim	10	0.97	0.05	1.38	34.9	0.012	0.010	0.040	0	0.46
Milk—whole	17	0.93	0.95	1.32	33.8	0.014	0.010	0.046	0	3.83
Buttermilk	12	0.94	0.25	1.35	33.0	0.014	0.010	0.044	0	1.04
Milk—instant nonfat dry	102	9.96	0.21	14.80	349.0	0.088	0.117	0.496	0	5.00
Canned skim milk—evaporated	22	2.11	0.06	3.22	82.0	0.078	0.013	0.088	0	1.11
Canned whole milk—evaporated	38	1.91	2.20	2.81	73.9	0.054	0.014	0.090	0	8.33
Carob flavor mix—powder	106	0.47	0.05	26.50	0	1.300	0.002	0	4.020	0
Chocolate milk—1%	18	0.92	0.28	2.96	32.5	0.068	0.010	0.047	0.425	0.79
Chocolate milk—2%	20	0.91	0.57	2.95	32.2	0.068	0.010	0.046	0.425	1.93
Chocolate milk—whole	24	0.90	0.96	2.94	31.8	0.068	0.010	0.046	0.425	3.52
Hot cocoa—with whole milk	25	1.03	1.03	2.93	33.8	0.088	0.012	0.049	0.340	3.74
Instant breakfast w/2% milk	25	1.52	0.47	3.50	31.0	0.807	0.040	0.048	0	1.82
Instant breakfast w/1% milk	23	1.51	0.25	3.50	31.3	0.807	0.040	0.048	0	1.00
Instant breakfast w/skim milk	22	1.55	0.04	3.50	31.4	0.804	0.039	0.041	0	0.40
Instant breakfast w/whole milk	28	1.51	0.82	3.47	30.4	0.807	0.040	0.047	0	3.33
Egg nog	38	1.08	2.12	3.84	36.8	0.057	0.010	0.054	0	16.60
Kefir	20	1.13	0.55	1.07	42.6	0.060	0.055	0.054	0	1.22
Malt powder—chocolate flavored	107	1.49	1.08	24.80	17.6	0.648	0.049	0.057	0.540	1.35
Malted milk powder	117	3.12	2.30	21.50	85.0	0.209	0.143	0.260	0.405	5.40
Malted milk drink—chocolate	25	1.00	0.95	3.19	32.5	0.064	0.014	0.047	0.043	3.64
Chocolate milkshake	36	0.96	1.05	5.80	32.0	0.088	0.016	0.069	0.035	3.70
Strawberry milkshake	32	0.95	0.80	5.35	32.0	0.030	0.013	0.055	0.024	3.10
Vanilla milkshake	32	0.98	0.84	5.09	34.5	0.026	0.013	0.052	0.019	3.20
Ovaltine powder—chocolate flavored	102	2.00	0.85	23.70	134.0	6.190	0.719	0.772	0.013	0

(continued)

DAIRY PRODUCTS (continued)

	kcal	Protein (g)	Lipid (g)	CHO (g)	Ca (mg)	Fe (mg)	B_1 (mg)	B_2 (mg)	Fiber (g)	Cholesterol (mg)
Ovaltine powder—malt flavored	104	2.53	0.24	23.60	106.0	5.820	0.772	1.010	0.040	0
Ovaltine drink—chocolate flavored	24	1.02	0.94	3.12	41.9	0.510	0.067	0.104	0.001	3.53
Ovaltine drink—malt flavored	24	1.06	0.89	3.10	39.7	0.480	0.072	0.124	0.003	3.53
Milk—goat	20	1.00	1.17	1.27	37.9	0.014	0.014	0.039	0	3.25
Milk—sheep	31	1.70	1.99	1.52	54.8	0.028	0.018	0.100	0	0
Milk—soybean	9	0.78	0.54	0.51	1.2	0.163	0.046	0.020	0	0
Ice cream—regular-vanilla	57	1.02	3.05	6.76	37.5	0.026	0.011	0.070	0	12.60
Ice cream—rich-vanilla	67	0.79	4.54	6.13	28.9	0.019	0.008	0.054	0	16.90
Ice cream—soft-serve	62	1.15	3.69	6.28	38.7	0.070	0.013	0.073	0	25.00
Creamsicle ice cream bar	44	0.52	1.33	7.56	19.8	0	0.009	0.034	0	0
Drumstick ice cream bar	88	1.23	4.68	10.20	31.7	0.047	0.009	0.043	0	0
Fudgesicle ice cream bar	35	1.48	0.08	7.22	50.0	0.039	0.012	0.070	0	0
Ice milk	40	1.12	1.22	6.28	38.0	0.039	0.016	0.075	0	3.90
Ice milk—soft serve—3% fat	36	1.30	0.75	6.22	44.4	0.045	0.019	0.088	0	2.10
Yogurt—coffee-vanilla	24	1.40	0.35	3.90	48.5	0.020	0.012	0.057	0	1.42
Yogurt—lowfat with fruit	29	1.24	0.31	5.37	43.0	0.020	0.010	0.050	0	1.25
Yogurt—lowfat-plain	18	1.49	0.43	2.00	51.8	0.022	0.012	0.060	0	1.75
Yogurt—nonfat milk	16	1.62	0.05	2.17	56.5	0.025	0.014	0.066	0	0.50
Yogurt—whole milk	17	0.98	0.92	1.32	34.3	0.014	0.008	0.040	0	3.68

VEGETABLES

	kcal	Protein (g)	Lipid (g)	CHO (g)	Ca (mg)	Fe (mg)	B_1 (mg)	B_2 (mg)	Fiber (g)	Cholesterol (mg)
Alfalfa sprouts	9	1.13	0.200	1.07	9.5	0.272	0.021	0.036	1.030	0
Artichoke hearts—marinated	28	0.680	0.250	2.18	6.5	0.270	0.010	0.029	1.780	0
Asparagus—raw spears	6	0.865	0.063	1.05	6.4	0.193	0.032	0.035	0.395	0
Asparagus—canned spears	5	0.606	0.184	0.70	3.9	0.177	0.017	0.025	0.454	0
Bamboo shoots—sliced—raw	8	0.738	0.088	1.47	3.8	0.143	0.043	0.020	0.738	0
Bamboo shoots—sliced, canned	5	0.489	0.113	0.91	2.2	0.090	0.007	0.007	0.706	0
Bean sprouts—fresh raw	9	0.861	0.050	1.68	3.8	0.258	0.024	0.035	0.736	0
Bean sprouts—boiled	6	0.576	0.025	1.19	3.4	0.185	0.014	0.029	0.572	0
Bean sprouts—stir fried	14	1.220	0.059	3.00	3.7	0.549	0.040	0.050	0.777	0
Black beans—cooked	37	2.500	0.152	6.72	7.8	0.593	0.069	0.017	2.540	0
Green beans—raw uncooked	9	0.515	0.034	2.02	10.6	0.363	0.024	0.030	0.644	0
Green beans—fresh—cooked	10	0.535	0.082	2.24	13.2	0.363	0.021	0.027	0.737	0
Green beans—frozen—cooked	8	0.386	0.038	1.73	12.8	0.233	0.014	0.021	0.880	0
Green beans—canned/drained	6	0.326	0.028	1.28	7.6	0.256	0.004	0.016	0.378	0
Red kidney beans—dry	94	6.690	0.234	16.90	40.5	2.330	0.150	0.062	6.160	0
Lima beans—dry large	96	6.080	0.194	18.00	22.9	2.130	0.144	0.057	8.600	0
Lima beans—fresh—cooked	35	1.930	0.090	6.70	9.0	0.695	0.040	0.027	2.670	0
Lima beans—dry small	98	5.790	0.397	18.20	18.4	2.270	0.136	0.048	8.500	0
Lima beans—canned/drained	27	1.530	0.100	5.20	8.0	0.487	0.010	0.013	2.420	0

(continued)

VEGETABLES (continued)

	kcal	Protein (g)	Lipid (g)	CHO (g)	Ca (mg)	Fe (mg)	B_1 (mg)	B_2 (mg)	Fiber (g)	Cholesterol (mg)
Beans/w/franks—canned	40	1.900	1.860	4.37	13.6	0.490	0.016	0.016	1.950	1.7
Pork & beans—canned	32	1.500	0.413	5.95	17.4	0.470	0.013	0.017	1.560	1.9
Navy beans—dry, cooked	40	2.460	0.162	7.77	19.9	0.703	0.057	0.017	2.490	0
Pinto beans—dry, cooked	39	2.320	0.148	7.28	13.6	0.741	0.053	0.026	3.230	0
Refried beans—canned	30	1.770	0.303	5.24	13.2	0.500	0.014	0.016	2.470	0
Soybeans—dry	118	10.400	5.650	8.55	78.5	4.450	0.248	0.247	1.570	0
White beans—dry	95	5.990	0.334	17.70	36.0	2.190	0.210	0.059	0.766	0
White beans—dry, cooked	40	2.550	0.182	7.32	20.7	0.808	0.067	0.017	2.230	0
Yellow wax beans—raw	9	0.515	0.034	2.02	10.6	0.294	0.024	0.030	0.644	0
Yellow wax beans—raw	10	0.535	0.082	2.24	13.2	0.363	0.021	0.027	0.726	0
Yellow wax beans—frozen	8	0.386	0.038	1.73	12.8	0.233	0.014	0.021	0.880	0
Beets—cooked	9	0.300	0.014	1.90	3.1	0.176	0.009	0.004	0.539	0
Beets—pickled slices	18	0.227	0.028	4.63	3.1	0.116	0.006	0.014	0.587	0
Broccoli—raw chopped	8	0.844	0.097	1.49	13.5	0.251	0.019	0.034	0.934	0
Broccoli—raw spears	8	0.845	0.098	1.49	13.5	0.250	0.018	0.034	0.935	0
Broccoli—frozen cooked spears	8	0.879	0.034	1.51	14.5	0.173	0.015	0.023	0.826	0
Brussels sprouts—raw	12	0.960	0.084	2.54	11.6	0.396	0.039	0.026	1.260	0
Brussels sprouts—cooked	11	1.090	0.145	2.45	10.2	0.342	0.030	0.023	1.220	0
Brussels sprouts—frozen cooked	12	1.030	0.112	2.36	7.0	0.210	0.029	0.032	1.230	0
Cabbage—raw, shredded	7	0.340	0.049	1.52	13.0	0.162	0.015	0.009	0.680	0
Cabbage—cooked	6	0.272	0.070	1.35	9.5	0.110	0.016	0.016	0.661	0
Bok choy—raw, shredded	4	0.425	0.057	0.62	30.0	0.227	0.011	0.020	0.486	0
Bok choy—cooked	3	0.442	0.045	0.51	26.3	0.295	0.009	0.018	0.454	0
Red cabbage—raw	8	0.393	0.073	1.74	14.6	0.142	0.018	0.009	0.648	0
Red cabbage—cooked	6	0.299	0.057	1.32	10.6	0.102	0.010	0.006	1.567	0
Carrot—whole, raw	12	0.291	0.055	2.87	7.5	0.142	0.028	0.017	1.906	0
Carrot—grated, raw	12	0.289	0.052	2.88	7.7	0.142	0.027	0.016	0.907	0
Carrots—sliced, cooked	13	0.309	0.050	2.97	8.7	0.176	0.010	0.016	0.992	0
Carrots—frozen, cooked	10	0.338	0.031	2.34	8.2	0.136	0.008	0.010	1.050	0
Carrots—canned, drained	7	0.183	0.054	1.57	7.4	0.181	0.005	0.009	0.435	0
Carrot juice	11	0.267	0.041	2.63	6.7	0.130	0.026	0.015	0.385	0
Cauliflower—raw	7	0.561	0.051	1.39	7.9	0.164	0.022	0.016	0.720	0
Cauliflower—cooked	7	0.530	0.050	1.31	7.8	0.119	0.018	0.018	0.622	0
Cauliflower—frozen, cooked	5	0.457	0.061	1.06	4.9	0.116	0.010	0.015	0.535	0
Celery—raw—chopped	5	0.189	0.033	1.03	10.4	0.137	0.009	0.009	0.472	0
Swiss chard—raw	5	0.510	0.057	1.06	14.5	0.510	0.011	0.025	0.512	0
Swiss chard—cooked	6	0.533	0.023	1.17	16.5	0.642	0.010	0.024	0.616	0
Collards—fresh	5	0.445	0.062	1.07	33.0	0.299	0.009	0.018	0.590	0
Collards—fresh, cooked	4	0.313	0.043	0.75	22.0	0.116	0.005	0.012	0.798	0
Collards—frozen, cooked	10	0.840	0.115	2.02	59.5	0.317	0.013	0.033	0.794	0
Corn—kernels raw	24	0.913	0.335	5.38	0.6	0.147	0.057	0.017	1.220	0
Corn on the cob—cooked	31	0.943	0.363	7.14	0.6	0.173	0.061	0.020	1.190	0
Corn—cooked from frozen	23	0.857	0.020	5.80	0.6	0.085	0.020	0.020	1.190	0
Corn—canned, drained	23	0.743	0.283	5.26	1.4	0.142	0.009	0.014	0.398	0
Corn—canned cream style	21	0.494	0.119	5.14	0.9	0.108	0.007	0.015	0.354	0
Cucumber slices w/peel	4	0.153	0.037	0.82	4.0	0.079	0.009	0.006	0.329	0
Eggplant—cooked	8	0.236	0.066	1.88	1.7	0.099	0.022	0.006	1.060	0
Escarole/curly endive—chopped	5	0.354	0.057	0.95	14.7	0.235	0.023	0.022	0.369	0
Garbanzo/chickpeas—dry	103	5.470	1.720	17.20	29.9	1.770	0.135	0.060	5.390	0

(continued)

VEGETABLES (continued)

	kcal	Protein (g)	Lipid (g)	CHO (g)	Ca (mg)	Fe (mg)	B_1 (mg)	B_2 (mg)	Fiber (g)	Cholesterol (mg)
Garbanzo/chickpeas—cooked	47	2.500	0.735	7.78	13.8	0.819	0.033	0.018	1.920	0
Jerusalem artichoke—raw	22	0.567	0.004	4.95	4.0	0.964	0.057	0.017	0.369	0
Kale—fresh, chopped	14	0.935	0.198	2.84	38.0	0.482	0.031	0.037	1.650	0
Kohlrabi—raw slices	8	0.482	0.028	1.76	6.9	0.113	0.014	0.006	0.405	0
Kohlrabi—cooked	8	0.510	0.030	1.96	7.0	0.113	0.011	0.006	0.395	0
Leeks—chopped raw	17	0.425	0.085	4.00	16.7	0.594	0.017	0.008	0.668	0
Leeks—cooked, chopped	9	0.230	0.057	2.16	8.5	0.310	0.007	0.006	0.927	0
Lentils—dry	96	7.960	0.273	16.20	14.6	2.550	0.135	0.069	3.400	0
Lentils—cooked from dry	33	2.560	0.106	5.73	5.3	0.944	0.048	0.020	1.430	0
Lentils—sprouted, raw	30	2.540	0.156	6.30	7.0	0.909	0.065	0.036	1.150	0
Lettuce—butterhead	4	0.367	0.062	0.66	9.5	0.085	0.017	0.017	0.397	0
Lettuce—iceberg	4	0.286	0.054	0.59	5.4	0.142	0.013	0.009	0.347	0
Lettuce—romaine	5	0.459	0.057	0.67	10.2	0.312	0.028	0.028	0.482	0
Mushrooms—raw sliced	7	0.593	0.119	1.32	1.4	0.352	0.029	0.127	0.508	0
Mushrooms—cooked	8	0.614	0.134	1.46	1.7	0.494	0.020	0.085	0.625	0
Mushrooms—canned, drained	7	0.530	0.082	1.40	3.1	0.224	0.017	0.063	0.596	0
Mustard greens—fresh	7	0.764	0.057	1.39	29.4	0.414	0.023	0.031	0.764	0
Mustard greens—cooked	4	0.640	0.068	0.60	21.0	0.316	0.012	0.018	0.587	0
Okra pods—cooked	9	0.530	0.048	2.04	17.9	0.128	0.037	0.016	0.624	0
Okra slices—cooked	11	0.589	0.085	2.32	27.1	0.190	0.028	0.035	0.709	0
Onions—chopped, raw	10	0.335	0.074	2.07	7.1	0.105	0.017	0.003	0.454	0
Onion slices—raw	10	0.335	0.074	2.08	7.2	0.105	0.017	0.003	0.454	0
Onion—dehydrated flakes	91	2.530	0.122	23.70	72.9	0.446	0.022	0.018	2.510	0
Onion rings—frozen, heated	115	1.520	7.570	10.80	8.8	0.482	0.079	0.040	0.240	0
Parsley—freeze dried	81	8.910	1.420	11.90	40.5	15.200	0.304	0.648	22.000	0
Parsley—fresh chopped	9	0.624	0.085	1.96	36.9	1.760	0.023	0.031	1.550	0
Parsnips—sliced raw	21	0.341	0.085	5.09	10.0	0.167	0.026	0.014	1.280	0
Fresh peas—uncooked	23	1.530	0.113	4.10	7.0	0.416	0.075	0.037	1.380	0
Peas—cooked	24	1.520	0.060	4.43	7.8	0.438	0.073	0.042	1.360	0
Peas—frozen, cooked	22	1.460	0.078	4.04	6.7	0.443	0.080	0.050	1.280	0
Peas—edible pods—fresh	12	0.794	0.057	2.15	12.1	0.589	0.043	0.023	0.794	0
Split peas—dry	97	6.970	0.328	17.10	15.5	1.250	0.206	0.061	4.030	0
Peas + carrots—frozen, cooked	14	0.875	0.120	2.87	6.4	0.266	0.064	0.020	1.170	0
Green chili pepper—raw	11	0.557	0.057	2.68	5.0	0.340	0.026	0.026	0.504	0
Red chili peppers—raw/chopped	11	0.567	0.057	2.68	4.9	0.340	0.026	0.026	0.454	0
Jalapeno peppers—canned chopped	7	0.225	0.170	1.39	7.5	0.792	0.008	0.014	0.850	0
Baked potato with skin	31	0.653	0.028	7.16	2.8	0.386	0.030	0.009	0.660	0
Baked potato—flesh only	26	0.556	0.029	6.10	1.5	0.100	0.030	0.006	0.436	0
Potato skin—oven baked	56	1.220	0.029	13.20	9.8	1.080	0.035	0.034	1.130	0
Potato + peel—microwaved	30	0.692	0.028	6.83	3.1	0.350	0.034	0.009	0.660	0
Peeled potato—boiled	24	0.485	0.029	5.67	2.1	0.088	0.028	0.005	0.426	0
French fries—oven heated	63	0.980	2.480	9.64	2.3	0.380	0.035	0.009	0.567	0
French fries—frozen—vegetable oil	90	1.140	4.690	11.20	5.7	0.215	0.050	0.008	0.567	0
Cottage-fried potatoes	62	0.975	2.320	9.64	2.8	0.425	0.034	0.009	0.567	0
Hash-brown potatoes	30	0.343	1.980	3.02	1.1	0.115	0.010	0.003	0.567	0

(continued)

VEGETABLES (continued)

	kcal	Protein (g)	Lipid (g)	CHO (g)	Ca (mg)	Fe (mg)	B_1 (mg)	B_2 (mg)	Fiber (g)	Cholesterol (mg)
Mashed potatoes prep/milk	22	0.548	0.166	4.98	7.4	0.077	0.025	0.011	0.405	0.5
Mashed potatoes—milk & margarine	30	0.533	1.200	4.74	7.3	0.074	0.024	0.014	0.405	0.5
Potato pancakes	88	1.730	4.700	9.85	7.8	0.451	0.039	0.035	0.563	34.7
Potatoes au gratin mix	26	0.653	1.170	3.65	23.5	0.090	0.006	0.023	0.487	1.4
Scalloped potatoes—recipe	24	0.813	1.040	3.05	16.2	0.163	0.020	0.026	0.289	3.4
Potato chips	148	1.590	10.000	14.70	7.0	0.339	0.040	0.006	1.360	0
Potato flour	100	2.260	0.226	22.60	9.3	4.880	0.119	0.040	0.317	0
Pumpkin—canned	10	0.311	0.080	2.28	7.4	0.394	0.007	0.015	0.519	0
Red radishes	4	0.170	0.151	1.01	5.7	0.082	0.001	0.013	0.624	0
Rutabaga—cooked cubes	10	0.314	0.053	2.19	12.0	0.133	0.020	0.010	0.434	0
Sauerkraut—canned liquid	5	0.258	0.040	1.21	8.7	0.417	0.006	0.006	0.529	0
Soybeans—mature, raw	37	3.700	1.900	3.17	19.4	0.599	0.096	0.033	0.656	0
Spinach—cooked from fresh	7	0.843	0.074	1.06	38.4	1.010	0.027	0.067	0.702	0
Summer squash—raw slices	6	0.334	0.061	1.23	5.7	0.130	0.018	0.010	0.425	0
Zucchini squash—cooked	5	0.181	0.014	1.11	3.6	0.099	0.012	0.012	0.567	0
Acorn squash—boiled/mashed	10	0.190	0.023	2.49	7.5	0.159	0.028	0.002	0.680	0
Butternut squash/baked—cube	12	0.256	0.026	2.97	11.6	0.170	0.020	0.005	0.794	0
Spaghetti squash—baked/boiled	8	0.187	0.073	1.83	6.0	0.095	0.010	0.006	0.794	0
Winter squash—boiled	10	0.319	0.050	2.40	5.2	0.136	0.018	0.006	0.794	0
Sweet potato—baked in skin	29	0.487	0.032	6.89	8.0	0.129	0.020	0.036	0.850	0
Candied sweet potatoes	39	0.246	0.920	7.91	7.3	0.324	0.005	0.012	0.545	0
Tofu (soybean curd)	22	2.290	1.360	0.53	29.7	1.520	0.023	0.015	0.343	0
Tomato—fresh whole	6	0.251	0.060	1.23	2.1	0.136	0.017	0.014	0.415	0
Tomatoes—whole canned	6	0.265	0.070	1.22	7.4	0.171	0.013	0.009	0.298	0
Tomato sauce—canned	9	0.376	0.047	2.04	3.9	0.218	0.019	0.016	0.425	0
Tomato paste—canned	24	1.070	0.249	5.33	9.9	0.848	0.044	0.054	1.210	0
Tomato juice—canned	5	0.215	0.017	1.20	2.6	0.164	0.013	0.009	0.220	0
Turnip cubes—raw	8	0.255	0.028	1.76	8.5	0.085	0.011	0.009	0.587	0
Mixed vegetables—frozen, cooked	17	0.812	0.043	3.70	7.2	0.232	0.020	0.034	1.120	0
Vegetable juice cocktail	6	0.178	0.026	1.29	3.1	0.119	0.012	0.008	0.178	0
Water chestnuts—raw	30	0.398	0.027	6.77	3.2	0.170	0.040	0.057	0.869	0
Watercress—fresh	3	0.650	0.033	0.37	33.4	0.050	0.025	0.033	0.719	0
White yams—raw	34	0.438	0.049	7.90	8.7	0.153	0.032	0.009	0.822	0

SALAD BAR

	kcal	Protein (g)	Lipid (g)	CHO (g)	Ca (mg)	Fe (mg)	B_1 (mg)	B_2 (mg)	Fiber (g)	Cholesterol (mg)
Alfalfa sprouts	8.59	1.130	0.196	1.070	9.45	0.272	0.021	0.036	1.030	0
Artichoke hearts, marinated	28.00	0.680	2.250	2.180	6.50	0.270	0.010	0.029	1.780	0
Asparagus	6.35	0.867	0.062	1.050	6.35	0.193	0.032	0.035	0.432	0
Avocado	45.70	0.563	4.340	2.100	3.07	0.284	0.030	0.035	2.720	0
Bacon, regular	163.00	8.640	14.000	0.164	2.98	0.482	0.195	0.080	0	23.9
Bean sprouts	8.50	0.861	0.050	1.680	3.82	0.258	0.024	0.035	0.7365	0

(continued)

SALAD BAR (continued)

	kcal	Protein (g)	Lipid (g)	CHO (g)	Ca (mg)	Fe (mg)	B_1 (mg)	B_2 (mg)	Fiber (g)	Cholesterol (mg)
Beets	8.67	0.300	0.013	1.900	3.00	0.176	0.009	0.004	0.567	0
Beets, canned, diced	9.00	0.260	0.040	2.040	4.34	0.517	0.003	0.012	0.590	0
Broccoli, raw	7.73	0.844	0.097	1.490	13.50	0.251	0.019	0.034	0.934	0
Cabbage	6.48	0.340	0.049	1.520	13.00	0.162	0.015	0.009	0.680	0
Cabbage, red	7.70	0.393	0.073	1.740	14.60	0.142	0.018	0.009	0.648	0
Carrots, grated	12.40	0.289	0.052	2.880	7.73	0.142	0.027	0.016	0.907	0
Cauliflower	6.80	0.561	0.051	1.390	7.94	0.164	0.022	0.016	0.720	0
Celery	4.54	0.189	0.030	1.030	10.40	0.137	0.009	0.009	0.472	0
Chicken salad	96.70	3.820	8.900	0.469	5.92	0.239	0.012	0.028	0.109	17.3
Crab, cooked	23.90	5.050	0.561	0.140	12.90	0.104	0.012	0.044	0	18.0
Croutons, dry bread cubes	105.00	3.690	1.040	20.500	35.00	1.020	0.099	0.099	0.085	0
Cucumber slices	3.69	0.153	0.037	0.824	3.99	0.079	0.009	0.006	0.329	0
Egg, chopped	40.40	3.520	2.790	0.338	13.80	0.475	0.014	0.133	0	113
Escarole/curly endive	4.82	0.354	0.057	0.953	14.70	0.235	0.023	0.022	0.369	0
Garbanzo/chickpeas, cooked	46.50	2.500	0.735	7.780	13.80	0.819	0.033	0.018	1.920	0
Green pepper, sweet	6.80	0.244	0.130	1.500	1.70	0.357	0.024	0.014	0.454	0
Ham salad	51.50	5.000	3.000	0.880	2.00	0.280	0.244	0.072	0	16
Ham, minced	74.20	4.620	5.860	0.526	2.70	0.216	0.203	0.054	0	20.2
Leeks	17.30	0.425	0.085	4.000	16.70	0.594	0.017	0.008	0.688	0
Lettuce, butterhead	3.69	0.366	0.062	0.658	9.47	0.085	0.017	0.017	0.370	0
Lettuce, iceberg	3.69	0.287	0.054	0.592	5.37	0.142	0.013	0.009	0.370	0
Lettuce, loose leaf	5.11	0.369	0.085	0.992	19.20	0.397	0.014	0.023	0.391	0
Lettuce, Romaine	4.54	0.459	0.057	0.673	10.20	0.312	0.028	0.028	0.482	0
Lobster meat	27.80	5.800	0.168	0.364	17.20	0.111	0.020	0.019	0	20.3
Mushrooms, raw	7.09	0.593	0.119	1.320	1.42	0.352	0.029	0.127	0.508	0
Onions	9.57	0.335	0.074	2.070	7.09	0.105	0.017	0.003	0.454	0
Parmesan cheese, grated	129.00	11.800	8.500	1.060	389.00	0.270	0.013	0.109	0	22.0
Peas, cooked	22.30	1.460	0.078	4.040	6.73	0.443	0.080	0.050	1.280	0
Sesame seed kernels, dried	167.00	7.480	15.500	2.660	37.20	2.210	0.204	0.024	1.950	0
Shrimp, boiled	28.00	5.930	0.306	0	11.00	0.876	0.009	0.009	0	55.3
Spinach, fresh	6.23	0.810	0.099	0.992	28.00	0.770	0.022	0.054	0.947	0
Sunflower seeds, dry	162.00	6.460	14.000	5.320	32.90	1.920	0.650	0.070	1.970	0
Tomatoes	5.51	0.252	0.061	1.230	1.89	0.135	0.017	0.014	0.416	0
Tuna salad	53.00	4.550	2.630	2.670	4.84	0.282	0.009	0.019	0.340	3.73
Turkey meat	41.30	5.270	2.030	0.149	11.40	0.358	0.025	0.064	0	11.9

VARIETY

	kcal	Protein (g)	Lipid (g)	CHO (g)	Ca (mg)	Fe (mg)	B_1 (mg)	B_2 (mg)	Fiber (g)	Cholesterol (mg)
Chips & crackers										
Doritos—nacho flavor	139	2.20	6.79	18.00	17.0	0.399	0.040	0.030	1.10	0
Doritos—taco flavor	140	2.60	6.59	17.60	44.9	0.699	0.080	0.090	1.10	0
Potato chips—sour cream & onion	153	2.40	9.48	14.60	21.0	0.474	0.040	0.055	1.35	1.0
Wheat cracker—thin	124	3.19	4.96	17.70	10.6	1.060	0.142	0.106	1.84	0
Whole wheat crackers	124	3.19	5.32	17.70	10.6	1.850	0.070	0.106	2.94	0

(continued)

VARIETY (continued)

	kcal	Protein (g)	Lipid (g)	CHO (g)	Ca (mg)	Fe (mg)	B_1 (mg)	B_2 (mg)	Fiber (g)	Cholesterol (mg)
Condiments										
Catsup	30	0.52	0.11	7.17	6.2	0.228	0.026	0.020	0.45	0
Mustard	21	1.34	1.25	1.81	23.8	0.567	0.024	0.057	0.11	0
Soy sauce	14	1.46	0.02	2.40	4.7	0.567	0.014	0.036	0	0
Deli meats										
Bologna—beef	89	3.32	8.04	0.56	3.7	0.394	0.016	0.036	0	16.0
Bratwurst	92	4.05	7.90	0.84	13.8	0.292	0.070	0.064	0	17.8
Keilbasa sausage	88	3.76	7.70	0.61	12.0	0.414	0.064	0.061	0	18.5
Knockwurst sausage	87	3.37	7.88	0.05	2.9	0.258	0.097	0.040	0	16.3
Liverwurst	93	4.00	8.10	0.63	7.9	1.810	0.077	0.291	0	44.1
Pepperoni sausage	140	5.94	12.50	0.80	2.8	0.397	0.09	0.07		9.79
Polish sausage	92	3.99	8.13	0.46	3.0	0.409	0.142	0.042	0	20.0
Salami—beef	72	4.17	5.69	0.70	2.47	0.567	0.036	0.073	0	17.3
Salami—pork & beef	72	3.94	5.70	0.64	3.68	0.755	0.068	0.106	0	18.5
Salami—turkey	55	4.62	3.89	0.15	5.47	0.463	0.029	0.075	0	22.9
Salami—dry—beef & pork	120	6.49	9.75	0.74	2.84	0.425	0.170	0.082	0	22.7
Turkey pastrami	37	5.22	1.75	0.43	2.49	0.403	0.022	0.075	0	14.9
Mexican foods										
Beef taco	75.2	4.94	4.80	3.67	30.9	0.469	0.01	0.049	0.407	16.2
Beef enchilada	69.0	3.09	3.26	3.69	60.2	0.418	0.017	0.039	0.465	8.93
Cheese enchilada	78.0	3.12	4.2	3.78	108.0	0.324	0.015	0.050	0.465	10.2
Chicken enchilada	63.6	3.38	2.48	3.69	60.5	0.359	0.018	0.036	0.465	9.10
Corn tortilla, enriched, regular	61.4	1.89	0.964	12.30	39.7	0.567	0.047	0.028	2.27	0
Corn torilla, enriched, thin	61.0	1.64	0.95	12.30	39.8	0.567	0.046	0.028	2.26	0
Corn tortilla, fried	82.2	2.08	2.84	12.30	39.7	0.567	0.047	0.028	2.27	0
Enchirito	60.4	3.15	2.75	3.31	51.5	0.410	0.015	0.037	0.748	9.18
Flour tortilla	84	2.07	2.15	15.50	17.0	0.440	0.102	0.062	0.800	0
Retried beans, canned	30.3	1.77	0.303	5.24	13.2	0.500	0.014	0.016	2.47	0
Nuts & seeds										
Almonds—dried, chopped	167	5.65	14.80	5.78	75.5	1.040	0.060	0.220	3.36	0
Almonds—whole toasted	167	5.77	14.40	6.48	80.0	1.400	0.037	0.170	3.99	0
Sunflower seeds—dry	162	6.46	14.00	5.32	32.9	1.920	0.650	0.070	1.97	0
Oils & shortening										
Cocoa butter oil	251	0	28.40	0	0	0	0	0	0	0
Corn oil	251	0	28.40	0	0	0.001	0	0	0	0
Cottonseed oil	251	0	28.40	0	0	0	0	0	0	0
Olive oil	251	0	28.40	0	0.1	0.109	0	0	0	0
Palm oil	251	0	28.40	0	0.1	0.003	0	0	0	0
Palm kernel oil	251	0	28.40	0	0	0	0	0	0	0
Peanut oil	251	0	28.40	0	0	0.008	0	0	0	0
Safflower oil	251	0	28.40	0	0	0	0	0	0	0
Sesame oil	250	0	28.40	0	0	0	0	0	0	0
Soybean oil	251	0	28.40	0	0	0.007	0	0	0	0
Sunflower oil	251	0	28.40	0	0	0	0	0	0	0
Walnut oil	251	0	28.40	0	0	0	0	0	0	0
Wheat germ oil	250	0	28.40	0	0	0	0	0	0	0
Vegetable shortening	251	0	28.40	0	0	0	0	0	0	0

(continued)

VARIETY (continued)

	kcal	Protein (g)	Lipid (g)	CHO (g)	Ca (mg)	Fe (mg)	B_1 (mg)	B_2 (mg)	Fiber (g)	Cholesterol (mg)
Pasta & noodles										
Spaghetti, cooked firm, hot	41	1.42	0.142	8.53	3.1	0.454	0.051	0.028	0.482	0
Spaghetti, cooked tender, hot	31	1.01	0.111	6.48	3.0	0.405	0.04	0.022	0.425	0
Whole wheat spaghetti, cooked	35	1.53	0.113	7.49	4.3	0.244	0.048	0.020	1.040	0
Spaghetti + sauce + cheese, canned	22	0.68	0.227	4.42	4.5	0.318	0.040	0.032	0.284	0.3
Spaghetti + sauce + cheese, homemade	30	1.02	1.02	4.20	9.07	0.260	0.028	0.020	0.284	0.9
Spaghetti + sauce + meat, canned	30	1.36	1.13	4.42	6.01	0.374	0.017	0.020	0.312	2.6
Spaghetti + sauce + meat, homemade	38	2.17	1.37	4.46	14.20	0.423	0.029	0.034	0.314	10.2
Spaghetti sauce, homemade	23	0.77	1.25	2.95	6.70	0.380	0.026	0.017	0.343	0
Spaghetti sauce, canned	31	0.52	1.35	4.52	7.97	0.184	0.016	0.017	0.343	0
Spaghetti meat sauce,	30	1.03	1.30	3.72	4.95	0.385	0.028	0.022	0.193	2.3
Spaghetti sauce, dry, packet	79	1.70	0.28	18.20	48.20	0.765	NA	0.162	0.057	0
Spaghetti sauce + mushrooms, packet	85	2.84	2.55	13.90	113.00	0.510	NA	0.136	0.085	0
Egg noodles, cooked	35	1.17	0.35	6.60	3.19	0.400	0.039	0.023	0.624	8.9
Chow mein noodles, dry	139	3.72	6.93	16.40	8.82	0.252	0.032	0.019	1.100	3.2
Spinach noodles, dry	108	3.97	1.08	20.20	11.60	1.290	0.278	0.133	1.930	0
Spinach noodles, cooked	32	1.13	0.36	5.97	3.37	0.429	0.043	0.027	0.569	0
Chicken + noodles, recipe	43	2.60	2.13	3.07	3.07	0.278	0.006	0.020	0.142	12.2
Chicken + noodles, frozen	32	2.17	1.30	2.49	15.70	0.393	0.009	0.018	0.022	8.0
Noodles-ramen-beef, cooked	28	0.76	0.94	4.17	NA	NA	NA	NA	0.500	NA
Noodles, ramen, chicken, cooked	25	0.76	0.85	3.63	NA	NA	NA	NA	0.512	NA
Noodles, ramen, oriental	26	0.74	1.07	3.83	NA	NA	NA	NA	0.512	NA
Lasagna, frozen entree	38	2.32	1.71	2.61	34.00	0.343	0.026	0.045	0.194	12.4
Pizza										
Pizza—cheese	69	3.54	2.13	9.21	52.00	0.378	0.080	0.069	0.510	13.2
Pizza—mozzarella	80	7.60	4.67	0.89	207.00	0.076	0.006	0.097	0	15.0
Pizza—Canadian bacon	52	6.82	2.36	0.38	3.00	0.229	0.231	0.055	0	16.3
Pizza—pepperoni	140	5.94	12.50	0.81	2.80	0.397	0.090	0.070	0	9.8
Pizza—onion	10	0.34	0.07	2.07	7.10	1.105	0.017	0.003	0.450	0
Popcorn										
Popcorn—plain, air popped	106	3.50	1.42	21.30	3.50	0.709	0.106	0.035	4.600	0
Popcorn—cooked in oil/salted	142	2.32	7.99	15.50	7.70	0.696	0.026	0.052	3.090	0
Popcorn—syrup-coated	109	1.60	0.81	24.30	1.60	0.405	0.106	0.016	0.810	0
Rice										
Brown—dry	102	2.13	0.54	21.90	9.04	0.510	0.096	0.014	0.965	0
Brown—cooked	34	0.709	0.17	7.23	3.40	0.170	0.026	0.006	0.483	0
White—regular, dry	103	1.90	0.11	22.80	6.74	0.828	0.125	0.009	0.340	0
White—regular, cooked	31	0.567	0.03	6.86	2.84	0.397	0.03	0.003	0.102	0
White—converted, dry	105	2.10	0.15	23.00	17.00	0.828	0.124	0.010	0.624	0
White—converted, cooked	30	0.599	0.02	6.60	5.35	0.227	0.03	0.003	0.180	0

(continued)

VARIETY (continued)

	kcal	Protein (g)	Lipid (g)	CHO (g)	Ca (mg)	Fe (mg)	B_1 (mg)	B_2 (mg)	Fiber (g)	Cholesterol (mg)
Rice (continued)										
White—instant, dry	106	2.13	0.06	23.40	1.42	1.300	0.125	0.008	0.737	0
White—instant, prepared	31	0.624	0.03	6.86	0.85	0.227	0.037	0.003	0.216	0
Wild—cooked	26	1.02	0.06	5.39	1.42	0.312	0.031	0.045	0.709	0
Rice bran	78	3.77	5.44	14.40	21.50	5.500	0.64	0.070	6.150	0
Rice polish	75	3.43	3.62	16.40	19.40	4.560	0.521	0.051	0.680	0
Salad dressings										
Blue cheese salad dressing	143	1.37	14.80	2.09	22.90	0.057	0.003	0.028	0.020	7.6
Caesars salad dressing	126	2.66	12.70	0.67	44.40	0.239	0.007	0.025	0.050	33.9
French dressing	150	0.16	16.00	1.81	3.55	0.113	0	0	0.220	0
Italian dressing—low calorie	15	0.02	1.18	1.37	0.59	0.059	0	0	0.080	1.7
Mayonnaise	203	0.31	22.60	0.77	5.67	0.168	0.005	0.012	0	16.8
Imitation mayonnaise	66	0	5.67	3.78	0	0	0	0	0	7.6
Ranch salad dressing	104	0.86	10.70	1.31	28.40	0.075	0.010	0.040	0	11.1
Russian salad dressing	140	0.45	14.50	3.00	5.44	0.174	0.014	0.014	0.080	18.4
1000 island dressing	107	0.26	10.10	4.30	3.52	0.170	0.006	0.009	0.060	7.3
1000 island dressing—low calorie	45	0.22	3.00	4.58	3.12	1.174	0.006	0.008	0.340	3.4
Vinegar & oil dressing	124	0	14.20	0	0	0	0	0	0	0
Salads, prepared										
Chicken salad w/celery	97	3.82	8.90	0.47	5.92	0.239	0.012	0.028	0.110	17.3
Cole slaw	20	0.36	0.74	3.52	12.80	0.166	0.019	0.017	0.570	2.3
Egg salad	68	2.91	6.01	0.45	14.50	0.525	0.019	0.070	0	97.4
Ham salad spread	62	2.46	4.39	3.01	2.24	0.168	0.123	0.034	0.030	10.4
Macaroni salad—no cheese	75	0.54	6.66	3.52	5.50	0.229	0.020	0.014	0.270	4.9
Potato salad w/mayo + eggs	41	0.76	2.32	3.16	5.44	0.185	0.022	0.017	0.420	19.3
Tuna salad	53	4.55	2.53	2.67	4.84	0.282	0.009	0.019	0.340	3.7
Waldorf salad	85	0.72	8.33	2.62	8.82	0.196	0.020	0.013	0.720	4.3
Sandwiches										
Avocado & cheese—white	64	2.02	4.00	5.39	43.1	0.418	0.057	0.059	0.98	4.4
Avocado & cheese—whole wheat	62	2.14	3.97	5.24	37.8	0.477	0.047	0.05	1.76	4.3
BLT —whole wheat	68	2.49	3.77	6.45	11.4	0.570	0.077	0.043	1.55	4.1
BUT—white	70	2.30	3.77	6.70	18.2	0.489	0.092	0.055	0.43	4.2
Grilled cheese—wheat	91	4.22	5.37	7.10	87.4	0.565	0.057	0.076	1.59	11.8
Grilled cheese—part WW	95	4.39	5.82	6.59	103.0	0.526	0.067	0.093	0.61	13.3
Grilled cheese—white	97	4.22	5.79	6.88	103.0	0.441	0.068	0.092	0.30	13.3
Chicken salad—wheat	80	3.00	4.25	8.13	14.7	0.679	0.066	0.046	1.88	6.2
Chicken salad—white	85	2.83	4.63	8.05	22.7	0.552	0.080	0.060	0.39	7.1
Corn dog	84	2.55	5.10	6.97	8.7	0.495	0.072	0.043	0.03	9.5
Corned beef & swiss on rye	83	5.26	4.59	4.90	63.8	0.768	0.044	0.078	0.97	16.4
English muffin (egg/cheese/bacon)	74	3.70	3.70	6.37	40.5	0.637	0.095	0.103	0.32	43.8
Egg salad—wheat	79	2.60	4.56	7.44	17.0	0.744	0.063	0.059	1.67	48.8
Egg salad—soft white	83	2.41	4.90	7.25	24.5	0.636	0.075	0.074	0.30	41.6
Ham—rye bread	59	3.84	2.09	6.10	12.0	0.474	0.182	0.073	1.24	7.1
Ham—whole wheat	59	3.79	2.04	6.84	12.4	0.617	0.164	0.060	1.54	6.1

(continued)

VARIETY (continued)

	kcal	Protein (g)	Lipid (g)	CHO (g)	Ca (mg)	Fe (mg)	B_1 (mg)	B_2 (mg)	Fiber (g)	Cholesterol (mg)
Sandwiches (continued)										
Ham—soft white	61	3.74	2.08	6.60	18.6	0.504	0.186	0.073	0.29	6.7
Ham & swiss—rye	68	4.65	3.23	5.08	63.5	0.389	0.147	0.079	0.99	10.8
Ham & cheese—wheat	67	4.20	3.23	5.72	40.5	0.527	0.136	0.066	1.27	9.7
Ham & cheese—soft white	69	4.20	3.36	5.43	48.0	0.428	0.152	0.078	0.23	10.6
Ham salad—wheat	75	2.45	4.02	7.83	11.5	0.569	0.104	0.045	1.52	5.6
Ham salad—white	78	2.25	4.26	7.71	17.5	0.454	0.119	0.057	0.28	6.2
Hotdog/frankfurter & bun	87	2.80	5.10	7.04	19.6	0.570	0.095	0.062	0.40	7.6
Patty melt—gound beef/ rye	91	5.09	6.07	3.96	36.5	0.533	0.040	0.072	0.81	17.1
Peanut butter & jam—whole wheat	92	3.40	3.85	12.30	15.4	0.751	0.070	0.045	2.29	0
Peanut butter & jam—white	98	3.29	4.14	12.80	23.4	0.632	0.085	0.059	0.85	0
Reuben grilled	58	3.43	3.38	3.53	43.6	0.633	0.030	0.052	0.80	10.4
Roast beef—whole wheat	64	4.00	2.52	6.71	12.3	0.760	0.061	0.054	1.53	6.2
Roast beef—white	67	3.97	2.63	6.46	18.5	0.665	0.072	0.066	0.27	6.9
Tuna salad—wheat	72	3.29	3.29	8.03	13.0	0.667	0.057	0.040	1.74	5.5
Tuna salad—white	76	3.18	3.47	7.92	19.6	0.555	0.068	0.052	0.44	6.2
Turkey—whole wheat	62	4.09	2.33	6.67	11.6	0.554	0.056	0.044	1.53	6.0
Turkey—white	64	4.07	2.42	6.41	17.8	0.435	0.066	0.055	0.27	6.7
Turkey & ham—rye	58	3.74	2.12	6.18	12.3	0.743	0.060	0.079	1.23	8.4
Turkey & ham—whole wheat	59	3.71	2.07	6.90	12.6	0.846	0.060	0.064	1.54	7.2
Turkey & ham—white	60	3.65	2.10	6.67	18.8	0.762	0.071	0.078	0.28	8.0
Turkey & ham & cheese on rye	68	4.22	3.46	5.04	44.2	0.616	0.050	0.083	0.99	12.1
Turkey & ham & cheese—wheat	67	4.14	3.25	5.77	40.5	0.716	0.051	0.070	1.27	10.6
Turkey & ham & cheese—white	69	4.13	3.38	5.48	48.3	0.636	0.059	0.082	0.23	11.6
Sauces										
Bordelaise sauce	24	0.33	1.46	1.10	3.80	0.179	0.008	0.010	0.01	3.8
Hot chili sauce, red pepper	5	0.25	0.17	1.10	2.51	0.137	0.003	0.026	2.29	0
Teriyaki sauce	24	1.69	0.09	4.52	6.30	0.488	0.008	0.020	0	0
Seafood										
Anchovy—raw	37	5.78	1.37	0	41.7	0.921	0.016	0.073	0	19.6
Frog legs—raw meat	21	4.65	0.085	0	5.1	0.539	0.040	0.070	0	14.2
Lobster meat—cooked	28	5.80	0.17	0.36	17.2	0.111	0.020	0.019	0	20.3
Scampi—fried in crumbs	69	6.07	3.49	3.26	19.0	0.357	0.037	0.039	0.04	50.2
Shrimp—boiled	28	5.93	0.31	0	11.0	0.876	0.009	0.009	0	55.3
Squid (calamari)—fried in flour	50	5.10	2.12	2.20	11.0	0.287	0.016	0.130	0	73.7
Soups										
Cream of celery	20	0.38	1.27	2.00	9.04	0.141	0.007	0.011	0.09	3.2
Chicken, chunky	20	1.43	0.75	1.95	2.71	0.195	0.010	0.020	0.03	3.4
Chicken + dumpling	23	1.30	1.28	1.39	3.34	0.144	0.004	0.017	0.10	7.6
Chicken gumbo	13	0.60	0.32	1.89	5.53	0.201	0.006	0.009	0.05	0.9
Chicken-noodle—chunky	14	1.50	0.70	0.24	2.84	0.170	0.009	0.020	0.09	2.1
Chili with beans	32	1.62	1.56	3.38	13.20	0.973	0.014	0.030	0.91	4.8
Clam chowder—New England	19	1.08	0.75	1.90	21.40	0.169	0.008	0.027	0.11	2.5
Minestrone—chunky	15	0.60	0.33	2.45	7.20	0.209	0.006	0.014	0.12	0.6

(continued)

VARIETY (continued)

	kcal	Protein (g)	Lipid (g)	CHO (g)	Ca (mg)	Fe (mg)	B_1 (mg)	B_2 (mg)	Fiber (g)	Cholesterol (mg)
Soups (continued)										
Cream of mushroom	29	0.46	2.15	2.10	7.23	0.119	0.007	0.019	0.06	0.4
Mushroom—barley	14	0.43	0.51	1.69	2.82	0.113	0.006	0.020	0.17	0
Onion—canned	13	0.87	0.40	1.89	6.10	0.156	0.008	0.006	0.11	0
Oyster stew	14	0.49	0.89	0.94	4.96	0.227	0.005	0.008	0	3.1
Pea—prepared w/milk	27	1.40	0.79	3.59	19.30	0.224	0.017	0.030	0.07	2.0
Cream of potato	17	0.39	0.53	2.59	4.52	0.107	0.008	0.008	0.10	1.5
Split pea + ham	22	1.31	0.47	3.17	3.90	0.253	0.014	0.011	0.19	0.8
Tomato—canned	19	0.47	0.43	3.75	3.05	0.396	0.020	0.011	0.11	0
Tomato-beef-noodle	32	1.00	0.97	4.78	3.95	0.252	0.019	0.020	0.03	0.9
Tomato bisque prepared w/milk	22	0.71	0.75	3.32	21.00	0.099	0.013	0.030	0.01	2.5
Turkey—chunky	16	1.23	0.53	1.69	6.00	0.229	0.010	0.029	0.12	1.1
Turkey noodle	16	0.88	0.45	1.95	2.60	0.212	0.017	0.014	0.03	1.1
Cream vegetable—dry mix	126	2.27	6.84	14.80	1.42	0.539	1.470	0.127	0.22	1.2
Vegetable	16	0.49	0.45	2.77	4.96	0.249	0.012	0.010	0.37	0
Miscellaneous										
Garlic cloves	42	1.80	0.14	9.38	51.30	0.482	0.057	0.030	0.47	0
Gelatin salad/desert	17	0.43	0	3.99	0.50	0.024	0.002	0.002	0.02	0
Quiche lorraine	97	2.09	7.73	4.67	34.00	0.226	0.018	0.052	0.09	45.9
Spinach souffle	45	2.29	3.84	0.59	47.90	0.279	0.019	0.064	0.79	38.4

PART 2

Nutritive Values for Alcoholic and Nonalcoholic Beverages

The nutritive values for alcoholic and nonalcoholic beverages are expressed in 1-ounce (28.4-g) portions. We have also included the nutritive values for the minerals calcium, iron, magnesium, phosphorus, and potassium and the vitamins thiamine (B_1), riboflavin (B_2), niacin, and cobalamin (B_{12}). The alcoholic beverages contain no cholesterol or fat.

ALCOHOLIC BEVERAGES (1 OUNCE)

	kcal	Protein (g)	CHO (g)	Minerals					Vitamins			
				Ca (mg)	Fe (mg)	Mg (mg)	P (mg)	K (mg)	B_1 (mg)	B_2 (mg)	Niacin (mg)	B_{12} (mg)
Beer, regular	12	0.072	1.1	1.4	0.009	1.83	3.50	7.09	0.002	0.007	0.128	0.005
Beer, light	8	0.057	0.4	1.4	0.011	1.42	3.44	5.13	0.003	0.008	0.111	0.002
Brandy	69	0	10.6	2.5	0.012		1.01	1.01	0.002	0.002	0.004	0
Champagne	22	0.043	0.6	1.6	0.093	2.40	1.90	22.60	0	0.003	0.019	0
Dessert wine, dry	36	0.057	1.2	2.3	0.068	2.55	2.55	26.20	0.005	0.005	0.060	0
Dessert wine, sweet	44	0.057	3.3	2.3	0.057	2.55	2.64	26.20	0.005	0.005	0.060	0
Gin, rum, vodka, scotch, whiskey, 80 proof	64	0	0	0	0.010	0	0	1.01	0	0	0	0

(continued)

ALCOHOLIC BEVERAGES (1 OUNCE) (continued)

	kcal	Protein (g)	CHO (g)	Minerals Ca (mg)	Fe (mg)	Mg (mg)	P (mg)	K (mg)	Vitamins B$_1$ (mg)	B$_2$ (mg)	Niacin (mg)	B$_{12}$ (mg)
Gin, rum, vodka, scotch, whiskey, 86 proof	71	0	0	0	0.012	0	1.16	0.55	0.002	0.002	0.004	0
Gin, rum, vodka, scotch, whiskey, 90 proof	74	0	0	0	0.010	0	0	0.86	0	0	0	0
Sherry, dry	28	0.024	0.3	2.1	0.052	1.96	2.60	17.80	0.002	0.002	0.024	0
Sherry, medium	40	0.066	2.3	2.3	0.071	2.27	1.89	23.60	0.002	0.008	0.035	0
Vermouth, dry	34	0.028	1.6	2.0	0.096	1.42	1.89	11.30	NA	NA	0.011	0
Vermouth, sweet	44	0.014	4.5	1.7	0.099	1.13	1.65	8.50	NA	NA	0.011	0
Wine, dry white	19	0.029	0.2	2.6	0.093	2.62	1.67	17.40	0	0.001	0.019	0
Wine, medium white	19	0.028	0.2	2.5	0.085	3.03	3.84	22.60	0.001	0.001	0.019	0
Wine, red	20	0.055	0.5	2.2	0.122	3.60	3.84	31.50	0.001	0.008	0.023	0.004
Wine, rosé	20	0.055	0.4	2.4	0.108	2.74	4.08	28.10	0.001	0.004	0.020	0.002
Creme de menthe	105	0	11.8	0	0.023	0	0	0	0	0	0.001	0
Bloody mary	22	0.153	0.9	1.9	0.105	2.10	4.02	41.40	0.010	0.006	0.123	0
Bourbon and soda	26	0	0	1.0	0.244	0.24	0.48	0.48	0	0	0.005	0
Daiquiri	52	0	1.9	0.9	0.043	0.47	1.89	6.14	0.004	0.	0.012	0
Manhattan	64	0	0.9	0.5	0.025	0.01	1.99	7.46	0.003	0.001	0.026	0
Martini	63	0	0.1	0.4	0.024	0.40	0.81	5.26	0	0	0.004	0
Pina colada	53	0.120	8.0	2.2	0.062		2.01	20.10	0.008	0.004	0.033	0
Screwdriver	23	0.160	2.5	2.1	0.023	2.26	3.86	43.30	0.018	0.004	0.046	0
Tequila	31	0.099	2.4	1.7	0.077	1.98	2.80	29.30	0.010	0.005	0.054	0
Tom collins	16	0.013	0.4	1.3	NA	0.38	0.12	2.30	0	0	0.004	0
Whiskey sour	42	0	3.7	0.3	0.021	0.26	1.60	5.08	0.003	0.002	0.006	0
Coffee + cream liqueur	93	0.784	5.9	4.2	0.036	0.60	13.90	9.05	0	0.016	0.022	0
Coffee liqueur	95	0	13.3	0.5	0.016	0.54	1.64	8.18	0.001	0.003	0.040	0

NONALCOHOLIC BEVERAGES (1 OUNCE)

	kcal	Protein (g)	CHO (g)	Minerals Ca (mg)	Fe (mg)	Mg (mg)	P (mg)	K (mg)	Vitamins B$_1$ (mg)	B$_2$ (mg)	Niacin (mg)	B$_{12}$ (mg)
Hot cocoa with whole milk	25	1.030	2.9	33.8	0.088	6.350	30.60	54.400	0.012	0.049	0.041	0.099
Cocoa mix + water—diet	7	0.561	1.3	13.3	0.110	4.870	19.80	59.800	0.006	0.030	0.024	0
Coffee—brewed	0.2	0.016	0.1	0.5	0.113	1.590	0.32	15.400	0	0.002	0.063	0
Coffee—instant dry powder	1.4	0.016	0.3	0.8	0.019	1.100	2.05	67.70	0	0	0.061	0
Coffee—capuchino	9.2	0.059	1.6	1.0	0.022	1.330	3.84	17.600	0	0	0.048	0
Coffee—Swiss mocha	7.7	0.078	1.3	1.1	0.036	1.360	4.37	17.900	0	0	0.039	0
Coffee whitener—												
nondairy,	38.5	0.284	3.2	2.6	0.009	0.060	18.20	54.1	0	0	0	0
liquid powder	155	1.360	15.6	6.3	0.326	1.200	120.00	230.0	0	0.047	0	0
Cola beverage, regular	12	0	3.0	0.7	0.009	0.230	3.52	0.306	0	0	0	0
Diet cola—w/ aspartame	0	0	0	1.0	0.009	0.319	2.40	0	0.001	0.007	0	0

(continued)

NONALCOHOLIC BEVERAGES (1 OUNCE) (continued)

				Minerals					Vitamins			
	kcal	Protein (g)	CHO (g)	Ca (mg)	Fe (mg)	Mg (mg)	P (mg)	K (mg)	B_1 (mg)	B_2 (mg)	Niacin (mg)	B_{12} (mg)
Club soda	0	0	0	1.4	0.012	0.319	0	0.479	0	0	0	0
Cream soda	15	0	3.8	1.5	0.015	0.229	0	0.306	0	0	0	0
Diet soda-avg assorted	0	0	0.0	1.1	0.011	0.200	3.03	0.559	0	0	0	0
Egg nog—commercial	38	1.080	3.8	36.8	0.057	5.250	31.00	46.900	0.010	0.054	0.030	0.127
Five Alive citrus	13	0.135	3.1	1.7	0.021	1.950	2.70	34.000	0.015	0.003	0.060	0
Fruit flavored soda pop	13	0	3.2	1.1	0.020	0.305	0.15	1.520	0	0	0.002	0
Fruit punch drink—canned	13	0.015	3.4	2.1	0.058	0.610	0.31	7.160	0.006	0.006	0.006	0
Gatorade	5	0	1.3	2.8	NA	NA	0	2.840	NA	NA	NA	0
Ginger ale	10	0.008	2.5	0.9	0.051	0.232	0.08	0.387	0	0	0	0
Grape soda carbonated	12	0	3.2	0.9	0.024	0.305	0	0.229	0	0	0	0
Kool-Aid w/ NutraSweet	0	0	0	0	0	0.028	0	0	0	0	0	0
Kool-Aid w/sugar added	12	0	3.0	0	0	0	0	0	0	0	0	0
Lemon-lime soda	12	0	3.0	0.7	0.019	0.154	0.08	0.308	0	0	0.004	0
Lemonade drink from dry	11	0	2.9	7.6	0.016	0.322	3.65	3.540	0	0	0.004	0
Lemonade frozen conc	51	0.078	13.3	1.9	0.205	1.420	2.46	19.200	0.007	0.027	0.020	0
Limeade frozen conc	53	0.052	14.0	1.4	0.029	7.800	1.69	16.800	0.003	0.003	0.028	0
Chocolate milkshake	36	0.962	5.8	32.0	0.088	4.700	28.90	56.800	0.016	0.069	0.046	0.097
Strawberry milkshake	32	0.952	5.4	32.0	0.030	3.600	28.40	51.700	0.013	0.055	0.050	0.088
Vanilla milkshake	32	0.982	5.1	34.5	0.026	3.500	29.00	49.300	0.013	0.052	0.052	0.101
Orange drink/ carbonated	14	0	3.5	1.5	0.018	0.305	0.31	0.686	0	0	0	0
Pepper-type soda	12	0	2.9	0.9	0.010	0.077	3.16	0.154	0	0	0	0
Root beer	12	0.008	3.0	1.5	0.014	0.306	0.15	0.230	0	0	0	0
Pineapple grapefruit drink	13	0.068	3.3	2.0	0.087	1.700	1.59	17.500	0.009	0.005	0.076	0
Pineapple orange drink	14	0.352	3.3	1.5	0.076	1.590	1.13	13.200	0.009	0.005	0.059	0
Tang orange juice crystals	13	0.170	0.06	3.1	4.57	0.002	0.02	0.008	0	0	0	0
Tonic water/Quinine water	10	0	2.5	0.4	0.019	0.077	0	0.077	0	0	0	0
Tea-brewed	0	0.001	0.1	0	0.006	0.796	0.16	10.500	0	0.004	0.012	0
Herbal tea, brewed	0	0	0	0.6	0.022	0.319	0	2.390	0.003	0.001	0	0
Perrier water	0	0	0	3.8	0	0.148	0	0	0	0	0	0
Poland Springs bottled water	0	0	0	0.4	0.001	0.239	0	0	0	0	0	0

Note: Alcoholic beverages contain no fat or cholesterol; light beer contains 0.5 g fiber and regular beer contains 1.2 g fiber per 8 oz. serving. All of the other nonmixed alcoholic beverages have no fiber.

Note: Other nonalcoholic beverages are listed in the sections on fruits and vegetables.

PART 3

Nutritive Values For Specialty and Fast-Food Items

Nutrient information was kindly provided by the manufacturer or its representative, and is reproduced from their literature. Unlike Parts 1 and 2, nutritive values are not given for 1-ounce portions but for actual amounts of the foods sold commercially. To make a direct comparison of the kcal values and the various nutrients, we recommend that the weight of the food and its nutrients be expressed relative to 1-ounce (28.4-g) portions.

Arby's

Market Fresh™ Salads	Serving Weight (g)	kcal	kcals from fat	Fat – Total (g)	Saturated Fat (g)	Trans Fat (g)	Cholesterol (mg)	Sodium (mg)	Total CHO (g)	Dietary Fiber (g)	Sugars (g)	Proteins (g)
Light Buttermilk Ranch Dressing	64	112	57	6	1	0.14	1	472	13	1	5	1
Almonds, Toasted Sliced	14	81	76	8	1	0.01	0	0	2	1	0	4
Buttermilk Ranch Dressing	64	325	304	34	5	0.67	28	657	4	0	2	1
Chicken Club Salad	366	487	229	25	8	0.5	178	1220	31	4	3	32
Garlic & Cheese Croutons	14	77	42	5	1	0.05	1	116	7	0	0	2
Martha's Vineyard Salad™	330	277	71	8	4	0	72	451	24	4	17	26
Raspberry Vinaigrette	64	194	123	14	2	0	0	387	18	0	16	0
Southwest Ranch Dressing	64	296	279	31	5	0	21	692	4	0	1	1
Santa Fe Salad™	365	477	189	21	6	0.5	53	1131	42	6	6	29
Santa Fe Salad™ w/ Grilled Chicken	350	283	77	9	4	0	72	521	21	6	8	29
Tortilla Strips	14	71	27	3	0	0	0	25	9	1	0	1

Market Fresh™ Sandwiches & Wraps	Serving Weight (g)	kcal	kcals from fat	Fat – Total (g)	Saturated Fat (g)	Trans Fat (g)	Cholesterol (mg)	Sodium (mg)	Total CHO (g)	Dietary Fiber (g)	Sugars (g)	Proteins (g)
Corned Beef Reuben Wrap	280	577	264	29	8	0.5	83	1721	42	1	6	38
Roast Turkey Reuben Wrap	280	581	241	27	6	0	94	1301	43	1	6	48
Roast Ham & Swiss Sandwich	359	705	279	31	8	0.5	63	2103	75	5	19	36
Chicken Salad w/ Pecans Sandwich	322	769	351	39	10	0	74	1240	79	9	17	30
Chicken Salad w/ Pecans Wrap	277	638	342	38	10	1	74	1199	48	8	3	30
Corned Beef Reuben Sandwich	309	606	293	33	9	0.5	83	1849	55	3	6	34
Roast Beef & Swiss Sandwich	339	777	372	41	13	1.5	89	1743	73	5	16	37
Roast Turkey & Swiss Sandwich	359	725	270	30	8	0.5	91	1788	75	5	17	45
Roast Turkey Ranch & Bacon Sandwich	382	834	341	38	11	0.5	109	2258	75	5	17	49
Roast Turkey Ranch & Bacon Wrap	317	700	332	37	11	1	109	2215	44	4	3	49
Roast Turkey Reuben Sandwich	309	611	270	30	8	0.5	94	1429	56	3	6	44
Southwest Chicken Wrap	254	567	265	29	9	1	88	1451	42	4	3	36
Ultimate BLT Sandwich	294	779	407	45	11	0.5	51	1571	75	6	18	23
Ultimate BLT Wrap	249	648	398	44	11	1	51	1530	45	5	4	23

(continued)

Shakes & Desserts	Serving Weight (g)	kcal	kcals from fat	Fat – Total (g)	Saturated Fat (g)	Trans Fat (g)	Cholesterol (mg)	Sodium (mg)	Total CHO (g)	Dietary Fiber (g)	Sugars (g)	Proteins (g)
Strawberry Banana Swirl Shake	482	567	140	16	9	0.5	39	425	87	0	79	15
Apple Turnover	128	377	146	16	5	6.5	0	201	65	2	41	4
Cherry Turnover	128	377	137	15	5	6	0	201	65	2	41	4
Chocolate Chip Cookie	45	202	89	10	4	2	15	213	26	1	16	2
Chocolate Shake – Large	510	660	154	17	10	0.5	43	455	110	1	106	17
Chocolate Shake – Regular	397	507	121	13	8	0	34	357	83	0	81	13
Jamocha Shake – Large	510	647	154	17	10	0.5	43	509	107	1	102	17
Jamocha Shake – Regular	397	498	121	13	8	0	34	393	81	0	78	13
Strawberry Shake – Large	510	646	154	17	10	0.5	43	464	107	1	101	16
Strawberry Shake – Regular	397	498	121	13	8	0	34	363	81	0	77	13
Vanilla Shake – Large	468	555	154	17	10	0.5	43	445	83	0	82	16
Vanilla Shake – Regular	369	437	121	13	8	0	34	350	66	0	65	13

Arby's Chicken Naturals®	Serving Weight (g)	kcal	kcals from fat	Fat – Total (g)	Saturated Fat (g)	Trans Fat (g)	Cholesterol (mg)	Sodium (mg)	Total CHO (g)	Dietary Fiber (g)	Sugars (g)	Proteins (g)
Popcorn Chicken – Large	184	531	233	26	6	1	59	1666	39	3	0	35
Popcorn Chicken Shakers™	240	585	239	27	6	1	59	2795	51	3	9	36
Popcorn Chicken – Regular	126	365	160	18	4	0.5	40	1145	27	2	0	24
BBQ Dipping Sauce	28	44	1	0	0	0	0	343	11	0	8	0
Buffalo Dipping Sauce	28	10	5	1	0	0	0	790	2	0	1	0
Chicken Bacon & Swiss – Crispy	214	624	264	29	7	0	68	1320	52	2	13	36
Chicken Bacon & Swiss – Grilled	209	462	151	17	4	0	25	1333	38	2	9	38
Chicken Cordon Bleu Sandwich – Crispy	243	650	283	31	6	0.5	74	1548	49	2	11	40
Chicken Cordon Bleu Sandwich – Grilled	238	488	169	19	4	0	32	1561	35	2	7	42
Chicken Fillet Sandwich – Crispy	238	576	266	30	5	0	52	901	50	3	11	30
Chicken Fillet Sandwich – Grilled	233	414	153	17	3	0	9	913	36	3	7	32
Chicken Tenders – 3 piece	131	379	166	18	3	0	42	1188	28	2	0	25
Chicken Tenders – 5 piece	218	630	277	31	5	0	70	1977	47	3	0	42
Honey Mustard Dipping	28	129	106	12	2	0	9	151	6	0	5	0

Arby's® Toasted Subs	Serving Weight (g)	kcal	kcals from fat	Fat – Total (g)	Saturated Fat (g)	Trans Fat (g)	Cholesterol (mg)	Sodium (mg)	Total CHO (g)	Dietary Fiber (g)	Sugars (g)	Proteins (g)
Classic Italian Toasted Sub	379	828	410	46	13	0.5	89	2496	69	3	5	37
French Dip & Swiss Toasted Sub	337	622	180	20	7	1.5	79	3397	68	3	2	37
Philly Beef Toasted Sub	281	739	331	37	9	1	85	1881	64	3	4	32
Turkey Bacon Club Toasted Sub	341	619	159	18	4	0	82	2052	65	3	4	42

(continued)

Sides & Sidekickers®	Serving Weight (g)	kcal	kcals from fat	Fat – Total (g)	Saturated Fat (g)	Trans Fat (g)	Cholesterol (mg)	Sodium (mg)	Total CHO (g)	Dietary Fiber (g)	Sugars (g)	Proteins (g)
Mozzarella Sticks – Regular (4)	137	426	254	28	13	1	45	1370	38	2	5	18
Bronco Berry Dipping Sauce®	57	122	0	0	0	0	0	36	30	0	28	0
Cheddar Fries – Medium	170	465	253	28	6	2	2	1311	51	5	0	6
Cheddar Cheese Sauce – side	21	30	18	2	1	0.5	1	181	2	0	0	0
Cool Ranch Sour Cream Dipping Sauce	43	158	142	16	4	0	0	277	2	0	1	1
Curly Fries – Large	198	631	337	37	7	1	0	1476	73	7	0	8
Curly Fries – Medium	125	397	212	24	4	0	0	928	46	4	0	5
Curly Fries – Small	106	338	181	20	4	0	0	791	39	4	0	4
Homestyle Fries – Large	213	566	331	37	7	1	0	1029	82	6	1	6
Homestyle Fries – Medium	142	377	221	25	4	0.5	0	686	55	4	1	4
Homestyle Fries	142	377	221	25	4	0.67	0	686	55	4	1	4
Homestyle Fries – Small	113	302	177	20	4	0.5	0	549	44	3	1	3
Jalapeno Bites® – Large (10)	220	611	383	43	18	1.5	56	1052	58	4	5	11
Jalapeno Bites® – Regular (5)	110	305	191	21	9	1	28	526	29	2	3	5
Ketchup Packet	14	13	0	0	0	0	0	158	3	0	3	0
Loaded Potato Bites® – Large (10)	224	707	398	44	14	1.5	27	1601	54	5	0	23
Loaded Potato Bites® – Reg (5)	112	353	199	22	7	0.5	13	800	27	2	0	11
Mozzarella Sticks – Large (8)	273	849	507	56	26	2	90	2730	75	4	9	36
Onion Petals – Large	283	828	511	57	9	1	2	831	88	5	18	10
Onion Petals – Regular	113	331	205	23	4	0	1	332	35	2	7	4
Potato Cakes (2)	100	246	166	18	4	1	0	391	26	2	0	2
Potato Cakes (3)	150	369	249	28	5	1.5	0	587	39	3	0	3
Tangy Southwest Sauce®	57	333	312	35	5	0.5	29	371	5	0	4	1

Other	Serving Weight (g)	kcal	kcals from fat	Fat – Total (g)	Saturated Fat (g)	Trans Fat (g)	Cholesterol (mg)	Sodium (mg)	Total CHO (g)	Dietary Fiber (g)	Sugars (g)	Proteins (g)
Spicy Cajun Fish Sandwich	246	603	287	32	7	0	68	883	61	3	9	21
Fish Sandwich	239	543	225	25	6	0	55	956	61	3	9	21

Arby's® Roast Beef Sandwiches & Melts	Serving Weight (g)	kcal	kcals from fat	Fat – Total (g)	Saturated Fat (g)	Trans Fat (g)	Cholesterol (mg)	Sodium (mg)	Total CHO (g)	Dietary Fiber (g)	Sugars (g)	Proteins (g)
Kids Meal – Junior Roast Beef Sandwich	125	272	92	10	4	0	29	740	34	2	5	16
Arby's Melt	146	302	110	12	4	1	30	921	36	2	5	16
Arby's Sauce	14	15	1	0	0	0	0	177	4	0	1	0
Bacon Beef 'n Cheddar Sandwich	212	521	239	27	9	1.5	64	1573	45	2	9	27

(continued)

Arby's® Roast Beef Sandwiches & Melts	Serving Weight (g)	kcal	kcals from fat	Fat – Total (g)	Saturated Fat (g)	Trans Fat (g)	Cholesterol (mg)	Sodium (mg)	Total CHO (g)	Dietary Fiber (g)	Sugars (g)	Proteins (g)
BBQ Bacon 'n Jack 2for	169	360	141	16	5	0.5	38	1175	42	2	10	19
Beef 'n Cheddar Sandwich	195	445	185	21	6	1.5	51	1274	44	2	8	22
French Dip & Swiss Sandwich	224	473	160	18	7	1	79	1679	38	3	2	32
Ham & Swiss Melt Sandwich	138	275	51	6	2	0	27	1118	35	1	6	18
Horsey Sauce	14	62	45	5	1	0	5	173	3	0	1	0
Large Roast Beef Sandwich	281	547	256	28	12	1.5	102	1869	41	3	6	42
Medium Roast Beef Sandwich	210	415	186	21	9	1	73	1379	34	2	5	31
Regular Roast Beef	154	320	123	14	5	0.5	44	953	34	2	5	21
Mayonnaise Packet	14	105	103	11	2	0	9	74	0	0	0	0
Sourdough Ham Melt	165	380	118	13	3	0	31	1280	39	2	5	19
Sourdough Roast Beef Melt	166	355	126	14	5	1	30	1047	40	2	4	18
Super Roast Beef	198	398	174	19	6	0.5	44	1060	40	2	10	21
Swiss Melt	146	303	111	12	4	1	29	919	37	2	6	16
SpicyThree Pepper Sauce®	14	22	8	1	0	0	0	140	3	0	3	0

Kids Meal	Serving Weight (g)	kcal	kcals from fat	Fat – Total (g)	Saturated Fat (g)	Trans Fat (g)	Cholesterol (mg)	Sodium (mg)	Total CHO (g)	Dietary Fiber (g)	Sugars (g)	Proteins (g)
Kids Meal – Junior Roast Beef Sandwich	125	272	92	10	4	0	29	740	34	2	5	16
Fruit Cup	57	35	2	0	0	0	0	0	9	1	8	0
Market Fresh™Mini Ham & Cheese Sandwich	112	228	43	5	1	0	23	916	28	2	6	14
Market Fresh™ Mini Turkey & Cheese Sandwich	112	235	40	4	1	0	33	798	28	2	6	17
Kids Meal – Chicken Tenders – 2 piece	100	289	127	14	2	0	32	907	21	1	0	19

Breakfast	Serving Weight (g)	kcal	kcals from fat	Fat – Total (g)	Saturated Fat (g)	Trans Fat (g)	Cholesterol (mg)	Sodium (mg)	Total CHO (g)	Dietary Fiber (g)	Sugars (g)	Proteins (g)
Bacon & Egg Croissant	120	337	195	22	10	0	187	651	23	1	3	11
Bacon Biscuit	95	340	191	21	6	0	13	1028	29	1	3	9
Bacon, Egg & Cheese Biscuit	158	461	251	28	8	0	169	1446	30	1	4	17
Bacon, Egg & Cheese Croissant	133	378	202	22	10	0	198	850	23	1	3	14
Bacon, Egg & Cheese Sourdough	173	437	146	16	5	0	174	1220	40	2	5	20
Bacon, Egg, & Cheese Wrap	193	515	257	29	8	0.5	165	1367	50	2	2	16
Biscuit-Plain	82	273	139	15	4	0	1	786	28	1	3	5
Blueberry Muffin	85	320	108	12	2	0	20	490	49	1	26	4
Breakfast Syrup	28	78	0	0	0	0	0	25	20	0	11	0
Chicken Biscuit	132	417	203	23	5	0	17	1240	39	1	3	15
Croissant	57	190	90	10	6	0	30	190	21	1	2	3
Egg & Cheese Sourdough	164	392	112	12	3	0	166	1058	40	2	5	17
French Toastix	124	312	119	13	2	0	0	492	44	1	11	6
Sausage, Egg & Cheese Biscuit	185	557	340	38	11	0	187	1579	30	1	3	18
Sausage, Egg & Cheese Sourdough	191	514	246	27	8	0	186	1232	40	2	5	19

(continued)

Breakfast (continued)	Serving Weight (g)	kcal	kcals from fat	Fat – Total (g)	Saturated Fat (g)	Trans Fat (g)	Cholesterol (mg)	Sodium (mg)	Total CHO (g)	Dietary Fiber (g)	Sugars (g)	Proteins (g)
Ham & Cheese Croissant	113	274	108	12	7	0	53	842	22	1	3	13
Ham Biscuit	125	316	151	17	4	0	13	1240	29	1	4	13
Ham, Egg & Cheese Biscuit	188	437	211	23	6	0	169	1658	31	1	4	20
Ham, Egg & Cheese Croissant	213	434	216	24	10	0	343	1282	25	1	4	22
Ham, Egg & Cheese Sourdough	296	679	318	35	11	0	354	2104	42	2	6	34
Ham, Egg, & Cheese Wrap	242	568	275	31	10	1	183	1929	51	2	3	24
Sausage & Egg Croissant	147	433	284	32	13	0	206	784	23	1	3	12
Sausage Biscuit	122	436	279	31	9	0	32	1160	28	1	3	10
Sausage Gravy Biscuit	238	961	614	68	14	0	12	3755	107	1	19	7
Sausage Patty	51	210	180	20	7	0	40	480	0	0	0	6
Sausage, Egg & Cheese Croissant	160	475	290	32	13	0	216	982	23	1	3	15
Sausage, Egg & Cheese Wrap	239	689	404	45	15	1	202	1849	50	2	2	21

Burger King

Core Menu Items August 7, 2007

Nutrition: Menu Items	Serving Size (g)	kcal	Total Fat (g)	Saturated Fat (g)	Trans Fat (g)	Cholesterol (mg)	Sodium (mg)	Total CHO (g)	Dietary Fiber (g)	Total Sugars (g)	Protein (9)
Whopper Sandwiches											
WHOPPER® Sandwich	290	670	39	11	1.5	51	1020	51	3	11	28
w/o mayo	269	510	22	9	1	80	880	51	3	11	28
WHOPPER® Sandwich with Cheese	315	760	47	16	1.5	115	1450	52	3	11	33
w/o mayo	294	600	30	14	1.5	100	1310	52	3	11	32
DOUBLE WHOPPER® Sandwich	373	900	57	19	2	175	1090	51	3	11	47
w/o mayo	352	740	39	17	2	160	950	51	3	11	47
DOUBLE WHOPPER® Sandwich w/Cheese	398	990	64	24	2.5	195	1520	52	3	11	52
w/o mayo	376	830	47	22	2	180	1380	52	3	11	52
TRIPLE WHOPPER® Sandwich	456	1130	74	27	3	255	1160	51	3	11	67
w/o mayo	434	980	57	24	2.5	240	1020	51	3	11	66
TRIPLE WHOPPER® Sandwich w/Cheese	480	1230	82	32	3.5	275	1590	52	3	11	71
w/o mayo	459	1070	65	29	3	260	1450	52	3	11	71
WHOPPER JR.® Sandwich	158	370	21	6	0.5	50	570	31	2	6	15
w/o mayo	147	290	12	4.5	0	40	490	31	2	6	15
WHOPPER JR.® Sandwich with Cheese	170	410	24	8	1	60	780	32	2	6	18
w/o mayo	149	330	16	7	0.5	55	710	31	2	6	17
Bacon (1 Strip)	2.5	15	1	0	0	5	50	0	0	0	1
Fire-Grilled Burgers	**Serving Size (g)**	**kcal**	**Total Fat (g)**	**Saturated Fat (g)**	**Trans Fat (g)**	**Cholesterol (mg)**	**Sodium (mg)**	**Total CHO (g)**	**Dietary Fiber (g)**	**Total Sugars (g)**	**Protein (9)**
Hamburger	121	290	12	4.5	0	40	560	30	1	6	15
Cheeseburger	133	330	16	7	0.5	55	780	31	1	6	17
Double Hamburger	164	410	21	9	1	85	600	30	1	6	25
Double Cheeseburger	189	500	29	14	1.5	105	1030	31	1	6	30
Bacon Cheeseburger	138	360	18	8	0.5	60	870	31	1	6	19
Bacon Double Cheeseburger	194	530	31	14	1.5	110	1130	32	1	6	32
BK™ Double Stacker	190	610	39	16	1.5	125	1100	32	1	5	34

BK™ Triple Stacker	250	800	54	23	2	185	1450	33	1	5	48
BK™ Quad Stacker	311	1000	68	30	3	240	1800	34	1	6	62
The Angus Steak Burger	273	640	33	10	1.5	185	1260	55	3	10	33
Chicken, Fish, & Veggie	**Serving Size (g)**	**kcal**	**Total Fat (g)**	**Saturated Fat (g)**	**Trans Fat (g)**	**Cholesterol (mg)**	**Sodium (mg)**	**Total CHO (g)**	**Dietary Fiber (g)**	**Total Sugars (g)**	**Protein (9)**
TENDERGRILL® Chicken Sandwich	258	450	10	2	0	75	1210	53	4	9	37
with Mayo	258	510	19	3.5	0.5	75	1180	49	4	7	37
w/o Sauce	244	400	7	1.5	0	70	1090	49	4	7	36
TENDERCRISP® Chicken Sandwich	313	790	44	8	4	70	1640	68	5	9	33
Original Chicken Sandwich	219	660	40	8	2.5	70	1440	52	4	5	24
w/o Mayo	190	450	17	4	2	50	1250	52	4	5	23
CHICK'N CRISP™ Sandwich	144	480	31	5	2	45	870	36	1	4	15
w/o Mayo	122	320	13	2.5	1.5	30	730	36	1	4	15
CHICKEN TENDERS® Kid's Meal 4 pc	62	170	10	2.5	1.5	25	480	11	0	0	9
CHICKEN TENDERS® 5 pc	77	210	12	3	2	35	600	13	0	0	12
CHICKEN TENDERS® Big Kid's Meal 6 pc	92	250	15	3.5	2.5	40	720	16	0	0	14
CHICKEN TENDERS® 8 pc	123	340	20	5	3	55	960	21	<1	1	19
Barbecue Dipping Sauce (1oz)	28	40	0	0	0	0	310	11	0	10	0
Honey Mustard Dipping Sauce (1 oz)	28	90	6	1	0	10	180	8	0	7	0
Sweet and Sour Dipping Sauce (1 oz)	28	45	0	0	0	0	55	11	0	10	0
Ranch Dipping Sauce (1 oz)	28	140	15	2.5	0	5	95	1	0	1	1
BK™ CHICKEN FRIES 6 pc	85	260	15	3.5	3	35	650	18	2	1	12
9pc	128	390	23	5	4.5	50	980	26	3	1	18
12 pc	170	520	31	7	6	65	1300	35	4	2	25
Buffalo Dipping Sauce (1oz)	28	80	8	1.5	0	5	350	2	0	1	0
BKBIG FISH® Sandwich	249	640	32	6	2.5	65	1450	67	3	9	24
w/o Tartar Sauce	220	470	13	3	2	50	1240	65	3	7	23
BK VEGGIE® Burger**	215	420	16	2.5	0	10	1100	46	7	8	23
w/ Cheese	228	470	20	5	0	20	1320	47	7	9	25
w/o Mayo	205	340	8	1	0	0	1030	46	7	8	23

(continued)

Side Orders	Serving Size (g)	kcal	Total Fat (g)	Saturated Fat (g)	Trans Fat (g)	Cholesterol (mg)	Sodium (mg)	Total CHO (g)	Dietary Fiber (g)	Total Sugars (g)	Protein (g)
MOTT'S® Strawberry Flavored Apple Sauce	113	90	0	0	0	0	0	23	<1	21	0
Onion Rings-Small	43	140	7	1.5	1	0	210	18	2	2	2
Onion Rings-Medium	91	310	15	3.5	2.5	0	440	37	3	4	4
Onion Rings-Large	130	440	22	4.5	4	0	620	53	5	6	6
Onion Rings-King	150	500	25	5	4.5	0	720	62	5	7	7
Zesty Onion Ring Dipping Sauce (1 oz)	28	150	15	2.5	0	15	210	3	<1	2	0
CHEESY TOTS™-Small (6 pc)	77	210	12	4.5	2	20	650	20	2	1	7
CHEESY TOTS™-Medium (9 pc)	115	320	18	7	3	30	970	30	2	2	10
CHEESY TOTS™-Large (12 pc)	153	430	24	9	4	40	1300	40	3	2	14
French Fries-Small (Salted)	74	230	13	3	3	0	380	26	2	1	2
French Fries-Medium (Salted)	116	360	20	4.5	4.5	0	590	41	4	1	4
French Fries-Large (Salted)	160	500	28	6	6	0	820	57	5	1	5
French Fries-King (Salted)	194	600	33	8	7	0	990	69	6	2	6
French Fries-Small (Salt not added	74	230	13	3	3	0	240	26	2	1	2
French Fries-Medium (Salt not added)	116	360	20	4.5	4.5	0	380	41	4	1	4
French Fries-Large (Salt not added)	160	500	28	6	6	0	530	57	5	1	5
French Fries-King (Salt not added)	194	600	33	8	7	0	640	69	6	2	6
Salads (w/out dressing or garlic parmesan croutons)	**Serving Size (g)**	**kcal**	**Total Fat (g)**	**Saturated Fat (g)**	**Trans Fat (g)**	**Cholesterol (mg)**	**Sodium (mg)**	**Total CHO (g)**	**Dietary Fiber (g)**	**Total Sugars (g)**	**Protein (g)**
Side Garden Salad	98	15	0	0	0	0	0	3	1	1	1
TENDERGRILL™ Chicken Garden Salad	292	240	9	3.5	0	80	720	8	4	3	33
TENDERCRISP™ Chicken Garden Salad	306	410	22	6	3.5	70	1080	26	5	5	29
Garden Salad (no chicken)	184	90	5	2.5	0	15	125	7	3	3	5

Salad Dressings & Toppings & Condiments	Serving Size (g)	kcal	Total Fat (g)	Saturated Fat (g)	Trans Fat (g)	Cholesterol (mg)	Sodium (mg)	Total CHO (g)	Dietary Fiber (g)	Total Sugars (g)	Protein (g)
KEN'S® Light Italian Dressing (2 oz)	57	120	11	1.5	0	0	440	5	0	4	0
KEN'S® Ranch Dressing (2oz)	57	190	20	3	0	20	560	2	0	1	1
KEN'S® Creamy Caesar Dressing (2 oz)	57	210	21	4	0	25	610	4	0	3	3
KEN'S® Honey Mustard Dressing (2 oz)	57	270	23	3	0	20	520	15	0	14	1
KEN'S® Fat Free Ranch Dressing (2 oz)	57	60	0	0	0	0	740	15	2	5	0
Salads (w/out dressing or garlic parmesan croutons)	**Serving Size (g)**	**kcal**	**Total Fat (g)**	**Saturated Fat (g)**	**Trans Fat (g)**	**Cholesterol (mg)**	**Sodium (mg)**	**Total CHO (g)**	**Dietary Fiber (g)**	**Total Sugars (g)**	**Protein (g)**
Garlic Parmesan Croutons	14	60	2	0	0	0	120	9	0	1	1
Ketchup (Packet)	10	10	0	0	0	0	125	3	0	2	0
Mayonnaise (Packet)	12	80	9	0.5	0	10	75	1	0	0	0
Dessert	**Serving Size (g)**	**kcal**	**Total Fat (g)**	**Saturated Fat (g)**	**Trans Fat (g)**	**Cholesterol (mg)**	**Sodium (mg)**	**Total CHO (g)**	**Dietary Fiber (g)**	**Total Sugars (g)**	**Protein (g)**
Dutch Apple Pie	108	300	13	3	3	0	270	45	1	23	2
HERSHEY®'S Sundae Pie	79	310	19	12	0	10	220	32	1	22	3
Breakfast	**Serving Size (g)**	**kcal**	**Total Fat (g)**	**Saturated Fat (g)**	**Trans Fat (g)**	**Cholesterol (mg)**	**Sodium (mg)**	**Total CHO (g)**	**Dietary Fiber (g)**	**Total Sugars (g)**	**Protein (g)**
CROISSAN'WICH® Egg & Cheese	115	300	17	6	2	145	740	26	<1	5	12
CROISSAN'WICH® Sausage & Cheese	106	370	25	9	2	50	810	23	<1	4	14
CROISSAN'WICH® Sausage, Egg & Cheese	159	470	32	11	2.5	180	1060	26	<1	5	19
CROISSAN'WICH® Ham, Egg & Cheese	149	340	18	6	2	160	1230	26	1	6	18
CROISSAN'WICH® Bacon, Egg & Cheese	122	340	20	7	2	155	890	26	<1	5	15

(continued)

Breakfast	Serving Size (g)	kcal	Total Fat (g)	Saturated Fat (g)	Trans Fat (g)	Cholesterol (mg)	Sodium (mg)	Total CHO (g)	Dietary Fiber (g)	Total Sugars (g)	Protein (g)
DOUBLE CROISSAN'WICH™ w/ Sausage, Egg, & Cheese	215	680	51	18	3	220	1590	26	1	6	29
DOUBLE CROISSAN'WICH™ w/ Bacon, Egg, & Cheese	142	430	27	10	2	175	1250	27	<1	6	21
DOUBLE CROISSAN'WICH™ w/ Ham, Egg, & Cheese	196	420	23	9	2	185	2210	27	1	7	27
DOUBLE CROISSAN'WICH™ w/ Sausage, Bacon, Egg & Cheese	179	550	39	14	2.5	200	1420	27	1	6	25
DOUBLE CROISSAN'WICH™ w/Ham, Bacon, Egg & Cheese	169	420	24	9	2	180	1600	27	1	7	24
DOUBLE CROISSAN'WICH™ w/ Ham, Sausage, Egg & Cheese	206	550	37	14	2.5	205	2040	27	1	6	28
Enormous Omelet Sandwich	266	730	45	16	1	330	1940	44	2	8	37
Ham Omelet Sandwich	139	330	14	5	0	90	1130	35	1	9	16
Sausage Biscuit	118	390	26	8	5	35	1020	28	1	2	12
Ham, Egg, & Cheese Biscuit	156	390	22	7	5	145	1410	31	1	4	16
Sausage, Egg, & Cheese Biscuit	183	530	37	12	6	175	1490	31	1	4	20
Bacon, Egg & Cheese Biscuit	146	410	25	8	5	150	1320	31	1	4	16
Hash Browns – Small	84	260	17	4.5	5	0	500	25	2	0	2
Hash Browns – Medium	140	430	28	8	9	0	830	42	4	0	4
Hash Browns – Large	202	620	40	11	13	0	1200	60	6	1	5
CHEESY TOTS™ - See Side Orders											

Cini-minis	108	390	18	5	4	20	560	51	2	19	7
Vanilla Icing (for Cini-minis)	28	110	3	0.5	0.5	0	40	21	0	20	0
French Toast Sticks (3 piece)	65	240	13	2.5	2	0	260	26	1	6	4
French Toast Sticks (5 piece)	109	390	22	4.5	3	0	440	43	2	9	7
French Toast Kid's Meal (with syrup)	494	680	24	6	3	10	590	100	3	55	15
Grape Jam	12	30	0	0	0	0	0	7	0	6	0
Strawberry Jam	12	30	0	0	0	0	0	7	0	6	0
Breakfast Syrup	28	80	0	0	0	0	20	21	0	14	0

Footnote for "Saturated Fat (g)": Does Not Include Trans Fat*

Footnote for BK VEGGIE® Burger**: **Burger King Corporation makes no claim that the BK VEGGIE* Burger or any other of its products meets the requirements of a vegan or vegetarian diet.*

The patty is cooked in the microwave.

Footnote for "Salt not added-French Fries": To reduce sodium, you can order French fries without added salt

Carl's Jr.

Charbroiled Burgers	Serving Size (g)	kcal	kcals from fat	Total Fat (g)	Saturated Fat (g)	Cholesterol (mg)	Sodium (mg)	Total CHO (g)	Dietary Fiber (g)	Sugars (g)	Protein (g)
The Original Six Dollar Burger™	430	1010	600	68	27	150	1980	60	3	18	40
The Western Bacon Six Dollar Burger™	382	1130	600	66	28	150	2540	83	4	19	47
The Bacon Cheese Six Dollar Burger™	409	1070	670	76	30	170	1910	50	3	10	46
The Guacamole Bacon Six Dollar Burger™	447	1140	760	85	29	160	2010	54	6	11	43
The Double Six Dollar Burger™	602	1520	990	111	47	265	2760	60	3	18	69
The Low Carb Six Dollar Burger™	267	490	330	37	15	130	1290	6	2	4	33
Famous Star™ with Cheese	278	660	340	39	12	85	1260	53	3	10	27
Super Star® with Cheese	385	930	520	59	21	160	1600	54	3	10	47
Philly Cheesesteak Burger	297	830	480	55	17	125	1510	52	3	9	40
Western Bacon Cheeseburger®	241	710	290	33	12	85	1480	70	3	15	32
Double Western Bacon Cheeseburger™	323	970	470	52	21	155	1820	71	3	15	52
Jalapeño Burger™	286	720	410	45	8	90	1320	50	3	10	27
Big Hamburger	209	470	160	17	6	60	1060	54	3	13	24
Kid's hamburger	195	460	160	17	6	60	1060	53	2	13	24

Chicken & Other Choices	Serving Size (g)	kcal	kcals from fat	Total Fat (g)	Saturated Fat (g)	Cholesterol (mg)	Sodium (mg)	Total CHO (g)	Dietary Fiber (g)	Sugars (g)	Protein (g)
Charbroiled BBQ Chicken™ Sandwich	239	360	40	4.5	1	60	1150	48	4	12	34
Charbroiled Chicken Club™ Sandwich	264	550	210	25	7	95	1410	43	4	9	40
Charbroiled Santa Fe Chicken™ Sandwich	264	610	290	32	8	100	1540	43	4	10	37
Bacon Swiss Crispy Chicken™ Sandwich	318	720	310	35	8	85	1750	64	3	9	35
Chicken Breast Strips (3 pieces)	129	420	220	25	3.5	50	1210	28	1	1	23
Chicken Breast Strips (5 pieces)	215	710	370	41	6	80	2020	46	2	1	38
Spicy Chicken Sandwich	213	560	260	30	6	40	1480	59	2	7	15
Carl's Catch™ Fish Sandwich	291	660	280	31	5	30	1290	75	3	14	22

Sides	Serving Size (g)	kcal	kcals from fat	Total Fat (g)	Saturated Fat (g)	Cholesterol (mg)	Sodium (mg)	Total CHO (g)	Dietary Fiber (g)	Sugars (g)	Protein (g)
French Fries (Kids)	79	250	110	12	2.5	0	150	32	3	0	4
French Fries (Small)	92	290	120	14	3	0	180	37	3	0	5
French Fries (Medium)	147	460	200	22	4.5	0	280	59	5	1	7
French Fries (Large)	198	620	260	29	6	0	380	80	7	1	10
Onion Rings	128	430	190	21	4	0	550	53	2	5	6
Fried Zucchini	139	320	170	19	5	0	850	31	0	0	6
Fish & Chips	258	630	250	28	5	10	990	68	3	4	26
CrissCut® Fries	139	410	220	24	5	0	950	43	4	0	5
Chicken Stars™ (4 pieces)	57	170	100	11	3	25	320	10	1	0	9
Chicken Stars™ (6 pieces)	85	260	150	16	4	35	470	14	1	1	13
Chicken Stars™ (9 pieces)	127	380	220	24	6	55	710	21	1	1	20

Salads – Without Dressings	Serving Size (g)	kcal	kcals from fat	Total Fat (g)	Saturated Fat (g)	Cholesterol (mg)	Sodium (mg)	Total CHO (g)	Dietary Fiber (g)	Sugars (g)	Protein (g)
Charbroiled Chicken Salad	417	260	60	7	3.5	75	710	16	5	8	34
Side Salad	139	50	20	2.5	1.5	5	60	5	2	3	3

Salad Dressings – 2 Oz Packets	Serving Size (g)	kcal	kcals from fat	Total Fat (g)	Saturated Fat (g)	Cholesterol (mg)	Sodium (mg)	Total CHO (g)	Dietary Fiber (g)	Sugars (g)	Protein (g)
House Dressing	57	220	200	22	3.5	20	440	2	0	2	1
Blue Cheese Dressing	57	320	310	34	7	20	410	1	0	1	2
Thousand Island Dressing	57	250	20	2	3.5	20	480	7	0	3	0
Low Fat Balsamic Dressing	57	35	15	1.5	0	0	480	5	0	3	0

Breakfast	Serving Size (g)	kcal	kcals from fat	Total Fat (g)	Saturated Fat (g)	Cholesterol (mg)	Sodium (mg)	Total CHO (g)	Dietary Fiber (g)	Sugars (g)	Protein (g)
Breakfast Burger™	309	830	420	47	15	275	1580	65	3	13	37
Sourdough Breakfast Sandwich	193	460	190	21	9	280	1050	39	2	4	28
Sunrise Croissant™ Sandwich	172	560	370	41	15	290	970	27	1	5	20
Bacon & Egg Burrito	208	570	300	33	11	515	990	37	1	1	30
Loaded Breakfast Burrito	328	820	460	51	16	595	1530	52	2	3	38
Steak & Egg Burrito	322	660	320	35	13	545	1690	44	0	4	40
French Toast Dips® - No Syrup (5 pcs)	129	430	160	18	2.5	0	530	58	1	15	9
Hash Brown Nuggets	108	330	190	21	4.5	0	460	32	3	1	3

Desserts	Serving Size (g)	kcal	kcals from fat	Total Fat (g)	Saturated Fat (g)	Cholesterol (mg)	Sodium (mg)	Total CHO (g)	Dietary Fiber (g)	Sugars (g)	Protein (g)
Chocolate Chip Cookie	71	350	160	18	7	20	330	46	1	27	3
Chocolate Cake	85	300	100	12	3	30	350	48	1	37	3
Strawberry Swirl Cheesecake	99	290	150	17	9	55	230	30	0	20	6

Hand-Scooped Ice Cream Shakes & Malts™	Serving Size (g)	kcal	kcals from fat	Total Fat (g)	Saturated Fat (g)	Cholesterol (mg)	Sodium (mg)	Total CHO (g)	Dietary Fiber (g)	Sugars (g)	Protein (g)
Vanilla Shake	397	710	300	33	23	100	230	86	0	76	14
Chocolate Shake	397	710	300	33	23	100	290	85	1	71	14
Strawberry Shake	397	700	300	33	23	100	240	84	0	75	14
OREO® Cookie Shake	397	720	340	37	24	100	350	79	1	64	16
Vanilla Malt	414	780	310	35	24	105	300	99	0	84	17
Chocolate Malt	414	780	310	35	24	105	360	98	1	79	17
Strawberry Malt	414	770	310	35	24	105	310	97	0	83	17
OREO® Cookie Malt	414	790	350	39	25	105	420	91	1	72	18

Dairy Queen

Burgers	Serving Size (g)	kcal	kcals from fat	Total Fat (g)	Saturated Fat (g)	Trans Fat (g)	Cholesterol (mg)	Sodium (mg)	Total CHO (g)	Dietary Fiber (g)	Sugars (g)	Proteins (g)	Percent Daily Value Vitamin A	Percent Daily Value Vitamin C	Percent Daily Value Calcium	Percent Daily Value Iron
DQ® Homestyle® Burger	142	350	130	14	7	0.5	50	400	33	1	8	17	6	0	4	15
DQ® Homestyle® Cheeseburger	156	400	160	18	9	0.5	65	640	34	1	9	19	12	0	10	15
DQ® Homestyle® Double Cheeseburger	226	640	310	34	18	1	130	950	34	1	9	34	15	0	20	25
DQ® Homestyle® Bacon Double Cheeseburger	245	730	370	41	21	1	150	1270	35	1	9	41	15	0	20	25
DQ® Ultimate® Burger	259	780	430	48	22	1.5	155	1110	33	1	8	41	20	20	20	45
1/4 lb. FlameThrower® GrilllBurgerTM	245	780	480	54	14	3	90	1490	41	2	9	33	20	15	25	20
1/2 lb. FlameThrower® GrilllBurgerTM	344	1030	650	73	23	4	145	2020	41	2	9	53	25	15	30	30
Classic GrilllBurgerTM	212	470	200	23	7	2.5	40	1020	42	2	12	24	20	6	15	20
Classic GrilllBurgerTM with Cheese	231	560	270	30	11	2.5	60	1160	42	2	12	29	25	6	30	20
1/2 lb. GrilllBurgerTM	297	670	330	37	12	3.5	80	1310	42	2	12	42	20	6	15	30
1/2 lb. GrilllBurgerTM with Cheese	330	820	430	49	19	3.5	115	1510	47	2	12	51	25	6	45	30
Bacon Cheddar GrilllBurgerTM	229	650	330	37	13	2.5	80	1480	41	2	11	36	10	0	30	20
Mushroom Swiss GrilllBurgerTM	210	630	350	40	11	3	65	950	39	2	8	29	4	0	30	20

Hot Dogs	Serving Size (g)	kcal	kcals from fat	Total Fat (g)	Saturated Fat (g)	Trans Fat (g)	Cholesterol (mg)	Sodium (mg)	Total CHO (g)	Dietary Fiber (g)	Sugars (g)	Proteins (g)	Percent Daily Value Vitamin A	Percent Daily Value Vitamin C	Percent Daily Value Calcium	Percent Daily Value Iron
All-Beef Hot Dog	115	300	130	15	6	0	30	870	30	1	5	11	4	0	8	15
All-Beef Chili Cheese Dog	150	380	220	24	11	0.5	55	1100	24	1	4	16	10	2	15	10

Sandwiches/Baskets	Serving Size (g)	kcal	kcals from fat	Total Fat (g)	Saturated Fat (g)	Trans Fat (g)	Cholesterol (mg)	Sodium (mg)	Total CHO (g)	Dietary Fiber (g)	Sugars (g)	Proteins (g)	Percent Daily Value Vitamin A	Percent Daily Value Vitamin C	Percent Daily Value Calcium	Percent Daily Value Iron
Crispy Chicken Sandwich	198	540	260	29	5	2.5	45	700	47	1	6	23	10	6	4	25
Grilled Chicken Sandwich	177	350	140	16	2.5	0	55	780	49	1	6	23	10	6	4	10
Chicken Strip BasketTM, 4-piece*	446	1030	480	54	9	10	75	2400	105	8	7	37	2	2	15	40
Chicken Strip BasketTM, 6-piece*	531	1270	600	67	11	12	110	2910	121	10	8	51	2	2	15	50

Salads	Serving Size (g)	kcal	kcals from fat	Total Fat (g)	Saturated Fat (g)	Trans Fat (g)	Cholesterol (mg)	Sodium (mg)	Total CHO (g)	Dietary Fiber (g)	Sugars (g)	Proteins (g)	Percent Daily Value Vitamin A	Percent Daily Value Vitamin C	Percent Daily Value Calcium	Percent Daily Value Iron
Crispy Chicken Salad – no dressing	424	420	200	22	7	2	70	960	90	6	9	28	130	80	80	25
Grilled Chicken Salad – no dressing	424	270	100	11	5	0	80	1160	92	4	9	32	130	80	70	15
Side Salad – no dressing	Serving Size (g)	kcal	kcals from fat	Total Fat (g)	Saturated Fat (g)	Trans Fat (g)	Cholesterol (mg)	Sodium (mg)	Total CHO (g)	Dietary Fiber (g)	Sugars (g)	Proteins (g)	Percent Daily Value Vitamin A	Percent Daily Value Vitamin C	Percent Daily Value Calcium	Percent Daily Value Iron
Salad Dressings	Serving Size (g)	kcal	kcals from fat	Total Fat (g)	Saturated Fat (g)	Trans Fat (g)	Cholesterol (mg)	Sodium (mg)	Total CHO (g)	Dietary Fiber (g)	Sugars (g)	Proteins (g)	Percent Daily Value Vitamin A	Percent Daily Value Vitamin C	Percent Daily Value Calcium	Percent Daily Value Iron
DQ® Honey Mustard Dressing	57	260	190	21	3.5	0	20	370	18	0	11	1	0	0	2	6
DQ® Blue Cheese Dressing	57	210	180	20	4	0	5	700	4	0	2	2	2	0	6	0
DQ® Ranch Dressing	57	310	300	33	5	0	25	390	3	0	2	1	0	0	2	0
Fat Free Italian Dressing	43	10	0	0	0	0	0	390	3	0	1	0	0	0	0	0
Fries/Onion Rings	Serving Size (g)	kcal	kcals from fat	Total Fat (g)	Saturated Fat (g)	Trans Fat (g)	Cholesterol (mg)	Sodium (mg)	Total CHO (g)	Dietary Fiber (g)	Sugars (g)	Proteins (g)	Percent Daily Value Vitamin A	Percent Daily Value Vitamin C	Percent Daily Value Calcium	Percent Daily Value Iron
DQ® Small French Fries	140	360	150	16	3	2.5	0	760	50	5	0	4	0	2	2	6
DQ® Medium French Fries	196	510	210	23	4	3.5	0	1070	70	7	1	6	0	4	2	8
DQ® Large French Fries	280	730	290	33	6	5	0	1530	100	10	1	8	0	6	4	10
DQ® Regular Onion Rings	113	470	270	30	6	7	0	740	45	3	7	6	0	30	4	6
DQ® Large Onion Rings	142	590	330	37	7	9	0	930	56	4	9	7	0	15	4	8
Cones	Serving Size (g)	kcal	kcals from fat	Total Fat (g)	Saturated Fat (g)	Trans Fat (g)	Cholesterol (mg)	Sodium (mg)	Total CHO (g)	Dietary Fiber (g)	Sugars (g)	Proteins (g)	Percent Daily Value Vitamin A	Percent Daily Value Vitamin C	Percent Daily Value Calcium	Percent Daily Value Iron
DQ® Vanilla Soft Serve, 1/2 cup	94	150	45	5	3	0	15	70	22	0	19	3	6	0	15	4
DQ® Chocolate Soft Serve, 1/2 cup	94	150	45	5	3.5	0	15	75	22	0	17	4	10	0	10	4

(continued)

Cones	Serving Size (g)	kcal	kcals from fat	Total Fat (g)	Saturated Fat (g)	Trans Fat (g)	Cholesterol (mg)	Sodium (mg)	Total CHO (g)	Dietary Fiber (g)	Sugars (g)	Proteins (g)	Percent Daily Value Vitamin A	Percent Daily Value Vitamin C	Percent Daily Value Calcium	Percent Daily Value Iron
Small Vanilla Cone	142	240	70	7	4.5	0	20	115	32	0	27	6	10	2	20	6
Medium Vanilla Cone	199	340	90	10	6	0	30	160	54	0	38	8	15	2	25	8
Large Vanilla Cone	284	480	130	15	9	0.5	45	230	76	0	55	11	20	2	35	10
Small Chocolate Cone	142	240	70	7	5	0	20	115	32	0	25	6	15	0	15	8
Medium Chocolate Cone	199	340	90	10	7	0	30	160	54	0	34	9	15	2	25	10
Small Dipped Cone	156	340	140	16	10	1	20	120	36	1	31	6	10	2	20	8
Medium Dipped Cone	220	490	210	23	15	1.5	30	170	61	1	43	8	15	2	25	10
Large Dipped Cone	312	670	280	31	21	2.5	40	210	83	0	62	13	8	0	30	15
Royal Treats®	**Serving Size (g)**	**kcal**	**kcals from fat**	**Total Fat (g)**	**Saturated Fat (g)**	**Trans Fat (g)**	**Cholesterol (mg)**	**Sodium (mg)**	**Total CHO (g)**	**Dietary Fiber (g)**	**Sugars (g)**	**Proteins (g)**	**Percent Daily Value Vitamin A**	**Percent Daily Value Vitamin C**	**Percent Daily Value Calcium**	**Percent Daily Value Iron**
Banana Split	374	530	120	14	10	0	30	180	98	3	77	8	15	35	25	10
Peanut Buster® Parfait	304	710	270	30	16	0	30	380	96	2	74	16	15	2	35	20
Brownie Earthquake™	304	740	250	28	15	0	60	370	149	1	87	10	15	2	25	15
Malts, Shakes, and Arctic Rush™	**Serving Size (g)**	**kcal**	**kcals from fat**	**Total Fat (g)**	**Saturated Fat (g)**	**Trans Fat (g)**	**Cholesterol (mg)**	**Sodium (mg)**	**Total CHO (g)**	**Dietary Fiber (g)**	**Sugars (g)**	**Proteins (g)**	**Percent Daily Value Vitamin A**	**Percent Daily Value Vitamin C**	**Percent Daily Value Calcium**	**Percent Daily Value Iron**
Small Chocolate Malt	427	650	140	15	10	0	50	310	112	0	96	14	20	2	45	15
Medium Chocolate Malt	567	900	190	21	13	0.5	65	460	157	0	134	19	30	4	60	20
Large Chocolate Malt	854	1300	280	31	20	1	95	670	224	0	191	28	45	4	100	30
Small Chocolate Shake	406	560	130	14	9	0	45	280	95	0	82	12	20	2	45	15
Medium Chocolate Shake	550	780	180	20	13	0.5	60	380	133	0	115	17	30	4	60	20
Large Chocolate Shake	811	1130	260	29	19	1	90	500	188	0	163	25	45	4	90	25
Small Arctic Rush™ Slush	453	240	0	0	0	0	0	0	48	0	48	0	0	0	0	0
Medium Arctic Rush™ Slush	595	310	0	0	0	0	0	0	63	0	63	0	0	0	0	0
MooLatté® Frozen Blended Coffee	**Serving Size (g)**	**kcal**	**kcals from fat**	**Total Fat (g)**	**Saturated Fat (g)**	**Trans Fat (g)**	**Cholesterol (mg)**	**Sodium (mg)**	**Total CHO (g)**	**Dietary Fiber (g)**	**Sugars (g)**	**Proteins (g)**	**Percent Daily Value Vitamin A**	**Percent Daily Value Vitamin C**	**Percent Daily Value Calcium**	**Percent Daily Value Iron**
Cappuccino MooLatté® – 16 oz.	411	500	170	18	15	0	30	170	73	0	65	7	15	2	25	6
Cappuccino MooLatté® – 24 oz.	602	710	220	24	18	0.5	50	260	107	0	95	11	20	2	40	10

Mocha MooLatté® – 16 oz.	427	590	210	23	15	0	30	200	84	0	74	8	15	2	25	10
Mocha MooLatté® – 24 oz.	623	840	280	31	20	0.5	45	300	121	1	106	12	20	2	40	15
French Vanilla MooLatté® – 16 oz.	433	570	160	18	14	0	30	170	90	0	76	7	15	2	25	6
French Vanilla MooLatté® – 24 oz.	623	770	210	24	18	0.5	45	260	123	0	106	11	20	2	40	10
Caramel MooLatté® – 16 oz.	448	630	170	19	16	0	35	260	103	0	50	8	15	2	30	6
Caramel MooLatté® – 24 oz.	651	840	280	31	20	0.5	45	300	121	1	106	12	20	2	40	15
Sundaes	**Serving Size (g)**	**kcal**	**kcals from fat**	**Total Fat (g)**	**Saturated Fat (g)**	**Trans Fat (g)**	**Cholesterol (mg)**	**Sodium (mg)**	**Total CHO (g)**	**Dietary Fiber (g)**	**Sugars (g)**	**Proteins (g)**	**Percent Daily Value Vitamin A**	**Percent Daily Value Vitamin C**	**Percent Daily Value Calcium**	**Percent Daily Value Iron**
Small Strawberry Sundae	192	280	60	7	4.5	0	20	130	50	1	45	5	10	45	20	6
Medium Strawberry Sundae	248	370	90	10	7	0	30	170	63	1	56	7	15	45	25	8
Large Strawberry Sundae	333	510	130	15	9	0	45	240	83	1	73	10	20	45	40	10
Small Chocolate Sundae	163	280	60	7	4.5	0	20	130	49	0	42	5	10	2	20	8
Medium Chocolate Sundae	234	410	90	10	7	0	30	190	72	0	61	7	15	2	25	10
Large Chocolate Sundae	333	580	130	15	9	0	45	262	100	0	86	10	20	2	35	15
Novelties	**Serving Size (g)**	**kcal**	**kcals from fat**	**Total Fat (g)**	**Saturated Fat (g)**	**Trans Fat (g)**	**Cholesterol (mg)**	**Sodium (mg)**	**Total CHO (g)**	**Dietary Fiber (g)**	**Sugars (g)**	**Proteins (g)**	**Percent Daily Value Vitamin A**	**Percent Daily Value Vitamin C**	**Percent Daily Value Calcium**	**Percent Daily Value Iron**
DQ® Sandwich	85	190	45	5	3	0	10	95	32	1	18	4	2	0	8	2
Chocolate Dilly® Bar	87	240	140	15	9	0	15	70	24	1	20	4	6	0	10	0
Buster Bar®	148	480	280	31	15	0	20	220	45	2	35	11	8	0	20	6
StarKiss®	85	80	0	0	0	0	0	10	21	0	21	0	0	0	0	0
DQ® Fudge Bar – no sugar added	66	50	0	0	0	0	0	70	13	0	3	4	6	0	10	0
DQ® Vanilla Orange Bar – no sugar added	66	60	0	0	0	0	0	40	17	0	2	2	2	0	6	0
Blizzard® Treats	**Serving Size (g)**	**kcal**	**kcals from fat**	**Total Fat (g)**	**Saturated Fat (g)**	**Trans Fat (g)**	**Cholesterol (mg)**	**Sodium (mg)**	**Total CHO (g)**	**Dietary Fiber (g)**	**Sugars (g)**	**Proteins (g)**	**Percent Daily Value Vitamin A**	**Percent Daily Value Vitamin C**	**Percent Daily Value Calcium**	**Percent Daily Value Iron**
Small Oreo®† Cookies Blizzard®	283	560	190	21	10	0	40	430	83	1	64	11	20	2	35	15
Medium Oreo®† Cookies Blizzard®	334	690	230	26	12	0.5	45	560	103	1	77	13	20	2	40	15
Large Oreo®† Cookies Blizzard®	500	1000	330	37	18	1.0	70	770	148	2	113	19	30	4	60	25
Small Choc. Chip Cookie Dough Blizzard®	319	720	250	28	14	3.0	50	370	105	1	78	12	30	2	35	15
Medium Choc. Chip Cookie Dough Blizzard®	446	1030	360	40	20	4.5	70	530	151	1	112	17	40	4	50	20

(continued)

Blizzard® Treats	Serving Size (g)	kcal	kcals from fat	Total Fat (g)	Saturated Fat (g)	Trans Fat (g)	Cholesterol (mg)	Sodium (mg)	Total CHO (g)	Dietary Fiber (g)	Sugars (g)	Proteins (g)	Percent Daily Value Vitamin A	Percent Daily Value Vitamin C	Percent Daily Value Calcium	Percent Daily Value Iron
Small Banana Split Blizzard®	297	460	130	14	9	0	40	210	73	1	62	10	20	10	35	10
Medium Banana Split Blizzard®	382	580	150	17	11	0.5	50	260	97	1	91	12	25	15	40	15
Large Banana Split Blizzard®	527	810	210	23	15	1.0	70	360	134	1	113	16	30	25	60	
Small Reese's®†† Peanut Butter Cup Blizzard®	305	600	190	21	16	0	40	220	87	0	76	14	25	0	40	10
Medium Reese's®†† Peanut Butter Cup Blizzard®	383	790	250	28	22	0.5	50	280	114	0	99	18	30	0	50	15
Large Reese's®†† Peanut Butter Cup Blizzard®	514	1050	340	38	29	1	70	370	152	0	133	25	45	0	70	20
Small Strawberry CheeseQuake™ Blizzard®	283	530	190	21	13	1	85	320	76	<1	62	10	30	0	40	10
Medium Strawberry CheeseQuake™ Blizzard®	376	730	260	29	18	1	120	440	105	<1	84	13	40	0	50	15
Large Strawberry CheeseQuake™ Blizzard®	510	990	350	39	24	1.5	160	600	143	<1	114	18	55	0	70	20
DQ® Blizzard® Cakes	**Serving Size (g)**	**kcal**	**kcals from fat**	**Total Fat (g)**	**Saturated Fat (g)**	**Trans Fat (g)**	**Cholesterol (mg)**	**Sodium (mg)**	**Total CHO (g)**	**Dietary Fiber (g)**	**Sugars (g)**	**Proteins (g)**	**Percent Daily Value Vitamin A**	**Percent Daily Value Vitamin C**	**Percent Daily Value Calcium**	**Percent Daily Value Iron**
Oreo® Cookies Blizzard® Cake,**8", 1/8 of Cake	220	490	180	20	12	1	30	250	67	1	51	8	15	0	25	10
Reese's® PB Cup Blizzard® Cake,**8", 1/8 of Cake	220	490	180	20	13	0	30	190	67	1	54	9	15	0	25	10
Chocolate Xtreme Blizzard® Cake,**8", 1/8 of Cake	249	660	280	31	20	1.5	40	340	85	2	68	10	20	0	25	15
DQ® Cakes	**Serving Size (g)**	**kcal**	**kcals from fat**	**Total Fat (g)**	**Saturated Fat (g)**	**Trans Fat (g)**	**Cholesterol (mg)**	**Sodium (mg)**	**Total CHO (g)**	**Dietary Fiber (g)**	**Sugars (g)**	**Proteins (g)**	**Percent Daily Value Vitamin A**	**Percent Daily Value Vitamin C**	**Percent Daily Value Calcium**	**Percent Daily Value Iron**
8" Round Cake, **1/8 of Cake	209	410	140	16	11	1	30	220	60	<1	47	8	15	2	25	8

**Includes four or six breaded chicken strips, small French fries, Texas toast and gravy. **Undecorated*

www.dairyqueen.com

Hardee's

Breakfast	Serving Size (g)	kcal	kcals from Fat	Total Fat (g)	Saturated Fat (g)	Cholesterol (mg)	Sodium (mg)	Total CHO (g)	Dietary Fiber (g)	Sugars (g)	Protein (g)
Loaded Breakfast Burrito	258	780	460	51	20	495	1620	38	2	2	40
Made from Scratch Biscuit	109	370	210	23	5	0	890	35	0	3	5
Egg Biscuit	152	450	260	29	6	205	940	35	0	4	11
Bacon Biscuit	120	430	250	28	7	10	1110	35	0	4	8
Sausage Biscuit	142	530	340	38	10	30	1240	36	0	4	11
Country Ham Biscuit	144	440	240	26	6	35	1710	36	0	3	14
Breaded Chicken Fillet Biscuit	226	600	310	34	7	55	1680	50	1	3	24
Breaded Country Steak Biscuit	180	620	370	41	11	35	1360	44	0	3	16
Breaded Pork Chop Biscuit	222	690	380	42	8	40	1330	48	1	4	29
Sausage & Egg Biscuit	185	610	390	44	11	235	1290	36	0	4	17
Country Steak & Egg Biscuit	223	690	420	47	11	235	1800	44	0	4	22
Bacon, Egg & Cheese Biscuit	174	560	340	38	11	225	1360	37	0	4	16
Ham, Egg & Cheese Biscuit	220	560	320	35	10	245	1800	37	0	5	23
Loaded Omelet Biscuit	198	640	400	44	14	245	1510	37	0	5	21
Monster Biscuit	212	710	460	51	17	70	2250	37	0	4	24
Biscuits "N" Gravy	251	530	310	34	8	10	1550	47	0	6	8
Sunrise Croissant with Ham	164	430	230	26	10	250	1050	28	0	5	23
Sunrise Croissant with Bacon	138	450	260	29	12	240	900	28	0	5	19
Sunrise Croissant with Sausage	161	550	340	38	15	265	1030	29	0	5	22
Sunrise Croissant	57	210	90	10	4	5	200	26	0	4	4
Frisco Breakfast Sandwich	185	420	180	20	7	240	1340	37	2	2.7	24
Loaded Omelet	89	270	190	21	9	245	620	2	0	2	16
Loaded Biscuit "N" Gravy Breakfast Bowl	326	770	490	54	14	245	1950	49	1	7	20
Low Carb Breakfast Bowl	208	620	450	50	21	325	1380	6	2	2	36
Pancake Platter	135	300	45	5	1	25	830	55	2	12	8
Big Country Breakfast Platter – Country Ham	377	970	470	53	12	460	2600	90	3	12	33
Big Country Breakfast Platter – Bacon	355	980	500	56	13	435	2080	90	3	13	28
Big Country Breakfast Platter – Sausage	374	1060	570	64	15	455	2140	91	4	13	30
Big Country Breakfast Platter – Chicken	458	1140	540	61	13	480	2580	105	4	12	44
Big Country Breakfast Platter – Breaded Pork Chop	455	1220	620	68	13	465	2230	102	4	13	48
Big Country Breakfast Platter – Country Steak	412	1150	610	68	16	455	2260	98	4	12	36
Hash Rounds – small	83	260	150	16	4	0	360	25	2	1	3
Hash Rounds – medium	114	350	200	22	5	0	490	34	3	1	4

Lunch & Dinner	Serving Size (g)	kcal	kcals from Fat	Total Fat (g)	Saturated Fat (g)	Cholesterol (mg)	Sodium (mg)	Total CHO (g)	Dietary Fiber (g)	Sugars (g)	Protein (g)
1/3 LB** Thickburger	349	910	570	64	21	110	1560	53	3	13	30
1/3 LB** Cheeseburger	254	680	350	39	19	90	1450	52	2	11	29
1/3 LB** Mushroom 'N' Swiss Thickburger	276	720	380	42	21	100	1570	48	2	7	35
1/3 LB** Bacon Cheese Thickburger	334	910	570	64	24	115	1550	50	3	10	33
1/3 LB** Low Carb Thickburger	245	420	280	32	12	115	1010	5	2	3	30

(continued)

Lunch & Dinner	Serving Size (g)	kcal	kcals from Fat	Total Fat (g)	Saturated Fat (g)	Cholesterol (mg)	Sodium (mg)	Total CHO (g)	Dietary Fiber (g)	Sugars (g)	Protein (g)
1/2 LB** Six Dollar Burger	412	1060	660	73	28	150	1950	58	3	18	40
1/2 LB** Grilled Sourdough Thickburger	381	1030	690	77	28	155	1910	42	2.8	5.4	42
2/3 LB** Double Thickburger	471	1250	810	90	35	195	2160	54	3	13	51
2/3 LB** Double Bacon Cheese Thickburger	463	1300	870	97	38	205	2200	50	3	10	54
2/3 LB** Monster Thickburger	413	1420	970	108	43	230	2770	46	2	9	60
Charbroiled Chicken Club Sandwich	277	560	270	30	8	95	1430	32	3	7	39
Charbroiled BBQ Chicken Sandwich	242	340	40	4	1	60	1070	40	3	13	33
Low Carb Charbroiled Chicken Club Sandwich	250	370	190	21	7	90	1170	10	2	5	35
Big Chicken Fillet Sandwich	351	800	330	37	6	90	1890	76	3	9	41
Spicy Chicken Sandwich	159	470	230	25	5	40	1220	46	2	6	13
Regular Roast Beef	137	330	150	16	7	40	860	29	2	2	19
Big Roast Beef	199	470	210	23	10	60	1290	38	2	3	29
Hot Ham 'N' Cheese	191	420	170	18	10	55	1600	39	2	4	30
Big Hot Ham 'N' Cheese	244	520	210	24	13	85	2190	40	2	4	40
Hot Dog	152	420	270	30	12	55	1200	22	1	4	16
1/4 LB** Double Cheeseburger	186	510	240	26	5	90	1120	38	1	9	28
1/4 LB** Double Hamburger	161	420	170	19	5	70	670	37	1	9	23
Cheeseburger	131	350	140	16	4	45	780	36	1	8	17
Hamburger	118	310	110	12	4	35	560	36	1	8	14
3 Piece Chicken Strips	145	380	190	21	4	55	1360	27	1	1	22
5 Piece Chicken Strips	241	630	310	34	6	90	2260	45	2	1	37
Kids Meal - Hamburger	197	560	210	24	6	35	710	67	4	8	18
Kids Meal - Cheeseburger	210	600	250	27	6	45	930	68	4	8	21
Kids Meal -2 Chicken Strips	175	500	230	25	5	35	1050	50	3	1	19

Sides	Serving Size (g)	kcal	kcals from Fat	Total Fat (g)	Saturated Fat (g)	Cholesterol (mg)	Sodium (mg)	Total CHO (g)	Dietary Fiber (g)	Sugars (g)	Protein (g)
American Cheese slice (large)	16	60	45	5	4	15	260	1	0	1	3
American Cheese slice (small)	12	50	35	4	3	10	200	1	0	0	2
Swiss Cheese slice	16	50	35	4	3	15	230	0	0	0	4
Bacon - 2 strips	9	45	30	4	1	10	150	0	0	0	3
Au Jus Sauce	85	10	0	0	0	0	320	2	0	1	0
Fried Chicken Breast	148	370	130	15	4	75	1190	29	0	0	29
Fried Chicken Wing	66	200	70	8	2	30	740	23	0	0	10
Fried Chicken Thigh	121	330	130	15	4	60	1000	30	0	0	19
Fried Chicken Leg	69	170	60	7	2	45	570	15	0	0	13
French Fries-Kids	79	250	100	12	3	0	150	32	3	0	4
French Fries-Small	126	390	170	19	4	0	240	51	4	1	6
French Fries-Medium	166	520	220	24	5	0	320	67	5	1	8
French Fries-Large	193	610	260	28	6	0	370	78	6	1	10
Crispy Curls - Small	109	340	150	17	4	0	840	43	4	0	4
Crispy Curls - Medium	132	410	180	20	5	0	1020	52	4	0	5
Crispy Curls - Large	153	480	210	23	6	0	1190	60	5	0	6
Cole Slaw (small = 1 serving)	113	170	90	10	2	10	140	20	2	16	1
Mashed Potatoes (small = 1 serving)	142	90	15	2	0	0	410	17	0	1	1
Peach Cobbler	180	280	60	7	2	0	230	56	1	45	1
Chicken Gravy	43	20	5	1	0	0	220	3	0	1	0

(continued)

Sides—*continued*	Serving Size (g)	kcal	kcals from Fat	Total Fat (g)	Saturated Fat (g)	Cholesterol (mg)	Sodium (mg)	Total CHO (g)	Dietary Fiber (g)	Sugars (g)	Protein (g)
Honey Mustard - Dipping Sauce	28	110	80	9	1.5	10	220	6	0	4	0
Ranch Dressing - Dipping Sauce	28	160	150	16	3	15	240	2	0	1	0
BBQ Sauce - Dipping Sauce	28	45	0	0	0	0	290	10	1	7	1
Sweet N Sour - Dipping Sauce	28	45	0	0	0	0	85	10	0	9	0
Mayonnaise (Packet)	12	90	80	9	1.5	5	70	1	0	0	0
Hot Sauce (Packet)	7	0	0	0	0	0	210	0	0	0	0
Horseradish Sauce (Packet)	7	25	20	2	0	5	35	1	0	1	0
Ketchup (Packet)	9	10	0	0	0	0	105	2	0	2	0
Desserts	**Serving Size (g)**	**kcal**	**kcals from Fat**	**Total Fat (g)**	**Saturated Fat (g)**	**Cholesterol (mg)**	**Sodium (mg)**	**Total CHO (g)**	**Dietary Fiber (g)**	**Sugars (g)**	**Protein (g)**
Chocolate Chip Cookie	68	290	100	11	5	20	270	44	0	26	4
Apple Turnover	85	290	140	15	5	5	350	36	1	11	2
Single Scoop Ice Cream Cone†	126	285	120	13	8	47	140	37	0	26	6
Single Scoop Ice Cream Bowl†	113	235	115	13	8	47	85	27	0	22	5
Vanilla Shake (Hand-Dipped) (regular)	16 fl oz	710	300	33	23	100	240	87	0	73	14
Chocolate Shake (Hand-Dipped) (regular)	16 fl oz	700	300	34	24	100	290	85	1	55	15
Strawberry Shake (Hand-Dipped) (regular)	16 fl oz	700	300	33	23	100	240	86	0	76	14
Hardee's Vanilla Malt (Hand-Dipped) 16 fl oz	16 fl oz	770	310	35	24	105	320	97	0.4	79	17
Hardee's Strawberry Malt (Hand-Dipped) 16 fl oz	16 fl oz	775	310	35	24	105	310	98	0.4	84	17
Hardee's Chocolate Malt (Hand-Dipped) 16 fl oz	16 fl oz	780	320	35	24	105	355	97	1.6	79	17

Jack In the Box

Breakfast	Serving Weight (g)	kcal	kcals from fat	Fat – Total (g)	Saturated Fat (g)	Trans Fat (g)	Cholesterol (mg)	Sodium (mg)	Potassium (mg)	Total CHO (g)	Dietary Fiber (g)	Sugars (g)	Protein (g)
Bacon, Egg & Cheese Biscuit	149	430	220	25	8	5	220	1100	140	34	1	3	17
Bacon Breakfast Jack®	113	300	120	14	5	0.5	215	730	180	29	1	4	16
Blueberry French Toast Sticks (4)	121	450	180	20	4.5	4.5	0	550	115	59	3	15	8
Breakfast Jack®	125	290	110	12	4.5	0	220	760	210	29	1	4	17
Chicken Biscuit	154	450	220	24	6	6	30	980	170	42	2	2	15
Ciabatta Breakfast Sandwich	278	710	320	36	10	1	440	1730	440	63	3	4	36
Extreme Sausage® Sandwich	213	670	430	48	17	1.5	290	1300	370	31	2	5	29
Hash Brown (1)	57	150	90	10	2.5	3	0	230	190	13	2	0	1
Meaty Breakfast Burrito	183	480	260	29	10	1	350	1210	300	29	2	1	25
Original French Toast Sticks (4)	121	470	210	23	5	5	25	450	120	58	4	14	7
Sausage Biscuit	131	440	260	29	8	5	35	870	340	32	2	3	12
Sausage Breakfast Jack®	154	450	250	28	10	1	245	840	250	29	1	4	20
Sausage Croissant	174	580	350	39	13	4	255	770	260	37	2	5	21
Sausage, Egg & Cheese Biscuit	234	740	490	55	17	6	280	1430	310	35	2	3	27
Spicy Chicken Biscuit	169	460	200	22	5	7	40	1020	260	44	2	2	21
Supreme Croissant	151	450	230	25	9	3.5	235	860	240	36	1	5	20
Ultimate Breakfast Sandwich	249	570	240	27	10	1	445	1700	370	49	2	8	34
Burgers	**Serving Weight (g)**	**kcal**	**kcals from fat**	**Fat – Total (g)**	**Saturated Fat (g)**	**Trans Fat (g)**	**Cholesterol (mg)**	**Sodium (mg)**	**Potassium (mg)**	**Total CHO (g)**	**Dietary Fiber (g)**	**Sugars (g)**	**Protein (g)**
Bacon Ultimate Cheeseburger	338	1090	700	77	30	3	140	2040	540	53	2	12	46
Bacon 'n' Cheese Ciabatta Burger	395	1120	690	76	28	3	135	1670	660	66	4	9	45
Hamburger	118	310	130	14	6	1	40	600	250	30	1	6	16
Hamburger with Cheese	131	350	160	17	8	1	50	790	270	30	1	7	18
Hamburger Deluxe	169	370	190	21	7	1	45	560	330	31	2	6	17
Hamburger Deluxe with Cheese	194	460	250	28	11	1	70	930	360	33	2	7	21
Jumbo Jack®	261	600	310	35	12	1.5	45	940	380	51	3	11	21
Jumbo Jack® with Cheese	286	690	370	42	16	1.5	70	1310	410	54	3	12	25
Junior Bacon Cheeseburger	131	430	230	25	9	1	60	820	270	30	1	6	20
Single Bacon 'n' Cheese Ciabatta Burger	308	870	490	54	18	1.5	90	1550	490	66	4	8	31
Sirloin Cheese Burger (Real Swiss & Grilled Onions)	421	1070	630	71	25	1.5	180	1850	680	61	4	10	53

Sirloin Bacon 'n' Cheese Burger (American Cheese & Red Onions)	422	1120	660	73	24	2.5	190	2620	790	63	4	11	54
Sourdough Jack®	245	710	460	51	18	3	75	1230	430	36	3	7	27
Sourdough Ultimate Cheeseburger	291	950	660	73	29	4.5	125	1360	490	36	2	7	38
Ultimate Cheeseburger	323	1010	640	71	28	3	125	1580	480	53	2	12	40
Shakes & Desserts	**Serving Weight (g)**	**kcal**	**kcals from fat**	**Fat – Total (g)**	**Saturated Fat (g)**	**Trans Fat (g)**	**Cholesterol (mg)**	**Sodium (mg)**	**Potassium (mg)**	**Total CHO (g)**	**Dietary Fiber (g)**	**Sugars (g)**	**Protein (g)**
Cheesecake	103	310	140	16	9	1	55	220	180	34	0	23	7
Chocolate Ice Cream Shake – 16oz cup	414	880	400	45	31	2	135	330	840	107	1	94	14
Chocolate Ice Cream Shake – 24oz cup	576	1230	520	58	39	2.5	190	470	1220	159	2	141	19
Chocolate Overload Cake	93	300	60	7	1.5	0	40	350	260	57	2	34	4
Egg Nog Shake – 16oz cup (seasonal only)	414	870	400	44	31	2	135	280	750	103	0	78	13
Egg Nog Shake – 24oz cup (seasonal only)	576	1210	510	57	39	3	190	390	1040	152	1	110	18
OREO® Cookie Ice Cream Shake – 16oz cup	404	910	440	49	32	2	135	420	750	102	1	80	14
OREO® Cookie Ice Cream Shake – 24oz cup	556	1290	600	67	42	2.5	190	650	1030	148	2	115	20
Strawberry Ice Cream Shake – 16oz cup	417	880	400	44	31	2	135	290	750	105	0	88	13
Strawberry Ice Cream Shake – 24oz cup	582	1220	510	57	39	2.5	190	390	1030	155	1	131	18
Vanilla Ice Cream Shake – 16oz cup	379	790	400	44	31	2	135	280	750	83	0	70	13
Vanilla Ice Cream Shake – 24oz cup	506	1050	510	57	39	2.5	190	380	1030	112	1	94	18
Salads	**Serving Weight (g)**	**kcal**	**kcals from fat**	**Fat – Total (g)**	**Saturated Fat (g)**	**Trans Fat (g)**	**Cholesterol (mg)**	**Sodium (mg)**	**Potassium (mg)**	**Total CHO (g)**	**Dietary Fiber (g)**	**Sugars (g)**	**Protein (g)**
Asian Chicken Salad (with Grilled Chicken)*	365	160	15	1.5	0	0	65	380	870	18	5	11	22
Asian Chicken Salad (with Crispy Chicken)*	394	330	120	13	3	3	40	650	830	34	7	11	21
Chicken Club Salad (with Grilled Chicken)*	373	320	140	16	6	0	105	780	830	11	4	5	34
Chicken Club Salad (with Crispy Chicken)*	402	480	250	27	9	3	80	1060	800	28	6	5	33

Nutritional data does not include dressing or condiments.

(continued)

Snacks & Extras	Serving Weight (g)	kcal	kcals from fat	Fat – Total (g)	Saturated Fat (g)	Trans Fat (g)	Cholesterol (mg)	Sodium (mg)	Potassium (mg)	Total CHO (g)	Dietary Fiber (g)	Sugars (g)	Protein (g)
Side Salad*	123	50	25	3	1.5	0	10	60	260	5	2	2	3
Southwest Chicken Salad (with Grilled Chicken)*	430	320	110	12	6	0	90	760	950	27	7	5	31
Southwest Chicken Salad (with Crispy Chicken)*	459	480	210	23	8	3	70	1040	920	44	9	5	30
Bacon Cheddar Potato Wedges	257	720	430	48	15	12	45	1360	950	52	4	2	21
Beef Monster Taco®	112	240	130	15	5	2	20	390	220	20	3	4	8
Egg Roll (1)	57	130	60	6	2	1	5	310	140	15	2	1	5
Egg Rolls (2)	170	400	170	19	6	3	15	920	430	44	6	4	14
Fruit Cup	198	90	5	0	0	0	0	20	400	22	2	18	1
Mozzarella Cheese Sticks (3)	71	240	110	12	5	2	25	420	60	21	1	1	11
Mozzarella Cheese Sticks (6)	138	483	244	27	11	4	46	1018	210	39	2	1	20
Natural Cut Fries – small	124	340	160	17	4	5	0	620	860	41	5	1	5
Natural Cut Fries – medium	166	450	210	23	5	7	0	830	1150	54	6	1	6
Natural Cut Fries – large	236	640	300	33	8	10	0	1180	1630	77	9	1	9
Onion Rings (8)	119	500	270	30	6	10	0	420	140	51	3	3	6
Regular Beef Taco	76	160	70	8	3	1	15	270	190	15	2	4	5
Sampler Trio	236	750	350	39	14	7	85	1760	440	65	5	4	35
Spicy Chicken Bites (7)	93	290	130	14	3	3	45	660	270	21	3	1	18
Spicy Chicken Bites (16)	213	650	290	33	7	7	100	1500	630	49	6	1	41
Seasoned Curly Fries – small	84	270	140	15	3	5	0	590	390	30	3	1	4
Seasoned Curly Fries – medium	125	400	200	23	5	7	0	890	580	45	5	1	6
Seasoned Curly Fries – large	170	550	280	31	6	10	0	1200	790	60	6	1	8
Stuffed Jalapenos (3)	72	230	110	13	6	2	20	690	105	22	2	2	7
Stuffed Jalapenos (7)	168	530	270	30	13	4.5	45	1600	240	51	4	5	15

www.jackinthebox.com

McDonald's

Sandwiches	Serving Size	kcal	kcals from Fat	Total Fat (g)	% Daily Value**	Saturated Fat (g)	% Daily Value**	Trans Fat (g)	Cholesterol (mg)	% Daily Value**	Sodium (mg)	% Daily Value**	CHO (g)	% Daily Value**	Dietary Fiber (g)	% Daily Value**	Sugars (g)	Protein (g)	Vitamin A % DV	Vitamin C % DV	Calcium % DV	Iron % DV
Hamburger	3.5 oz (100 g)	250	80	9	13	3.5	16	0.5	25	9	520	22	31	10	2	6	6	12	0	2	10	15
Cheeseburger	4 oz (114 g)	300	110	12	19	6	28	0.5	40	13	750	31	33	11	2	7	6	15	6	2	20	15
Double Cheeseburger	5.8 oz (165 g)	440	210	23	35	11	54	1.5	80	26	1150	48	34	11	2	8	7	25	10	2	25	20
Quarter Pounder®+	6 oz (169 g)	410	170	19	29	7	37	1	65	22	730	30	37	12	3	10	8	24	2	4	15	20
Quarter Pounder® with Cheese+	7 oz (198 g)	510	230	26	40	12	61	1.5	90	30	1190	50	40	13	3	12	9	29	10	4	30	25
Double Quarter Pounder® with Cheese++	9.8 oz (279 g)	740	380	42	65	19	96	2.5	155	52	1380	57	40	13	3	12	9	48	10	4	30	35
Big Mac®	7.5 oz (214 g)	540	260	29	45	10	51	1.5	75	25	1040	43	45	15	3	13	9	25	6	2	25	25
Big N' Tasty®	7.2 oz (206 g)	460	220	24	37	8	42	1.5	70	23	720	30	37	12	3	12	8	24	6	8	15	25
Big N' Tasty® with Cheese	7.7 oz (220 g)	510	250	28	43	11	54	1.5	85	28	960	40	38	13	3	12	8	27	10	8	20	25
Filet-O-Fish®	5.1 oz (143 g)	380	160	18	28	4	20	1	35	12	660	28	38	13	2	8	5	15	2	0	15	10
McChicken®	5.2 oz (147 g)	360	150	16	25	3.5	18	1	40	14	790	33	40	13	1	5	5	14	0	2	10	15
Premium Grilled Chicken Classic Sandwich	7.9 oz (226 g)	420	90	10	15	2	11	0	70	23	1190	50	51	17	3	13	11	32	4	10	8	20
Premium Crispy Chicken Classic Sandwich	8.1 oz (229 g)	500	150	17	26	3.5	16	1.5	50	16	1330	55	61	20	3	13	10	27	4	10	8	20
Premium Grilled Chicken Club Sandwich	9.1 oz (260 g)	570	190	21	32	7	35	0	100	34	1720	72	52	17	4	14	12	44	8	10	20	20
Premium Crispy Chicken Club Sandwich	9.3 oz (263 g)	660	250	28	43	8	41	1.5	80	27	1860	77	63	21	4	14	11	39	8	10	20	20
Premium Grilled Chicken Ranch BLT Sandwich	8.6 oz (246 g)	520	140	16	24	4	21	0	90	30	1760	73	53	18	3	14	13	40	4	10	10	20
Premium Crispy Chicken Ranch BLT Sandwich	8.8 oz (249 g)	600	200	23	35	5	27	1.5	70	23	1900	79	64	21	3	14	12	35	4	10	8	20
Ranch Snack Wrap™ with Crispy Chicken	4.1 oz (115 g)	330	140	16	25	4.5	24	1	30	10	780	32	32	11	2	6	2	14	2	2	10	10
Ranch Snack Wrap™ with Grilled Chicken	4.3 oz (122 g)	270	90	10	15	4	19	0	45	15	830	34	26	9	1	4	2	18	2	2	10	10
Honey Mustard Snack Wrap™ with Crispy Chicken	4.1 oz (117 g)	320	130	15	22	4.5	22	1	30	10	750	31	34	11	1	6	4	14	2	2	10	10
Honey Mustard Snack Wrap™ with Grilled Chicken	4.4 oz (124 g)	260	80	9	13	3.5	18	0	45	15	800	33	27	9	1	4	4	18	2	2	10	10

(continued)

Sandwiches (continued)	Serving Size	kcal	kcals from Fat	Total Fat (g)	% Daily Value**	Saturated Fat (g)	% Daily Value**	Trans Fat (g)	Cholesterol (mg)	% Daily Value**	Sodium (mg)	% Daily Value**	CHO (g)	% Daily Value**	Dietary Fiber (g)	% Daily Value**	Sugars (g)	Protein (g)	Vitamin A % DV	Vitamin C % DV	Calcium % DV	Iron % DV
Chipotle BBQ Snack Wrap™ with Crispy Chicken	4.2 oz (118 g)	320	130	14	22	4.5	22	1	25	9	780	32	35	12	2	6	4	14	4	2	10	10
Chipotle BBQ Snack Wrap™ with Grilled Chicken	4.4 oz (125 g)	260	80	8	13	3.5	18	0	45	14	820	34	28	9	1	5	5	18	4	2	10	10
French Fries	**Serving Size**	**kcal**	**kcals from Fat**	**Total Fat (g)**	**% Daily Value****	**Saturated Fat (g)**	**% Daily Value****	**Trans Fat (g)**	**Cholesterol (mg)**	**% Daily Value****	**Sodium (mg)**	**% Daily Value****	**CHO (g)**	**% Daily Value****	**Dietary Fiber (g)**	**% Daily Value****	**Sugars (g)**	**Protein (g)**	**Vitamin A % DV**	**Vitamin C % DV**	**Calcium % DV**	**Iron % DV**
Small French Fries	2.6 oz (74 g)	250	120	13	20	2.5	13	3.5	0	0	140	6	30	10	3	12	0	2	0	6	2	4
Medium French Fries	4 oz (114 g)	380	180	20	31	4	20	5	0	0	220	9	47	16	5	19	0	4	0	10	2	6
Large French Fries	6 oz (170 g)	570	270	30	47	6	30	8	0	0	330	14	70	23	7	28	0	6	0	15	2	10
Ketchup Packet	1 pkg (10 g)	15	0	0	0	0	0	0	0	0	110	5	3	1	0	0	2	0	2	2	0	0
Salt Packet	1 pkg (0.7 g)	0	0	0	0	0	0	0	0	0	270	11	0	0	0	0	0	0	0	0	0	0
Chicken McNuggets®/ Chicken Selects® Premium Breast Strips/Sauces	**Serving Size**	**kcal**	**kcals from Fat**	**Total Fat (g)**	**% Daily Value****	**Saturated Fat (g)**	**% Daily Value****	**Trans Fat (g)**	**Cholesterol (mg)**	**% Daily Value****	**Sodium (mg)**	**% Daily Value****	**CHO (g)**	**% Daily Value****	**Dietary Fiber (g)**	**% Daily Value****	**Sugars (g)**	**Protein (g)**	**Vitamin A % DV**	**Vitamin C % DV**	**Calcium % DV**	**Iron % DV**
Chicken McNuggets® (4 piece)	2.3 oz (64 g)	170	90	10	15	2	11	1	25	8	450	19	10	3	0	0	0	10	2	2	0	2
Chicken McNuggets® (6 piece)	3.4 oz (96 g)	250	130	15	22	3	16	1.5	35	12	670	28	15	5	0	0	0	15	2	2	2	4
Chicken McNuggets® (10 piece)	5.6 oz (160 g)	420	220	24	37	5	27	2.5	60	21	1120	47	26	9	0	0	0	25	4	2	2	6
Barbeque sauce	1 pkg (28 g)	50	0	0	0	0	0	0	0	0	260	11	12	4	0	0	10	0	2	0	0	0
Honey	1 pkg (14 g)	50	0	0	0	0	0	0	0	0	0	0	12	4	0	0	11	0	0	0	0	0
Hot Mustard Sauce	1 pkg (28 g)	60	20	2.5	4	0	0	0	5	1	250	10	9	3	2	8	6	1	0	0	0	2
Sweet 'N Sour Sauce	1 pkg (28 g)	50	0	0	0	0	0	0	0	0	150	6	12	4	0	0	10	0	2	0	0	0
Chicken Selects® Premium Breast Strips (3 pc)	4.7 oz (133 g)	380	180	20	30	3.5	19	2.5	55	18	930	39	28	9	0	0	0	23	0	4	2	4
Chicken Selects® Premium Breast Strips (5 pc)	7.8 oz (221 g)	630	300	33	51	6	31	4.5	90	30	1550	65	46	15	0	0	0	39	0	6	4	8
Spicy Buffalo Sauce	1.5 oz (43 g)	70	60	7	11	1	5	0	0	0	960	40	1	0	2	6	0	0	6	2	0	2
Creamy Ranch Sauce	1.5 oz (43 g)	200	200	22	33	3.5	17	0	10	3	320	13	2	1	0	0	1	0	0	0	2	0

Tangy Honey Mustard Sauce	1.5 oz (43 g)	70	20	2.5	4	0	0	0	5	2	170	7	13	4	0	0	9	1	0	0	0	0
Southwestern Chipotle Barbeque Sauce	1.5 oz (43 g)	70	0	0	0	0	0	0	0	0	260	11	18	6	1	3	13	0	4	0	2	4
Salads	**Serving Size**	**kcal**	**kcals from Fat**	**Total Fat (g)**	**% Daily Value****	**Saturated Fat (g)**	**% Daily Value****	**Trans Fat (g)**	**Cholesterol (mg)**	**% Daily Value****	**Sodium (mg)**	**% Daily Value****	**CHO (g)**	**% Daily Value****	**Dietary Fiber (g)**	**% Daily Value****	**Sugars (g)**	**Protein (g)**	**Vitamin A % DV**	**Vitamin C % DV**	**Calcium % DV**	**Iron % DV**
Southwest Salad with Grilled Chicken	12.3 oz (350 g)	320	90	9	15	3	14	0	70	24	970	40	30	10	7	27	11	30	130	50	15	15
Southwest Salad with Crispy Chicken	12.4 oz (352 g)	400	150	16	25	4	20	1.5	50	17	1110	46	41	14	7	27	10	25	130	50	15	15
Southwest Salad (without chicken)	8.1 oz (230 g)	140	40	4.5	7	2	9	0	10	3	150	6	20	7	6	24	5	6	130	45	15	10
Asian Salad with Grilled Chicken	12.7 oz (362 g)	300	90	10	15	1	6	0	65	21	890	37	23	8	5	21	12	32	130	90	15	15
Asian Salad with Crispy Chicken	12.9 oz (365 g)	380	150	17	26	2.5	12	1.5	45	15	1030	43	33	11	5	21	12	27	130	80	15	15
Asian Salad (without chicken)	8.6 oz (243 g)	150	70	7	11	0.5	3	0	0	0	35	1	15	5	5	21	9	8	130	70	15	15
Bacon Ranch Salad with Grilled Chicken	11.2 oz (321 g)	260	90	9	15	4	21	0	90	30	1010	42	12	4	3	13	5	33	130	50	15	10
Bacon Ranch Salad with Crispy Chicken	11.4 oz (323 g)	350	150	16	25	5	27	1.5	70	23	1150	48	23	8	3	13	4	28	130	50	15	10
Bacon Ranch Salad (without chicken)	7.8 oz (223 g)	140	70	7	11	3.5	18	0	25	9	300	12	10	3	3	13	4	9	130	50	15	8
Caesar Salad with Grilled Chicken	10.9 oz (311 g)	220	60	6	10	3	15	0	75	25	890	37	12	4	3	13	5	30	130	50	20	10
Caesar Salad with Crispy Chicken	11 oz (313 g)	300	120	13	20	4	21	1.5	55	18	1020	43	22	7	3	13	4	25	130	50	20	10
Caesar Salad (without chicken)	7.5 oz (213 g)	90	35	4	6	2.5	12	0	10	4	180	7	9	3	3	13	4	7	130	50	20	8
Side Salad	3.1 oz (87 g)	20	0	0	0	0	0	0	0	0	10	0	4	1	1	6	2	1	45	25	2	4
Butter Garlic Croutons	0.5 oz (14 g)	60	15	1.5	3	0	0	0	0	0	140	6	10	3	1	2	0	2	0	0	2	4
Snack Size Fruit & Walnut Salad	1 pkg (163 g)	210	70	8	13	1.5	7	0	5	2	60	2	31	10	2	9	25	4	0	170	8	2

(continued)

Salad Dressings	Serving Size	kcal	kcals from Fat	Total Fat (g)	% Daily Value**	Saturated Fat (g)	% Daily Value**	Trans Fat (g)	Cholesterol (mg)	% Daily Value**	Sodium (mg)	% Daily Value**	CHO (g)	% Daily Value**	Dietary Fiber (g)	% Daily Value**	Sugars (g)	Protein (g)	Vitamin A % DV	Vitamin C % DV	Calcium % DV	Iron % DV
Newman's Own® Creamy Southwest Dressing	1.5 fl oz (44 ml)	100	50	6	9	1	5	0	20	7	340	14	11	4	0	0	3	1	0	0	2	2
Newman's Own® Creamy Caesar Dressing	2 fl oz (59 ml)	190	170	18	28	3.5	17	0	20	7	500	21	4	1	0	0	2	2	0	0	6	0
Newman's Own® Low Fat Balsamic Vinaigrette	1.5 fl oz (44 ml)	40	25	3	4	0	0	0	0	0	730	30	4	1	0	0	3	0	0	4	0	0
Newman's Own® Low Fat Family Recipe Italian Dressing	1.5 fl oz (44 ml)	60	20	2.5	4	0	0	0	0	0	730	30	8	3	0	0	1	1	0	0	0	0
Newman's Own® Low Fat Sesame Ginger Dressing	1.5 fl oz (44 ml)	90	20	2.5	4	0	0	0	0	0	740	31	15	5	0	0	10	1	0	0	0	0
Newman's Own® Ranch Dressing	2 fl oz (59 ml)	170	130	15	23	2.5	12	0	20	6	530	22	9	3	0	0	4	1	0	0	4	0
Breakfast	**Serving Size**	**kcal**	**kcals from Fat**	**Total Fat (g)**	**% Daily Value****	**Saturated Fat (g)**	**% Daily Value****	**Trans Fat (g)**	**Cholesterol (mg)**	**% Daily Value****	**Sodium (mg)**	**% Daily Value****	**CHO (g)**	**% Daily Value****	**Dietary Fiber (g)**	**% Daily Value****	**Sugars (g)**	**Protein (g)**	**Vitamin A % DV**	**Vitamin C % DV**	**Calcium % DV**	**Iron % DV**
Egg McMuffin®	4.8 oz (139 g)	300	110	12	19	5	24	0	260	87	820	34	30	10	2	8	3	18	10	0	30	20
Sausage McMuffin®	3.9 oz (114 g)	370	200	22	34	8	42	0	45	15	850	35	29	10	2	8	2	14	6	2	25	15
Sausage McMuffin® with Egg	5.7 oz (164 g)	450	250	27	42	10	51	0	285	95	920	38	30	10	2	8	2	21	10	2	30	20
English Muffin	2 oz (57 g)	140	15	1.5	2	0	0	0	0	0	260	11	27	9	2	7	2	5	0	0	15	10
Bacon, Egg & Cheese Biscuit (Regular Size Biscuit)	5.1 oz (144 g)	450	230	25	39	11	53	0	245	82	1360	57	36	12	2	7	3	18	10	0	15	15
Bacon, Egg & Cheese Biscuit (Large Size Biscuit)	5.7 oz (162 g)	520	270	30	46	13	67	0	245	82	1520	63	43	14	3	12	4	19	15	0	15	20
Biscuit with Egg (Regular Size Biscuit)	5.6 oz (159 g)	500	290	32	50	12	60	0	250	83	1130	47	35	12	2	6	2	17	6	0	10	20
Sausage Biscuit with Egg (Large Size Biscuit)	6.2 oz (177 g)	570	330	37	57	15	74	0	250	83	1280	53	42	14	3	11	3	18	10	0	10	20
Sausage Biscuit (Large Size Biscuit)	4 oz (113 g)	410	240	27	41	10	51	0	30	10	1040	43	33	11	2	6	2	11	0	0	6	15
Biscuit (Regular Size)	4.6 oz (131 g)	480	280	31	48	13	65	0	30	10	1190	50	39	13	3	11	3	11	4	0	8	15
Biscuit (Large Size)	2.5 oz (72 g)	250	100	11	17	5	24	0	0	0	700	29	32	11	2	6	2	4	0	0	6	10

Bacon, Egg & Cheese McGriddles®	3.2 oz (90 g)	320	140	16	25	8	38	0	0	0	850	36	39	13	3	11	3	5	4	0	6	15
Sausage, Egg & Cheese McGriddles®	6.1 oz (173 g)	460	190	21	33	9	43	0	245	82	1360	56	48	16	2	8	16	19	10	0	20	15
Sausage McGriddles®	7.1 oz (202 g)	560	290	32	49	12	62	0	265	88	1360	56	48	16	2	8	15	20	10	0	20	15
Big Breakfast® (Regular Size Biscuit)	5 oz (141 g)	420	200	22	34	8	40	0	35	11	1030	43	44	15	2	8	15	11	0	0	8	10
Big Breakfast® (Large Size Biscuit)	9.2 oz (262 g)	720	410	46	71	16	78	2.5	555	185	1500	63	49	16	3	13	3	27	15	20	15	25
Deluxe Breakfast (Reg. Size Biscuit) w/o Syrup & Margarine	9.9 oz (280 g)	790	460	51	78	18	92	2.5	555	185	1660	69	55	18	4	18	3	28	15	2	15	30
Deluxe Breakfast (Large Size Biscuit) w/o Syrup & Margarine	14.6 oz (413 g)	1070	490	55	84	18	88	2.5	575	192	2090	87	109	36	6	23	17	36	15	2	25	40
Sausage Burrito	15.2 oz (431 g)	1140	530	59	91	20	101	2.5	575	192	2250	94	115	38	7	28	17	36	15	2	30	40
Hotcakes and Sausage (2 pats margarine & syrup)	3.9 oz (111 g)	300	140	16	25	7	33	0.5	130	43	830	35	26	9	1	4	2	12	10	2	15	15
Hotcakes (2 pats margarine & syrup)	9.3 oz (264 g)	780	300	33	51	9	46	4	50	17	1020	42	106	35	3	10	48	15	2	0	15	15
Sausage Patty	7.9 oz (223 g)	610	160	18	27	4	19	4	20	7	680	28	105	35	3	10	47	9	2	0	15	15
Scrambled Eggs (2)	1.4 oz (41 g)	170	140	15	23	5	27	0	30	10	340	14	1	0	0	0	0	7	0	0	2	2
Hash Browns	3.3 oz (96 g)	170	100	11	17	4	19	0	520	174	180	7	1	0	0	0	0	15	15	0	6	10
Grape Jam	1.9 oz (53 g)	140	70	8	13	1.5	8	2	0	0	290	12	15	5	2	7	0	1	0	2	0	2
Strawberry Preserves	0.5 oz (14 g)	35	0	0	0	0	0	0	0	0	0	0	9	3	0	0	9	0	0	2	0	0
Desserts/Shakes	Serving Size	kcal	kcals from Fat	Total Fat (g)	% Daily Value**	Saturated Fat (g)	% Daily Value**	Trans Fat (g)	Cholesterol (mg)	% Daily Value**	Sodium (mg)	% Daily Value**	CHO (g)	% Daily Value**	Dietary Fiber (g)	% Daily Value**	Sugars (g)	Protein (g)	Vitamin A % DV	Vitamin C % DV	Calcium % DV	Iron % DV
Fruit 'n Yogurt Parfait»	5.3 oz (149 g)	160	20	2	3	1	5	0	5	2	85	4	31	10	1	3	21	4	0	15	15	4
Fruit 'n Yogurt Parfait (without granola)»	5 oz (142 g)	130	15	2	3	1	5	0	5	2	55	2	25	8	0	0	19	4	0	15	10	2
Apple Dippers	1 pkg (68 g)	35	0	0	0	0	0	0	0	0	0	0	8	3	0	0	6	0	0	310	4	0
Low Fat Caramel Dip	0.8 oz (21 g)	70	5	0.5	1	0	0	0	5	1	35	2	15	5	0	0	9	0	0	0	2	0
Vanilla Reduced Fat Ice Cream Cone	3.2 oz (90 g)	150	35	3.5	6	2	11	0	15	5	60	2	24	8	0	0	18	4	6	0	10	2
Kiddie Cone	1 oz (29 g)	45	10	1	2	0.5	4	0	5	2	20	1	8	3	0	0	6	1	2	0	4	0
Strawberry Sundae	6.3 oz (178 g)	280	60	6	10	4	20	0	25	8	95	4	49	16	1	6	45	6	10	4	20	0
Hot Caramel Sundae	6.4 oz (182 g)	340	70	8	12	5	25	0	30	10	160	7	60	20	1	6	44	7	10	0	25	0
Hot Fudge Sundae	6.3 oz (179 g)	330	90	10	15	7	35	0	25	8	180	8	54	18	2	8	48	8	10	0	25	6
Peanuts (for Sundaes)	0.3 oz (7 g)	45	30	3.5	5	0.5	3	0	0	0	0	0	2	1	1	2	0	2	0	0	0	0
Swamp Sludge McFlurry® (12 fl oz cup)	10 oz (283 g)	510	150	16	25	9	47	1	50	16	180	8	80	27	1	3	69	12	20	0	40	6

(continued)

Desserts/Shakes (continued)	Serving Size	kcal	kcals from Fat	Total Fat (g)	% Daily Value**	Saturated Fat (g)	% Daily Value**	Trans Fat (g)	Cholesterol (mg)	% Daily Value**	Sodium (mg)	% Daily Value**	CHO (g)	% Daily Value**	Dietary Fiber (g)	% Daily Value**	Sugars (g)	Protein (g)	Vitamin A % DV	Vitamin C % DV	Calcium % DV	Iron % DV
Swamp Sludge McFlurry® (16 fl oz cup)	13.5 oz (383 g)	710	200	23	35	13	65	1.5	65	22	250	11	110	37	1	5	95	16	25	0	50	8
McFlurry® with M&M'S® Candies (12 fl oz cup)	12.3 oz (348 g)	620	180	20	30	12	59	1	55	19	190	8	96	32	1	3	85	14	20	0	45	6
McFlurry® with OREO® Cookies (12 fl oz cup)	11.9 oz (337 g)	560	150	16	25	9	43	2	50	17	250	10	88	29	0	0	71	14	20	0	45	10
Minty Mudd Bath Triple Thick® Shake (12 fl oz cup)	266 g	430	90	10	15	6	30	0.5	40	13	150	6	75	25	0	0	63	10	15	0	30	4
Minty Mudd Bath Triple Thick® Shake (16 fl oz cup)	355 g	570	120	13	21	8	40	1	50	17	210	9	101	34	0	0	84	13	20	0	45	4
Minty Mudd Bath Triple Thick® Shake (21 fl oz cup)	472 g	760	160	18	27	11	54	1	70	23	270	11	134	45	0	0	112	17	30	0	60	6
Minty Mudd Bath Triple Thick® Shake (32 fl oz cup)	710 g	1150	240	27	41	16	81	2	100	34	410	17	201	67	0	0	169	26	40	0	90	8
Chocolate Triple Thick® Shake (12 fl oz cup)	333 ml	440	90	10	16	6	31	0.5	40	13	190	8	76	25	1	3	63	10	15	0	35	8
Chocolate Triple Thick® Shake (16 fl oz cup)	444 ml	580	120	14	21	8	41	1	50	17	250	11	102	34	1	4	84	13	20	0	45	10
Chocolate Triple Thick® Shake (21 fl oz cup)	583 ml	770	160	18	28	11	55	1	70	23	330	14	134	45	1	5	111	18	30	0	60	15
Chocolate Triple Thick® Shake (32 fl oz cup)	888 ml	1160	240	27	42	16	82	2	100	34	510	21	203	68	2	7	168	27	40	0	90	20
Strawberry Triple Thick® Shake (12 fl oz cup)	333 ml	420	90	10	15	6	30	0.5	40	13	130	5	73	24	0	0	63	10	15	2	30	2
Strawberry Triple Thick® Shake (16 fl oz cup)	444 ml	560	120	13	20	8	40	1	50	17	170	7	97	32	0	0	84	13	20	2	45	2
Strawberry Triple Thick® Shake (21 fl oz cup)	583 ml	740	160	18	27	11	53	1	70	23	230	10	128	43	0	0	111	17	30	2	60	2
Strawberry Triple Thick® Shake (32 fl oz cup)	888 ml	1110	240	26	41	16	80	2	100	34	350	15	194	65	0	0	168	25	40	4	90	4
Vanilla Triple Thick® Shake (12 fl oz cup)	333 ml	420	90	10	15	6	30	0.5	40	13	140	6	72	24	0	0	54	9	15	0	30	2
Vanilla Triple Thick® Shake (16 fl oz cup)	444 ml	550	120	13	20	8	40	1	50	17	190	8	96	32	0	0	72	13	20	0	45	2
Vanilla Triple Thick® Shake (21 fl oz cup)	583 ml	740	160	18	27	11	53	1	70	23	250	10	128	43	0	0	96	17	30	0	60	2

Vanilla Triple Thick® Shake (32 fl oz cup)	888 ml	1110	240	26	41	16	80	2	100	34	370	16	193	64	0	0	145	25	40	0	90	2
Baked Apple Pie	2.7 oz (76 g)	270	110	12	19	3.5	16	5	0	0	190	8	36	12	4	17	14	3	2	10	2	8
Cinnamon Melts	4 oz (114 g)	460	170	19	30	9	43	0	15	5	370	15	66	22	3	11	32	6	4	0	6	15
McDonaldland® Chocolate Chip Cookies	2 oz (56 g)	270	100	11	17	6	32	0	35	12	170	7	39	13	1	5	19	3	4	0	2	10
McDonaldland® Cookies	2 oz (57 g)	250	70	8	12	2	9	2.5	0	0	270	11	42	14	1	4	14	4	0	0	0	10
Chocolate Chip Cookie	1 cookie (33 g)	160	70	7	12	2.5	12	1.5	10	3	90	4	22	7	1	3	15	2	4	0	2	8
Oatmeal Raisin Cookie	1 cookie (33 g)	150	50	6	9	1.5	7	1.5	10	3	135	6	22	7	1	3	13	2	4	0	2	4
Sugar Cookie	1 cookie (32 g)	150	60	6	10	1.5	7	2	5	2	110	5	21	7	0	0	11	2	6	0	2	4

** Contains less than 2% of the Daily Value of these nutrients*

† Available at participating McDonald's

+ Based on the weight before cooking 4 oz. (113.4g)

++ Based on the weight before cooking 8 oz. (226.8g)

§ The values represent the sodium derived from ingredients plus water. Sodium content of the water is based on the value listed for municipal water in the USDA National Nutrient Database. The actual amount of sodium may be higher or lower depending upon the sodium content of the water where the beverage is dispensed.

» Made with low fat yogurt

*** Percent Daily Values (DV) are based on a 2,000 calorie diet. Your daily values may be higher or lower depending on your calorie needs.*

Sonic

Burgers	Serving Weight (g)	kcal	kcals from Fat	Total Fat (g)	Saturated Fat (g)	Trans Fat (g)	Cholesterol (mg)	Sodium (mg)	CHO (g)	Dietary Fiber (g)	Sugars (g)	Protein (g)	Vitamin A % DV	Vitamin C % DV	Calcium % DV	Iron % DV
Sonic® Burger (w/ Mustard)	235	540	230	25	9	2	60	730	52	4	9	24	6%	10%	15%	30%
Sonic® Burger (w/ Ketchup)	235	540	230	25	9	2	60	730	54	4	10	24	6%	10%	15%	30%
Sonic® Cheeseburger (w/ Mayonnaise)	260	700	380	42	14	2	85	1020	55	4	10	27	8%	10%	15%	30%
Sonic® Cheeseburger (w/ Mustard)	253	600	280	31	12	2	75	1050	54	4	10	27	10%	10%	25%	30%
Sonic® Cheeseburger (w/ Ketchup)	260	610	280	31	12	2	75	1120	57	4	13	28	10%	10%	25%	30%
Sonic® Bacon Cheeseburger	273	770	420	47	16	2	100	1280	55	4	10	32	15%	15%	25%	30%
Super Sonic® Cheeseburger (w/ Mayonnaise)	337	970	570	63	24	3.5	165	1420	56	4	11	45	10%	10%	25%	30%
Super Sonic® Cheeseburger (w/ Mustard)	330	870	470	52	23	3.5	155	1440	55	4	11	45	15%	10%	40%	35%
Super Sonic® Cheeseburger (w/ Ketchup	337	880	470	52	23	3.5	155	1520	59	4	14	45	15%	10%	40%	35%
Jr. Burger	117	320	140	16	5	1	35	610	29	2	7	15	20%	15%	40%	35%
Jr. Cheeseburger	135	380	190	21	9	1.5	55	930	30	2	8	18	4%	4%	10%	10%
Dixie Burger	249	640	330	37	11	2	70	790	53	4	9	24	8%	4%	20%	10%
Dixie cheeseburger	267	710	380	42	14	2	85	1110	55	4	10	27	6%	10%	15%	30%
Thousand Island Jr. Cheeseburger	137	440	250	28	10	1.5	60	700	29	2	6	17	10%	10%	25%	30%
California Cheeseburger	260	670	340	38	13	2	80	1050	56	4	11	27	10%	0%	20%	10%
Super Sonic® Jalapeno Cheeseburger	286	860	470	52	23	3.5	155	1310	53	3	10	45	15%	10%	25%	30%
Thousand Island Cheeseburger	260	660	330	37	13	2	85	1110	56	4	11	28	15%	2%	35%	35%
Jalapeno Cheeseburger	209	600	270	30	12	2	75	910	52	3	9	27	15%	10%	25%	30%
Jalapeno Burger	191	530	230	25	9	2	60	590	50	3	8	24	8%	2%	25%	25%
Green Chili Cheeseburger	281	610	280	31	12	2	75	1050	55	4	10	27	2%	2%	15%	25%

Chili Cheeseburger	220	640	310	34	14	2	85	970	54	4	9	30	10%	25%	25%	30%
Hickory Cheeseburger	230	620	270	30	12	2	75	1150	60	4	15	27	10%	6%	25%	30%
Jr. Double Cheeseburger	190	570	320	36	16	2.5	110	1290	32	2	8	30	15%	4%	30%	15%
Add Ons	**Serving Weight (g)**	**kcal**	**kcals from Fat**	**Total Fat (g)**	**Saturated Fat (g)**	**Trans Fat (g)**	**Cholesterol (mg)**	**Sodium (mg)**	**CHO (g)**	**Dietary Fiber (g)**	**Sugars (g)**	**Protein (g)**	**Vitamin A % DV**	**Vitamin C % DV**	**Calcium % DV**	**Iron % DV**
Cheese	18	60	45	5	3	0	20	310	2	0	1	3	6%	0%	10%	0%
Bacon	13	70	50	5	2	0	15	260	0	0	0	4	0%	0%	0%	2%
Chili	33	50	35	3.5	1.5	0	10	160	2	1	1	3	6%	2%	2%	2%
Jalapeno	21	5	0	0	0	0	0	280	1	1	0	0	2%	0%	2%	2%
Green Chiles	28	5	0	0	0	0	0	5	1	0	0	0	0%	15%	0%	0%
Slaw	28	45	30	3	0.5	0	5	45	4	1	1	0	4%	80%	2%	0%
Grilled Onions	28	25	10	1.5	0	0	0	200	2	1	2	0	4%	0%	0%	2%
Kids' Meal	**Serving Weight (g)**	**kcal**	**kcals from Fat**	**Total Fat (g)**	**Saturated Fat (g)**	**Trans Fat (g)**	**Cholesterol (mg)**	**Sodium (mg)**	**CHO (g)**	**Dietary Fiber (g)**	**Sugars (g)**	**Protein (g)**	**Vitamin A % DV**	**Vitamin C % DV**	**Calcium % DV**	**Iron % DV**
Jr. Burger	117	320	140	16	5	1	35	610	29	2	7	15	4%	4%	10%	10%
Jr. Cheeseburger	135	380	190	21	9	1.5	55	930	30	2	8	18	8%	4%	20%	10%
Corn Dog	73	250	130	15	4	1.5	15	80	23	2	8	5	0%	0%	15%	6%
Grilled Cheese	118	390	150	17	8	1.5	35	1010	45	2	7	14	15%	0%	30%	10%
Chicken Strips (2)	72	210	100	11	2	2	35	430	13	1	0	14	0%	0%	2%	4%
Toaster® Sandwiches	**Serving Weight (g)**	**kcal**	**kcals from Fat**	**Total Fat (g)**	**Saturated Fat (g)**	**Trans Fat (g)**	**Cholesterol (mg)**	**Sodium (mg)**	**CHO (g)**	**Dietary Fiber (g)**	**Sugars (g)**	**Protein (g)**	**Vitamin A % DV**	**Vitamin C % DV**	**Calcium % DV**	**Iron % DV**
Chicken Club Toaster® Sandwich	265	690	310	35	10	3	80	1900	64	4	11	32	15%	6%	25%	15%
Bacon Cheeseburger Toaster® Sandwich	251	690	330	37	14	3	90	1410	58	3	13	31	15%	10%	30%	20%

(continued)

Fresh Tastes® Salads	Serving Weight (g)	kcal	kcals from Fat	Total Fat (g)	Saturated Fat (g)	Trans Fat (g)	Cholesterol (mg)	Sodium (mg)	CHO (g)	Dietary Fiber (g)	Sugars (g)	Protein (g)	Vitamin A % DV	Vitamin C % DV	Calcium % DV	Iron % DV
Grilled Chicken Salad	351	310	130	14	6	1	95	1050	19	4	8	28	110%	40%	25%	10%
Jumbo Popcorn Chicken® Salad	354	490	250	28	9	4	60	1440	39	5	8	22	110%	40%	30%	10%
Santa Fe Chicken Salad	399	370	140	15	6	1	95	1140	29	6	8	30	120%	50%	25%	10%
Hidden Valley® Ranch Dressings	Serving Weight (g)	kcal	kcals from Fat	Total Fat (g)	Saturated Fat (g)	Trans Fat (g)	Cholesterol (mg)	Sodium (mg)	CHO (g)	Dietary Fiber (g)	Sugars (g)	Protein (g)	Vitamin A % DV	Vitamin C % DV	Calcium % DV	Iron % DV
Original Ranch Dressing	57	260	250	28	4.5	0	20	490	0	0	0	0	0%	0%	0%	0%
Original Light Ranch Dressing	57	120	60	7	1	0	15	740	14	0	5	1	0%	0%	2%	0%
Honey Mustard	57	240	190	21	3	0	15	300	14	0	12	1	0%	0%	0%	0%
Fat Free Golden Italian	57	50	0	0	0	0	0	600	13	0	4	0	0%	0%	0%	0%
Southwest Ranch	57	120	60	7	1	0	15	770	15	0	5	1	4%	0%	0%	0%
Thousand Island	57	250	230	25	4	0	30	590	9	0	7	1	15%	4%	0%	0%
Wraps	*Serving Weight (g)*	*kcal*	*kcals from Fat*	*Total Fat (g)*	*Saturated Fat (g)*	*Trans Fat (g)*	*Cholesterol (mg)*	*Sodium (mg)*	*CHO (g)*	*Dietary Fiber (g)*	*Sugars (g)*	*Protein (g)*	*Vitamin A % DV*	*Vitamin C % DV*	*Calcium % DV*	*Iron % DV*
Grilled Chicken Wrap	247	380	100	11	2.5	1	75	1300	44	4	3	27	8%	8%	25%	15%
Chicken Strip Wrap	234	480	180	20	4	3	40	1170	56	5	3	20	8%	8%	25%	15%
FRITOS® Chili Cheese Wrap	239	670	340	38	12	1.5	50	1260	66	6	3	22	25%	4%	40%	20%

Chicken	Serving Weight (g)	kcal	kcals from Fat	Total Fat (g)	Saturated Fat (g)	Trans Fat (g)	Cholesterol (mg)	Sodium (mg)	CHO (g)	Dietary Fiber (g)	Sugars (g)	Protein (g)	Vitamin A % DV	Vitamin C % DV	Calcium % DV	Iron % DV
Chicken Strip Dinner (4)	382	920	390	43	8	8	70	1730	97	9	8	36	2%	15%	15%	20%
Grilled Chicken On Ciabatta with Mayonnaise	213	410	160	18	3	0.5	80	980	34	2	5	29	6%	6%	10%	15%
Breaded Chicken On Ciabatta	215	540	260	29	5	2.5	55	1190	47	4	5	24	8%	6%	10%	15%
Jumbo Popcorn Chicken® – Snack	113	370	190	21	4	4	40	1270	27	2	0	19	0%	0%	4%	6%
Jumbo Popcorn Chicken® – Large	170	560	290	32	6	6	65	1910	41	3	0	28	0%	0%	6%	8%
Ranch Sauce	28	150	140	16	2.5	0	10	210	1	0	1	0	0%	0%	0%	0%
Honey Mustard Sauce	28	90	70	7	1	0	10	190	7	0	5	0	0%	0%	0%	0%
BBQ Sauce	28	45	0	0	0	0	0	390	11	0	7	0	2%	0%	0%	2%
Coneys	**Serving Weight (g)**	**kcal**	**kcals from Fat**	**Total Fat (g)**	**Saturated Fat (g)**	**Trans Fat (g)**	**Cholesterol (mg)**	**Sodium (mg)**	**CHO (g)**	**Dietary Fiber (g)**	**Sugars (g)**	**Protein (g)**	**Vitamin A % DV**	**Vitamin C % DV**	**Calcium % DV**	**Iron % DV**
Extra-Long Chili Cheese Coney	237	600	290	33	11	1	75	1700	54	4	7	24	10%	2%	15%	25%
Corn Dog	73	250	130	15	4	1.5	15	80	23	2	8	5	0%	0%	15%	6%
Extra-Long Slaw Dog	280	670	340	38	12	1	80	1770	60	4	8	24	15%	120%	20%	25%
Other Items																
FRITOS® Chili Pie	275	940	570	64	18	1	65	1540	72	6	3	25	30%	4%	35%	10%
Fish Sandwich	245	640	280	31	5	3	35	1180	69	5	10	22	2%	2%	15%	25%
Breaded Pork Fritter Sandwich	274	720	330	36	7	3.5	45	1010	71	5	12	27	6%	6%	15%	30%
Burrito	120	370	180	20	7	1	15	520	37	3	13	11	4%	0%	4%	15%
Burrito Deluxe	144	400	200	22	8	1.5	25	640	36	3	13	13	10%	2%	6%	20%
Tacos	118	310	160	18	6	2	25	370	30	4	1	12	10%	0%	15%	8%

(continued)

Sides	Serving Weight (g)	kcal	kcals from Fat	Total Fat (g)	Saturated Fat (g)	Trans Fat (g)	Cholesterol (mg)	Sodium (mg)	CHO (g)	Dietary Fiber (g)	Sugars (g)	Protein (g)	Vitamin A % DV	Vitamin C % DV	Calcium % DV	Iron % DV
Onion Rings – Regular	156	500	250	28	5	6	0	210	55	4	13	6	0%	0%	40%	8%
Onion Rings – Large	227	720	370	41	7	8	0	300	79	5	18	9	0%	0%	60%	10%
Tater Tots – Regular	84	220	120	14	2.5	3	0	600	23	3	0	2	0%	2%	0%	4%
Tater Tots – Large	126	330	180	20	3.5	4	0	890	35	4	0	3	0%	4%	2%	6%
Tater Tots - SONIC Size	168	440	240	27	4.5	6	0	1190	46	5	0	3	0%	6%	2%	8%
French Fries – Regular	75	210	90	10	2	2	0	260	28	4	0	3	0%	15%	2%	4%
French Fries – Large	98	280	120	13	2.5	3	0	340	37	5	1	4	0%	15%	2%	6%
French Fries - SONIC Size	134	380	160	18	3.5	4	0	470	50	7	1	5	0%	20%	2%	8%
French Fries w/cheese – Regular	93	280	140	15	5	2.5	20	570	29	4	1	6	6%	15%	10%	4%
French Fries w/cheese – Large	125	380	190	21	7	3	25	810	39	5	2	8	8%	15%	15%	6%
French Fries w/cheese – SONIC Size	170	510	250	28	10	4	35	1090	53	7	3	11	10%	20%	20%	8%
French Fries w/chili & cheese – Regular	122	300	160	18	6	2.5	25	530	31	5	1	9	10%	15%	15%	8%
French Fries w/chili & cheese – Large	186	440	240	27	10	3.5	40	820	43	6	2	14	15%	20%	20%	10%
French Fries w/chili & cheese – SONIC Size	262	620	330	37	13	4.5	55	1160	58	9	3	20	25%	25%	25%	15%
Tater Tots w/cheese – Regular	102	290	170	19	6	3	20	910	25	3	1	5	6%	2%	10%	4%
Tater Tots w/cheese – Large	153	430	250	28	8	4.5	25	1360	37	4	1	7	8%	4%	15%	6%
Tater Tots w/cheese – SONIC Size	204	570	340	38	11	6	35	1820	49	5	2	9	10%	6%	20%	8%
Tater Tots w/chili & cheese – Regular	131	310	190	21	7	3	25	860	26	3	1	8	10%	4%	10%	6%
Tater Tots w/chili & cheese – Large	193	440	250	28	7	4.5	20	1220	40	5	2	8	10%	6%	4%	10%
Tater Tots w/chili & cheese – SONIC Size	296	680	420	47	15	6	55	1880	55	7	2	18	25%	8%	25%	15%
Mozzarella Sticks	135	410	190	21	9	2.5	40	1040	35	2	1	19	10%	0%	35%	4%
Ched 'R' Bites	108	360	190	21	9	2	40	910	28	2	0	17	10%	0%	40%	0%
Ched 'R' Peppers	112	290	150	17	6	2.5	20	1040	28	2	1	8	8%	0%	15%	4%

Sonic Blast®	Serving Weight (g)	kcal	kcals from Fat	Total Fat (g)	Saturated Fat (g)	Trans Fat (g)	Cholesterol (mg)	Sodium (mg)	CHO (g)	Dietary Fiber (g)	Sugars (g)	Protein (g)	Vitamin A % DV	Vitamin C % DV	Calcium % DV	Iron % DV
Oreo® Sonic Blast® – Regular (14 oz)	390	660	250	28	18	1	60	220	94	1	84	8	15%	0%	30%	10%
Oreo® Sonic Blast® – Large (20 oz)	559	960	360	40	25	1	85	310	139	2	124	12	20%	0%	45%	15%
M&M's® Sonic Blast® – Regular (14 oz)	390	660	250	28	18	1	60	220	95	1	84	8	15%	0%	30%	10%
M&M's® Sonic Blast® – Large (20 oz)	559	960	360	40	25	1	85	310	139	2	124	12	20%	0%	45%	15%
Reese's Peanut Butter Cups® Sonic Blast® - Regular (14 oz)	387	620	200	22	14	0.5	65	270	96	1	79	10	15%	0%	30%	8%
Reese's Peanut Butter Cups® Sonic Blast® - Large (20 oz)	555	900	270	30	19	1	90	400	142	2	115	15	20%	0%	40%	10%
Butterfinger® Sonic Blast® – Regular (14 oz)	389	670	280	31	19	1	60	250	89	1	77	9	10%	0%	25%	8%
Butterfinger® Sonic Blast® – Large (20 oz)	557	980	400	45	26	1.5	85	360	131	1	112	13	15%	0%	35%	10%
Shakes	**Serving Weight (g)**	**kcal**	**kcals from Fat**	**Total Fat (g)**	**Saturated Fat (g)**	**Trans Fat (g)**	**Cholesterol (mg)**	**Sodium (mg)**	**CHO (g)**	**Dietary Fiber (g)**	**Sugars (g)**	**Protein (g)**	**Vitamin A % DV**	**Vitamin C % DV**	**Calcium % DV**	**Iron % DV**
Vanilla Shake – Regular (14 oz)	417	540	180	20	12	1	75	230	82	0	72	8	15%	0%	30%	8%
Vanilla Shake – Large (20 oz)	603	780	260	29	18	1	105	330	118	0	104	11	20%	0%	45%	10%
Chocolate Shake – Regular (14 oz)	433	610	170	19	12	0.5	70	300	101	0	84	7	15%	0%	30%	8%
Chocolate Shake – Large (20 oz)	637	920	240	27	16	1	100	470	156	0	129	11	20%	0%	40%	10%
Strawberry Shake – Regular (14 oz)	430	580	170	19	12	0.5	70	220	94	1	79	8	15%	15%	30%	8%
Strawberry Shake – Large (20 oz)	631	860	240	27	16	1	100	320	143	1	118	11	20%	25%	40%	15%

(continued)

Shakes (continued)	Serving Weight (g)	kcal	kcals from Fat	Total Fat (g)	Saturated Fat (g)	Trans Fat (g)	Cholesterol (mg)	Sodium (mg)	CHO (g)	Dietary Fiber (g)	Sugars (g)	Protein (g)	Vitamin A % DV	Vitamin C % DV	Calcium % DV	Iron % DV
Banana Shake – Regular (14 oz)	436	550	170	19	12	0.5	70	220	87	1	73	8	15%	6%	30%	8%
Banana Shake – Large (20 oz)	637	790	240	27	17	1	100	310	127	2	106	11	20%	10%	40%	10%
Pineapple Shake – Regular (14 oz)	430	570	170	19	12	0.5	70	230	92	0	76	7	15%	80%	30%	8%
Pineapple Shake – Large (20 oz)	631	840	240	27	16	1	100	330	138	0	113	10	20%	160%	40%	10%
Peanut Butter Shake-Regular (14 oz)	426	710	330	37	15	0.5	70	330	87	0	73	11	15%	0%	30%	8%
Peanut Butter Shake-Large-20 oz)	623	1120	570	63	22	1	100	540	128	0	107	18	20%	0%	40%	10%
Peanut Butter Fudge Shake-Reg (14 oz)	430	680	280	31	15	0.5	70	300	92	1	77	9	15%	0%	30%	8%
Peanut Butter Fudge Shake-Large (20 oz)	610	990	430	47	22	1	100	450	128	1	108	14	20%	0%	40%	10%
Hot Fudge Shake-Regular (14 oz)	431	640	220	24	16	0.5	70	270	97	1	81	7	15%	0%	30%	10%
Hot Fudge Shake-Large (20 oz)	633	980	330	37	25	1	100	420	148	2	123	10	20%	0%	40%	15%
Malts	**Serving Weight (g)**	**kcal**	**kcals from Fat**	**Total Fat (g)**	**Saturated Fat (g)**	**Trans Fat (g)**	**Cholesterol (mg)**	**Sodium (mg)**	**CHO (g)**	**Dietary Fiber (g)**	**Sugars (g)**	**Protein (g)**	**Vitamin A % DV**	**Vitamin C % DV**	**Calcium % DV**	**Iron % DV**
Vanilla Malt – Regular (14 oz)	420	550	190	21	13	1	75	240	84	0	73	8	15%	0%	30%	420
Vanilla Malt – Large (20 oz)	609	810	270	30	19	1	110	350	122	0	107	12	20%	0%	45%	609
Chocolate Malt – Regular (14 oz)	436	630	180	20	12	0.5	70	310	102	0	86	8	15%	0%	30%	436
Chocolate Malt – Large (20 oz)	643	950	260	28	17	1	100	490	160	0	132	11	20%	0%	40%	643
Strawberry Malt – Regular (14 oz)	433	590	180	20	12	0.5	70	230	96	1	80	8	15%	15%	30%	433
Strawberry Malt – Large (20 oz)	637	890	260	28	17	1	100	340	147	1	121	12	20%	25%	45%	637
Banana Malt – Regular (14 oz)	439	560	180	20	12	0.5	70	230	89	1	75	8	15%	6%	30%	439

Banana Malt – Large (20 oz)	643	820	260	29	17	1	100	330	131	2	109	12	20%	10%	45%	643
Pineapple Malt – Regular (14 oz)	433	590	180	20	12	0.5	70	240	93	0	78	8	15%	80%	30%	433
Pineapple Malt – Large (20 oz)	637	870	260	28	17	1	100	350	142	0	116	11	20%	160%	40%	637

CreamSlush® Treat	Serving Weight (g)	kcal	kcals from Fat	Total Fat (g)	Saturated Fat (g)	Trans Fat (g)	Cholesterol (mg)	Sodium (mg)	CHO (g)	Dietary Fiber (g)	Sugars (g)	Protein (g)	Vitamin A % DV	Vitamin C % DV	Calcium % DV	Iron % DV
Strawberry CreamSlush® Treat – Regular (14 oz)	441	450	100	12	7	0	45	150	84	1	72	5	8%	15%	20%	441
Strawberry CreamSlush® Treat – Large (20 oz)	578	620	130	15	9	0.5	55	200	118	1	99	7	10%	25%	25%	578
Orange CreamSlush® Treat – Regular (14 oz)	437	430	110	13	8	0	45	160	77	0	70	5	8%	0%	20%	437
Orange CreamSlush® Treat – Large (20 oz)	569	580	150	17	10	0.5	60	210	104	0	94	6	10%	0%	25%	569
Cherry CreamSlush® Treat – Regular (14 oz)	437	440	110	13	8	0	45	160	77	0	71	5	8%	0%	20%	437
Cherry CreamSlush® Treat – Large (20 oz)	569	590	150	17	10	0.5	60	210	105	0	96	6	10%	0%	25%	569
Grape CreamSlush® Treat – Regular (14 oz)	437	430	110	13	8	0	45	160	76	0	70	5	8%	0%	20%	437
Grape CreamSlush® Treat – Large (20 oz)	569	580	150	17	10	0.5	60	220	103	0	94	7	10%	0%	25%	569
Watermelon CreamSlush® Treat – Regular (14 oz)	437	440	110	13	8	0	45	160	77	0	70	5	8%	0%	20%	437
Watermelon CreamSlush® Treat – Large (20 oz)	570	590	150	17	10	0.5	60	210	105	0	94	7	10%	0%	25%	570
Blue Coconut CreamSlush® Treat – Regular (14 oz)	437	430	110	13	8	0	45	160	76	0	69	5	8%	0%	20%	437
Blue Coconut CreamSlush® Treat – Large (20 oz)	569	580	150	17	10	0.5	60	210	102	0	92	7	10%	0%	25%	569

(continued)

CreamSlush® Treat (continued)	*Serving Weight (g)*	*kcal*	*kcals from Fat*	*Total Fat (g)*	*Saturated Fat (g)*	*Trans Fat (g)*	*Cholesterol (mg)*	*Sodium (mg)*	*CHO (g)*	*Dietary Fiber (g)*	*Sugars (g)*	*Protein (g)*	*Vitamin A % DV*	*Vitamin C % DV*	*Calcium % DV*	*Iron % DV*
Lemon CreamSlush® Treat – Regular (14 oz)	446	430	110	13	8	0	45	160	77	0	69	5	8%	8%	20%	446
Lemon CreamSlush® Treat – Large (20 oz)	587	590	150	17	10	0.5	60	210	104	0	92	7	10%	15%	25%	587
Lemon-Berry CreamSlush® Treat – Regular (14 oz)	450	460	100	12	7	0	45	150	85	1	73	5	8%	20%	20%	450
Lemon-Berry CreamSlush® Treat – Large (20 oz)	596	630	130	15	9	0.5	55	200	119	1	99	7	10%	40%	25%	596
Lime CreamSlush® Treat – Regular (14 oz)	444	430	110	13	8	0	45	160	77	0	69	5	8%	4%	20%	444
Lime CreamSlush® Treat – Large (20 oz)	583	580	150	17	10	0.5	60	210	104	0	92	7	10%	8%	25%	583
Cream Pie Shakes	*Serving Weight (g)*	*kcal*	*kcals from Fat*	*Total Fat (g)*	*Saturated Fat (g)*	*Trans Fat (g)*	*Cholesterol (mg)*	*Sodium (mg)*	*CHO (g)*	*Dietary Fiber (g)*	*Sugars (g)*	*Protein (g)*	*Vitamin A % DV*	*Vitamin C % DV*	*Calcium % DV*	*Iron % DV*
Banana Cream Pie Shake – Regular (14 oz)	477	690	210	23	15	1	65	230	113	1	96	8	15%	6%	30%	8%
Banana Cream Pie Shake – Large (20 oz)	698	1000	280	31	19	1.5	90	300	171	3	146	11	20%	10%	40%	10%
Coconut Cream Pie Shake – Regular (14 oz)	458	680	220	24	15	1	70	240	108	1	94	8	15%	0%	30%	8%
Coconut Cream Pie Shake – Large (20 oz)	665	990	290	32	20	1.5	100	330	162	1	144	11	20%	0%	40%	10%
Chocolate Cream Pie Shake – Regular (14 oz)	475	750	210	23	15	1	65	310	127	1	107	8	10%	0%	30%	8%

Chocolate Cream Pie Shake – Large (20 oz)	698	1130	270	30	19	1.5	90	470	200	1	169	11	15%	0%	40%	10%
Strawberry Cream Pie Shake – Regular (14 oz)	472	720	210	23	15	1	65	240	120	1	101	8	10%	15%	30%	8%
Strawberry Cream Pie Shake – Large (20 oz)	692	1070	270	30	19	1.5	90	330	187	2	158	11	15%	25%	40%	15%
Floats/Blended Floats	*Serving Weight (g)*	*kcal*	*kcals from Fat*	*Total Fat (g)*	*Saturated Fat (g)*	*Trans Fat (g)*	*Cholesterol (mg)*	*Sodium (mg)*	*CHO (g)*	*Dietary Fiber (g)*	*Sugars (g)*	*Protein (g)*	*Vitamin A % DV*	*Vitamin C % DV*	*Calcium % DV*	*Iron % DV*
Coca-Cola® Float/ Blended Float – Regular (14 oz)	355	290	70	8	5	0	30	95	54	0	50	3	6%	0%	10%	4%
Coca-Cola® Float/ Blended Float – Large (20 oz)	501	430	110	12	7	0	45	140	77	0	71	5	8%	0%	20%	4%
Diet Coke® Float/ Blended Float – Regular (14 oz)	348	220	70	8	5	0	30	100	33	0	29	3	6%	0%	10%	4%
Diet Coke® Float/ Blended Float – Large (20 oz)	492	330	110	12	7	0	45	150	50	0	44	5	8%	0%	20%	4%
Dr. Pepper® Float/ Blended Float – Regular (14 oz)	407	310	70	8	5	0	30	120	58	0	54	3	6%	0%	10%	4%
Dr. Pepper® Float/ Blended Float – Large (20 oz)	502	420	110	12	7	0	45	170	76	0	70	5	8%	0%	20%	4%
Diet Dr. Pepper® Float/ Blended Float – Regular (14 oz)	348	220	70	8	5	0	30	130	33	0	29	3	6%	0%	10%	4%
Diet Dr. Pepper® Float/ Blended Float – Large (20 oz)	492	330	110	12	7	0	45	190	50	0	44	5	8%	0%	20%	4%
Barq's® Root Beer Float/Blended Float – Regular (14 oz)	356	300	70	8	5	0	30	110	56	0	52	3	6%	0%	10%	4%
Barq's® Root Beer Float/Blended Float – Large (20 oz)	503	440	110	12	7	0	45	160	80	0	74	5	8%	0%	20%	4%

(continued)

Desserts	Serving Weight (g)	kcal	kcals from Fat	Total Fat (g)	Saturated Fat (g)	Trans Fat (g)	Cholesterol (mg)	Sodium (mg)	CHO (g)	Dietary Fiber (g)	Sugars (g)	Protein (g)	Vitamin A % DV	Vitamin C % DV	Calcium % DV	Iron % DV
Junior Banana Split	139	200	40	4.5	3.5	0	10	60	38	1	27	2	6%	60%	15%	4%
Hot Fudge Cake Sundae	280	530	200	23	14	0	50	310	75	2	58	5	2%	30%	4%	2%
Banana Fudge	293	480	160	18	13	0	35	170	72	2	57	4	6%	0%	15%	30%
Single Topping Sundaes	**Serving Weight (g)**	**kcal**	**kcals from Fat**	**Total Fat (g)**	**Saturated Fat (g)**	**Trans Fat (g)**	**Cholesterol (mg)**	**Sodium (mg)**	**CHO (g)**	**Dietary Fiber (g)**	**Sugars (g)**	**Protein (g)**	**Vitamin A % DV**	**Vitamin C % DV**	**Calcium % DV**	**Iron % DV**
Hot Fudge	253	440	160	18	13	0	35	170	63	1	52	4	6%	0%	15%	6%
Peanut Butter	248	510	280	31	12	0	35	230	53	0	44	8	6%	0%	15%	4%
Peanut Butter Fudge	250	470	220	25	13	0	35	200	58	1	48	6	6%	0%	15%	4%
Strawberry	252	380	120	13	9	0	35	120	61	1	49	4	6%	15%	15%	4%
Chocolate	255	410	120	13	9	0	35	190	67	0	55	4	6%	0%	15%	4%
Pineapple	252	370	120	13	9	0	35	125	58	0	47	4	6%	80%	15%	4%
Nuts Add-on	3.5	20	15	1.5	0	0	0	0	1	0	0	1	0%	0%	0%	0%
Cones and Dishes	**Serving Weight (g)**	**kcal**	**kcals from Fat**	**Total Fat (g)**	**Saturated Fat (g)**	**Trans Fat (g)**	**Cholesterol (mg)**	**Sodium (mg)**	**CHO (g)**	**Dietary Fiber (g)**	**Sugars (g)**	**Protein (g)**	**Vitamin A % DV**	**Vitamin C % DV**	**Calcium % DV**	**Iron % DV**
Vanilla Cone	133	180	60	6	4	0	25	80	30	0	22	2	4%	0%	10%	2%
Vanilla Dish	184	240	80	9	5	0	35	100	36	0	32	3	6%	0%	15%	4%
Real Fruit Slushes	**Serving Weight (g)**	**kcal**	**kcals from Fat**	**Total Fat (g)**	**Saturated Fat (g)**	**Trans Fat (g)**	**Cholesterol (mg)**	**Sodium (mg)**	**CHO (g)**	**Dietary Fiber (g)**	**Sugars (g)**	**Protein (g)**	**Vitamin A % DV**	**Vitamin C % DV**	**Calcium % DV**	**Iron % DV**
Lemon Real Fruit Slush – Small (14 oz)	399	200	0	0	0	0	0	30	53	0	50	0	0%	8%	0%	0%
Lemon Real Fruit Slush – Large (32 oz)	921	460	0	0	0	0	0	70	124	0	117	0	0%	20%	0%	2%

Lemon-Berry Real Fruit Slush – Small (14 oz)	401	210	0	0	0	0	0	30	55	0	52	0	0%	15%	0%	0%
Lemon-Berry Real Fruit Slush – Large (32 oz)	925	500	0	0	0	0	0	75	132	1	121	1	0%	40%	0%	2%
Lime Real Fruit Slush – Small (14 oz)	397	200	0	0	0	0	0	30	52	0	50	0	0%	4%	0%	0%
Lime Real Fruit Slush – Large (32 oz)	915	460	0	0	0	0	0	70	123	0	117	0	0%	10%	0%	2%
Strawberry Real Fruit Slush – Small (14 oz)	392	210	0	0	0	0	0	30	55	0	52	0	0%	6%	0%	0%
Strawberry Real Fruit Slush – Large (32 oz)	898	490	0	0	0	0	0	75	129	1	120	1	0%	20%	0%	2%

Slushes	Serving Weight (g)	kcal	kcals from Fat	Total Fat (g)	Saturated Fat (g)	Trans Fat (g)	Cholesterol (mg)	Sodium (mg)	CHO (g)	Dietary Fiber (g)	Sugars (g)	Protein (g)	Vitamin A % DV	Vitamin C % DV	Calcium % DV	Iron % DV
Cherry Slush – Small (14 oz)	391	200	0	0	0	0	0	30	53	0	53	0	0%	0%	0%	0%
Cherry Slush – Large (32 oz)	895	470	0	0	0	0	0	70	124	0	124	0	0%	0%	0%	0%
Grape Slush – Small (14 oz)	391	190	0	0	0	0	0	35	52	0	52	0	0%	0%	0%	0%
Grape Slush – Large (32 oz)	895	460	0	0	0	0	0	80	121	0	121	0	0%	0%	0%	0%
Orange Slush – Small (14 oz)	390	200	0	0	0	0	0	30	52	0	51	0	0%	0%	0%	0%
Orange Slush – Large (32 oz)	894	460	0	0	0	0	0	75	122	0	120	0	0%	0%	0%	0%
Blue Coconut Slush – Small (14 oz)	390	190	0	0	0	0	0	30	52	0	51	0	0%	0%	0%	0%
Blue Coconut Slush – Large (32 oz)	894	450	0	0	0	0	0	70	121	0	118	0	0%	0%	0%	2%
Watermelon Slush – Small (14 oz)	391	200	0	0	0	0	0	30	53	0	51	0	0%	0%	0%	0%
Watermelon Slush – Large (32 oz)	895	470	0	0	0	0	0	75	124	0	120	0	0%	0%	0%	0%
Green Apple Slush – Small (14 oz)	391	200	0	0	0	0	0	30	54	0	53	0	0%	0%	0%	0%

(continued)

Slushes (continued)	Serving Weight (g)	kcal	kcals from Fat	Total Fat (g)	Saturated Fat (g)	Trans Fat (g)	Cholesterol (mg)	Sodium (mg)	CHO (g)	Dietary Fiber (g)	Sugars (g)	Protein (g)	Vitamin A % DV	Vitamin C % DV	Calcium % DV	Iron % DV
Green Apple Slush – Large (32 oz)	897	490	0	0	0	0	0	75	129	0	124	0	0%	0%	0%	0%
Bubble Gum Slush – Small (14 oz)	391	190	0	0	0	0	0	35	52	0	51	0	0%	0%	0%	0%
Bubble Gum Slush – Large (32 oz)	895	460	0	0	0	0	0	85	121	1	120	0	0%	0%	0%	0%
Breakfast Foods	**Serving Weight (g)**	**kcal**	**kcals from Fat**	**Total Fat (g)**	**Saturated Fat (g)**	**Trans Fat (g)**	**Cholesterol (mg)**	**Sodium (mg)**	**CHO (g)**	**Dietary Fiber (g)**	**Sugars (g)**	**Protein (g)**	**Vitamin A % DV**	**Vitamin C % DV**	**Calcium % DV**	**Iron % DV**
Breakfast Bistro – Bacon, Egg & Cheese	156	470	250	27	9	1	320	1370	35	2	6	21	15%	0%	20%	20%
Breakfast Bistro – Ham, Egg & Cheese	175	430	190	21	7	1	325	1640	35	2	6	25	15%	0%	20%	20%
Breakfast Bistro – Sausage, Egg & Cheese	183	560	330	37	12	1.5	340	1320	35	2	6	22	15%	0%	20%	20%
BREAKFAST TOASTER® – Sausage, Egg & Cheese	202	630	350	39	13	1.5	340	1380	46	2	7	23	15%	0%	25%	20%
BREAKFAST TOASTER® – Bacon, Egg & Cheese	175	540	270	30	10	1.5	325	1440	46	2	7	22	15%	0%	25%	15%
BREAKFAST TOASTER® – Ham, Egg & Cheese	194	500	210	23	7	1.5	325	1700	46	2	7	26	15%	0%	25%	15%
Breakfast Burritos – Sausage, Egg & Cheese	167	470	270	30	11	1.5	325	1040	38	3	2	19	15%	0%	40%	20%
Breakfast Burritos – Bacon, Egg & Cheese	157	450	240	27	10	1.5	320	1140	38	3	2	20	15%	0%	40%	15%
Breakfast Burritos – Ham, Egg & Cheese	183	440	210	23	8	1.5	330	1530	37	3	2	25	15%	0%	40%	20%
Super Sonic® Breakfast Burrito	216	550	310	35	11	2.5	325	1240	47	4	2	19	20%	4%	40%	25%

French Toast Sticks (4)	136	500	230	26	5	4.5	25	580	59	2	12	8	0%	0%	10%	15%
Syrup	28	80	0	0	0	0	0	0	21	0	19	0	0%	0%	0%	0%
Fruit Smoothies	Serving Weight (g)	kcal	kcals from Fat	Total Fat (g)	Saturated Fat (g)	Trans Fat (g)	Cholesterol (mg)	Sodium (mg)	CHO (g)	Dietary Fiber (g)	Sugars (g)	Protein (g)	Vitamin A % DV	Vitamin C % DV	Calcium % DV	Iron % DV
Strawberry Fruit Smoothie – Regular (14 oz)	435	460	0	0	0	0	0	180	113	8	91	1	160%	240%	150%	8%
Strawberry-Banana Fruit Smoothie – Regular (14 oz)	415	440	0	0	0	0	0	160	108	3	76	1	150%	160%	150%	10%
Tropical Fruit Smoothie – Regular (14 oz)	420	500	0	0	0	0	0	170	124	4	98	1	150%	270%	140%	10%

http://www.sonicdrivein.com/pdfs/menu/SonicNutritionGuide.pdf

Taco Bell "Fresco" Style* Nutrition Guide

Our most popular "Fresco" Style Items Under 10 Grams of Fat	Serving Size (g)	kcal	kcals from Fat	Total Fat (g)	% Daily Value**	Saturated Fat (g)	% Daily Value**	Trans Fat (g)	Cholesterol (mg)	% Daily Value**	Sodium (mg)	% Daily Value**	CHO	% Daily Value**	Dietary Fiber (g)	% Daily Value**	Sugars (g)	Protein (g)	Vitamin A % DV	Vitamin C % DV	Calcium % DV	Iron % DV
Crunchy Taco	92	150	70	8	12	2.5	13	0	20	7	370	15	13	4	3	12	1	7	6	4	4	6
Crunchy TACO SUPREME®	106	150	70	8	12	2.5	13	0	20	7	370	15	14	5	3	12	2	7	6	8	4	6
Soft Taco – Beef	113	180	70	7	11	3	15	0	20	7	650	27	21	7	3	12	2	8	6	4	8	10
Soft Taco Supreme® – Beef	128	190	70	7	11	3	15	0	20	7	650	27	22	7	3	12	3	9	6	8	8	10
Ranchero Chicken Soft Taco	135	170	35	4	6	1.5	8	0	25	8	730	30	21	7	3	12	3	12	8	8	8	10
Grilled Steak Soft Taco	128	160	40	4.5	7	1.5	8	0	20	7	550	23	20	7	2	8	3	10	4	10	8	10
Bean Burrito	213	320	60	7	11	2.5	13	0.5	0	0	1200	50	54	18	9	36	4	12	10	10	15	25
7-Layer Burrito	248	380	80	8	12	2.5	13	0.5	0	0	1190	50	62	21	9	36	4	13	6	10	15	25
Chili Cheese Burrito	149	270	70	8	12	3	15	0	15	5	930	39	39	13	4	16	3	10	6	4	15	20
1/2 lb.† Cheesy Bean & Rice Burrito	198	330	70	7	11	2	10	0	0	0	1080	45	55	18	6	24	4	10	8	6	15	20
Enchirito® – Beef	206	230	80	8	12	3.5	18	0.5	20	7	1300	54	34	11	7	28	3	12	20	15	10	15
MexiMelt®	120	190	70	7	11	3	15	0	20	7	710	30	22	7	3	12	3	8	8	6	8	10
Steak Grilled Taquitos	135	260	60	7	11	2.5	13	0	20	7	830	35	37	12	3	12	3	13	4	4	10	20
Mexican Rice	138	120	25	3	5	0.5	3	0	0	0	760	32	23	8	2	8	1	3	15	10	2	8
Pintos 'n Cheese	135	100	20	2	3	0.5	3	0.5	0	0	640	27	19	6	7	28	1	6	10	10	4	8
Tacos	Serving Size (g)	kcal	kcals from Fat	Total Fat (g)	% Daily Value**	Saturated Fat (g)	% Daily Value**	Trans Fat (g)	Cholesterol (mg)	% Daily Value**	Sodium (mg)	% Daily Value**	CHO	% Daily Value**	Dietary Fiber (g)	% Daily Value**	Sugars (g)	Protein (g)	Vitamin A % DV	Vitamin C % DV	Calcium % DV	Iron % DV
Crunchy Taco	78	170	90	10	15	3.5	18	0	25	8	350	15	13	4	3	12	1	8	4	2	8	6
Crunchy TACO SUPREME®	113	210	120	13	20	6	30	0	40	13	370	15	15	5	3	12	2	9	10	6	10	6
DOUBLE DECKER® Taco Supreme®	191	370	150	17	26	7	35	1	40	13	820	34	40	13	7	28	4	14	10	6	15	20
Soft Taco – Beef	99	200	80	9	14	4	20	0	25	8	630	26	21	7	3	12	2	10	4	2	10	10
Soft Taco Supreme® – Beef	135	250	120	13	20	6	30	0.5	40	13	650	27	23	8	3	12	3	11	10	6	15	15
Ranchero Chicken Soft Taco	135	270	130	14	22	4	20	0	35	12	820	34	21	7	2	8	3	14	6	6	15	10
Grilled Steak Soft Taco	128	270	150	16	25	4.5	23	0	35	12	660	28	20	7	2	8	3	12	4	6	10	15
GORDITAS																						
Gordita Supreme® – Beef	153	310	140	16	25	6	30	0.5	40	13	620	26	29	10	3	12	6	14	8	6	15	15
Gordita Supreme® – Chicken	153	290	110	12	18	5	25	0	45	15	650	27	28	9	2	8	6	17	8	8	15	10

Gordita Supreme® – Steak	153	290	120	13	20	5	25	0	40	13	530	22	28	9	2	8	6	15	6	6	10	15
Gordita Baja® – Beef	153	340	170	19	29	5	25	0	35	12	780	33	29	10	4	16	6	13	8	4	10	15
Gordita Baja® – Chicken	153	320	140	16	25	3.5	18	0	40	13	800	33	28	9	3	12	6	17	8	6	10	10
Gordita Baja® – Steak	153	320	150	17	26	4	20	0	35	12	690	29	27	9	3	12	5	15	6	4	10	15
Gordita Nacho Cheese – Beef	153	300	130	14	22	4	20	1.5	25	8	770	32	31	10	3	12	6	12	4	6	10	15
Gordita Nacho Cheese – Chicken	153	280	100	11	17	2.5	13	1	25	8	800	33	29	10	2	8	6	16	4	8	10	10
Gordita Nacho Cheese – Steak	153	270	100	12	18	3	13	1	20	7	680	28	29	10	2	8	6	14	2	6	8	15
CHALUPAS																						
Chalupa Supreme – Beef	153	380	210	23	35	7	35	0.5	40	13	620	26	30	10	3	12	4	14	8	6	15	15
Chalupa Supreme – Chicken	153	360	180	20	31	5	25	0	45	15	650	27	29	10	2	8	4	17	8	8	15	10
Chalupa Supreme – Steak	153	360	180	21	32	6	30	0	40	13	530	22	28	9	2	8	4	15	6	6	10	15
Chalupa Baja – Beef	153	410	240	27	42	6	30	0	35	12	780	33	30	10	4	16	4	13	8	4	10	15
Chalupa Baja – Chicken	153	390	210	23	35	4	20	0	40	13	800	33	29	10	3	12	4	17	8	6	10	10
Chalupa Baja – Steak	153	390	220	24	37	4.5	23	0	35	12	690	29	28	9	3	12	3	15	6	4	10	15
Chalupa Nacho Cheese – Beef	153	370	190	22	34	4.5	23	1.5	20	7	770	32	32	11	3	12	4	12	4	6	10	15
Chalupa Nacho Cheese – Chicken	153	350	160	18	28	3	15	1	25	8	790	33	30	10	2	8	4	16	4	8	10	10
Chalupa Nacho Cheese – Steak	153	340	170	19	29	3.5	18	1.5	20	7	680	28	30	10	2	8	4	14	2	6	8	15
BURRITOS																						
Bean Burrito	198	340	80	9	14	3.5	18	0.5	5	2	1190	50	54	18	8	32	4	13	10	8	20	25
7-Layer Burrito	283	490	170	18	28	7	35	1	25	8	1350	56	65	22	9	36	5	17	10	25	25	30
Burrito Supreme® – Beef	248	410	150	17	26	8	40	1	40	13	1340	56	51	17	7	28	5	17	15	10	20	25
Burrito Supreme® – Chicken	248	390	120	13	20	6	30	0.5	45	15	1360	57	49	16	6	24	5	20	15	15	20	25
Burrito Supreme® – Steak	248	380	130	14	22	7	35	0.5	40	13	1250	52	49	16	6	24	5	18	15	15	20	25
Fiesta Burrito – Beef	184	370	120	13	20	5	25	0	25	8	1200	50	49	16	4	16	4	14	8	4	20	25
Fiesta Burrito – Chicken	184	350	90	10	15	3.5	18	0	30	10	1220	51	47	16	3	12	4	18	8	4	20	20
Fiesta Burrito – Steak	184	340	100	11	17	4	20	0	25	8	1110	46	47	16	3	12	3	15	6	4	20	20
Grilled Stuft Burrito – Beef	325	680	270	30	46	10	50	1	55	18	2120	88	76	25	9	36	6	27	15	4	30	40
Grilled Stuft Burrito – Chicken	325	640	210	23	35	7	35	0.5	65	22	2160	90	73	24	7	28	6	34	10	6	30	35
Grilled Stuft Burrito – Steak	325	630	220	25	38	8	40	1	55	18	1930	80	72	24	7	28	5	30	10	8	30	40
BIG BELL VALUE MENU®																						
Grande Soft Taco	206	430	180	20	31	8	40	1.5	45	15	1440	60	43	14	5	20	5	19	8	2	20	25
DOUBLE DECKER® Taco	156	320	120	13	20	5	25	0.5	25	8	810	34	38	13	6	24	2	14	6	2	15	15
Spicy Chicken Soft Taco	113	170	50	6	9	2	10	0	25	8	580	24	20	7	2	8	2	10	8	4	10	10
Spicy Chicken Burrito	191	400	150	17	26	4	20	0	30	10	1190	50	48	16	3	12	4	14	10	4	15	20
1/2 lb.† Beef Combo Burrito	241	430	160	18	28	8	40	1	45	15	1630	68	51	17	8	32	4	21	15	6	20	30

(continued)

	Serving Size (g)	kcal	kcals from Fat	Total Fat (g)	% Daily Value**	Saturated Fat (g)	% Daily Value**	Trans Fat (g)	Cholesterol (mg)	% Daily Value**	Sodium (mg)	% Daily Value**	CHO	% Daily Value**	Dietary Fiber (g)	% Daily Value**	Sugars (g)	Protein (g)	Vitamin A % DV	Vitamin C % DV	Calcium % DV	Iron % DV
1/2 lb.† Beef & Potato Burrito	252	520	210	23	35	7	35	1	30	10	1720	72	66	22	6	24	4	15	15	6	15	25
1/2 lb.† Cheesy Bean & Rice Burrito	227	470	180	20	31	6	30	1.5	15	5	1400	58	58	19	6	24	5	13	8	4	20	25
Cheesy Fiesta Potatoes	138	290	150	17	26	4	20	1.5	15	5	830	35	30	10	3	12	2	4	6	2	6	6
Caramel Apple Empanada	85	290	120	14	22	2.5	13	1.5	5	2	300	13	37	12	1	4	13	3	2	15	4	6
SPECIALTIES																						
Crunchwrap Supreme®	254	560	220	24	37	8	40	1.5	35	12	1430	60	68	23	5	20	7	17	8	8	25	30
Spicy Chicken CRUNCHWRAP SUPREME®	254	540	200	23	35	7	35	1.5	40	13	1360	57	67	22	4	16	7	19	10	8	30	30
Mexican Pizza	216	530	270	30	46	8	40	1	40	13	1000	42	46	15	7	28	3	20	10	8	35	20
Enchirito® – Beef	213	340	150	17	26	9	45	1	50	17	1420	59	34	11	7	28	3	18	25	10	30	20
Enchirito® – Chicken	213	320	120	13	20	7	35	0.5	50	17	1450	60	33	11	6	24	3	22	25	15	30	15
Enchirito® – Steak	213	310	130	14	22	7	35	1	45	15	1330	55	33	11	6	24	3	20	25	15	30	15
MexiMelt®	128	280	130	14	22	7	35	0.5	40	13	860	36	22	7	3	12	2	15	10	4	25	15
Fiesta Taco Salad	548	840	400	45	69	11	55	1.5	65	22	1780	74	80	27	15	60	10	30	25	20	45	40
Fiesta Taco Salad without Shell	479	470	220	24	37	10	50	1.5	65	22	1510	63	41	14	13	52	9	23	25	20	30	25
Chicken Fiesta Taco Salad	548	800	340	38	58	8	40	1	75	25	1830	76	77	26	13	52	10	37	25	25	40	35
Chicken Fiesta Taco Salad without Shell	479	430	160	18	28	6	30	1	75	25	1560	65	38	13	11	44	9	30	25	25	30	20
Express Taco Salad	479	610	290	32	49	10	50	1.5	65	22	1420	59	56	19	14	56	8	25	20	20	30	25
Steak Grilled Taquitos with Guacamole	170	380	150	17	26	6	30	0	35	12	1040	43	41	14	4	16	4	17	4	30	20	20
Steak Grilled Taquitos with Salsa	170	320	100	11	17	5	25	0	35	12	1030	43	39	13	3	12	5	16	10	6	25	20
Steak Grilled Taquitos with Sour Cream	170	390	170	19	29	10	50	0.5	60	20	900	38	39	13	2	8	5	17	10	2	25	20
Chicken Quesadilla	184	520	250	28	43	12	60	0.5	75	25	1420	59	59	13	3	12	4	28	10	2	45	20
Steak Quesadilla	184	520	260	28	43	13	65	1	70	23	1300	54	54	13	3	12	4	26	10	0	45	20
Zesty Chicken BORDER BOWL®	418	640	310	35	54	6	30	1	30	10	1800	75	75	20	10	40	4	22	15	15	15	25
Zesty Chicken BORDER BOWL® without Dressing	376	440	130	15	23	2.5	13	0.5	30	10	1540	64	64	19	10	40	3	21	15	15	15	20
Southwest Steak BORDER BOWL®	443	600	220	24	37	6	30	1	55	18	2120	88	88	23	9	36	3	28	20	15	20	35
NACHOS AND SIDES																						
Nachos	99	330	180	21	32	3.5	18	2	5	2	530	22	32	11	2	8	3	4	0	0	8	4

Nachos Supreme	195	450	230	26	40	7	35	1.5	35	12	800	33	41	14	7	28	3	12	8	8	10	10
Nachos BellGrande®	308	770	390	44	68	9	45	3	35	12	1280	53	77	26	12	48	5	19	8	8	20	20
Pintos 'n Cheese	128	150	50	6	9	3	15	0.5	15	5	670	28	19	6	7	28	1	9	10	6	15	8
Mexican Rice	131	170	60	7	11	3	15	0	15	5	790	33	23	8	1	4	1	6	15	6	10	8
Cinnamon Twists	35	170	60	7	11	0	0	0	0	0	200	8	26	9	1	4	12	1	0	0	0	2
REGIONAL MENU ITEMS																						
Cheese Quesadilla	142	470	240	26	40	12	60	0.5	50	17	1100	46	39	13	2	8	4	19	10	2	45	20
Chili Cheese Burrito	156	370	140	16	25	8	40	0.5	40	13	1060	44	40	13	3	12	3	16	10	0	30	20
Tostada	170	230	90	10	15	3.5	18	0.5	15	5	730	30	27	9	7	28	2	11	10	8	20	10

***Percent daily values are based on a 2,000 calorie diet.*

** "Fresco" Style fat reduction varies per menu item and not all menu items will meet a 25% reduction in fat.*

† 1/2 lb. claim based on average weight. Individual product weights necessarily vary.

http://www.yum.com/nutrition/documents/tb_nutrition.pdf

Wendy's

Garden Sensations® Salads Flavor-Packed Entrée Salads* Prepared Fresh Daily	kcal	Total Fat (g)	Saturated Fat (g)	Trams Fat (g)	Cholesterol (mg)	Sodium (mg)	Total CHO (g)	Dietary Fiber (g)	Sugars (g)	Protein (g)
Mandarin Chicken® Salad	170	2.5	0.5	0	60	520	16	3	12	21
Crispy Noodles	70	2.5	0	0	0	190	10	0	0	1
Roasted Almonds	130	11	1	0	0	70	4	2	1	5
Oriental Sesame Dressing	170	9	1.5	0	0	430	19	0	17	1
Chicken Caesar Salad	180	6	2.5	0	70	660	8	3	3	25
Homestyle Garlic Croutons	70	2.5	0	0	0	125	9	0	0	2
Caesar Dressing	120	13	2.5	0	20	220	1	0	0	1
Chicken BLT Salad	330	18	9	0	105	1050	11	4	5	33
Homestyle Garlic Croutons	70	2.5	0	0	0	125	9	0	0	2
Honey Mustard Dressing	250	23	3.5	0	20	330	9	0	9	1
Southwest Taco Salad	430	22	12	1	80	1090	30	8	9	30
Reduced Fat Acidifi ed Sour Cream	50	4	2.5	0	10	30	2	0	1	1
Seasoned Tortilla Strips	110	5	1	0	0	160	13	1	0	2
Ancho Chipotle Ranch Dressing	90	8	1.5	0	10	270	3	0	2	1
Additional Salad Dressings										
Fat Free French	70	0	0	0	0	190	17	0	14	0
Reduced Fat Creamy Ranch**	90	7	1.5	0	10	400	6	1	3	1
Low Fat Honey Mustard**	100	2.5	0	0	0	300	19	0	14	0
Italian Vinaigrette	130	11	1.5	0	0	360	8	0	7	0
Creamy Ranch	200	20	3.5	0	15	400	4	0	2	1
Blue Cheese**	260	27	4.5	0	35	480	2	0	1	2
Thousand Island**	230	22	3.5	0	20	400	7	0	5	1

** Toppings and Salad Dressings listed separately.*

*** Not available in all locations.*

Side Selections Numerous Options for a Balanced Meal	kcal	Total Fat (g)	Saturated Fat (g)	Trams Fat (g)	Cholesterol (mg)	Sodium (mg)	Total CHO (g)	Dietary Fiber (g)	Sugars (g)	Protein (g)
Side Salad	35	0	0	0	0	25	8	2	4	1
Caesar Side Salad	80	4.5	2	0	10	240	6	2	1	6
Mandarin Orange Cup	80	0	0	0	0	15	19	1	17	1
Low Fat Strawberry Flavored Yogurt	140	1.5	1	0	5	90	27	0	24	6
Granola Topping	110	4.5	0.5	0	0	0	15	1	6	2
Plain Baked Potato (avg. wgt. 10oz.)	270	0	0	0	0	25	61	7	3	7
Sour Cream & Chives Baked Potato	320	4	2.5	0	10	55	63	7	4	9
Buttery Best Spread	50	6	1	0	0	90	0	0	0	0
Small Chili	220	6	2.5	0	35	780	23	5	6	17
Large Chili	330	9	3.5	0.5	55	1170	35	8	9	25
Hot Chili Seasoning	5	0	0	0	0	270	2	0	1	0
Saltine Crackers	25	0.5	0	0	0	95	4	0	0	0
Cheddar Cheese, Shredded	70	6	3.5	0	15	110	1	0	0	4
Kid's Meal French Fries*	210	10	1.5	0	0	210	26	3	0	3
Small French Fries*	330	16	2.5	0.5	0	340	42	4	0	4
Medium French Fries*	420	20	3	1	0	430	53	5	0	6
Large French Fries*	520	24	3.5	1	0	550	69	7	0	7

**Recommended portion sizes. French fries are individually portioned at every restaurant. Variations will exist from restaurant to restaurant.*

Beverages and Frosty™ Refreshments for Everyone's Thirst	kcal	Total Fat (g)	Saturated Fat (g)	Trams Fat (g)	Cholesterol (mg)	Sodium (mg)	Total CHO (g)	Dietary Fiber (g)	Sugars (g)	Protein (g)
Milk, 2% Reduced Fat Milk	120	4.5	3	0	20	125	12	0	11	7
Milk, 1% Low Fat Chocolate	170	2.5	1.5	0	15	200	28	0	26	8
Diet Coke®, Small Cup	0	0	0	0	0	15+	0	0	0	0
Sprite®, Small Cup	130	0	0	0	0	30+	34	0	34	0
Coca-Cola®, Small Cup	140	0	0	0	0	0+	37	0	37	0
Dasani® Water	0	0	0	0	0	0	0	0	0	0
Chocolate Frosty Junior	160	4	2.5	0	15	75	28	0	21	4
Chocolate Frosty Small	330	8	5	0	35	150	56	0	42	8
Chocolate Frosty Medium	430	11	7	0	45	200	74	0	55	10
Vanilla Frosty Junior	150	4	2.5	0	20	90	26	0	21	4
Vanilla Frosty Small	310	8	5	0	35	180	52	0	43	8
Vanilla Frosty Medium	410	10	6	0.5	45	240	68	0	57	11
Vanilla Frosty Float with Coca-Cola*	410	8	5	0	35	190+	78	0	69	8
Chocolate Frosty Fix 'N Mix	170	4	2.5	0	20	80	29	0	22	4
Vanilla Frosty Fix 'N Mix	160	4	2.5	0	20	95	27	0	22	4
Oreo® Cookie Crumbles*	100	4	1.5	0	0	115	15	1	9	1
Butterfi nger® Candy Crumbles*	130	5	2.5	0	0	65	20	1	13	2
M&M® Candy Crumbles*	140	6	3.5	0	5	15	20	1	18	1

Sandwiches Made when you order it using each sandwich's standard toppings	kcal	Total Fat (g)	Saturated Fat (g)	Trams Fat (g)	Cholesterol (mg)	Sodium (mg)	Total CHO (g)	Dietary Fiber (g)	Sugars (g)	Protein (g)
Jr. Hamburger	230	8	3	0	25	500	26	1	5	13
Jr. Cheeseburger	270	11	5	0.5	35	710	26	1	6	15
Jr. Cheeseburger Deluxe	300	14	5	0.5	40	760	28	2	7	15
Jr. Bacon Cheeseburger	310	16	6	0.5	45	690	26	1	5	17
Hamburger, Kids' Meal	220	8	3	0	25	500	25	1	5	13
Cheeseburger, Kids' Meal	260	11	5	0.5	35	710	26	1	5	15
Ham & Cheese Sandwich, Kids' Meal	200	5	2.5	0	30	810	25	1	4	13
Turkey & Cheese Sandwich, Kids' Meal	210	6	2.5	0	25	830	27	1	4	12
Single w/Everything	430	20	7	1	65	900	37	2	9	25
Double w/Everything and Cheese	700	40	16	2.5	140	1500	38	2	9	48
Triple w/Everything and Cheese	980	59	25	3.5	215	2090	38	2	9	70
Baconator™	830	51	22	2.5	170	1920	35	1	8	57
Ultimate Chicken Grill Sandwich	320	7	1.5	0	70	950	36	2	8	28
Spicy Chicken Fillet Sandwich	440	16	2.5	0	60	1320	46	3	6	28
Homestyle Chicken Fillet Sandwich	430	16	2.5	0	45	1140	48	2	6	25
Chicken Club Sandwich	540	25	7	0.5	75	1410	49	2	7	33
Crispy Chicken Sandwich	320	14	2.5	0	30	660	34	1	4	15
Black Forest Ham & Swiss Frescata®	460	19	6	0	60	1470	50	4	8	27
Roasted Turkey & Swiss Frescata	470	20	6	0	60	1520	51	4	4	25
Frescata Club	440	17	3.5	0	50	1600	49	4	5	23

Crispy Chicken Nuggets Crispy All-White Meat for Full Flavor Dipping	kcal	Total Fat (g)	Saturated Fat (g)	Trams Fat (g)	Cholesterol (mg)	Sodium (mg)	Total CHO (g)	Dietary Fiber (g)	Sugars (g)	Protein (g)
4 Piece Kids' Meal Chicken Nuggets	190	12	2	0	30	420	10	0	0	10
5 Piece Chicken Nuggets	230	15	3	0	35	520	12	0	0	12
10 Piece Chicken Nuggets	460	30	6	0	70	1040	24	0	0	24
Barbecue Nugget Sauce	45	0	0	0	0	170	10	0	8	1
Sweet & Sour Nugget Sauce	50	0	0	0	0	120	13	0	11	0
Honey Mustard Nugget Sauce	130	12	2	0	10	220	6	0	5	0
Heartland Ranch Dipping Sauce	160	17	2.5	0	15	220	1	0	1	0

http://www.wendys.com/food/pdf/us/nutrition.pdf

Appendix B Energy Expenditure in Household, Occupational, Recreational, and Sports Activities[a,b]

HOW TO USE APPENDIX B

Refer to the column that comes closest to your present body mass. Multiply the number in this column by the number of minutes you spend in an activity. Suppose that an individual weighing 80.0 kg (176 lb) spends 45 minutes working out with free weights. To determine the energy cost of participation, multiply the caloric value per minute (6.8 kcal) by 45 to obtain the 45-minute gross expenditure of 306 kcal. If the same individual does aerobic dance for 60 minutes, the gross (value includes resting energy expenditure) energy expended would be calculated as 7.8 kcal × 60 minutes, or 468 kcal.

[a] All values for energy expenditure expressed in kilocalories per minute.

YOUR BODY WEIGHT

Activity	kg lb	47 104	50 110	53 117	56 123	59 130	62 137	65 143	68 150
Archery		3.1	3.3	3.4	3.6	3.8	4.0	4.2	4.4
Backpacking									
without load		5.7	6.1	6.4	6.8	7.1	7.5	7.9	8.2
with 11 pound load		6.1	6.5	6.8	7.2	7.6	8.0	8.4	8.8
with 22 pound load		6.6	7.0	7.4	7.8	8.3	8.7	9.1	9.5
with 44 pound load		7.0	7.4	7.8	8.2	8.7	9.1	9.6	10.0
Badminton									
leisure		4.6	4.9	5.1	5.4	5.7	6.0	6.3	6.6
tournament		7.0	7.3	7.7	8.1	8.6	9.0	9.4	9.9
Baking, general (F)		1.6	1.8	1.9	2.0	2.1	2.2	2.3	2.4
Baseball									
fielder		2.8	3.0	3.2	3.4	3.6	3.8	4.0	4.1
pitcher		4.2	4.5	4.8	5.0	5.3	5.6	5.9	6.2
Basketball									
competition		7.1	7.4	7.9	8.3	8.7	9.2	9.6	10.1
practice		6.5	6.9	7.3	7.7	8.1	8.6	9.0	9.4
Baton twirling		6.3	6.8	7.3	7.6	8.1	8.5	8.9	9.3
Billiards ("pool")		2.0	2.1	2.2	2.4	2.5	2.6	2.7	2.9
Bookbinding		1.8	1.9	2.0	2.1	2.2	2.4	2.5	2.6
Bowling		4.4	4.8	5.2	5.4	5.7	6.0	6.3	6.6
Boxing									
in ring, match		10.4	11.1	11.8	12.4	13.1	13.8	14.4	15.1
sparring, practice		6.5	6.9	7.3	7.7	8.1	8.6	9.0	9.4
Calisthenics, warm-ups		3.4	3.7	4.0	4.2	4.4	4.7	4.9	5.1
Canoeing									
leisure (2.5 mph)		2.1	2.2	2.3	2.5	2.6	2.7	2.9	3.0
racing ("fast")		4.8	5.2	5.5	5.8	6.1	6.4	6.7	7.0
Car washing		3.3	3.5	3.7	3.9	4.1	4.3	4.5	4.8
Card playing		1.2	1.3	1.3	1.4	1.5	1.6	1.6	1.7
Carpentry, general		2.4	2.6	2.8	2.9	3.1	3.2	3.4	3.5
Carpet sweeping (F)		2.2	2.3	2.4	2.5	2.7	2.8	2.9	3.1
Carpet sweeping (M)		2.3	2.4	2.5	2.7	2.8	3.0	3.1	3.3
Circuit resistance training									
Free weights		4.0	4.3	4.5	4.8	5.0	5.3	5.5	5.8
Hydra-Fitness		6.2	6.6	7.0	7.4	7.8	8.2	8.6	9.0
Nautilus		4.3	4.6	4.9	5.2	5.5	5.8	6.0	6.3
Universal		5.3	5.8	6.2	6.5	6.9	7.2	7.5	7.9
Cleaning (F)		2.9	3.1	3.3	3.5	3.7	3.8	4.0	4.2
Cleaning (M)		2.7	2.9	3.1	3.2	3.4	3.6	3.8	3.9
Coal mining									
drilling coal, rock		4.4	4.7	5.0	5.3	5.5	5.8	6.1	6.4
erecting supports		4.1	4.4	4.7	4.9	5.2	5.5	5.7	6.0
shoveling coal		5.1	5.4	5.7	6.0	6.4	6.7	7.0	7.3
Cooking (F)		2.1	2.3	2.4	2.5	2.7	2.8	2.9	3.1
Cooking (M)		2.3	2.4	2.5	2.7	2.8	3.0	3.1	3.3
Cricket									
batting		3.9	4.2	4.4	4.6	4.9	5.1	5.4	5.6
bowling		4.2	4.5	4.8	5.0	5.3	5.6	5.9	6.1
fielding		3.7	3.9	4.1	4.3	4.8	4.8	5.0	5.3

Note: Symbols (M) and (F) denote experiments for males and females, respectively.

71 157	74 163	77 170	80 176	83 183	86 190	89 196	92 203	95 209	98 216
4.6	4.8	5.0	5.2	5.4	5.6	5.8	6.0	6.2	6.4
8.6	9.0	9.3	9.7	10.0	10.4	10.8	11.1	11.5	11.9
9.2	9.5	9.9	10.3	10.7	11.1	11.5	11.9	12.3	12.6
9.9	10.4	10.8	11.2	11.6	12.0	12.5	12.9	13.3	13.7
10.4	10.9	11.3	11.8	12.2	12.6	13.1	13.5	14.0	14.4
6.9	7.2	7.5	7.8	8.1	8.3	8.6	8.9	9.2	9.5
10.4	10.8	11.2	11.6	12.1	12.5	12.9	13.4	13.8	14.3
2.5	2.6	2.7	2.8	2.9	3.0	3.1	3.2	3.3	3.4
4.3	4.5	4.7	4.9	5.1	5.2	5.4	5.6	5.8	6.0
6.4	6.7	7.0	7.2	7.5	7.8	8.0	8.3	8.6	8.9
10.5	10.9	11.4	11.8	12.3	12.7	13.1	13.6	14.0	14.5
9.8	10.2	10.6	11.0	11.5	11.9	12.3	12.7	13.1	13.5
9.5	9.7	9.9	10.1	10.4	10.6	10.8	11.0	11.2	11.4
3.0	3.1	3.2	3.4	3.5	3.6	3.7	3.9	4.0	4.1
2.7	2.8	2.9	3.0	3.2	3.3	3.4	3.5	3.6	3.7
6.9	7.2	7.5	7.7	8.1	8.4	8.6	8.9	9.2	9.5
15.8	16.4	17.1	17.8	18.4	19.1	19.8	20.4	21.1	21.8
9.8	10.2	10.6	11.0	11.5	11.9	12.3	12.7	13.1	13.5
5.3	5.5	5.8	6.0	6.2	6.5	6.7	6.9	7.1	7.3
3.1	3.3	3.4	3.5	3.7	3.8	3.9	4.0	4.2	4.3
7.3	7.6	7.9	8.2	8.5	8.9	9.2	9.5	9.8	10.1
5.0	5.2	5.5	5.7	5.7	5.9	6.1	6.3	6.5	6.9
1.8	1.9	1.9	2.0	2.1	2.2	2.2	2.3	2.4	2.5
3.7	3.8	4.0	4.2	4.3	4.5	4.6	4.8	4.9	5.1
3.2	3.3	3.5	3.6	3.7	3.9	4.0	4.1	4.3	4.4
3.4	3.6	3.7	3.8	4.0	4.1	4.3	4.4	4.6	4.7
6.1	6.3	6.6	6.8	7.1	7.4	7.6	7.9	8.1	8.4
9.4	9.7	10.2	10.5	10.9	11.4	11.7	12.1	12.5	12.9
6.6	6.8	7.1	7.4	7.7	8.0	8.2	8.5	8.8	9.1
8.3	8.6	8.9	9.3	9.6	10.0	10.3	10.7	11.0	11.4
4.4	4.6	4.8	5.0	5.1	5.3	5.5	5.7	5.9	6.1
4.1	4.3	4.5	4.6	4.8	5.0	5.2	5.3	5.5	5.7
6.7	7.0	7.2	7.5	7.8	8.1	8.4	8.6	8.9	9.2
6.2	6.5	6.8	7.0	7.3	7.6	7.8	8.1	8.4	8.6
7.7	8.0	8.3	8.6	9.0	9.3	9.6	9.9	10.3	10.6
3.2	3.3	3.5	3.6	3.7	3.9	4.0	4.1	4.3	4.4
3.4	3.6	3.7	3.8	4.0	4.1	4.3	4.4	4.6	4.7
5.9	6.1	6.4	6.6	6.9	7.1	7.4	7.6	7.9	8.1
6.4	6.7	6.9	7.2	7.5	7.7	8.0	8.3	8.6	8.8
5.6	5.9	6.2	6.5	6.8	7.1	7.4	7.7	8.0	8.3

(continued)

YOUR BODY WEIGHT (continued)

Activity	kg lb	47 104	50 110	53 117	56 123	59 130	62 137	65 143	68 150
Croquet		2.8	3.0	3.1	3.3	3.5	3.7	3.8	4.0
Cycling									
leisure, 5.5 mph		3.0	3.2	3.4	3.6	3.8	4.0	4.2	4.4
leisure, 9.4 mph		4.8	5.0	5.3	5.6	5.9	6.2	6.5	6.8
racing, fast		8.0	8.5	9.0	9.5	10.0	10.5	11.0	11.5
Dancing									
aerobic, easy		4.3	4.8	5.2	5.6	5.9	6.2	6.4	6.7
aerobic, medium		4.8	5.2	5.5	5.8	6.1	6.4	6.7	7.0
aerobic, intense		6.3	6.7	7.1	7.5	7.9	8.3	8.7	9.2
ballroom		2.4	2.6	2.7	2.9	3.0	3.2	3.3	3.5
choreographed		5.0	5.2	5.5	5.8	6.1	6.4	6.7	7.0
"twist," "lambada"		8.0	8.4	8.9	9.4	9.9	10.4	10.9	11.4
modern		3.4	3.6	3.8	4.0	4.3	4.5	4.7	4.9
Digging trenches		6.8	7.3	7.7	8.1	8.6	9.0	9.4	9.9
Drawing (standing)		1.7	1.8	1.9	2.0	2.1	2.2	2.3	2.4
Eating (sitting)		1.1	1.2	1.2	1.3	1.4	1.4	1.5	1.6
Electrical work		2.7	2.9	3.1	3.2	3.4	3.6	3.8	3.9
Farming									
bam cleaning		6.3	6.8	7.2	7.6	8.0	8.4	8.8	9.2
driving harvester		1.9	2.0	2.1	2.2	2.4	2.5	2.6	2.7
driving tractor		1.8	1.9	2.0	2.1	2.2	2.3	2.4	2.5
feeding cattle		4.2	4.3	4.5	4.8	5.0	5.3	5.5	5.8
feeding animals		3.1	3.3	3.4	3.6	3.8	4.0	4.2	4.4
forking straw bales		6.7	6.9	7.3	7.7	8.1	8.6	9.0	9.4
milking by hand		2.5	2.7	2.9	3.0	3.2	3.3	3.5	3.7
milking by machine		1.1	1.2	1.2	1.3	1.4	1.4	1.5	1.6
shoveling grain		4.2	4.3	4.5	4.8	5.0	5.3	5.5	5.8
Fencing									
competition		7.2	7.6	8.1	8.5	9.0	9.4	9.9	10.8
practice		3.6	3.9	4.2	4.4	4.6	4.9	5.1	5.3
Field hockey		6.5	6.7	7.1	7.5	7.9	8.3	8.7	9.1
Fishing		3.0	3.1	3.3	3.5	3.7	3.8	4.0	4.2
Food shopping (F)		3.0	3.1	3.3	3.5	3.7	3.8	4.0	4.2
Football, competition		6.2	6.6	7.0	7.4	7.8	8.2	8.6	9.0
Forestry									
ax chopping, fast		14.0	14.9	15.7	16.6	17.5	18.4	19.3	20.2
ax chopping, slow		4.0	4.3	4.5	4.8	5.0	5.3	5.5	5.8
barking trees		5.8	6.2	6.5	6.9	7.3	7.6	8.0	8.4
carrying logs		8.7	9.3	9.9	10.4	11.0	11.5	12.1	12.6
felling trees		6.2	6.6	7.0	7.4	7.8	8.2	8.6	9.0
hoeing		4.2	4.6	4.8	5.1	5.4	5.6	5.9	6.2
planting by hand		5.1	5.5	5.8	6.1	6.4	6.8	7.1	7.4
sawing by hand		5.7	6.1	6.5	6.8	7.2	7.6	7.9	8.3
sawing, power		3.5	3.8	4.0	4.2	4.4	4.7	4.9	5.1
stacking firewood		4.2	4.4	4.7	4.9	5.2	5.5	5.7	6.0
trimming trees		6.1	6.5	6.8	7.2	7.6	8.0	8.4	8.8
weeding		3.4	3.6	3.8	4.0	4.2	4.5	4.7	4.9
Frisbee		4.7	5.0	5.3	5.5	5.9	6.2	6.4	6.8
Furriery		3.9	4.2	4.4	4.6	4.9	5.1	5.4	5.6

71	74	77	80	83	86	89	92	95	98
157	163	170	176	183	190	196	203	209	216
4.2	4.4	4.5	4.7	4.9	5.1	5.3	5.4	5.6	5.8
4.5	4.7	4.9	5.1	5.3	5.5	5.7	5.9	6.1	6.3
7.1	7.4	7.7	8.0	8.3	8.6	8.9	9.2	9.5	9.8
12.0	12.5	13.0	13.5	14.0	14.5	15.0	15.5	16.1	16.6
6.9	7.2	7.5	7.8	8.1	8.4	8.8	9.1	9.4	9.7
7.3	7.6	7.9	8.2	8.5	8.9	9.2	9.5	9.8	10.1
9.6	10.0	10.4	10.8	11.2	11.6	12.0	12.4	12.8	13.2
3.6	3.8	3.9	4.1	4.2	4.4	4.5	4.7	4.8	5.0
7.3	7.6	7.9	8.2	8.5	8.9	9.2	9.5	9.8	10.1
11.9	12.4	12.9	13.4	13.9	14.4	15.0	15.5	16.0	16.5
5.1	5.3	5.6	5.8	6.0	6.2	6.4	6.7	6.9	7.1
10.3	10.7	11.2	11.6	12.0	12.5	12.9	13.3	13.8	14.2
2.6	2.7	2.8	2.9	3.0	3.1	3.2	3.3	3.4	3.5
1.6	1.7	1.8	1.8	1.9	2.0	2.0	2.1	2.2	2.3
4.1	4.3	4.5	4.6	4.8	5.0	5.2	5.3	5.5	5.7
9.6	10.0	10.4	10.8	11.2	11.6	12.0	12.4	12.8	13.2
2.8	3.0	3.1	3.2	3.3	3.4	3.6	3.7	3.8	3.9
2.6	2.7	2.8	3.0	3.1	3.2	3.3	3.4	3.5	3.6
6.0	6.3	6.5	6.8	7.1	7.3	7.6	7.8	8.1	8.3
4.6	4.8	5.0	5.2	5.4	5.6	5.8	6.0	6.2	6.4
9.8	10.2	10.6	11.0	11.5	11.9	12.3	12.7	13.1	13.5
3.8	4.0	4.2	4.3	4.5	4.6	4.8	5.0	5.1	5.3
1.6	1.7	1.8	1.8	1.9	2.0	2.0	2.1	2.2	2.3
6.0	6.3	6.5	6.8	7.1	7.3	7.6	7.8	8.1	8.3
11.2	11.7	12.1	12.6	13.1	13.5	14.0	14.4	14.9	15.5
5.6	5.8	6.1	6.3	6.5	6.8	7.0	7.2	7.4	7.7
9.5	9.9	10.3	10.7	11.1	11.5	11.9	12.3	12.7	13.1
4.4	4.6	4.8	5.0	5.1	5.3	5.5	5.7	5.9	6.1
4.4	4.6	4.8	5.0	5.1	5.3	5.5	5.7	5.9	6.1
9.4	9.8	10.2	10.6	11.0	11.4	11.7	12.1	12.5	12.9
21.1	22.0	22.9	23.8	24.7	25.5	26.4	27.3	28.2	29.1
6.0	6.3	6.5	6.8	7.1	7.3	7.6	7.8	8.1	8.3
8.7	9.1	9.5	9.8	10.2	10.6	10.9	11.3	11.7	12.1
13.2	13.8	14.3	14.9	15.4	16.0	16.6	17.1	17.7	18.2
9.4	9.8	10.2	10.6	11.0	11.4	11.7	12.1	12.5	12.9
6.5	6.7	7.0	7.3	7.6	7.8	8.1	8.4	8.6	8.9
7.7	8.1	8.4	8.7	9.0	9.4	9.7	10.0	10.4	10.7
8.7	9.0	9.4	9.8	10.1	10.5	10.9	11.2	11.6	12.0
5.3	5.6	5.8	6.0	6.2	6.5	6.7	6.9	7.1	7.4
6.2	6.5	6.8	7.0	7.3	7.6	7.8	8.1	8.4	8.6
9.2	9.5	9.9	10.3	10.7	11.1	11.5	11.9	12.3	12.6
5.1	5.3	5.5	5.8	6.0	6.2	6.4	6.6	6.8	7.1
7.1	7.4	7.7	8.0	8.2	8.5	8.8	9.1	9.4	9.7
5.9	6.1	6.4	6.6	6.9	7.1	7.4	7.6	7.9	8.1

(continued)

YOUR BODY WEIGHT (continued)

Activity	kg lb	47 104	50 110	53 117	56 123	59 130	62 137	65 143	68 150
Gardening									
digging		5.9	6.3	6.7	7.1	7.4	7.8	8.2	8.6
hedging		3.3	3.9	4.1	4.3	4.5	4.8	5.0	5.2
mowing		5.3	5.6	5.9	6.3	6.6	6.9	7.3	7.6
raking		2.5	2.7	2.9	3.0	3.2	3.3	3.5	3.7
Golf		4.0	4.3	4.5	4.8	5.0	5.3	5.5	5.8
Gymnastics		3.0	3.3	3.5	3.7	3.9	4.1	4.3	4.5
Handball		6.9	7.2	7.7	8.1	8.5	9.0	9.4	9.8
orse-grooming		6.0	6.4	6.8	7.2	7.6	7.9	8.3	8.7
Horseback riding									
galloping		6.4	6.9	7.3	7.7	8.1	8.5	8.9	9.3
trotting		5.2	5.5	5.8	6.2	6.5	6.8	7.2	7.5
walking		1.9	2.1	2.2	2.3	2.4	2.5	2.7	2.8
Horseshoes		3.3	3.4	3.5	3.7	3.9	4.1	4.3	4.5
Housework									
mopping floors		2.8	3.1	3.3	3.5	3.7	3.8	4.0	4.2
dusting		3.0	3.3	3.4	3.6	3.8	4.0	4.2	4.4
laundry		3.1	3.4	3.5	3.7	3.9	4.1	4.3	4.5
washing windows		3.2	3.5	3.6	3.8	4.0	4.2	4.4	4.6
vacuuming		3.0	3.3	3.4	3.6	3.8	4.0	4.2	4.4
Hunting		4.1	4.4	4.7	4.9	5.2	5.5	5.7	6.0
Ice hockey		7.4	7.7	8.2	8.6	9.1	9.6	10.0	10.5
Ironing clothes		1.6	1.7	1.7	1.8	1.9	2.0	2.1	2.2
Judo		9.2	9.8	10.3	10.9	11.5	12.1	12.7	13.3
Jumping rope									
70 per min		7.6	8.1	8.6	9.1	9.6	10.0	10.5	11.0
80 per min		7.7	8.2	8.7	9.2	9.7	10.2	10.7	11.2
125 per min		8.3	8.9	9.4	9.9	10.4	11.0	11.5	12.0
145 per min		9.3	9.9	10.4	11.0	11.6	12.2	12.8	13.4
Karate		9.5	9.8	10.3	10.9	11.5	12.1	12.7	13.3
Kendo		9.3	9.7	10.2	10.8	11.4	12.0	12.6	13.2
Knitting, sewing		1.1	1.1	1.2	1.2	1.3	1.4	1.4	1.5
Lacrosse		7.0	7.4	7.9	8.3	8.7	9.2	9.6	10.1
Locksmith		2.8	2.9	3.0	3.2	3.4	3.5	3.7	3.9
Lying at ease		1.0	1.1	1.2	1.2	1.3	1.4	1.4	1.5
Machine-tooling									
machining		2.3	2.4	2.5	2.7	2.8	3.0	3.1	3.3
operating lathe		2.5	2.6	2.8	2.9	3.1	3.2	3.4	3.5
operating punch press		4.2	4.4	4.7	4.9	5.2	5.5	5.7	6.0
tapping and drilling		3.2	3.3	3.4	3.6	3.8	4.0	4.2	4.4
welding		2.4	2.6	2.8	2.9	3.1	3.2	3.4	3.5
working sheet metal		2.3	2.4	2.5	2.7	2.8	3.0	3.1	3.3
Marching, rapid		6.7	7.1	7.5	8.0	8.4	8.8	9.2	9.7
Mountain climbing		7.4	7.9	8.4	8.9	9.4	9.9	10.3	10.8
Motorcycle riding		6.5	6.9	7.3	7.7	8.1	8.5	8.9	9.3

71	74	77	80	83	86	89	92	95	98
157	163	170	176	183	190	196	203	209	216
8.9	9.3	9.7	10.1	10.5	10.8	11.2	11.6	12.0	12.3
5.5	5.7	5.9	6.2	6.4	6.6	6.9	7.1	7.3	7.5
8.0	8.3	8.6	9.0	9.3	9.6	10.0	10.3	10.6	11.0
3.8	4.0	4.2	4.3	4.5	4.6	4.8	5.0	5.1	5.3
6.0	6.3	6.5	6.8	7.1	7.3	7.6	7.8	8.1	8.3
4.7	4.9	5.1	5.3	5.5	5.7	5.9	6.1	6.3	6.5
10.3	10.7	11.2	11.5	12.0	12.5	12.9	13.3	13.7	14.2
9.1	9.5	9.9	10.2	10.6	11.0	11.4	11.8	12.2	12.5
9.7	10.1	10.6	11.0	11.4	11.8	12.2	12.6	13.0	13.4
7.8	8.1	8.5	8.8	9.1	9.5	9.8	10.1	10.5	10.8
2.9	3.0	3.2	3.3	3.4	3.5	3.6	3.8	3.9	4.0
4.7	4.9	5.1	5.3	5.5	5.7	5.9	6.1	6.3	6.5
4.4	4.6	4.8	5.0	5.2	5.4	5.6	5.8	6.0	6.2
4.6	4.7	4.9	5.1	5.3	5.5	5.7	5.9	6.1	6.3
4.7	4.9	5.1	5.3	5.5	5.7	5.9	6.1	6.3	6.5
4.8	5.0	5.2	5.4	5.6	5.8	6.0	6.2	6.4	6.6
4.6	4.8	5.0	5.2	5.4	5.6	5.8	6.0	6.2	6.4
6.2	6.5	6.7	7.0	7.2	7.5	7.8	8.0	8.2	8.5
11.0	11.5	12.0	12.5	13.1	13.6	14.1	14.6	15.1	15.7
2.3	2.4	2.5	2.6	2.7	2.8	2.9	3.0	3.1	3.2
13.8	14.4	15.0	15.6	16.2	16.8	17.4	17.9	18.5	19.1
11.5	12.0	12.5	13.0	13.4	13.9	14.4	14.9	15.4	15.9
11.6	12.1	12.6	13.1	13.6	14.1	14.6	14.6	15.6	16.1
12.6	13.1	13.6	14.2	14.7	15.2	15.8	16.3	16.8	17.3
14.0	14.6	15.2	15.8	16.4	16.9	17.5	18.1	18.7	19.3
13.8	14.4	15.0	15.6	16.2	16.8	17.4	17.9	18.5	19.1
13.7	14.3	14.9	15.5	16.1	16.7	17.3	17.8	18.4	19.0
1.6	1.6	1.7	1.8	1.8	1.9	2.0	2.0	2.1	2.2
10.4	10.7	11.0	11.2	11.5	11.8	12.1	12.4	12.7	13.0
4.0	4.2	4.4	4.6	4.7	4.9	5.1	5.2	5.4	5.6
1.6	1.6	1.7	1.8	1.8	1.9	2.0	2.0	2.1	2.2
3.4	3.6	3.7	3.8	4.0	4.1	4.3	4.4	4.6	4.7
3.7	3.8	4.0	4.2	4.3	4.5	4.6	4.8	4.9	5.1
6.2	6.5	6.8	7.0	7.3	7.6	7.8	8.1	8.4	8.6
4.6	4.8	5.0	5.2	5.4	5.6	5.8	6.0	6.2	6.4
3.7	3.8	4.0	4.2	4.3	4.5	4.6	4.8	4.9	5.1
3.4	3.6	3.7	3.8	4.0	4.1	4.3	4.4	4.6	4.7
10.1	10.5	10.9	11.4	11.8	12.2	12.6	13.1	13.5	13.9
11.3	11.7	12.2	12.7	13.2	13.7	14.1	14.6	15.0	15.6
9.7	10.1	10.5	10.9	11.3	11.7	12.1	12.5	12.9	13.3

(continued)

YOUR BODY WEIGHT (continued)

Activity	kg lb	47 104	50 110	53 117	56 123	59 130	62 137	65 143	68 150
Music playing									
accordion (sitting)		1.5	1.6	1.7	1.8	1.9	2.0	2.1	2.2
cello (sitting)		2.0	2.1	2.2	2.3	2.4	2.5	2.7	2.8
conducting		1.9	2.0	2.1	2.2	2.3	2.4	2.5	2.7
drums (sitting)		3.1	3.3	3.5	3.7	3.9	4.1	4.3	4.5
flute (sitting)		1.7	1.8	1.9	2.0	2.1	2.2	2.3	2.4
horn (sitting)		1.4	1.5	1.5	1.6	1.7	1.8	1.9	2.0
organ (sitting)		2.6	2.7	2.8	3.0	3.1	3.3	3.4	3.6
piano (sitting)		1.9	2.0	2.1	2.2	2.4	2.5	2.6	2.7
trumpet (standing)		1.5	1.6	1.6	1.7	1.8	1.9	2.0	2.1
violin (sitting)		2.2	2.3	2.4	2.5	2.7	2.8	2.9	3.1
woodwind (sitting)		1.5	1.6	1.7	1.8	1.9	2.0	2.1	2.2
Paddleball		8.5	8.9	9.4	10.0	10.5	11.0	11.6	12.1
Paddle tennis		8.4	8.6	9.1	9.6	10.1	10.7	11.1	11.7
Painting									
inside projects		1.6	1.7	1.8	1.9	2.0	2.1	2.2	2.3
outside projects		3.7	3.9	4.1	4.3	4.5	4.8	5.0	5.2
scraping		3.1	3.2	3.3	3.5	3.7	3.9	4.1	4.3
Planting seedings		3.3	3.5	3.7	3.9	4.1	4.3	4.6	4.8
Plastering		3.7	3.9	4.1	4.4	4.6	4.8	5.1	5.3
Printing press work		1.7	1.8	1.9	2.0	2.1	2.2	2.3	2.4
Racquetball		8.4	8.9	9.4	10.0	10.5	11.0	11.6	12.1
Roller skating, leisure		5.3	5.8	6.2	6.5	6.9	7.3	7.3	8.0
Rope jumping									
110 rpm		6.7	7.1	7.5	7.9	8.4	8.8	9.2	9.7
120 rpm		6.4	6.8	7.3	7.7	8.1	8.5	8.9	9.3
130 rpm		6.0	6.4	6.8	7.1	7.5	7.7	8.3	8.7
Rowing									
machine, moderate		5.7	6.0	6.3	6.7	7.0	7.4	7.7	8.1
machine, race pace		8.6	8.9	9.4	10.0	10.5	11.0	11.6	12.1
skull, leisure		4.7	5.0	5.3	5.5	5.9	6.2	6.4	6.8
skull, race pace		8.7	8.9	9.4	10.0	10.5	11.0	11.6	12.1
Running, cross-country		7.8	8.2	8.6	9.1	9.6	10.1	10.6	11.1
Running, on flat surface									
11 min, 30 s per mile		6.3	6.8	7.2	7.6	8.0	8.4	8.8	9.2
9 min per mile		9.1	9.7	10.2	10.8	11.4	12.0	12.5	13.1
8 min per mile		9.8	10.8	11.3	11.9	12.5	13.1	13.6	14.2
7 min per mile		10.7	12.2	12.7	13.3	13.9	14.5	15.0	15.6
6 min per mile		11.8	13.9	14.4	15.0	15.6	16.2	16.7	17.3
5 min, 30 s per mile		13.6	14.5	15.3	16.2	17.1	17.9	18.8	19.7
Sailing, leisure		2.1	2.2	2.3	2.5	2.6	2.7	2.9	3.0
Scrubbing floors		5.1	5.5	5.8	6.1	6.4	6.8	7.1	7.4
Scuba diving		10.9	11.2	11.5	11.8	12.1	12.4	12.7	13.0
Shoe repair, general		2.2	2.3	2.4	2.5	2.7	2.8	2.9	3.1
Sitting quietly		1.0	1.1	1.1	1.2	1.2	1.3	1.4	1.4
Skateboarding		5.6	5.8	6.2	6.5	6.9	7.2	7.5	7.9
Skiing, hard snow									
level, moderate speed		5.6	6.0	6.3	6.7	7.0	7.4	7.7	8.1
level, walking speed		6.7	7.2	7.6	8.0	8.4	8.9	9.3	9.7
uphill, "fast" speed		12.9	13.7	14.5	15.3	16.2	17.0	17.8	18.6

71 157	74 163	77 170	80 176	83 183	86 190	89 196	92 203	95 209	98 216
2.3	2.4	2.5	2.6	2.7	2.8	2.8	2.9	3.0	3.1
2.9	3.0	3.2	3.3	3.4	3.5	3.6	3.8	3.9	4.0
2.8	2.9	3.0	3.1	3.2	3.4	3.5	3.6	3.7	3.8
4.7	4.9	5.1	5.3	5.5	5.7	5.9	6.1	6.3	6.6
2.5	2.6	2.7	2.8	2.9	3.0	3.1	3.2	3.3	3.4
2.1	2.1	2.2	2.3	2.4	2.5	2.6	2.7	2.8	2.8
3.8	3.9	4.1	4.2	4.4	4.6	4.7	4.9	5.0	5.2
2.8	3.0	3.1	3.2	3.3	3.4	3.6	3.7	3.8	3.9
2.2	2.3	2.4	2.5	2.6	2.7	2.8	2.9	2.9	3.0
3.2	3.3	3.5	3.6	3.7	3.9	4.0	4.1	4.3	4.4
2.3	2.4	2.5	2.6	2.7	2.8	2.8	2.9	3.0	3.1
12.6	13.2	13.7	14.2	14.8	15.3	15.8	16.4	16.9	17.4
12.2	12.7	13.2	13.7	14.2	14.2	15.2	15.8	16.3	16.8
2.4	2.5	2.6	2.7	2.8	2.9	3.0	3.1	3.2	3.3
5.5	5.7	5.9	6.2	6.4	6.6	6.9	7.1	7.3	7.5
4.5	4.7	4.9	5.0	5.2	5.4	5.6	5.8	6.0	6.2
5.0	5.2	5.4	5.6	5.8	6.0	6.2	6.4	6.7	6.9
5.5	5.8	6.0	6.2	6.5	6.7	6.9	7.2	7.4	7.6
2.5	2.6	2.7	2.8	2.9	3.0	3.1	3.2	3.3	3.4
12.6	13.2	13.7	14.2	14.8	15.3	15.8	16.4	16.9	17.4
8.3	8.6	9.0	9.3	9.7	10.1	10.4	10.8	11.1	11.4
10.1	10.5	10.5	11.3	11.8	12.2	12.6	13.1	13.5	13.9
9.8	10.1	10.6	10.9	11.4	11.8	12.2	12.6	13.0	13.4
9.1	9.4	9.8	10.2	10.6	11.0	11.3	11.7	12.1	12.5
8.5	8.9	9.3	9.7	10.1	10.6	11.1	11.6	12.1	12.6
12.6	13.2	13.7	14.2	14.8	15.3	15.8	16.4	16.9	17.4
7.2	7.6	8.0	8.4	8.8	9.2	9.6	10.0	10.4	10.8
12.6	13.2	13.7	14.2	14.8	15.3	15.8	16.4	16.9	17.4
11.6	12.1	12.6	13.0	13.5	14.0	14.5	15.0	15.5	16.0
9.6	10.0	10.5	10.9	11.3	11.7	12.1	12.5	12.9	13.3
13.7	14.3	14.9	15.4	16.0	16.6	17.2	17.8	18.3	18.9
14.8	15.4	16.0	16.5	17.1	17.7	18.3	18.9	19.4	20.0
16.2	16.8	17.4	17.9	18.5	19.1	19.7	20.3	20.8	21.4
17.9	18.5	19.1	19.6	20.2	20.8	21.4	22.0	22.5	23.1
20.5	21.4	22.3	23.1	24.0	24.9	25.7	26.6	27.5	28.3
3.1	3.3	3.4	3.5	3.7	3.8	3.9	4.1	4.2	4.3
7.7	8.1	8.4	8.7	9.0	9.4	9.7	10.0	10.4	10.7
13.3	13.6	13.9	14.2	14.5	14.8	15.1	15.4	15.7	16.0
3.2	3.3	3.5	3.6	3.7	3.9	4.0	4.1	4.3	4.4
1.5	1.6	1.6	1.7	1.7	1.8	1.9	1.9	2.0	2.1
8.3	8.6	8.9	9.3	9.6	10.0	10.3	10.7	11.0	11.4
8.4	8.8	9.2	9.5	9.9	10.2	10.6	10.9	11.3	11.7
10.2	10.6	11.0	11.4	11.9	12.3	12.7	13.2	13.6	14.0
19.5	20.3	21.1	21.9	22.7	23.6	24.4	25.2	26.0	26.9

(continued)

YOUR BODY WEIGHT (continued)

Activity	kg / lb	47 / 104	50 / 110	53 / 117	56 / 123	59 / 130	62 / 137	65 / 143	68 / 150
Skiing, soft snow									
leisure (F)		4.6	4.9	5.2	5.5	5.8	6.1	6.4	6.7
leisure (M)		5.2	5.6	5.9	6.2	6.5	6.9	7.2	7.5
Skindiving									
considerable motion		13.0	13.8	14.6	15.5	16.3	17.1	17.9	18.8
moderate motion		9.7	10.3	10.9	11.5	12.2	12.8	13.4	14.0
Snorkeling		4.3	4.6	4.9	5.2	5.5	5.8	6.0	6.3
Snowshoeing, soft snow		7.8	8.3	8.8	9.3	9.8	10.3	10.8	11.3
Snowmobiling		3.4	3.7	4.0	4.2	4.4	4.7	4.9	5.1
Soccer		6.5	6.8	7.3	7.7	8.1	8.5	8.9	9.3
Softball		3.3	3.5	3.7	3.9	4.1	4.3	4.5	4.7
Squash		10.0	10.6	11.2	11.9	12.5	13.1	13.8	14.4
Standing quietly (M)		1.3	1.4	1.4	1.5	1.6	1.7	1.8	1.8
Steel mill, working in									
fettling		4.3	4.5	4.7	5.0	5.3	5.5	5.8	6.1
forging		4.7	5.0	5.3	5.6	5.9	6.2	6.5	6.8
hand rolling		6.4	6.9	7.3	7.7	8.1	8.5	8.9	9.3
merchant mill rolling		6.8	7.3	7.7	8.1	8.6	9.0	9.4	9.9
removing slag		8.4	8.9	9.4	10.0	10.5	11.0	11.6	12.1
tending furnace		5.9	6.3	6.7	7.1	7.4	7.8	8.2	8.6
tipping molds		4.3	4.6	4.9	5.2	5.4	5.7	6.0	6.3
Surfing		3.9	4.1	4.3	4.5	4.8	5.0	5.3	5.5
Stock clerking		2.5	2.7	2.9	3.0	3.2	3.3	3.5	3.7
Swimming, fitness swims									
back stroke		7.9	8.5	9.0	9.5	10.0	10.5	11.0	11.5
breast stroke		7.6	8.1	8.6	9.1	9.6	10.0	10.5	11.0
butterfly			8.6	9.1	9.6	10.1	10.7	11.1	11.7
crawl, fast		7.3	7.8	8.3	8.7	9.2	9.7	10.1	10.6
crawl, slow		6.0	6.4	6.8	7.2	7.6	7.9	8.3	8.7
side stroke		5.7	6.1	6.5	6.8	7.2	7.6	7.9	8.3
treading, fast		8.0	8.5	9.0	9.5	10.0	10.5	11.1	11.6
treading, normal		2.9	3.1	3.3	3,5	3.7	3.8	4.0	4.2
Table tennis (ping pong)		3.2	3.4	3.6	3.8	4.0	4.2	4.4	4.6
Tailoring									
cutting		2.0	2.1	2.2	2.3	2.4	2.5	2.7	2.8
hand-sewing		1.5	1.6	1.7	1.8	1.9	2.0	2.1	2.2
machine-sewing		2.2	2.3	2.4	2.5	2.7	2.8	2.9	3.1
pressing		2.9	3.1	3.3	3.5	3.7	3.8	4.0	4.2
Tennis									
competition		6.9	7.3	7.8	8.2	8.7	9.1	9.5	9.9
recreational		5.1	5.5	5.8	6.1	6.4	6.8	7.1	7.4
Typing									
electric (computer)		1.3	1.4	1.4	1.5	1.6	1.7	1.8	1.8
manual		1.5	1.6	1.6	1.7	1.8	1.9	2.0	2.1
Volleyball									
competition		5.9	7.3	7.8	8.2	8.7	9.1	9.5	10.0
recreational		2.4	2.5	2.7	2.8	3.0	3.1	3.3	3.4

71 157	74 163	77 170	80 176	83 183	86 190	89 196	92 203	95 209	98 216
7.0	7.3	7.5	7.8	8.1	8.4	8.7	9.0	9.3	9.6
7.9	8.2	8.5	8.9	9.2	9.5	9.9	10.2	10.5	10.9
19.6	20.4	21.3	22.1	22.9	23.7	24.6	25.4	26.2	27.0
14.6	15.2	15.9	16.5	17.1	17.7	18.3	19.0	19.6	20.2
6.6	6.8	7.1	7.4	7.7	8.0	8.2	8.5	8.8	9.1
11.8	12.3	12.8	13.3	13.8	14.3	14.8	15.3	15.8	16.3
5.3	5.5	5.8	6.0	6.2	6.5	6.7	6.9	7.1	7.3
9.8	10.1	10.6	10.9	11.4	11.8	12.2	12.6	13.0	13.4
4.9	5.1	5.3	5.5	5.7	5.9	6.1	6.3	6.5	6.7
15.1	15.7	16.3	17.0	17.6	18.2	18.9	19.5	20.1	20.8
1.9	2.0	2.1	2.2	2.2	2.3	2.4	2.5	2.6	2.6
6.3	6.6	6.9	7.1	7.4	7.7	7.9	8.2	8.5	8.7
7.1	7.4	7.7	8.0	8.3	8.6	8.9	9.2	9.5	9.8
9.7	10.1	10.6	11.0	11.4	11.8	12.2	12.6	13.0	13.4
10.3	10.7	11.2	11.6	12.0	12.5	12.9	13.3	13.8	14.2
12.6	13.2	13.7	14.2	14.8	15.3	15.8	16.4	16.9	17.4
8.9	9.3	9.7	10.1	10.5	10.8	11.2	11.6	12.0	12.3
6.5	6.8	7.1	7.4	7.6	7.9	8.2	8.5	8.7	9.0
5.7	6.0	6.3	6.5	6.8	7.0	7.2	7.4	7.6	7.9
3.8	4.0	4.2	4.3	4.5	4.6	4.8	5.0	5.1	5.3
12.0	12.5	13.0	13.5	14.0	14.5	15.0	15.5	16.1	16.6
11.5	12.0	12.5	13.0	13.4	13.9	14.4	14.9	15.4	15.9
12.2	12.7	13.2	13.7	14.2	14.2	15.2	15.8	16.3	16.8
11.1	11.5	12.0	12.5	12.9	13.4	13.9	14.4	14.8	15.3
9.1	9.5	9.9	10.2	10.6	11.0	11.4	11.8	12.2	12.5
8.7	9.0	9.4	9.8	10.1	10.5	10.9	11.2	11.6	12.0
12.1	12.6	13.1	13.6	14.1	14.6	15.1	15.6	16.2	16.7
4.4	4.6	4.8	5.0	5.1	5.3	5.5	5.7	5.9	6.1
4.8	5.0	5.2	5.4	5.6	5.8	6.1	6.3	6.5	6.7
2.9	3.0	3.2	3.3	3.4	3.5	3.6	3.8	3.9	4.0
2.3	2.4	2.5	2.6	2.7	2.8	2.8	2.9	3.0	3.1
3.2	3.3	3.5	3.6	3.7	3.9	4.0	4.1	4.3	4.4
4.4	4.6	4.8	5.0	5.1	5.3	5.5	5.7	5.9	6.1
10.2	10.6	11.1	11.5	11.9	12.4	12.8	13.2	13.7	14.1
7.7	8.1	8.4	8.7	9.0	9.4	9.7	10.0	10.4	10.7
1.9	2.0	2.1	2.2	2.2	2.3	2.4	2.5	2.6	2.6
2.2	2.3	2.4	2.5	2.6	2.7	2.8	2.9	2.9	3.0
3.6	3.7	3.9	4.0	4.2	4.3	4.5	4.6	4.8	4.9
10.5	10.9	11.4	11.8	12.3	12.7	13.1	13.6	14.0	14.5

(continued)

YOUR BODY WEIGHT (continued)

Activity	kg lb	47 104	50 110	53 117	56 123	59 130	62 137	65 143	68 150
Walking, leisure									
outdoors									
asphalt road		3.8	4.0	4.2	4.5	4.7	5.0	5.2	5.4
fields and hillsides		3.9	4.1	4.3	4.6	4.8	5.1	5.3	5.6
grass track		3.8	4.1	4.3	4.5	4.8	5.0	5.3	5.5
plowed field		3.6	3.9	4.1	4.3	4.5	4.8	5.0	5.2
Walking, treadmill									
level									
2.0 mph		2.4	2.6	2.8	3.0	3.1	3.3	3.4	3.6
2.5 mph		3.0	3.2	3.4	3.6	3.8	4.0	4.2	4.4
3.0 mph		3.6	3.8	4.0	4.2	4.4	4.6	4.8	5.0
3.5 mph		4.0	4.3	4.6	4.8	5.1	5.3	5.6	6.1
4.0 mph		4.6	4.9	5.2	5.4	5.7	6.0	6.3	6.6
Wallpapering		2.3	2.4	2.5	2.7	2.8	3.0	3.1	3.3
Water polo, recreation		7.0	7.4	7.7	8.1	8.5	8.9	9.3	9.7
Water polo, competition		9.4	9.9	10.4	11.0	11.5	12.0	12.5	13.1
Water-skiing		5.6	6.0	6.4	6.7	7.1	7.5	7.8	8.2
Watch repairing		1.2	1.3	1.3	1.4	1.5	1.6	1.6	1.7
Whitewater rafting, recreational		4.1	4.4	4.6	4.9	5.2	5.4	5.7	6.0
Window cleaning		2.9	3.0	3.1	3.3	3.5	3.7	3.8	4.0
Wind surfing		3.3	3.5	3.7	3.9	4.1	4.3	4.6	4.8
Wrestling, competition		9.1	9.7	10.3	10.8	11.4	12.0	12.6	13.2
Writing (sitting)		1.4	1.5	1.5	1.6	1.7	1.8	1.9	2.0
Yoga		2.9	3.1	3.3	3.5	3.7	3.8	4.0	4.2

71	74	77	80	83	86	89	92	95	98
157	163	170	176	183	190	196	203	209	216
5.7	5.9	6.2	6.4	6.6	6.9	7.1	7.4	7.6	7.8
5.8	6.1	6.3	6.6	6.8	7.1	7.3	7.5	7.8	8.0
5.8	6.0	6.2	6.5	6.7	7.0	7.2	7.5	7.7	7.9
5.5	5.7	5.9	6.2	6.4	6.6	6.9	7.1	7.3	7.5
3.7	3.9	4.1	4.2	4.4	4.5	4.7	4.9	5.0	5.2
4.5	4.7	4.9	5.1	5.3	5.5	5.7	5.9	6.1	6.3
5.3	5.5	5.7	5.9	6.2	6.5	6.7	6.9	7.1	7.3
6.1	6.4	6.6	6.9	7.1	7.4	7.7	7.9	8.2	8.4
6.9	7.2	7.5	7.8	8.1	8.4	8.7	8.9	9.2	9.5
3.4	3.6	3.7	3.8	4.0	4.1	4.3	4.4	4.6	4.7
10.1	10.5	10.9	11.3	11.7	12.1	12.5	12.9	13.3	13.7
13.6	14.1	14.7	15.2	15.7	16.3	16.8	17.3	17.9	18.4
8.7	9.1	9.4	9.8	10.1	10.5	10.9	11.2	11.6	12.0
1.8	1.9	1.9	2.0	2.1	2.2	2.2	2.3	2.4	2.5
6.2	6.5	6.7	7.0	7.3	7.5	7.8	8.1	8.3	8.6
4.2	4.4	4.5	4.7	4.9	5.1	5.3	5.4	5.6	5.8
5.0	5.2	5.4	5.6	5.8	6.0	6.2	6.4	6.7	6.9
13.8	14.3	14.9	15.5	16.1	16.7	17.2	17.8	18.4	19.0
2.1	2.1	2.2	2.3	2.4	2.5	2.6	2.7	2.8	2.8
4.4	4.6	4.8	5.0	5.1	5.3	5.5	5.7	5.9	6.1

Appendix C Assessment of Energy and Nutrient Intake: Three-Day Dietary Survey

The three-day dietary survey represents a relatively simple yet accurate method to determine the nutritional quality and total calories of food consumed daily. The key to successfully accomplish these goals requires a daily log of food intake for three days that represent your normal eating pattern (including at least one weekend).

Experiments have shown that calculations of caloric intake made from records of daily food consumption are usually within 10% of the number of calories actually consumed. For example, suppose a bomb calorimeter determined that your daily food intake equaled 2130 kcal. If you kept a three-day dietary history and estimated your calorie intake, the daily value would likely be within 10% of the actual value (1920 and 2350 kcal).

Use four items to measure food: (1) plastic ruler, (2) standard measuring cup, (3) measuring spoons, and (4) balance or weighing scale. Use Appendix A or consult one of several sources that list the nutritional content of foods including: Pennington JAT, Douglass JP. Bowes & Church's food values of portions commonly used. 18th ed. Baltimore: Lippincott Williams & Wilkins, 2005. You may also wish to consult the following URL: http://nat.crgq.com/ mainnat.html.

Measure or weight each of the food items in your diet. This represents the only reliable way to obtain an accurate estimate of the size of a food portion. Be sure to do the following:

- List specific types, brands, and method of preparation.

Example	*List as:*
Milk	8 fl oz, 2% milk
1/2 chicken breast	3 oz breast, baked, without skin
Margarine	1 tsp. Fleishmann's Light Margarine

- Use these guidelines to estimate cooked portion sizes for these food categories:

Meat and Fish
Measure the portion of meat or fish by thickness, length, and width, or record weight on the scale.

Vegetables, Potatoes, Rice, Cereals, Salads
Measure the portion in a measuring cup or record weight on the scale.

Cream or Sugar Added to Coffee or Tea
Measure with measuring spoons before adding to the drink, or record weight on the scale.

Fluids and Bottled Drinks
Check the labels for volume or empty the container into the measuring cup. If you weigh the fluid, be sure to subtract the weight of the cup or glass. Sugar-free soft drinks usually have kcal values listed on their labels.

Cookies, Cakes, Pies
Measure the diameter and thickness with a ruler, or weigh on the scale. Evaluate frosting or sauces separately.

Fruits
Cut them in half before eating and measure the diameters, or weight them on the scale. For fruits that must be peeled or have rinds or cores, be sure to subtract the weight of the non-edible portion from the total weight of the food. Do this for items such as oranges, apples, and bananas.

Jam, Salad Dressing, Catsup, Mayonnaise
Measure the condiment with the measuring spoon or weigh the portion on the scale.

Record all the foods you consume using the blank 3-day food logs on the pages of this appendix. We encourage you to keep the sheets with you and record the pertinent information about the foods as you consume them.

DIRECTIONS FOR COMPUTING YOUR THREE-DAY DIETARY SURVEY

Step 1 Prepare a table (similar to Table C.1) indicating the intake of food items during a day. Include the amount (g or oz); caloric value; and carbohydrate, lipid, and protein content; the minerals Ca and Fe; and vitamins C, B_1 (thiamine), and B_2 (riboflavin); fiber; and cholesterol.

Step 2 List each food you consume for breakfast, lunch, dinner, between-meal eating, and snacks. Include food items that are used in preparing the meal (e.g., butter, oils, margarine, bread crumbs, egg coating, etc.).

Step 3 Weigh, measure or approximate the size of each portion of food that you eat. Record these values on your daily record chart (e.g., 3 oz of salad oil, 1/8 piece of 80 diameter apple pie, etc.).

Step 4 Record your daily calorie and nutrient intake on a chart similar to Table C.1, which was recorded for a 21-year-old college student. Record the daily totals for the caloric and nutrient headings on the "Daily and Average Daily Summary Chart" (Table C.2). When you've completed your three-day survey, compute the three-day total by adding up the values for days 1, 2, and 3; then divide by 3 to determine the daily average of each nutrient category.

Step 5 Using each of the average daily nutrient values, calculate the percentage of the RDA consumed for that particular nutrient and graph your results as shown in Figure C.1 An example for calculating the percentage of the RDA is shown in Table C.3, along with the specific RDA values for men and women.

Step 6 Be as accurate and honest as possible. Do not include unusual or atypical days in your dietary survey (e.g., days that you are sick, special occasions such as birthdays, or eating out at restaurants unless that is normal for you).

Step 7 Remember that the protein RDA equals 0.8 g protein per kilogram of body mass (1 kg = 2.2 lb).

Step 8 Compute the percentage of your total calories supplied from carbohydrate, lipid, and protein.

For example, if total average daily caloric intake is 2450 kcal/day, and 1600 kcal are from carbohydrates, the daily percentage of total calories from carbohydrates equals: $1600/2450 \times 100 = 65\%$

Step 9 While there is no specific RDA for lipid or carbohydrate, a prudent recommendation is that lipid should not exceed more than 30% of your total caloric intake; for active men and women, carbohydrates should be approximately 60% of the total calories ingested.

For example, if 50% of your average daily calories comes from lipid, you are taking in 167% of the recommended value ("RDA") for this nutrient: [50% divided by 30% (recommended percentage) × 100 = 167%]

Step 10 As was the case for lipid and carbohydrate, no RDA exists for average daily caloric intake. Any recommendation for energy intake must consider body fat level and current daily energy expenditure. However, average values for daily caloric intake have been published for the typical young adult and equal about 2100 kcal for young women and 3000 kcal for young men. Thus, for graphing purposes in Figure C.1, you can evaluate your average daily caloric intake against the "average" values for your sex and age.

If you eat a food item not listed in Appendix A, try to make an intelligent guess as to its composition and amount consumed. It is better to overestimate the amount of food consumed than to underestimate or to make no estimation at all. If you go to a restaurant for dinner, or to a friend's house where it may be inappropriate to measure the food, then omit this day from the counting procedure and resume record keeping the following day.

Record-keeping for 3 days is extremely important so an accurate appraisal can be made of the average daily energy and nutrient intake. **Be sure to record everything you eat.** If you are not completely honest, you are wasting your time. Most people find it easier to keep accurate records if they record food items while preparing a meal or immediately afterwards when eating snack items.

For example, if you are a 20-year-old female and you consume an average of 2400 kcal daily, your energy intake would equal 114% of the average ("RDA") for your age and sex. [2400 kcal divided by 2100 kcal (average) × 100 = 114%]. This does not mean that you need to go on a diet and reduce food intake to bring you in line with the average U.S. value. To the contrary, your higher-than-average caloric intake may be required to power your active lifestyle that contributes to maintaining a desirable body mass and body composition.

TABLE C.1 Sample One-Day Caloric and Nutrient Intake for a 21-year-old College Student

Food Item	Amount	kcal	Protein (g)	CHO (g)	Lipid (g)	Ca (mg)	Fe (g)	Fiber (g)	Cholesterol (mg)	Thiam[a] (mg)	Ribofl[a] (mg)
Breakfast											
Eggs, hard boiled	2 (2 oz ea)	160	14.1	1.4	11.2	55.2	1.9	0.0	452	0.06	0.53
Orange juice	8 oz	104	0.9	86.4	0.5	72.4	0.8	0.9	0.0	0.20	0.06
Corn flakes	1 cup/1 oz	110	2.3	24.4	0.5	1.0	1.8	0.6	0.0	0.37	0.42
Skim milk	8 oz	80	7.8	10.6	0.6	279.2	0.1	0.0	3.7	0.08	0.32
Snack											
None											
Lunch											
Tuna fish (oil pack)	2 oz	112	16.5	0.0	68.0	7.8	0.8	0.0	10.0	0.02	0.06
White bread (toast)	2 pieces	168	5.3	31.4	2.5	81.2	1.8	1.3	0.0	0.24	0.21
Mayonnaise	1 oz	203	0.3	0.8	22.6	5.7	0.2	0.0	16.8	0.01	0.01
Skim milk	8 oz	80	7.8	10.6	0.6	279.2	0.1	0.0	3.7	0.08	0.32
Plums	4 (2 oz ea)	128	1.8	29.5	1.4	10.3	0.2	4.4	0.0	0.10	0.22
Snack											
Chocolate milkshake	8 oz	288	7.7	46.4	8.4	256	0.7	0.3	29.6	0.13	0.55
Dinner											
Sirloin steak, lean	8 oz	456	64.8	0.0	20.2	18.6	5.8	0.0	173.6	0.21	0.47
French fries, veg. oil	6 oz	540	6.8	67.2	28.1	34.2	1.3	3.4	0.0	0.30	0.05
Cole slaw	4 oz	80	1.4	14.1	3.0	51.2	0.7	2.3	9.2	0.08	0.07
Italian bread	2 oz	156	5.1	32.0	1.0	9.4	1.5	0.9	0.0	0.23	0.13
Light beer	8 oz	96	0.6	8.8	0.0	11.2	0.1	0.5	0.0	0.02	0.06
Snack											
Yogurt, whole milk	6 oz	102	5.9	7.9	5.5	205.8	0.1	0.0	22.1	0.05	0.24
Daily Total		**2863**	**149.1**	**371.5**	**174.1**	**1378.4**	**17.2**	**14.6**	**720.7**	**2.18**	**3.72**

[a]*Thiam, thiamin; Ribofl, riboflavin.*

TABLE C.2 Daily and Average Summary Chart of the Intake of Calories and Specific Food Nutrients

Day	kcal	Protein[a] (g)	Lipid[a] (g)	CHO[a] (g)	Ca (mg)	Fe (mg)	Thiamine (mg)	Riboflavin (mg)	Fiber (mg)	Cholesterol (mg)
#1										
#2										
#3										
Three-day total										
Average Daily Value[b]										

[a]*Use the following caloric transformations to convert your average daily grams of carbohydrate (CHO), lipid, and protein to average daily calories:*

1 g CHO = 4 kcal

1 g Lipid = 9 kcal

1 g Protein = 4 kcal

[b]*Use the Average Daily Value to determine the percentage of the RDA for your graph. See Table 1 for sample calculations. Figure C.1 shows a bar graph for the nutrient values as a percentage of the average or recommended value for each item.*

TABLE C.3 RDA Values for Selected Nutrients Including Sample Computations for Deriving the Percent of RDA from Your Dietary Survey. Values Listed in Table C.1 are 100% Values for Graphing your Dietary Survey

Age	kcal[a]	Protein (g/kg)	Ca (mg)	Fe (mg)	Men Thiamine (mg)	Riboflavin (mg)	Fiber[a] (g)	Cholesterol[a] (mg)
19–22	3000	0.8	1200	10	1.5	1.7	30	300
23–50	2700	0.8	800	10	1.5	1.7	30	300
Age	kcal[a]	Protein (g/kg)	Ca (mg)	Fe (mg)	Women Thiamine (mg)	Riboflavin (mg)	Fiber[a] (g)	Cholesterol[a] (mg)
19–22	2100	0.8	1200	15	1.1	1.3	30	300
23–50	2000	0.8	800	15	1.1	1.3	30	300

Source: Recommended Dietary Allowances, Revised 1989, Washington, DC: Food and Nutrition Board, National Academy of Sciences-National Research Council, 1989.

[a]*No RDA exists for daily caloric intake or for the intake of fiber or cholesterol. Values for caloric intake represent an average for adult Americans, while fiber and cholesterol values are recommended as being prudent for maintaining good health.*

How to Determine the Percentage of the RDA from Your Dietary Survey

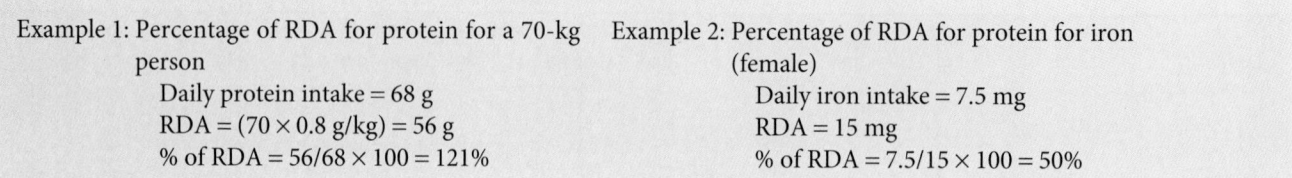

Example 1: Percentage of RDA for protein for a 70-kg person
Daily protein intake = 68 g
RDA = (70 × 0.8 g/kg) = 56 g
% of RDA = 56/68 × 100 = 121%

Example 2: Percentage of RDA for protein for iron (female)
Daily iron intake = 7.5 mg
RDA = 15 mg
% of RDA = 7.5/15 × 100 = 50%

FIGURE C.1
Example of a bar graph to illustrate the food and nutrient intake expressed as a percentage of recommended values.

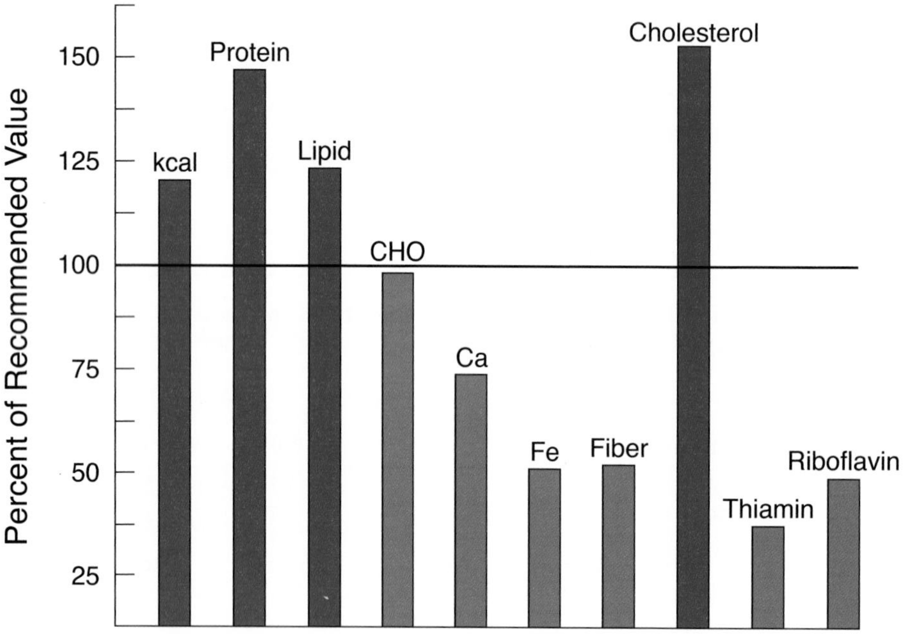

100% Value Represents

kcal:	3000 kcal for men age 19–22
	2700 kcal for men age 23–50
	2100 kcal for women age 19–22
	2000 kcal for women age 23–50
Lipid:	30% of total calories
CHO:	60% of total calories
Fiber:	30 g
Cholesterol:	300 mg

Sample Food Record

Time	Place	Amount	Description (including preparation)	Comments/Questions
8 AM	Home	3/4 cup	Kellogg's Corn Flakes	
		1/2 cup	Skim milk	Breakfast
		1 large	Orange	
		8 fl. oz	Coffee, black	
		2 tsp	White sugar	
11:30 AM	Away	1/2 cup	Tuna, water packed	Lunch
		2 Tbls	Mayonnaise, light	
		2 slices	White bread	
		1 cup	Campbell's tomato soup	
		4 rounds	Melba toast (crackers)	
		1 oz.	Potato chips, Lay's	
		1 piece	Apple pie	
3:00 PM	Away	1 large	Apple, red delicious	Snack
6:00 PM	Home	4 oz.	Chicken breast, baked, no skin	Dinner
		1 medium	Baked potato, flesh and ski	
		3 tsp	Light margarine	
		1 cup	Broccoli, steamed, plain	
		1 cup	Salad lettuce, romaine	
		3 whole	Cherry tomatoes	
		5 slices	Cucumber	1/4 inch each
		2 Tbls	Ranch dressing, regular	
		2 cups	Water	
8:30 PM	Home	3 cups	Popcorn, air popped, plain	Snack
		12 oz. can	Orange soda, regular	
		1	Donut, chocolate	Dunkin Donut
10:00 PM		2 cups	Ice cream, chocolate	Rich but good
10:45 PM		4 oz.	Chocolate bar, regular	Hershey's
11:10 PM		1 large	Apple, Macintosh	
11:30 PM		6 oz.	Apple cider	Hot
11:35 PM		1 small	Cookie, chocolate chip	

3-Day Food Record **Day 1**

Time	Place	Amount	Description (including preparation)	Comments/Questions

3-Day Food Record **Day 2**

Time	Place	Amount	Description (including preparation)	Comments/Questions

3-Day Food Record **Day 3**

Time	Place	Amount	Description (including preparation)	Comments/Questions

Appendix D Body Composition Assessment[a]

This appendix contains the age- and sex-specific equations to predict body fat percentage based on three girth measurements. There are four charts, one each for young and older men and women. In our experience, it is important to calibrate the tape measure prior to its use. Use a meter stick as the standard and check the markings on the cloth tape at 10-cm increments. A cloth tape is preferred over a metal one because little skin compression occurs when applying a cloth tape to the skin's surface at a relatively constant tension.

To use the charts, measure the three girths at the sites indicated in Figure 13.11, which shows the anatomic landmarks. The specific equation to predict percentage body fat with its corresponding constant is presented at the bottom of each of the four charts (Charts 2 to 5).

CHART 1 Body Sites Measured by the Circumference Method

		Site Measured		
Age (years)	Sex	A	B	C
18–26	M	Right upper arm	Abdomen	Right forearm
	F	Abdomen	Right thigh	Right forearm
27–50	M	Buttocks	Abdomen	Right forearm
	F	Abdomen	Right thigh	Right calf

CHART 2 Conversion Constants to Predict Percentage Body Fat for Young Men

Upper Arm			Abdomen			Forearm		
in	cm	Constant A	in	cm	Constant B	in	cm	Constant C
7.00	17.78	25.91	21.00	53.34	27.56	7.00	17.78	38.01
7.25	18.41	26.83	21.25	53.97	27.88	7.25	18.41	39.37
7.50	19.05	27.76	21.50	54.61	28.21	7.50	19.05	40.72
7.75	19.68	28.68	21.75	55.24	28.54	7.75	19.68	42.08
8.00	20.32	29.61	22.00	55.88	28.87	8.00	20.32	43.44
8.25	20.95	30.53	22.25	56.51	29.20	8.25	20.95	44.80
8.50	21.59	31.46	22.50	57.15	29.52	8.50	21.59	46.15
8.75	22.22	32.38	22.75	57.78	29.85	8.75	22.22	47.51
9.00	22.86	33.31	23.00	58.42	30.18	9.00	22.86	48.87
9.25	23.49	34.24	23.25	59.05	30.51	9.25	23.49	50.23
9.50	24.13	35.16	23.50	59.69	30.84	9.50	24.13	51.58
9.75	24.76	36.09	23.75	60.32	31.16	9.75	24.76	52.94
10.00	25.40	37.01	24.00	60.96	31.49	10.00	25.40	54.30
10.25	26.03	37.94	24.25	61.59	31.82	10.25	26.03	55.65
10.50	26.67	38.86	24.50	62.23	32.15	10.50	26.67	57.01
10.75	27.30	39.79	24.75	62.86	32.48	10.75	27.30	58.37
11.00	27.94	40.71	25.00	63.50	32.80	11.00	27.94	59.73
11.25	28.57	41.64	25.25	64.13	33.13	11.25	28.57	61.08

CHART 2 Conversion Constants to Predict Percentage Body Fat for Young Men (continued)

Upper Arm			Abdomen			Forearm		
in	cm	Constant A	in	cm	Constant B	in	cm	Constant C
11.50	29.21	42.56	25.50	64.77	33.46	11.50	29.21	62.44
11.75	29.84	43.49	25.75	65.40	33.79	11.75	29.84	63.80
12.00	30.48	44.41	26.00	66.04	34.12	12.00	30.48	65.16
12.25	31.11	45.34	26.25	66.67	34.44	12.25	31.11	66.51
12.50	31.75	46.26	26.50	67.31	34.77	12.50	31.75	67.87
12.75	32.38	47.19	26.75	67.94	35.10	12.75	32.38	69.23
13.00	33.02	48.11	27.00	68.58	35.43	13.00	33.02	70.59
13.25	33.65	49.04	27.25	69.21	35.76	13.25	33.65	71.94
13.50	34.29	49.96	27.50	69.85	36.09	13.50	34.29	73.30
13.75	34.92	50.89	27.75	70.48	36.41	13.75	34.92	74.66
14.00	35.56	51.82	28.00	71.12	36.74	14.00	35.56	76.02
14.25	36.19	52.74	28.25	71.75	37.07	14.25	36.19	77.37
14.50	36.83	53.67	28.50	72.39	37.40	14.50	36.83	78.73
14.75	37.46	54.59	28.75	73.02	37.73	14.75	37.46	80.09
15.00	38.10	55.52	29.00	73.66	38.05	15.00	38.10	81.45
15.25	38.73	56.44	29.25	74.29	38.38	15.25	38.73	82.80
15.50	39.37	57.37	29.50	74.93	38.71	15.50	39.37	84.16
15.75	40.00	58.29	29.75	75.56	39.04	15.75	40.00	85.52
16.00	40.64	59.22	30.00	76.20	39.37	16.00	40.64	86.88
16.25	41.27	60.14	30.25	76.83	39.69	16.25	41.27	88.23
16.50	41.91	61.07	30.50	77.47	40.02	16.50	41.91	89.59
16.75	42.54	61.99	30.75	78.10	40.35	16.75	42.54	90.95
17.00	43.18	62.92	31.00	78.74	40.68	17.00	43.18	92.31
17.25	43.81	63.84	31.25	79.37	41.01	17.25	43.81	93.66
17.50	44.45	64.77	31.50	80.01	41.33	17.50	44.45	95.02
17.75	45.08	65.69	31.75	80.64	41.66	17.75	45.08	96.38
18.00	45.72	66.62	32.00	81.28	41.99	18.00	45.72	97.74
18.25	46.35	67.54	32.25	81.91	42.32	18.25	46.35	99.09
18.50	46.99	68.47	32.50	82.55	42.65	18.50	46.99	100.45
18.75	47.62	69.40	32.75	83.18	42.97	18.75	47.62	101.81
19.00	48.26	70.32	33.00	83.82	43.30	19.00	48.26	103.17
19.25	48.89	71.25	33.25	84.45	43.63	19.25	48.89	104.52
19.50	49.53	72.17	33.50	85.09	43.96	19.50	49.53	105.88
19.75	50.16	73.10	33.75	85.72	44.29	19.75	50.16	107.24
20.00	50.80	74.02	34.00	86.36	44.61	20.00	50.80	108.60
20.25	51.43	74.95	34.25	86.99	44.94	20.25	51.43	109.95
20.50	52.07	75.87	34.50	87.63	45.27	20.50	52.07	111.31
20.75	52.70	76.80	34.75	88.26	45.60	20.75	52.70	112.67
21.00	53.34	77.72	35.00	88.90	45.93	21.00	53.34	114.02
21.25	53.97	78.65	35.25	89.53	46.25	21.25	53.97	115.38
21.50	54.61	79.57	35.50	90.17	46.58	21.50	54.61	116.74
21.75	55.24	80.50	35.75	90.80	46.91	21.75	55.24	118.10
22.00	55.88	81.42	36.00	91.44	47.24	22.00	55.88	119.45
			36.25	92.07	47.57			
			36.50	92.71	47.89			
			36.75	93.34	48.22			
			37.00	93.98	48.55			

(continued)

CHART 2 Conversion Constants to Predict Percentage Body Fat for Young Men (continued)

Upper Arm			Abdomen			Forearm		
in	cm	Constant A	in	cm	Constant B	in	cm	Constant C
			37.25	94.61	48.88			
			37.50	95.25	49.21			
			37.75	95.88	49.54			
			38.00	96.52	49.86			
			38.25	97.15	50.19			
			38.50	97.79	50.52			
			38.75	98.42	50.85			
			39.00	99.06	51.18			
			39.25	99.69	51.50			
			39.50	100.33	51.83			
			39.75	100.96	52.16			
			40.00	101.60	52.49			
			40.25	102.23	52.82			
			40.50	102.87	53.14			
			40.75	103.50	53.47			
			41.00	104.14	53.80			
			41.25	104.77	54.13			
			41.50	105.41	54.46			
			41.75	106.04	54.78			
			42.00	106.68	55.11			

Note: Percent Fat = Constant A + Constant B – Constant C – 10.2

CHART 3 Conversion Constants to Predict Percentage Body Fat for Older Men

Buttocks			Abdomen			Forearm		
in	cm	Constant A	in	cm	Constant B	in	cm	Constant C
28.00	71.12	29.34	25.50	64.77	22.84	7.00	17.78	21.01
28.25	71.75	29.60	25.75	65.40	23.06	7.25	18.41	21.76
28.50	72.39	29.87	26.00	66.04	23.29	7.50	19.05	22.52
28.75	73.02	30.13	26.25	66.67	23.51	7.75	19.68	23.26
29.00	73.66	30.39	26.50	67.31	23.73	8.00	20.32	24.02
29.25	74.29	30.65	26.75	67.94	23.96	8.25	20.95	24.76
29.50	74.93	30.92	27.00	68.58	24.18	8.50	21.59	25.52
29.75	75.56	31.18	27.25	69.21	24.40	8.75	22.22	26.26
30.00	76.20	31.44	27.50	69.85	24.63	9.00	22.86	27.02
30.25	76.83	31.70	27.75	70.48	24.85	9.25	23.49	27.76
30.50	77.47	31.96	28.00	71.12	25.08	9.50	24.13	28.52
30.75	78.10	32.22	28.25	71.75	25.29	9.75	24.76	29.26
31.00	78.74	32.49	28.50	72.39	25.52	10.00	25.40	30.02
31.25	79.37	32.75	28.75	73.02	25.75	10.25	26.03	30.76
31.50	80.01	33.01	29.00	73.66	25.97	10.50	26.67	31.52
31.75	80.64	33.27	29.25	74.29	26.19	10.75	27.30	32.27
32.00	81.28	33.54	29.50	74.93	26.42	11.00	27.94	33.02
32.25	81.91	33.80	29.75	75.56	26.64	11.25	28.57	33.77
32.50	82.55	34.06	30.00	76.20	26.87	11.50	29.21	34.52
32.75	83.18	34.32	30.25	76.83	27.09	11.75	29.84	35.27

(continued)

CHART 3 Conversion Constants to Predict Percentage Body Fat for Older Men (*continued*)

Buttocks			Abdomen			Forearm		
in	cm	Constant A	in	cm	Constant B	in	cm	Constant C
33.00	83.82	34.58	30.50	77.47	27.32	12.00	30.48	36.02
33.25	84.45	34.84	30.75	78.10	27.54	12.25	31.11	36.77
33.50	85.09	35.11	31.00	78.74	27.76	12.50	31.75	37.53
33.75	85.72	35.37	31.25	79.37	27.98	12.75	32.38	38.27
34.00	86.36	35.63	31.50	80.01	28.21	13.00	33.02	39.03
34.25	86.99	35.89	31.75	80.64	28.43	13.25	33.65	39.77
34.50	87.63	36.16	32.00	81.28	28.66	13.50	34.29	40.53
34.75	88.26	36.42	32.25	81.91	28.88	13.75	34.92	41.27
35.00	88.90	36.68	32.50	82.55	29.11	14.00	35.56	42.03
35.25	89.53	36.94	32.75	83.18	29.33	14.25	36.19	42.77
35.50	90.17	37.20	33.00	83.82	29.55	14.50	36.83	43.53
35.75	90.80	37.46	33.25	84.45	29.78	14.75	37.46	44.27
36.00	91.44	37.73	33.50	85.09	30.00	15.00	38.10	45.03
36.25	92.07	37.99	33.75	85.72	30.22	15.25	38.73	45.77
36.50	92.71	38.25	34.00	86.36	30.45	15.50	39.37	46.53
36.75	93.34	38.51	34.25	86.99	30.67	15.75	40.00	47.28
37.00	93.98	38.78	34.50	87.63	30.89	16.00	40.64	48.03
37.25	94.61	39.04	34.75	88.26	31.12	16.25	41.27	48.78
37.50	95.25	39.30	35.00	88.90	31.35	16.50	41.91	49.53
37.75	95.88	39.56	35.25	89.53	31.57	16.75	42.54	50.28
38.00	96.52	39.82	35.50	90.17	31.79	17.00	43.18	51.03
38.25	97.15	40.08	35.75	90.80	32.02	17.25	43.81	51.78
38.50	97.79	40.35	36.00	91.44	32.24	17.50	44.45	52.54
38.75	98.42	40.61	36.25	92.07	32.46	17.75	45.08	53.28
39.00	99.06	40.87	36.50	92.71	32.69	18.00	45.72	54.04
39.25	99.69	41.13	36.75	93.34	32.91	18.25	46.35	54.78
39.50	100.33	41.39	37.00	93.98	33.14			
39.75	100.96	41.66	37.25	94.61	33.36			
40.00	101.60	41.92	37.50	95.25	33.58			
40.25	102.23	42.18	37.75	95.88	33.81			
40.50	102.87	42.44	38.00	96.52	34.03			
40.75	103.50	42.70	38.25	97.15	34.26			
41.00	104.14	42.97	38.50	97.79	34.48			
41.25	104.77	43.23	38.75	98.42	34.70			
41.50	105.41	43.49	39.00	99.06	34.93			
41.75	106.04	43.75	39.25	99.69	35.15			
42.00	106.68	44.02	39.50	100.33	35.38			
42.25	107.31	44.28	39.75	100.96	35.59			
42.50	107.95	44.54	40.00	101.60	35.82			
42.75	108.58	44.80	40.25	102.23	36.05			
43.00	109.22	45.06	40.50	102.87	36.27			
43.25	109.85	45.32	40.75	103.50	36.49			
43.50	110.49	45.59	41.00	104.14	36.72			
43.75	111.12	45.85	41.25	104.77	36.94			
44.00	111.76	46.12	41.50	105.41	37.17			
44.25	112.39	46.37	41.75	106.04	37.39			
44.50	113.03	46.64	42.00	106.68	37.62			
44.75	113.66	46.89	42.25	107.31	37.87			
45.00	114.30	47.16	42.50	107.95	38.06			
45.25	114.93	47.42	42.75	108.58	38.28			
45.50	115.57	47.68	43.00	109.22	38.51			
45.75	116.20	47.94	43.25	109.85	38.73			
46.00	116.84	48.21	43.50	110.49	38.96			
46.25	117.47	48.47	43.75	111.12	39.18			
46.50	118.11	48.73	44.00	111.76	39.41			

(continued)

CHART 3 Conversion Constants to Predict Percentage Body Fat for Older Men (*continued*)

Buttocks in	Buttocks cm	Constant A	Abdomen in	Abdomen cm	Constant B	Forearm in	Forearm cm	Constant C
46.75	118.74	48.99	44.25	112.39	39.63			
47.00	119.38	49.26	44.50	113.03	39.85			
47.25	120.01	49.52	44.75	113.66	40.08			
47.50	120.65	49.78	45.00	114.30	40.30			
47.75	121.28	50.04						
48.00	121.92	50.30						
48.25	122.55	50.56						
48.50	123.19	50.83						
48.75	123.82	51.09						
49.00	124.46	51.35						

Note: Percent Fat = Constant A + Constant B − Constant C − 15.0

CHART 4 Conversion Constants to Predict Percentage Body Fat for Young Women

Abdomen in	Abdomen cm	Constant A	Thigh in	Thigh cm	Constant B	Forearm in	Forearm cm	Constant C
20.00	50.80	26.74	14.00	35.56	29.13	6.00	15.24	25.86
20.25	51.43	27.07	14.25	36.19	29.65	6.25	15.87	26.94
20.50	52.07	27.41	14.50	36.83	30.17	6.50	16.51	28.02
20.75	52.70	27.74	14.75	37.46	30.69	6.75	17.14	29.10
21.00	53.34	28.07	15.00	38.10	31.21	7.00	17.78	30.17
21.25	53.97	28.41	15.25	38.73	31.73	7.25	18.41	31.25
21.50	54.61	28.74	15.50	39.37	32.25	7.50	19.05	32.33
21.75	55.24	29.08	15.75	40.00	32.77	7.75	19.68	33.41
22.00	55.88	29.41	16.00	40.64	33.29	8.00	20.32	34.48
22.25	56.51	29.74	16.25	41.27	33.81	8.25	20.95	35.56
22.50	57.15	30.08	16.50	41.91	34.33	8.50	21.59	36.64
22.75	57.78	30.41	16.75	42.54	34.85	8.75	22.22	37.72
23.00	58.42	30.75	17.00	43.18	35.37	9.00	22.86	38.79
23.25	59.05	31.08	17.25	43.81	35.89	9.25	23.49	39.87
23.50	59.69	31.42	17.50	44.45	36.41	9.50	24.13	40.95
23.75	60.32	31.75	17.75	45.08	36.93	9.75	24.76	42.03
24.00	60.96	32.08	18.00	45.72	37.45	10.00	25.40	43.10
24.25	61.59	32.42	18.25	46.35	37.97	10.25	26.03	44.18
24.50	62.23	32.75	18.50	46.99	38.49	10.50	26.67	45.26
24.75	62.86	33.09	18.75	47.62	39.01	10.75	27.30	46.34
25.00	63.50	33.42	19.00	48.26	39.53	11.00	27.94	47.41
25.25	64.13	33.76	19.25	48.89	40.05	11.25	28.57	48.49
25.50	64.77	34.09	19.50	49.53	40.57	11.50	29.21	49.57
25.75	65.40	34.42	19.75	50.16	41.09	11.75	29.84	50.65
26.00	66.04	34.76	20.00	50.80	41.61	12.00	30.48	51.73
26.25	66.67	35.09	20.25	51.43	42.13	12.25	31.11	52.80
26.50	67.31	35.43	20.50	52.07	42.65	12.50	31.75	53.88
26.75	67.94	35.76	20.75	52.70	43.17	12.75	32.38	54.96
27.00	68.58	36.10	21.00	53.34	43.69	13.00	33.02	56.04
27.25	69.21	36.43	21.25	53.97	44.21	13.25	33.65	57.11
27.50	69.85	36.76	21.50	54.61	44.73	13.50	34.29	58.19
27.75	70.48	37.10	21.75	55.24	45.25	13.75	34.92	59.27
28.00	71.12	37.43	22.00	55.88	45.77	14.00	35.56	60.35

(continued)

CHART 4 Conversion Constants to Predict Percentage Body Fat for Young Women (continued)

Abdomen			Thigh			Forearm		
in	cm	Constant A	in	cm	Constant B	in	cm	Constant C
28.25	71.75	37.77	22.25	56.51	46.29	14.25	36.19	61.42
28.50	72.39	38.10	22.50	57.15	46.81	14.50	36.83	62.50
28.75	73.02	38.43	22.75	57.78	47.33	14.75	37.46	63.58
29.00	73.66	38.77	23.00	58.42	47.85	15.00	38.10	64.66
29.25	74.29	39.10	23.25	59.05	48.37	15.25	38.73	65.73
29.50	74.93	39.44	23.50	59.69	48.89	15.50	39.37	66.81
29.75	75.56	39.77	23.75	60.32	49.41	15.75	40.00	67.89
30.00	76.20	40.11	24.00	60.96	49.93	16.00	40.64	68.97
30.25	76.83	40.44	24.25	61.59	50.45	16.25	41.27	70.04
30.50	77.47	40.77	24.50	62.23	50.97	16.50	41.91	71.12
30.75	78.10	41.11	24.75	62.86	51.49	16.75	42.54	72.20
31.00	78.74	41.44	25.00	63.50	52.01	17.00	43.18	73.28
31.25	79.37	41.78	25.25	64.13	52.53	17.25	43.81	74.36
31.50	80.01	42.11	25.50	64.77	53.05	17.50	44.45	75.43
31.75	80.64	42.45	25.75	65.40	53.57	17.75	45.08	76.51
32.00	81.28	42.78	26.00	66.04	54.09	18.00	45.72	77.59
32.25	81.91	43.11	26.25	66.67	54.61	18.25	46.35	78.67
32.50	82.55	43.45	26.50	67.31	55.13	18.50	46.99	79.74
32.75	83.18	43.78	26.75	67.94	55.65	18.75	47.62	80.82
33.00	83.82	44.12	27.00	68.58	56.17	19.00	48.26	81.90
33.25	84.45	44.45	27.25	69.21	56.69	19.25	48.89	82.98
33.50	85.09	44.78	27.50	69.85	57.21	19.50	49.53	84.05
33.75	85.72	45.12	27.75	70.48	57.73	19.75	50.16	85.13
34.00	86.36	45.45	28.00	71.12	58.26	20.00	50.80	86.21
34.25	86.99	45.79	28.25	71.75	58.78			
34.50	87.63	46.12	28.50	72.39	59.30			
34.75	88.26	46.46	38.75	73.02	59.82			
35.00	88.90	46.79	29.00	73.66	60.34			
35.25	89.53	47.12	29.25	74.29	60.86			
35.50	90.17	47.46	29.50	74.93	61.38			
35.75	90.80	47.79	29.75	75.56	61.90			
36.00	91.44	48.13	30.00	76.20	62.42			
36.25	92.07	48.46	30.25	76.83	62.94			
36.50	92.71	48.80	30.50	77.47	63.46			
36.75	93.34	49.13	30.75	78.10	63.98			
37.00	93.98	49.46	31.00	78.74	64.50			
37.25	94.61	49.80	31.25	79.37	65.02			
37.50	95.25	50.13	31.50	80.01	65.54			
37.75	95.88	50.47	31.75	80.64	66.06			
38.00	96.52	50.80	32.00	81.28	66.58			
38.25	97.15	51.13	32.25	81.91	67.10			
38.50	97.79	51.47	32.50	82.55	67.62			
38.75	98.42	51.80	32.75	83.18	68.14			
39.00	99.06	52.14	33.00	83.82	68.66			
39.25	99.69	52.47	33.25	84.45	69.18			
39.50	100.33	52.81	33.50	85.09	69.70			
39.75	100.96	53.14	33.75	85.72	70.22			
40.00	101.60	53.47	34.00	86.36	70.74			

Note: Percent Fat = Constant A + Constant B − Constant C − 19.6

CHART 5 Conversion Constants to Predict Percentage Body Fat for Older Women

Abdomen			Thigh			Forearm		
in	cm	Constant A	in	cm	Constant B	in	cm	Constant C
25.00	63.50	29.69	14.00	35.56	17.31	10.00	25.40	14.46
25.25	64.13	29.98	14.25	36.19	17.62	10.25	26.03	14.82
25.50	64.77	30.28	14.50	36.83	17.93	10.50	26.67	15.18
25.75	65.40	30.58	14.75	37.46	18.24	10.75	27.30	15.54
26.00	66.04	30.87	15.00	38.10	18.55	11.00	27.94	15.91
26.25	66.67	31.17	15.25	38.73	18.86	11.25	28.57	16.27
26.50	67.31	31.47	15.50	39.37	19.17	11.50	29.21	16.63
26.75	67.94	31.76	15.75	40.00	19.47	11.75	29.84	16.99
27.00	68.58	32.06	16.00	40.64	19.78	12.00	30.48	17.35
27.25	69.21	32.36	16.25	41.27	20.09	12.25	31.11	17.71
27.50	69.85	32.65	16.50	41.91	20.40	12.50	31.75	18.08
27.75	70.48	32.95	16.75	42.54	20.71	12.75	32.38	18.44
28.00	71.12	33.25	17.00	43.18	21.02	13.00	33.02	18.80
28.25	71.75	33.55	17.25	43.81	21.33	13.25	33.65	19.16
28.50	72.39	33.84	17.50	44.45	21.64	13.50	34.29	19.52
28.75	73.02	34.14	17.75	45.08	21.95	13.75	34.92	19.88
29.00	73.66	34.44	18.00	45.72	22.26	14.00	35.56	20.24
29.25	74.29	34.73	18.25	46.35	22.57	14.25	36.19	20.61
29.50	74.93	35.03	18.50	46.99	22.87	14.50	36.83	20.97
29.75	75.56	35.33	18.75	47.62	23.18	14.75	37.46	21.33
30.00	76.20	35.62	19.00	38.26	23.49	15.00	38.10	21.69
30.25	76.83	35.92	19.25	48.89	23.80	15.25	38.73	22.05
30.50	77.47	36.22	19.50	49.53	24.11	15.50	39.37	22.41
30.75	78.10	36.51	19.75	50.16	24.42	15.75	40.00	22.77
31.00	78.74	36.81	20.00	50.80	24.73	16.00	40.64	23.14
31.25	79.37	37.11	20.25	51.43	25.04	16.25	41.27	23.50
31.50	80.01	37.40	20.50	52.07	25.35	16.50	41.91	23.86
31.75	80.64	37.70	20.75	52.70	25.66	16.75	42.54	24.22
32.00	81.28	38.00	21.00	53.34	25.97	17.00	43.18	24.58
32.25	81.91	38.30	21.25	53.97	26.28	17.25	43.81	24.94
32.50	82.55	38.59	21.50	54.61	26.58	17.50	44.45	25.31
32.75	83.18	38.89	21.75	55.24	26.89	17.75	45.08	25.67
33.00	83.82	39.19	22.00	55.88	27.20	18.00	45.72	26.03
33.25	84.45	39.48	22.25	56.51	27.51	18.25	46.35	26.39
33.50	85.09	39.78	22.50	57.15	27.82	18.50	46.99	26.75
33.75	85.72	40.08	22.75	57.78	28.13	18.75	47.62	27.11
34.00	86.36	40.37	23.00	58.42	28.44	19.00	48.26	27.47
34.25	86.99	40.67	23.25	59.05	28.75	19.25	48.89	27.84
34.50	87.63	40.97	23.50	59.69	29.06	19.50	49.53	28.20
34.75	88.26	41.26	23.75	60.32	29.37	19.75	50.16	28.56
35.00	88.90	41.56	24.00	60.96	29.68	20.00	50.80	28.92
35.25	89.53	41.86	24.25	61.59	29.98	20.25	51.43	29.28
35.50	90.17	42.15	24.50	62.23	30.29	20.50	52.07	29.64
35.75	90.80	42.45	24.75	62.86	30.60	20.75	52.70	30.00
36.00	91.44	42.75	25.00	63.50	30.91	21.00	53.34	30.37
36.25	92.07	43.05	25.25	64.13	31.22	21.25	53.97	30.73
36.50	92.71	43.34	25.50	64.77	31.53	21.50	54.61	31.09
36.75	93.35	43.64	25.75	65.40	31.84	21.75	55.24	31.45
37.00	93.98	43.94	26.00	66.04	32.15	22.00	55.88	31.81
37.25	94.62	44.23	26.25	66.67	32.46	22.25	56.51	32.17
37.50	95.25	44.53	26.50	67.31	32.77	22.50	57.15	32.54
37.75	95.89	44.83	26.75	67.94	33.08	22.75	57.78	32.90
38.00	96.52	45.12	27.00	68.58	33.38	23.00	58.42	33.26
38.25	97.16	45.42	27.25	69.21	33.69	23.25	59.05	33.62

(continued)

CHART 5 Conversion Constants to Predict Percentage Body Fat for Older Women (continued)

Abdomen			Thigh			Forearm		
in	cm	Constant A	in	cm	Constant B	in	cm	Constant C
38.50	97.79	45.72	27.50	69.85	34.00	23.50	59.69	33.98
38.75	98.43	46.01	27.75	70.48	34.31	23.75	60.32	34.34
39.00	99.06	46.31	28.00	71.12	34.62	24.00	60.96	34.70
39.25	99.70	46.61	28.25	71.75	34.93	24.25	61.59	35.07
39.50	100.33	46.90	28.50	72.39	35.24	24.50	62.23	35.43
39.75	100.97	47.20	28.75	73.02	35.55	24.75	62.86	35.79
40.00	101.60	47.50	29.00	73.66	35.86	25.00	63.50	36.15
40.25	101.24	47.79	29.25	74.29	36.17			
40.50	102.87	48.09	29.50	74.93	36.48			
40.75	103.51	48.39	29.75	75.56	36.79			
41.00	104.14	48.69	30.00	76.20	37.09			
41.25	104.78	48.98	30.25	76.83	37.40			
41.50	105.41	49.28	30.50	77.47	37.71			
41.75	106.05	49.58	30.75	78.10	38.02			
42.00	106.68	49.87	31.00	78.74	38.33			
42.25	107.32	50.17	31.25	79.37	38.64			
42.50	107.95	50.47	31.50	80.01	38.95			
42.75	108.59	50.76	31.75	80.64	39.26			
43.00	109.22	51.06	32.00	81.28	39.57			
43.25	109.86	51.36	32.25	81.91	39.88			
43.50	110.49	51.65	32.50	82.55	40.19			
43.75	111.13	51.95	32.75	83.18	40.49			
44.00	111.76	52.25	33.00	83.82	40.80			
44.25	112.40	52.54	33.25	84.45	41.11			
44.50	113.03	52.84	33.50	85.09	41.42			
44.75	113.67	53.14	33.75	85.72	41.73			
45.00	114.30	53.44	34.00	86.36	42.04			

Note: Percentage Fat = Constant A + Constant B − Constant C − 18.4

Appendix E Body Composition Characteristics of Athletes in Different Sports[a,b]

Sport	Sex	N	Age (y)	Stature (cm)	Mass (kg)	Body Fat (%)	Reference Number
Ballet							
	F	34	21.9	168.0	54.4	16.9	3
			±4.3	±6.8	±6.0	±4.7	
Baseball and softball							
Baseball	M		27.4	183.1	88.0	12.6	39
Softball	F	14	22.6	167.1	59.6	19.1	41
			±4.1	±6.1	±5.8	±5.0	
Basketball	F	49	19.3	176.5	±6.8	19.2	34
			±1.4	±8.8	±6.7	±4.6	
	M	10	20.9	194.3	87.5	10.5	27
			±1.3	±10.2	±7.2	±3.8	
Biathlon	F	9	25.1	165.9	59.0	15.0	2
			±5.3	±7.1	±7.1	±2.2	
Bicycling	M	11	22.2	176.4	±8.5	10.5	40
			±3.6	±7.1	±6.4	±2.4	
Field events							
Decathlon	M	3	22.5	186.3	84.1	8.4	40
			±2.2	±1.4	±9.2	±5.1	
Pentathlon	F	9	21.5	175.4	±5.4	11.0	15
			±3.1	±3.0	±5.7	±3.3	
Throwing	F	9	18.8	173.9	80.8	27.0	38
			±3.0	±6.9	±21.1	±8.4	
Discus	M	7	28.3	186.1	104.7	16.4	6
			±5.0	±2.6	±13.2	±4.3	
Shot	M	5	27.0	188.2	112.5	16.5	6
			±3.9	±3.6	±7.3	±4.3	
Jumping	F	13	17.4	173.6	57.1	12.9	33
			±0.9	±8.0	±6.0	±2.5	
	M	16	17.6	181.7	±9.2	8.5	33
			±0.8	±6.1	±7.2	±2.1	
Hammer, elite	M	10	24.8	187.3	104.2	15.1	20
			±3.2	±3.1	±9.1	±4.2	
Shotput, elite	M	10	23.5	187.0	112.3	14.8	20
			±4.2	±4.0	±6.2	±3.4	
Discus, elite	M	10	23.5	191.7	108.2	13.2	20
			±4.5	±4.7	±6.9	±4.6	
Javelin, elite	M	10	21.9	186.0	90.6	8.5	20
			±3.7	±5.1	±6.1	±3.2	
Field hockey	F	13	19.8	159.8	58.1	21.3	31
			±1.4	±5.5	±6.6	±7.2	
Football							
Defensive backs, Pro	M	26	24.5	182.5	84.8	9.6	37
			±3.2	±4.5	±5.2	±4.2	
College	M	15		178.3	77.3	11.5	18
College	M	12		179.9	83.1	8.8	
College	M	15		183.0	83.7	9.6	
Pro, current	M	26		182.5	84.8	9.6	
Pro, older	M	25		183.0	91.2	10.7	

(continued)

Sport	Sex	N	Age (y)	Stature (cm)	Mass (kg)	Body Fat (%)	Reference Number
Football, *continued*							
Offensive backs and wide receivers, Pro	M	40	24.7 ±3.0	183.8 ±4.1	90.7 ±8.4	9.4 ±4.0	37
College	M	15		179.7	79.8	12.4	36
College	M	29		181.8	84.1	9.5	18
College	M	18		185.6	86.1	9.9	
Pro, current	M	40		183.8	90.7	9.4	
Pro, older	M	25		183.0	91.7	10.0	
Line backers, Pro	M	28	24.2 ±2.4	188.6 ±2.9	102.2 ±6.3	14.0 ±4.6	37
College	M	7		180.1	87.2	13.4	36
College	M	17		186.1	97.1	13.1	18
College	M	17		185.6	98.8	13.2	
Pro, current	M	28		188.6	102.2	14.0	
Offensive line, Pro	M	38	24.7 ±3.2	193.0 ±3.5	112.6 ±6.8	15.6 ±3.8	37
College	M	13		186.0	99.2	19.1	36
College	M	23		187.5	107.6	19.5	18
College	M	25		191.1	106.5	15.3	
Pro, current	M	38		193.0	112.6	15.6	
Defensive line, Pro	M	32	25.7 ±3.4	192.4 ±6.5	117.1 ±10.3	18.2 ±5.4	37
College	M	15		186.6	97.8	18.5	36
College	M	8		188.8	114.3	19.5	18
College	M	13		191.1	109.3	14.7	
Pro, current	M	32		192.4	117.1	18.2	
Pro, older	M	25		185.7	97.1	14.0	
Quarterbacks, Pro	M	16	24.1 ±2.7	185.0 ±5.4	90.1 ±11.3	14.4 ±6.5	37
Total Team							
College	M	65		182.5	88.0	15.0	36
College	M	91		184.9	97.3	13.9	18
College	M	88		186.6	96.6	11.4	
Pro, current	M	164		188.1	101.5	13.4	
Pro, older	M	25		183.1	91.2	10.4	
Dallas-Jets	M	107		188.2	100.4	12.6	
Gymnastics							
	F	44	19.4 ±1.1	160.6 ±4.4	53.7 ±5.9	15.3 ±4.0	30
	F	97	15.7 ±1.1	162.4 ±5.6	54.0 ±6.5	8.2	5
	M	19		168.7 ±6.7	±5.8 ±4.3	±.5 ±2.4	32
Lacrosse	F	17	24.4 ±4.5	166.3 ±7.5	±0.6 ±7.3	19.3 ±5.7	41
	M	26	26.7 ±4.2	177.6 ±5.5	74.0 ±8.6	12.3 ±4.3	40
Orienteering	M	7	25.9 ±8.5	176.2 ±6.8	±4.7 ±5.0	10.7 ±2.9	40
Racket sports							
Badminton	F	6	23.0 ±5.3	167.7 ±2.5	±1.5 ±2.6	21.0 ±2.1	41
	M	7	24.5 ±3.6	180.0 ±5.2	71.2 ±5.6	12.8 ±3.1	40
Tennis	F	7	21.3	164.7	59.6	22.4	31

(continued)

Sport	Sex	N	Age (y)	Stature (cm)	Mass (kg)	Body Fat (%)	Reference Number
Racket sports, *continued*							
			±0.9	±4.2	±4.6	±2.0	
	M	9		179.1	73.8	11.3	32
				±4.5	±7.3	±5.2	
Squash	M	9	22.6	177.5	71.9	11.2	40
			±6.8	±4.1	±8.3	±3.7	
Rowers	M	18	20.6	185.8	86.3	12.2	13
			±1.9	±2.2	±6.4	±4.1	
Skating							
Ice hockey	M	27	24.9	182.9	85.6	9.2	1
			±3.6	±6.1	±7.1	±4.6	
Speed skating	F	9	19.7	165.0	±1.2	16.5	23
			±3.0	±6.0	±6.9	±4.1	
	M	6	22.2	178.0	73.3	7.4	23
			±4.1	±7.1	±7.1	±2.5	
Skiing							
(Nordic)	F	5	23.5	164.5	56.9	16.1	29
			±4.7	±3.3	±1.1	±1.6	
Alpine	F	6	19.6	165.0	±3.6	16.6	35
	F	5	20.2	164.7	±0.1	18.5	12
	M	8	19.8	173.0	72.6	±.5	35
	M	5	21.2	175.5	73.0	7.2	12
	M	11	22.8	179.0	71.8	7.2	29
			±1.9	±5.0	±5.4	±1.9	
Soccer	F	11	22.1	164.9	±1.2	22.0	41
			±4.1	±5.6	±8.6	±6.8	
	M	19		176.8	72.4	9.5	32
				±6.6	±8.9	±4.9	
Swimming	F	9	13.5	164.5	53.3	17.2	19
			±0.9	±7.4	±5.3	±3.6	
	F	13	16.4	168.8	57.9	15.6	
			±0.9	±7.1	±5.5	±4.0	
	F	19	19.2	169.6	56.0	16.1	
			±0.8	±4.7	±3.1	±3.7	
	M	27		178.3	71.0	8.8	32
				±6.4	±5.9	±3.2	
Channel swimmers	M	11	38.2	173.8	87.5	22.4	24
			±10.2	±7.4	±10.4	±7.5	
Track events							
Distance runners	F	15	27	161.0	47.2	14.3	8
				±4.0	±4.6	±3.3	
	M	20		177.0	±3.1	4.7	22
				±6.0	±4.8	±3.1	
Masters and competitors	M	11	40–49	180.7	±3.1	4.7	21
		5	50–59	174.2	±7.2	10.9	
		6	±0–69	175.4	±7.1	11.3	
		3	70.8	175.6	±6.7	13.6	
Sprinters and hurdlers	F	8	15.8	166.5	54.0	10.9	38
			±2.7	±9.3	±8.4	±3.6	
	M	5	28.4	179.9	±6.8	8.3	40
			±0.1	±0.7	±0.9	±5.2	
Walkers	F	4	24.9	163.4	51.7	18.1	41
			±6.3	±3.9	±4.8	±4.4	
Walkers	M	3	20.3	178.4	±6.1	7.3	40
			±2.0	±2.1	±1.8	±1.3	

(continued)

Sport	Sex	N	Age (y)	Stature (cm)	Mass (kg)	Body Fat (%)	Reference Number
Track events, *continued*							
Triathlon	F	16	24.2	162.1	55.2	16.5	16
			±4.3	±6.3	±4.6	±1.4	
	M	14	36.0	176.4	73.3	12.5	17
			±9.9	±8.6	±8.6	±5.9	
	M	8	29.6	180.0	73.9	7.9	26
			±2.6	±2.4	±2.1	±0.5	
Volleyball	F	14	21.6	178.3	70.5	17.9	25
			±0.8	±4.2	±5.5	±3.6	
	M	11	20.9	185.3	78.3	9.8	40
			±3.7	±10.2	±12.0	±2.9	
Weight lifting and body building							
Power lift	F	10	25.2	164.6	±8.6	21.5	10
			±6.0	±3.7	±3.6	±1.3	
	M	13	24.8	173.5	80.8	9.1	11
			±1.6	±2.8	±3.2	±1.2	
Body builders	F	10	30.4	165.2	56.5	13.5	10
			±8.2	±5.6	±0.9	±1.5	
	F	10	27.0	160.8	53.8	13.2	7
	M	16	28.0	175.1	86.2	12.5	4
			±1.8	±1.7	±3.1	±3.4	
	M	18	27.8	177.1	82.4	9.3	11
			±1.8	±1.1	±1.0	±0.8	
	M	14	31.6	170.8	83.8	10.9	14
			±6.7	±5.6	±9.2	±2.4	
Wrestling[c]							
Adult	M	37	19.6	174.6	74.8	8.8	28
			±1.34	±7.0	±12.2	±4.1	
Adolescent	M	409	16.2	171.0	±3.2	11.0	9
			±1.0	±7.1	±10.0	±4.0	
Sumo seki-tori)	M	37	21.1	178.9	115.9	26.1	14
			±3.6	±5.2	±27.4	±6.4	

[a]*Values reported as means ± SD.*
[b]*Modified from Sinning, W.E.: Body composition in athletes. In Human Body Composition. Roche AF, et al, eds. Human Kinetics, Champaign, IL, 1996.*
[c]*Note: consult our web page (http://www.lww.com/mkk) for the recent NCAA policy about minimal wrestling weight certification.*

References

1. Agre JC, et al. Professional ice hockey players: Physiologic, anthropometric, and musculoskeletal characteristics. *Arch Phys Med Rehab* 1988;69:188.
2. Bacharach DW, et al. Relationship of blood urea nitrogen to training intensity of elite female biathlon skiers. *J Strength Cond Res* 1996;10:105.
3. Calabrese LH, et al. Menstrual abnormalities, nutrition patterns, and body composition in female classical ballet dancers. *Phys Sportsmed* 1983;11:86.
4. Cordain L, et al. Variability of body composition assessment in men exhibiting extreme muscular hypertrophy. *J Strength Cond Res* 1995;9:85.
5. Eckerson JM, et al. Validity of bioelectrical impedence equations for estimating fat-free weight in high school female gymnasts. *Med Sci Exerc Sports* 1997;29:962.
6. Fahey TD, et al. Body composition and $V{\cdot}O_{2max}$ of exceptional weight trained athletes. *J Appl Physiol* 1975;39:559.
7. Freedson PF, et al. Physique, body composition, and psychological characteristics of competitive female body builders. *Phys Sportsmed* 1983;11:85.
8. Graves JE, et al. Body composition of elite female distance runners. *Int J Sports Med* 1987;8:96.
9. Housh TJ, et al. Validity of anthropometric estimations of body composition in high school wrestlers. *Res Q Exerc Sport* 1989;60:239.
10. Johnson GO, et al. A physiological profile comparison of female body builders and power lifters. *J Sports Med Phys Fitness* 1990;30:361.
11. Katch VL, et al. Muscular development and lean body weight in body builders and weight lifters. *Med Sci Sports* 1980;12:340.
12. Katch FI. Body composition of elite male and female alpine skiers. Unpublished data. University of Massachusetts, 1998.
13. Katch FI. Physiological characteristics of lightweight and heavyweight male collegiate rowers. Unpublished data. University of Massachusetts, 1999.
14. Kondo M, et al. Upper limit of fat-free mass in humans: a study on Japanese Sumo wrestlers. *Am J Human Biol* 1994;6:613.
15. Krahenbuhl GS, et al. Characteristics of national and world class female pentathletes. *Med Sci Sports*, 1979;11:20.
16. Leake CN, and Carter, J.E. Comparison of body composition and somatotype of trained female triathletes. *J Sports Sci* 1991;9:125.
17. Lofton M, et al. Peak physiological function and performance of recreational triathletes. *J Sports Med Phys Fitness* 1988;28:33.
18. McArdle WD, et al. *Exercise Physiology.* 4th edition. Baltimore: Williams & Wilkins, 1996:590.
19. Meleski BW, et al. Size, physique and body composition of competitive female swimmers 11 through 20 years of age. *Human Biol* 1982;54:609.
20. Morrow JR, et al. Anthropometric strength, and performance characteristics of American world class throwers. *J Sports Med Phys Fitness* 1982;22:73.
21. Pollock ML, et al. Physiological characteristics of champion American track athletes 40 to 75 years of age. *J Gerontol* 1974;29:645.
22. Pollock ML, et al. Body composition of elite class distance runners. *Ann New York Acad Sci* 1977;301:361.
23. Pollock ML, et al. Comparison of male and female speedskating candidates. In: DM Landers (ed). *Sports and Elite Performance.* Champaign, IL: Human Kinetics, 143–152.
24. Pugh LG, et al. A physiological study of channel swimming. *Clin Sci* 1955;19:257.
25. Puhl J, et al. Physical and physiological characteristics of elite volleyball players. *Res Q Exerc Sport* 1982;53:257.
26. Rowbottom DG, et al. Training adaptation and biological changes among well-trained male triathletes. *Med Sci Sports Exerc* 1997;29:1233.
27. Siders WA, et al. Effects of participation in a collegiate sport season on body composition. *J Sports Med Phys Fitness* 1991;31:571.
28. Sinning WE. Body composition assessment of college wrestlers. *Med Sci Sports* 1974;6:139.
29. Sinning WE, et al. Body composition and somatotype of male and female Nordic skiers. *Res Q* 1977;48:741.
30. Sinning WE. Anthropometric estimation of body density, fat, and lean body weight in women gymnasts. *Med Sci Sports* 1978;10:243.
31. Sinning WE, and Wilson JR. Validity of "generalized" equations for body composition analysis in women athletes. *Res Q Exerc Sports* 1984;55:153.
32. Sinning WE, et al. Validity of generalized equations for body composition analysis in male athletes. *Med Sci Sports Exerc* 1985;17:124.
33. Thorland WG, et al. Body composition and somatotype characteristics of junior olympic athletes. *Med Sci Sports Exerc* 1981;13:332.
34. Walsh FK, et al. Estimation of body composition of female intercollegiate basketball players. *Phys Sportsmed* 1984;12:74.
35. White A, and Johnson S. Physiological comparison of international, national, and regional alpine skiers. *Int J Sports Med* 1991;12:374.
36. Wickkiser JD, and Kelly JM. The body composition of a college football team. Med *Sci Sports* 1975;7:199.
37. Wilmore JH, et al. Football pro's strengths and CV weaknesses charted. *Phys Sportsmed* 1976;4:45.
38. Wilmore JH, et al. Body physique and composition of the female distance runner. *Ann New York Acad Sci* 1977;301:764.
39. Wilmore JH. Body composition in sport and exercise: Directions for future research. *Med Sci Sports Exerc* 1983;15:21.
40. Withers RT, et al. Relative body fat and anthropometric prediction of body density of male athletes. *Eur J Appl Physiol* 1987;56:191.
41. Withers RT, et al. Relative body fat and anthropometric prediction of body density of female athletes. *Eur J Appl Physiol* 1987;56:169.

Appendix F Three-Day Physical Activity Log

A three-day log of physical activities provides a relatively simple yet accurate way to assess average daily energy expenditure.

Step 1 Review Table 1 which provides an example of a daily physical activity log for one of your textbook authors. Note that the list includes mostly typical activities of daily living.

Step 2 Record your daily physical activities on each of the log entry forms for three typical days. Be specific for the beginning and ending times of activity; round off to the nearest minute.

Step 3 Consolidate the information from the three log entry forms (Step 2) to the Master Log in Table 2. If you devote more than 120 minutes to one of the recreational and sports activities, check the 120 minute box. For typical household activities, list activities by minutes and hours.

Step 4 Determine your basal metabolic rate (BMR) in $kcal \cdot h^{-1}$ as follows:

Men

BMR ($kcal \cdot h^{-1}$) = 38 $kcal \cdot m^2 \cdot h^{-1}$ × surface area[a] (m^2)

Women

BMR ($kcal \cdot h^{-1}$) = 38 $kcal \cdot m^2 \cdot h^{-1}$ × surface area[a] (m^2)

Example of BMR Calculations
Data: Male
Age, 40y
Stature, 182 cm (72 in)
Body mass, 86.4 kg (190 lb)
Body surface area[a] = 2.08 m^2
$kcal \cdot m^2 \cdot h^{-1}$ = 38.0

Calculations
a. $kcal \cdot h^{-1} = 38.0 \times 2.08 = 79.0$
b. $kcal \cdot min^{-1} = 79.0 \div 60 = 1.3$

Step 5 Determine energy expenditure ($kcal \cdot min^{-1}$) for each of the activities in the Master Log (Table 2). Use Appendix B to determine caloric expenditure per minute. The values represent gross values plus resting. If an activity is not included, list one most similar to yours. The bottom of the Daily Log form includes a box to record daily total kcal.

Step 6 Multiply energy expenditure for each activity by the number of minutes of participation.

Step 7 Sum the total energy expenditure for each activity, including the value for sleep, to arrive at your TOTAL daily energy expenditure.

Step 8 Repeat Steps 5–7 for Days 2 and 3. Calculate average daily calorie by summing the total calories expended for three days and divide by 3.

Total energy expenditure (kcal) = Day 1 kcal 1 Day 2 kcal 1 Day 3 kcal
= ___ kcal + ___ kcal + ___ kcal

Average daily energy expenditure 3= Total kcal ÷ 3
= _____ kcal ÷ 3

[a]Compute body surface area (BSA, m^2) as: Body mass, $kg^{0.425}$ × stature, $cm^{0.725}$ × 0.007184
Example: Body Mass=162 lb (73.5 kg); stature = 5′9″ (175.3 cm)
BSA, $m^2 = 73.5^{0.425} \times 175.3^{0.725} \times 0.007184$
$= 6.210 \times 42.332 \times 0.007184$
$= 1.89$

TABLE F.1 Example of Daily Physical Activity Log. [Column 5 Lists Activities Similar to those in Column 1.]

Activity	Begin Time	End Time	Total Minutes	Similar Activity[a]	$kcal \cdot min^{-1}$	Total kcal
Wake, bathroom use	6:45AM	6:53AM	8	Standing quietly	2.3	18.4
Go back to bed	6:53	7:30	38	BMR	1.3	48.1
Eat breakfast	7:30	7:50	10	Eating, sitting	2.0	40.0
Use bathroom	7:50	8:00	10	Standing quietly	2.3	23.0
Dress	8:00	8:06	6	Standing quietly	2.3	13.8
Drive to school	8:06	8:17	11	Sitting quietly	2.0	22.0
Walk to office	8:17	8:25	8	Walking, normal pace	6.9	55.8
Work in office, pick up mail	8:25	10:00	95	Writing, sitting	2.5	237.5
Up/down stairs	10:00	10:10	10	11 min 30 s pace	11.7	117.0
Work in office	10:10	12:10PM	120	Writing, sitting	2.5	300.0
Go to locker	12:10PM	12:12	2	Walking, normal pace	6.9	13.8
Get dressed	12:12	12:16	4	Standing quietly	2.3	9.2
Walk to track	12:16	12:20	4	Walk, normal pace	6.9	27.6
Wait for friend	12:20	12:30	10	Standing quietly	2.3	23.0
Run to park, back	12:30	2:00	90	8-min mile pace	17.2	1553.0
Walk to locker	2:00	2:04	4	Walk, normal pace	6.9	27.6
Shower, dress	2:04	2:20	16	Quiet standing	2.3	36.8
Walk to office	2:20	2:24	4	Walk, normal pace	6.9	27.6
Meeting/lunch	2:24	3:00	36	Eating, sitting	2.0	72.0
Work in office	3:00	5:05	125	Writing, sitting	2.5	312.5
Walk to library	5:05	5:12	7	Walk, normal pace	6.9	48.3
Work in library	5:12	6:05	53	Writing, sitting	2.5	132.5
Walk to dean	6:05	6:10	5	Walk, normal pace	6.9	34.5
Meeting, dean	6:10	6:35	25	Writing, sitting	2.5	62.5
Walk to office	6:35	6:43	8	Walk, normal pace	6.9	55.2
Walk to car	6:43	6:51	8	Walk, normal pace	6.9	55.2
Drive home	6:51	7:03	12	Sitting quietly	1.8	21.6
Change clothes	7:03	7:07	4	Standing quietly	2.3	9.2
Wash-up	7:07	7:11	4	Standing quietly	2.3	9.2
Cook dinner	7:11	8:00	49	Cooking	4.1	200.9
Watch TV	8:00	8:30	30	Sitting quietly	1.8	54.0
Eat dinner	8:30	9:00	30	Eating, sitting	2.0	60.0
Mail letter	9:00	9:05	5	Walk, normal pace	6.9	34.5
Listen to stereo	9:05	9:30	25	Sitting quietly	1.8	45.0
Watch TV	9:30	10:30	60	Sitting quietly	1.8	108.0
Wash-up	10:30	10:38	8	Standing quietly	2.3	18.4
Read in bed	10:38	11:15	37	Lying at ease	1.9	70.3
						DAILY TOTAL = 4583

[a]*When you cannot match a specific activity with a table value in Appendix B, select a similar activity and base the kcal value on that activity.*

DAY 2. Physical Activity Log

Activity	Begin Time	End Time	Total Minutes	Similar Activity[a]	kcal · min^{-1}	Total kcal

DAILY TOTAL =

DAY 3. Physical Activity Log

Activity	Begin Time	End Time	Total Minutes	Similar Activity[a]	$kcal \cdot min^{-1}$	Total kcal

DAILY TOTAL =

TABLE F.2 Master Log of Physical Activity

Activity	Day 1	Day 2	Day 3	Minutes 0–10	10–20	20–30	30–40	40–50	50–60	60–70	70–80	80–90	90–100	100–110	110–120	kcal
Aerobics	☐	☐	☐	☐	☐	☐	☐	☐	☐	☐	☐	☐	☐	☐	☐	____
Basketball	☐	☐	☐	☐	☐	☐	☐	☐	☐	☐	☐	☐	☐	☐	☐	____
Fitness Center	☐	☐	☐	☐	☐	☐	☐	☐	☐	☐	☐	☐	☐	☐	☐	____
Rowing Machine	☐	☐	☐	☐	☐	☐	☐	☐	☐	☐	☐	☐	☐	☐	☐	____
Stair Master	☐	☐	☐	☐	☐	☐	☐	☐	☐	☐	☐	☐	☐	☐	☐	____
Stationary Bike	☐	☐	☐	☐	☐	☐	☐	☐	☐	☐	☐	☐	☐	☐	☐	____
Treadmill	☐	☐	☐	☐	☐	☐	☐	☐	☐	☐	☐	☐	☐	☐	☐	____
Weight Lifting	☐	☐	☐	☐	☐	☐	☐	☐	☐	☐	☐	☐	☐	☐	☐	____
____________	☐	☐	☐	☐	☐	☐	☐	☐	☐	☐	☐	☐	☐	☐	☐	____
____________	☐	☐	☐	☐	☐	☐	☐	☐	☐	☐	☐	☐	☐	☐	☐	____
____________	☐	☐	☐	☐	☐	☐	☐	☐	☐	☐	☐	☐	☐	☐	☐	____
____________	☐	☐	☐	☐	☐	☐	☐	☐	☐	☐	☐	☐	☐	☐	☐	____
Cycling	☐	☐	☐	☐	☐	☐	☐	☐	☐	☐	☐	☐	☐	☐	☐	____
Field Hockey	☐	☐	☐	☐	☐	☐	☐	☐	☐	☐	☐	☐	☐	☐	☐	____
Hiking	☐	☐	☐	☐	☐	☐	☐	☐	☐	☐	☐	☐	☐	☐	☐	____
Jogging/Running	☐	☐	☐	☐	☐	☐	☐	☐	☐	☐	☐	☐	☐	☐	☐	____
Soccer	☐	☐	☐	☐	☐	☐	☐	☐	☐	☐	☐	☐	☐	☐	☐	____
Softball	☐	☐	☐	☐	☐	☐	☐	☐	☐	☐	☐	☐	☐	☐	☐	____
Swimming	☐	☐	☐	☐	☐	☐	☐	☐	☐	☐	☐	☐	☐	☐	☐	____
Racket Sports	☐	☐	☐	☐	☐	☐	☐	☐	☐	☐	☐	☐	☐	☐	☐	____
Martial Arts	☐	☐	☐	☐	☐	☐	☐	☐	☐	☐	☐	☐	☐	☐	☐	____
____________	☐	☐	☐	☐	☐	☐	☐	☐	☐	☐	☐	☐	☐	☐	☐	____
____________	☐	☐	☐	☐	☐	☐	☐	☐	☐	☐	☐	☐	☐	☐	☐	____
____________	☐	☐	☐	☐	☐	☐	☐	☐	☐	☐	☐	☐	☐	☐	☐	____
____________	☐	☐	☐	☐	☐	☐	☐	☐	☐	☐	☐	☐	☐	☐	☐	____
____________	☐	☐	☐	☐	☐	☐	☐	☐	☐	☐	☐	☐	☐	☐	☐	____
	☐	☐	☐	☐	☐	☐	☐	☐	☐	☐	☐	☐	☐	☐	☐	____

Activity	Day 1	Day 2	Day 3	Minutes 0–10	10–20	20–30	30–40	40–50	50–60	Hours 1	2	3	4	5	6	7	8	kcal
Sleep	☐	☐	☐	☐	☐	☐	☐	☐	☐	☐	☐	☐	☐	☐	☐	☐	☐	____
Walking	☐	☐	☐	☐	☐	☐	☐	☐	☐	☐	☐	☐	☐	☐	☐	☐	☐	____
Resting	☐	☐	☐	☐	☐	☐	☐	☐	☐	☐	☐	☐	☐	☐	☐	☐	☐	____
Personal Hygiene	☐	☐	☐	☐	☐	☐	☐	☐	☐	☐	☐	☐	☐	☐	☐	☐	☐	____
Watch TV	☐	☐	☐	☐	☐	☐	☐	☐	☐	☐	☐	☐	☐	☐	☐	☐	☐	____
Attend Class	☐	☐	☐	☐	☐	☐	☐	☐	☐	☐	☐	☐	☐	☐	☐	☐	☐	____
Homework	☐	☐	☐	☐	☐	☐	☐	☐	☐	☐	☐	☐	☐	☐	☐	☐	☐	____
Computer	☐	☐	☐	☐	☐	☐	☐	☐	☐	☐	☐	☐	☐	☐	☐	☐	☐	____
Eating	☐	☐	☐	☐	☐	☐	☐	☐	☐	☐	☐	☐	☐	☐	☐	☐	☐	____
____________	☐	☐	☐	☐	☐	☐	☐	☐	☐	☐	☐	☐	☐	☐	☐	☐	☐	____
____________	☐	☐	☐	☐	☐	☐	☐	☐	☐	☐	☐	☐	☐	☐	☐	☐	☐	____
____________	☐	☐	☐	☐	☐	☐	☐	☐	☐	☐	☐	☐	☐	☐	☐	☐	☐	____
____________	☐	☐	☐	☐	☐	☐	☐	☐	☐	☐	☐	☐	☐	☐	☐	☐	☐	____
____________	☐	☐	☐	☐	☐	☐	☐	☐	☐	☐	☐	☐	☐	☐	☐	☐	☐	____

Index

Page numbers in *italics* indicate figures. Page numbers ending in "t" indicate tables.

C

F

G

N

Q

R

S

T

Y

Z